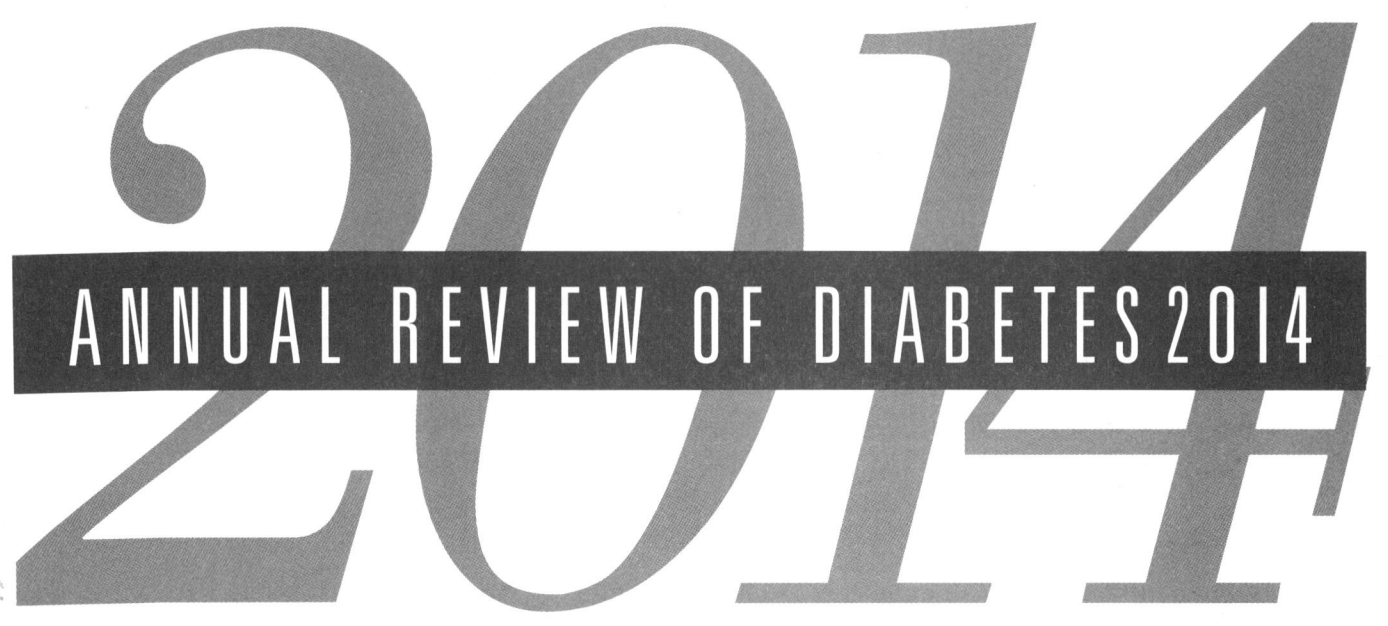

ANNUAL REVIEW OF DIABETES 2014

THE BEST OF THE AMERICAN DIABETES ASSOCIATION'S SCHOLARLY JOURNALS

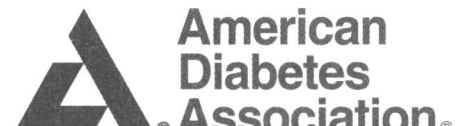

American Diabetes Association®

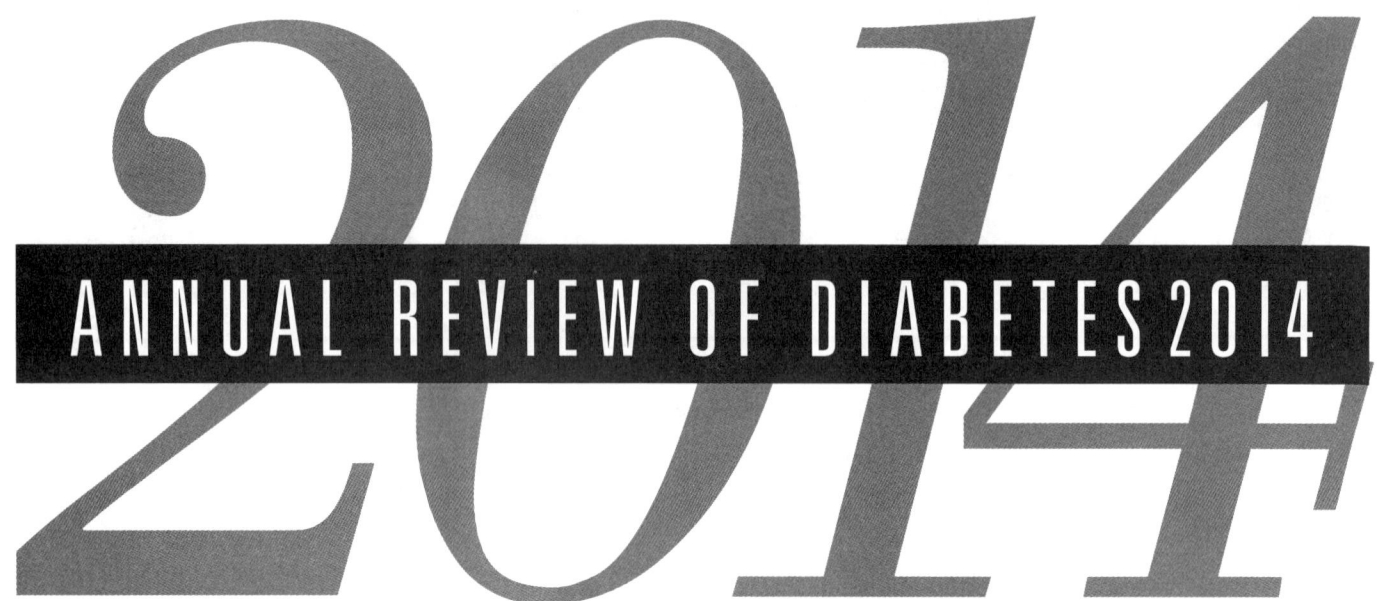

ANNUAL REVIEW OF DIABETES 2014

Printed in Canada
1 3 5 7 9 10 8 6 4 2

The suggestions and information contained in this publication are generally consistent with the *Clinical Practice Recommendations* and other policies of the American Diabetes Association, but they do not represent the policy or position of the Association or any of its boards or committees. Reasonable steps have been taken to ensure the accuracy of the information presented. However, the American Diabetes Association cannot ensure the safety or efficacy of any product or service described in this publication. Individuals are advised to consult a physician or other appropriate health care professional before undertaking any diet or exercise program or taking any medication referred to in this publication. Professionals must use and apply their own professional judgment, experience, and training and should not rely solely on the information contained in this publication before prescribing any diet, exercise, or medication. The American Diabetes Association—its officers, directors, employees, volunteers, and members—assumes no responsibility or liability for personal or other injury, loss, or damage that may result from the suggestions or information in this publication.

♾ The paper in this publication meets the requirements of the ANSI Standard Z39.48-1992 (permanence of paper).

ADA titles may be purchased for business or promotional use or for special sales. To purchase more than 50 copies of this book at a discount, or for custom editions of this book with your logo, contact the American Diabetes Association at the address below, at booksales@diabetes.org, or by calling 703-299-2046.

American Diabetes Association
1701 North Beauregard Street
Alexandria, Virginia 22311

DOI: 10.2337/9781580405515

ANNUAL REVIEW OF DIABETES 2014

EPIDEMIOLOGY & PATHOGENESIS

Identification of Serum Metabolites Associated With Risk of Type 2 Diabetes Using a Targeted Metabolomic Approach

Anna Floegel,[1] Norbert Stefan,[2] Zhonghao Yu,[3] Kristin Mühlenbruch,[4] Dagmar Drogan,[1] Hans-Georg Joost,[5] Andreas Fritsche,[2] Hans-Ulrich Häring,[2] Martin Hrabĕ de Angelis,[6] Annette Peters,[7] Michael Roden,[8,9] Cornelia Prehn,[6] Rui Wang-Sattler,[3] Thomas Illig,[3,10] Matthias B. Schulze,[4] Jerzy Adamski,[6] Heiner Boeing,[1] and Tobias Pischon[1,11]

Metabolomic discovery of biomarkers of type 2 diabetes (T2D) risk may reveal etiological pathways and help to identify individuals at risk for disease. We prospectively investigated the association between serum metabolites measured by targeted metabolomics and risk of T2D in the European Prospective Investigation into Cancer and Nutrition (EPIC)-Potsdam (27,548 adults) among all incident cases of T2D ($n = 800$, mean follow-up 7 years) and a randomly drawn subcohort ($n = 2,282$). Flow injection analysis tandem mass spectrometry was used to quantify 163 metabolites, including acylcarnitines, amino acids, hexose, and phospholipids, in baseline serum samples. Serum hexose; phenylalanine; and diacyl-phosphatidylcholines C32:1, C36:1, C38:3, and C40:5 were independently associated with increased risk of T2D and serum glycine; sphingomyelin C16:1; acyl-alkyl-phosphatidylcholines C34:3, C40:6, C42:5, C44:4, and C44:5; and lysophosphatidylcholine C18:2 with decreased risk. Variance of the metabolites was largely explained by two metabolite factors with opposing risk associations (factor 1 relative risk in extreme quintiles 0.31 [95% CI 0.21–0.44], factor 2 3.82 [2.64–5.52]). The metabolites significantly improved T2D prediction compared with established risk factors. They were further linked to insulin sensitivity and secretion in the Tübingen Family study and were partly replicated in the independent KORA (Cooperative Health Research in the Region of Augsburg) cohort. The data indicate that metabolic alterations, including sugar metabolites, amino acids, and choline-containing phospholipids, are associated early on with a higher risk of T2D.
Diabetes 62:639–648, 2013

From the [1]Department of Epidemiology, German Institute of Human Nutrition Potsdam-Rehbruecke, Nuthetal, Germany; the [2]Department of Internal Medicine IV, Divisions of Endocrinology, Diabetology, Nephrology, Vascular Disease, and Clinical Chemistry, University of Tübingen, Tübingen, Germany; the [3]Research Unit of Molecular Epidemiology, Helmholtz Zentrum München, German Research Center for Environmental Health, Neuherberg, Germany; the [4]Department of Molecular Epidemiology, German Institute of Human Nutrition Potsdam-Rehbruecke, Nuthetal, Germany; the [5]Department of Pharmacology, German Institute of Human Nutrition Potsdam–Rehbruecke, Nuthetal, Germany; the [6]Institute of Experimental Genetics, Helmholtz Zentrum München, German Research Center for Environmental Health, Neuherberg, Germany; the [7]Institute of Epidemiology II, Helmholtz Zentrum München, German Research Center for Environmental Health, Neuherberg, Germany; the [8]Institute of Clinical Diabetology, German Diabetes Center, Leibniz Center for Diabetes Research at Heinrich Heine University, Düsseldorf, Germany; the [9]Department of Metabolic Diseases, University Clinics, Düsseldorf, Germany; the [10]Hannover Unified Biobank, Hannover Medical School, Hannover, Germany; and the [11]Molecular Epidemiology Group, Max Delbrück Center for Molecular Medicine (MDC) Berlin-Buch, Berlin, Germany.
Corresponding author: Anna Floegel, anna.floegel@dife.de.

Received 22 April 2012 and accepted 22 July 2012.
DOI: 10.2337/db12-0495
This article contains Supplementary Data online at http://diabetes.diabetesjournals.org/lookup/suppl/doi:10.2337/db12-0495/-/DC1.
See accompanying commentary, p. 349.

Type 2 diabetes (T2D) is characterized by impaired insulin sensitivity of several tissues and inadequate insulin secretion from β-cells (1). A detailed understanding of the pathophysiology of T2D is a prerequisite for the development of preventive strategies. In particular, the identification of early metabolic alterations is promising in the study of etiological pathways and may further help to identify high-risk individuals. A number of biomarkers have been proposed as indicators for the estimation of T2D risk, such as fasting plasma glucose and glycated hemoglobin A_{1c} (HbA$_{1c}$) (2), triglycerides (3), HDL cholesterol (4), inflammatory markers (5), adiponectin (5,6), liver enzymes (7), and fetuin-A (8). However, most biomarkers fail to grasp the complexity of T2D etiology (3). Design and advancement of high-throughput analytical techniques determined the emergence of metabolomics, which is the simultaneous study of numerous low-molecular weight compounds, namely metabolites. Metabolites represent intermediates and end products of metabolic pathways that reflect more rapidly physiological dysfunctions than current biomarkers and, thus, may mirror earlier stages of T2D (9). Cross-sectional studies have linked alterations in metabolic profiles with obesity (10), glucose tolerance (11), and prevalent diabetes (12–14). The most prominent metabolic shifts involved blood acylcarnitines and branched-chain amino acids (BCAAs). Recently, observations from a prospective study found that a set of five amino acids was predictive for T2D, representing pioneering work in the emerging field of systems epidemiology (15).

In the current study, we investigated whether a targeted metabolomic approach involving a broader spectrum of metabolites and a larger number of study participants may help to identify metabolites associated with the risk of T2D and the mechanisms involved. Therefore, we profiled 163 serum metabolites in originally healthy individuals who were consecutively followed up for incident T2D in two large-scale prospective cohort studies in Germany and studied cross-sectional relationships of the identified metabolites with insulin sensitivity and secretion in precisely phenotyped participants. In addition, we evaluated the usefulness of the metabolites for T2D risk prediction compared with the German Diabetes Risk Score (DRS) (16) and established biomarkers.

RESEARCH DESIGN AND METHODS

European Prospective Investigation into Cancer and Nutrition-Potsdam study. The European Prospective Investigation into Cancer and Nutrition (EPIC)-Potsdam is part of the ongoing multicenter EPIC study and comprises 27,548 participants from the general population in the area of Potsdam in eastern Germany who were mainly 35–65 years of age at time of recruitment between 1994 and 1998 (17). At baseline, participants underwent an examination by qualified staff, including medical history, blood pressure measurement, and anthropometry (18). Participants also completed sociodemographic and lifestyle questionnaires and a validated food frequency questionnaire. In addition, 30 mL blood were drawn (random sampling) and immediately processed (19). Only participants with morning appointments were asked to fast overnight. Blood was fractionated into serum, plasma, buffy coat, and erythrocytes; aliquotted into straws of 0.5 mL each; and stored in tanks of liquid nitrogen at −196°C until analysis. Besides metabolomic profiling, other biomarkers have been measured in baseline blood samples as described previously (7,20,21). Every 2–3 years, follow-up questionnaires were sent to participants to identify incident cases of T2D, with response rates of ~95% (22,23). Once a participant was identified as a potential case, disease status was further verified with medical records, including the correct diagnosis (International Classification of Diseases, 10th revision, E11, non–insulin-dependent diabetes), the date of the diagnosis, and the means of diagnosis confirmation. This verification was achieved by sending a standard inquiry form to the treating physician. Consent was obtained from all study participants a priori, and the study was approved by the ethics committee of the Medical Society of the State of Brandenburg.

We constructed a case-cohort study within EPIC-Potsdam, including all incident cases of T2D of the full cohort identified up to 31 August 2005 (n = 849, mean follow-up 7 years), and a subcohort (n = 2,500) randomly drawn from the EPIC-Potsdam study population. Because the subcohort was representative of the full cohort, it included 2,415 noncases and 85 cases of incident T2D (i.e., internal cases). The remaining 764 cases did not belong to the subcohort (external cases). By randomly selecting the subcohort and using the appropriate statistic for this study design, the biomarkers only needed to be measured in the case-cohort sample; however, the results are expected to be generalizable to the full cohort (7). The case-cohort design was previously chosen based on its advantages, including a reduced chance of selection bias for the control group (24).

For the present analysis, we further excluded participants with prevalent T2D at baseline (n = 110), with missing or nonverified data on incident or prevalent T2D (n = 13), with missing blood samples or biomarker measurements (n = 64), and with missing covariate information (n = 80). Thus, the analytical sample included 2,282 individuals of the subcohort and 800 individuals with incident T2D.

Cooperative Health Research in the Region of Augsburg study. The Cooperative Health Research in the Region of Augsburg (KORA) study consists of population-based surveys and follow-up periods in the area of Augsburg in southern Germany. A total of 4,261 individuals between 25 and 74 years of age participated in the S4 survey between 1999 and 2001 (25). In the KORA cohort, blood was drawn into serum gel tubes after a fasting period of at least 8 h. Blood samples were rested for coagulation for 30 min at room temperature; serum was obtained by centrifugation at 2,750g at 15°C for 10 min and stored in a freezer at −80°C. A total of 3,080 individuals took part in the F4 follow-up survey during the years 2006–2008 (26). The identification of incident T2D was based on an oral glucose tolerance test (OGTT) or a validated physician diagnosis (27). All KORA participants gave written informed consent, and the KORA study was approved by the ethics committee of the Bavarian medical association.

A subcohort of 876 S4 participants 55–74 years of age without T2D at baseline and with metabolomics data available was included in the current study. Of them, 91 developed incident T2D during the 7-year follow-up.

Tübingen Family study for T2D. The Tübingen Family (TüF) study is in an ongoing investigation of the pathophysiology of T2D in southern Germany (28). Individuals meeting at least one of the following criteria were included in the study: a family history of T2D, a BMI >27 kg/m², and previous impaired glucose tolerance or gestational diabetes mellitus. They were considered healthy according to a physical examination and routine laboratory tests. Written informed consent was obtained from all participants, and the medical ethics committee of the University of Tübingen approved the protocol.

All individuals underwent a 75-g OGTT. Venous plasma samples were drawn at 0, 30, 60, 90, and 120 min for plasma glucose, insulin, C-peptide, and metabolomic analyses (minute 0). Insulin sensitivity was calculated from the OGTT (29). The plasma glucose and C-peptide areas under the curve (AUCs) during the OGTT were calculated by applying the trapezoid method. Insulin secretion was calculated from $AUC_{C-peptide}/AUC_{glucose}$. The present analysis included 76 Caucasians from the TüF study who had measurements of insulin sensitivity and insulin secretion as well as metabolomics data available.

Serum metabolite concentrations. Serum concentrations of metabolites were determined with the Absolute*IDQ* p150 and p180 Kits (Biocrates Life Sciences AG, Innsbruck, Austria) using the flow injection analysis tandem mass spectrometry (FIA-MS/MS) technique (30). The metabolomic method simultaneously quantified 163 metabolites, including 41 acylcarnitines (Cx:y), 14 amino acids, 1 hexose (sum of six-carbon monosaccharides without distinction of isomers), 92 glycerophospholipids (lyso-, diacyl-, and acyl-alkyl-phosphatidylcholines), and 15 sphingomyelins. To ensure valid measurements, metabolites below the limit of detection (n = 30) and those with very high analytical variance (n = 6) in our samples were excluded, leaving 127 metabolites for the present analysis.

Metabolomic measurements were performed in the Genome Analysis Center at the Helmholtz Zentum München. Sample preparation was done according to the manufacturer's protocol (Biocrates user's manual UM-P150) and has been described previously (30). In brief, after centrifugation, 10 μL serum were inserted into a filter on a 96-well sandwich plate, which already contained stable isotope-labeled internal standards. Amino acids were derivated with 5% phenylisothiocyanate reagent. Metabolites and internal standards were extracted with 5 mmol/L ammonium acetate in methanol. The solution was then centrifuged through a filter membrane and diluted with mass spectrometry running solvent. Final extracts were analyzed by FIA-MS/MS, and metabolites were quantified in μmol/L by appropriate internal standards. The method has been validated, and analytical specifications were provided in the Biocrates manual AS-P150. The manufacturer selected the metabolites based on the robustness of their measurements. The uncertainty of the measurements was <10% for most of the metabolites. Regarding accuracy, all included metabolites were found in the range of 80–115% of their theoretical values. The median analytical variance of EPIC-Potsdam samples was a 7.3% within-plate coefficient of variation and a 11.3% between-plates coefficient of variation (31). To account for run-order effects, serum samples were randomly analyzed together, regardless of the case status. We have shown previously that most of the metabolites had moderate to high intraclass correlation coefficients measured in participants over a 4-month period, indicating reasonable reliability of the measurements (31).

Statistical analysis

Step 1: Identification of metabolites associated with T2D risk in EPIC-Potsdam. Cox proportional hazards regression with weighting as suggested by Prentice (32) and robust sandwich covariance estimates to account for the case-cohort design were used to calculate multivariable-adjusted hazard ratios as a measure of relative risk (RR) and 95% CI, with age as the underlying time scale from recruitment to study exit (T2D diagnosis or censoring) of each participant. We considered z score–standardized metabolite concentrations (mean 0 [SD 1]) as the exposure variable and calculated a multivariable-adjusted model to select metabolites associated with T2D risk. This model was adjusted for age, sex, alcohol intake from beverages (nonconsumers; women >0–6, 6–12, and >12 g/day; and men >0–12, 12–24, and >24 g/day), smoking (never, former, current ≤20 cigarettes/day, current >20 cigarettes/day), cycling and sports (h/week), education (no degree/vocational training, trade/technical school, university degree), coffee intake (cups/day), red meat intake (g/day), whole-grain bread intake (g/day), prevalent hypertension (yes/no), BMI (kg/m²), and waist circumference (cm). Because the metabolomic approach is exploratory, the P values from Cox regression were corrected for multiple testing (n = 127) using the Bonferroni-Holm procedure (33), and a corrected P < 0.05 (two-sided testing) was considered significant to select metabolites.

We next calculated a model that included the covariates and all the identified metabolites and used stepwise Cox regression to select the independent predictors. To also account for the intercorrelation of some of the metabolites, we conducted a principal component analysis (PCA). In brief, the PCA aggregates the individual metabolites based on their degree of correlation with one another to a smaller number of metabolite factors (principal components). These metabolite factors are extracted in a way that explains the major fraction of the variance of individual metabolites. We included all metabolites associated with T2D risk in the PCA, based the PCA on the correlation matrix of metabolites, and used an orthogonal rotation procedure with the varimax method. We retained two metabolite factors according to the scree test and because they accounted for most of the observed variance. Thus, the proportion of explained variance of factor 1 and factor 2 were 34.2 and 16.1%, respectively. To investigate the association between metabolite factors and T2D risk, we estimated RR and 95% CI across quintiles of metabolite factors, particularly choosing quintiles of metabolite factors to facilitate the interpretation. We also investigated a possible effect modification of sex or fasting status on the association between metabolite factors and T2D risk by including multiplicative interaction terms into the models. We then repeated the PCA to include only fasting blood samples in order to evaluate whether the metabolite factors were different from those obtained from random blood samples. Finally, we calculated hazard rates of T2D during different periods of follow-up and tested whether they were different with a test of heterogeneity (34).

Step 2: Additional analyses, risk prediction, and replication in KORA. For significant metabolites found in step 1, we calculated multivariable-adjusted models with additional adjustment for blood glucose, HbA_{1c}, HDL cholesterol, and triglycerides. We also adjusted for the amino acids phenylalanine, tyrosine, and isoleucine, which have been found to be associated with T2D risk (35). Using data of the EPIC-Potsdam subcohort, we calculated Spearman partial correlation coefficients between identified metabolites and established T2D biomarkers. Data of the TüF study were used to calculate Spearman partial correlation coefficients between identified metabolites and measures of insulin sensitivity and secretion. We calculated measures of discrimination and calibration in different multivariable-adjusted logistic regression models using the DRS (16) as the reference model and adding established T2D biomarkers and the identified metabolites. Receiver operating characteristic (ROC) AUCs were compared using the DeLong test (36).

The results were replicated in the prospective KORA study, and metabolite factors were recalculated in KORA using the linear factor equations retrieved from the PCA in the EPIC-Potsdam sample. The risk estimates from EPIC-Potsdam and KORA were combined using a meta-analytical approach (37). Power calculation suggested a detectable RR per SD of 1.26 (38). Additionally, multivariable-adjusted RRs of T2D were calculated for the amino acids that were recently identified by Wang et al. (35) and that were also measured in the EPIC-Potsdam study. The statistical analyses were conducted with SAS version 9.2 (SAS Institute, Inc, Cary, NC) and in the R statistical environment (www.r-project.org).

RESULTS

Baseline characteristics of the EPIC-Potsdam sample are presented in Table 1. Of all the metabolites measured using a targeted metabolomic approach, 34 were significantly associated with T2D risk in the EPIC-Potsdam study after correction for multiple testing (Supplementary Table 1). These relations were also independent of relevant dietary and lifestyle factors as well as anthropometry and hypertension. Among these 34 metabolites, 14 were identified to be significantly associated with T2D risk independent of

the others (Table 2). Specifically, hexose, phenylalanine, and diacyl-phosphatidylcholines C32:1, C36:1, C38:3, and C40:5 were significantly positively associated with T2D risk, whereas glycine, sphingomyelin C16:1, lysophosphatidylcholine C18:2, and acyl-alkyl-phosphatidylcholines C34:3, C40:6, C42:5, C44:4, and C44:5 were significantly inversely related to T2D risk. Using PCA, we identified two metabolite factors that included multiple metabolites and explained most of their variation (Fig. 1). These metabolite factors showed significant and opposing associations with T2D risk. When comparing extreme quintiles, metabolite factor 1, which mainly contains acyl-alkyl-phosphatidylcholines, sphingomyelins, and lysophosphatidylcholines, was associated with a significant 69% reduced risk of T2D (RR 0.31 [95% CI 0.21–0.44]) (Table 3), whereas metabolite factor 2, consistent of diacyl-phosphatidylcholines, BCAA and aromatic amino acids, propionylcarnitine, and hexose, was associated with a significant 3.82-fold increased risk of T2D (3.82 [2.64–5.52]). When we restricted the PCA to fasting samples ($n = 429$), very similar metabolite factors could be generated with only minor differences in factor loadings (Supplementary Table 2). We also estimated the joint effects of both metabolite factors by summing them (factor 1 received a negative sign because it was inversely associated with T2D risk) and calculating RR of T2D across quintiles of combined factors. The RR (95% CI) of T2D from quintile 1 to quintile 5 of summed metabolite factors was as follows: 1.0, 1.47 (0.96–2.24), 2.29 (1.54–3.38), 2.67 (1.79–4.0), and 6.69 (4.50–9.96) (*P* for trend <0.0001).

Adjustment for established T2D biomarkers only marginally affected the magnitude of risk association for most

TABLE 1
Baseline characteristics of the EPIC-Potsdam case-cohort sample (1994–1998)

	Subcohort ($n = 2,282$)	Incident T2D cases ($n = 800$)	*P* for difference[†]
Age (years)[‡]	49.5 (8.9)	54.7 (7.3)	<0.0001
Women (%)[‡]	62.0	42.2	<0.0001
BMI (kg/m²)	26.1 (0.09)	30.1 (0.15)	<0.0001
Waist circumference, men (cm)[§]	93.7 (0.34)	103.6 (0.46)	<0.0001
Waist circumference, women (cm)[§]	80.6 (0.30)	93.4 (0.62)	<0.0001
Prevalent hypertension	49.5	70.8	<0.0001
Education			
No degree/vocational training	37.1	45.6	<0.0001
Trade/technical school	24.0	25.4	0.412
University degree	39.0	29.0	<0.0001
Smoking status			
Never	46.9	36.2	<0.0001
Former	33.0	42.3	<0.0001
Current	20.1	21.5	0.472
Among smokers, cigarettes/day	12.6 (0.43)	16.0 (0.74)	<0.0001
Physical activity (h/week)[¶]	2.8 (0.07)	2.2 (0.13)	<0.0001
Alcohol intake from beverages (g/day)	14.8 (0.41)	14.5 (0.71)	0.761
Coffee consumption (cups/day)	2.8 (0.04)	2.7 (0.08)	0.148
Whole-grain bread intake (g/day)	45.9 (1.11)	38.2 (1.91)	0.0003
Red meat intake (g/day)	43.3 (0.61)	48.9 (1.06)	<0.0001
Biomarkers			
Glucose (mg/dL)	88.1 (0.53)	107.0 (0.92)	<0.0001
HbA_{1c} (%)[‖]	5.42 (0.01)	6.30 (0.03)	<0.0001
HDL cholesterol (mg/dL)	47.5 (0.25)	40.9 (0.43)	<0.0001
Triglycerides (mg/dL)	114.8 (2.12)	177.2 (3.65)	<0.0001

Data are age- and sex-adjusted mean (SE) for continuous variables or % for categorical variables. †*P* for difference comparing incident cases of T2D with noncases of the subcohort. ‡Unadjusted mean (SD) or %. §Age-adjusted mean (SE). ¶Average of cycling and sports during summer and winter seasons. ‖Data were only available for $n = 2,900$.

TABLE 2
Mean serum concentrations of identified metabolites and their association with risk of T2D in EPIC-Potsdam

	Subcohort (n = 2,282) (µmol/L)	Cases (n = 800) (µmol/L)	RR per SD (95% CI)					
			Basic model[†]	+ Glucose[‡]	+ HbA$_{1c}$[‡]	+ HDL chol[‡]	+ Triglycerides[‡]	+ Glucose + HbA$_{1c}$ + HDL chol + Triglycerides[‡]
Hexose	4,698 (984)	5,783 (2,167)	2.36 (2.06–2.71)	1.62 (1.37–1.91)	2.11 (1.82–2.44)	2.43 (2.11–2.79)	2.34 (2.04–2.69)	1.51 (1.28–1.80)
Phenylalanine	56.4 (12.0)	61.0 (12.9)	1.35 (1.22–1.49)	1.24 (1.12–1.37)	1.37 (1.23–1.52)	1.34 (1.21–1.49)	1.30 (1.16–1.44)	1.25 (1.12–1.39)
Glycine	256 (77.2)	227 (59.6)	0.73 (0.64–0.83)	0.81 (0.71–0.92)	0.81 (0.71–0.93)	0.74 (0.65–0.84)	0.74 (0.65–0.84)	0.89 (0.78–1.01)
SM C16:1	17.6 (3.86)	17.4 (4.02)	0.80 (0.72–0.88)	0.82 (0.73–0.92)	0.74 (0.67–0.83)	0.87 (0.78–0.97)	0.79 (0.71–0.88)	0.91 (0.80–1.03)
PC ae C34:3	8.51 (2.48)	7.01 (2.02)	0.64 (0.56–0.72)	0.70 (0.61–0.80)	0.67 (0.58–0.77)	0.72 (0.63–0.82)	0.66 (0.58–0.74)	0.92 (0.78–1.07)
PC ae C40:6	5.52 (1.43)	5.03 (1.34)	0.77 (0.69–0.86)	0.81 (0.72–0.92)	0.83 (0.74–0.94)	0.82 (0.73–0.92)	0.76 (0.67–0.85)	0.94 (0.82–1.08)
PC ae C42:5	2.35 (0.54)	2.06 (0.46)	0.71 (0.63–0.79)	0.76 (0.67–0.86)	0.82 (0.72–0.92)	0.76 (0.68–0.86)	0.73 (0.64–0.82)	0.96 (0.83–1.12)
PC ae C44:4	0.38 (0.10)	0.33 (0.09)	0.76 (0.67–0.85)	0.77 (0.68–0.87)	0.84 (0.75–0.96)	0.82 (0.72–0.93)	0.77 (0.68–0.87)	0.97 (0.84–1.12)
PC ae C44:5	1.77 (0.48)	1.53 (0.43)	0.71 (0.63–0.80)	0.74 (0.65–0.84)	0.81 (0.71–0.91)	0.77 (0.68–0.87)	0.74 (0.65–0.83)	0.95 (0.82–1.09)
PC aa C32:1	16.9 (9.76)	20.4 (11.3)	1.18 (1.08–1.29)	1.12 (1.02–1.24)	1.12 (1.02–1.23)	1.23 (1.11–1.36)	1.12 (1.02–1.22)	1.15 (1.03–1.29)
PC aa C36:1	57.3 (15.6)	62.1 (17.2)	1.18 (1.08–1.30)	1.18 (1.07–1.30)	1.09 (0.98–1.21)	1.26 (1.14–1.39)	1.07 (0.96–1.19)	1.25 (1.10–1.41)
PC aa C38:3	55.4 (14.8)	65.3 (18.2)	1.37 (1.24–1.51)	1.35 (1.22–1.50)	1.31 (1.18–1.45)	1.38 (1.25–1.52)	1.24 (1.11–1.38)	1.38 (1.22–1.55)
PC aa C40:5	11.4 (3.49)	12.8 (4.17)	1.18 (1.08–1.29)	1.21 (1.10–1.33)	1.12 (1.02–1.24)	1.21 (1.10–1.32)	1.07 (0.96–1.18)	1.19 (1.06–1.32)
LysoPC a C18:2	35.2 (13.7)	29.6 (11.1)	0.74 (0.66–0.84)	0.72 (0.64–0.81)	0.77 (0.68–0.88)	0.79 (0.70–0.90)	0.72 (0.63–0.81)	0.84 (0.73–0.96)

Data are mean (SD) metabolite concentrations. a, acyl; aa, diacyl; ae, acyl-alkyl; chol, cholesterol; PC, phosphatidylcholine; SM, sphingomyelin. †Metabolites were selected by stepwise Cox proportional hazard regression modified by the Prentice method after standardizing metabolite concentrations to a mean of 0 (SD 1) and including all metabolites associated with T2D risk as well as relevant covariates. RRs for the basic model were then calculated in a continuous model adjusted for age, sex, alcohol intake from beverages (nonconsumers; women >0–6, 6–12, and >12 g/day; men >0–12, 12–24, and >24 g/day), smoking (never, former, current ≤20 cigarettes/day, current >20 cigarettes/day), physical activity (cycling and sports in h/week), education (low, medium, high), coffee intake (cups/day), red meat intake (g/day), whole-grain bread intake (g/day), prevalent hypertension (yes/no), BMI (kg/m^2), and waist circumference (cm). ‡Adjustment according to the basic model with additional adjustment for specified biomarkers.

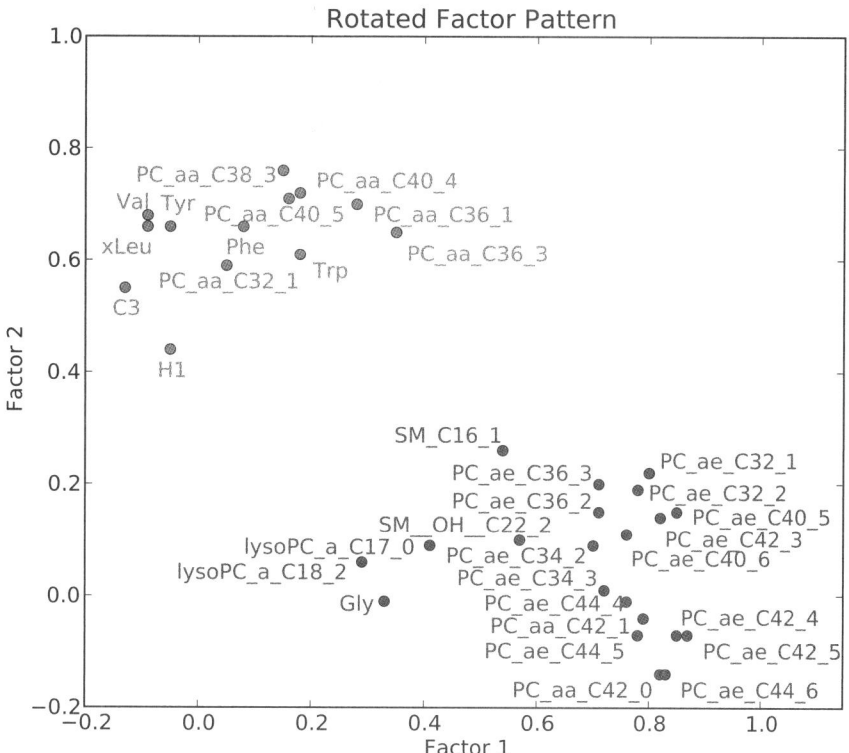

FIG. 1. Two metabolite factors associated with risk of T2D. Presented is a two-dimensional factor loading plot obtained from PCA. For simple interpretation, metabolites that cluster together in the plot are related to one another. Metabolites presented in blue are associated with decreased risk of T2D, whereas metabolites presented in red are associated with increased risk of T2D. More specifically, the factor loadings represent the correlation coefficients of individual metabolites with corresponding metabolite factors and may range from −1 to 1. They were identified by PCA based on the correlation matrix of all metabolites significantly associated with risk of T2D in the EPIC-Potsdam study. An orthogonal varimax rotation was used, and two factors were retained because they accounted for >50% of the observed variance. a, acyl; aa, diacyl; ae, acyl-alkyl; C3, propionylcarnitine; Gly, glycine; H1, hexose; PC, phosphatidylcholine; Phe, phenylalanine; SM, sphingomyelin; Trp, tryptophan; Tyr, tyrosine; Val; valine; xLeu, isoleucine.

of the metabolites (Table 2). An exception was that the inverse association between acyl-alkyl-phosphatidylcholines and sphingomyelin C16:1 and T2D risk was attenuated and no longer significant after adjustment for blood glucose, HbA_{1c}, HDL cholesterol, and triglycerides. The positive association between hexose and T2D risk was considerably weakened but remained significant after adjustment for plasma glucose. When we also adjusted for phenylalanine, tyrosine, and isoleucine, the associations for metabolite factor 1 were unchanged. The associations for metabolite factor 2, which included these three amino acids, were weakened but remained significant (data not shown).

We further observed that metabolites were linked to established T2D biomarkers (Supplementary Table 3). Specifically, metabolite factor 1, which was inversely associated with T2D risk, was negatively correlated to plasma glucose, HbA_{1c}, and triglycerides and positively related to HDL cholesterol and adiponectin. Metabolite factor 2, which was positively associated with T2D risk, was positively correlated with triglycerides and liver enzymes. Data from the TüF study revealed that acyl-alkyl-phosphatidylcholines, lysophosphatidylcholine C18:2, and glycine were positively associated with insulin sensitivity, whereas hexose and diacyl-phosphatidylcholines were inversely related to insulin sensitivity (Table 4). Furthermore, phenylalanine was positively associated with insulin secretion, whereas hexose, sphingomyelin C16:1, and acyl-alkyl-phosphatidylcholines were inversely related to insulin secretion. The

potential of identified metabolites to discriminate between T2D cases and noncases was comparable to that of the DRS (16) (ROC AUC 0.849 and 0.847, respectively, P for difference = 0.838) (Fig. 2). When the metabolites were added to established risk prediction models of T2D, discrimination was slightly but significantly improved up to a ROC AUC of 0.912, and these models were well calibrated (Fig. 2 and Supplementary Table 4). Replication in KORA revealed significant associations with T2D risk for metabolite factor 2 and hexose (Table 3 and Supplementary Table 5). In KORA, similar trends as in EPIC-Potsdam were seen for metabolite factor 1, acyl-alkyl-phosphatidylcholines, glycine, lysophosphatidylcholine C18:2, and sphingomyelin C16:1, with borderline significance. Although the risk estimates for diacyl-phosphatidylcholines were considerably lower in KORA than in EPIC-Potsdam, there was no significant heterogeneity between studies. We also calculated the RR of T2D for the BCAA and aromatic amino acids, which have recently been reported to be associated with T2D risk in the Framingham Offspring cohort and the Malmö Diet and Cancer study, to facilitate the comparison (35). In EPIC-Potsdam, isoleucine, valine, tyrosine, and phenylalanine were positively associated with T2D risk (RR per SD 1.30 [95% CI 1.17–1.43], 1.27 [1.16–1.40], 1.31 [1.18–1.45], 1.35 [1.22–1.49], respectively); leucine was not measured in EPIC-Potsdam. When combining isoleucine, tyrosine, and phenylalanine, the RR of T2D from lowest to highest quartile was 1.0, 1.13 (0.82–1.54), 1.45 (1.07–1.98), and 2.18 (1.62–2.95), respectively (P for trend < 0.0001).

TABLE 3
RR of T2D by quintiles of metabolite factors

	EPIC-Potsdam		Replication in KORA	
	Cases (N)	RR (95% CI)*	Cases (N)	RR (95% CI)*
Factor 1†				
Quintile 1	296	1.00	37	1.00
Quintile 2	194	0.61 (0.46–0.80)	15	0.59 (0.31–1.33)
Quintile 3	148	0.50 (0.37–0.67)	20	0.60 (0.31–1.14)
Quintile 4	95	0.37 (0.27–0.51)	12	0.56 (0.27–1.21)
Quintile 5	67	0.31 (0.21–0.44)	7	0.49 (0.17–1.25)
P for trend		2.95×10^{-13}		1.00×10^{-1}
Factor 2†				
Quintile 1	51	1.00	6	1.00
Quintile 2	102	1.23 (0.82–1.85)	9	1.38 (0.45–4.25)
Quintile 3	149	1.72 (1.17–2.51)	15	1.50 (0.52–4.32)
Quintile 4	191	1.80 (1.24–2.63)	18	1.81 (0.62–5.23)
Quintile 5	307	3.82 (2.64–5.52)	43	4.95 (1.96–12.48)
P for trend		6.64×10^{-18}		1.10×10^{-5}

a, acyl; aa, diacyl; ae, acyl-alkyl; PC, phosphatidylcholine; SM, sphingomyelin. *Relative risks were calculated with multivariate Cox regression (using the Prentice method to account for the case-cohort design in EPIC-Potsdam) across quintiles of metabolite factors after standardizing metabolite concentrations to a mean of 0 (SD 1). The model was adjusted for age, sex, alcohol intake from beverages (nonconsumers; women >0–6, 6–12, and >12 g/day; men >0–12, 12–24, and >24 g/day), smoking (never, former, current ≤20 cigarettes/day, current >20 cigarettes/day), physical activity (cycling and sports in h/week), education (low, medium, high), coffee intake (cups/day), red meat intake (g/day), whole-grain bread intake (g/day), prevalent hypertension (yes/no), BMI (kg/m²), and waist circumference (cm). †By conducting a PCA with orthogonal varimax rotation of all metabolites associated with T2D risk in EPIC-Potsdam, two metabolite factors could be identified that explained >50% of the variation of the metabolites. The corresponding linear factor equations (which equal the summed products of each metabolite's standardized concentration and corresponding factor loading) were as follows: Factor 1 = $(0.80 \times$ PC ae C32:1$) + (0.78 \times$ PC ae C32:2$) + (0.70 \times$ PC ae C34:2$) + (0.72 \times$ PC ae C34:3$) + (0.71 \times$ PC ae C36:2$) + (0.71 \times$ PC ae C36:3$) + (0.85 \times$ PC ae C40:5$) + (0.76 \times$ PC ae C40:6$) + (0.82 \times$ PC ae C42:3$) + (0.85 \times$ PC ae C42:4$) + (0.87 \times$ PC ae C42:5$) + (0.76 \times$ PC ae C44:4$) + (0.78 \times$ PC ae C44:5$) + (0.83 \times$ PC ae C44:6$) + (0.82 \times$ PC aa C42:0$) + (0.79 \times$ PC aa C42:1$) + (0.54 \times$ SM C16:1$) + (0.57 \times$ SM OH C22:2$) + (0.41 \times$ lysoPC a C17:0$)$. Factor 2 = $(0.55 \times$ propionylcarnitine$) + (0.66 \times$ phenylalanine$) + (0.61 \times$ tryptophan$) + (0.66 \times$ tyrosine$) + (0.68 \times$ valine$) + (0.66 \times$ isoleucine$) + (0.59 \times$ PC aa C32:1$) + (0.70 \times$ PC aa C36:1$) + (0.65 \times$ PC aa C36:3$) + (0.76 \times$ PC aa C38:3$) + (0.72 \times$ PC aa C40:4$) + (0.71 \times$ PC aa C40:5$) + (0.44 \times$ hexose$)$.

We conducted several sensitivity analyses. In EPIC-Potsdam, a small proportion of the participants (14.3%) had fasted. The proportion of incident T2D cases was equally distributed among fasting and nonfasting participants (26.8% and 26.7%, respectively). Additional adjustment for fasting status did not change the results. Further, we did not observe an effect modification of fasting status on the association between metabolite factors 1 and 2 and T2D risk (P for interaction = 0.115 and 0.688, respectively). We observed no interaction with sex (P = 0.407 and 0.441, respectively), and in both men and women, the risk associations were similar. Hazard rates of T2D in different periods of follow-up were not different (factor 1 P = 0.126, factor 2 P = 0.994), indicating that follow-up time did not affect the association between metabolite factors and risk of T2D. To ensure that the metabolite changes preceded the onset of T2D and were not attributed to prediabetic conditions, we repeated the analysis, excluding all cases of T2D that occurred shortly after the baseline examination

TABLE 4
Correlation between metabolites associated with T2D risk and measures of insulin sensitivity and secretion in the TüF study

	Insulin sensitivity	Insulin secretion
Hexose	−0.52	−0.39
Phenylalanine	−0.08	0.24
Glycine	0.34	0.08
SM C16:1	0.01	−0.13
PC ae C34:3	0.15	−0.24
PC ae C40:6	0.25	−0.08
PC ae C42:5	0.11	−0.24
PC ae C44:4	0.08	−0.21
PC ae C44:5	0.12	−0.30
PC aa C32:1	−0.15	−0.02
PC aa C36:1	−0.05	−0.09
PC aa C38:3	−0.24	0.01
PC aa C40:5	0.07	0.12
LysoPC a C18:2	0.36	−0.14
Factor 1†	0.23	−0.27
Factor 2‡	−0.15	0.00

Data are partial Spearman correlation coefficients. Insulin sensitivity was adjusted for age and sex; insulin secretion was adjusted for age, sex, and insulin sensitivity. Insulin sensitivity and insulin secretion were estimated from OGTTs in the TüF study ($n = 76$). a, acyl; aa, diacyl; ae, acyl-alkyl; PC, phosphatidylcholine; SM, sphingomyelin. †Factor 1 = $(0.82 \times$ PC aa C42:0$) + (0.79 \times$ PC aa C42:1$) + (0.80 \times$ PC ae C32:1$) + (0.78 \times$ PC ae C32:2$) + (0.70 \times$ PC ae C34:2$) + (0.72 \times$ PC ae C34:3$) + (0.71 \times$ PC ae C36:2$) + (0.71 \times$ PC ae C36:3$) + (0.85 \times$ PC ae C40:5$) + (0.76 \times$ PC ae C40:6$) + (0.82 \times$ PC ae C42:3$) + (0.85 \times$ PC ae C42:4$) + (0.87 \times$ PC ae C42:5$) + (0.76 \times$ PC ae C44:4$) + (0.78 \times$ PC ae C44:5$) + (0.83 \times$ PC ae C44:6$) + (0.54 \times$ SM C16:1$) + (0.57 \times$ SM OH C22:2$) + (0.41 \times$ lysoPC a C17:0$)$. ‡Factor 2 = $(0.55 \times$ propionylcarnitine$) + (0.66 \times$ phenylalanine$) + (0.61 \times$ tryptophan$) + (0.66 \times$ tyrosine$) + (0.68 \times$ valine$) + (0.66 \times$ isoleucine$) + (0.59 \times$ PC aa C32:1$) + (0.70 \times$ PC aa C36:1$) + (0.65 \times$ PC aa C36:3$) + (0.76 \times$ PC aa C38:3$) + (0.72 \times$ PC aa C40:4$) + (0.71 \times$ PC aa C40:5$) + (0.44 \times$ hexose$)$.

during the first 2 years of follow-up ($n = 208$). The risk associations were slightly lower, but not markedly different.

DISCUSSION

In this prospective investigation using a targeted metabolomic approach at population level, we found increased concentrations of hexose; phenylalanine; and diacyl-phosphatidylcholines C32:1, C36:1, C38:3, and C40:5 and reduced concentrations of glycine; sphingomyelin C16:1; acyl-alkyl-phosphatidylcholines C34:3, C40:6, C42:5, C44:4, and C44:5; and lysophosphatidylcholine C18:2 to be independently predictive of T2D in EPIC-Potsdam. The results agree with data from cross-sectional studies showing that patients with T2D had increased concentrations of sugar metabolites (13), acylcarnitines (14), and BCAA (13) and reduced concentrations of glycine (12). We were able to further replicate the results of Wang et al. (35), who recently reported that BCAA and aromatic amino acids predicted T2D in the prospective Framingham Offspring cohort and the Malmö Diet and Cancer study. In agreement with Wang et al. (35), we found higher concentrations of phenylalanine, isoleucine, tyrosine, and valine to be associated with increased risk of T2D and glycine to be associated with reduced risk of T2D. However, in the present study, BCAA and aromatic amino acids were linked to each other, and only phenylalanine was independently associated with T2D risk when accounting for the other metabolites. BCAAs may serve as substrates

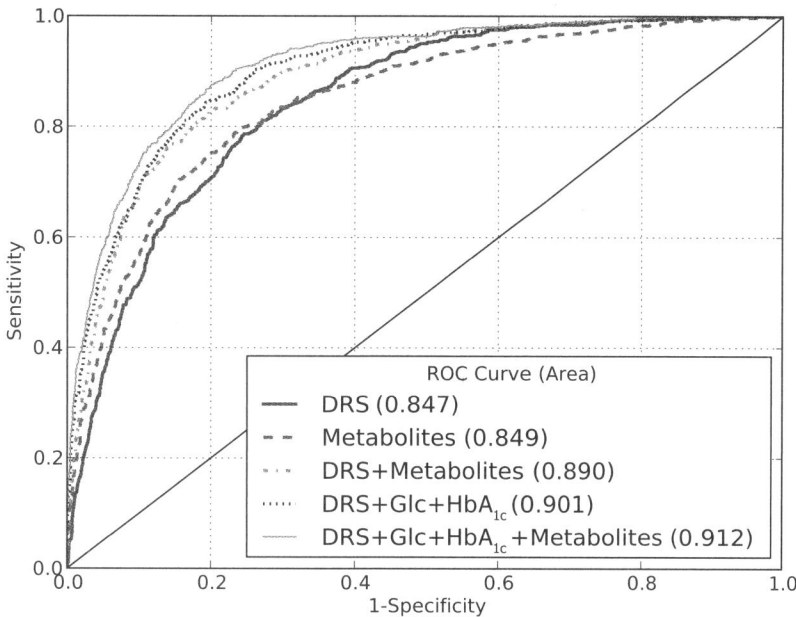

FIG. 2. Relative contribution of metabolites to predict T2D in EPIC-Potsdam. Presented are ROC curves comparing different multivariable-adjusted models to predict T2D, including the DRS, the identified metabolites, glucose (Glc), and HbA$_{1c}$. The DRS (16) combines information on several diabetes risk factors, such as diet, lifestyle, and anthropometry, to estimate risk of developing T2D. The DRS is computed according to the following formula: DRS = (7.4 × waist circumference [cm]) − (2.4 × height [cm]) + (4.3 × age [years]) + (46 × hypertension [self-report]) + (49 × red meat [each 150 g/day]) − (9 × whole-grain bread [each 50 g/day]) − (4 × coffee [each 150 g/day]) − (20 × moderate alcohol [between 10 and 40 g/day]) − (2 × physical activity [h/week]) + (24 × former smoker) + (64 × current heavy smoker [≥ 20 cigarettes/day]). Metabolites are hexose; phenylalanine; glycine; sphingomyelin C16:1; diacyl-phosphatidylcholines C32:1, C36:1, C38:3, and C40:5; acyl-alkyl-phosphatidylcholines C34:3, C40:6, C42:5, C44:4, and C44:5; and lysophosphatidylcholine C18:2.

for the glucose-alanine cycle in skeletal muscle. Through alanine aminotransferase–catalyzed transamination reactions, this may result in increased substrate availability for hepatic gluconeogenesis, thereby increasing hepatic glucose production (39). Conversely, glycine is a gluconeogenic amino acid; therefore, reduced serum glycine may also reflect increased gluconeogenesis. Alternative theories suggest that glycine depletion may reflect glutathione consumption driven by oxidative stress (40) or abundance of incompletely oxidized fuels that are excreted as urinary acylglycine conjugates (41–43). The frequently observed increase of BCAA in subjects with insulin resistance is also believed to be the result of reduced activities of key BCAA catabolic enzymes in liver and adipose tissue (44). Furthermore, amino acids may directly cause muscular insulin resistance by disrupting insulin signaling (45).

The positive association between hexose and T2D risk remained significant after adjustment for glucose. This observation could be an artifact from the different methods used to measure hexose and glucose. However, it has to be noted that hexose represented not only glucose but also the sum of all six-carbon monosaccharides. Previous studies have shown that in addition to glucose, fructose levels were elevated in individuals with T2D (12) and that intake of fructose was positively associated with risk of insulin resistance and T2D (46). In insulin-resistant conditions, the body aims to compensate for decreased glucose uptake of peripheral tissues through increased pancreatic insulin secretion (1). However, at the stage of overt insulin resistance, this system will eventually be exhausted, as caused by β-cell dysfunction and, subsequently, insulin secretion decreases (1). Phenylalanine, which was positively correlated to insulin secretion in the

present study, may be involved in pathways to compensate early stages of insulin resistance through stimulation of insulin secretion. In contrast, increased hexose concentrations may indicate manifest insulin resistance and defect of β-cells.

It is noteworthy that we observed significant associations between choline-containing phospholipids (i.e., diacyl-, acyl-alkyl-, and lysophosphatidylcholines and sphingomyelins) and T2D risk. Diacyl-phosphatidylcholines consist of glycerol linked to phosphocholine and two fatty acid residues, and removal of one fatty acid produces lysophosphatidylcholines. The corresponding acyl-alkyl-phosphatidylcholines comprise an ether linkage to one alkyl chain and one polyunsaturated fatty acid (47). Sphingomyelins are built of a ceramide core linked to one fatty acid and a phosphocholine or phosphoethanolamine (Fig. 3). Together, these phospholipids make up the main constituent of cellular membranes and may be involved in cellular signal transduction (48). In addition, they represent a major fraction of the human plasma lipidome because they are most abundant in all lipoproteins (49). Diacyl-phosphatidylcholines are particularly essential for hepatic secretion of triglyceride-rich VLDL particles and HDL (48), whereas acyl-alkyl-phosphatidylcholines may act as serum antioxidants to prevent lipoprotein oxidation (50). Their hepatic synthesis requires dietary choline (48). It was previously shown that choline-deficient mice on a high-fat diet showed reduced phosphatidylcholine biosynthesis and accumulated hepatic fat, but at the same time, they had reduced fasting insulin and improved glucose tolerance (51). In addition, impaired hepatic phosphatidylcholine biosynthesis led to reduced levels of plasma triglycerides and HDL cholesterol in vivo (52).

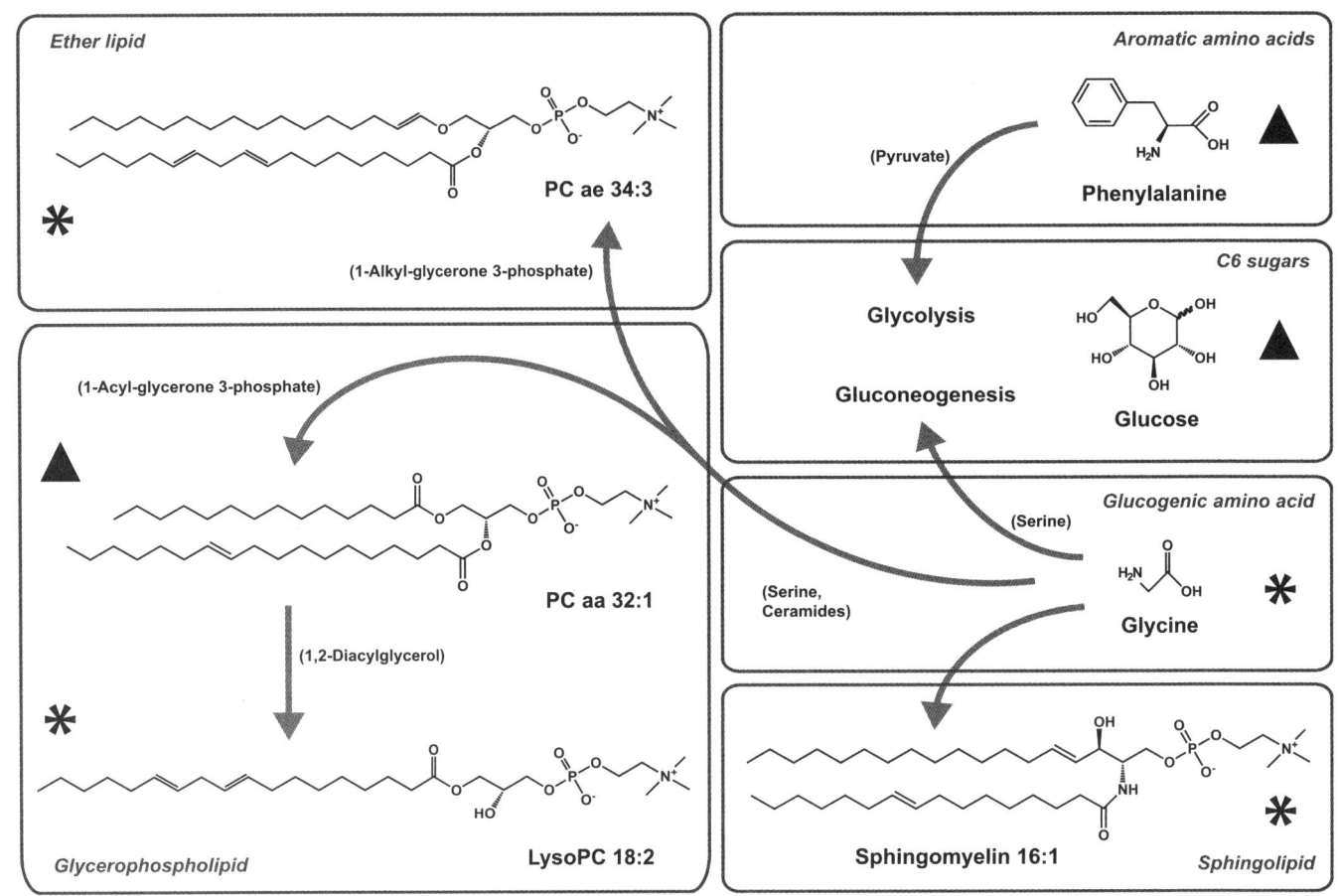

FIG. 3. Examples of metabolites associated with risk of T2D. ▲Metabolites with an increased risk (hexose, phenylalanine, and diacyl-phosphatidylcholines [PCs] C32:1, C36:1, C38:3, and C40:5). *Metabolites with a decreased risk (glycine; sphingomyelin C16:1; acyl-alkyl-PCs C34:3, C40:6, C42:5, C44:4, and C44:5; and lysophosphatidylcholine C18:2). Note that the mass spectrometric assay used does not distinguish molecular lipids and sugar types among hexoses. Therefore, formulas are given for a molecule corresponding to molecular mass and composition. Positions of double bonds and chain length may vary if more than one acid residue is present. Arrows represent many reactions, and key intermediates are given in the brackets. aa, diacyl; ae, acyl-alkyl. (A high-quality color representation of this figure is available in the online issue.)

Accordingly, phosphatidylcholines and sphingomyelins were positively related to plasma HDL cholesterol in the present study. Furthermore, acyl-alkyl-phosphatidylcholines were inversely correlated to plasma triglycerides, opposite to diacyl-phosphatidylcholines, and higher levels of acyl-alkyl-phosphatidylcholines but not diacyl-phosphatidylcholines were linked to improved insulin sensitivity and reduced insulin secretion. Previous studies reported that acyl-alkyl-phosphatidylcholine levels were lower in obese subjects and subjects with insulin resistance (50,53). These mechanisms may contribute to the antithetical association between two phosphatidylcholine subclasses and T2D risk found in the present study and may indicate a key role of the type of linkage between phospholipid core and fatty acid residue. Furthermore, those phosphatidylcholines containing fatty acids with a lower number of carbons and double bonds were positively associated with T2D risk, contrary to those with a higher number of carbons and double bonds. Similar observations have recently been reported for fatty acid compositions of erythrocyte membrane phospholipids (54) and triglycerides (55), suggesting that lipids with a shorter chain length and saturated fatty acid residues may trigger development of T2D, whereas those containing longer chains and unsaturated fatty acids may offer protection.

In summary, the present data suggest that the identified metabolites could be part of different pathways involved in the early genesis of T2D. Therefore, these novel candidates could be useful in clinical practice to identify high-risk individuals earlier in order to delay or prevent disease onset. Furthermore, serum metabolites in this study predicted risk of T2D in a similar manner to a combination of classic risk factors; thus, their measurement may be a useful approach to predict T2D risk for individuals in the future. The metabolites could also serve as markers for specific metabolic pathways that are deranged and, thereby, allow the implementation of individualized preventive and therapeutic strategies. However, future investigations are warranted to calculate in detail the individual risks and to better understand the metabolic effects of these biomarkers and their biological mechanisms.

The primary strength of this study is that, to our knowledge, we were among the first to adopt a targeted metabolomic approach at population level and included a large sample from three independent, well-described study populations. Furthermore, our targeted metabolomic platform covered a wide variety of metabolites with known identity and quantitative measurements. Because we used a prospective design with consecutive follow-up, we were able to investigate time-dependent exposure-disease associations.

The study, however, had several limitations. First, because we used independent study populations, the conditions of biosample collection, storage, and preparation were not necessarily the same, which may be a source of variation. In the KORA and TüF studies, fasting blood samples were collected from all participants, whereas in EPIC-Potsdam only a small proportion of participants provided fasting blood samples. Nevertheless, we did not observe an effect modification of fasting status on the association between metabolite factors and T2D risk, and we could reproduce very similar metabolite factors comparing fasting to nonfasting samples. Furthermore, the metabolomic analyses were based on serum samples in the EPIC-Potsdam and KORA studies but on plasma samples in the TüF study. As previously reported (56), the correlation between these serum and plasma metabolites was high; however, the absolute metabolite concentrations were higher in serum, which could lead to systematic changes. Second, the analytical method detected most of the metabolites with high specificity; however, it may not have detected all possible interferences among metabolites. Of the metabolites that we identified, diacyl-phosphatidylcholine C38:3 and sphingomyelin C16:1 may be interfering compounds for sphingomyelin C24:1 and diacyl-phosphatidylcholine C30:2, respectively. Third, we only had a limited number of incident T2D cases available from KORA. We may not have had sufficient statistical power, and the replication results have to be interpreted with caution. Fourth, there is a chance that reverse causation may explain the results, implying that overt diabetic conditions that were undiagnosed may have caused these metabolite changes. When we accounted for this issue, the results remained robust. Last, because this was an observational study, we cannot prove causality but only show associations. However, the identified metabolites were also correlated to established T2D biomarkers as well as to measures of insulin sensitivity and secretion in a different population, which underlines the biological plausibility of the results.

In conclusion, this prospective investigation using metabolomics data of independent study populations identified sugar metabolites, amino acids, and choline-containing phospholipids to be independently associated with risk of T2D. Beyond the classic pathways, these candidates point toward a novel role of phospholipid and lipoprotein metabolism in T2D pathophysiology. Future studies should further elucidate the biological mechanisms.

ACKNOWLEDGMENTS

The current study was supported by a grant from the Federal Ministry of Education and Research, Germany (Bundesministerium für Bildung und Forschung), to the German Center for Diabetes Research (Förderkennzeichen 01GI0922 to D.Z.D.). N.S. is supported by a Heisenberg professorship from the Deutsche Forschungsgemeinschaft.

No potential conflicts of interest relevant to this article were reported.

A.Fl., H.B., and T.P. designed the study. A.Fl., N.S., Z.Y., and K.M. analyzed the data. A.Fl., N.S., Z.Y., K.M., D.D., H.-G.J., A.Fr., H.-U.H., M.H.A., A.P., M.R., C.P., R.W.-S., T.I., M.B.S., J.A., H.B., and T.P. discussed the data and interpreted the results. A.Fl. wrote the first draft of the manuscript. N.S., Z.Y., K.M., D.D., H.-G.J., A.Fr., H.-U.H., M.H.A., A.P., M.R., C.P., R.W.-S., T.I., M.B.S., J.A., H.B., and T.P. provided their expertise and contributed to the writing of the manuscript. A.Fr., A.P., T.I., and H.B. collected the data. C.P. and J.A. conducted and supervised the metabolomic measurements. All authors take full responsibility for the contents of the manuscript. A.Fl. is the guarantor of this work and, as such, had full access to all the data in the study and takes responsibility for the integrity of the data and the accuracy of the data analysis.

The authors thank all the study participants of EPIC-Potsdam, KORA, and TüF. Special thanks go to Sven Knüppel and Wolfgang Bernigau (Department of Epidemiology, German Institute of Human Nutrition Potsdam-Rehbruecke) for statistical advice and to Martin Floegel (Max Born Institute for Non-Linear Optics, Berlin) for his support in figure formatting.

REFERENCES

1. DeFronzo RA. Banting Lecture. From the triumvirate to the ominous octet: a new paradigm for the treatment of type 2 diabetes mellitus. Diabetes 2009;58:773–795
2. Peters AL, Davidson MB, Schriger DL, Hasselblad V; Meta-analysis Research Group on the Diagnosis of Diabetes Using Glycated Hemoglobin Levels. A clinical approach for the diagnosis of diabetes mellitus: an analysis using glycosylated hemoglobin levels. JAMA 1996;276:1246–1252
3. Herder C, Baumert J, Zierer A, et al. Immunological and cardiometabolic risk factors in the prediction of type 2 diabetes and coronary events: MONICA/KORA Augsburg case-cohort study. PLoS ONE 2011;6:e19852
4. Abu-Qamar M, Wilson A. Evidence-based decision-making: the case for diabetes care. Int J Evid Based Healthc 2007;5:254–260
5. Swellam M, Sayed Mahmoud And M, Abdel-Fatah Ali A. Clinical implications of adiponectin and inflammatory biomarkers in type 2 diabetes mellitus. Dis Markers 2009;27:269–278
6. Li S, Shin HJ, Ding EL, van Dam RM. Adiponectin levels and risk of type 2 diabetes: a systematic review and meta-analysis. JAMA 2009;302:179–188
7. Ford ES, Schulze MB, Bergmann MM, Thamer C, Joost HG, Boeing H. Liver enzymes and incident diabetes: findings from the European Prospective Investigation into Cancer and Nutrition (EPIC)-Potsdam Study. Diabetes Care 2008;31:1138–1143
8. Stefan N, Fritsche A, Weikert C, et al. Plasma fetuin-A levels and the risk of type 2 diabetes. Diabetes 2008;57:2762–2767
9. Bain JR, Stevens RD, Wenner BR, Ilkayeva O, Muoio DM, Newgard CB. Metabolomics applied to diabetes research: moving from information to knowledge. Diabetes 2009;58:2429–2443
10. Newgard CB, An J, Bain JR, et al. A branched-chain amino acid-related metabolic signature that differentiates obese and lean humans and contributes to insulin resistance. Cell Metab 2009;9:311–326
11. Wopereis S, Rubingh CM, van Erk MJ, et al. Metabolic profiling of the response to an oral glucose tolerance test detects subtle metabolic changes. PLoS ONE 2009;4:e4525
12. Fiehn O, Garvey WT, Newman JW, Lok KH, Hoppel CL, Adams SH. Plasma metabolomic profiles reflective of glucose homeostasis in non-diabetic and type 2 diabetic obese African-American women. PLoS ONE 2010;5:e15234
13. Suhre K, Meisinger C, Döring A, et al. Metabolic footprint of diabetes: a multiplatform metabolomics study in an epidemiological setting. PLoS ONE 2010;5:e13953
14. Adams SH, Hoppel CL, Lok KH, et al. Plasma acylcarnitine profiles suggest incomplete long-chain fatty acid beta-oxidation and altered tricarboxylic acid cycle activity in type 2 diabetic African-American women. J Nutr 2009; 139:1073–1081
15. Hu FB. Metabolic profiling of diabetes: from black-box epidemiology to systems epidemiology. Clin Chem 2011;57:1224–1226
16. Schulze MB, Hoffmann K, Boeing H, et al. An accurate risk score based on anthropometric, dietary, and lifestyle factors to predict the development of type 2 diabetes. Diabetes Care 2007;30:510–515
17. Boeing H, Korfmann A, Bergmann MM. Recruitment procedures of EPIC-Germany. European Investigation into Cancer and Nutrition. Ann Nutr Metab 1999;43:205–215
18. Kroke A, Bergmann MM, Lotze G, Jeckel A, Klipstein-Grobusch K, Boeing H. Measures of quality control in the German component of the EPIC study. European Prospective Investigation into Cancer and Nutrition. Ann Nutr Metab 1999;43:216–224

19. Boeing H, Wahrendorf J, Becker N. EPIC-Germany—a source for studies into diet and risk of chronic diseases. European Investigation into Cancer and Nutrition. Ann Nutr Metab 1999;43:195–204

20. Weikert C, Stefan N, Schulze MB, et al. Plasma fetuin-A levels and the risk of myocardial infarction and ischemic stroke. Circulation 2008;118:2555–2562

21. Montonen J, Drogan D, Joost HG, et al. Estimation of the contribution of biomarkers of different metabolic pathways to risk of type 2 diabetes. Eur J Epidemiol 2011;26:29–38

22. Bergmann MM, Bussas U, Boeing H. Follow-up procedures in EPIC-Germany—data quality aspects. European Prospective Investigation into Cancer and Nutrition. Ann Nutr Metab 1999;43:225–234

23. Schienkiewitz A, Schulze MB, Hoffmann K, Kroke A, Boeing H. Body mass index history and risk of type 2 diabetes: results from the European Prospective Investigation into Cancer and Nutrition (EPIC)-Potsdam Study. Am J Clin Nutr 2006;84:427–433

24. Rothman KJ, Greenland S, Lash TL. Case-control studies. In *Modern epidemiology*. 3rd ed. Rothman KJ, Greenland S, Eds. Philadelphia, Lippincott-Williams & Wilkins, 2008, p. 111–127

25. Meisinger C, Strassburger K, Heier M, et al. Prevalence of undiagnosed diabetes and impaired glucose regulation in 35-59-year-old individuals in Southern Germany: the KORA F4 Study. Diabet Med 2010;27:360–362

26. Rathmann W, Strassburger K, Heier M, et al. Incidence of type 2 diabetes in the elderly German population and the effect of clinical and lifestyle risk factors: KORA S4/F4 cohort study. Diabet Med 2009;26:1212–1219

27. Kowall B, Rathmann W, Strassburger K, Meisinger C, Holle R, Mielck A. Socioeconomic status is not associated with type 2 diabetes incidence in an elderly population in Germany: KORA S4/F4 cohort study. J Epidemiol Community Health 2011;65:606–612

28. Stefan N, Kantartzis K, Machann J, et al. Identification and characterization of metabolically benign obesity in humans. Arch Intern Med 2008;168:1609–1616

29. Matsuda M, DeFronzo RA. Insulin sensitivity indices obtained from oral glucose tolerance testing: comparison with the euglycemic insulin clamp. Diabetes Care 1999;22:1462–1470

30. Römisch-Margl W, Prehn C, Bogumil R, Röhring C, Suhre K, Adamski J. Procedure for tissue sample preparation and metabolite extraction for high throughput targeted metabolomics. Metabolomics 11 March 2011 [Epub ahead of print]

31. Floegel A, Drogan D, Wang-Sattler R, et al. Reliability of serum metabolite concentrations over a 4-month period using a targeted metabolomic approach. PLoS ONE 2011;6:e21103

32. Prentice RL. Design issues in cohort studies. Stat Methods Med Res 1995;4:273–292

33. Holm S. A simple sequentially rejective multiple test procedure. Scand J Stat 1979;6:65–70

34. Hardy RJ, Thompson SG. Detecting and describing heterogeneity in meta-analysis. Stat Med 1998;17:841–856

35. Wang TJ, Larson MG, Vasan RS, et al. Metabolite profiles and the risk of developing diabetes. Nat Med 2011;17:448–453

36. DeLong ER, DeLong DM, Clarke-Pearson DL. Comparing the areas under two or more correlated receiver operating characteristic curves: a non-parametric approach. Biometrics 1988;44:837–845

37. Higgins JP, Thompson SG, Deeks JJ, Altman DG. Measuring inconsistency in meta-analyses. BMJ 2003;327:557–560

38. Hsieh FY, Lavori PW. Sample-size calculations for the Cox proportional hazards regression model with nonbinary covariates. Control Clin Trials 2000;21:552–560

39. Ruderman NB. Muscle amino acid metabolism and gluconeogenesis. Annu Rev Med 1975;26:245–258

40. Sekhar RV, McKay SV, Patel SG, et al. Glutathione synthesis is diminished in patients with uncontrolled diabetes and restored by dietary supplementation with cysteine and glycine. Diabetes Care 2011;34:162–167

41. Koves TR, Ussher JR, Noland RC, et al. Mitochondrial overload and incomplete fatty acid oxidation contribute to skeletal muscle insulin resistance. Cell Metab 2008;7:45–56

42. Muoio DM, Neufer PD. Lipid-induced mitochondrial stress and insulin action in muscle. Cell Metab 2012;15:595–605

43. Vianey-Liaud C, Divry P, Gregersen N, Mathieu M. The inborn errors of mitochondrial fatty acid oxidation. J Inherit Metab Dis 1987;10(Suppl 1):159–200

44. She P, Van Horn C, Reid T, Hutson SM, Cooney RN, Lynch CJ. Obesity-related elevations in plasma leucine are associated with alterations in enzymes involved in branched-chain amino acid metabolism. Am J Physiol Endocrinol Metab 2007;293:E1552–E1563

45. Tremblay F, Brûlé S, Hee Um S, et al. Identification of IRS-1 Ser-1101 as a target of S6K1 in nutrient- and obesity-induced insulin resistance. Proc Natl Acad Sci U S A 2007;104:14056–14061

46. Montonen J, Järvinen R, Knekt P, Heliövaara M, Reunanen A. Consumption of sweetened beverages and intakes of fructose and glucose predict type 2 diabetes occurrence. J Nutr 2007;137:1447–1454

47. Magnusson CD, Haraldsson GG. Ether lipids. Chem Phys Lipids 2011;164:315–340

48. Cole LK, Vance JE, Vance DE. Phosphatidylcholine biosynthesis and lipoprotein metabolism. Biochim Biophys Acta 2012;182:754–761

49. Quehenberger O, Dennis EA. The human plasma lipidome. N Engl J Med 2011;365:1812–1823

50. Wallner S, Schmitz G. Plasmalogens the neglected regulatory and scavenging lipid species. Chem Phys Lipids 2011;164:573–589

51. Raubenheimer PJ, Nyirenda MJ, Walker BR. A choline-deficient diet exacerbates fatty liver but attenuates insulin resistance and glucose intolerance in mice fed a high-fat diet. Diabetes 2006;55:2015–2020

52. Jacobs RL, Devlin C, Tabas I, Vance DE. Targeted deletion of hepatic CTP: phosphocholine cytidylyltransferase alpha in mice decreases plasma high density and very low density lipoproteins. J Biol Chem 2004;279:47402–47410

53. Pietiläinen KH, Sysi-Aho M, Rissanen A, et al. Acquired obesity is associated with changes in the serum lipidomic profile independent of genetic effects—a monozygotic twin study. PLoS ONE 2007;2:e218

54. Kröger J, Zietemann V, Enzenbach C, et al. Erythrocyte membrane phospholipid fatty acids, desaturase activity, and dietary fatty acids in relation to risk of type 2 diabetes in the European Prospective Investigation into Cancer and Nutrition (EPIC)-Potsdam Study. Am J Clin Nutr 2011;93:127–142

55. Rhee EP, Cheng S, Larson MG, et al. Lipid profiling identifies a triacylglycerol signature of insulin resistance and improves diabetes prediction in humans. J Clin Invest 2011;121:1402–1411

56. Yu Z, Kastenmüller G, He Y, et al. Differences between human plasma and serum metabolite profiles. PLoS ONE 2011;6:e21230

Inhibition of Class I Histone Deacetylases Unveils a Mitochondrial Signature and Enhances Oxidative Metabolism in Skeletal Muscle and Adipose Tissue

Andrea Galmozzi,[1] Nico Mitro,[2] Alessandra Ferrari,[1] Elise Gers,[1] Federica Gilardi,[1] Cristina Godio,[1] Gaia Cermenati,[2] Alice Gualerzi,[3] Elena Donetti,[3] Dante Rotili,[4] Sergio Valente,[4] Uliano Guerrini,[5] Donatella Caruso,[1] Antonello Mai,[4] Enrique Saez,[6] Emma De Fabiani,[1] and Maurizio Crestani[1]

Chromatin modifications are sensitive to environmental and nutritional stimuli. Abnormalities in epigenetic regulation are associated with metabolic disorders such as obesity and diabetes that are often linked with defects in oxidative metabolism. Here, we evaluated the potential of class-specific synthetic inhibitors of histone deacetylases (HDACs), central chromatin-remodeling enzymes, to ameliorate metabolic dysfunction. Cultured myotubes and primary brown adipocytes treated with a class I–specific HDAC inhibitor showed higher expression of Pgc-1α, increased mitochondrial biogenesis, and augmented oxygen consumption. Treatment of obese diabetic mice with a class I– but not a class II–selective HDAC inhibitor enhanced oxidative metabolism in skeletal muscle and adipose tissue and promoted energy expenditure, thus reducing body weight and glucose and insulin levels. These effects can be ascribed to increased Pgc-1α action in skeletal muscle and enhanced PPARγ/PGC-1α signaling in adipose tissue. In vivo ChIP experiments indicated that inhibition of HDAC3 may account for the beneficial effect of the class I–selective HDAC inhibitor. These results suggest that class I HDAC inhibitors may provide a pharmacologic approach to treating type 2 diabetes. *Diabetes* 62:732–742, 2013

Abnormalities in epigenetic regulation have been associated with multiple metabolic disorders, such as cardiovascular disease, obesity, and type 2 diabetes (1,2). Histone deacetylases (HDACs) regulate gene transcription by compacting chromatin and making it less accessible to transcriptional activators. Eighteen mammalian HDACs have been described, divided into four classes. While class I HDACs (HDACs 1, 2, 3, and 8) are broadly expressed and localize to the nucleus (3), class II HDACs (HDACs 4, 5, 6, 7, 9, and 10) can shuttle between cytoplasm and nucleus and exhibit minimal histone deacetylase activity (4,5). Class III HDACs (sirtuins) are good metabolic sensors (6); little is known about HDAC11, the single class IV HDAC in mammals (7).

Class II HDACs have been associated with the regulation of cardiac and skeletal muscle physiology (8,9). Genetic deletion of class II HDACs in skeletal muscle increases myocyte enhancer factor (MEF)2 activity and promotes the formation of slow-twitch type I fibers, rich in mitochondria and with high oxidative capacity. Less is known about the role of class I HDACs in skeletal muscle physiology, but cardiac-specific deletion of HDAC3 also results in increased expression of fatty acid oxidation and oxidative phosphorylation genes, though HDAC3 deletion is also associated with cardiac hypertrophy with deleterious consequences (10,11).

A recent report showed that sodium butyrate, an HDAC pan-inhibitor, has beneficial effects in mice with diet-induced obesity (12). To explore the promise of HDACs as targets in metabolic disorders, here we evaluated the therapeutic potential of selective class I and II HDAC synthetic inhibitors in obese diabetic mice. We found that class I, but not class II, HDAC inhibitors promote oxidative metabolism in *db/db* mice, reduce body weight, increase energy expenditure, and enhance insulin sensitivity, suggesting that class I HDAC inhibitors may be useful in conditions associated with suppressed oxidative metabolism, such as type 2 diabetes.

RESEARCH DESIGN AND METHODS

Reagents. Suberoyl anilide hydroxamic acid (SAHA) was from Cayman. MS275 and MC1568 were synthesized in-house. Anti–acetyl-H3, anti-HDAC1, anti-cytochrome C (CytC), and anti–rabbit IgG (Cell Signaling); anti–acetyl-tubulin, anti–α-tubulin, anti–β-actin, anti-Tfam, and anti–mouse IgG (Sigma-Aldrich); anti-HDAC3 and anti–peroxisome proliferator–activated receptor (PPAR)γ (Santa Cruz); and anti-HDAC3 (ChIP), anti–uncoupling protein (UCP)1, and anti-LCAD (Abcam) antibodies were used. Anti-electron transfer chain

From the [1]Laboratorio "Giovanni Galli" di Biochimica e Biologia Molecolare del Metabolismo e Spettrometria di Massa, Università degli Studi di Milano, Milan, Italy; the [2]Laboratorio "Giovanni Armenise-Harvard Foundation," Università degli Studi di Milano, Milan, Italy; the [3]Laboratorio di Immunoistochimica degli Epiteli, Dipartimento di Morfologia Umana e Scienze Biomediche "Città Studi," Università degli Studi di Milano, Milan, Italy; the [4]Dipartimento di Chimica e Tecnologie del Farmaco, Istituto Pasteur-Fondazione Cenci Bolognetti, Sapienza Università di Roma, Rome, Italy; the [5]Unit of Magnetic Resonance Imaging, Dipartimento di Scienze Farmacologiche e Biomolecolari, Università degli Studi di Milano, Milan, Italy; and the [6]Department of Chemical Physiology and The Skaggs Institute for Chemical Biology, The Scripps Research Institute, La Jolla, California.

Corresponding authors: Maurizio Crestani, maurizio.crestani@unimi.it, and Emma De Fabiani, emma.defabiani@unimi.it.

Received 28 April 2012 and accepted 25 August 2012.

DOI: 10.2337/db12-0548

This article contains Supplementary Data online at http://diabetes.diabetesjournals.org/lookup/suppl/doi:10.2337/db12-0548/-/DC1.

A.Ga., N.M., E.D.F., and M.C. contributed equally to this work.

A.Ga. and C.G. are currently affiliated with the Department of Chemical Physiology, The Scripps Research Institute, La Jolla, California.

F.G. is currently affiliated with the Center for Integrative Genomics, University of Lausanne, Lausanne, Switzerland.

See accompanying commentary, p. 685.

complexes (MitoProfile Total OXPHOS Rodent WB Antibody Cocktail) were from Mitosciences.

Cell culture. C2C12 cells were maintained in Dulbecco's modified Eagle's medium–10% FBS and differentiated in Dulbecco's modified Eagle's medium–2% horse serum. Cells were treated with SAHA (5 μmol/L), MS275 (5 μmol/L), MC1568 (5 μmol/L), or vehicle for 60 h. No toxicity was detected. Small interfering RNAs (Sigma-Aldrich) were transfected (30 nmol/L) into C2C12 myoblasts for 48 h prior to analysis. Adenoviruses expressing control or PPARγ coactivator (Pgc)-1α shRNAs were used to infect C2C12 myotubes at day 4 of differentiation. Myotubes were treated 24 h after infection and analyzed 16 h later. Primary brown preadipocytes were prepared from P0–P4 B6 mice as previously described (13).

Analysis of mitochondria. C2C12 myotubes were stained with 200 nmol/L MitoTracker Green FM or 400 nmol/L MitoTracker Red CM-H$_2$XRos (Invitrogen) for 30 min, 37°C, and then stained with Hoechst 33258. Fluorescence was measured with an EnVision (Perkin-Elmer). For electron microscopy, cells were processed as previously described (14). Ultrathin sections (200 nm) were evaluated using a JEM 1010 TEM (Jeol). Bioptic fragments from gastrocnemius (2 × 2 mm) were fixed in 3% glutaraldehyde in 0.1 mol/L Sorensen buffer, pH 7.4, overnight at 4°C and Araldite embedded. Two micron semithin sections were stained with toluidine blue. Ultrathin sections (60 nm) were stained with lead citrate and uranyl acetate and examined with a Jeol CX100 TEM (Jeol).

Gene expression and chromatin immunoprecipitation. Real time quantitative PCR (qPCR) was performed as previously described (15). For measurement of mitochondrial DNA, genomic qPCR was performed on 12S mitochondrial DNA and normalized to a nuclear Cyp7a1 sequence. Primer sequences are available upon request. Microarray analysis was performed by Genopolis (Milan, Italy). Differentially expressed genes were identified using Linear Models for Microarray Data. Chromatin immunoprecipitations (ChIPs) were performed as previously described (16) on C2C12 myotubes treated for 60 h. For in vivo ChIP, tissues were minced and fixed in 0.5% paraformaldehyde for 10 min and processed as previously described (17).

Oxygen consumption. Cells (5 × 10^5) were detached; resuspended in PBS containing 25 mmol/L glucose, 1 mmol/L sodium pyruvate, and 2% fatty acid–free BSA; and transferred to a Clark-type oxygen electrode chamber at 37°C. After recording of basal respiration, uncoupled respiration was determined with oligomycin (2.5 μg/mL), and maximal respiration was induced with 2.4 μmol/L carbonyl cyanide 4-(trifluoromethoxy)phenylhydrazone. Data were normalized to protein content.

Animal studies. Nine-week-old male C57BLKS/J-Lepr$^{db/db}$ mice (The Jackson Laboratory) were randomized into groups according to glucose levels and body weight and treated with 25 mg/kg i.p. SAHA, 10 mg/kg i.p. MS275, 6.5 mg/kg i.p. MC1568, or vehicle every other day. Compounds were dissolved in DMSO. Doses were based on pilot experiments (3–5 db/db mice per group). For blood chemistry analysis, animals were fasted for 16 h. Glycemia was determined using an Accu-Chek glucometer (Roche); commercial kits were used for other parameters (plasma triglyceride, Sentinel; NEFA-HR, Wako; ALT or AST Reagent, Teco Diagnostics; and Diagnostic Cholesterol, ABX Pentra). Insulin levels were determined with an AlphaLISA Immunoassay (Perkin-Elmer). Cholesterol distribution in lipoprotein fractions was determined by fast-protein liquid chromatography (FPLC). Lipids in vastus lateralis were extracted with the Folch method (18). Total triglycerides were quantified as described above using [^{3}H]-triolein as a standard. In glucose tolerance tests, mice were fasted for 16 h, and glucose levels were determined at the indicated times after injection of 2 g/kg i.p. glucose. At day 15 of treatment, oxygen consumption, heat production, and activity were measured over 3 days using the Oxymax System (Columbus Instruments). Mice were individually housed and allowed to acclimate with free access to food and water. Data were analyzed using the OxymaxWin, version 3.32, software as previously described (19). At day 20 of treatment, mice underwent a cold challenge (4°C for 2 h); rectal body temperature was measured every 20 min. Studies were conducted in accordance with European Commission regulations (European Union Directive 63/2010) and Italian regulations (decree no. 116, 27 January 1992) and with approval of The Scripps Research Institute's Institutional Animal Care and Use Committee.

Magnetic resonance imaging. At day 18 of treatment, mice were anesthetized and analyzed in a 4.7 Tesla Avance II magnetic resonance imaging (MRI) scanner (Bruker Corporation). After a gradient-echo scout, 16 axial 1-mm-thick T1-weighted slices were placed in the abdominal region spanning from kidneys to bladder inclusive. The field of view was 30 × 30 mm^2 with a matrix of 128 × 128 pixels. Four averages of a spin echo sequence with time to echo 10 ms and time of repetition 400 ms were acquired in 3′25″. The slice immediately frontal with respect to the ilium bone was chosen for visceral fat estimation and was computed as follows: (fat area)/(slice area). Areas were measured with Photoshop (Adobe Systems).

Histology. Skeletal muscle and adipose tissue were fixed with Carnoy solution/chloroform and embedded in paraffin, and 8-μm sections were stained with hematoxylin-eosin. For succinate dehydrogenase staining, slides were incubated for 30 min at 37°C in nitroblue tetrazolium–succinate solution. Quantification of dark fibers was performed counting multiple images ($n = 14$ for control, $n = 6$ for SAHA, and $n = 16$ for MS275) of nonconsecutive sections (four mice per group). Images were taken at ×20 magnification. For alkaline phosphatase staining, slides were incubated with borate buffer, pH 8.8, at 37°C for 1 h, fixed, and mounted. Esterase staining was performed by incubating slides at 37°C for 1 h in pararosaniline and sodium nitrite solution. For mitochondrial staining, white adipose tissue (WAT) sections were incubated with 200 nmol/L MitoTracker Green FM for 10 min and then washed and mounted. Fluorescence intensity was quantified using ImageJ.

Immunohistochemistry. Sections of WAT (8 μm) were deparaffinized, and antigen retrieval was performed with 0.05 mol/L NH$_4$Cl for 30 min, room temperature. Endogenous peroxidase activity was blocked with 1% H$_2$O$_2$ for 20 min. Blocking was performed in 1% BSA–0.1% Triton for 1 h. Anti-Mac1 (AbD Serotec) or anti-UCP1 (Abcam) was applied (1:300) overnight at 4°C. Incubation with biotinylated secondary antibodies (1:3000) followed. Histochemical reactions were performed using diaminobenzidine and sections counterstained with hematoxylin-eosin. Crown-like structures (Mac1 positive) were counted from multiple images ($n = 14$ for control, $n = 9$ for SAHA, and $n = 16$ for MS275) of nonconsecutive sections (four mice per group) taken at ×10 magnification.

Statistics. Statistical analyses were performed with Student t test or one-way ANOVA followed by Dunnett posttest as indicated, using Prism 5.0b (GraphPad Software).

RESULTS

Inhibition of class I HDACs promotes mitochondrial biogenesis. For evaluation of whether synthetic class I or class II HDAC inhibitors can enhance mitochondrial function, C2C12 myotubes were treated with the HDAC pan-inhibitor SAHA, a class I HDAC selective inhibitor (MS275), or a class II HDAC selective inhibitor (MC1568) (20–22). Concentrations were chosen based on dose-response curves (0.5–50 μmol/L) used to determine an effective, nontoxic, and selective concentration for each inhibitor based on the hyperacetylated state of histone H3 (a class I HDAC substrate) and α-tubulin (a class II HDAC substrate) (Supplementary Fig. 1A). After 60 h of treatment, global or class I HDAC inhibition resulted in increased mitochondrial density and activity, while inhibition of class II HDACs had no effect on these parameters (Fig. 1A and Supplementary Fig. 1B). These increases were accompanied by robust increases in mitochondrial DNA (Fig. 1A). Transmission electron microscopy confirmed that SAHA and MS275 induced mitochondrial biogenesis. Treatment with SAHA or MS275 resulted in an increase in mitochondrial density and greater electron opacity of the matrix typical of metabolically active cells. Cells treated with the class II HDAC inhibitor MC1568 showed mitochondria similar to those of controls (Fig. 1B).

Transcriptome analysis revealed that global or class I–selective HDAC inhibition increased expression of several key mitochondria-related transcription factors, such as Tfam, Tfb1m, and the coactivator Pgc-1α (Fig. 1C and D), as well as the levels of multiple genes involved in glucose and lipid metabolism (Supplementary Fig. 1D). These changes in gene expression and mitochondrial density translated to differences in oxidative metabolism, as global and class I–selective HDAC inhibitors induced a 20% increase in basal respiration (Fig. 1E). In the presence of oligomycin, only cells treated with SAHA showed a small but consistent increase (~15%) in oxygen consumption, while MS275 treatment increased maximal respiratory capacity by ~30%. SAHA treatment showed a tendency to increase maximal respiratory capacity but to

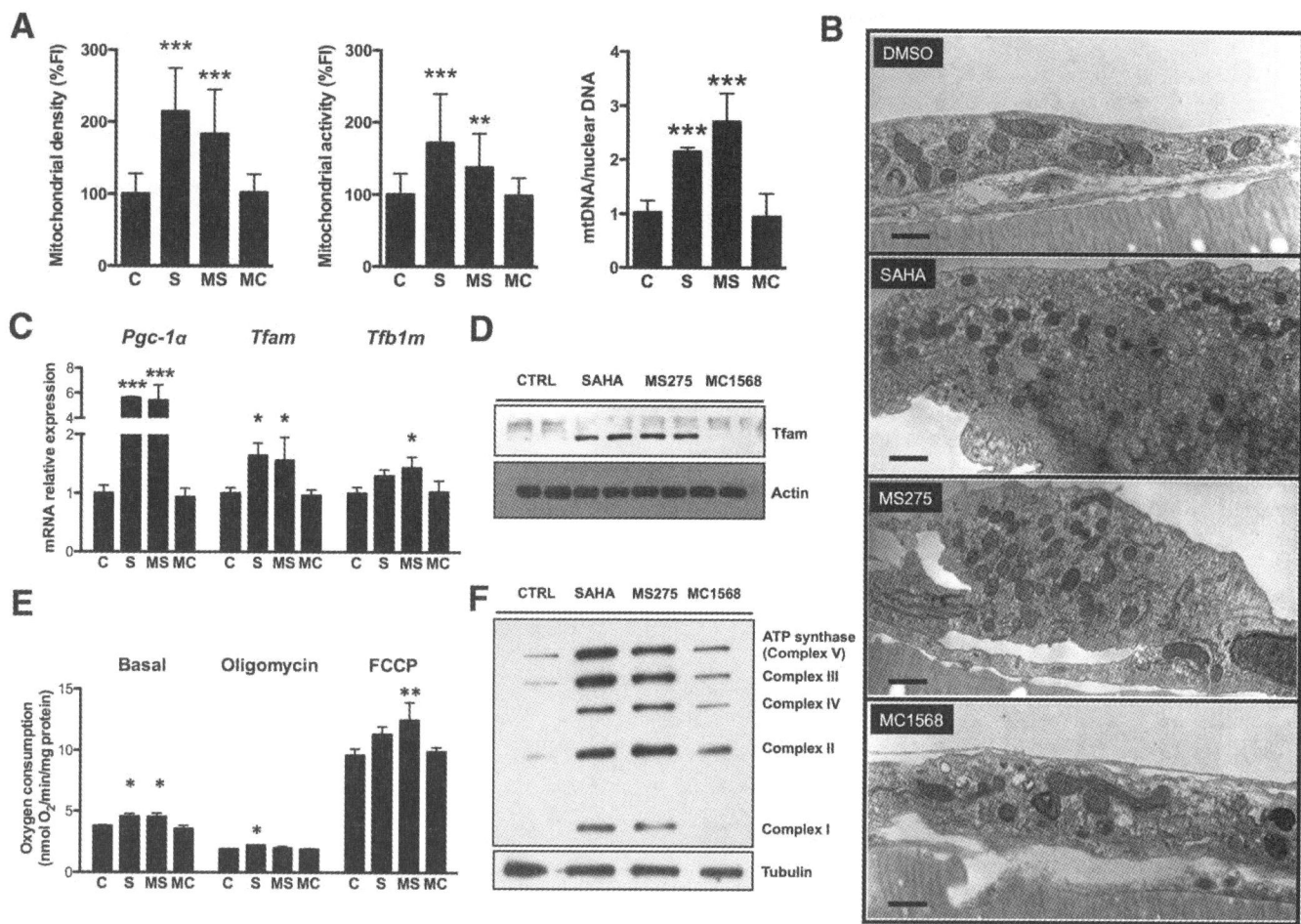

FIG. 1. Inhibition of class I HDACs promotes mitochondrial biogenesis and oxidative metabolism in C2C12 myotubes. *A*: Quantification of mito-chondrial density, activity, and mitochondrial DNA (mtDNA) in C2C12 myotubes after treatment with 5 μmol/L SAHA, 5 μmol/L MS275, 5 μmol/L MC1568, or vehicle. Fluorescence intensity (FI) of mitochondrial probes was normalized to a nuclear stain (Hoechst 33258). *B*: Representative electron microphotographs of ultrathin sections of C2C12 monolayers. The ultrastructural appearance of mitochondria in vehicle-treated cells was characterized by a dense matrix and well-organized cristae with dilated intracristae spaces in the typical condensed conformation of metabolically active cells (44). Treatment with SAHA or MS275 resulted in an increase in mitochondrial density and greater electron opacity of the matrix to the detriment of the development and organization of cristae. Cells treated with the class II HDAC inhibitor MC1568 showed rod-like mitochondria similar to those of controls (bars = 500 nm). *C*: Expression of genes associated with mitochondrial biogenesis (24 h) (*C*) and Western blot analysis of mitochondrial transcription factor A (Tfam) in C2C12 myotubes treated for 48 h with HDAC inhibitors (*D*). *E*: Measurement of oxygen con-sumption at the basal level and in the presence of oligomycin (2.5 μg/mL) or carbonyl cyanide 4-(trifluoromethoxy)phenylhydrazone (FCCP) (2.4 μmol/L) in C2C12 myotubes treated for 60 h with HDAC inhibitors. *F*: Western blot analysis of mitochondrial complexes I–V of the electron transfer chain in C2C12 myotubes treated with HDAC inhibitors for 48 h. Data are presented as means ± SD. *$P < 0.05$, **$P < 0.01$, ***$P < 0.001$ vs. control. C and CTRL, control; MC, MC1568; MS, MS275; S, SAHA.

a lesser extent (~20%). These changes were accompanied by corresponding increases in mitochondrial complex proteins (Fig. 1*F*). No differences were seen with the class II HDAC inhibitor. These results indicate that inhibition of class I HDACs reprograms myotubes toward a more oxidative state.

Class I–selective HDAC inhibitors ameliorate obesity and diabetes. Next, we tested the physiologic relevance of HDAC inhibition in a model of obesity and diabetes, the *db/db* mouse. At the doses used (25 mg/kg SAHA, 10 mg/kg MS275, and 6.5 mg/kg MC1568 administered every other day for a 23-day period), the compounds reached skeletal muscle and retained their class-selective inhibitory activity (Supplementary Fig. 2*A*). Mice treated with MS275 showed a significant reduction of body weight (Fig. 2*A* and Supplementary Fig. 2*B*), in spite of similar food intake (Supplementary Fig. 2*B*). Interestingly, we observed a dramatic reduction of fasting glycemia, of circulating

insulin, and of the homeostasis model assessment of in-sulin resistance index in animals treated with SAHA or MS275 but not in those treated with the class II HDAC inhibitor (Fig. 2*B* and *C* and Supplementary Fig. 2*C*). Moreover, global or class I–selective HDAC inhibition improved glucose clearance during glucose tolerance tests (Fig. 2*D*). Circulating triglycerides and nonesterified fatty acids were also decreased in SAHA and MS275 groups (Fig. 2*E*). MS275 completely cleared the lipids that accu-mulate in the liver of *db/db* mice, while SAHA had a sig-nificant but milder effect (Fig. 2*F*). The reduced hepatic steatosis was mirrored by decreased plasma trans-aminases, confirming that no toxic effects were observed with these compounds (Supplementary Fig. 2*D* and *E*). Interestingly, we did not observe any significant differ-ences in hepatic gene expression or mitochondrial con-tent, which suggests that the lack of hepatic steatosis is likely a reflection of the effect of MS275 in tissues other

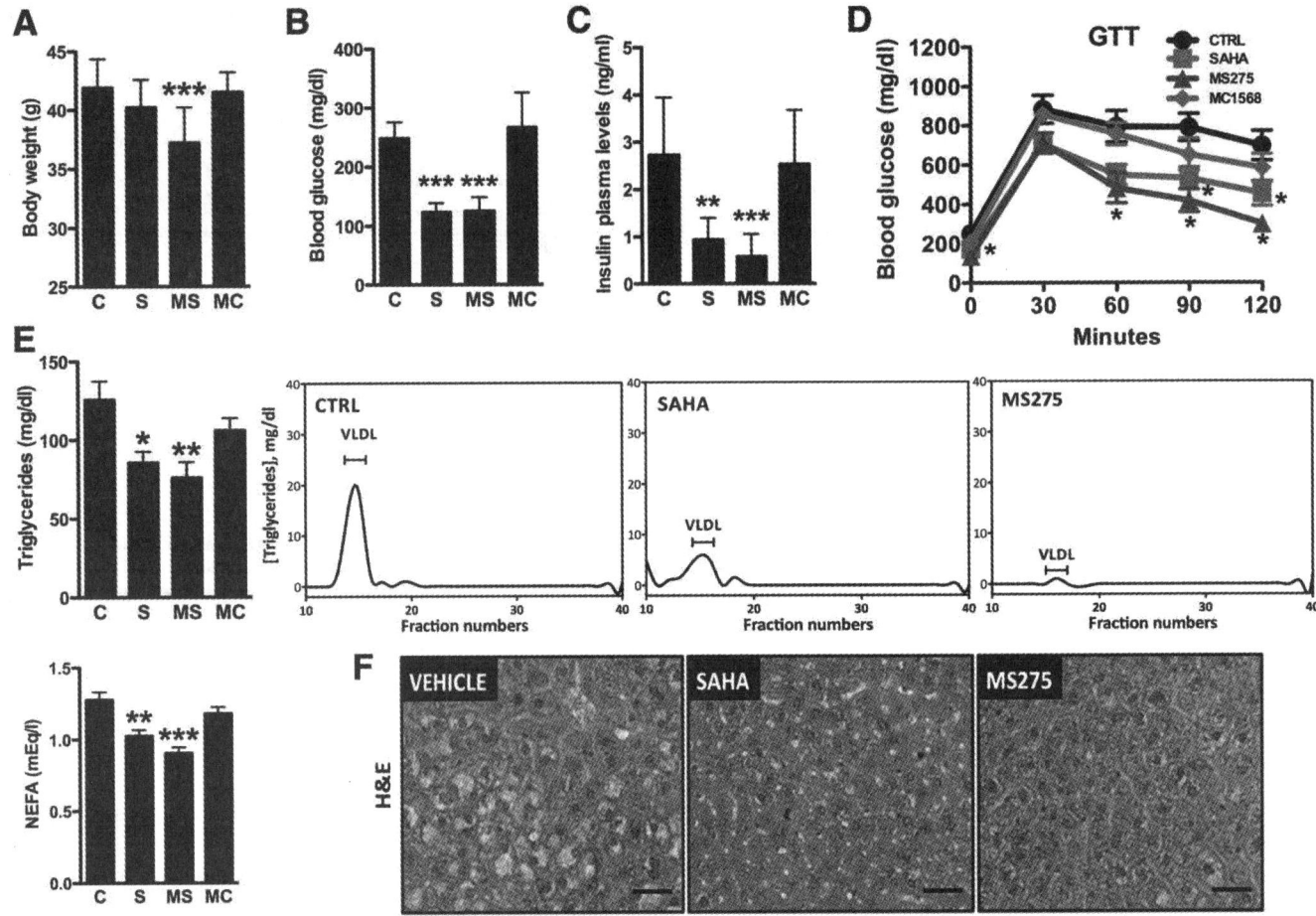

FIG. 2. MS275 ameliorates insulin resistance in *db/db* mice. *A*: Body weight of *db/db* mice treated with vehicle or HDAC inhibitors for 23 days (*n* = 10 per group). *B* and *C*: Fasting plasma glucose and insulin levels measured at day 23 of the treatment. *D*: Glucose tolerance test (GTT) performed on day 8 of treatment. *E*: Fasting serum triglycerides, nonesterified fatty acids (NEFA), and FPLC profile of plasma triglycerides of *db/db* mice treated with vehicle, SAHA, MS275, or MC1568. (FPLC samples are pools of 10 mice.) *F*: Hematoxylin-eosin (H&E) stain of liver sections from *db/db* mice treated with HDAC inhibitors. Data are presented as means ± SEM. *$P < 0.05$, **$P < 0.01$, ***$P < 0.001$ vs. control. C and CTRL, control; MC, MC1568; MS, MS275; S, SAHA. (A high-quality color representation of this figure is available in the online issue.)

than liver (Supplementary Fig. 2*F* and *G*). MC1568 had no effect on any parameter, indicating that inhibition of class I HDACs underlies the observed improvements in metabolic profile.

Class I HDAC inhibitors induce oxidative metabolism in skeletal muscle. To explore the molecular basis of the beneficial effects of SAHA and MS275 on metabolic parameters, we measured the expression of metabolic genes in skeletal muscle. In gastrocnemius, SAHA and MS275 increased expression of transcription factors and cofactors that regulate mitochondrial function (e.g., *Pgc-1α*, *Pgc-1β*, *Tfam*, and *Tfb1m*) (Fig. 3*A*) and of genes involved in glucose (*Glut4* and *Pk*) and lipid metabolism (*Acadl*), TCA cycle (*Idh3α* and *Suclg1*), and oxidative phosphorylation (*CytC*, *Cox6a1*, and *Etfdh*) (Fig. 3*B*). Similar effects were observed in the vastus lateralis and soleus (Supplementary Fig. 3*A* and *D*). Changes in gene expression translated to differences in protein levels (e.g., Tfam, Acadl [Fig. 3*C*]). Furthermore, succinate dehydrogenase staining demonstrated that mice treated with MS275, and to a lesser degree with SAHA, had an increased number of dark fibers, indicating greater oxidative capacity (Fig. 3*D*). Mitochondrial complex I and II proteins were also increased (Supplementary Fig. 3*B*). Electron microscopy

provided suggestions of differences in mitochondrial content, but these were not conclusive (Fig. 3*E*). No changes were detected in ectopic lipid levels (Supplementary Fig. 3*C*), perhaps because the extreme obesity of *db/db* mice did not allow detection of modest changes. Absence of toxicity was confirmed by lack of increased alkaline phosphatase or esterase staining (Supplementary Fig. 4*A*). Notably, while *Tnn1* mRNA levels increased in soleus, no concomitant changes in mRNA levels of contractile proteins characteristic of type I and II myofibers occurred in gastrocnemius or vastus lateralis (Supplementary Fig. 4*B*). These findings indicate that inhibition of class I HDACs in skeletal muscle contributes to ameliorating the phenotype of *db/db* mice at least in part by increasing expression of genes involved in fatty acid oxidation and glucose clearance.

Inhibition of class I HDACs promotes energy expenditure in *db/db* mice. Since the oxidative pattern of gene expression induced by global and class I–selective HDAC inhibitors has been associated with increased energy expenditure, we assessed energy balance in *db/db* mice treated with SAHA or MS275. Animals treated for 15 days with the class I–selective HDAC inhibitor showed increased oxygen consumption and carbon dioxide release

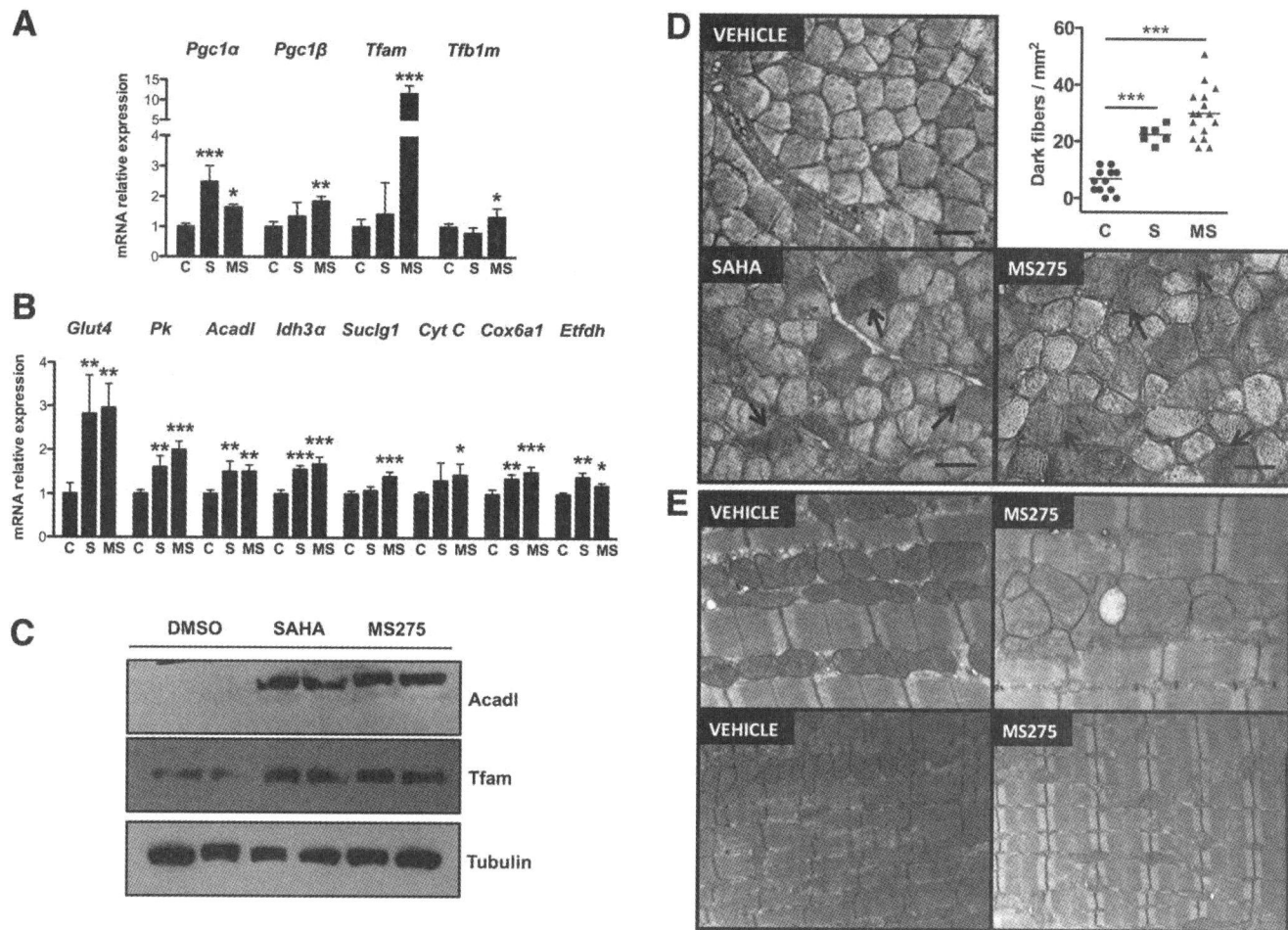

FIG. 3. Inhibition of class 1 HDACs promotes oxidative metabolism in skeletal muscle. mRNA expression levels of mitochondrial biogenesis–associated (*A*) and metabolic pathway (*B*) genes in skeletal muscle of *db/db* mice treated with HDAC inhibitors. *C*: Western blot analysis of Acadl and Tfam in skeletal muscle of *db/db* mice after treatment with HDAC inhibitors. *D*: Succinate dehydrogenase staining and quantification of dark fibers (arrows) in gastrocnemius sections (bars = 100 µm). *E*: Representative electron microphotographs of ultrathin sections of gastrocnemius from mice treated with vehicle or MS275 (magnification: *upper panels*, ×15,000; *lower panels*, ×8,000). Data are presented as means ± SD. *P < 0.05, **P < 0.01, ***P < 0.001 vs. control. C, control; MS, MS275; S, SAHA. (A high-quality color representation of this figure is available in the online issue.)

during the dark cycle, while only a trend for increased oxygen consumption was observed during the light cycle (Fig. 4*A* and *B* and Supplementary Fig. 5*A*). Nonetheless, these changes were sufficient to reduce the respiratory exchange ratio (RER) during both light and dark cycles, an indication that these mice use lipids preferentially as fuel (Fig. 4*C*). Heat production was also 12% greater in the MS275-treated group (Fig. 4*D*), while locomotor activity did not change (Supplementary Fig. 5*B*). SAHA had no significant effect on oxygen consumption, but treated mice showed a mild but significant reduction of RER during the day (Fig. 4*A*–*D*).

HDAC3 regulates oxidative metabolism in a Pgc-1α–dependent manner. To explore the mechanism whereby class I HDAC inhibition promotes mitochondrial biogenesis, oxidative metabolism, and increased energy expenditure, we evaluated the contribution of Pgc-1α to these effects. C2C12 myotubes infected with shRNA against Pgc-1α lost the ability to increase oxidative gene expression upon SAHA or MS275 exposure (Fig. 5*A*), indicating that Pgc-1α is a primary mediator of the effect of class I HDAC inhibition on oxidative gene expression.

Absence of Rip140 did not abolish the response to treatment with SAHA or MS275 (Supplementary Fig. 6*A* and *B*), suggesting that Rip140 is not a central mediator of the effect of these compounds.

Next, we sought to understand how class I HDAC inhibition enhances *Pgc-1α* expression. Two class I HDACs are recruited onto two different regions of the *Pgc-1α* promoter: Hdac1 represses Creb-mediated *Pgc-1α* transcription (23), while Hdac3, together with Hdac4, Hdac5, and the nuclear corepressor NCoR, is recruited onto members of the Mef2 family to repress transcriptional activation of *Pgc-1α* (24,25) (Fig. 5*B*). We found that a 70% reduction of Hdac3 (Fig. 5*C*) is sufficient to mimic the effect of class I HDAC inhibitors on the expression of *Pgc-1α*, *Glut4*, *Tfam*, and *Idh3α* (Fig. 5*D*). In contrast, similar silencing of Hdac1 had no effect on expression of these genes (Supplementary Fig. 6*C* and *D*). ChIP showed that treatment with SAHA or MS275 reduced Hdac3 recruitment onto the Mef-binding site in the *Pgc-1α* promoter (Fig. 5*E*). The presence of Hdac3 in the cAMP-responsive element region was barely detectable and was unaffected by compound treatment. Similar results were obtained

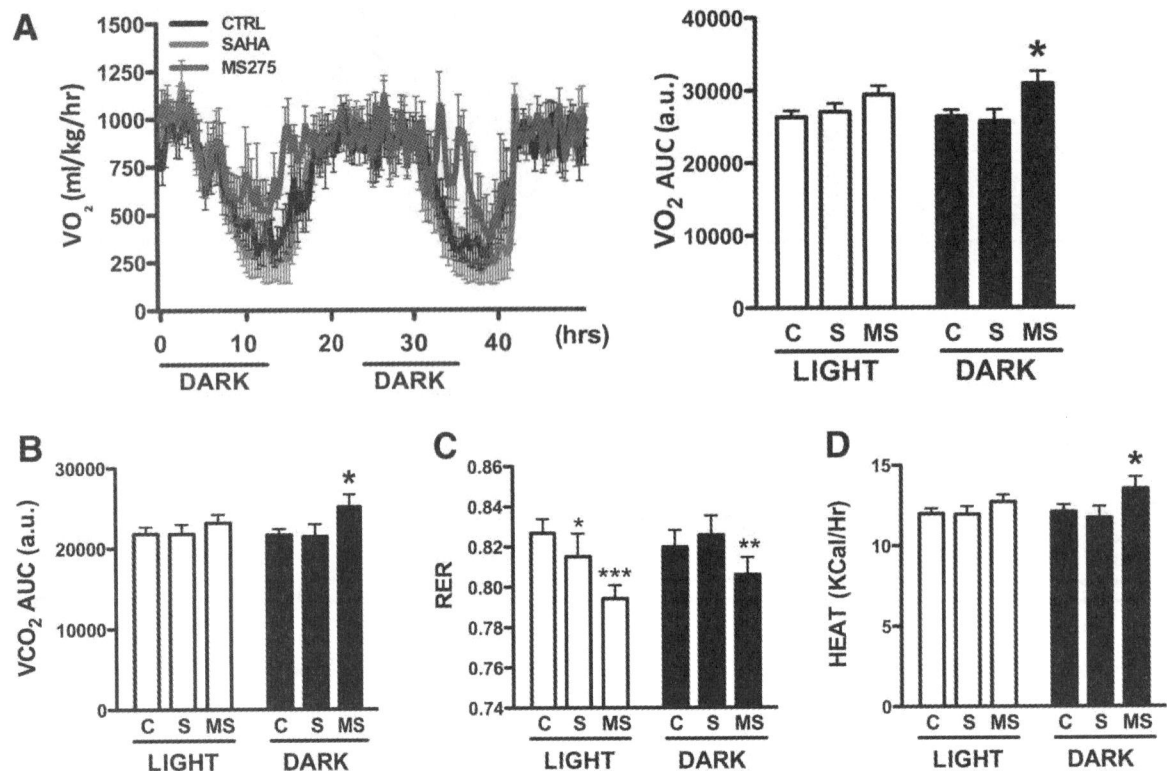

FIG. 4. Effect of HDAC inhibitors on energy balance in *db/db* mice. Oxygen consumption (*A* and *B*), RER (*C*), and heat production (*D*) in *db/db* mice treated every other day with vehicle, 25 mg/kg SAHA, or 10 mg/kg MS275 for 2 weeks prior to analysis. All parameters were measured over three days using five individually housed *db/db* male mice per group. Statistical comparison of repeated measurements was made using ANOVA. Data are presented as means ± SEM. *$P < 0.05$, **$P < 0.01$, ***$P < 0.001$ vs. control group. a.u., arbitrary units; AUC, area under the curve; C and CTRL, control; MS, MS275; S, SAHA.

when ChIP was performed in skeletal muscle extracts derived from *db/db* mice treated with SAHA or MS275: both compounds decreased Hdac3 recruitment on the *Pgc-1α* promoter in vivo, though MS275 had a greater effect (Fig. 5*F*). These results suggest that the beneficial effects of class I HDAC inhibition in muscle are primarily due to Hdac3 inhibition that results in increased *Pgc-1α* expression.

Inhibition of class I HDACs promotes uncoupled metabolism in brown adipose tissue. As observed for skeletal muscle, the compounds retained their class-selective inhibitory activity in the brown adipose tissue (BAT) of treated animals (Fig. 6*E*). BAT of obese diabetic animals treated with SAHA or MS275 showed a significant reduction in cell size (Fig. 6*A*). MRI analysis showed a 13.6 and 15.7% increase of interscapular BAT in SAHA- and MS275-treated animals, respectively (Fig. 6*B*). *db/db* mice treated with MS275, but not SAHA, maintained body temperature better during an acute cold challenge, indicating that the increased BAT mass is functional (Fig. 6*C*). Expression of classical markers of brown fat (e.g., *Ucp1*, *Elovl3*, *Dio2*, *Cidea*, *Prdm16*, and the β3-adrenergic receptor *Adrb3*) was robustly increased (Fig. 6*D* and *E*). MS275 upregulated the expression of *Ppary*, *Pgc-1α*, *Pgc-1β*, and mitochondrial biogenesis markers (e.g., *Tfam*, *Tfb1m*, and *CytC*) (Fig. 6*F*). The effects of SAHA were less pronounced, which may partially explain why animals treated with this compound did not show an increase in heat production (Fig. 4*D*). Similar to the in vivo scenario, primary brown adipocytes differentiated in vitro and treated with MS275 or SAHA showed higher levels of *Pgc-1α*, *Ucp1*, *Adrb3*, *Tfam*, and

PPARγ mRNA (Fig. 6*G*) and increased mitochondrial DNA content (Fig. 6*H*). As a consequence, treated primary brown adipocytes showed higher basal, uncoupled, and maximal respiratory capacity (Fig. 6*I*).

In analogy to skeletal muscle, we performed ChIP in BAT and found significantly diminished amounts of Hdac3 associated with the region containing the PPAR-responsive element of the *Pgc-1α* promoter in animals treated with MS275 (Fig. 6*J*). This observation suggests that Hdac3 inhibition, and its consequent dissociation from the promoter, may be primarily responsible for *Pgc-1α* induction in mice treated with MS275.

WAT treated with a class I HDAC inhibitor acquires brown fat features. White adipocyte size was reduced in *db/db* mice treated with the class I–selective HDAC inhibitor (Fig. 7*A* and Supplementary Fig. 7*A*), and MRI analysis also showed an 18% reduction of WAT in these animals (Supplementary Fig. 7*B*). These findings were associated with increased expression of genes that regulate lipid metabolism (Fig. 7*B*). *Ppary* expression was also dramatically upregulated, as was that of its direct targets (Fig. 7*C*). Class I HDAC inhibition also resulted in changes of *Pgc-1α*, *Tfam*, and *CytC* transcripts (Fig. 7*D*) and increased mitochondrial content (Fig. 7*E*) and density (Supplementary Fig. 7*C*), indicating a greater oxidative state in WAT. In addition, as may be expected from increased Ppary signaling, expression of inflammatory markers was robustly suppressed after SAHA or MS275 administration (Supplementary Fig. 7*D*). Immunohistochemical analysis confirmed reduced macrophage infiltration into WAT (Fig. 7*A* and Supplementary Fig. 7*E*).

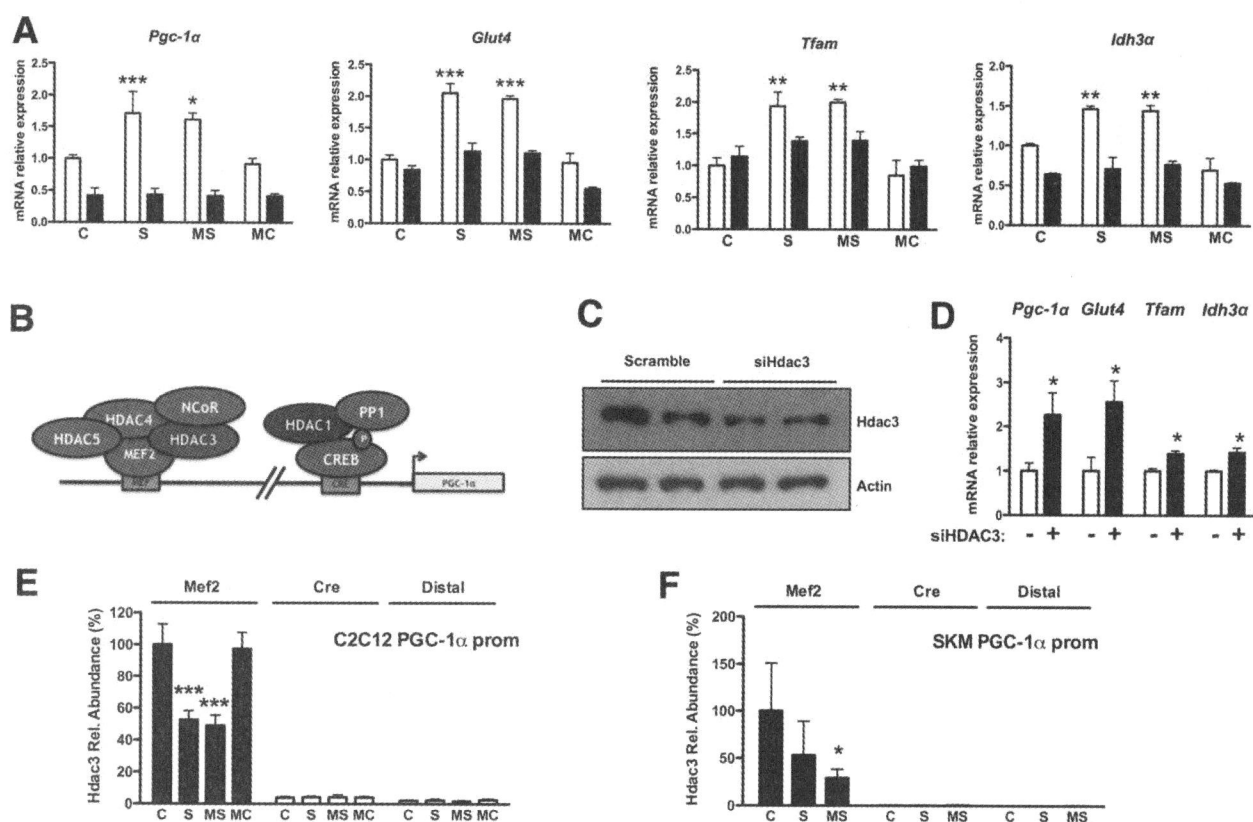

FIG. 5. HDAC3 ablation mimics the effect of class I HDAC inhibitors in a PGC-1α–dependent manner. *A*: *Pgc-1α*, *Glut4*, *Tfam*, and *Idh3α* expression in C2C12 myotubes infected with adenoviruses expressing shRNA against Pgc-1α (■) or scramble control (□). Note that the effect of HDAC inhibitors is lost in the absence of Pgc-1α. *B*: Schematic representation of the HDACs known to be present on the *Pgc-1α* promoter (prom). *C*: Hdac3 protein levels in C2C12 myoblasts transfected with small interfering RNA against Hdac3 or control. *D*: Gene expression profile after silencing Hdac3 in C2C12 myotubes. *E* and *F*: Hdac3 ChIP of C2C12 myotubes or skeletal muscle (SKM) of *db/db* mice treated with HDAC inhibitors. Bars represent presence of Hdac3 on the *Pgc-1α* promoter within the Mef2 or the cAMP-responsive element regions shown in *B*. A distal region was used as a negative control. Data are presented as means ± SD. *$P < 0.05$, **$P < 0.01$, ***$P < 0.001$ vs. control. C, control; MC, MC1568; MS, MS275; Rel., relative; S, SAHA. (A high-quality color representation of this figure is available in the online issue.)

Surprisingly, inhibition of class I HDACs also resulted in a dramatic increase in the expression of genes normally associated with brown fat (Fig. 7*F* and Supplementary Table 1). *Ucp1* (~50-fold increase), *Cidea*, *Dio2*, *Adrb3*, *C/ebpβ*, and other markers characteristic of brown adipocytes were robustly induced in WAT treated with MS275 and, to a lesser extent, with SAHA (Fig. 7*A* and *G*). As reported in other cases of "browning" of white adipose depots (26–29), the class I inhibitor appears to transcriptionally reprogram WAT toward a more oxidative phenotype characterized by a strong upregulation of Ucp1 expression.

DISCUSSION

In spite of provocative genetics data that demonstrate a role for class I and II HDACs in muscle physiology, significantly less is known about the ability of modulators of these HDAC classes to regulate systemic metabolism. Recent studies used the natural short-chain fatty acid sodium butyrate to show that this dual class I/II HDAC inhibitor increases insulin sensitivity and energy expenditure in high-fat–fed mice (12,30,31). However, sodium butyrate has a cornucopia of cellular effects, many of which are independent of its ability to block HDAC function (32). Conclusive association between chemical inhibition of

specific HDAC classes and systemic energy metabolism has thus been lacking. In this study, we have used a pan-inhibitor and class I– or class II–selective synthetic HDAC inhibitors to establish the contribution of specific HDACs to whole-body metabolism.

In vitro, class I HDAC inhibition enhanced expression of critical mitochondrial regulators resulting in increased mitochondrial biogenesis and greater oxygen consumption in muscle cells and primary brown adipocytes. The lack of an effect of the class II HDAC inhibitor was surprising; however, class II HDACs are thought to have minimal deacetylase activity and to behave primarily as bridging molecules that recruit catalytically active HDAC complexes and other corepressors (33). Hence, it is possible that chemical inhibition of class II HDACs is not sufficient to interfere with assembly of silencing complexes.

Pgc-1α mediates the effects of class I HDAC inhibition, as silencing of Pgc-1α abolished the effect of these compounds on oxidative gene expression and genetic knockdown of Hdac3 recapitulated the effects seen with the chemical inhibitor of class I HDACs on *Pgc-1α* expression. We have shown in vitro and in vivo that the class I–selective inhibitor induces Pgc-1α transcription by blunting Hdac3 recruitment onto the Pgc-1α promoter, thus driving oxidative gene expression in skeletal muscle and BAT and browning of WAT.

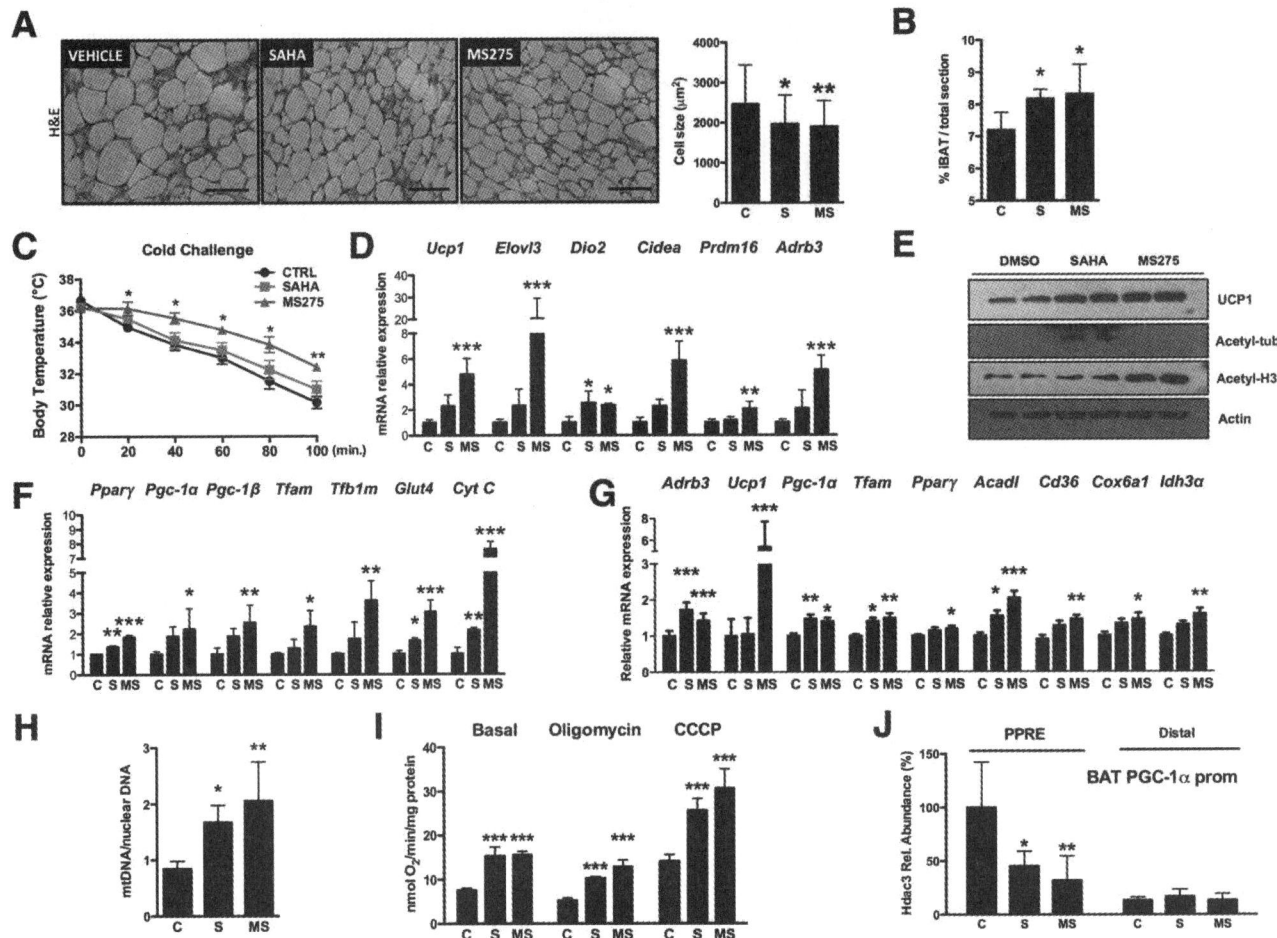

FIG. 6. Class I HDAC inhibition enhances oxidative metabolism in brown fat. *A*: Hematoxylin-eosin (H&E) stain of BAT from *db/db* mice treated with HDAC inhibitors (bar = 100 μm) and quantification of brown adipocyte cell size. *B*: Magnetic resonance analysis of interscapular BAT (iBAT) in *db/db* mice treated for 15 days with HDAC inhibitors. *C*: Body temperature of *db/db* mice treated with vehicle, SAHA, or MS275 and exposed to temperature of 4°C. Expression of classical markers of brown fat (*D*) and Western blot analysis of Ucp1 and HDAC targets, acetyl-tubulin, and acetyl-histone H3 (*E*). *F*: mRNA level of genes related to mitochondrial biogenesis or selected metabolic pathways in animals treated with vehicle, SAHA, or MS275. Note that MS275 has a more pronounced effect than SAHA on all genes examined. *G*: mRNA level of genes related to mitochondrial biogenesis or adrenergic response in primary brown adipocytes differentiated in vitro and treated with 1 μmol/L SAHA, 1 μmol/L MS275, or vehicle. *H*: Quantification of mitochondrial DNA (mtDNA) in primary brown adipocytes after treatment with 1 μmol/L SAHA, 1 μmol/L MS275, or vehicle. *I*: Measurement of oxygen consumption at the basal level and in the presence of oligomycin (2.5 μg/mL) or carbonyl cyanide 3-chlorophenylhydrazone (CCCP) (2.4 μmol/L) in primary brown adipocytes treated for 24 h with HDAC inhibitors. *J*: Hdac3 ChIP assay BAT of *db/db* mice treated with HDAC inhibitors. Bars represent presence of Hdac3 on the *Pgc-1α* promoter (prom) within the PPAR-responsive element (PPRE) region. A distal region was used as a negative control. Data are presented as means ± SD. C and CTRL, control; MS, MS275; Rel., relative; S, SAHA. *$P < 0.05$, **$P < 0.01$, ***$P < 0.001$ vs. control. (A high-quality color representation of this figure is available in the online issue.)

Treatment of *db/db* mice with SAHA or MS275 resulted in enhanced glucose tolerance and insulin sensitivity, clearance of liver lipids, and decreased plasma triglycerides and free fatty acids. Given the large mass of skeletal muscle, its contribution to glucose clearance is likely to be comparable in mice treated with either SAHA or MS275, perhaps explaining why glucose and insulin levels were similarly decreased in these two groups. The reduction in hepatic steatosis contrasts with the accumulation of liver lipids seen in liver-specific Hdac3-null mice (34). This difference may be ascribed to the effect of global versus local HDAC3 inhibition: in diabetic mice, systemic HDAC3 inhibition (i.e., MS275 treatment) increases peripheral oxidative metabolism and energy expenditure, thus preventing hepatic lipid buildup. The increased PPARγ activity that we observed in WAT of MS275-treated mice also likely means that the capacity of this tissue to remove from the

circulation and store excess fatty acids is enhanced, further preventing ectopic lipid deposition. The greater effect of the class I HDAC inhibitor relative to SAHA may be due to the fact that MS275 treatment resulted in significantly more dramatic changes in gene expression in adipose tissue. This could be a reflection of lower adipose tissue exposure to SAHA, perhaps a result of its pharmacokinetic profile (the in vivo half-life of SAHA is significantly shorter than that of MS275: 2 vs. 80 h) (35). This result suggests that robust suppression of class I HDACs in both skeletal muscle and adipose tissue is necessary to obtain the full metabolic benefit of inhibition of class I HDACs.

MS275 potentiates BAT function by increasing expression of markers of oxidative and uncoupled metabolism. These changes underlie the increased heat production and may contribute to the improvement of circulating lipid levels, as BAT plays a major role in triglyceride clearance

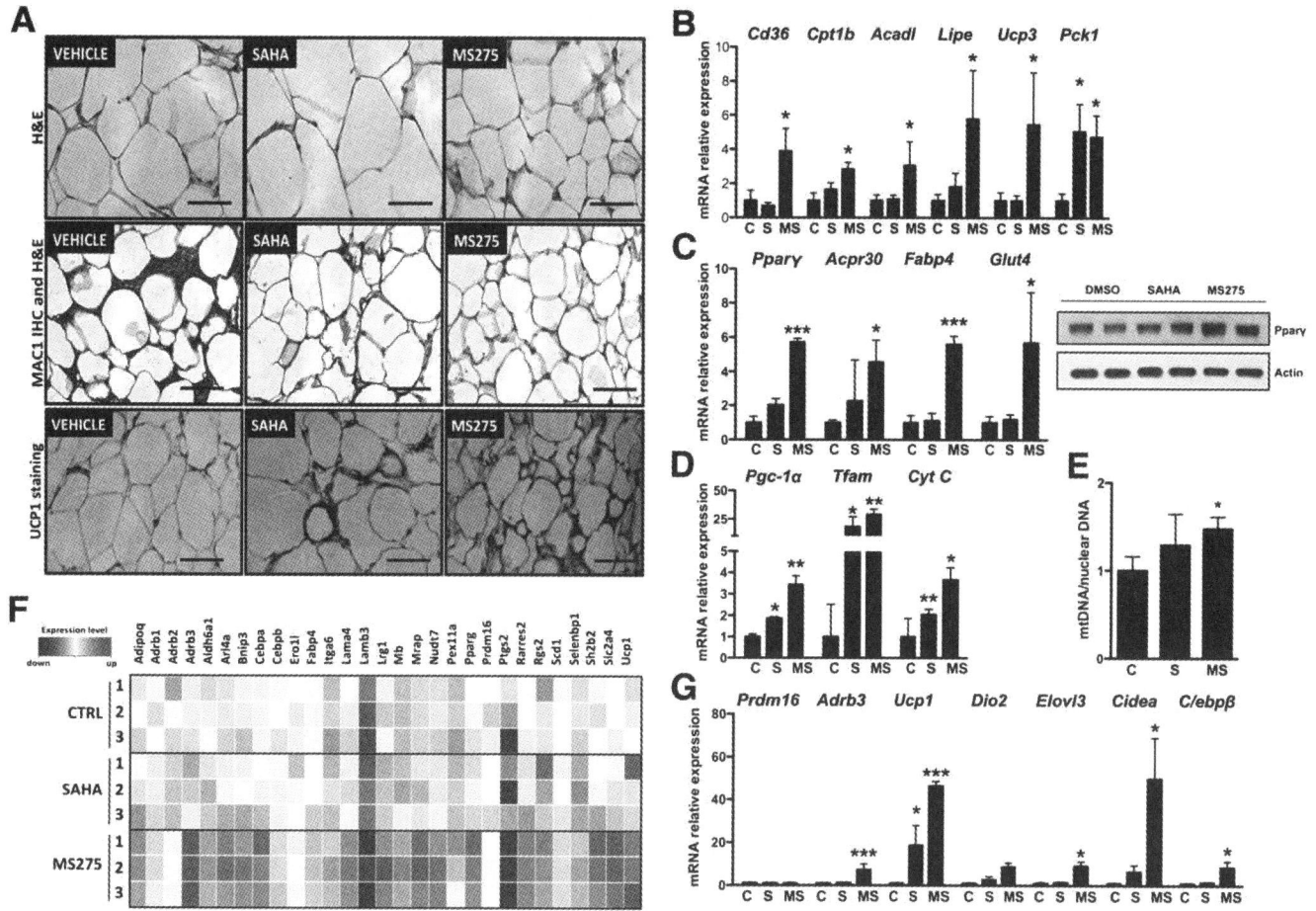

FIG. 7. Inhibition of class I HDACs in WAT promotes oxidative metabolism, reduces inflammation, and induces the acquisition of brown fat features. *A: top panel*, hematoxylin-eosin (H&E) stain of WAT from *db/db* mice treated with HDAC inhibitors (bars = 100 μm); *middle panel*, Mac1 immunohistochemistry (IHC) confirms reduced macrophage infiltration (bars = 100 μm); and *bottom panel*, UCP1 staining in sections of WAT from treated *db/db* mice confirms the "browning" of WAT prompted by inhibition of class I HDACs (bars = 100 μm). *B*: Expression of genes involved in lipid metabolism and mitochondrial function. *C*: Increased expression of *Ppar*γ and its direct targets in WAT of animals treated with MS275. *D*: Expression profile of genes involved in mitochondrial function after HDAC inhibitor treatment. *E*: Quantification of mitochondrial DNA in WAT after 23 days of treatment with SAHA, MS275, or vehicle. *F*: Heat map revealing the expression in MS275-treated WAT of multiple genes associated with BAT. *G*: Real time qPCR analysis showing that class I HDAC inhibition induces the expression of brown fat markers in white adipocytes. Data are presented as means ± SD. *$P < 0.05$, **$P < 0.01$, ***$P < 0.001$ vs. control. C and CTRL, control; MS, MS275; S, SAHA. (A high-quality digital representation of this figure is available in the online issue.)

(36,37). In vivo ChIP experiments indicate that inhibition of Hdac3 may be responsible for the beneficial effects of MS275 treatment in BAT.

MS275 treatment suppressed inflammatory markers and macrophage infiltration into white adipose, yet its most dramatic effect in WAT was its ability to induce robust expression of markers of BAT. This browning occurred in the absence of a change in expression of Prdm16, a major determinant of interscapular brown fat development (38). Consistent with work showing that chronic treatment of primary white adipocytes with Pparγ ligands results in the acquisition of brown adipocyte features in the absence of Prdm16 expression (26), we found that treatment with the class I HDAC inhibitor increased Pparγ expression and that of its targets in WAT. Increased Pparγ signaling in WAT could be a major determinant of the improvement of metabolic parameters seen in MS275-treated mice, for increased expression or enhanced activity of Pparγ exclusively in WAT has profound effects on systemic insulin sensitivity and lipid homeostasis (19,39). In analogy with our results in muscle and BAT, it is likely that enhanced

Pparγ activity in WAT upon MS275 treatment is due to inhibition of Hdac3, as this HDAC has been shown to associate with Pparγ to block its function, though we cannot exclude the possibility of contribution of other class I HDACs to this effect (40).

Mice lacking the nuclear corepressor NCoR1 in either skeletal muscle or adipose tissue exhibit a phenotype similar to animals treated with MS275 (41,42). NCoR1 participates in transcriptional repression together with silencing mediator for retinoid and thyroid hormone receptors (SMRTs) and Hdac3 (43); thus, these observations are consistent with the notion that interfering with Hdac3 activity improves skeletal muscle and adipose tissue function.

Our results highlight the pivotal role of class I HDAC activity in the regulation of energy homeostasis. We have shown that pharmacologic inhibition of class I HDACs in the context of obesity and diabetes potentiates mitochondrial function and oxidative capacity in skeletal muscle and adipose tissue. These observations suggest that synthetic class I HDAC inhibitors may have promise in the treatment of obesity and associated disorders.

ACKNOWLEDGMENTS

This work was supported by grants from the European Union (FP6 LSHM-CT2006-037498 to M.C.), Fondazione Cariplo (2008.2511 to M.C.), the Giovanni Armenise-Harvard Foundation (to N.M.), the Italian Ministry of University (PRIN 2008 ZTN724 to E.D.F.), the American Diabetes Association (to E.S.), and the National Institutes of Health (DK-081003 to E.S.).

No potential conflicts of interest relevant to this article were reported.

A.Ga. and N.M. conceived the study, designed the experimental plan, performed most of the experiments, analyzed data, and wrote and edited the manuscript. A.F. isolated primary brown adipocytes, measured oxygen consumption, performed immunoblots and some molecular experiments, and read and edited the manuscript. E.G, F.G., and C.G. participated in the initial elaboration of the project and read and edited the manuscript. G.C. performed some biological and biochemical experiments and read and edited the manuscript. A.Gu. and E.D. performed electron microscopy analysis, contributed to image interpretation, and read and edited the manuscript. D.R. and S.V. synthesized MS275 and MC1568 and read and edited the manuscript. U.G. provided expertise for MRI experiments and read and edited the manuscript. D.C. provided suggestions for some biological experiments and read and edited the manuscript. A.M. synthesized MS275 and MC1568 and read and edited the manuscript. E.S. conceived the study, designed the experimental plan, analyzed data, wrote the manuscript, and edited the manuscript. E.D.F. and M.C. conceived the study, designed the experimental plan, analyzed data, wrote the manuscript, supervised the entire work, and edited the manuscript. E.D.F. and M.C. are the guarantors of this work and, as such, had full access to all the data in the study and take responsibility for the integrity of the data and the accuracy of the data analysis.

The authors thank Dr. Anastasia Kralli (Scripps Research Institute) and Dr. Mark Montminy (Salk Institute, La Jolla, CA) for adenoviruses expressing shRNA against Pgc-1α, Dr. Malcolm Parker (Imperial College of London) and Dr. Asha Seth (Imperial College of London) for providing RIP140-null cells, Dr. Franco Salerno (Istituto Neurologico "Carlo Besta") for help in histological analysis of muscle sections, Marianna Gaman (Università degli Studi di Milano) and Paolo Monti (Università degli Studi di Milano) for electron microscopy, Dr. Anastasia Kralli (Scripps Research Institute) and Mari Gantner (Scripps Research Institute) for help with oxygen consumption measurements, and Erika Fiorino (Università degli Studi di Milano) for help in the setup of primary brown adipocytes. The authors also thank Dr. Anastasia Kralli (Scripps Research Institute) and Dr. Malcolm Parker (Imperial College of London) for discussion and comments on the manuscript. The authors thank Elda Desiderio Pinto (Università degli Studi di Milano) for administrative management.

REFERENCES

1. Franks PW, Ling C. Epigenetics and obesity: the devil is in the details. BMC Med 2010;8:88
2. Ling C, Groop L. Epigenetics: a molecular link between environmental factors and type 2 diabetes. Diabetes 2009;58:2718–2725
3. de Ruijter AJ, van Gennip AH, Caron HN, Kemp S, van Kuilenburg AB. Histone deacetylases (HDACs): characterization of the classical HDAC family. Biochem J 2003;370:737–749
4. Lahm A, Paolini C, Pallaoro M, et al. Unraveling the hidden catalytic activity of vertebrate class IIa histone deacetylases. Proc Natl Acad Sci USA 2007;104:17335–17340
5. Haberland M, Montgomery RL, Olson EN. The many roles of histone deacetylases in development and physiology: implications for disease and therapy. Nat Rev Genet 2009;10:32–42
6. Guarente L. Sirtuins as potential targets for metabolic syndrome. Nature 2006;444:868–874
7. Gao L, Cueto MA, Asselbergs F, Atadja P. Cloning and functional characterization of HDAC11, a novel member of the human histone deacetylase family. J Biol Chem 2002;277:25748–25755
8. McKinsey TA, Zhang C-L, Lu J, Olson EN. Signal-dependent nuclear export of a histone deacetylase regulates muscle differentiation. Nature 2000;408:106–111
9. Potthoff MJ, Wu H, Arnold MA, et al. Histone deacetylase degradation and MEF2 activation promote the formation of slow-twitch myofibers. J Clin Invest 2007;117:2459–2467
10. Montgomery RL, Potthoff MJ, Haberland M, et al. Maintenance of cardiac energy metabolism by histone deacetylase 3 in mice. J Clin Invest 2008; 118:3588–3597
11. Sun Z, Singh N, Mullican SE, et al. Diet-induced lethality due to deletion of the Hdac3 gene in heart and skeletal muscle. J Biol Chem 2011;286:33301–33309
12. Gao Z, Yin J, Zhang J, et al. Butyrate improves insulin sensitivity and increases energy expenditure in mice. Diabetes 2009;58:1509–1517
13. Klein J, Fasshauer M, Ito M, Lowell BB, Benito M, Kahn CR. β(3)-adrenergic stimulation differentially inhibits insulin signaling and decreases insulin-induced glucose uptake in brown adipocytes. J Biol Chem 1999;274:34795–34802
14. Guareschi S, Cova E, Cereda C, et al. An over-oxidized form of superoxide dismutase found in sporadic amyotrophic lateral sclerosis with bulbar onset shares a toxic mechanism with mutant SOD1. Proc Natl Acad Sci USA 2012;109:5074–5079
15. De Fabiani E, Mitro N, Gilardi F, Caruso D, Galli G, Crestani M. Coordinated control of cholesterol catabolism to bile acids and of gluconeogenesis via a novel mechanism of transcription regulation linked to the fasted-to-fed cycle. J Biol Chem 2003;278:39124–39132
16. Mitro N, Godio C, De Fabiani E, et al. Insights in the regulation of cholesterol 7alpha-hydroxylase gene reveal a target for modulating bile acid synthesis. Hepatology 2007;46:885–897
17. Villena JA, Hock MB, Chang WY, Barcas JE, Giguère V, Kralli A. Orphan nuclear receptor estrogen-related receptor alpha is essential for adaptive thermogenesis. Proc Natl Acad Sci USA 2007;104:1418–1423
18. Folch J, Lees M, Sloane Stanley GH. A simple method for the isolation and purification of total lipides from animal tissues. J Biol Chem 1957;226:497–509
19. Waki H, Park KW, Mitro N, et al. The small molecule harmine is an antidiabetic cell-type-specific regulator of PPARgamma expression. Cell Metab 2007;5:357–370
20. Hess-Stumpp H, Bracker TU, Henderson D, Politz O. MS-275, a potent orally available inhibitor of histone deacetylases—the development of an anticancer agent. Int J Biochem Cell Biol 2007;39:1388–1405
21. Mai A, Massa S, Rotili D, et al. Synthesis and biological properties of novel, uracil-containing histone deacetylase inhibitors. J Med Chem 2006;49:6046–6056
22. Nebbioso A, Manzo F, Miceli M, et al. Selective class II HDAC inhibitors impair myogenesis by modulating the stability and activity of HDAC-MEF2 complexes. EMBO Rep 2009;10:776–782
23. Canettieri G, Morantte I, Guzmán E, et al. Attenuation of a phosphorylation-dependent activator by an HDAC-PP1 complex. Nat Struct Biol 2003; 10:175–181
24. Grégoire S, Xiao L, Nie J, et al. Histone deacetylase 3 interacts with and deacetylates myocyte enhancer factor 2. Mol Cell Biol 2007;27:1280–1295
25. Handschin C, Rhee J, Lin J, Tarr PT, Spiegelman BM. An autoregulatory loop controls peroxisome proliferator-activated receptor gamma coactivator 1alpha expression in muscle. Proc Natl Acad Sci USA 2003;100:7111–7116
26. Petrovic N, Walden TB, Shabalina IG, Timmons JA, Cannon B, Nedergaard J. Chronic peroxisome proliferator-activated receptor gamma (PPARgamma) activation of epididymally derived white adipocyte cultures reveals a population of thermogenically competent, UCP1-containing adipocytes molecularly distinct from classic brown adipocytes. J Biol Chem 2010;285:7153–7164
27. Cao L, Choi EY, Liu X, et al. White to brown fat phenotypic switch induced by genetic and environmental activation of a hypothalamic-adipocyte axis. Cell Metab 2011;14:324–338
28. Yadav H, Quijano C, Kamaraju AK, et al. Protection from obesity and diabetes by blockade of TGF-β/Smad3 signaling. Cell Metab 2011;14:67–79
29. Seale P, Conroe HM, Estall J, et al. Prdm16 determines the thermogenic program of subcutaneous white adipose tissue in mice. J Clin Invest 2011; 121:96–105

30. Davie JR. Inhibition of histone deacetylase activity by butyrate. J Nutr 2003;133(Suppl.):2485S–2493S
31. Li H, Gao Z, Zhang J, et al. Sodium butyrate stimulates expression of fibroblast growth factor 21 in liver by inhibition of histone deacetylase 3. Diabetes 2012;61:797–806
32. Haberland M, Carrer M, Mokalled MH, Montgomery RL, Olson EN. Redundant control of adipogenesis by histone deacetylases 1 and 2. J Biol Chem 2010;285:14663–14670
33. Fischle W, Dequiedt F, Hendzel MJ, et al. Enzymatic activity associated with class II HDACs is dependent on a multiprotein complex containing HDAC3 and SMRT/N-CoR. Mol Cell 2002;9:45–57
34. Knutson SK, Chyla BJ, Amann JM, Bhaskara S, Huppert SS, Hiebert SW. Liver-specific deletion of histone deacetylase 3 disrupts metabolic transcriptional networks. EMBO J 2008;27:1017–1028
35. Minucci S, Pelicci PG. Histone deacetylase inhibitors and the promise of epigenetic (and more) treatments for cancer. Nat Rev Cancer 2006;6:38–51
36. Bartelt A, Bruns OT, Reimer R, et al. Brown adipose tissue activity controls triglyceride clearance. Nat Med 2011;17:200–205
37. Cannon B, Nedergaard J. Brown adipose tissue: function and physiological significance. Physiol Rev 2004;84:277–359
38. Seale P, Bjork B, Yang W, et al. PRDM16 controls a brown fat/skeletal muscle switch. Nature 2008;454:961–967
39. Sugii S, Olson P, Sears DD, et al. PPARgamma activation in adipocytes is sufficient for systemic insulin sensitization. Proc Natl Acad Sci USA 2009; 106:22504–22509
40. Fajas L, Egler V, Reiter R, et al. The retinoblastoma-histone deacetylase 3 complex inhibits PPARgamma and adipocyte differentiation. Dev Cell 2002;3:903–910
41. Li P, Fan W, Xu J, et al. Adipocyte NCoR knockout decreases PPARγ phosphorylation and enhances PPARγ activity and insulin sensitivity. Cell 2011;147:815–826
42. Yamamoto H, Williams EG, Mouchiroud L, et al. NCoR1 is a conserved physiological modulator of muscle mass and oxidative function. Cell 2011; 147:827–839
43. Guenther MG, Barak O, Lazar MA. The SMRT and N-CoR corepressors are activating cofactors for histone deacetylase 3. Mol Cell Biol 2001;21:6091–6101
44. Hackenbrock CR, Rehn TG, Weinbach EC, Lemasters JJ. Oxidative phosphorylation and ultrastructural transformation in mitochondria in the intact ascites tumor cell. J Cell Biol 1971;51:123–137

A Lipidomics Analysis of the Relationship Between Dietary Fatty Acid Composition and Insulin Sensitivity in Young Adults

C. Lawrence Kien,[1,2] Janice Y. Bunn,[3] Matthew E. Poynter,[2] Robert Stevens,[4,5,6] James Bain,[4,5,6] Olga Ikayeva,[4,5,6] Naomi K. Fukagawa,[2] Catherine M. Champagne,[7] Karen I. Crain,[2] Timothy R. Koves,[4,5,6] and Deborah M. Muoio[4,5,6]

Relative to diets enriched in palmitic acid (PA), diets rich in oleic acid (OA) are associated with reduced risk of type 2 diabetes. To gain insight into mechanisms underlying these observations, we applied comprehensive lipidomic profiling to specimens collected from healthy adults enrolled in a randomized, crossover trial comparing a high-PA diet to a low-PA/high-OA (HOA) diet. Effects on insulin sensitivity (S_I) and disposition index (DI) were assessed by intravenous glucose tolerance testing. In women, but not men, S_I and DI were higher during HOA. The effect of HOA on S_I correlated positively with physical fitness upon enrollment. Principal components analysis of either fasted or fed-state metabolites identified one factor affected by diet and heavily weighted by the PA/OA ratio of serum and muscle lipids. In women, this factor correlated inversely with S_I in the fasted and fed states. Medium-chain acylcarnitines emerged as strong negative correlates of S_I, and the HOA diet was accompanied by lower serum and muscle ceramide concentrations and reductions in molecular biomarkers of inflammatory and oxidative stress. This study provides evidence that the dietary PA/OA ratio impacts diabetes risk in women. *Diabetes* 62:1054–1063, 2013

W estern-style diets that are high in fat content have been linked to increased risk of type 2 diabetes (1,2). The two most prevalent fatty acids (FAs) in this diet are palmitic acid (PA; C16:0) and oleic acid (OA; C18:1), each present in approximately equal amounts as a percentage of dietary energy. Although total dietary fat consumption is comparably high in Mediterranean countries, epidemiological studies show that these populations have a paradoxically low prevalence of type 2 diabetes and cardiovascular disease (1,2). Owing to liberal use of olive oil, the typical Mediterranean diet is rich in OA and low in PA (3–5). Numerous studies in cultured cells suggest that exposure to high PA disrupts insulin action and provokes proinflammatory signaling events, whereas OA mitigates these adverse responses (6–8). However, exposure of cells to high concentrations of PA may not reflect normal physiology, raising doubts about the clinical relevance of such experiments (9).

Progress toward a clearer understanding of the role of specific dietary FA in conferring cardioprotective and/or antidiabetic benefits requires carefully controlled dietary intervention studies. Although previous dietary trials have attempted to elucidate the distinct metabolic properties of PA and OA (10,11), most of these studies relied on prescribed diets and/or did not actually measure the impact of the experimental diets on the FA composition of circulating and cellular lipids. As a result, the current literature on this topic is conflicted and difficult to interpret. In this study, we present new findings testing the hypothesis that replacing dietary PA with OA would impact insulin sensitivity. Because a previous study found sex differences in lipid metabolism (12), we also sought to consider sex as a factor that might influence metabolic responses to a change in dietary FA composition.

RESEARCH DESIGN AND METHODS

Subjects, screening, and overall design. This study was approved by institutional committees associated with the University of Vermont General Clinical Research Center (GCRC).

Healthy men ($n = 9$) and women ($n = 9$), aged 18–40 years, with a BMI >18 and <30 were recruited for this study. These 18 volunteers constituted the cohort for all results in this article, except for studies of muscle protein expression and muscle ceramide content performed in an additional 10 volunteers (5 women and 5 men), who also participated in the same protocol (see Supplementary Data).

Exclusion criteria included regular aerobic exercise training, dyslipidemia (13), and evidence of type 2 diabetes or insulin resistance (14). Women were enrolled if they did not receive hormonal forms of contraception and manifested normal ovulation based both on a urine luteinizing hormone test and serum concentrations of estradiol and progesterone.

Screening indicated a habitual intake of 37% kcal total fat, 14.5% saturated fat, and 12% monounsaturated fat, consistent with the usual American diet (15). After screening, all subjects ingested a low-fat/low-PA, baseline/control diet for 7 days (protein, 19.7% kcal; carbohydrate, 51.6% kcal; fat, 28.4% kcal; PA, 5.3% kcal; and OA, 15.9% kcal) (13). On the morning of day 8 of the baseline/control diet, fasting blood and muscle tissue were collected at 0700 h (16), and 3 h after a breakfast (one-third daily kcal), muscle biopsy and blood collection were repeated. Then, the subjects participated in a crossover study of 3-wk diet periods, consisting of a diet resembling the habitual diet and high in PA (HPA; fat, 40.4% kcal; PA, 16.0% kcal; and OA, 16.2% kcal) or a diet low in PA and high in OA (HOA; 40.1% kcal; 2.4% kcal; and 28.8% kcal, respectively) (Supplementary Table 1). These diets were separated by a 1-week period on the baseline/control diet. Repeat blood collection and muscle biopsy in the fasted and fed state were carried out on the 22nd day of each experimental diet (HPA and HOA). Further details concerning the diets were described previously (16) and in the Supplementary Data.

In women, postexperimental diet evaluations took place in the luteal phase of the cycle prior to menstruation. On the first day of the baseline diet and at the end of the HPA and HOA diets, body composition was assessed, including upper

From the [1]Department of Pediatrics, University of Vermont, Burlington, Vermont; the [2]Department of Medicine, University of Vermont, Burlington, Vermont; the [3]Department of Medical Biostatistics, University of Vermont, Burlington, Vermont; the [4]Stedman Nutrition and Metabolism Center, Duke University, Durham, North Carolina; the [5]Department of Medicine, Duke University, Durham, North Carolina; the [6]Department of Pharmacology and Cancer Biology, Duke University, Durham, North Carolina; and the [7]Pennington Biomedical Research Center, Baton Rouge, Louisiana.
Corresponding author: C. Lawrence Kien, cl.kien@uvm.edu.
Received 23 March 2012 and accepted 5 October 2012.
DOI: 10.2337/db12-0363
This article contains Supplementary Data online at http://diabetes .diabetesjournals.org/lookup/suppl/doi:10.2337/db12-0363/-/DC1.

body (android), truncal, legs, and lower body (gynoid) regions (GE Lunar Prodigy Densitometer, Version 5.6; GE Healthcare) (17). On the 21st day of each experimental diet, after an overnight fast in the GCRC, we completed a frequently sampled intravenous glucose tolerance test (18). We used a modified version of the MINMOD program (18) to estimate the following parameters: glucose effectiveness (Sg), the capacity of glucose to mediate its own disposal; acute insulin response to glucose (AIRg); insulin sensitivity index (S_I), the capacity of insulin to promote glucose disposal; and disposition index (DI): AIRg * S_I (19). The usual range of S_I is ~0–15 × 10^{-4} ($min^{-1}/\mu U/$ mL), with the MINMOD program generating values for S_I that have been multiplied by 10^4. While verifying the adequacy of the data from the intravenous glucose tolerance test, we noted that some women seemed to exhibit lower nadirs for blood glucose concentration during one of the diets. Since we knew that some of these women were more physically fit than others, we elected to explore the correlation of peak oxygen consumption with cycling exercise (VO_{2peak}) with diet change in S_I. VO_{2peak} was measured at screening (20). Physical activity was assessed daily using an ActiGraph Activity Monitor, worn at the waist (catalog number GT1M; ActiGraph, Pensacola, FL).

Metabolic measurements. Glucose concentration was measured using a YSI 2300 Stat Plus glucose analyzer (YSI Inc., Yellow Springs, OH), and serum insulin concentration was measured by radioimmunoassay (Linco Research Inc., St. Charles, MO) (GCRC Core Laboratory). Standard radioimmunoassay kits and a Wallac Wizard 1470-010 automatic γ counter (PerkinElmer) were used for assays of leptin and adiponectin (Linco RIA kits; Linco Research Inc.). β-Hydroxybutyrate was measured by a standard method (Wako, Richmond, VA). Ceramides were extracted and analyzed based on the methods of Merrill et al. (21) using flow-injection tandem mass spectrometry. Nonesterified FA (NEFA) and total FA (free plus esterified) in serum were assessed by capillary gas chromatography/mass spectrometry (22). Fasting and fed, muscle, and serum concentrations of acylcarnitines (AC) and amino acids were measured by direct-injection electrospray tandem mass spectrometry (23). Muscle organic acids were quantified as previously described (24).

FA composition and concentration of skeletal muscle diacylglycerol, triacylglycerol, and phospholipids. The FA composition of diacylglycerol (DAG) and triacylglycerol (TAG) as well as serum and muscle phospholipids was analyzed by gas chromatography using recently described methods (16).

Bio-Plex analysis of signaling cascades active in muscle. Bio-Rad Bio-Plex phosphoprotein assays (Bio-Rad, Hercules, CA) and Bio-Plex total target assays (Luminex xMAP technology; Luminex) were used to detect the activity (phosphorylation) of inhibitor of κBα (IκBα), nuclear factor-κBp65, c-Jun N-terminal kinase (JNK), Akt, and insulin-receptor substrate-1 (IRS-1) in lysates derived from 5–10 mg of muscle biopsy samples.

Serum concentration (pg/mL) of interleukin-6, interleukin-10, tumor necrosis factor-α, and ferritin (all measured on the n = 18 cohort). Serum cytokine concentrations were measured after the HPA and HOA diets in the fasting and fed states. Custom Bio-Plex (Bio-Rad, Hercules, CA) 3-plex kits were designed containing coupled beads and antibodies recognizing human interleukin-6 (IL-6), IL-10, and tumor necrosis factor-α (TNF-α). All assays were performed in duplicate according to the manufacturer's instructions. Because of the interrelationships of physical fitness, iron status, insulin sensitivity, and oxidant stress (25–28), serum ferritin was measured and related to diet change (Fletcher Allen Health Center, direct chemiluminescence assay; Siemens ADVIA Centaur Ferritin; Siemens Healthcare Global).

Statistics. All data are expressed as mean ± SEM. Analyses were performed with SAS, version 9.2 (SAS Institute). This study used a two-treatment, two-period, two-sequence crossover design. Diet effects were analyzed using a repeated-measures ANOVA, including sequence and treatment effects, with the baseline value as a covariate, when available. Because sex-specific responses to the diets were anticipated (12), men and women were analyzed both as a group and separately. For some analyses, we used the same model using ranks. All correlations reported are Spearman rank correlations.

Principal components analysis (PCA) was used to reduce the dimensionality of both the fasting and fed data and to aid in explaining the highest variance within the overall dataset. Orthogonal rotation was used to aid in the interpretation of the components. Diet differences in component scores were examined using the repeated-measures ANOVA methods described above. In addition, select components were included as time-varying covariates in the analysis to examine the relationship between dependent variables of interest and the component scores. Additional details are provided in the Supplementary Data.

RESULTS

Body composition, physical fitness, and physical activity. The diets did not affect body weight, BMI, or whole-body composition (Table 1). In men and women combined, the HPA diet period was associated with greater android adiposity (percent fat) (P = 0.037) and a trend for higher truncal adiposity (P = 0.068). A similar trend (P = 0.060) for increased android adiposity was observed when women (but not men) were analyzed separately. However, there was no diet effect on total or regional fat mass in men and women together or separately (Supplementary Table 2). Compared with women, men exhibited higher VO_{2peak} (mL/kg/min) at screening (49.11 ± 3.71 vs. 36.22 ± 4.32) and lower percent body fat after the baseline diet (Table 1). In both men and women, physical activity correlated positively with VO_{2peak}, regardless of the diet (r = 0.66–0.87; P < 0.02).

Comprehensive analyses of circulating and cellular lipids. A major goal of this study was to compare the effects of the two diets on the quantity and quality of circulating and intracellular lipid pools. Because lipid metabolism fluctuates dramatically in response to acute changes in nutrient and/or hormonal status, biological specimens were collected in both the fasted and postprandial states. The heat maps in Fig. 1A and B provide compelling evidence that even a short-term change in dietary fats can have broad-ranging effects on circulating as well as muscle lipids. Thus, when comparing the HOA to the HPA diet, the PA/OA ratio was increased in nearly every lipid pool analyzed including muscle TAG, DAG, and

TABLE 1
Demographic and metabolic characteristics

	Men			Women		
	Baseline	HPA	HOA	Baseline	HPA	HOA
HOMA-IR	2.02 ± 0.14	1.8 ± 0.14	1.92 ± 0.18	2.12 ± 0.15	2.61 ± 0.58	1.86 + 0.14
Body fat (%)	17.8 ± 2.7*	17.5 ± 3.1	17.3 ± 3	30.6 ± 3.1	30.1 ± 3	29.6 ± 3.1
FFM (kg)	64.4 ± 3	63.3 ± 2.8	63.5 ± 2.9	46.5 ± 1.5	46 ± 1.6	46.2 ± 1.5
Fasting insulin (pmol/L)	69.0 ± 4.8	61.0 ± 4.9	66.4 ± 6.1	73.8 ± 4.1†	91.5 ± 21.8	65 ± 5
Fasting glucose (mmol/L)	4.57 ± 0.07	4.61 ± 0.14	4.54 ± 0.07	4.49 ± 0.17	4.51 ± 0.14	4.49 ± 0.06
DI		1,089.1 ± 139.7	1,071.1 ± 143.8		1,137 ± 198‡	1,661 ± 324
AIRg (min/mU/mL)		227.9 ± 36.7	250.3 ± 41.6		330.8 ± 53.4	325.5 ± 68.3
Sg (min^{-1})		0.021 ± 0.001	0.021 ± 0.002		0.020 ± 0.002	0.021 ± 0.002
S_I × 10^{-4} (min^{-1}/mU/mL)		5.48 ± 0.77	5.31 ± 1.05		3.96 ± 0.7§	6.46 ± 1.38

Mean ± SEM for the first cohort mentioned in the text; n = 9 men, n = 9 women. FFM, fat-free mass; HOMA-IR, homeostatic model assessment of insulin resistance index (14); Sg, glucose effectiveness (capacity of glucose to mediate its own disposal). *P = 0.007, men versus women. †P = 0.03 versus HOA. ‡P = 0.02 versus HOA. §P = 0.036 versus HOA.

phosphatidylcholine (PC) (Fig. 1A and B). The impact of the diets on the FA composition of lipids was universally evident in every subject, and in general, this effect was more robust in the fed than the fasted state. Notably, the diet also affected the PA/OA ratio measured in circulating NEFAs, which are derived principally from lipolysis of adipose tissue TAG (Fig. 1C). Likewise, the pronounced diet-induced shift in the PA/OA ratio of mitochondrial-derived AC metabolites, both in the circulation and in muscle (Fig. 1E and F), indicates that the diets had a strong influence on the types of FA undergoing β-oxidation, not only in the fed state but also during fasting. Data in Fig. 1C–F are shown for men and women combined, but for most variables, similar results were found for men and women separately (see Supplementary Data).

Diet effects on insulin secretion and S_I. Because sex-specific responses to the diets were anticipated a priori

(12), men and women were analyzed both as a group and separately. Both the DI and S_I were similar between men and women regardless of the diet condition. When the diet effect on DI was analyzed by repeated-measures ANOVA, the diet group by sex interaction approached statistical significance ($P = 0.06$). In women only, the DI was 46% higher during HOA ($P = 0.02$) (Table 1 and Fig. 2A). The diet group by sex interaction for S_I was not significant using normal distribution statistics ($P = 0.109$), but trended toward significance when calculated with rank-transformed data ($P = 0.079$). Analysis of men and women separately showed that eight of nine female subjects manifested higher S_I when consuming the HOA diet (Fig. 2B; $P = 0.03$), whereas in men, only four of nine showed a higher S_I on the same diet (Fig. 2C and Supplementary Table 3). In women, the average increase in S_I during the HOA diet was 63% ($P = 0.036$, NS, men) (Fig. 2D and

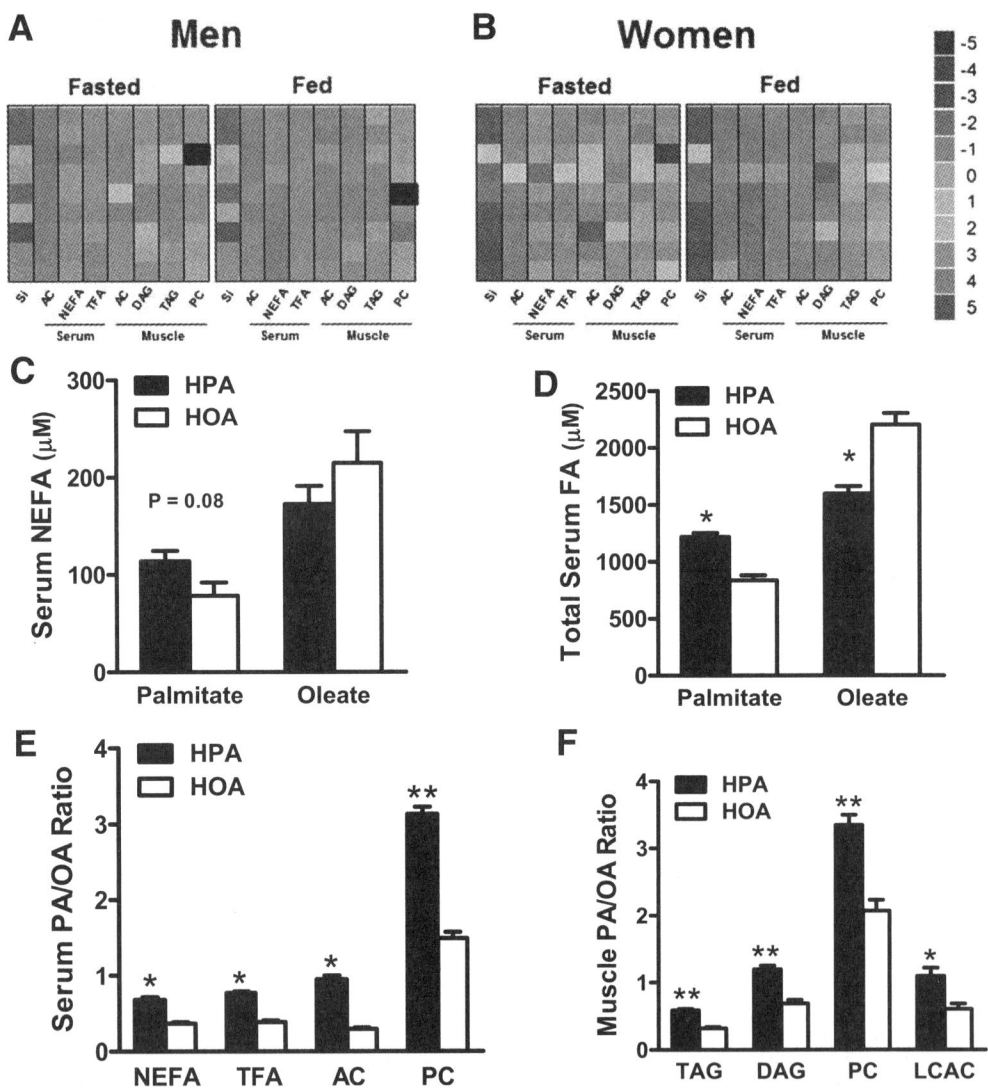

FIG. 1. The FA composition of the diet is reflected in a broad range of circulating and intramuscular lipids (see text for abbreviations, except where indicated). A and B: Heat maps depicting diet-induced changes in the PA/OA ratio of blood and muscle lipids according to the scale on the right (total FA [TFA]). Change scores were calculated from absolute values of log base 5 transformed PA/OA data in the fasted or fed state on the HPA versus HOA diet (HPA/HOA). Each square represents an individual subject, and black indicates a missing value. S_I reflects insulin sensitivity measured in the fasted state. Results in men and women were combined to show diet effects on serum concentrations (μmol/L) of nonesterified PA and OA (C); serum concentration (μmol/L) of total PA and OA (D); the PA/OA ratio in serum NEFA, TFA, AC, and PC (E); and the PA/OA ratio in skeletal muscle lipid metabolites (F): TAG, DAG, PC, and LCAC. *$P \leq 0.001$, **$P \leq 0.01$ denote diet effect.

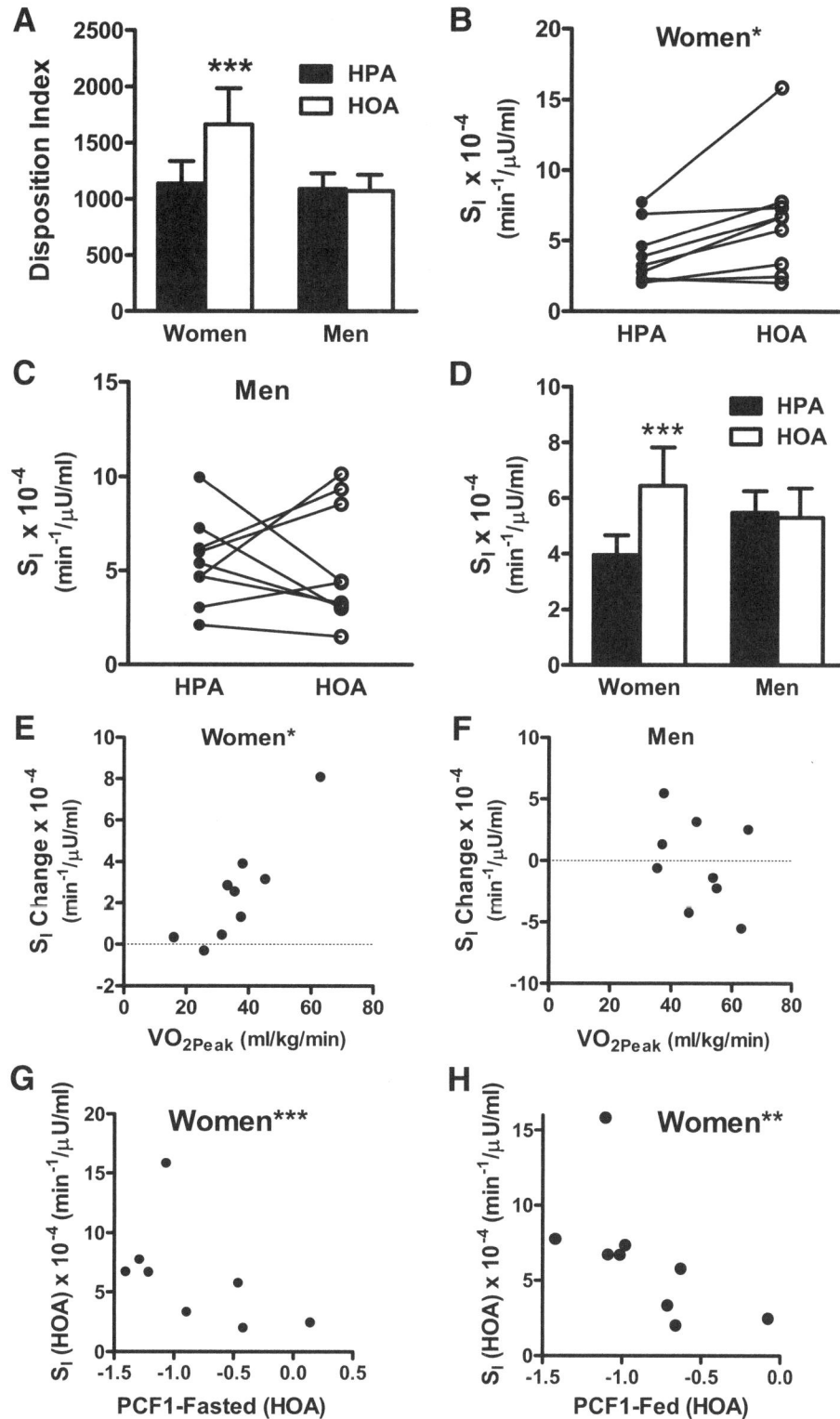

FIG. 2. The HOA diet improved insulin secretion and sensitivity in women. *A*: DI. *B* and *C*: Insulin sensitivity index (S_I) in individual women and men measured during the HOA and HPA diets. *D*: S_I. Relationship between diet-induced change in S_I (HOA − HPA) (S_I Change) and VO_{2peak} in women (*E*) and men (*F*) (*Spearman r = 0.90; $P \leq 0.001$). In women, during the HOA diet, S_I correlated inversely with PCF1-Fasted (*G*) (***r = −0.786, P = 0.021) and PCF1-Fed (*H*) (**r = −0.850, P = 0.004). ***$P \leq 0.05$ denotes a diet effect.

Table 1). In women, but not men, we identified a strong rank correlation between VO_{2peak} and the diet-induced change in S_I (Spearman r = 0.90; P = 0.001) (Fig. 2*E* and *F*). Thus, the most impressive gains in S_I during the HOA diet

occurred in women who were most physically fit at the inception of the study. Importantly, the diet effect on S_I and the relationship between S_I and VO_{2peak} were maintained (P = 0.027 and P = 0.007, respectively) even after exclusion of one female subject who demonstrated the most robust change in S_I. Additional details pertaining to the relationship between the S_I response to the diets and baseline characteristics of male and female subjects are provided in the Supplementary Data.

PCA. The dimension reduction strategy of PCA was used to reduce all metabolites measured, including those in serum/plasma, muscle, and urine, into a smaller number of orthogonal variables. This analysis was performed separately for fasted and fed conditions. PCA identified 31 factors among 329 total variables measured in the fasted state. Only one of these factors, Principal Components Factor1-Fasted (PCF1-Fasted) was affected by diet in both men and women ($P < 0.0001$) and almost uniformly reflected the PA/OA ratio of serum and muscle lipids (Supplementary Table 3). PCA identified 31 factors among 277 variables measured in the fed state. PCF1-Fed was affected by diet in both men and women ($P < 0.0001$) and again reflected the PA/OA ratio of lipids (Supplementary Table 4). PA contributed a positive loading score and OA a negative score; thus, F1 was higher during the HPA compared with the HOA diet ($P < 0.0001$). These computer-generated factors provided an unbiased, composite index of systemic FA composition that was then used to evaluate the relationship between the PA/OA content of biological lipids and glucose homeostasis. In women but not men, both PCF1-Fasted and PCF1-Fed correlated inversely with S_I assessed during the HOA diet ($r = -0.786$, $P = 0.021$; and $r = -0.850$, $P = 0.004$, respectively) (Fig. 2F and G). Inclusion of PCF1-Fed in an ANCOVA model abrogated the diet effect on S_I in women, whereas this relationship was maintained after adjusting for PCF1-Fasted. In aggregate, these findings suggest that the diet effects on S_I in women were related to and possibly mediated by the PA/OA ratio of serum and muscle lipids.

Diet-induced changes in candidate mediators of insulin resistance. To gain mechanistic insights into the insulin-sensitizing effect of the HOA diet in women, we initially focused our analysis on systemic lipid metabolites that have been linked to insulin resistance, including ceramides and AC. In women (Fig. 3A) and men (Fig. 4A), total ceramide concentrations in serum were higher during the HPA diet in both the fasting and fed states; and nearly every ceramide species measured in serum increased in response to the HPA diet (Supplementary Table 5). However, we did not detect an inverse correlation between circulating ceramides and S_I. By contrast, S_I in women measured during the HPA diet correlated inversely with serum concentration of medium chain AC (MCAC) (Fig. 3B) and with the serum medium-chain to long-chain AC ratio (MCAC/LCAC) (Fig. 3C). In women (Fig. 3D), the serum MCAC/LCAC ratio was higher after the HPA diet compared with HOA. These diet effects were not evident in men (Fig. 4).

We next examined concentrations in muscle of specific metabolites that are known markers and/or suspected mediators of insulin resistance, including TAG, DAG, AC, and ceramides (29,30). In women, muscle TAG measured in the fed state was higher during the HOA diet ($P = 0.05$; Fig. 3E), whereas muscle DAG content was unaffected by diet (Fig. 3F). Notably, the diet-induced change in the OA content of intramuscular TAG correlated positively with VO_{2peak} ($r = 0.667$; $P = 0.05$), again suggesting an interaction between diet and physical fitness in women. Muscle MCAC levels in the fed state were 58% higher during the HPA compared with the HOA diet in women (Fig. 3G) but not in men (Fig. 4G).

Muscle ceramides were measured in a separate cohort of five men and five women. In men, fasting levels of total muscle ceramides were 23% higher during HPA compared with HOA diet ($P = 0.023$) (Fig. 4H), whereas in women, similar fractional increases in total muscle ceramides (19 to 20%) did not reach statistical significance (Fig. 3H). In this second cohort, S_I increased during the HOA diet in all five women ($P = 0.043$).

Diet-induced changes in molecular markers of insulin resistance and inflammation. In female subjects, we found no evidence of a diet effect on phosphorylated Akt (pAkt) relative to total Akt or serine phosphorylation of IRS-1 (pIRS-1 [Ser636/Ser639]) relative to total IRS-1. However, in men, both pAkt (Ser473) and the pAkt/total Akt ratio measured in the fed state were higher during the HOA diet compared with the HPA diet (both $P \le 0.01$), and these values increased in all five men. It is noteworthy that these measures were made in specimens collected 3 h after feeding, which might not reflect muscle signaling changes occurring during the acute-phase insulin response. In women, muscle levels of phosphorylated c-Jun N-terminal kinase (pJNK) (Thr183/Tyr185) were lower after the HOA diet compared with the HPA diet during the fasted state ($P = 0.02$, using ranks) (Fig. 5A and B), but we observed no diet effect on pJNK in men (Fig. 6A and B).

Assessment of systemic inflammatory tone. In both women and men, serum concentrations of IL-10 and TNF-α were unaffected by the diets. Notably, however, six of the nine women had a higher fasting IL-6 concentration during the HPA diet ($P = 0.05$, using ranks) (Fig. 5C). Additionally, serum ferritin concentration was higher during the HPA diet in all nine women ($P = 0.014$; $P = 0.007$ using ranks), and the mean concentration was 35% higher on the HPA compared with the HOA diet ($P = 0.014$; Fig. 5D). In men, IL-6 and ferritin were unaffected by diet (Fig. 6).

DISCUSSION

This study provides direct evidence that replacing dietary palmitate with oleate can benefit clinically relevant measures of metabolic wellness in healthy individuals. In women, a diet-induced shift favoring less saturation and more monounsaturation of cellular lipids (lower PA/OA ratio) was associated with improvements in both DI and S_I. All women were studied in the postluteal phase of the menstrual cycle, verified by measurements of estrogen and progesterone. Considering that estrogen can alter expression of genes linked to regulation of lipid oxidation (31,32), these results may not necessarily be generalizable to nonovulating women. Whereas a diet effect on S_I was evident in women, results in men were variable, implying that sex influences the interplay between dietary FA composition and clinical outcomes. However, due to insufficient power, we are unable to form firm conclusions regarding gender specificity.

Both candidate and unbiased lipidomic profiling approaches were used to gain a comprehensive view of how the experimental diets impacted systemic lipid composition. Remarkably, we found that a relatively short-term change in the quality and quantity of specific dietary FA affected the FA composition of nearly every class of biological lipids evaluated in blood and muscle biopsy specimens. We also targeted several prominent lipid metabolites previously implicated as mediators and/or strong markers of insulin resistance. Notably, the HPA diet increased circulating levels and muscle content of

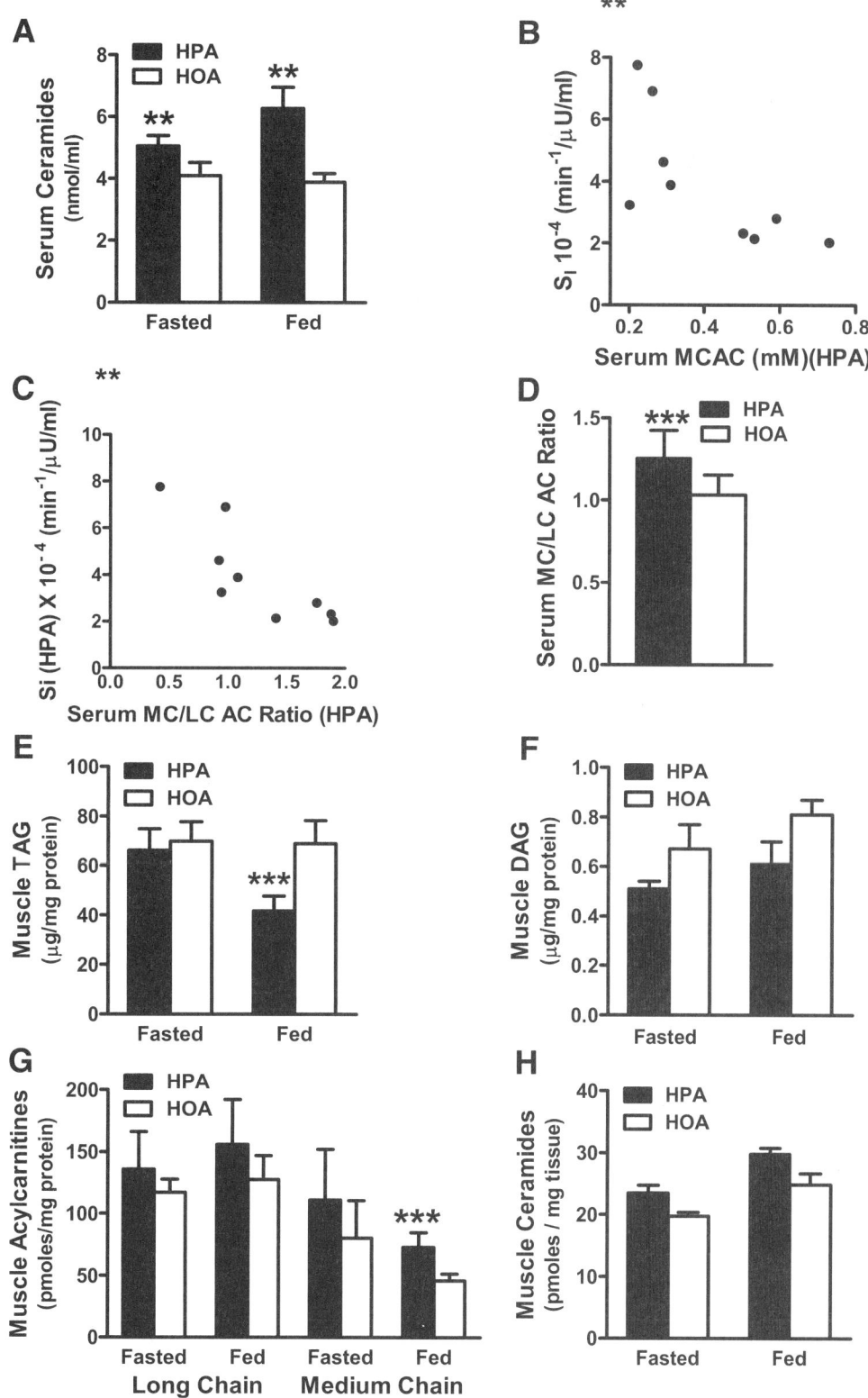

FIG. 3. Dietary FA composition affected lipid biomarkers of insulin resistance in women. *A*: Serum ceramide concentrations measured in the fasting and fed states. *B*: Relationship between S_I and MCAC measured in the fed state during the HPA diet (**$r = -0.783$, $P = 0.013$). *C*: Relationship between S_I and the serum MCAC/LCAC measured in the fed state during the HPA diet (**$r = -0.867$, $P = 0.002$). *D*: Serum MCAC/LCAC ratio in the fed state. Muscle biopsy specimens harvested in the fasted and fed states were used to quantify intramuscular concentrations of TAG (*E*), DAG (*F*), and LCAC and MCAC (*G*) and total ceramides (*H*). **$P \leq 0.01$, ***$P \leq 0.05$ denote a diet effect.

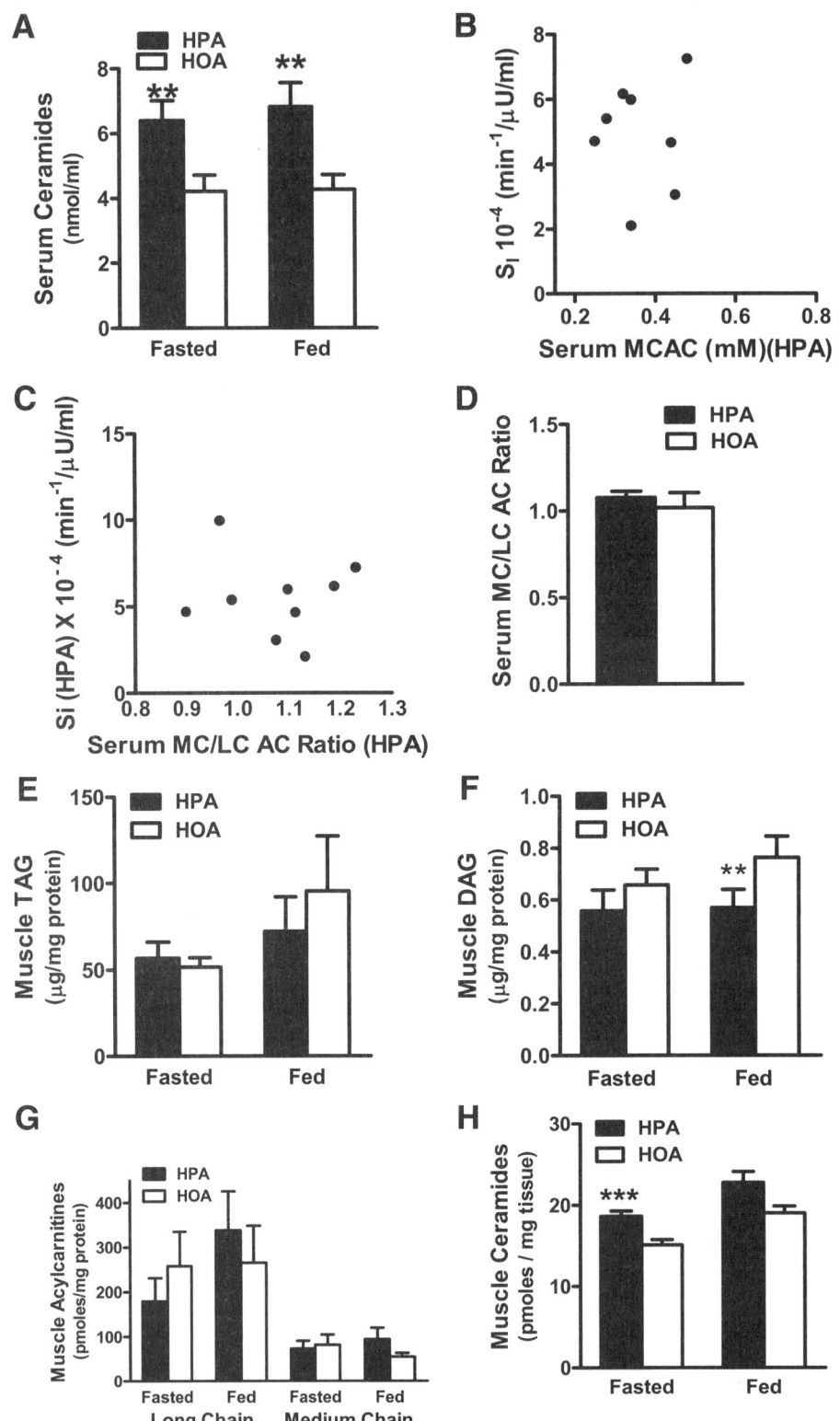

FIG. 4. Dietary FA composition affected lipid biomarkers of insulin resistance in men. *A*: Serum ceramide concentrations measured in the fasting and fed states. *B*: Relationship between S_I and MCAC measured in the fed state during the HPA diet ($r = -0.33, P = 0.38$). *C*: Relationship between S_I and the serum MCAC/LCAC measured in the fed state during the HPA diet ($r = 0.05, P = 0.90$). *D*: Serum MCAC/LCAC ratio in the fed state. Muscle biopsy specimens harvested in the fasted and fed states were used to quantify intramuscular concentrations of TAG (*E*), DAG (*F*), and LCAC and MCAC (*G*) and total ceramides (*H*). **$P \leq 0.01$, ***$P \leq 0.05$ denote a diet effect.

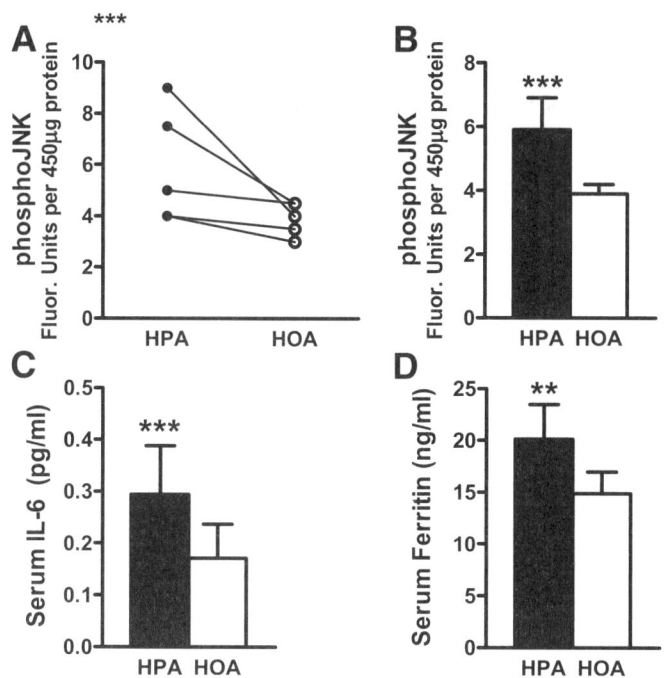

FIG. 5. Dietary FA composition affected molecular markers of insulin resistance and oxidant stress in women. Skeletal muscle biopsies harvested in the fasted state were used to assess pJNK using the Bio-Plex phosphoprotein assay (Bio-Rad); results are shown for individual women (*A*) and group averages measured after each diet (*B*). Blood samples harvested in the fasted state were used to measure serum IL-6 (*C*) and serum ferritin (*D*). **$P \leq 0.01$, ***$P \leq 0.05$ denote a diet effect.

metabolites might serve as markers of mitochondrial stress and/or cellular events that are known to influence insulin action (29). For example, accumulation of lipid-derived medium chain acyl-CoAs might reflect a mitochondrial environment that is conducive to the production of reactive oxygen species (ROS) (36), perturbations in cellular redox balance (30), and/or inhibition of pyruvate dehydrogenase (37,38).

Fitting with potential shifts in cellular stress, we speculate that the HOA diet lowered oxidant and inflammatory stress in women but not men. In support of this possibility, we found that serum concentrations of IL-6 and ferritin were lower in women during the HOA diet. Circulating levels of IL-6 are elevated in patients with obesity and/or type 2 diabetes, although the role of this cytokine as a direct mediator of insulin resistance remains controversial (39,40). Ferritin, best known as a major iron storage protein, is also recognized as an acute-phase protein (41). Its expression is upregulated by cytokines and ROS during conditions of infection and ramped inflammation (28). Under these conditions, the robust increase in circulating ferritin serves to reduce iron bioavailability, thereby mitigating ROS production and oxidant damage (28). Because iron intake was identical during the two diets and the treatment order was randomized, we surmise that increased ferritin levels in women consuming the HPA diet might reflect heightened oxidative and/or inflammatory stress. It is also important to consider that the distinct antioxidant properties of the vegetable oils used to formulate the HOA and HPA diets might have contributed to the overall effects of the two experimental regimens (42). Notably, however, with the exception of the virgin olive oil added to the HPA diet, the oils used in this study were highly purified (see Supplementary Data).

Although the molecular mechanisms linking lipid dysregulation, inflammation, and/or oxidative stress to insulin resistance are still unfolding, strong evidence implicates a role for JNK1, a member of the mitogen-activated family of serine kinases that serves as a major hub for several discrete signaling pathways involved in monitoring metabolic stress (30,43). In both cultured cells and animal models, JNK1 is activated in response to IL-6, TNF-α, ROS, endoplasmic reticulum stress, and exposure to surplus lipids, resulting in serine phosphorylation and consequent inhibition of IRS-1 (30,43). Most compelling, prolonged high-fat feeding increases JNK phosphorylation in rodents, and genetic ablation of JNK1 protects against obesity-induced insulin resistance (43). Likewise, in the current study, the insulin-sensitizing properties of the HOA diet in women were accompanied by a reduction in muscle levels of pJNK. Our findings suggest that a shift in the FA composition of the diet was sufficient to modulate JNK activity, which in turn contributed to corresponding changes in insulin action. At this stage, we are uncertain as to whether JNK was responding to fluctuations in ROS production, inflammatory tone, endoplasmic reticulum stress (44), and/or other lipid-sensitive signaling molecules. Perhaps subtle perturbations in multiple pathways converged at the JNK nexus.

Interestingly, in women but not men, physical fitness was identified as a strong, positive modifier of changes in cellular lipid composition as well as S_I. These results suggest that the extent to which dietary FAs penetrate cellular lipids and affect glucose homeostasis in women depends on physical activity. Because exercise promotes

ceramides, thus resembling abnormal ceramide metabolism observed in subjects with insulin resistance and/or type 2 diabetes (33). These exciting results provide the first demonstration that a shift in dietary FA composition can actually alter systemic and cellular ceramide metabolism in humans. Surprisingly, however, our analysis failed to detect a convincing association between ceramides and S_I, suggesting that short-term changes in these lipid molecules do not necessarily influence insulin action.

Intriguingly, in women, the HPA diet also increased muscle and blood concentrations of MCAC measured in the fed state. Moreover, the circulating concentration of MCAC in the fed state emerged as a strong negative correlate of S_I when women were consuming the HPA diet. Earlier studies likewise identified a link between insulin resistance and MCAC assessed in human muscle and primary human skeletal myocytes (34). Most MCAC are generated in the mitochondrial matrix and originate from medium-chain acyl-CoA intermediates of the β-oxidation pathway. Accordingly, we measured muscle mRNA abundance of medium-chain acyl-CoA dehydrogenase but did not find a diet effect on expression of this gene (not shown), pointing to other explanations for the HPA diet-induced rise in MCAC content.

Yet unclear is whether the AC can act as signaling molecules or if these metabolites are strictly reporting on changes in mitochondrial substrate flux and/or load. Although convincing evidence that AC play a direct role in mediating insulin resistance is lacking, support for this possibility comes from a recent study showing that exposure of RAW264.7 cells to low micromolar concentrations of MCAC stimulated activity of the stress-sensitive transcription factor nuclear factor-κB (35). Alternatively, these

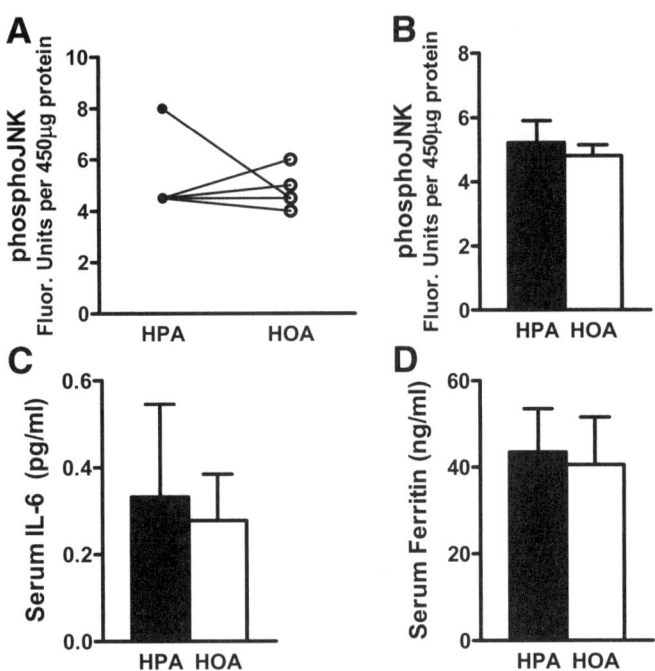

FIG. 6. Dietary FA composition did not affect molecular markers of insulin resistance and oxidant stress in men. Skeletal muscle biopsies harvested in the fasted state were used to assess pJNK using the Bio-Plex phosphoprotein assay; results are shown for individual men (*A*) and group averages measured after each diet (*B*). Blood samples harvested in the fasted state were used to measure serum IL-6 (*C*) and serum ferritin (*D*).

metabolic wellness, a common assumption is that physically inactive individuals have the most to gain by improving dietary habits. Instead, we found that the most active, physically fit women gained the greatest benefit from replacing PA with OA, suggesting that exercise and dietary OA acted synergistically on a common molecular target. Whereas a previous study found that OA increases the energy cost of exercise (20), perhaps by promoting mitochondrial uncoupling (45), investigations to delineate the distinct uncoupling properties of specific FAs have produced conflicting results (46,47). Exercise also decreases the saturation index of muscle lipids and promotes synthesis, storage, and turnover of intramuscular TAG (48,49). Thus, the strong interaction between diet and physical activity might relate to adaptations in muscle lipid droplet metabolism (50). Hinting at this possibility, we found that diet-induced changes in the fractional OA content of muscle TAG correlated positively with VO$_{2peak}$ in women.

In summary, this investigation supports the notion that palmitate imposes a heavy metabolic burden on subcellular machinery, including muscle mitochondria, which was most evident in women during the period after consumption of an HPA meal. In simple terms, when women were consuming the HPA meals, we found less FA safely sequestered into muscle TAG and more FA routed toward the production of AC and ceramides. In women, the metabolic effects of the HPA diet were dependent on physical fitness and associated with decreased insulin sensitivity and insulin secretion. Still uncertain is whether the results of this study point toward sexually dimorphic responses to the experimental diets or, alternatively, if larger cohorts, longer exposures, and/or interventions in populations at

risk for diabetes might reveal comparable effects in men and women. These are important questions that highlight the need for additional dietary trials to better establish the efficacy of replacing palmitate with oleate as a nutritional strategy to combat chronic metabolic disease.

ACKNOWLEDGMENTS

This study was supported by National Institutes of Health Grants R01-DK-073284 and R01-DK-082803, and these studies were conducted at The University of Vermont GCRC, funded by grant RR-00109 from the National Center for Research Resources, National Institutes of Health, U.S. Public Health Service.

No potential conflicts of interest relevant to this article were reported.

C.L.K., J.Y.B., and D.M.M. researched the data, contributed to discussion, and wrote the manuscript. M.E.P. and T.R.K. researched the data and contributed to discussion. R.S., J.B., O.I., and K.I.C. researched the data. N.K.F. and C.M.C. contributed to discussion. C.L.K. is the guarantor of this work and, as such, had full access to all the data in the study and takes responsibility for the integrity of the data and the accuracy of the data analysis.

Data on the effects of these diets on insulin sensitivity were presented in abstract form at The Obesity Society's 28th Annual Scientific Meeting, San Diego, California, 8–12 October 2010. In addition, at the same meeting, we presented a limited amount of data, described in this article, on the PA/OA ratio of muscle lipids as well as data showing the LDL-lowering effect of the HOA diet (not presented in this article) (Obesity 2010;18:S103). Finally, some of the data in this study were published in abstract form at the 72nd Scientific Sessions of the American Diabetes Association, Philadelphia, Pennsylvania, 8–12 June 2012.

The authors thank the staff of the University of Vermont GCRC for dietary, nursing, body composition, and exercise services, administration, and informatics support. The authors also thank the many subjects for patience and hard work in enduring the rigorous protocol; Dr. Julia Johnson, University of Massachusetts Medical School, for assistance with testing of ovulation status; and Julie Smith, MS, RD, The University of Vermont, for help with diet development under the overall supervision of C.L.K. and Emily Tarleton, MS, RD, LD, Bionutrition Manager at The University of Vermont GCRC, in consultation with C.M.C., Pennington Biomedical Research Center.

REFERENCES

1. Kien CL. Dietary interventions for metabolic syndrome: role of modifying dietary fats. Curr Diab Rep 2009;9:43–50
2. Astrup A, Dyerberg J, Elwood P, et al. The role of reducing intakes of saturated fat in the prevention of cardiovascular disease: where does the evidence stand in 2010? Am J Clin Nutr 2011;93:684–688
3. Esposito K, Maiorino MI, Ceriello A, Giugliano D. Prevention and control of type 2 diabetes by Mediterranean diet: a systematic review. Diabetes Res Clin Pract 2010;89:97–102
4. Gillingham LG, Harris-Janz S, Jones PJ. Dietary monounsaturated fatty acids are protective against metabolic syndrome and cardiovascular disease risk factors. Lipids 2011;46:209–228
5. Hu FB, van Dam RM, Liu S. Diet and risk of type II diabetes: the role of types of fat and carbohydrate. Diabetologia 2001;44:805–817
6. Coll T, Eyre E, Rodríguez-Calvo R, et al. Oleate reverses palmitate-induced insulin resistance and inflammation in skeletal muscle cells. J Biol Chem 2008;283:11107–11116
7. Yuzefovych L, Wilson G, Rachek L. Different effects of oleate vs. palmitate on mitochondrial function, apoptosis, and insulin signaling in L6 skeletal muscle cells: role of oxidative stress. Am J Physiol Endocrinol Metab 2010; 299:E1096–E1105

8. Wen H, Gris D, Lei Y, et al. Fatty acid-induced NLRP3-ASC inflammasome activation interferes with insulin signaling. Nat Immunol 2011;12:408–415

9. Li LO, Klett EL, Coleman RA. Acyl-CoA synthesis, lipid metabolism and lipotoxicity. Biochim Biophys Acta 2010;1801:246–251.

10. Vessby B, Uusitupa M, Hermansen K, et al.; KANWU Study. Substituting dietary saturated for monounsaturated fat impairs insulin sensitivity in healthy men and women: The KANWU Study. Diabetologia 2001;44:312–319

11. Tierney AC, McMonagle J, Shaw DI, et al. Effects of dietary fat modification on insulin sensitivity and on other risk factors of the metabolic syndrome—LIPGENE: a European randomized dietary intervention study. Int J Obes (Lond) 2011; 35:800–809

12. Kien CL, Bunn JY. Gender alters the effects of palmitate and oleate on fat oxidation and energy expenditure. Obesity (Silver Spring) 2008;16:29–33

13. Expert Panel on Detection, Evaluation, and Treatment of High Blood Cholesterol in Adults. Executive Summary of The Third Report of The National Cholesterol Education Program (NCEP) Expert Panel on Detection, Evaluation, And Treatment of High Blood Cholesterol In Adults (Adult Treatment Panel III). JAMA 2001;285:2486–2497

14. Stern SE, Williams K, Ferrannini E, DeFronzo RA, Bogardus C, Stern MP. Identification of individuals with insulin resistance using routine clinical measurements. Diabetes 2005;54:333–339

15. Roger VL, Go AS, Lloyd-Jones DM, et al.; American Heart Association Statistics Committee and Stroke Statistics Subcommittee. Heart disease and stroke statistics—2011 update: a report from the American Heart Association. Circulation 2011;123:e18–e209

16. Kien CL, Everingham KI, D Stevens R, Fukagawa NK, Muoio DM. Short-term effects of dietary fatty acids on muscle lipid composition and serum acylcarnitine profile in human subjects. Obesity (Silver Spring) 2011;19:305–311

17. Heymsfield SB, Smith R, Aulet M, et al. Appendicular skeletal muscle mass: measurement by dual-photon absorptiometry. Am J Clin Nutr 1990;52:214–218

18. Saad MF, Anderson RL, Laws A, et al. A comparison between the minimal model and the glucose clamp in the assessment of insulin sensitivity across the spectrum of glucose tolerance. Insulin Resistance Atherosclerosis Study. Diabetes 1994;43:1114–1121

19. Kahn SE, Prigeon RL, McCulloch DK, et al. Quantification of the relationship between insulin sensitivity and beta-cell function in human subjects. Evidence for a hyperbolic function. Diabetes 1993;42:1663–1672

20. Børsheim E, Kien CL, Pearl WM. Differential effects of dietary intake of palmitic acid and oleic acid on oxygen consumption during and after exercise. Metabolism 2006;55:1215–1221

21. Merrill AH Jr, Sullards MC, Allegood JC, Kelly S, Wang E. Sphingolipidomics: high-throughput, structure-specific, and quantitative analysis of sphingolipids by liquid chromatography tandem mass spectrometry. Methods 2005;36:207–224

22. Newgard CB, An J, Bain JR, et al. A branched-chain amino acid-related metabolic signature that differentiates obese and lean humans and contributes to insulin resistance. Cell Metab 2009;9:311–326

23. Koves TR, Li P, An J, et al. PPARgamma coactivator-1alpha -mediated metabolic remodeling of skeletal myocytes mimics exercise training and reverses lipid-induced mitochondrial inefficiency. J Biol Chem 2005;280:33588–33598

24. Jensen MV, Joseph JW, Ilkayeva O, et al. Compensatory responses to pyruvate carboxylase suppression in islet beta-cells. Preservation of glucose-stimulated insulin secretion. J Biol Chem 2006;281:22342–22351

25. Brown RT, McIntosh SM, Seabolt VR, Daniel WA Jr. Iron status of adolescent female athletes. J Adolesc Health Care 1985;6:349–352

26. Brownlie T 4th, Utermohlen V, Hinton PS, Haas JD. Tissue iron deficiency without anemia impairs adaptation in endurance capacity after aerobic training in previously untrained women. Am J Clin Nutr 2004;79:437–443

27. Rajpathak SN, Wylie-Rosett J, Gunter MJ, et al.; Diabetes Prevention Program (DPP) Research Group. Biomarkers of body iron stores and risk of developing type 2 diabetes. Diabetes Obes Metab 2009;11:472–479

28. Arosio P, Levi S. Cytosolic and mitochondrial ferritins in the regulation of cellular iron homeostasis and oxidative damage. Biochim Biophys Acta 2010;1800:783–792

29. Muoio DM. Intramuscular triacylglycerol and insulin resistance: guilty as charged or wrongly accused? Biochim Biophys Acta 2010;1801:281–288

30. Muoio DM, Newgard CB. Obesity-related derangements in metabolic regulation. Annu Rev Biochem 2006;75:367–401

31. D'Eon TM, Souza SC, Aronovitz M, Obin MS, Fried SK, Greenberg AS. Estrogen regulation of adiposity and fuel partitioning. Evidence of genomic and non-genomic regulation of lipogenic and oxidative pathways. J Biol Chem 2005;280:35983–35991

32. Kamei Y, Suzuki M, Miyazaki H, et al. Ovariectomy in mice decreases lipid metabolism-related gene expression in adipose tissue and skeletal muscle with increased body fat. J Nutr Sci Vitaminol (Tokyo) 2005;51:110–117

33. Haus JM, Kashyap SR, Kasumov T, et al. Plasma ceramides are elevated in obese subjects with type 2 diabetes and correlate with the severity of insulin resistance. Diabetes 2009;58:337–343

34. Kovalik JP, Slentz D, Stevens RD, et al. Metabolic remodeling of human skeletal myocytes by cocultured adipocytes depends on the lipolytic state of the system. Diabetes 2011;60:1882–1893

35. Adams SH, Hoppel CL, Lok KH, et al. Plasma acylcarnitine profiles suggest incomplete long-chain fatty acid beta-oxidation and altered tricarboxylic acid cycle activity in type 2 diabetic African-American women. J Nutr 2009; 139:1073–1081

36. Anderson EJ, Lustig ME, Boyle KE, et al. Mitochondrial H2O2 emission and cellular redox state link excess fat intake to insulin resistance in both rodents and humans. J Clin Invest 2009;119:573–581

37. Sugden MC, Holness MJ. Recent advances in mechanisms regulating glucose oxidation at the level of the pyruvate dehydrogenase complex by PDKs. Am J Physiol Endocrinol Metab 2003;284:E855–E862

38. Muoio DM, Noland RC, Kovalik JP, et al. Muscle-specific deletion of carnitine acetyltransferase compromises glucose tolerance and metabolic flexibility. Cell Metab 2012;15:764–777

39. Jové M, Planavila A, Laguna JC, Vázquez-Carrera M. Palmitate-induced interleukin 6 production is mediated by protein kinase C and nuclear-factor kappaB activation and leads to glucose transporter 4 down-regulation in skeletal muscle cells. Endocrinology 2005;146:3087–3095

40. Al-Khalili L, Bouzakri K, Glund S, Lönnqvist F, Koistinen HA, Krook A. Signaling specificity of interleukin-6 action on glucose and lipid metabolism in skeletal muscle. Mol Endocrinol 2006;20:3364–3375

41. Van Campenhout A, Van Campenhout C, Lagrou AR, et al. Impact of diabetes mellitus on the relationships between iron-, inflammatory- and oxidative stress status. Diabetes Metab Res Rev 2006;22:444–454

42. Hatipoğlu A, Kanbağli O, Balkan J, et al. Hazelnut oil administration reduces aortic cholesterol accumulation and lipid peroxides in the plasma, liver, and aorta of rabbits fed a high-cholesterol diet. Biosci Biotechnol Biochem 2004;68:2050–2057

43. Hirosumi J, Tuncman G, Chang L, et al. A central role for JNK in obesity and insulin resistance. Nature 2002;420:333–336

44. Fu S, Yang L, Li P, et al. Aberrant lipid metabolism disrupts calcium homeostasis causing liver endoplasmic reticulum stress in obesity. Nature 2011;473:528–531

45. Tonkonogi M, Krook A, Walsh B, Sahlin K. Endurance training increases stimulation of uncoupling of skeletal muscle mitochondria in humans by non-esterified fatty acids: an uncoupling-protein-mediated effect? Biochem J 2000;351:805–810

46. Borst P, Loos JA, Christ EJ, Slater EC. Uncoupling activity of long-chain fatty acids. Biochim Biophys Acta 1962;62:509–518

47. Esteves TC, Parker N, Brand MD. Synergy of fatty acid and reactive alkenal activation of proton conductance through uncoupling protein 1 in mitochondria. Biochem J 2006;395:619–628

48. Dobrzyn P, Pyrkowska A, Jazurek M, Szymanski K, Langfort J, Dobrzyn A. Endurance training-induced accumulation of muscle triglycerides is coupled to upregulation of stearoyl-CoA desaturase 1. J Appl Physiol 2010;109:1653–1661

49. Chabowski A, Zendzian-Piotrowska M, Nawrocki A, Gorski J. Not only accumulation, but also saturation status of intramuscular lipids is significantly affected by PPARgamma activation. Acta Physiol (Oxf) 2012;205:145–158

50. Amati F, Dubé JJ, Alvarez-Carnero E, et al. Skeletal muscle triglycerides, diacylglycerols, and ceramides in insulin resistance: another paradox in endurance-trained athletes? Diabetes 2011;60:2588–2597

Mitochondrial Function in Diabetes: Novel Methodology and New Insight

Liping Yu,[1] Brian D. Fink,[2] Judith A. Herlein,[2] and William I. Sivitz[2]

Interpreting mitochondrial function as affected by comparative physiologic conditions is confounding because individual functional parameters are interdependent. Here, we studied muscle mitochondrial function in insulin-deficient diabetes using a novel, highly sensitive, and specific method to quantify ATP production simultaneously with reactive oxygen species (ROS) at clamped levels of inner mitochondrial membrane potential ($\Delta\Psi$), enabling more detailed study. We used a 2-deoxyglucose (2DOG) energy clamp to set $\Delta\Psi$ at fixed levels and to quantify ATP production as 2DOG conversion to 2DOG-phosphate measured by one-dimensional ^{1}H and two-dimensional $^{1}H/^{13}C$ heteronuclear single quantum coherence nuclear magnetic resonance spectroscopy. These techniques proved far more sensitive than conventional ^{31}P nuclear magnetic resonance and allowed high-throughput study of small mitochondrial isolates. Over conditions ranging from state 4 to state 3 respiration, ATP production was lower and ROS per unit of ATP generated was greater in mitochondria isolated from diabetic muscle. Moreover, ROS began to increase at a lower threshold for inner membrane potential in diabetic mitochondria. Further, ATP production in diabetic mitochondria is limited not only by respiration but also by limited capacity to use $\Delta\Psi$ for ATP synthesis. In summary, we describe novel methodology for measuring ATP and provide new mechanistic insight into the dysregulation of ATP production and ROS in mitochondria of insulin-deficient rodents. *Diabetes* 62:1833–1842, 2013

A ccording to the widely accepted chemiosmotic theory, oxidative phosphorylation uses the electrochemical gradient across the inner mitochondrial membrane ($\Delta\Psi$) to drive ATP production (1). In this process, protons move inward with the charge gradient, driving the rotary component of ATP synthase in stepwise fashion to bind ADP, phosphorylate ADP, and release ATP to the matrix (2,3). Oxidative phosphorylation has been divided into three modules that independently control $\Delta\Psi$ (4). Each act in different fashions to either supply or consume $\Delta\Psi$ (Fig. 1). These modules include supply by respiration, consumption by proton leaks, and consumption for ATP synthesis.

Major metrics used to describe mitochondrial function include oxygen consumption (respiration), membrane potential, the rate of ATP production, and generation of

reactive oxygen species (ROS) in the form of superoxide. Respiration as measured in isolated mitochondria is proportional to electron transport. In recent work (5), we underscored the importance of considering mitochondrial ROS production not only as an isolated entity but also in relation to electron transport, the process from which electron leaks derive. We showed that absolute ROS production by muscle mitochondria of insulin-deficient rats was reduced, but it was substantially increased when viewed as a function of respiration (electron transport).

In this study, we further investigated the relationships between parameters of muscle mitochondrial function as affected by insulin deficiency. In particular, we examined ATP production in a way that provides new information about contributions of the modular components (Fig. 1) to the process. We also examined ROS production as affected at different levels of ATP production as respiration proceeds from state 4 to state 3.

To achieve our objectives, we developed a novel, highly sensitive, and specific ATP assay that can be performed with high throughput in samples obtained from small-volume mitochondrial isolates. ROS production can be assayed simultaneously. The purpose of this report is two-fold, to describe this assay and to provide new insight into mitochondrial function as affected by insulin-deficient diabetes.

RESEARCH DESIGN AND METHODS

Materials. Reagents were purchased as indicated or were from standard sources.

Animal studies. Male Sprague-Dawley rats were obtained from Harlan (Indianapolis, IN). Animals were fed standard chow (Harlan Tekland #7001) and maintained according to National Institutes of Health guidelines. The protocol was approved by our institutional Animal Care Committee. Rats were killed by incision of the left ventricle after injection of 100 mg/kg i.p. pentobarbital, a dose that does not affect mitochondrial respiration or potential (6).

Rats were made diabetic with intraperitoneal streptozotocin (STZ) 60 mg/kg. Controls received vehicle (saline). Rats were killed at ~1000 h, 2 h after removal of food. Gastrocnemius muscle was removed, washed, blotted, and weighed before preparation of mitochondria. Two animal protocols were followed (Fig. 2). Each included three groups of animals: STZ diabetic (STZ-DM), STZ diabetic treated with insulin (DM-INS), and controls (injected with saline as vehicle for STZ). Ages at onset of protocols 1 and 2 were 110 ± 0 and 98 ± 1 days, respectively, with no differences between groups within each protocol. Weight differentials between control and STZ-DM rats (an indicator of severity of diabetes) were similar for protocols 1 and 2. The duration of insulin treatment in protocol 2 was less by intent. Protocol 1 was performed to assess ATP and ROS production and their relationship with clamped membrane potential. Protocol 2 was performed to assess the effect of insulin-deficient diabetes on the capacity to use membrane potential (module 3 of Fig. 1). However, we included some short-duration insulin-treated diabetic rats in protocol 2, mainly to determine if this was sufficient to improve defective ATP production. Insulin-treated rats of protocol 1 received 4 units s.c. glargine insulin daily at 1600–1700 h. Insulin-treated rats of protocol 2 received 6 units s.c. of glargine insulin daily at 1600–1700 h. Although the rats of protocol 1 regained weight, glucose was not well-controlled, prompting the higher dose in protocol 2. Tail-vein glucose at euthanization was >500 mg/100 mL (values >600 were beyond the range of the glucose meter) in all STZ-DM rats as well as in the DM-INS rats in both protocols despite insulin therapy and weight gain (Fig. 2).

From the [1]NMR Core Facility and Department of Biochemistry, University of Iowa, Iowa City, Iowa; and the [2]Department of Internal Medicine and Endocrinology, University of Iowa and the Iowa City Veterans Affairs Medical Center, Iowa City, Iowa.

Corresponding author: William I. Sivitz, william-sivitz@uiowa.edu.

Received 23 August 2012 and accepted 3 December 2012.

DOI: 10.2337/db12-1152

This article contains Supplementary Data online at http://diabetes .diabetesjournals.org/lookup/suppl/doi:10.2337/db12-1152/-/DC1.

See accompanying commentary, p. 1826.

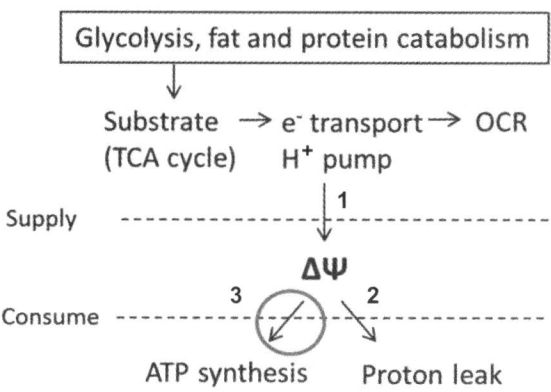

FIG. 1. Modular components regulating oxidative phosphorylation. Module 1 generates the charge gradient ($\Delta\Psi$) through proton pumping at respiratory complexes I, III, and IV. Module 2 consumes $\Delta\Psi$ through proton leak pathways including catalysis through uncoupling proteins, action of the mitochondrial permeability transition pore, or other specific or nonspecific processes. Module 3 (circle) consumes $\Delta\Psi$ for ATP synthesis. TCA, tricarboxylic acid; OCR, oxygen consumption rate.

Isolation of mitochondria. Muscle mitochondria were isolated as previously described (7–9). Mitochondrial protein was determined on homogenates by the Bradford technique using a kit from Bio-Rad (Hercules, CA). Mitochondria prepared in this fashion were highly pure, as indicated by the distribution of glyceraldehyde-3-phosphate dehydrogenase and porin in whole tissue and mitochondrial extracts (8). Mitochondrial integrity was assessed by cytochrome C release (Cytochrome c Oxidase Assay Kit; Sigma-Aldrich) in several preparations (seven each) for control, diabetic, and insulin-treated diabetic mitochondria. Values for intact mitochondria were 94.4 ± 4.8, 98.3 ± 2.4, and 94.3 ± 3.8%, respectively, which were well within an acceptable range compared with mitochondrial preparations from several sources (10).

Respiration and potential. Respiration and $\Delta\Psi$ were determined as we previously described (11,12) using a 600-μL respiratory chamber fitted with a tetraphenylphosphonium electrode. Mitochondria (0.5 mg/mL) were incubated in ionic respiratory buffer (120 mmol/L KCl, 5 mmol/L KH$_2$PO$_4$, 2 mmol/L MgCl$_2$, 1 mmol/L EGTA, 3 mmol/L HEPES [pH 7.2] with 0.3% fatty acid–free BSA).

Mitochondrial ROS production by fluorescent measurement. H$_2$O$_2$ production was assessed using the fluorescent probe 10-acetyl-3,7-dihydroxyphenoxazine (DHPA or Amplex Red; Invitrogen), a highly sensitive and stable substrate for horseradish peroxidase and a well-established probe for isolated mitochondria (13). Fluorescence was measured and quantification was performed as previously described (12). Addition of catalase, 500 units/mL, reduced fluorescence to below the detectable limit, indicating specificity for H$_2$O$_2$. Addition of substrates to respiratory buffer without mitochondria did not affect fluorescence.

2-Deoxyglucose as an ATP energy clamp. To assess mitochondrial functional parameters at fixed $\Delta\Psi$, we used excess 2-deoxyglucose (2DOG) (5 mmol/L) and hexokinase (HK; 5 units/mL) to generate an "ATP energy clamp" (Fig. 3A). The conversion of 2DOG to 2DOG phosphate (2DOGP) occurs rapidly and irreversibly, thereby effectively clamping ADP concentrations and $\Delta\Psi$ dependent on the amount of exogenous ADP added. This enables titration of membrane potential at different fixed values, whereas mitochondria transit from state 4 (no ADP, maximal potential) to state 3 (high levels of ADP resulting in reduced $\Delta\Psi$). The 2DOG clamp has been used in the past to assess mitochondrial-bound hexokinase activity at constant ADP (14), but not to assess mitochondrial physiology or ATP production as described herein.

Use of the 2DOG ATP energy clamp to quantify ATP production in isolated mitochondria and simultaneous assessment of H$_2$O$_2$ production. Mitochondria (0.1 mg/mL) were added to individual wells of 96-well plates in a total volume of 60 μL and incubated at 37°C in respiratory buffer plus 5 units/mL HK (Worthington Biochemical) and 5 mmol/L 2DOG or, in some experiments, [6-^{13}C]2DOG (Cambridge Isotope Laboratories, Andover MA) in the presence of ADP or ATP ranging from 0 to 1,000 μmol/L, depending on the particular experiment. After incubation for the desired time, the contents of the microplate wells were removed to tubes on ice containing 1 μL of 120 μmol/L oligomycin to inhibit ATP synthase. Tubes were then centrifuged 4 min at 14,000g to pellet the mitochondria. Supernatants were transferred to new tubes and held at −20°C until nuclear magnetic resonance (NMR) analysis. To prepare the NMR sample, 40 μL assay supernatant was added to a 5-mm (outer diameter) standard NMR tube (Norell) along with 50 μL deuterium oxide (D$_2$O) and 390 μL buffer consisting of 120 mmol/L KCl, 5 mmol/L KH$_2$PO$_4$, and 2 mmol/L MgCl$_2$ (pH 7.2).

ATP production rates were calculated based on the percent conversion of 2DOG to 2DOGP, the initial 2DOG concentration, incubation volume, and incubation time. To simultaneously assess H$_2$O$_2$ production, mitochondrial incubations were performed in the presence of DHPA as described.

NMR spectroscopy. NMR spectra were collected at 37°C on a Bruker Avance II 500 NMR spectrometer. The 2DOG and 2DOGP ^{1}H and ^{13}C NMR resonances were assigned through ^{1}H homonuclear two-dimensional DQF-COSY (15) and TOCSY (16,17) experiments and ^{1}H/^{13}C two-dimensional heteronuclear

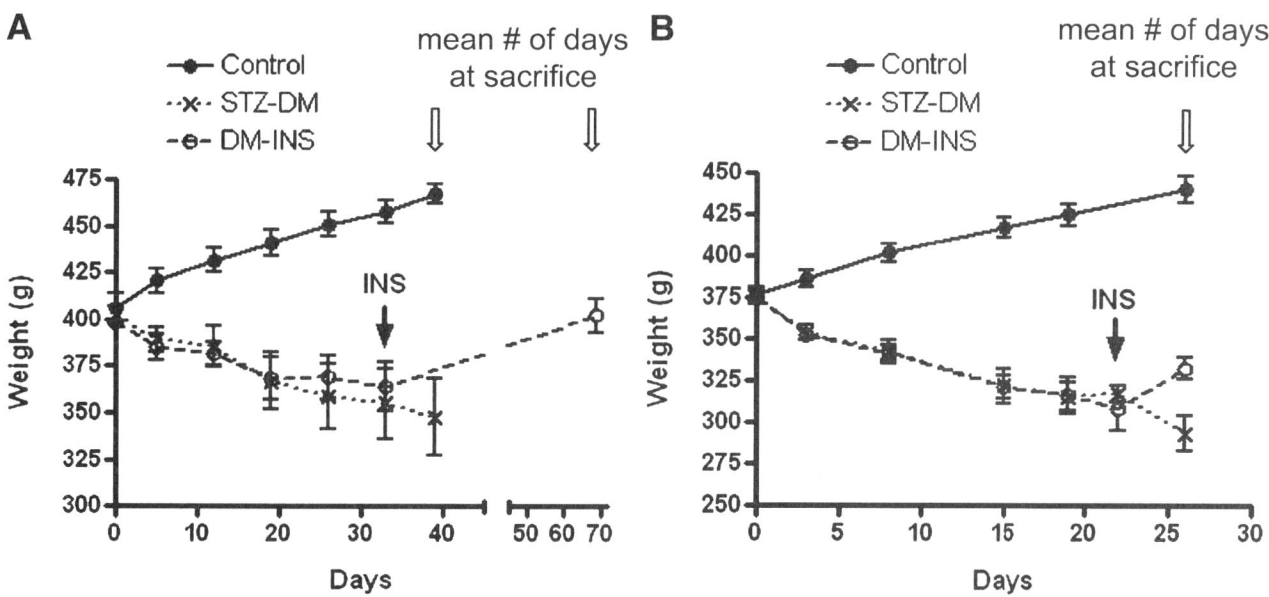

FIG. 2. Weight change (mean ± SE) after injection of STZ 60 mg/kg or vehicle (saline) on day 0 in control, STZ-DM, or DM-INS rats. Diabetes was diagnosed based on a glucose >300 mg/100 mL within 5 days of STZ. Lantus insulin (INS) was administered to the DM-INS rats daily starting at the day number indicated by the *arrow*. The last time points indicated (*open arrows*) represent the average day number at euthanization. *A*: Protocol 1. Rats were killed after the average number of days indicated (range, 34–43 days for control and STZ-DM; 66–68 for DM-INS; n = 8, 8, and 7 for control, STZ-DM, and DM-INS groups). *B*: Protocol 2. Rats were killed after the average number of days indicated (range, 21–35 days for all groups; n = 8, 7, and 7 for control, STZ-DM, and DM-INS groups).

A

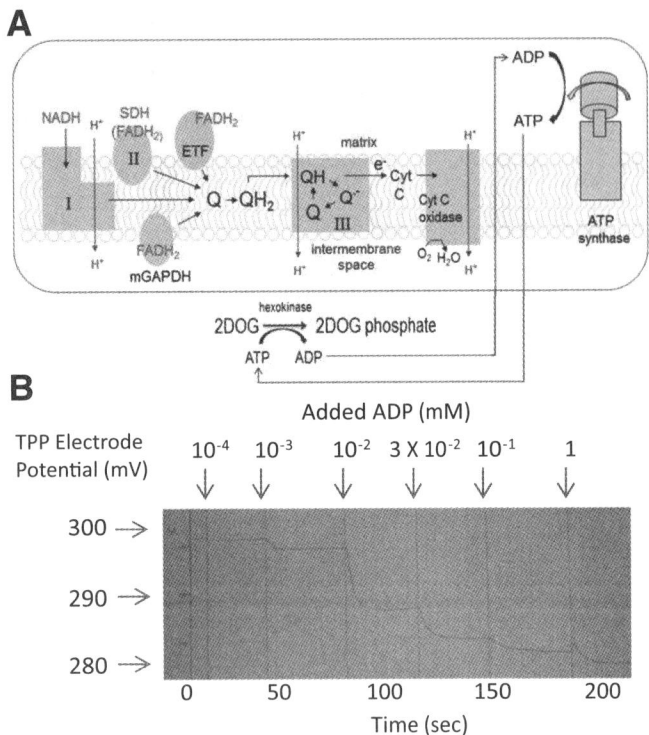

B

FIG. 3. The 2DOG energy clamp. *A*: Saturating amounts of 2DOG and hexokinase recycle ATP back to ADP by irreversibly converting 2DOG into 2DOGP. The resulting ADP availability is clamped at levels determined by the amount of ADP added. Complex numbers are indicated in Roman numerals. *B*: Representative tracing of inner membrane potential vs. time obtained by incubating normal rat gastrocnemius mitochondria (0.25 mg/mL) fueled by combined substrates including 5 mmol/L succinate plus 5 mmol/L glutamate plus 1 mmol/L malate. ADP was added in incremental amounts to generate the final total recycling nucleotide phosphate concentrations indicated. After each addition, a plateau potential was reached, consistent with recycling at a steady ADP concentration and generation of a stepwise transition from state 4 to state 3 respiration. Note that the potential shown on the *y*-axis represents negative values of electrode potential (not mitochondrial potential). The actual $\Delta\Psi$ follows a similar pattern after calculation using the Nernst equation based on the distribution of tetraphenylphosphonium (TPP), external and internal, to mitochondria. ETF, electron transport flavoprotein; Cyt C, cytochrome C.

multiple quantum coherence and heteronuclear multiple bond coherence experiments (18). Mitochondrial samples were studied by NMR spectroscopy by acquiring one-dimensional ^{1}H NMR spectra using unlabeled 2DOG or two-dimensional ^{1}H/^{13}C heteronuclear single quantum coherence (HSQC) NMR spectra (19) using ^{13}C-labeled 2DOG at C6-position, i.e., [6-^{13}C]2DOG, in NMR buffer containing 120 mmol/L KCl, 5 mmol/L KH$_2$PO$_4$, 2 mmol/L MgCl$_2$ (pH 7.2), and 90% H$_2$O/10% D$_2$O. The amounts of 2DOG and 2DOGP present in the NMR samples were quantitatively measured using the peak intensities of the assigned resonances of these compounds. The ^{1}H and ^{31}P chemical shifts are referenced to 2,2-dimethyl-2-silapentane-5-sulfonate and external 2% H$_3$PO$_4$ in D$_2$O (20), respectively. NMR spectra were processed with the NMRPipe package (21) and analyzed using NMRView software (22).

Other biochemical assays. Glucose was determined on tail-vein blood using a reagent strip and meter (OneTouch Ultra).

Statistics. Data were analyzed by ANOVA, linear regression, or second-order polynomial curve fitting as indicated in the figures or text. Rates of ATP and H$_2$O$_2$ production and respiration ($\pm$SE) are expressed per milligram of mitochondrial protein.

RESULTS

Effectiveness of the 2DOG ATP energy clamp. For this technique to work as predicted, sequential increases in ADP added to isolated mitochondria should reduce $\Delta\Psi$ in stepwise fashion. Figure 3*B* shows that with each addition

of ADP, $\Delta\Psi$ rapidly decreased to plateau levels. Adding ATP instead of ADP resulted in nearly identical data, which was as expected given the recycling effect of the clamp. Oxygen consumption increased as expected with each addition of ADP (data not shown) as respiration shifted toward state 3. When this experiment was performed with ATP but in the absence of HK, respiration did not increase and $\Delta\Psi$ did not decline, consistent with the lack of recycling to ADP.

Validation of coupling of conversion of 2DOG to 2DOGP for quantification of ATP production. To determine whether HK-mediated conversion of 2DOG to 2DOGP reflects ATP production, we examined the ^{31}P NMR spectrum of 0.85 mmol/L ATP dissolved in a buffer containing 5 mmol/L KH$_2$PO$_4$, 120 mmol/L KCl, 2 mmol/L MgCl$_2$, and 4.5 mmol/L 2DOG (pH 7.2) plus 10% D$_2$O in the absence or presence of HK. In the absence of HK, the ^{31}P NMR spectrum obtained, as expected, was composed of three peaks (α, β, γ) from ATP and one peak (Pi) from the buffer phosphate (Supplementary Fig. 1*A*). However, on addition of HK (5 units/mL), the ATP fully converted to ADP with concurrent formation of 2DOGP from 2DOG (Supplementary Fig. 1*B*). The Pi peak of the sample with HK present is shifted slightly toward right because of the slightly increased acidity (pH, 7.05) of the sample as a result of ATP hydrolysis during the conversion of 2DOG into 2DOGP.

Comparison of ^{1}H and ^{31}P NMR sensitivity. Traditionally, ATP production has been measured directly through detection of the ATP signals via ^{31}P NMR spectroscopy in which the three phosphate signals α, β, γ (Supplementary Fig. 1*A*) are well-resolved from each other and from other ^{31}P signals. However, because of the much smaller magnetogyric ratio of ^{31}P than ^{1}H nuclei, ^{31}P NMR is inherently much less sensitive than ^{1}H NMR. Moreover, the NMR probes routinely accessible in many NMR laboratories, including the triple resonance probe and broadband observe probe, provide significantly superior ^{1}H than ^{31}P signal sensitivity. As shown in Supplementary Fig. 2, for the samples prepared at the same concentration and the data collected with identical acquisition time, the ^{1}H NMR spectrum of 2DOGP provides a much improved signal-to-noise ratio, e.g., 580 for the 2α' proton (Supplementary Fig. 2*A*), than the ^{31}P NMR spectrum of ADP, which has a signal-to-noise ratio of 17 for either the α or the β phosphate group (Supplementary Fig. 2*B*). Therefore, detecting ATP via 2DOGP using ^{1}H NMR signals significantly reduces the detection limit for ATP and shortens the data acquisition time.

ATP production using one-dimensional ^{1}H NMR spectroscopy. Highly sensitive one-dimensional ^{1}H NMR was used effectively to monitor 2DOGP production from 2DOG. The ^{1}H NMR spectra of 2DOG and 2DOGP were clearly different (Fig. 4*A*). In particular, the resonances of H6β, H4α, H4β, and H5β protons of 2DOGP are resolved from 2DOG peaks. Moreover, the H2α protons at $\sim$1.7 ppm and H2β protons at $\sim$1.5 ppm are partially resolved from each other (Fig. 4*A*). Because this region (1.4–1.8 ppm) of the ^{1}H NMR spectra is generally free from other overlapping peaks among the mitochondrial samples tested, we used H2α protons at $\sim$1.7 ppm and H2β protons at $\sim$1.5 ppm to monitor their peak intensity changes as affected by various ADP concentrations in control (Fig. 4*B*) and STZ-diabetic (Fig. 4*C*) mitochondrial incubates. Figure 4*B* and *C* clearly shows that under identical experimental conditions, the control mitochondria produced substantially more 2DOGP (or ATP) than the diabetic mitochondria.

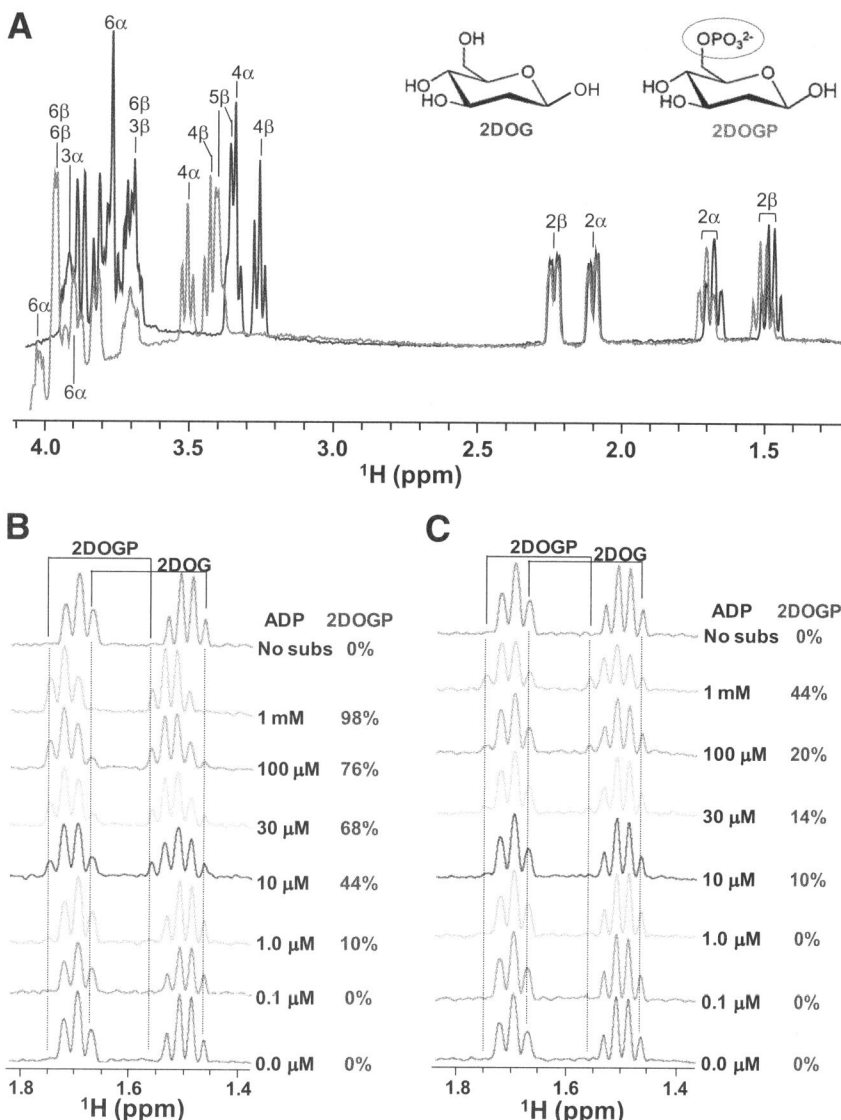

FIG. 4. Quantification of ATP production in control and diabetic mitochondria by one-dimensional ¹H NMR. *A*: Overlay of one-dimensional ¹H NMR spectra of 2DOG (blue) and 2DOGP (red). The resonance assignments are indicated. Regions of one-dimensional ¹H NMR spectra of 2DOG and 2DOGP of gastrocnemius mitochondrial samples isolated from a control (*B*) and diabetic (*C*) rat. Mitochondria (0.006 mg) were incubated in 60 μL of respiratory buffer with 5 mmol/L 2DOG, 5 units/mL hexokinase, and variable concentrations of ADP, and fueled with 5 mmol/L succinate plus 5 mmol/L glutamate plus 1 mmol/L malate for 20 min. Mitochondria were then precipitated and 40 μL supernatant was diluted into a final volume of 480 μL in NMR buffer. A total of 384 scans were collected for each sample. Quantification of the percent conversion of 2DOG into 2DOGP was performed by using the peak intensities of 2α and 2β protons of 2DOG and 2DOGP. ADP concentrations and the percent of 2DOGP converted from 2DOG are indicated to the right of the spectra. No subs = control with no added substrate or ADP.

ATP production using two-dimensional ¹H/¹³C NMR spectroscopy. The two-dimensional ¹H/¹³C heteronuclear multiple quantum coherence spectra of 2DOG and 2DOGP were assigned (Fig. 5*A*). The C6/H6 and C4/H4 cross-peaks of 2DOGP clearly were resolved from those of 2DOG. Using 2DOG with ¹³C-labeling only at C6 position, i.e., [6-¹³C] 2DOG, we can zoom-in to the C6 region (boxed in Fig. 5*A*) and collect high-resolution two-dimensional ¹H/¹³C HSQC NMR spectra of control versus diabetic mitochondrial samples (Fig. 5*B*). Clearly, the cross-peaks derived from 2DOGP are well-resolved from those of 2DOG. Moreover, the cross-peaks of the α- and β-anomeric forms of those compounds are now well-resolved. Therefore, the amount of 2DOGP being converted from 2DOG can be reliably quantified by measuring the peak intensities in the contour plot or via the one-dimensional slices through the relevant

cross-peaks (Fig. 5*B*). Because the C6/H6 cross-peak derived from the β-anomeric form of 2DOGP has the highest intensity, it is routinely chosen to quantify the amount of 2DOGP formed as a result of ATP production by mitochondria. Figure 5*B* clearly demonstrates that under identical experimental conditions, the diabetic mitochondrial sample produced much less 2DOGP or ATP than the control mitochondrial sample. This two-dimensional NMR method is sensitive, with a signal-to-noise ratio of 698 for the C6/H6 cross-peak of the β-anomeric form of 2DOGP (Supplementary Fig. 3) obtained by using a sample at the same concentration and with the same acquisition time as shown in Supplementary Fig. 2. Because of the narrow spectral width in the ¹³C-dimension, it only took 4.5 min to acquire the high-resolution two-dimensional spectrum for the concentrated sample shown in Fig. 5*B*. For a typical

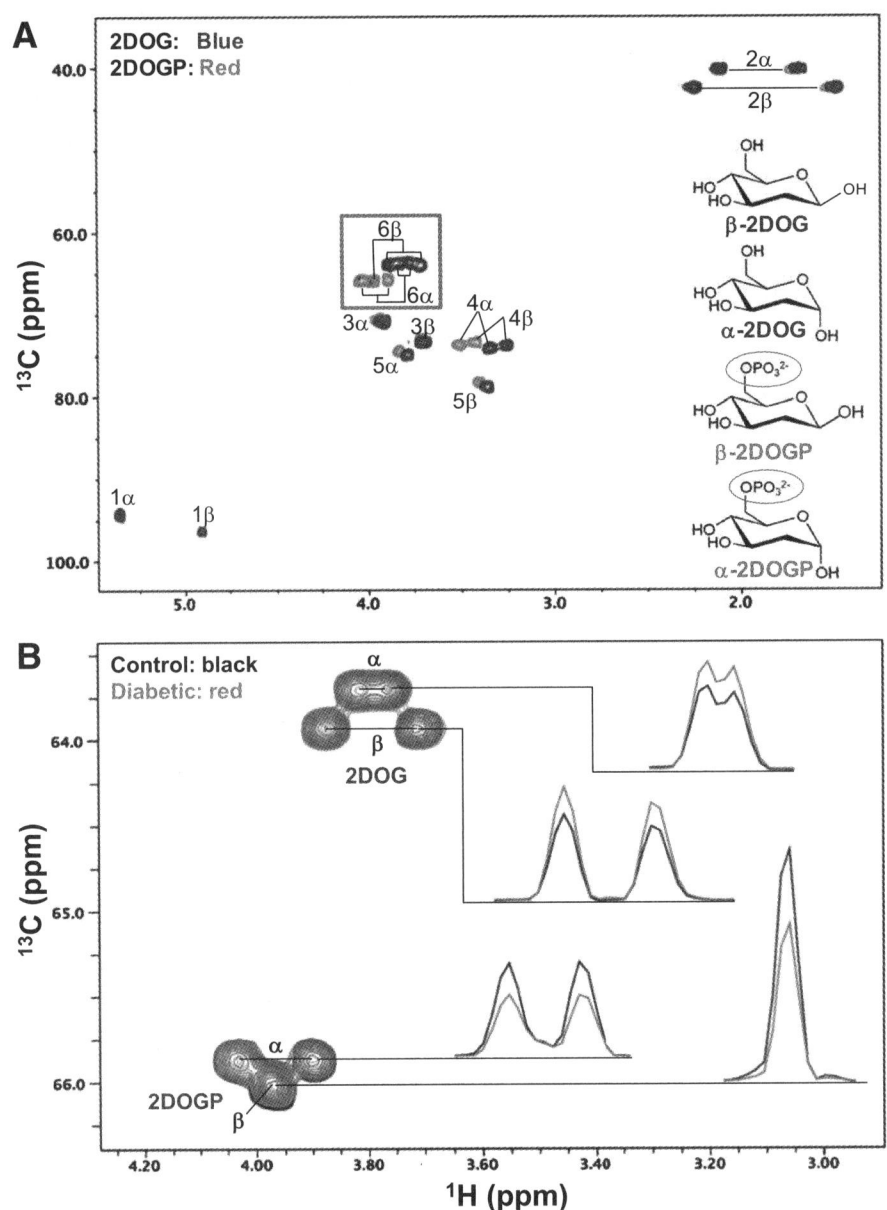

FIG. 5. Quantification of ATP production in control and diabetic mitochondria by two-dimensional $^1H/^{13}C$ NMR. *A*: Overlay of two-dimensional $^1H/^{13}C$ heteronuclear multiple quantum coherence spectra of unlabeled 2DOG (blue) and 2DOGP (red). The green box indicates the H6/C6 region of interest. The α- and β-anomeric structures of 2DOG and 2DOGP are included. The cross-peaks of the α- and β-anomeric forms are assigned. *B*: Overlay of two-dimensional $^1H/^{13}C$ HSQC spectra of the H6/C6 region of 2DOG and 2DOGP for samples that contain mitochondria from a control (black) rat and a diabetic (red) rat. Mitochondria (0.1 mg/mL) were incubated for 20 min in respiratory buffer containing 5.0 mmol/L [6-^{13}C]2DOG, 5 units/mL hexokinase, and 1 mmol/L ADP, and fueled with 5 mmol/L succinate, 5 mmol/L glutamate, and 1 mmol/L malate. Mitochondria were then precipitated by centrifugation and 50 μL D_2O was added to 450 μL supernatant for NMR studies. Each spectrum only took 4.5 min to acquire because the samples contained high concentrations of 2DOG and 2DOGP. The cross-peaks are labeled and one-dimensional slices through the cross-peaks are included.

mitochondrial NMR sample that contained ~0.42 mmol/L [6-^{13}C]2DOG initially, we acquired 15 complex t_1 increments with 16 scans per increment and a long recycle time of 4.4 s per scan, leading to a total acquisition time of 35 min (Supplementary Fig. 4). Most importantly, with the use of [6-^{13}C]2DOG, the acquired two-dimensional NMR spectra are clean, with no interference from background signals, even for samples that contain larger amounts of mitochondria or in the presence of different inhibitors used to assess mitochondrial function.

ATP detection limits. As shown in Supplementary Fig. 5*A–F*, we detected ATP production in mitochondrial

samples at a concentration of 0.01 mg/mL in an incubation volume of 60 μL or a sample of 0.6 μg mitochondria. Conventional ^{31}P NMR was insensitive even at the highest mitochondrial concentration (Supplementary Fig. 5*G* and *H*). **Time effect after addition of oligomycin and effect of shaking during incubation.** The time period between addition of oligomycin and completion of centrifugation to separate mitochondria (4 min) did not impact our results. In pilot experiments (Supplementary Fig. 6*A*), we removed mitochondria from the incubation mixture immediately (less than 30 s) after adding oligomycin by rapid filtration (versus centrifugation) and observed no difference in ATP production. Mitochondria were not routinely shaken or stirred during incubation in the plate reader. However, it is possible to intermittently shake the wells within the plate reader between fluorescent reading cycles. Shaking in this way did not alter ATP production (Supplementary Fig. 6B). **ATP production rates on different substrate and inhibitor combinations.** Our studies of diabetic and control mitochondria were performed using a combination of glutamate, malate, and succinate. However, as shown in Supplementary Fig. 7, our assay also can be used for different substrate conditions with the expected effects of the classic inhibitors, rotenone, oligomycin, and carbonyl cyanide p-[trifluoromethoxy]-phenyl-hydrazone.

ATP production rates in gastrocnemius mitochondria at clamped levels of ADP and potential. We measured ATP production by one-dimensional ^{1}H NMR as a function of added ADP for control, diabetic, and insulin-treated diabetic rats following protocol 1. As shown in Fig. 6A, for each amount of ADP added, diabetic mitochondria generated less ATP than controls. Mitochondria isolated from the insulin-treated diabetic rats produced amounts of ATP equivalent to controls. Plotting the same ATP data versus $\Delta\Psi$ (generated at each level of added ADP) again showed that the diabetic mitochondria produced less ATP compared with mitochondria of controls or from insulin-treated diabetic rats (Fig. 6B).

ROS production by gastrocnemius muscle of control and diabetic mitochondria. We examined the relationships between ROS production and inner membrane potential, as well as ROS production per unit ATP generated in gastrocnemius mitochondria of protocol 1 animals at various levels of clamped ADP (and, consequently, clamped, $\Delta\Psi$). The probe DHPA did not interfere with the ATP assay (Supplementary Fig. 8A), enabling concurrent assessment of ROS in the same 96-well plates. Both ATP and H_2O_2 concentrations increased in linear fashion during incubation (Supplementary Fig. 8). Respiration and $\Delta\Psi$ were assessed in parallel. Figure 7A depicts plateau levels of $\Delta\Psi$ as created by different concentrations of added ADP or ATP in STZ-DM, DM-INS, and control mitochondria. As expected, ROS production becomes very low at ADP

concentrations high enough to drive mitochondria toward state 3 respiration (Fig. 7B). However, it is clear that ROS production by STZ-DM mitochondria begins to increase at a lower $\Delta\Psi$ threshold compared with control or DM-INS mitochondria. As shown in Fig. 7C, respiration, at any given $\Delta\Psi$, is reduced in mitochondria of STZ-DM rats compared with controls and DM-INS. As shown in Fig. 7D, the reduced $\Delta\Psi$ threshold effect for ROS is more evident when ROS production is viewed in relation to electron transport activity (proportional to respiration). Finally, ROS production per ATP generated is significantly higher in diabetic mitochondria (Fig. 7E).

ATP production rates in gastrocnemius mitochondria as a function of membrane potential independent of [ADP]. Although Fig. 6B depicts ATP production at different potential, these levels of $\Delta\Psi$ were achieved by varying [ADP]. To assess ATP production as a function of module 3 in Fig. 1, it is necessary to manipulate potential apart from a means that is, itself, operative in module 3. Therefore, we varied potential through titration with different substrate concentrations at the same ADP concentration (100 μmol/L). We incubated mitochondria in the presence of combined substrates using a constant ratio of 5:5:1 for succinate to glutamate to malate, with values for succinate and glutamate of 0.5, 1.0, 2.0, and 4.0 mmol/L and values for malate of 0.1, 0.2, 0.4, and 0.8 mmol/L.

These experiments were performed in rats treated according to protocol 2 (Fig. 2), and ATP production was assessed using two-dimensional ^{1}H/^{13}C HSQC NMR. As indicated in Fig. 8A, ATP production is linear with time for 30 min under the conditions of study. Therefore, ATP production rates were assessed over 30 min in all experiments. ATP production was decreased in both STZ-DM and DM-INS mitochondria compared with controls at the higher substrate concentrations (Fig. 8B).

At approximately the same time and on the same mitochondrial preparations, respiration and potential were measured in our respiratory chamber with sequential additions of substrates to achieve the desired concentrations. Respiration and potential increased with each increase of substrates and stabilized at plateau levels

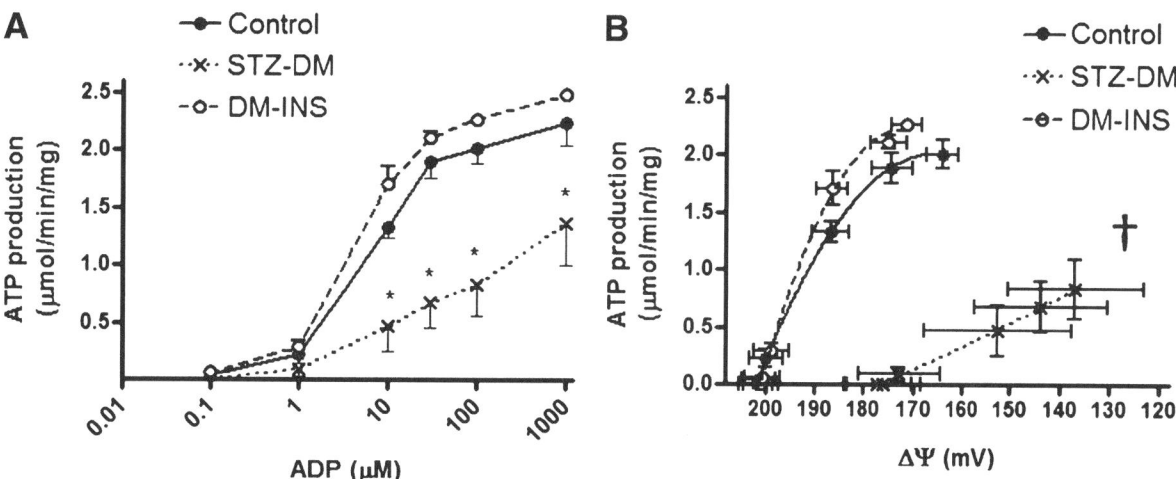

FIG. 6. Effect of STZ-DM and DM-INS on gastrocnemius muscle mitochondrial ATP production. *A*: ATP production rates as a function of ADP concentration for mitochondria isolated from control, STZ-DM, and DM-INS rats treated according to protocol 1 (Fig. 2; $n = 4$ per group). Mitochondria were incubated for 20 min and processed as described in the legend of Fig. 4. DHPA (20 μmol/L) was included in each well for simultaneous assessment of ROS (Fig. 7). *B*: ATP production rates for samples of *A* expressed as a function of $\Delta\Psi$. *P < 0.01 compared with control by two-way ANOVA; †*P* < 0.001 for difference in second-order polynomial curve fit models by F-test.

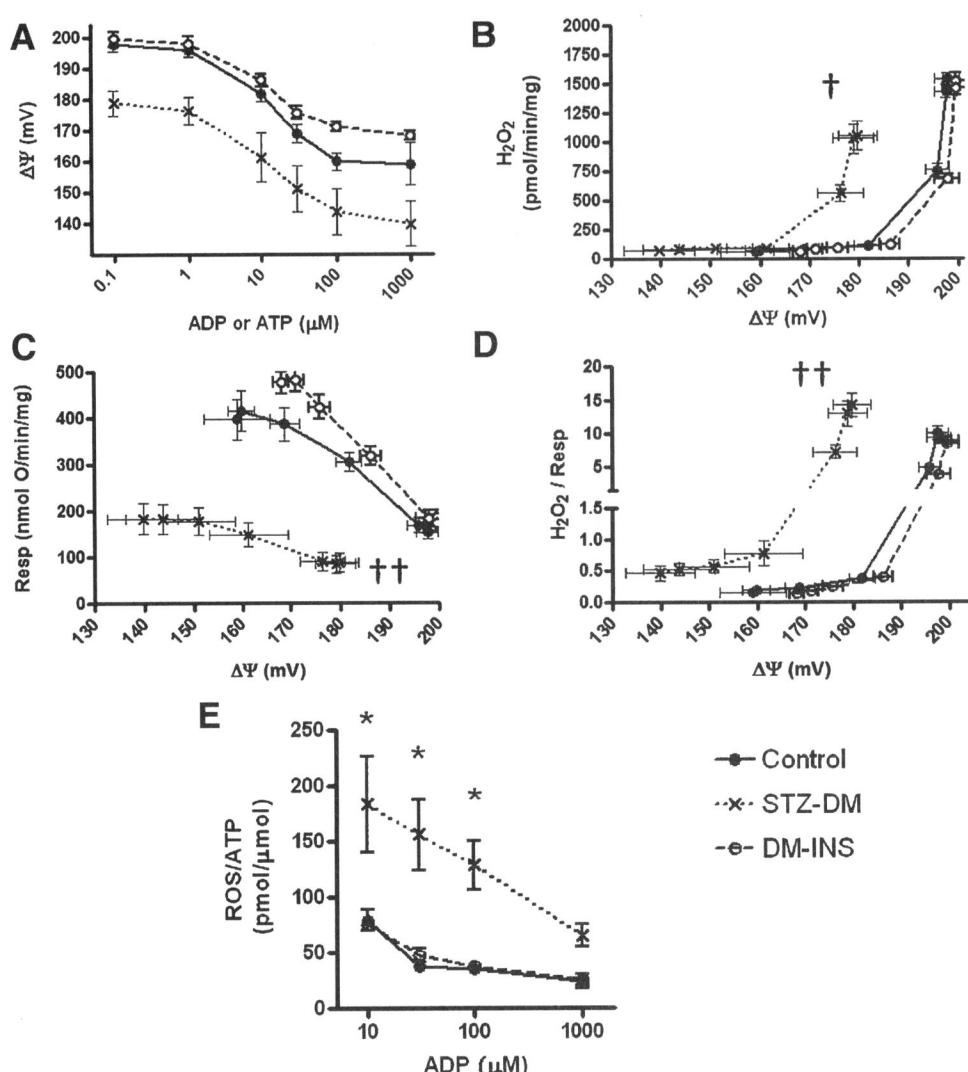

FIG. 7. Mitochondrial ROS production relative to $\Delta\Psi$ in control, STZ-DM, or DM-INS rats treated according to protocol 1 (Fig. 2). Mitochondria were incubated for 20 min as described in the legend of Fig. 4. The data in A–D include the mitochondrial incubates from the four rats (per group) depicted in Fig. 6 plus additional mitochondrial incubates from additional rats wherein ATP was added rather than ADP (same concentrations). Essentially, the same data were obtained using either adenine nucleotide (as expected given the recycling effect), so the results were combined (total $n = 8, 8, 7$ for control, STZ-DM, and DM-INS, respectively). A: $\Delta\Psi$ as a function of ADP or ATP concentration. B: Absolute H_2O_2 production as a function of $\Delta\Psi$. C: Respiration as a function of $\Delta\Psi$. D: H_2O_2 per oxygen consumed vs. $\Delta\Psi$. E: H_2O_2 produced per unit of ATP generated as a function of ADP added ($n = 4$ per group, all using ADP). Data of E do not include ADP concentrations <10 μmol/L because ATP formation is very low (Fig. 6) and H_2O_2 production is high, so that the denominator effect causes marked variability in the ratio. †$P < 0.05$ or ††$P < 0.01$ for difference in second-order polynomial curve fit models by F-test. *$P < 0.01$ compared with control by two-way ANOVA.

before the next addition, generating a range of potentials. Thus, we determined the relationship of ATP production to $\Delta\Psi$ in control, STZ-DM, and DM-INS rats under conditions in which ATP production was dependent on potential in a manner reflecting module 3 of Fig. 1. The results (Fig. 8C–E) revealed that ATP production, as expected, increased with potential. However, the slope of that relationship was reduced in the STZ-DM and DM-INS mitochondria compared with controls (Fig. 8F), indicating a reduced capacity to utilize increments in potential to generate ATP.

DISCUSSION

We applied novel methodology to enable a more detailed evaluation of mitochondrial function as affected by insulin-deficient diabetes. There are several advantages to our ATP

assay. First, the assay is performed under clamped $\Delta\Psi$, allowing assessment of ATP as a function of its direct driving force, $\Delta\Psi$. Second, our assay is sensitive enough to measure ATP production in small isolates of mitochondria. As indicated in Supplementary Figs. 2 and 3, the one-dimensional ^{1}H NMR method is 34-fold more sensitive and the two-dimensional ^{1}H/^{13}C HSQC NMR method is 41-fold more sensitive when compared with one-dimensional ^{31}P NMR for ATP detection. The high sensitivity of the two-dimensional NMR method is attributable to the fact that the chemical shifts of the two H6 protons of the β-anomeric form of 2DOGP are degenerate, resulting in detection of one single C6/H6 HSQC cross-peak with high intensity. Third, both the one-dimensional and two-dimensional NMR spectra are highly specific. In particular, the two-dimensional NMR method involves almost no interference from background signals. Fourth, there is good throughput

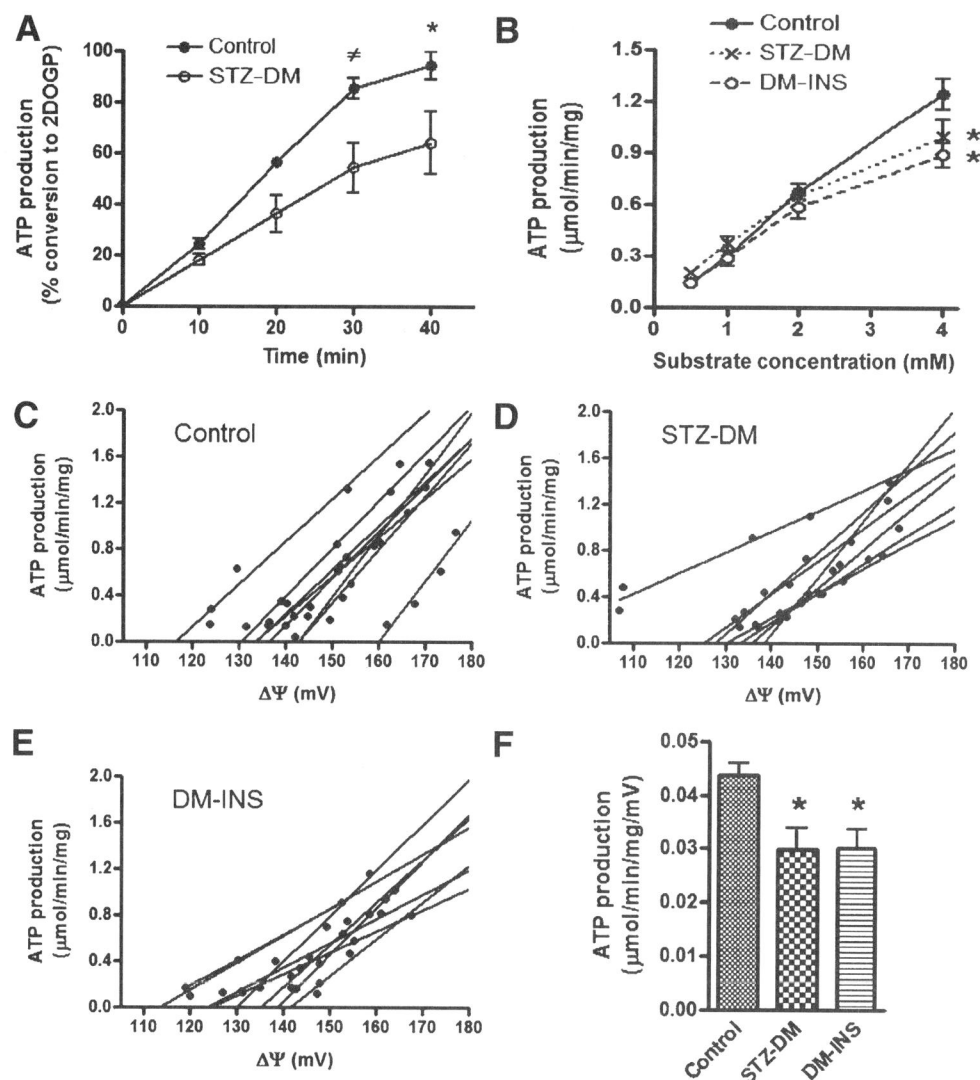

FIG. 8. Dependency of ATP production by gastrocnemius mitochondria on ΔΨ in control, STZ-DM, and DM-INS rats treated according to protocol 2 (Fig. 2). Membrane potential was modulated by incubating mitochondria in the presence of different substrate concentrations (combined succinate and glutamate each at 0.5, 1.0, 2.0, and 4.0 mmol/L, and malate at 0.1, 0.2. 0.4, and 0.8 mmol/L). *A*: Mitochondria were incubated in 96-well plates for 10, 20, 30, or 40 min in respiratory buffer containing 5 mmol/L [6-^{13}C]-2DOG and 5 units/mL HK in the presence of 4.0 mmol/L succinate, 4.0 mmol/L glutamate, and 0.8 mmol/L malate ($n = 4$ per group; $*P < 0.05$ or $\neq P < 0.01$ by two-way ANOVA compared with control). Similar linear, although lower, rates were observed for the lower substrate concentrations (not shown). Because ATP production was linear over the first 30 min, further studies (subsequent panels) were performed in mitochondria incubated for 30 min. *B*: ATP production as a function of substrate concentrations. The *x*-axis indicates only the concentrations of succinate and glutamate, although malate was included at 20% of the indicated values ($n = 8$, 7, and 7 for control, STZ-DM, and DM-INS mitochondria, respectively). $*P < 0.01$ compared with control by two-way ANOVA. *C–E*: In parallel experiments on the same mitochondrial preparations, mitochondria were incubated in our respiratory chamber at progressively increasing substrate concentrations (those used in the wells for ATP determination) to obtain values for ΔΨ. Data depict the relationship of ATP production to ΔΨ in control, STZ-DM, and DM-INS rats. Lines represent linear regression for each mitochondrial incubation. All regression analyses were significant ($P < 0.05$), with $r^2 > 0.9$. *F*: Slopes (mean ± SE) for the regressions in *C–E*. $*P < 0.05$ compared with control by one-way ANOVA and Tukey posttest.

because we can add mitochondria to multiple wells of a 96-well plate, incubate, spin-off the mitochondria, and save the samples that can be directly used for NMR analysis. Fifth, a powerful aspect of this technique is that we can assess mitochondrial ROS along with ATP formation rates simultaneously because the ROS probe (DHPA) does not interfere with the NMR signals of interest in either one-dimensional or two-dimensional NMR spectra. Moreover, DHPA does not interfere with ATP production (Supplementary Fig. 8*A*). It also may be possible to use TMRM or other probes to simultaneously assess potential, although preliminary experiments indicate that higher TMRM concentration may mildly reduce ATP production.

The methods described here have clear advantages over existing methods for ATP assay. Fluorescent and bioluminescent measurements are sensitive, but not specific, and are prone to background interference or variations in light emission (23). Phosphorous NMR is not sensitive enough and requires long acquisition times unless large numbers of mitochondria are used. High-performance liquid chromatography has been used when precise data are needed, but it is cumbersome. ATP:O ratios often are reported as indicative of ATP production because of these difficulties. However, this does not measure ATP and the ratio can be altered by any condition that affects uncoupling, ATP synthase, and respiration itself. Even compared with high-resolution respirometry with luminescent detection of ATP, our method has clear advantages. It is more specific, can be performed with far more throughput involving 96-well plates as compared with dual chambers, can measure ATP at clamped ADP and potential, and can simultaneously measure other fluorescent signals. Of course, the 2DOG technique could be used to clamp potential in the high-resolution respirometer. However, if this were performed, then one could not use reagents such as luciferase (24) or magnesium green (25) to assess ATP production because the 2DOG/hexokinase reaction would compete for ATP.

The energy clamp/ATP assay allowed us to perform novel studies, which was not previously possible. We show that gastrocnemius muscle mitochondria isolated from diabetic rats generate less ATP at any given clamped level of ADP availability (Fig. 6). Thus, the reduction in ATP production occurs throughout progression from state 4 to state 3 respiration. In addition, we investigated the capacity of ATP production to directly utilize $\Delta\Psi$ (Fig. 8C–F). Although respiration and proton leaks (modules 1 and 2) determine membrane potential, according to the chemiosmotic hypothesis, it is only potential itself that drives ATP synthase (1). So, the different dynamic relationship of ATP production relative to potential (manipulated independent of module 3) in the diabetic mitochondria (Fig. 8F) implies an inability of ATP synthase to effectively utilize potential for ATP synthesis. This is important because it implicates a functional defect within module 3 of oxidative phosphorylation.

With regard to ROS, we used the 2DOG energy clamp to provide novel information about the relationship of ROS production to $\Delta\Psi$ (Fig. 7). We and others recently reported (26,27) that absolute ROS production from muscle and heart mitochondria is not increased, or is decreased, in mitochondria of insulin-deficient diabetic rodents. In further work (5), we showed that ROS production expressed per unit of electron transport is actually increased in muscle and heart mitochondria. Here, we used the 2DOG clamp technology to provide new data indicating a $\Delta\Psi$ threshold effect (Fig. 7B and D) for ROS production, which is lower in diabetic mitochondria (move ROS at lower potential). In addition, we provide novel data indicating that, for any given level of added ADP, ROS per unit of ATP generated is increased (Fig. 7E) in diabetic mitochondria. In other words, the ROS "cost" of ATP production is markedly increased for mitochondria of STZ-diabetic rodents. With respect to this, we point out an important advantage of expressing ROS production per unit of respiration or per unit of ATP production. These metrics are independent of mitochondrial mass, simply because the units of mass in the numerators and denominators cancel. Finally, we show that the defective ATP production by diabetic mitochondria is reversible, at least with sufficient duration of treatment.

Why should insulin deficiency and insulin treatment impact ATP production? Decreased expression of several genes regulating ATP synthase as well as other genes involved in modules 1 and 3 of Fig. 1 have been reported in skeletal muscle and heart of insulin-deficient rodents and humans (28–31). Our studies, for the first time, implicate a functional defect at the level of module 3 contributing to reduced ATP production. This could occur because of a diabetes-induced decrease in expression of any component of ATP synthase, impaired ADP delivery to the mitochondrial matrix, or a perturbation in any factor regulating the activity of the ATP synthase complex. In fact, as recently reviewed

(32), a myriad of proteins, various ions, and membrane structure or folding all could alter ATP synthase.

Aside from defects in oxidative phosphorylation at the level of module 3, decreased respiration (module 1) clearly contributes by decreasing $\Delta\Psi$, but not to the capacity to utilize $\Delta\Psi$. Uncoupling (module 2) also could affect ATP production by reducing $\Delta\Psi$, but, again, not to the capacity to utilize $\Delta\Psi$. However, based on our past studies of insulin-deficient gastrocnemius mitochondria, uncoupling does not likely play a role in reducing mitochondrial ATP production, because proton conductance was, if anything, decreased (8). This is also consistent with a reported lack of change in uncoupling in heart mitochondria of insulin-deficient mice (27).

Karakelides et al. (28) assessed muscle mitochondrial ATP production by bioluminescence in units of μmol/min/g of tissue. ATP production was reduced in biopsy samples of subjects with type 1 diabetes after transient withdrawal of insulin therapy. Our results agree and extend observations to the direct utilization of $\Delta\Psi$ and to simultaneous measurement of ROS with ATP at clamped potential. Our results agree with the data of Kacerovsky et al. (33), who used in vivo saturation transfer to assess the exchange between phosphate and ATP by ^{31}P NMR. These investigators reported that insulin-stimulated unidirectional flux through ATP synthesis was reduced in eight type 1 diabetic subjects.

In protocol 2, we included short-duration insulin-treated rats to see if this would restore ATP production, as occurred after longer-duration insulin therapy in protocol 1. As shown (Fig. 8B), this was not the case. We can only speculate as to possible reasons. Multiple cellular pathways may require time to adjust as muscle converts from a catabolic (insulin-deficient) to an anabolic recovery state. Moreover, insulin strongly impacts fatty acid flux. Conceivably, this could alter mitochondrial lipid composition in a time-dependent manner, which might then alter the activity of ATP synthase or other mitochondrial membrane proteins.

We acknowledge some differences between protocols 1 and 2, but we doubt that these explain the lack of recovery with the shorter duration of insulin. Substrate concentrations used in the ATP production studies of protocol 1 (Fig. 6) and protocol 2 (Fig. 8B) were not exactly the same but were similar (5 mmol/L glutamate and succinate and 1 mmol/L malate in protocol 1 compared with maximal concentrations of 4, 4, and 0.8 mmol/L, respectively, in protocol 2), and, within each protocol, substrate concentrations were identical for all treatment groups. Also, we used one-dimensional NMR for protocol 1 but elected to proceed to the two-dimensional technique for the protocol 2 studies. However, both the one-dimensional and two-dimensional methods generated very clean signals with excellent sensitivity. The time period of diabetes (after STZ treatment until euthanization) was somewhat shorter in protocol 2 and the insulin dose was larger. However, we would expect those factors to favor rather than hinder the recovery of ATP production.

A limitation is that we did not come close to normalizing the glucose in our insulin-treated rats. However, that is difficult or impossible in STZ-DM, and we did observe substantial body weight recovery given adequate time. Another limitation is simply that isolated mitochondria, as opposed to in vivo techniques such as phosphocreatine and ATP resynthesis and ATP saturation transfer (34), do not consider the external environment. Conversely, studies of isolated mitochondria remain the only way to assess intrinsic mitochondrial properties altered by preexisting physiologic states. Moreover, our ATP methods have an advantage in that clamped ADP and potential are more physiologic than what occurs by conventional mitochondrial methods wherein ADP concentrations continuously decrease and $\Delta\Psi$ continuously increases after addition of ADP.

In summary, we report several novel findings. We show, for the first time, that the mechanism by which ATP production is reduced in mitochondria of insulin-deficient diabetic rats involves, at least in part, a functional defect in module 3 of oxidative phosphorylation. Defective ATP production by diabetic mitochondria is evident across a range from state 3 to 4 respiration. ROS production (absolute and per unit of electron transport) begins to increase in muscle mitochondria of insulin-deficient rats at a lower $\Delta\Psi$ threshold. The ROS "cost" of ATP production is greater in mitochondria from insulin-deficient rats. Defective ATP production is reversible in diabetic mitochondria by insulin treatment but, subject to limitations of our protocols, appears dependent on adequate duration of therapy. We describe a novel method for assessing ATP production that enables these studies and possesses advantages applicable to a myriad of future projects.

ACKNOWLEDGMENTS

This work was supported by Veterans Affairs Medical Research Funds, the National Institutes of Health (5R01HL073166), and by the Iowa Affiliate Fraternal Order of Eagles.

No potential conflicts of interest relevant to this article were reported.

L.Y. wrote the manuscript, participated in design, and conducted experiments. B.D.F. participated in design, conducted experiments, and reviewed and edited the manuscript. J.A.H. conducted experiments. W.I.S. wrote the manuscript, participated in design, and conducted experiments. W.I.S. is the guarantor of this work and, as such, had full access to all the data in the study and takes responsibility for the integrity of the data and the accuracy of the data analysis.

Parts of this study were presented at the 72nd Scientific Sessions of the American Diabetes Association, Philadelphia, Pennsylvania, 8–12 June 2012.

REFERENCES

1. Mitchell P. Coupling of phosphorylation to electron and hydrogen transfer by a chemi-osmotic type of mechanism. Nature 1961;191:144–148
2. Fillingame RH, Dmitriev OY. Structural model of the transmembrane Fo rotary sector of H+-transporting ATP synthase derived by solution NMR and intersubunit cross-linking in situ. Biochim Biophys Acta 2002;1565:232–245
3. von Ballmoos C, Cook GM, Dimroth P. Unique rotary ATP synthase and its biological diversity. Annu Rev Biophys 2008;37:43–64
4. Brand MD, Nicholls DG. Assessing mitochondrial dysfunction in cells. Biochem J 2011;435:297–312
5. Herlein JA, Fink BD, Henry DM, Yorek MA, Teesch LM, Sivitz WI. Mitochondrial superoxide and coenzyme Q in insulin-deficient rats: increased electron leak. Am J Physiol Regul Integr Comp Physiol 2011;301:R1616–R1624
6. Takaki M, Nakahara H, Kawatani Y, Utsumi K, Suga H. No suppression of respiratory function of mitochondrial isolated from the hearts of anesthetized rats with high-dose pentobarbital sodium. Jpn J Physiol 1997;47:87–92
7. Fink BD, Reszka KJ, Herlein JA, Mathahs MM, Sivitz WI. Respiratory uncoupling by UCP1 and UCP2 and superoxide generation in endothelial cell mitochondria. Am J Physiol Endocrinol Metab 2005;288:E71–E79
8. Herlein JA, Fink BD, O'Malley Y, Sivitz WI. Superoxide and respiratory coupling in mitochondria of insulin-deficient diabetic rats. Endocrinology 2009;150:46–55
9. Hong Y, Fink BD, Dillon JS, Sivitz WI. Effects of adenoviral overexpression of uncoupling protein-2 and -3 on mitochondrial respiration in insulinoma cells. Endocrinology 2001;142:249–256
10. Wojtczak L, Zaluska H, Wroniszewska A, Wojtczak AB. Assay for the intactness of the outer membrane in isolated mitochondria. Acta Biochim Pol 1972;19:227–234
11. Fink BD, Herlein JA, Almind K, Cinti S, Kahn CR, Sivitz WI. Mitochondrial proton leak in obesity-resistant and obesity-prone mice. Am J Physiol Regul Integr Comp Physiol 2007;293:R1773–R1780
12. O'Malley Y, Fink BD, Ross NC, Prisinzano TE, Sivitz WI. Reactive oxygen and targeted antioxidant administration in endothelial cell mitochondria. J Biol Chem 2006;281:39766–39775
13. Rhee SG, Chang TS, Jeong W, Kang D. Methods for detection and measurement of hydrogen peroxide inside and outside of cells. Mol Cells 2010;29:539–549
14. da-Silva WS, Gómez-Puyou A, de Gómez-Puyou MT, et al. Mitochondrial bound hexokinase activity as a preventive antioxidant defense: steady-state ADP formation as a regulatory mechanism of membrane potential and reactive oxygen species generation in mitochondria. J Biol Chem 2004;279:39846–39855
15. Rance M, Sørensen OW, Bodenhausen G, Wagner G, Ernst RR, Wüthrich K. Improved spectral resolution in cosy ^{1}H NMR spectra of proteins via double quantum filtering. Biochem Biophys Res Commun 1983;117:479–485
16. Braunschweiler L, Ernst RR. Coherence transfer by isotropic mixing: Application to proton correlation spectroscopy. J Magn Reson 1983;53:521–528
17. Bax A, Davis DG. MLEV-17-based two-dimensional homonuclear magnetization transfer spectroscopy. J Magn Reson 1985;65:355–360
18. Nyberg NT, Sørensen OW. Multiplicity-edited broadband HMBC NMR spectra. Magn Reson Chem 2006;44:451–454
19. Palmer AG, Cavanagh J, Wright PE, Rance M. Sensitivity improvement in proton-detected two-dimensional heteronuclear correlation NMR spectroscopy. J Magn Reson 1991;93:151–170
20. Olsson U, Lycknert K, Stenutz R, Weintraub A, Widmalm G. Structural analysis of the O-antigen polysaccharide from Escherichia coli O152. Carbohydr Res 2005;340:167–171
21. Delaglio F, Grzesiek S, Vuister GW, Zhu G, Pfeifer J, Bax A. NMRPipe: a multidimensional spectral processing system based on UNIX pipes. J Biomol NMR 1995;6:277–293
22. Johnson BA, Blevins RA. NMR View: A computer program for the visualization and analysis of NMR data. J Biomol NMR 1994;4:603–614
23. Manfredi G, Spinazzola A, Checcarelli N, Naini A. Assay of mitochondrial ATP synthesis in animal cells. Methods Cell Biol 2001;65:133–145
24. Lundin A. Use of firefly luciferase in ATP-related assays of biomass, enzymes, and metabolites. Methods Enzymol 2000;305:346–370
25. Chinopoulos C, Vajda S, Csanády L, Mándi M, Mathe K, Adam-Vizi V. A novel kinetic assay of mitochondrial ATP-ADP exchange rate mediated by the ANT. Biophys J 2009;96:2490–2504
26. Herlein JA, Fink BD, Sivitz WI. Superoxide production by mitochondria of insulin-sensitive tissues: mechanistic differences and effect of early diabetes. Metabolism 2010;59:247–257
27. Bugger H, Boudina S, Hu XX, et al. Type 1 diabetic akita mouse hearts are insulin sensitive but manifest structurally abnormal mitochondria that remain coupled despite increased uncoupling protein 3. Diabetes 2008;57:2924–2932
28. Karakelides H, Asmann YW, Bigelow ML, et al. Effect of insulin deprivation on muscle mitochondrial ATP production and gene transcript levels in type 1 diabetic subjects. Diabetes 2007;56:2683–2689
29. Basu R, Oudit GY, Wang X, et al. Type 1 diabetic cardiomyopathy in the Akita (Ins2WT/C96Y) mouse model is characterized by lipotoxicity and diastolic dysfunction with preserved systolic function. Am J Physiol Heart Circ Physiol 2009;297:H2096–H2108
30. Chowdhury SK, Zherebitskaya E, Smith DR, et al. Mitochondrial respiratory chain dysfunction in dorsal root ganglia of streptozotocin-induced diabetic rats and its correction by insulin treatment. Diabetes 2010;59:1082–1091
31. Johnson DT, Harris RA, French S, Aponte A, Balaban RS. Proteomic changes associated with diabetes in the BB-DP rat. Am J Physiol Endocrinol Metab 2009;296:E422–E432
32. Johnson JA, Ogbi M. Targeting the F1Fo ATP Synthase: modulation of the body's powerhouse and its implications for human disease. Curr Med Chem 2011;18:4684–4714
33. Kacerovsky M, Brehm A, Chmelik M, et al. Impaired insulin stimulation of muscular ATP production in patients with type 1 diabetes. J Intern Med 2011;269:189–199
34. Szendroedi J, Phielix E, Roden M. The role of mitochondria in insulin resistance and type 2 diabetes mellitus. Nat Rev Endocrinol 2011;8:92–103

Targeting Pyruvate Carboxylase Reduces Gluconeogenesis and Adiposity and Improves Insulin Resistance

Naoki Kumashiro,[1,2] Sara A. Beddow,[3] Daniel F. Vatner,[2] Sachin K. Majumdar,[2]
Jennifer L. Cantley,[1,2] Fitsum Guebre-Egziabher,[2] Ioana Fat,[2] Blas Guigni,[2] Michael J. Jurczak,[2]
Andreas L. Birkenfeld,[2] Mario Kahn,[2] Bryce K. Perler,[2] Michelle A. Puchowicz,[4]
Vara Prasad Manchem,[5] Sanjay Bhanot,[5] Christopher D. Still,[6] Glenn S. Gerhard,[6] Kitt Falk Petersen,[2]
Gary W. Cline,[2] Gerald I. Shulman,[1,2,7] and Varman T. Samuel[2,3]

We measured the mRNA and protein expression of the key gluconeogenic enzymes in human liver biopsy specimens and found that only hepatic pyruvate carboxylase protein levels related strongly with glycemia. We assessed the role of pyruvate carboxylase in regulating glucose and lipid metabolism in rats through a loss-of-function approach using a specific antisense oligonucleotide (ASO) to decrease expression predominantly in liver and adipose tissue. Pyruvate carboxylase ASO reduced plasma glucose concentrations and the rate of endogenous glucose production in vivo. Interestingly, pyruvate carboxylase ASO also reduced adiposity, plasma lipid concentrations, and hepatic steatosis in high fat–fed rats and improved hepatic insulin sensitivity. Pyruvate carboxylase ASO had similar effects in Zucker Diabetic Fatty rats. Pyruvate carboxylase ASO did not alter de novo fatty acid synthesis, lipolysis, or hepatocyte fatty acid oxidation. In contrast, the lipid phenotype was attributed to a decrease in hepatic and adipose glycerol synthesis, which is important for fatty acid esterification when dietary fat is in excess. Tissue-specific inhibition of pyruvate carboxylase is a potential therapeutic approach for nonalcoholic fatty liver disease, hepatic insulin resistance, and type 2 diabetes. *Diabetes* **62:2183–2194, 2013**

A key step in the pathogenesis of type 2 diabetes is the development of increased hepatic gluconeogenesis and fasting hyperglycemia (1–3). Hepatic gluconeogenesis is enzymatically regulated primarily by four gluconeogenic enzymes: phosphoenolpyruvate carboxykinase (PEPCK), fructose-1,6-bisphosphatase (FBP1), glucose-6-phosphatase (G6PC), and pyruvate carboxylase (4–7). Increased hepatic gluconeogenesis is often ascribed to transcriptional regulation of two key gluconeogenic enzymes, PEPCK and G6PC, through an intricate web of transcriptional factors and cofactors (8–12). Yet, despite the high degree of transcription regulation for these enzymes, the control they exert over gluconeogenic flux is relatively weak (13–16). We recently reported that hepatic expression of PEPCK and G6PC mRNA was not related to fasting hyperglycemia in two rodent models of type 2 diabetes and in patients with type 2 diabetes (17). Thus, we hypothesized that other mechanisms must account for increased hepatic gluconeogenesis and fasting hyperglycemia in type 2 diabetes.

Pyruvate carboxylase catalyzes the first committed step for gluconeogenesis and is well poised to regulate hepatic glucose production. Pyruvate carboxylase is allosterically activated by acetyl-CoA (18). However, increased expression of pyruvate carboxylase has been reported in rodent models of type 1 diabetes (19,20) and in obese Zucker Diabetic Fatty (ZDF) rats (21). Here, we performed a comprehensive assessment of hepatic gluconeogenic enzyme expression and discovered a strong association between pyruvate carboxylase protein expression and glycemia in humans. We then quantified the effect of pyruvate carboxylase on glucose and lipid metabolism in vivo in multiple rodent models by using a specific antisense oligonucleotide (ASO) to decrease pyruvate carboxylase expression selectively in liver and adipose tissue. Although chemical inhibitors of pyruvate carboxylase can acutely reduce glucose production (22), these compounds lack tissue specificity. ASOs primarily decrease expression in liver and adipose, but not in other key tissues such as pancreas, muscle, or neurons (23,24). Thus, this approach permits us to chronically decrease pyruvate carboxylase expression in select tissues of adult animals, without altering expression in tissues where this enzyme supports anaplerotic flux (e.g., β-cells, astrocytes), and also avoids any potentially confounding compensatory effects that may occur in germline gene-knockout rodent studies. We assessed the effects of pyruvate carboxylase ASO in several rodent models, quantifying changes in glucose metabolism, lipid metabolism, and insulin sensitivity in vivo.

RESEARCH DESIGN AND METHODS

Animals. Male Sprague-Dawley (SD) rats (160–180 g), ZDF rats (7 weeks old), and C57/BL6 mice (7 weeks old) were received from Charles River Laboratories (Wilmington, MA) and given at least 3 days to acclimate. Rats and mice were housed on a 12:12-h light/dark cycle and received food and water ad libitum. Chow consisted of regular rodent chow (60% carbohydrate, 10% fat, 30% protein calories) and a high-fat diet (Dyets 112245: 26% carbohydrate, 59% fat, 15% protein calories; Dyets, Inc., Bethlehem, PA). ZDF rats were fed Purina Laboratory Diet 5008 (56.4% carbohydrate, 16.7% fat, 26.8% protein calories). Body weight was monitored twice weekly.

From the [1]Howard Hughes Medical Institute, Yale University School of Medicine, New Haven, Connecticut; the [2]Department of Internal Medicine, Yale University School of Medicine, New Haven, Connecticut; the [3]Veterans Affairs Medical Center, West Haven, Connecticut; the [4]Department of Nutrition, Case Western Reserve University, Cleveland, Ohio; [5]ISIS Pharmaceuticals, Carlsbad, California; the [6]Weis Center for Research, Geisinger Clinic, Danville, Pennsylvania; and the [7]Department of Cellular & Molecular Physiology, Yale University School of Medicine, New Haven, Connecticut.

Corresponding author: Varman T. Samuel, varman.samuel@yale.edu.

Received 24 September 2012 and accepted 9 February 2013.

DOI: 10.2337/db12-1311

This article contains Supplementary Data online at http://diabetes .diabetesjournals.org/lookup/suppl/doi:10.2337/db12-1311/-/DC1.

ASOs were injected intraperitoneally at a dose of 75 mg/kg weekly for at least 4 weeks. For high fat–fed (HFF) rats, the ASO injection was started on the same day as the high-fat diet. For fasting experiments, rats were fasted overnight (~14 h). Rats underwent the placement of jugular venous catheters for blood sampling and carotid artery catheters for infusion ~10 days before the terminal studies. They recovered their presurgical weights by 5–7 days after the operation. All procedures were approved by the Yale University School of Medicine Institutional Animal Care and Use Committee.

Study population. All patients who were enrolled in the Bariatric Surgery Program of the Geisinger Center for Nutrition and Weight Management between October 2004 and October 2010 were offered the opportunity to participate in this study and some other studies (25). More than 90% of patients consented to participate. Patients underwent a preoperative assessment and preparation program of monthly visits, during which time a comprehensive set of clinical and laboratory measures were obtained. Although patients lost an average of ~9% body weight during the year before surgery, their weight remained relatively stable during the preoperative period between blood sampling and liver biopsy, with an average percentage change in body weight of 0.41%. The protocol was approved by the institutional review boards of the Geisinger Clinic and Yale University, and all participants provided written informed consent.

Liver biopsies. During the bariatric surgery, a wedge biopsy sample (250–300 mg) was obtained from the right lobe of the liver 10 cm to the left of the falciform ligament and flash frozen in liquid nitrogen for subsequent analysis.

Selection of ASOs. Rats and mice pyruvate carboxylase and control ASOs were designed and produced as previously described (26). The sequence 5-GCCAGACTTCATGGTAGCCG-3 (ISIS-330749) was selected for both rats and mice pyruvate carboxylase and the sequence 5-CCTTCCCTGAAGGT-TCCTCC-3 (ISIS-141923) was selected as the control ASO.

RT-PCR. RT-PCR was performed as previously described (26,27). Primer sequences are described in Supplementary Table 3.

Western blotting. For gluconeogenic enzymes, liver proteins were compartmentalized into three fractions, namely, a mitochondria-containing fraction, a cytoplasm fraction, and a microsomal fraction, as previously reported (27–29). G6PC was detected in the microsomal fraction, cytosolic PEPCK (C-PEPCK) and FBP1 were detected in the cytoplasmic fraction, and pyruvate carboxylase and mitochondrial PEPCK (M-PEPCK) were detected in the mitochondria-containing fraction. The sheep polyclonal C-PEPCK antibody was a gift from Daryl Granner (Vanderbilt University Medical Center). G6PC, pyruvate carboxylase, and M-PEPCK antibodies were purchased from Santa Cruz Biotechnology, Inc. (Santa Cruz, CA). FBP1 was purchased from Abcam, Inc. (Cambridge, MA).

For immunoprecipitation, the mitochondria fraction was extracted as above, but 50 mmol/L N-ethylmaleimide, 250 mmol/L nicotinamide, and 50 mmol/L sodium fluoride were added in the buffer. Mitochondria protein (1 mg) was mixed with 4 μg pyruvate carboxylase antibody and protein A/G (Santa Cruz Biotechnology, Inc.). Homogenization buffer was added up to 500 μL and incubated overnight. After overnight incubation, samples were washed three times with homogenization buffer containing 1% NP-40, and then 40 μL sample buffer was added and boiled for 5 min. Ubiquitin was detected using ubiquitin antibody (Covance, Inc., Dedham, MA) and then stripped and reprobed with pyruvate carboxylase antibody.

Whole cell lysates preparation, protein kinase C (PKC) translocation assay, and Western blotting for all the proteins were done as previously described (26,27,30).

Biochemical analysis and calculations. Plasma C-peptide was measured by radioimmunoassay kit (Millipore, Billerica, MA). Plasma lactate concentration was measured on Roche Cobas Mira Plus (Analytical Instruments, LLC, Golden Valley, MN) using the lactate reagent test kit (Pointe Scientific, Inc., Canton, MI). The others were measured as previously described (26,27).

Mixed-meal loading test. Chronically catheterized rats treated with ASOs were fasted overnight and given a mixed meal (15 kcal/kg body weight, Ensure Plus Ready-to-Drink Homemade Vanilla [Abbott Nutrition, Columbus, OH], 57% carbohydrate, 28% fat, 15% protein calories) through a gastric catheter. Blood was taken from the venous catheter at the indicated time in the results.

Pyruvate tolerance test. A pyruvate tolerance test was performed as previously described (30).

Hepatic lipid metabolites assay. Hepatic triglyceride and diacylglycerol contents were determined as previously described (26,27).

Mice body composition, metabolic parameters, and physical activity. Body composition was assessed by ^{1}H magnetic resonance spectroscopy using a Bruker Minispec analyzer mq10 (Bruker Optics, Inc., Billerica, MA). Metabolic parameters, energy expenditure, and food intake were measured using the comprehensive animal metabolic monitoring system (Columbus Instruments, Columbus, OH).

Hyperinsulinemic-euglycemic clamp studies. Hyperinsulinemic-euglycemic clamp studies were performed as previously described (26,31). Insulin was infused at 4 mU/kg per min for HFF rats and at 12 mU/kg per min for ZDF rats.

Lipid oxidation assay with primary hepatocytes. Methods were modified from the previous methods (32). Briefly, primary hepatocytes were isolated by the Yale Liver Center from HFF rats treated with control or pyruvate carboxylase ASO for 4 weeks. After recovery, cells were incubated with [1-^{13}C]oleate (GE Healthcare Biosciences, Piscataway, NJ) or [1-^{13}C]palmitate (PerkinElmer, Inc., San Jose, CA) in sealed flasks containing a center well supplied with a clean filter paper. After 1 h, incubations were quenched with 30% perchloric acid and 2 mol/L NaOH to collect [^{13}CO$_2$], which was quantified by scintillation counting. Perchloric acid-soluble ^{13}C-radioactivity (representing ketone bodies, acyl-carnitine, and Krebs cycle intermediates) was also quantified. Counts were normalized to protein content.

In vivo de novo lipogenesis assay (assessment of ^{2}H labeling in triglyceride palmitate). This assay was performed as described previously (26).

In vivo whole-body lipolysis assay. This assay was performed as described previously (26).

Glyceroneogenesis assay. This assay was done as previously described (33). The "% total newly made triglyceride-glycerol" was calculated using the Eq (33): [% total newly made triglyceride-glycerol = [^{2}H-labeling of triglyceride-glycerol/(^{2}H-labeling of plasma × n)] × 100], where ^{2}H-labeling of triglyceride-glycerol is the M1 isotopomer, the ^{2}H-labeling of plasma is the average labeling in a given rat, and n is the number of exchangeable hydrogens. Previous studies have experimentally measured this value as 4.25 in vivo (34).

Statistical analysis. Linear regression analysis of the data was performed using GraphPad Prism 5.0 software. Data were compared using the Student unpaired t test or ANOVA with the Tukey post hoc test between two groups or more than two groups, respectively. For the lipid oxidation assay, the average of control ASO group was set as 1 every time and the assay was repeated five times and compared using paired t test; each replicate was a separate animal. All data are expressed as mean ± SE, unless otherwise indicated. P values of less than 0.05 were considered significant.

RESULTS

Pyruvate carboxylase protein was increased parallel to glycemic level in humans.
We assessed mRNA and protein expression of four gluconeogenic enzymes in human liver biopsy samples obtained from 20 patients undergoing bariatric surgery (Table 1) in relation to measures of glycemia assessed by fasting plasma glucose concentration and hemoglobin A$_{1c}$ (HbA$_{1c}$). Although none of these patients had a prior diagnosis of type 2 diabetes, there was still a range of fasting plasma glucose concentrations and HbA$_{1c}$. The protein expression of the other gluconeogenic enzymes (mitochondrial and cytosolic PEPCK, FBP1, and G6PC) did not relate to fasting plasma glucose (data not shown) or HbA$_{1c}$ (Supplementary Fig. 2). Expression of pyruvate carboxylase mRNA expression also did not relate with measures of glycemia (Fig. 1A and B). In humans, three known isoforms of pyruvate carboxylase mRNA differ in the

TABLE 1
Characteristics of participants

Participants (N)	20
Sex (n)	
Female	14
Male	6
Age (years)	41.5 ± 2.7
BMI (kg/m^2)	48.4 ± 1.8
Fasting plasma glucose (mg/dL)	99.8 ± 4.0
Fasting plasma insulin (μU/mL)	23.3 ± 2.0
HbA$_{1c}$ (%)	5.8 ± 0.2
HOMA-IR [(mg/dL) × (μU/mL)]	5.4 ± 0.6
Alanine aminotransferase (IU/L)	30.8 ± 3.2
Aspartate aminotransferase (IU/L)	26.6 ± 2.1
LDL cholesterol (mmol/L)	2.84 ± 0.24
HDL cholesterol (mmol/L)	1.09 ± 0.04
Triglyceride (mmol/L)	1.73 ± 0.28

HOMA-IR, homeostatic model assessment of insulin resistance index.

first exon; however, expression of these isoforms also did not correlate with glycemia (Supplementary Fig. 1). In contrast, pyruvate carboxylase protein expression closely related to plasma glucose concentrations, accounting for 52% of the variation in HbA_{1c} (Fig. 1C and D). Thus, of all the key gluconeogenic enzymes, hepatic pyruvate carboxylase expression best relates to glycemia in humans.

Pyruvate carboxylase ASO treatment was well tolerated and decreased plasma glucose concentrations in regular chow-fed rats. To determine the extent to which pyruvate carboxylase controls endogenous glucose production in vivo, we treated regular chow-fed and HFF male SD rats with pyruvate carboxylase ASO. Pyruvate carboxylase ASO treatment decreased hepatic and adipose pyruvate carboxylase mRNA expressions ~80–90% in regular chow-fed and HFF rats. Hepatic and adipose pyruvate carboxylase protein expressions were decreased ~70–90% (Fig. 2). Pyruvate carboxylase mRNA expression was also slightly decreased in gastrocnemius and kidney cortex, but this did not reduce protein expression in these tissues (Supplementary Fig. 3). Interestingly, HFF per se increased hepatic pyruvate

carboxylase protein expression relative to regular chow-fed rats, without changes in mRNA expression, reminiscent of the observation in human liver. In the cohort of rats treated with a control ASO, we found that ubiquitination of pyruvate carboxylase was decreased in livers of HFF rats relative to regular chow-fed rats (Supplementary Fig. 4). This may decrease protein degradation in the ubiquitin-proteasome system and allow for accumulation of pyruvate carboxylase protein out of proportion with changes in mRNA expression.

Pyruvate carboxylase ASO treatment did not have any apparent toxicity; plasma transaminase and lactate concentrations were not different from control ASO-treated chow-fed or HFF rats (Supplementary Table 1). Pyruvate carboxylase ASO decreased fasting and ad lib–fed plasma glucose concentrations in regular chow-fed rats (Fig. 3A and C). Plasma glucose excursion after a mixed-meal tolerance test was slightly but significantly reduced, without alterations in the plasma insulin secretion (Fig. 3D and F). To assess the effect of pyruvate carboxylase ASO on glucose production from pyruvate, we performed a pyruvate

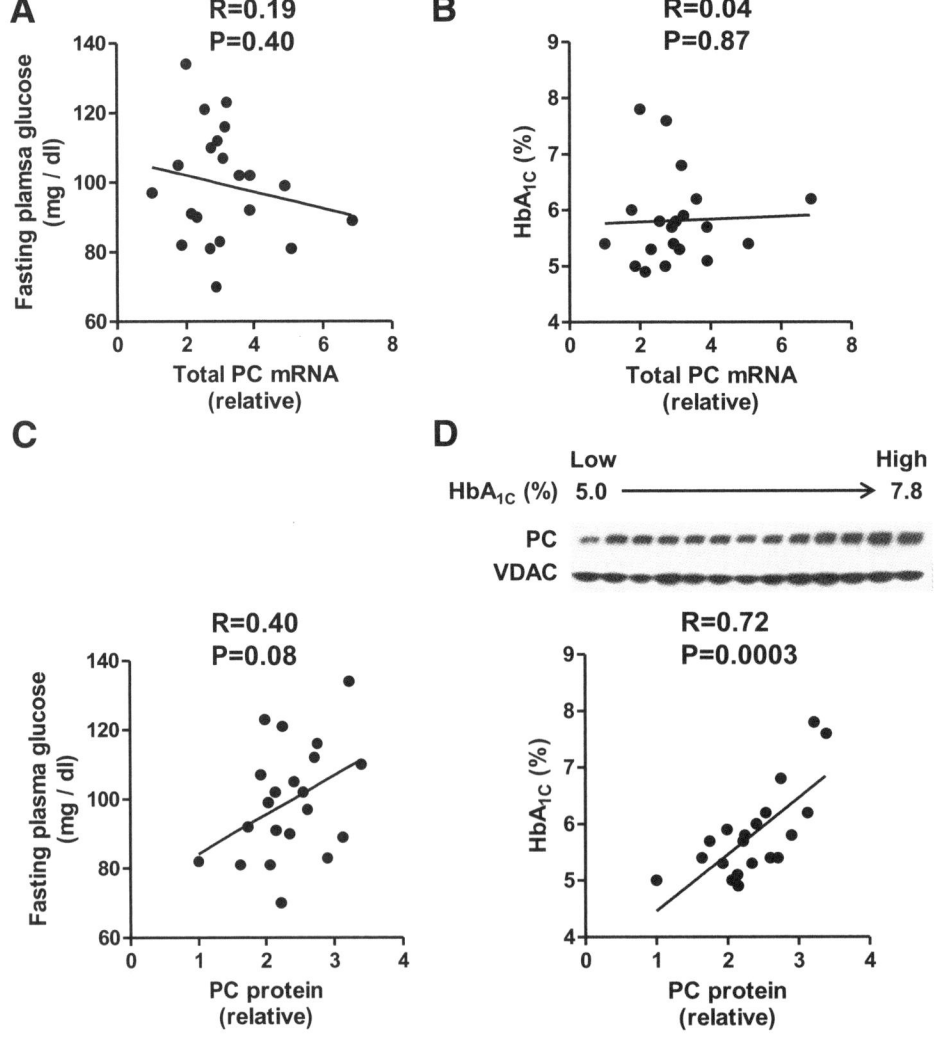

FIG. 1. Hepatic pyruvate carboxylase (PC) protein expression levels relate to glycemic levels in humans. Hepatic PC mRNA expression in human livers compared with fasting plasma glucose concentration (A) and HbA_{1c} (B). Hepatic PC protein expression in human livers compared with fasting plasma glucose concentration (C) and HbA_{1c}, along with representative bands (D). PC mRNA and protein are expressed as a relative increase to the lowest expression in the data set (n = 20). VDAC, voltage-dependent anion channel.

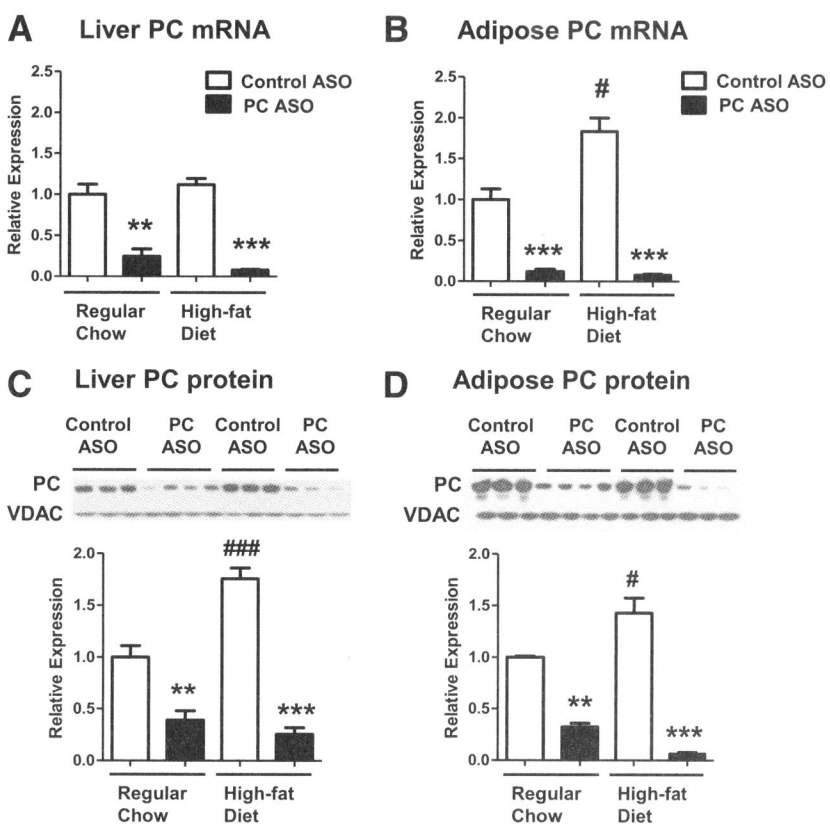

FIG. 2. Pyruvate carboxylase (PC) ASO decreased PC expression in liver and epididymal adipose tissue. PC mRNA in liver (*A*) and epididymal adipose tissue (*B*). PC protein, with representative bands, is shown in liver (*C*) and epididymal adipose tissue (*D*). **$P < 0.01$ and ***$P < 0.001$ compared with control ASO group in the same diet condition. #$P < 0.05$ and ###$P < 0.001$ compared with control ASO group in regular chow-fed condition (*n* = 3–4 per group in regular chow-fed condition; *n* = 9–10 per group in HFF condition). All rats were killed and tissues were taken at 4 weeks of treatment. VDAC, voltage-dependent anion channel.

tolerance test in regular chow-fed and HFF rats treated with a control ASO or pyruvate carboxylase ASO. We found that glucose excursion was significantly suppressed by pyruvate carboxylase ASO in the regular chow-fed condition (Fig. 3*G*). The decrease in glucose production was even more marked in HFF rats. Consistent with this observation in vivo, the glucose production from pyruvate in primary hepatocytes isolated from regular chow-fed SD rats was significantly reduced by pyruvate carboxylase suppression by pyruvate carboxylase ASO transfection (Supplementary Fig. 5). Taken together, pyruvate carboxylase ASO treatment reduced hepatic gluconeogenic capacity with a reduction in fasting and fed glucose concentration. This was well tolerated, without evidence for hepatotoxicity, lactic acidosis, or suppression of insulin secretion.

Pyruvate carboxylase ASO reduced adiposity and hepatic steatosis in HFF rats. Interestingly, pyruvate carboxylase ASO also protected HFF rats from weight gain (Fig. 4*A*) and adiposity (Fig. 4*B*). Unlike some lipoatrophic and lipodystrophic models, the reduction in adiposity was associated with a decrease in hepatic triglyceride content (Fig. 4*C*), which was not observed in the regular chow-fed condition (Supplementary Fig. 6). There was no change in skeletal muscle triglyceride content (Fig. 3*D*). Of note, pyruvate carboxylase ASO also reduced plasma fatty acids and cholesterol concentrations in regular chow-fed SD rats and in HFF SD rats (Supplementary Table 1).

To further characterize the mechanism whereby pyruvate carboxylase ASO protected animals from adiposity,

we treated HFF male C57BL/6 mice with pyruvate carboxylase ASO and assessed body composition by ^{1}H magnetic resonance spectroscopy and also whole-body energy expenditure and food intake in metabolic cages. As in HFF rats, pyruvate carboxylase ASO decreased body weight gain and fat mass over time. The reduction in weight gain was attributable to a decrease in fat mass; lean body mass was preserved (Supplementary Fig. 7*A* and *B*). Whole-body energy balance was assessed using metabolic cages at 5 weeks of treatment, before any significant difference in body weight, allowing us to assess energy balance without the confounding effects introduced with divergent body weights. Reduction in adiposity and hepatic triglyceride content occurred without any measurable increases in whole-body energy expenditure or reduction in food intake in the mice treated with pyruvate carboxylase ASO (Supplementary Fig. 7*C* and *D*).

Although these measurements were preformed when body weight was matched, we also analyzed the relationship between whole-body energy expenditure and body mass, which was similar between the groups by ANCOVA analysis (i.e., the slopes were not different between the groups [$P = 0.83$]), suggesting that pyruvate carboxylase ASO decreased adiposity without measurable changes in whole-body energy balance. In addition, there was no difference in the respiratory exchange ratio between pyruvate carboxylase and control ASO groups (0.836 ± 0.003 and 0.831 ± 0.005, respectively). Thus, in HFF rodents, decreasing pyruvate carboxylase expression in liver and

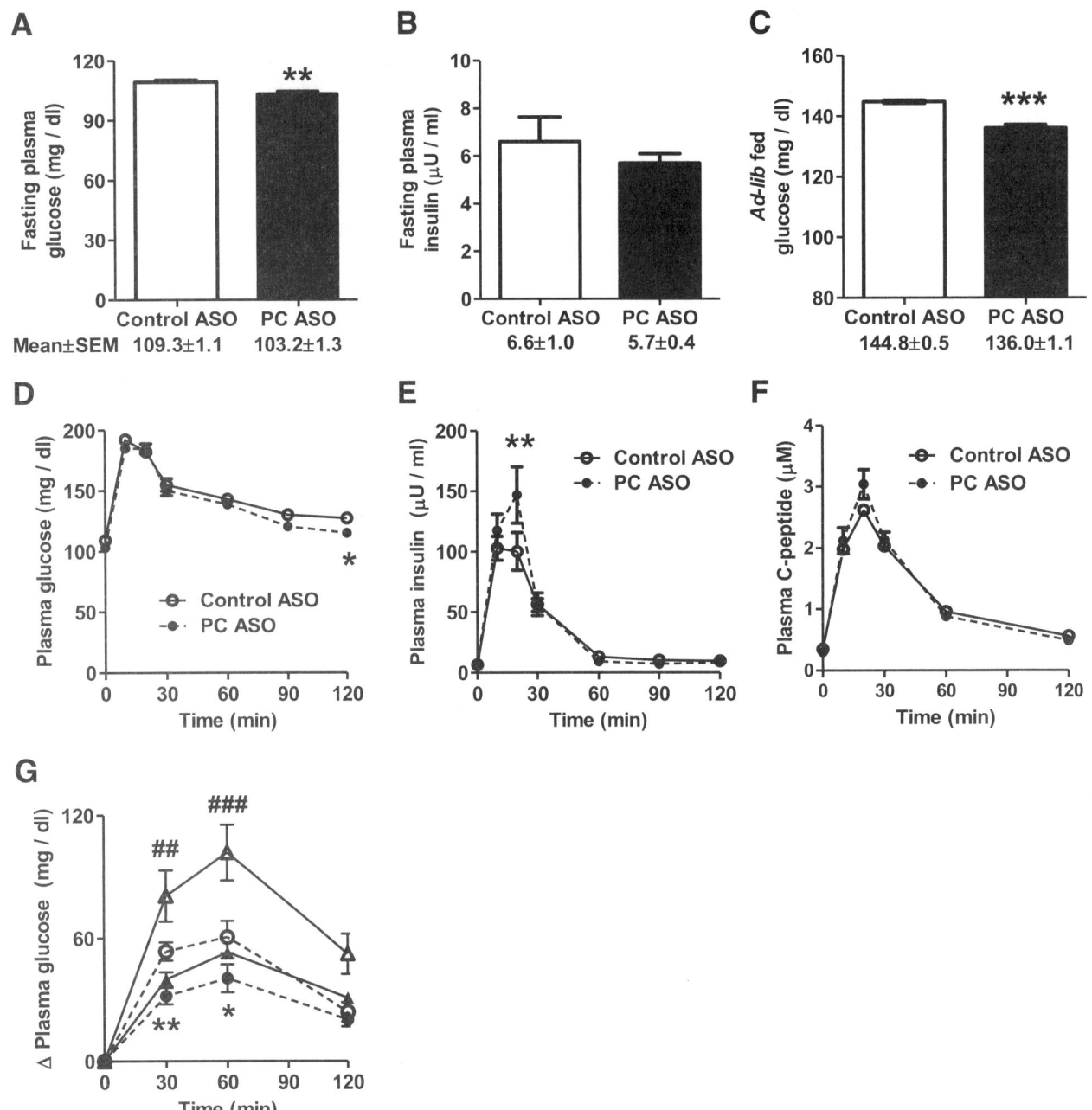

FIG. 3. Pyruvate carboxylase (PC) ASO decreased plasma glucose concentration and did not decrease insulin secretion. Fasting plasma glucose (*A*) and insulin concentration (*B*) in the regular chow-fed rats ($n = 7$–10 per group). *C*: Ad lib–fed plasma glucose concentration in the regular chow-fed rats ($n = 5$ per group). Results of mixed-meal tolerance test in the regular chow-fed rats for plasma glucose (*D*), plasma insulin (*E*), and plasma C-peptide (*F*) ($n = 7$–10). *G*: Pyruvate tolerance test in the regular chow-fed and HFF rats. ○ are control ASO and ● are PC ASO in regular chow-fed rats (both $n = 9$). △ are control ASO and ▲ are PC ASO in HFF rats (both $n = 8$). *$P < 0.05$, **$P < 0.01$, and ***$P < 0.001$ between control and PC ASO in regular chow-fed rats; ##$P < 0.01$ and ###$P < 0.001$ between control and PC ASO in HFF rats. Experiments were done at 4–5 weeks of treatment.

adipose tissue protects against hepatic steatosis and adiposity without affecting lean body mass or measurable changes in whole-body energy expenditure and food intake. **Pyruvate carboxylase ASO improved hepatic insulin sensitivity in HFF rats.** Hepatic steatosis has been associated with insulin resistance, at least partly by diacylglycerol (DAG)-mediated activation of PKCε and impairment of insulin signaling in rodents and humans (27,31,35). We performed hyperinsulinemic-euglycemic clamp studies in HFF rats to assess if pyruvate carboxylase ASO altered insulin

sensitivity (Fig. 5). Pyruvate carboxylase ASO reduced fasting plasma glucose concentrations and basal rates of hepatic glucose production without increasing plasma insulin concentration, as expected (Fig. 5*A*–*C*). Insulin-stimulated peripheral glucose metabolism, which largely reflects insulin-stimulated skeletal muscle glucose uptake, was unchanged (Fig. 5*D*-F), without any changes in muscle triglyceride content (Fig. 4*D*). In contrast, pyruvate carboxylase ASO improved hepatic insulin sensitivity as reflected by a ~50% reduction in hepatic glucose production and

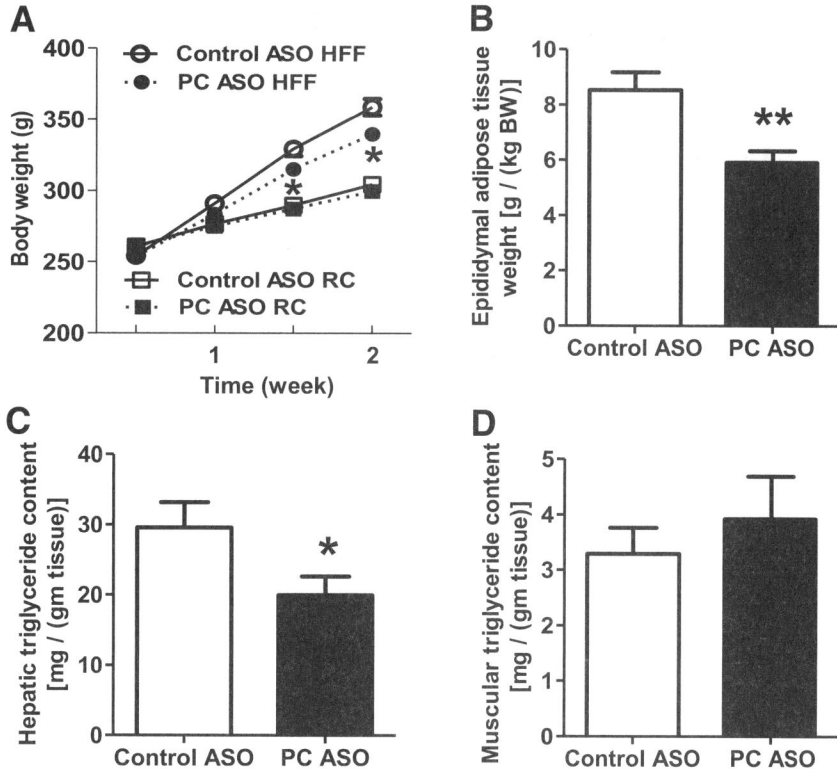

FIG. 4. Pyruvate carboxylase (PC) ASO reduced adiposity and hepatic steatosis in HFF rats. *A*: Body weight (BW) time course in regular chow-fed (*n* = 10–11 per group) and HFF rats (*n* = 12 per group). Epididymal adipose tissue weight (*B*), hepatic triglyceride content (*C*), and muscular triglyceride content (*D*) at 4 weeks of treatment in HFF rats (*n* = 9–10 per group). *P < 0.05 and **P < 0.01 compared with control ASO group in HFF condition. RC, regular chow.

greater suppression of endogenous glucose production compared with the control ASO–treated rats during the hyperinsulinemic-euglycemic clamp (Fig. 5*G* and *H*). To determine the mechanisms underlying the improvement in hepatic insulin sensitivity, we assessed hepatic DAG content, PKCε activation, and Akt phosphorylation. Pyruvate carboxylase ASO treatment decreased hepatic DAG content in cytosol and membrane fractions, decreased activation of PKCε, and increased insulin-mediated hepatic Akt Ser[367] phosphorylation (Fig. 6), a key node of the insulin-signaling pathway (35).

Pyruvate carboxylase ASO was also effective in ZDF rats. We also tested the efficacy of pyruvate carboxylase ASO in ZDF rats, a widely used preclinical model of type 2 diabetes. In chow-fed ZDF rats, pyruvate carboxylase ASO lowered the fasting plasma glucose concentration and rates of endogenous glucose production during basal and hyperinsulinemic periods, and suppression of endogenous glucose production by insulin was greater in pyruvate carboxylase ASO–treated rats than in control ASO–treated rats (Supplementary Fig. 8).

Reduction in glyceroneogenesis is the primary mechanism causing reduction in adiposity and hepatic steatosis. To further assess the mechanisms underlying the reduction in adiposity and hepatic steatosis, we performed a series of studies to quantify whole body lipolysis, lipid oxidation, de novo fatty acid synthesis, and glycerol synthesis in HFF rats (Supplementary Fig. 9). Pyruvate carboxylase is involved in adipogenesis (36–39); however, the adipose expressions of key genes associated with adipogenesis, such as peroxisome proliferator activated receptor (PPAR) γ, adiponectin, cluster of differentiation (CD) 36,

and adipocyte protein (aP) 2, were not altered by pyruvate carboxylase ASO (Supplementary Table 2). Pyruvate carboxylase ASO did slightly decrease adipose mRNA expression of adipocyte triglyceride lipase (ATGL) and patatin-like phospholipase domain-containing 3 (PNPLA3) (Supplementary Table 2), and also decreased plasma nonesterified fatty acid concentration (Supplementary Table 1). However, no difference occurred in the rates of whole-body lipolysis as assessed by glycerol turnover (Fig. 7*A*). There was no difference in the rates of fatty acid oxidation measured using primary hepatocytes isolated from control ASO or pyruvate carboxylase ASO–treated rats (Fig. 7*B* and *C*) or in the expression of genes regulating fatty acid oxidation in liver and adipose tissue (Supplementary Table 2).

We quantified hepatic de novo lipogenesis by measuring ^2H_2O incorporation into triglyceride palmitate in vivo. Neither the percentage of de novo fatty acid synthesis (Fig. 7*D*) nor the expression of lipogenic genes in liver (Supplementary Table 2) was altered. Adipose sterol regulatory element binding transcription factor 1c (SREBP1c) mRNA expression was decreased by pyruvate carboxylase ASO treatment, but the downstream genes, such as acetyl-CoA carboxylase 1 (ACC1) and fatty acid synthase (FAS), were not decreased (Supplementary Table 2). However, pyruvate carboxylase ASO decreased glycerol synthesis in liver and adipose tissue, as measured by the incorporation of ^2H_2O into triglyceride-glycerol (i.e., the glycerol backbone of a triglyceride molecule, Fig. 7*E* and *F*). This method quantifies total new glycerol synthesis, which includes glyceroneogenesis and formation of glycerol from glucose. In HFF conditions, however, glyceroneogenesis is thought important for the production of glycerol 3-phosphate (33)

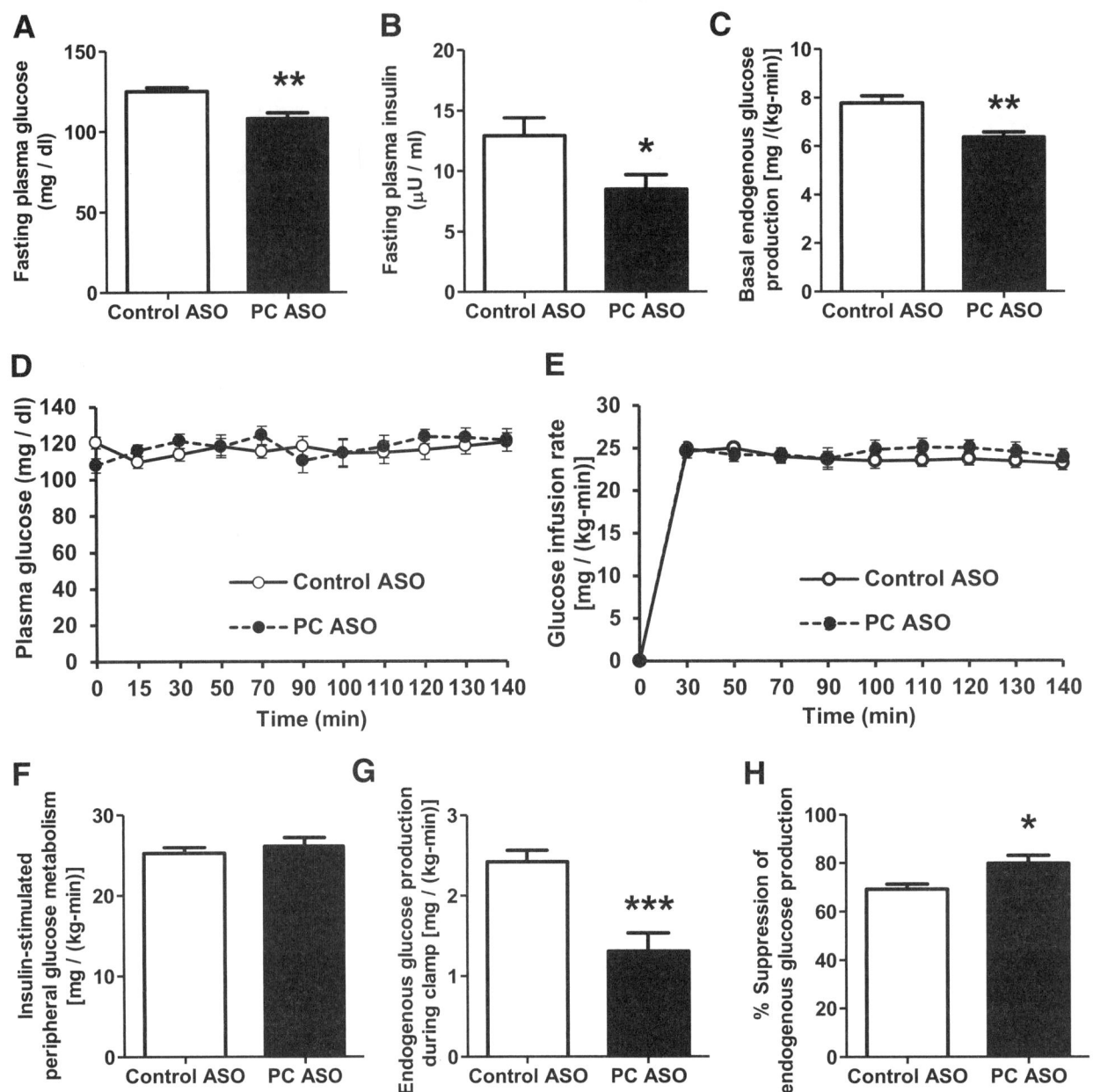

FIG. 5. Pyruvate carboxylase (PC) ASO improves hepatic insulin sensitivity in HFF rats. Fasting plasma glucose (*A*) and insulin concentration (*B*) (*n* = 9 per group). *C*: Basal endogenous glucose production (*n* = 9 per group). Plasma glucose concentration (*D*) and glucose infusion rate time course (*E*) during hyperinsulinemic-euglycemic (4 mU/kg per min) clamp, respectively (*n* = 7–8 per group). Insulin-stimulated peripheral glucose metabolism (*F*), endogenous glucose production (*G*), and percentage suppression of endogenous glucose production (*H*) during clamp (*n* = 7–8 per group). *$P < 0.05$, **$P < 0.01$, and ***$P < 0.001$ compared with control ASO group. Experiments were done at 4–5 weeks of treatment.

for the esterification and storage of fatty acids as triglyceride (Supplementary Fig. 9). Therefore, reduced glyceroneogenesis may be the primary mechanism accounting for the reduction in adiposity and hepatic steatosis in HFF rodents (Fig. 7*G*).

DISCUSSION

Patients with type 2 diabetes have increased gluconeogenesis (1,3,40,41). The molecular links between islet hormones and transcription of PEPCK and G6PC supported a view that increased gluconeogenesis was a consequence of increased transcription of these enzymes (9–12). However,

we previously reported that the expression of PEPCK and G6PC mRNA did not relate to fasting hyperglycemia in rodent models of type 2 diabetes or in humans with type 2 diabetes (17). We now extend this initial observation, demonstrating that increases in pyruvate carboxylase protein expression, but not mRNA expression, better relate to glycemia than expression of the other gluconeogenic enzymes. Using an ASO approach to reduce pyruvate carboxylase protein expression, we quantified the changes in glucose and lipid metabolism in vivo. We demonstrated that decreasing pyruvate carboxylase expression in liver and adipose tissue is well tolerated and effective in decreasing basal rates of endogenous glucose production and plasma glucose

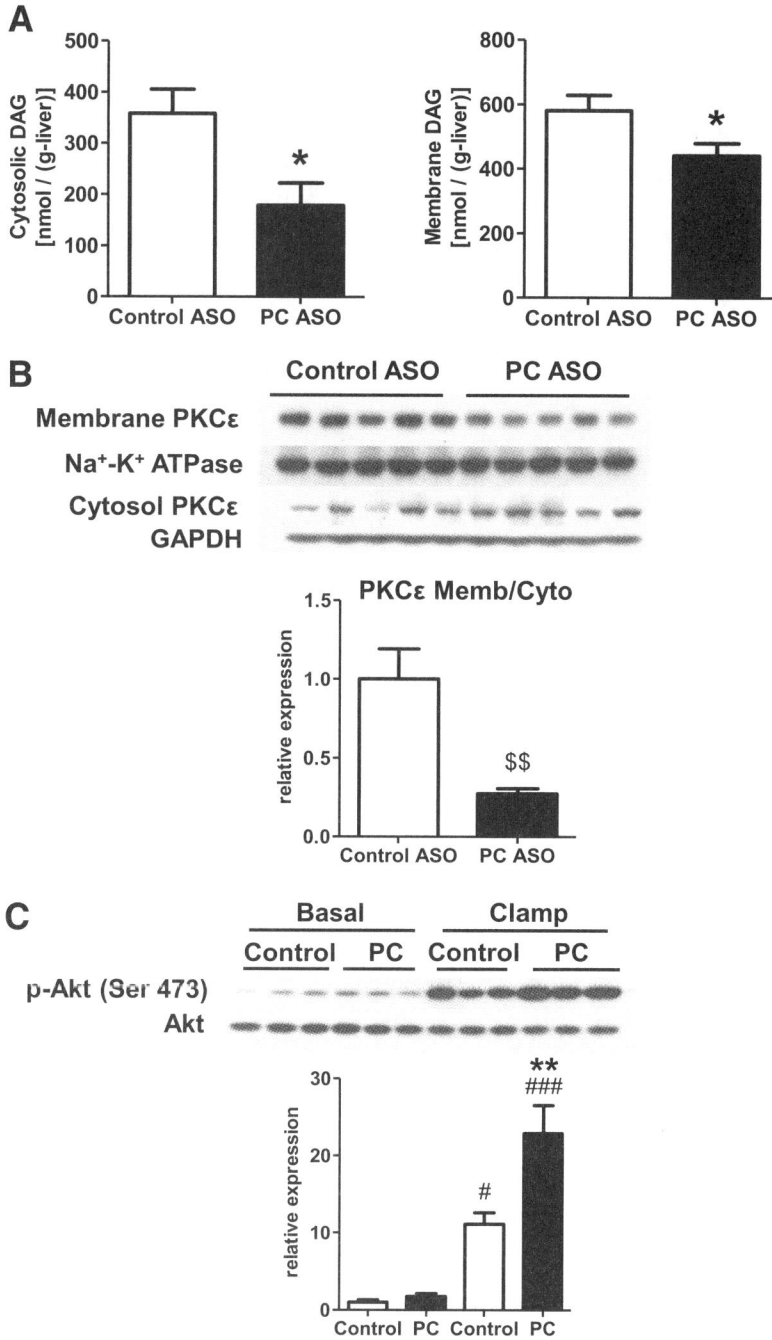

FIG. 6. Pyruvate carboxylase (PC) ASO decreased hepatic DAG content and PKCε activation and increased hepatic Akt phosphorylation in HFF rats. *A:* Hepatic DAG content (n = 9–10 per group). *P < 0.05 compared with control ASO group. *B:* PKCε activation. The average of control ASO group was set as 1 (n = 5 per group). GAPDH, glyceraldehyde-3-phosphate dehydrogenase. $$P$ < 0.001 compared with control ASO group. *C:* Akt phosphorylation (Ser^{473}). The average expression of control ASO group in the basal condition was set as 1 (n = 5 per group). #P < 0.05 and ###P < 0.001 compared with control ASO group in basal condition. **P < 0.01 compared with control ASO group in clamp condition. All tissues were taken at 4–5 weeks of treatment.

concentrations. In addition, we observed a reduction of adiposity and hepatic steatosis in HFF rats, with improvements in hepatic insulin sensitivity in HFF rats and ZDF rats. The changes in lipid metabolism are likely a consequence of decreased glycerol synthesis in liver and adipose tissue and highlight the importance of pyruvate carboxylase in supporting glyceroneogenesis in vivo.

We first quantified the expression of the key rate-controlling gluconeogenic enzymes in liver biopsy specimens obtained from human subjects undergoing elective surgery and related the expression of these enzymes to plasma glucose concentration and HbA$_{1c}$. Only pyruvate carboxylase protein expression correlated to glycemia in this cohort. The relationship between pyruvate carboxylase protein and HbA$_{1c}$ was stronger than the relationship with fasting plasma glucose concentrations, raising the possibility that hepatic pyruvate carboxylase expression impacts both fasting and postprandial glucose concentrations. Thus, HbA$_{1c}$

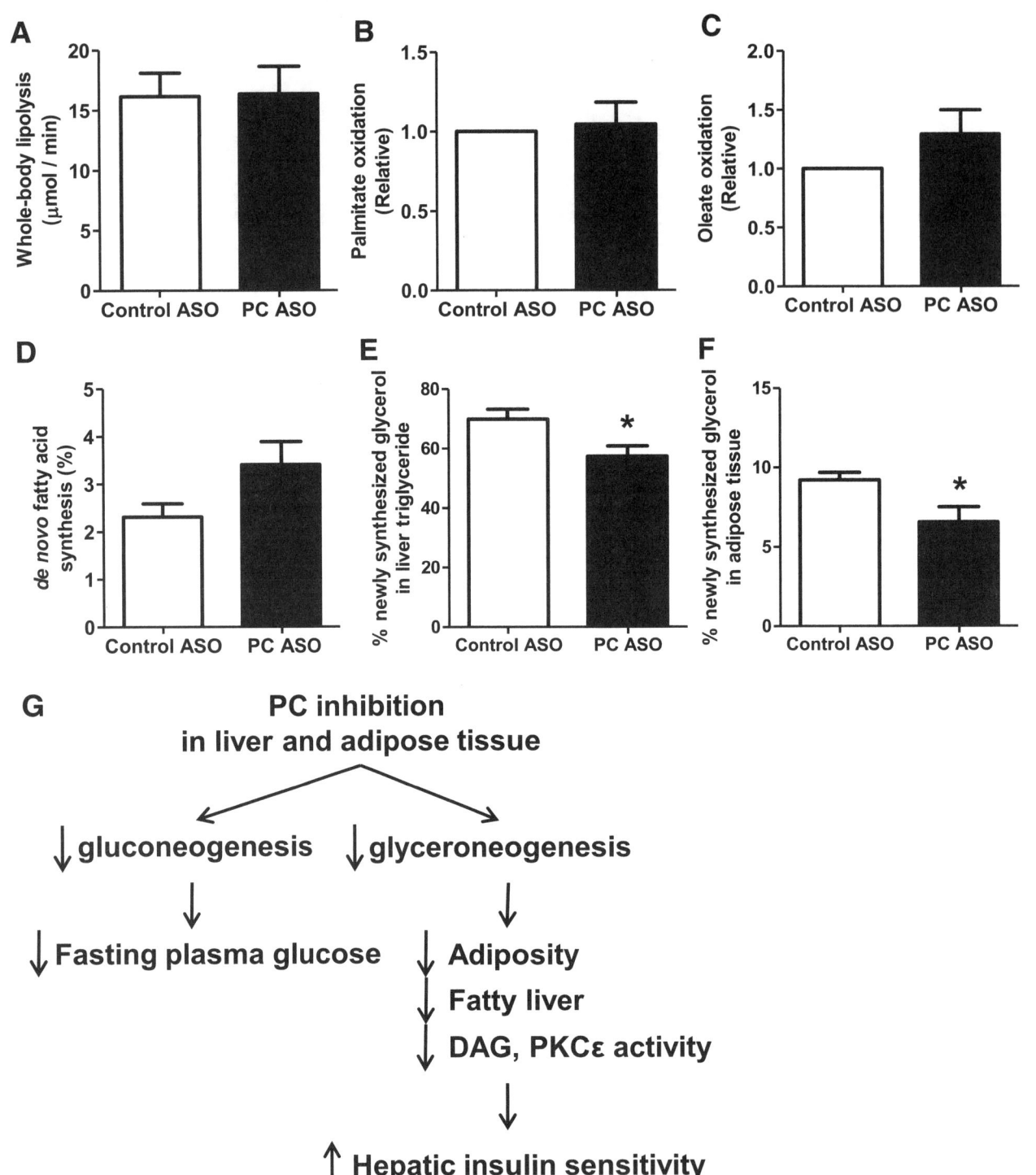

FIG. 7. Pyruvate carboxylase (PC) ASO reduced hepatic and adipose glycerol synthesis. *A*: Whole-body lipolysis as assessed by glycerol turnover in HFF rats (*n* = 8–9 per group). Palmitate oxidation (*B*) and oleate oxidation (*C*) assay with primary hepatocytes isolated from HFF-treated and ASO-treated rats (*n* = 5 per group). *D*: In vivo hepatic de novo fatty acid synthesis in HFF rats (*n* = 9–10 per group). Hepatic (*E*) and adipose glycerol synthesis (*F*) in HFF rats (*n* = 7–8 per group). *G*: Summary of this study. *$P < 0.05$ compared with control ASO group. All experiments were done at 4–5 weeks of treatment.

better relates to pyruvate carboxylase expression than fasting plasma glucose concentrations. However, it is also possible that a single fasting plasma glucose concentration does not accurately reflect long-term trends of fasting glycemia.

The increase in pyruvate carboxylase protein expression occurred without changes in mRNA, suggesting that other mechanisms affect protein abundance (e.g., posttranscriptional modification). We observed a similar disassociation between pyruvate carboxylase protein and mRNA abundance in HFF rodents compared with chow-fed rodents. We used this model to explore possible mechanisms accounting for the disassociation between pyruvate carboxylase mRNA and protein expression. Pyruvate carboxylase ubiquitination is decreased in HFF rat liver relative to chow-fed rat liver. This suggests that pyruvate carboxylase degradation in the ubiquitin-proteasome system is decreased, which may result in increased pyruvate carboxylase protein accumulation. This also may provide a possible mechanism that accounts for the increased hepatic pyruvate carboxylase flux that was recently reported in humans with nonalcoholic fatty liver disease (42).

To quantify the role of pyruvate carboxylase in controlling glucose and lipid metabolism, we used a loss-of-function approach. Although phenylalkanoic compounds can acutely reduce hepatic glucose production and plasma glucose concentration (22), these compounds lack tissue specificity and can potentially impair glucose-stimulated insulin secretion (43). Moreover, there are no reports of chronic inhibition of pyruvate carboxylase. ASOs have inherent tissue specificity, effectively silencing gene expression in liver and white adipose tissue but negligibly in muscle, brown adipose tissue, pancreas, brain, or stomach (23,24). This tissue specificity mirrors the two promoters that control pyruvate carboxylase expression (44). The proximal promoter element (P1) is primarily active in liver, adipose, kidney, and the mammary glands. In contrast, the distal promoter element (P2) maintains pyruvate carboxylase expression in many other tissues, including skeletal muscle, β-cells, and astrocytes. These discrete promoters may allow specific tissues to use pyruvate carboxylase as a common means to different ends: for glucose and lipid metabolism in P1-predominant tissues and anaplerosis in P2-predominant tissues. Thus, this approach permits us to assess the effects of decreasing pyruvate carboxylase expression in P1-selective tissues and also serves to vet tissue-targeted inhibition of pyruvate carboxylase expression and activity as a potential treatment for type 2 diabetes.

Decreasing pyruvate carboxylase expression decreased fasting plasma glucose concentrations in regular chow-fed SD rats, HFF SD rats, and ZDF rats. This was associated with a decrease in basal rates of hepatic glucose production in HFF SD rats and ZDF rats. Patients with pyruvate carboxylase deficiency can develop severe lactic acidosis at an early age (45). In contrast, the tissue-specific decrease in pyruvate carboxylase expression by ASO treatment did not result in any hepatotoxicity or lactic acidosis, although there was a small increase in plasma lactate concentrations in ZDF rats. Although ASOs do not decrease β-cell gene expression, we confirmed that insulin secretion was unaffected in mixed-meal tolerance tests in SD rats. Thus, tissue-specific inhibition of pyruvate carboxylase by ASO treatment effectively and safely lowers hepatic glucose production in multiple rodent models in chronic treatment.

Interestingly, pyruvate carboxylase inhibition also profoundly altered lipid metabolism. Pyruvate carboxylase ASO reduced adiposity and hepatic steatosis in HFF rodents. By comparison, liver-specific deletion of PEPCK and inhibition of G6PC resulted in hepatic steatosis (46,47), and inhibition of FBP1 resulted in hyperlipidemia (48). Adipose pyruvate carboxylase expression is reported to be induced during adipogenesis and increased by PPARγ agonists, but there are no data on how inhibition of pyruvate carboxylase may alter lipid metabolism (36–39). Metabolic cage studies in mice treated with pyruvate carboxylase ASO did not reveal increases in whole-body energy expenditure or a reduction in food intake, although it may be possible that changes specific to liver or adipose tissue are not reflected in measures of whole-body energy metabolism.

To better characterize the lipid phenotype, we performed a comprehensive set of studies assessing various components of lipid metabolism. There were no differences in lipolysis, fatty acid oxidation, or de novo fatty acid synthesis. However, we demonstrated that pyruvate carboxylase ASO treatment reduced adipose and hepatic glycerol synthesis in vivo, likely due to a decrease in glyceroneogenesis. Glyceroneogenesis plays a minor role in animals fed high-carbohydrate diets (i.e., low-fat), but its contribution to total glycerol 3-phosphate synthesis increases under fat-fed conditions, accounting for ~50–90% of glycerol 3-phosphate synthesis (33,49,50). This is consistent with our observation that the reduction in adiposity is primarily apparent in fat-fed rodents. Thus, when dietary lipid is in excess, the reduction in adipose and hepatic glycerol synthesis with pyruvate carboxylase ASO may impair lipid esterification and, consequently, lipid storage. In comparison, PEPCK is important for adipose glyceroneogenesis (51) but does not appear to be as essential for hepatic glyceroneogenesis because mice lacking PEPCK can still develop hepatic steatosis (46). By comparison, decreasing pyruvate carboxylase expression by ASO treatment protected mice and rats from adiposity and hepatic steatosis. The subsequent improvement in hepatic insulin sensitivity could be attributed to decreased DAG content and PKCε activation as well as improved insulin-stimulated Akt phosphorylation (31,35,52).

In conclusion, these are the first studies to demonstrate that increased hepatic pyruvate carboxylase protein expression is specifically and closely associated with plasma glycemia in humans, suggesting that hepatic pyruvate carboxylase is a key determinant of hepatic gluconeogenesis in humans. Pyruvate carboxylase ASO decreased liver and adipose expression of this enzyme and lowered plasma glucose concentrations and hepatic glucose production in vivo, without any apparent adverse toxicity. In addition, pyruvate carboxylase ASO decreased adiposity and hepatic steatosis in fat-fed rodents by decreasing adipose and hepatic glycerol synthesis. This, in turn, improved hepatic insulin signaling and hepatic insulin responsiveness. These studies suggest that pyruvate carboxylase is a key regulator of both gluconeogenesis and glyceroneogenesis. Through the latter, pyruvate carboxylase may also regulate lipid metabolism. Taken together these data demonstrate that tissue-specific inhibition of pyruvate carboxylase may be a potential strategy for treating many aspects of the metabolic syndrome and type 2 diabetes.

ACKNOWLEDGMENTS

This project was supported by grants from the United States Public Health Service (R24-DK-085638, R01-DK-40936, R01-AG-23686, R01-DK-088231, R01-DK-34989, UL1-RR-0241395, P30-DK-034989, P30-DK-45735), Manpei Suzuki Diabetes Foundation Fellowship (N.K.), a Distinguished Clinical Scientist Award (K.F.P.) and a Mentor-Based Postdoctoral Fellowship Grant (G.I.S.) from the American Diabetes Association, and a VA Merit Grant (5I01BX000901) (V.T.S.).

V.P.M. and S.B. are employees of ISIS and may own stock in the company. No other potential conflicts of interest relevant to this article were reported.

N.K., S.A.B., D.F.V., S.K.M., J.L.C., F.G.-E., I.F., B.G., M.J.J., A.L.B., M.K., B.K.P., M.A.P., K.F.P., G.W.C., G.I.S., and V.T.S. researched data and were involved in the analysis and interpretation of data. V.P.M. and S.B. designed, screened, and generated ASOs. C.D.S. and G.S.G. obtained liver biopsy specimens from humans. N.K., G.I.S., and V.T.S. wrote the manuscript. V.T.S. is the guarantor of this work and, as such, had full access to all the data in the study and takes responsibility for the integrity of the data and the accuracy of the data analysis.

Preliminary data from this study were presented at the 70th Scientific Sessions of the American Diabetes Association, Orlando, Florida, 25–29 June 2010, and at the 71st Scientific Sessions of the American Diabetes Association, San Diego, California, 24–28 June 2011.

The authors thank the volunteers for participating in this study, Daryl Granner (Vanderbilt University Medical Center) for his kind gift of C-PEPCK antibody, and Yanna Kosover, Jianying Dong, Kathy Harry, Dongyan Zhang, Toru Yoshimura, Shoichi Kanda, Derek M. Erion, Rebecca L. Pongratz, Codruta Todeasa, Maria Batsu, and Aida Groszmann (all of the Yale University School of Medicine) for their excellent technical support.

REFERENCES

1. Magnusson I, Rothman DL, Katz LD, Shulman RG, Shulman GI. Increased rate of gluconeogenesis in type II diabetes mellitus. A ^{13}C nuclear magnetic resonance study. J Clin Invest 1992;90:1323–1327

2. Maggs DG, Buchanan TA, Burant CF, et al. Metabolic effects of troglitazone monotherapy in type 2 diabetes mellitus. A randomized, double-blind, placebo-controlled trial. Ann Intern Med 1998;128:176–185

3. Hundal RS, Krssak M, Dufour S, et al. Mechanism by which metformin reduces glucose production in type 2 diabetes. Diabetes 2000;49:2063–2069

4. Utter MF, Keech DB. Formation of oxaloacetate from pyruvate and carbon dioxide. J Biol Chem 1960;235:PC17–PC18

5. Weber G, Cantero A. Glucose-6-phosphatase studies in fasting. Science 1954;120:851–852

6. Utter MF, Kurahashi K. Purification of oxalacetic carboxylase from chicken liver. J Biol Chem 1954;207:787–802

7. McGilvery RW, Mokrasch LC. Purification and properties of fructose-1,6-diphosphatase. J Biol Chem 1956;221:909–917

8. Jurado LA, Song S, Roesler WJ, Park EA. Conserved amino acids within CCAAT enhancer-binding proteins (C/EBP(alpha) and beta) regulate phosphoenolpyruvate carboxykinase (PEPCK) gene expression. J Biol Chem 2002;277:27606–27612

9. Koo SH, Flechner L, Qi L, et al. The CREB coactivator TORC2 is a key regulator of fasting glucose metabolism. Nature 2005;437:1109–1111

10. Nakae J, Kitamura T, Silver DL, Accili D. The forkhead transcription factor Foxo1 (Fkhr) confers insulin sensitivity onto glucose-6-phosphatase expression. J Clin Invest 2001;108:1359–1367

11. O'Brien RM, Noisin EL, Suwanichkul A, et al. Hepatic nuclear factor 3- and hormone-regulated expression of the phosphoenolpyruvate carboxykinase and insulin-like growth factor-binding protein 1 genes. Mol Cell Biol 1995;15:1747–1758

12. Yoon JC, Puigserver P, Chen G, et al. Control of hepatic gluconeogenesis through the transcriptional coactivator PGC-1. Nature 2001;413:131–138

13. Burgess SC, He T, Yan Z, et al. Cytosolic phosphoenolpyruvate carboxykinase does not solely control the rate of hepatic gluconeogenesis in the intact mouse liver. Cell Metab 2007;5:313–320

14. Le Lay J, Tuteja G, White P, Dhir R, Ahima R, Kaestner KH. CRTC2 (TORC2) contributes to the transcriptional response to fasting in the liver but is not required for the maintenance of glucose homeostasis. Cell Metab 2009;10:55–62

15. Ramnanan CJ, Edgerton DS, Rivera N, et al. Molecular characterization of insulin-mediated suppression of hepatic glucose production in vivo. Diabetes 2010;59:1302–1311

16. Sloop KW, Showalter AD, Cox AL, et al. Specific reduction of hepatic glucose 6-phosphate transporter-1 ameliorates diabetes while avoiding complications of glycogen storage disease. J Biol Chem 2007;282:19113–19121

17. Samuel VT, Beddow SA, Iwasaki T, et al. Fasting hyperglycemia is not associated with increased expression of PEPCK or G6Pc in patients with type 2 diabetes. Proc Natl Acad Sci U S A 2009;106:12121–12126

18. Jitrapakdee S, St Maurice M, Rayment I, Cleland WW, Wallace JC, Attwood PV. Structure, mechanism and regulation of pyruvate carboxylase. Biochem J 2008;413:369–387

19. Weinberg MB, Utter MF. Effect of streptozotocin-induced diabetes mellitus on the turnover of rat liver pyruvate carboxylase and pyruvate dehydrogenase. Biochem J 1980;188:601–608

20. Large V, Beylot M. Modifications of citric acid cycle activity and gluconeogenesis in streptozotocin-induced diabetes and effects of metformin. Diabetes 1999;48:1251–1257

21. Jitrapakdee S, Gong Q, MacDonald MJ, Wallace JC. Regulation of rat pyruvate carboxylase gene expression by alternate promoters during development, in genetically obese rats and in insulin-secreting cells. Multiple transcripts with 5′-end heterogeneity modulate translation. J Biol Chem 1998;273:34422–34428

22. Bahl JJ, Matsuda M, DeFronzo RA, Bressler R. In vitro and in vivo suppression of gluconeogenesis by inhibition of pyruvate carboxylase. Biochem Pharmacol 1997;53:67–74

23. Nagai Y, Yonemitsu S, Erion DM, et al. The role of peroxisome proliferator-activated receptor gamma coactivator-1 beta in the pathogenesis of fructose-induced insulin resistance. Cell Metab 2009;9:252–264

24. Sazani P, Gemignani F, Kang SH, et al. Systemically delivered antisense oligomers upregulate gene expression in mouse tissues. Nat Biotechnol 2002;20:1228–1233

25. Chu X, Erdman R, Susek M, et al. Association of morbid obesity with FTO and INSIG2 allelic variants. Arch Surg 2008;143:235–240; discussion 241

26. Kumashiro N, Yoshimura T, Cantley JL, et al. Role of patatin-like phospholipase domain-containing 3 on lipid-induced hepatic steatosis and insulin resistance in rats. Hepatology 2013;57:1763–1772

27. Kumashiro N, Erion DM, Zhang D, et al. Cellular mechanism of insulin resistance in nonalcoholic fatty liver disease. Proc Natl Acad Sci U S A 2011;108:16381–16385

28. Wiese TJ, Lambeth DO, Ray PD. The intracellular distribution and activities of phosphoenolpyruvate carboxykinase isozymes in various tissues of several mammals and birds. Comp Biochem Physiol B 1991;100:297–302

29. Petrescu I, Bojan O, Saied M, Bârzu O, Schmidt F, Kühnle HF. Determination of phosphoenolpyruvate carboxykinase activity with deoxyguanosine 5′-diphosphate as nucleotide substrate. Anal Biochem 1979;96:279–281

30. Kumashiro N, Tamura Y, Uchida T, et al. Impact of oxidative stress and peroxisome proliferator-activated receptor gamma coactivator-1alpha in hepatic insulin resistance. Diabetes 2008;57:2083–2091

31. Samuel VT, Liu ZX, Wang A, et al. Inhibition of protein kinase Cepsilon prevents hepatic insulin resistance in nonalcoholic fatty liver disease. J Clin Invest 2007;117:739–745

32. Birkenfeld AL, Lee HY, Guebre-Egziabher F, et al. Deletion of the mammalian INDY homolog mimics aspects of dietary restriction and protects against adiposity and insulin resistance in mice. Cell Metab 2011;14:184–195

33. Bederman IR, Foy S, Chandramouli V, Alexander JC, Previs SF. Triglyceride synthesis in epididymal adipose tissue: contribution of glucose and non-glucose carbon sources. J Biol Chem 2009;284:6101–6108

34. Turner SM, Murphy EJ, Neese RA, et al. Measurement of TG synthesis and turnover in vivo by 2H2O incorporation into the glycerol moiety and application of MIDA. Am J Physiol Endocrinol Metab 2003;285:E790–E803

35. Samuel VT, Shulman GI. Mechanisms for insulin resistance: common threads and missing links. Cell 2012;148:852–871

36. Jitrapakdee S, Vidal-Puig A, Wallace JC. Anaplerotic roles of pyruvate carboxylase in mammalian tissues. Cell Mol Life Sci 2006;63:843–854

37. Jitrapakdee S, Slawik M, Medina-Gomez G, et al. The peroxisome proliferator-activated receptor-gamma regulates murine pyruvate carboxylase gene expression in vivo and in vitro. J Biol Chem 2005;280:27466–27476

38. Wellen KE, Uysal KT, Wiesbrock S, Yang Q, Chen H, Hotamisligil GS. Interaction of tumor necrosis factor-alpha- and thiazolidinedione-regulated pathways in obesity. Endocrinology 2004;145:2214–2220

39. Wilson-Fritch L, Nicoloro S, Chouinard M, et al. Mitochondrial remodeling in adipose tissue associated with obesity and treatment with rosiglitazone. J Clin Invest 2004;114:1281–1289

40. Cobelli C, Mari A, Duner E, Mollo F, Nosadini R. On the estimation of absorption of subcutaneous injected insulin from plasma concentrations using mathematical models. Diabetologia 1984;26:314–316

41. Woerle HJ, Szoke E, Meyer C, et al. Mechanisms for abnormal postprandial glucose metabolism in type 2 diabetes. Am J Physiol Endocrinol Metab 2006;290:E67–E77

42. Sunny NE, Parks EJ, Browning JD, Burgess SC. Excessive hepatic mitochondrial TCA cycle and gluconeogenesis in humans with nonalcoholic fatty liver disease. Cell Metab 2011;14:804–810

43. Farfari S, Schulz V, Corkey B, Prentki M. Glucose-regulated anaplerosis and cataplerosis in pancreatic beta-cells: possible implication of a pyruvate/citrate shuttle in insulin secretion. Diabetes 2000;49:718–726

44. Jitrapakdee S, Booker GW, Cassady AI, Wallace JC. The rat pyruvate carboxylase gene structure. Alternate promoters generate multiple transcripts with the 5′-end heterogeneity. J Biol Chem 1997;272:20522–20530

45. Marin-Valencia I, Roe CR, Pascual JM. Pyruvate carboxylase deficiency: mechanisms, mimics and anaplerosis. Mol Genet Metab 2010;101:9–17

46. Burgess SC, Hausler N, Merritt M, et al. Impaired tricarboxylic acid cycle activity in mouse livers lacking cytosolic phosphoenolpyruvate carboxykinase. J Biol Chem 2004;279:48941–48949

47. Bandsma RH, Wiegman CH, Herling AW, et al. Acute inhibition of glucose-6-phosphate translocator activity leads to increased de novo lipogenesis and development of hepatic steatosis without affecting VLDL production in rats. Diabetes 2001;50:2591–2597

48. van Poelje PD, Potter SC, Chandramouli VC, Landau BR, Dang Q, Erion MD. Inhibition of fructose 1,6-bisphosphatase reduces excessive endogenous glucose production and attenuates hyperglycemia in Zucker diabetic fatty rats. Diabetes 2006;55:1747–1754

49. Chen JL, Peacock E, Samady W, et al. Physiologic and pharmacologic factors influencing glyceroneogenic contribution to triacylglyceride glycerol measured by mass isotopomer distribution analysis. J Biol Chem 2005; 280:25396–25402

50. Nye CK, Hanson RW, Kalhan SC. Glyceroneogenesis is the dominant pathway for triglyceride glycerol synthesis in vivo in the rat. J Biol Chem 2008;283:27565–27574

51. Millward CA, Desantis D, Hsieh CW, et al. Phosphoenolpyruvate carboxykinase (Pck1) helps regulate the triglyceride/fatty acid cycle and development of insulin resistance in mice. J Lipid Res 2010;51:1452–1463

52. Samuel VT, Liu ZX, Qu X, et al. Mechanism of hepatic insulin resistance in non-alcoholic fatty liver disease. J Biol Chem 2004;279:32345–32353

Circadian Regulation of Lipid Mobilization in White Adipose Tissues

Anton Shostak,[1] Judit Meyer-Kovac,[1] and Henrik Oster[1,2]

In mammals, a network of circadian clocks regulates 24-h rhythms of behavior and physiology. Circadian disruption promotes obesity and the development of obesity-associated disorders, but it remains unclear to which extent peripheral tissue clocks contribute to this effect. To reveal the impact of the circadian timing system on lipid metabolism, blood and adipose tissue samples from wild-type, ClockΔ19, and Bmal1$^{-/-}$ circadian mutant mice were subjected to biochemical assays and gene expression profiling. We show diurnal variations in lipolysis rates and release of free fatty acids (FFAs) and glycerol into the blood correlating with rhythmic regulation of two genes encoding the lipolysis pacemaker enzymes, adipose triglyceride (TG) lipase and hormone-sensitive lipase, by self-sustained adipocyte clocks. Circadian clock mutant mice show low and nonrhythmic FFA and glycerol blood content together with decreased lipolysis rates and increased sensitivity to fasting. Instead circadian clock disruption promotes the accumulation of TGs in white adipose tissue (WAT), leading to increased adiposity and adipocyte hypertrophy. In summary, circadian modulation of lipolysis rates regulates the availability of lipid-derived energy during the day, suggesting a role for WAT clocks in the regulation of energy homeostasis. **Diabetes 62:2195–2203, 2013**

Living organisms are influenced by rhythmic changes in the environment due to the Earth's rotation around its axis. In an attempt to optimally adapt to such recurring events, most species have evolved circadian clocks, internal timing systems controlling 24-h rhythms of behavior and physiology (1). In mammals, most, if not all, cells harbor their own molecular timer. Internal synchrony and thus overt behavioral and physiological rhythms are regulated via a hierarchical system of central and peripheral clocks. External time information is perceived by a master circadian pacemaker located in the hypothalamic suprachiasmatic nucleus, which relays timing cues to the rest of the body. In the suprachiasmatic nucleus and the periphery, the molecular clock machinery is based on interlocked transcriptional–translational feedback loops comprised of a set of clock genes. The basic helix–loop–helix transcription factors CLOCK and BMAL1 (ARNTL) induce expression of the negative regulators *Per1–3* and *Cry1/2* through binding to E-box promoter elements. With a delay of several hours,

PER/CRY protein complexes enter the nucleus and repress activity of CLOCK/BMAL1 heterodimers, thereby shutting down their own transcription. Further loops interact with this E-box–mediated transcription rhythm and stabilize its characteristic 24-h periodicity. Clock genes further regulate the activity of numerous tissue-specific output genes, thereby translating time-of-day information into physiologically meaningful signals (2).

Both rodent and human studies suggest a tight interaction between circadian clock regulation and energy homeostasis. Circadian disruption, either external (as seen for example in shift workers) or internal (e.g., in *Clock* gene mutant mice), can lead to obesity and the development of type 2 diabetes and metabolic syndrome (3–6). While appetite regulation appears mostly centrally controlled, recent animal studies indicate an additional role for peripheral tissue clocks in the control of energy metabolism. For instance, local circadian oscillators in liver and pancreas regulate glucose utilization, whereas cardiomyocyte clocks are involved in cardiac repolarization (6–8).

White adipose tissues (WATs) store large amounts of lipids in the form of triglycerides (TGs). During extended periods of energy shortage (e.g., fasting), the release of lipids from WAT mediated by the hydrolysis of TGs to free fatty acids (FFAs) and glycerol (lipolysis) becomes an important energy source for other organs. The timing of FFA release from adipose stores, however, has to be tightly controlled, as excess of circulating lipids may lead to lipotoxicity and promote cardiovascular disorders (9). In contrast, redundant deposition of TGs causes obesity, a risk factor for type 2 diabetes. Previous reports show that adipose tissues exhibit rhythmic clock gene expression in mice and man (10–12). Cell-based and animal studies suggest that clock genes are positive regulators of adipogenesis (13,14). It remains unclear, however, how circadian disruption may lead to increased adipose tissue deposition and obesity, as observed in human shift workers and in various clock gene mutant mice.

In this study, we analyze the role of white adipose clocks in lipid utilization in mice. We show that self-sustained local clocks regulate rhythmic FFA release from WAT stores, thus revealing a novel and peripherally regulated mechanism by which circadian disruption may impinge on energy homeostasis.

RESEARCH DESIGN AND METHODS

Experimental animals. Male wild-type (C57BL/6), congenic homozygous *Clock^{Δ19}* (15), *Bmal1$^{-/-}$* (16), and *PER2::LUCIFERASE* (17) mice of 2–4 months of age were used for all experiments. All animal experiments were done after ethical assessment and licensed by the Office of Consumer Protection and Food Safety of the State of Lower Saxony and in accordance with the German Law of Animal Welfare. Mice were housed in small groups of five or fewer under a 12-h light/12-h dark cycle (LD) or constant darkness (DD) conditions with food and water access ad libitum.

Fat pad cultures. Wild-type or *PER2::LUCIFERASE* mice (17) were LD entrained and killed by cervical dislocation at Zeitgeber time (ZT) 9 (i.e., 3 h

From the [1]Circadian Rhythms Group, Max Planck Institute for Biophysical Chemistry, Göttingen, Germany; and the [2]Medical Department I, University of Lübeck, Lübeck, Germany.

Corresponding author: Henrik Oster, henrik.oster@uksh.de.

Received 20 October 2012 and accepted 17 February 2013.

DOI: 10.2337/db12-1449

This article contains Supplementary Data online at http://diabetes .diabetesjournals.org/lookup/suppl/doi:10.2337/db12-1449/-/DC1.

See accompanying commentary, p. 2175.

before lights off). WAT and brown adipose tissue (BAT) samples were isolated and washed with 1× Hanks' balanced salt solution (PAA Laboratories, Cölbe, Germany). Tissues were divided into 20–30-mg pieces and cultured in colorless Dulbecco's modified Eagle's medium (DMEM; PAA Laboratories) supplemented with 10% FBS (PAA Laboratories) and 100 nmol/L luciferin sodium salt (Biosynth, Staad, Switzerland). For RNA extraction fat pads were removed at 6-h intervals, and total RNA was extracted and processed as described below. Bioluminescence recordings were performed using a Lumicycle luminometer (Actimetrics, Willmette, IL). Period and damping rate were calculated using the Lumicycle Analysis software (Actimetrics).

Quantitative real-time PCR. Mice were entrained to LD for at least 2 weeks, released into DD, and killed at 37, 43, 49, 55, and 61 h after lights off (corresponding to circadian times 1, 7, 13, and 19, respectively). For LD cohorts, mice were kept under LD and killed at ZT1, 7, 13, and 19. Epididymal fat was isolated, and total RNA was extracted using TRIzol reagent (Life Technologies, Darmstadt, Germany). cDNA synthesis was performed by High Capacity cDNA Reverse Transcription Kit (Life Technologies) using random hexamer primers. Quantitative real-time PCR was performed using iQ SYBR Green Supermix on an CFX96 thermocycler (Bio-Rad, Munich, Germany) according to the manufacturer's protocol. Relative gene expression was quantified using a $\Delta\Delta$ threshold cycle method and $Eef1\alpha$ as a reference gene (18). Primer sequences are listed in Supplementary Table 1.

Cloning of adipose TG lipase and hormone-sensitive lipase promoters and PCR mutagenesis. A 4.3-kb fragment containing the murine adipose TG lipase ($Atgl$) upstream sequence and the first intron were PCR-amplified from genomic DNA using Advantage 2 polymerase mix (Clontech, Mountain View, CA). PCR products were digested with $Hind$III (New England Biolabs, Ipswich, MA) and XhoI (New England Biolabs) and cloned into $Hind$III/XhoI–digested $pGL4$ vector (Promega, Madison, WI). A 4.5-kb fragment of the murine hormone-sensitive lipase (Hsl) promoter was PCR-amplified as described for $Atgl$. PCR products were cloned into the $pGL3$ vector by In-Fusion Cloning (Clontech). Inserts were confirmed by sequencing. E-box mutations to GGATCC were performed using a PCR mutagenesis kit (Agilent Technologies, Santa Clara, CA) and confirmed by sequencing. Primer sequences are listed in Supplementary Table 2.

Luciferase promoter assays. HEK293A and NIH-3T3 cells were maintained in DMEM (PAA Laboratories) supplemented with 10% FBS (PAA Laboratories) and antibiotics. One day prior to transfection, cells were plated onto 24-well plates at a density of 10^5 cells/well. HEK cells were cotransfected using PEI (Sigma-Aldrich, Hamburg, Germany) and 50 ng of $pGL3/4$ reporter plasmid in the presence of 200 ng of $Bmal1$, $Clock$, or $Cry1$ constructs. Empty $pcDNA3.1$ vector was used to make up the total amount of DNA to 0.7 µg/well. A total of 10 ng of a pRL-CMV $Renilla$ luciferase reporter vector (Promega) was added to each reaction as internal control. Two days later, cells were harvested and assayed using the Dual-Luciferase Reporter Assay System (Promega) on a TriStar LB941 luminometer (Berthold Technologies, Wildbach, Germany). NIH-3T3 cells were transfected using X-fect (Clontech) with 1 µg $pGL3$-Hsl, $pGL4$-$Atgl$, or $Bmal1$-luc (19) reporter plasmids. Two days later, cells were synchronized by 50% serum shock for 2 h. For luminescence recordings, cells were kept in colorless DMEM, 10% FBS, and 100 nmol/L luciferin sodium salt (Life Technologies).

Chromatin immunoprecipitation. Epididymal fat pads from wild-type and $Bmal1^{-/-}$ mice were isolated at ZT7 and ZT19, homogenized, and immediately cross linked in 1% formaldehyde. Chromatin was sonicated to obtain an average DNA length of ~400 bp (15-s on/20-s off cycles for 22 min) using a Bioruptor (Diagenode Inc.). Samples were incubated overnight at 4°C with BMAL1 antibody (N-20; Santa Cruz Biotechnology). After clearing, samples were incubated with A/G agarose beads (Thermo Scientific) for 1 h at 4°C followed by intensive washings. Afterward, samples were boiled for 10 min in 10% Chelex (Bio-Rad) with Proteinase K (150 µg/mL) and spun down. DNA-containing supernatant was collected for PCR. Quantitative real-time PCR was performed as described above, and values were normalized to percentage of input. Primer sequences are listed in Supplementary Table 3.

Lipolysis assays. Epididymal fat pads from were dissected at the given time points, cut into 10–25 mg samples, and incubated at 37°C in DMEM and 10% FBS with antibiotics. Glycerol release was measured from media aliquots using Free Glycerol Reagent (Sigma-Aldrich) and normalized to fat pad dry weight.

Blood glycerol and FFA measurements. Trunk blood was collected at circadian times/ZT 1, 7, 13, and 19 and was allowed to clot. Subsequently serum was isolated by centrifugation at 2,000g for 20 min at 4°C. Serum FFAs, TG/glycerol, and cholesterol levels were determined using a NEFA kit (Zen-Bio, Research Triangle Park, NC), serum TG determination kit (Sigma-Aldrich), and cholesterol assay kit (Cayman Chemical) according to the manufacturers' protocols.

Adipocyte histology. Freshly isolated epididymal WAT samples were fixed with 4% paraformaldehyde/PBS overnight. Samples were dehydrated with ascending alcohol concentrations and embedded in paraffin. Sections were cut at 6 µm and stained with hematoxylin-eosin. Adipocyte size was determined with Image J software (National Institutes of Health, Bethesda, MD).

Statistical analysis. All results are expressed as a mean ± SEM. For statistical comparison unpaired two-tailed Student t tests or two-way ANOVAs with Bonferroni posttests were performed using Prism 5 software (GraphPad Software). Analysis of circadian gene expression was performed with CircWave software (20) downloaded at http://www.euclock.org. P values <0.05 were considered significant.

RESULTS

Circadian Clock$^{\Delta 19}$ mutants show increased adiposity and blunted FFA and glycerol rhythms in blood. To gain more insights into the circadian regulation of lipid metabolism, we compared diurnal profiles of various lipid parameters in serum between circadian clock–deficient $Clock^{\Delta 19}$ and wild-type mice. Consistent with a previous report (4), $Clock^{\Delta 19}$ mice had significantly higher cholesterol levels in the blood, albeit no significant circadian variation was observed in either genotype (Fig. 1A). In contrast, serum TG levels were rhythmic, but indistinguishable between genotypes (Fig. 1B). Interestingly, FFA serum levels showed a robust circadian profile in wild-type animals ($P = 0.005$). This rhythm was abolished, and overall levels were decreased in $Clock^{\Delta 19}$ mutants ($P = 0.802$) (Fig. 1C), suggesting an involvement of the circadian clock machinery in the regulation of fatty acid release from TG stores. In line with this hypothesis, serum glycerol concentrations showed similar variations in wild-type serum, whereas in $Clock^{\Delta 19}$ mutants, levels were nonrhythmic and overall low ($P = 0.003$ vs. $P = 0.678$) (Fig. 1D). Comparable effects on FFA and glycerol levels were also observed under LD conditions (Fig. 1E and F) and in another clock-deficient mouse model, $Bmal1^{-/-}$ (Fig. 1G and H). Surprisingly, while blood TG and FFA levels were unaltered or low, $Clock^{\Delta 19}$ mutants at the same time exhibited higher overall body weight gain with increased adiposity (Fig. 2A and B and Supplementary Fig. 1A) together with hyperphagy, but unaltered overall activity (Supplementary Fig. 1B and C) (4). Histological analysis of WAT paraffin sections revealed increased WAT lipid accumulation and adipocyte hypertrophy in $Clock^{\Delta 19}$ mutant mice (Fig. 2C), suggesting that the $Clock$ mutation either promotes lipid accumulation or inhibits lipid mobilization in WAT.

Circadian regulation of genes involved in WAT lipid metabolism. Circadian clocks regulate local cellular physiology via transcriptional programs involving large numbers of tissue-specific clock-controlled genes (21). To test if molecular clocks are involved in regulating WAT physiology, we analyzed circadian variations in mRNAs of genes involved in WAT lipid metabolism. Genes were selected using the Gene Ontology database (http://www.geneontology.org) and expression data assembled on BioGPS (http://biogps.org) and compared with published literature (Supplementary Fig. 2A). Epididymal WAT transcript levels were assessed at the beginning of the rest phase (37 h in DD) and in the early subjective night (49 h in DD). For genes which showed significant regulation between both time points, we determined full circadian transcriptional profiles in $Clock^{\Delta 19}$ and wild-type mice. Of the genes associated with FFA transport and TG biosynthesis (i.e., the conversion of FFAs for storage in adipose lipid droplets), $Caveolin2$, the acyl-CoA synthetases $Acsl1$ and $Acsl4$ and the phosphatidate phosphatase $Lpin1$ showed significant differences in expression between

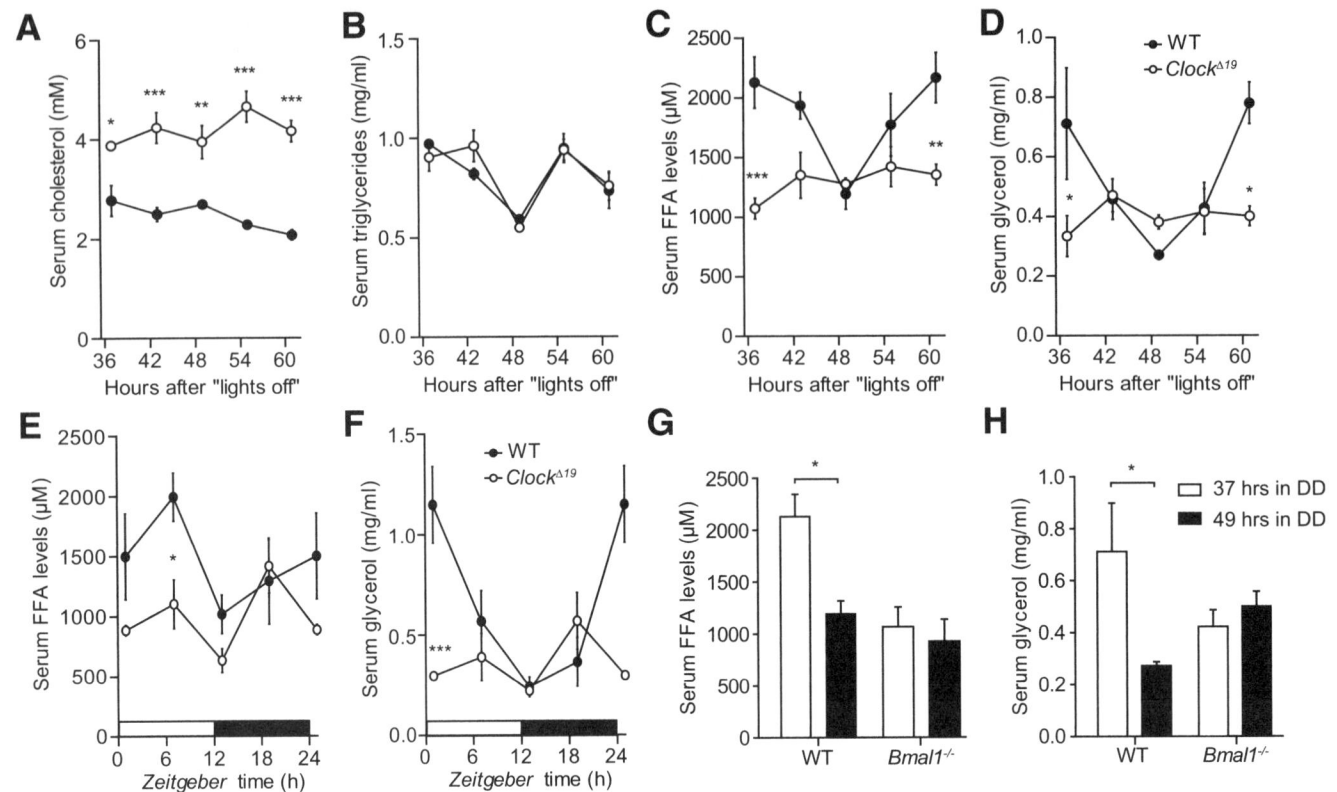

FIG. 1. Serum lipids change in *Clock*^Δ19 mice. Diurnal profiles of cholesterol (*A*), TGs (*B*), FFAs (*C*), and glycerol (*D*) in the serum of wild-type (WT; closed circles) and *Clock*^Δ19 (open circles) mice in DD (*n* = 3/time point). Time points indicate hours spent in DD after the last lights off. Diurnal profiles of FFAs (*E*) and glycerol (*F*) in the serum of wild-type (closed circles) and *Clock*^Δ19 (open circles) mice in LD conditions (*n* = 3–5/time point). Time-of-day dependent variations in serum FFA and glycerol levels in WT (black bars) and *Bmal1*^−/− (white bars) animals kept in DD (*n* = 3–5/time point). All data are shown as means ± SEM. *P < 0.05; **P < 0.01; ***P < 0.001 by two-way ANOVA with Bonferroni posttest.

37 and 49 h in DD (Fig. 3*A*). In *Clock*^Δ19 mutants, FFA transport/TG biosynthesis mRNAs were either unaffected (*Acsl4*, *Lpl*) or dampened and overall downregulated when compared with wild-type controls (Fig. 3*B* and *C* and Supplementary Fig. 2*B*). In contrast, the mRNAs of two rate-limiting lipolytic enzymes, *Atgl* (or *Pnpla2*) and *Hsl* (or *Lipe*), exhibited circadian variations in wild-type animals (Fig. 3*A*), while in *Clock*^Δ19 mutants, *Atgl* and *Hsl* mRNA levels (together with that of *Mgll*) were significantly reduced and arrhythmic (Fig. 4*A*) (*P* < 0.001 vs. *P* = 0.85

[*Atgl*] and *P* < 0.001 vs. *P* = 0.63 [*Hsl*], respectively), strongly correlating with the reduced and arrhythmic FFA/glycerol serum levels observed in these mice (Fig. 1). To test TG breakdown from WAT stores more directly, we performed lipolysis assays on fat pad explants at four different time points in DD and LD. In wild-types, glycerol excretion showed a rhythmic pattern, whereas dampened rhythmicity and a general downregulation of basal lipolysis rates were observed in explants of *Clock*^Δ19 mice (Fig. 4*B* and *C*) (*P* = 0.001 vs. *P* = 0.95 [DD] and *P* < 0.001 vs. *P* = 0.63

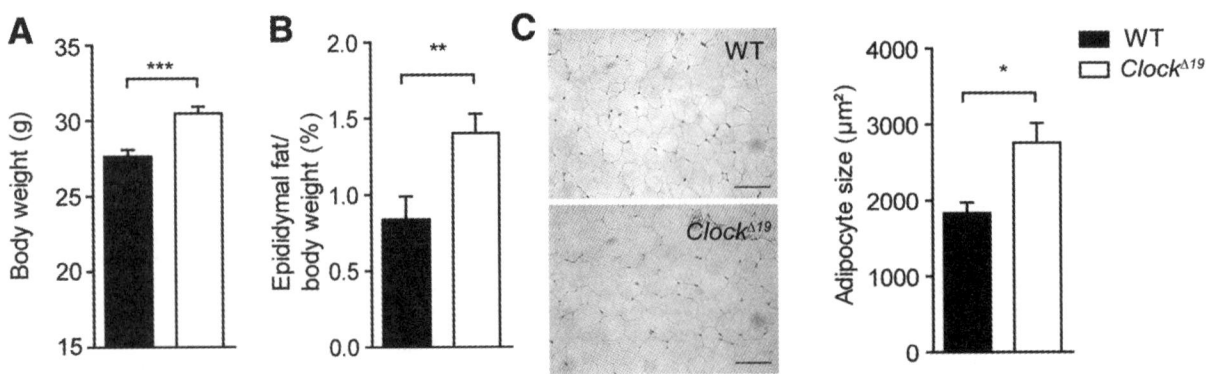

FIG. 2. Increased body weight and adiposity in *Clock*^Δ19 mice. Body weight (*A*) and adiposity (epididymal fat to body weight ratio) (*B*) in wild-type (WT; black bars) and *Clock*^Δ19 (white bars) mice fed standard chow for 10 weeks (*n* = 14). *C*: Representative sections and adipocyte size of epididymal WAT after 10 weeks of standard diet (scale bars, 100 μm; *n* = 3). *P < 0.05; **P < 0.01; ***P < 0.001 by unpaired *t* test. All data are shown as means ± SEM.

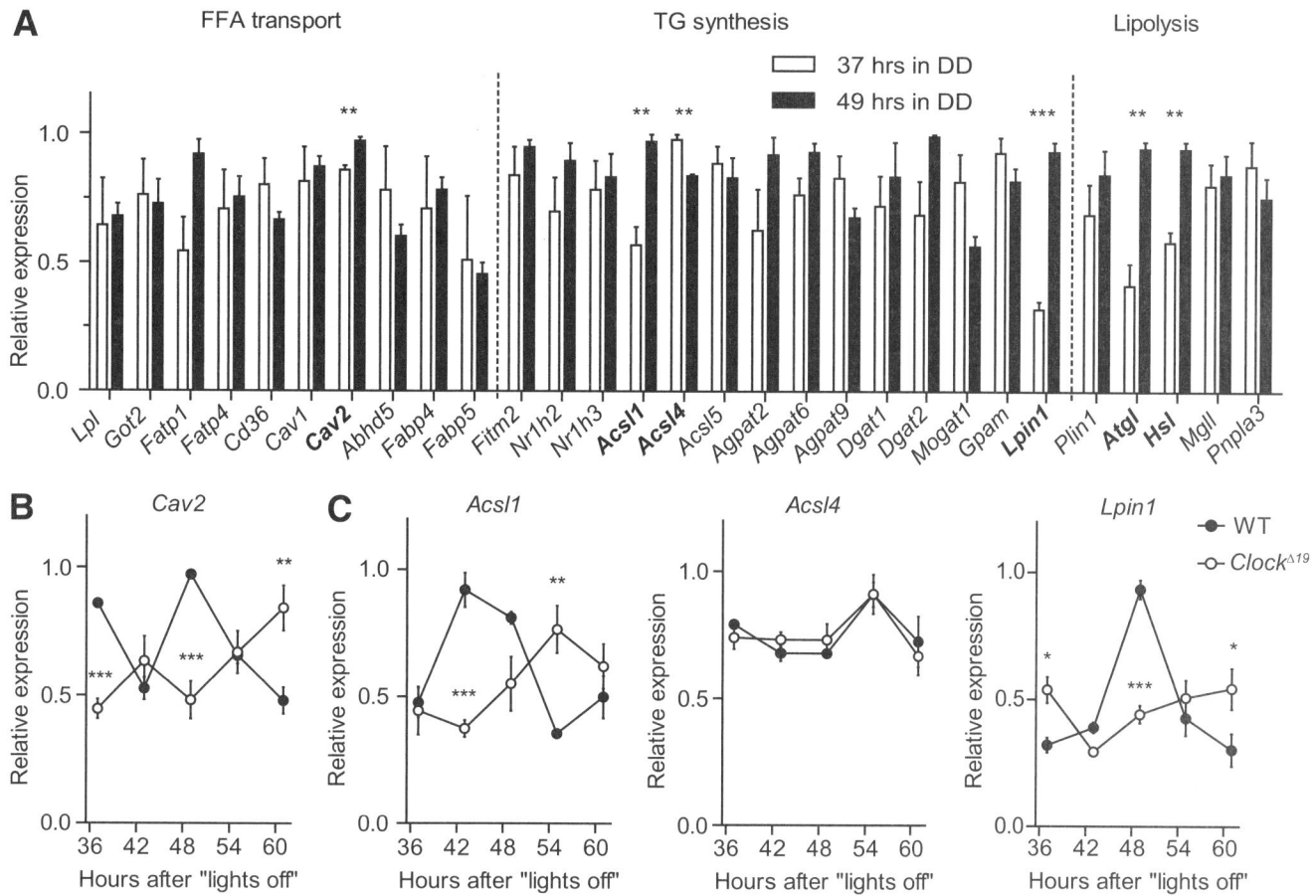

FIG. 3. Circadian clock controls TG metabolism in WAT. *A*: mRNA levels of genes involved in adipocyte TG metabolism from wild-type (WT) WAT samples isolated at two opposite circadian time points, 37 h (open bars) and 49 h (closed bars) in DD (*n* = 3 per time point [*P < 0.05; **P < 0.01 by unpaired *t* test]). Circadian expression profiles of candidate genes from (*A*) involved in FFA transport (*B*) and TG synthesis (*C*) in WAT samples from WT (closed circles) and *Clock*^*Δ19*^ (open circles) mice in DD (*n* = 3/time point [*P < 0.05; **P < 0.01; ***P < 0.001 by two-way ANOVA with Bonferroni posttest]). All data are shown as means ± SEM.

[LD], respectively). Of note, on the second day in DD, *Clock* mutants retained a rhythmic, though dampened, feeding profile (Supplementary Fig. 3*A*). Moreover, when animals were subjected to nighttime restricted feeding (i.e., food access between ZT12 and ZT24) under LD conditions, daytime *Atgl* and *Hsl* levels remained reduced in *Clock* mutant mice, indicating that *Atgl/Hsl* transcription does not merely reflect feeding rhythms (Supplementary Fig. 3*B*). Analogously, *Bmal1*^−/−^ mice showed lower expression levels of *Atgl* and *Hsl* (Fig. 4*D*) and *Bmal1*-deficient fat pads displayed lower lipolysis rates (Fig. 4*E*)

Adipose peripheral clocks regulate rhythmic expression of *Atgl* and *Hsl*. To further characterize the circadian regulation of adipose physiology, we analyzed WAT clock gene regulation in DD. Expression of *Bmal1*, *Per2*, and *Dbp* genes exhibited robust circadian variations in wild-type animals, which were significantly downregulated and arrhythmic (*Per2*, *Dbp*) or dampened (*Bmal1*) in *Clock*^*Δ19*^ mutant mice (Fig. 5*A*). To characterize the sustainability of molecular circadian rhythms in WAT and compare clock function between different fat depots, we cultured epididymal, perirenal, peritoneal, subcutaneous white, as well as intrascapular BAT fat explants from *PER2::LUCIFERASE* circadian reporter mice. All cultures showed sustained bioluminescence rhythms in the circadian range for several days (Fig. 5*B*

and Supplementary Fig. 4*A*) (17). The phases of luminescent oscillations were comparable between different depots and to those reported from other peripheral tissue explants (17,22) (Supplementary Fig. 4*B*). Periodogram analysis revealed endogenous periodicities of ~25 h; statistically significant differences in period were only observed between epididymal white fat and BAT (25.8 ± 0.2 vs. 24.7 ± 0.3 h; Supplementary Fig. 4*C*). Moreover, rhythm dampening was comparable among all adipose tissues tested (Supplementary Fig. 4*D*). To test if *Atgl* and *Hsl* transcription is clock-driven at the tissue level, we kept epididymal fat explants in culture for 36 h. We observed rhythmic *Atgl* and *Hsl* mRNA expression in wild-type fat pads (*P* < 0.001 and *P* = 0.006, respectively). Similar to what was observed in vivo, transcript variations were abolished, and overall levels were reduced in explants from *Clock*^*Δ19*^ mice (*P* > 0.8 for both genes) (Fig. 5*C*). Notably, the expression rhythms of the two lipolytic genes were in phase coherence with E-box–regulated genes such as *Per2* and in antiphase to *Bmal1* (compare Fig. 5*C* and *D*). Taken together, these data suggested a direct control of *Atgl* and *Hsl* expression by CLOCK and BMAL1.

BMAL1 and CLOCK regulate expression of *Atgl* and *Hsl* via E-boxes. We identified two canonical E-box sequences (CACGTG) in the first intron of *Atgl* (chr7:

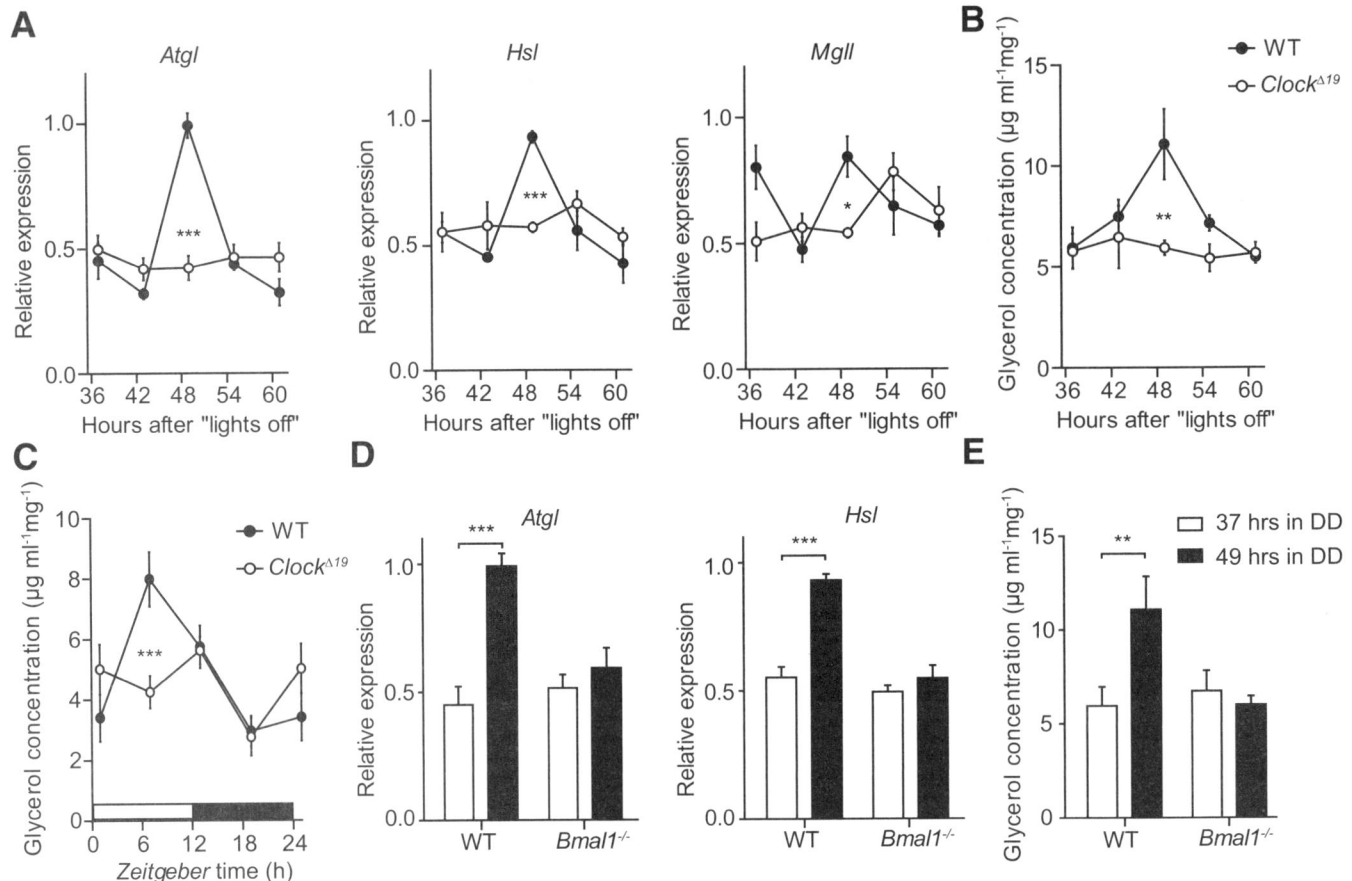

FIG. 4. Circadian clock regulates lipid mobilization in WAT. *A*: Circadian expression profiles of genes involved in lipolysis in adipose tissue from wild-type (WT; closed circles) and *Clock*$^{\Delta 19}$ (open circles) mice in DD (*n* = 3–4/time point). Profiles of glycerol excretion from WT (closed circles) and *Clock*$^{\Delta 19}$ (open circles) epididymal WAT fat-pad explants harvested in DD (*B*) and LD (*C*) (*n* = 6–14/time point). *D*: Expression of *Atgl* and *Hsl* in WAT of WT (black bars) and *Bmal1*$^{-/-}$ (white bars) animals at 37 and 49 h after lights off (*n* = 2–3/time point). *E*: Changes in glycerol excretion from WT (black bars) and *Bmal1*$^{-/-}$ (white bars) epididymal WAT fat-pad explants harvested at 37 and 49 h after lights off (*n* = 8/time point). All data are shown as means ± SEM. *$P < 0.05$; **$P < 0.01$; ***$P < 0.001$ by two-way ANOVA with Bonferroni posttest.

148642099–148642104, 148642860–148642866) and in the upstream region of *Hsl* (chr7: 26181156–26181161, 26181424–26181430). Genomic DNA fragments containing these *cis*-regulatory elements were used for luciferase-based transactivation assays in HEK293A cells (Fig. 6*A*). Cotransfection with *Clock* and *Bmal1* increased the activity of both *Atgl* and *Hsl* promoters by 6.5- and 2.3-fold, respectively (Fig. 6*B*). Activation was inhibited by cotransfection with *Cry1*, a negative E-box regulator. Moreover, mutation of the E-box proximal to the second exon of the *Atgl* gene (chr7: 148642860–148642866) abolished transcriptional activation by CLOCK/BMAL1 (Fig. 6*B*, *left*). Similar results were obtained upon mutation of both upstream E-boxes in the *Hsl* promoter (Fig. 6*B*, *right*). To confirm direct BMAL1 promoter binding in vivo, we performed chromatin immunoprecipitation (ChIP) on epididymal adipose tissue sampled at two different time points. ChIP analysis revealed time-of-day dependent occupancy of BMAL1 on *Dbp*, *Atgl*, and *Hsl* E-boxes, but not on 500-bp downstream regions in wild-type mice. In *Bmal1*-deficient animals, binding signal was markedly reduced (Fig. 6*C*). Finally, we transfected *Atgl-luc* and *Hsl-luc* constructs into NIH-3T3 cells and recorded bioluminescence for 48 h after serum shock synchronization. We observed a rhythmic bioluminescence signal for *Atgl-luc* and *Hsl-luc* antiphasic to *Bmal1-luc* (Supplementary

Fig. 4*E* and *F*), comparable to what has been reported for other E-box controlled genes such as *Per2* (23). Together, these results strongly suggest that circadian *Atgl* and *Hsl* transcription is directly regulated by CLOCK/BMAL1 via E-box activation at the adipose tissue level.

Defective lipolysis leads to fasting intolerance in Clock$^{\Delta 19}$ mutant mice. Lipolysis becomes an important energy source during the fasting (i.e., rest) phase of the day. In line with this, reduced FFA mobilization provokes aberrant physiological responses under fasting conditions (24). To test if fasting responses are impaired in *Clock*$^{\Delta 19}$ mutants, we food-deprived mutant and wild-type mice starting at the end of the light phase (ZT12). FFA and glycerol levels were upregulated in serum in response to 12- and 24-h starves (starting at the end of the normal rest phase, at ZT12) in wild-types, whereas the lipolytic response was severely dampened in *Clock*$^{\Delta 19}$ animals (Fig. 7*A* and *B*). Given that FFA release, and, thus, the availability of lipids as energy source, appeared impaired, we speculated that under fasting conditions, mutants may rely more heavily on carbohydrate or protein utilization (24). In line with this, liver glycogen stores in *Clock*$^{\Delta 19}$ mice were depleted much faster than in wild-types under fasting conditions (Fig. 7*C*). Moreover, after food removal, mutants showed lower rectal temperature when compared

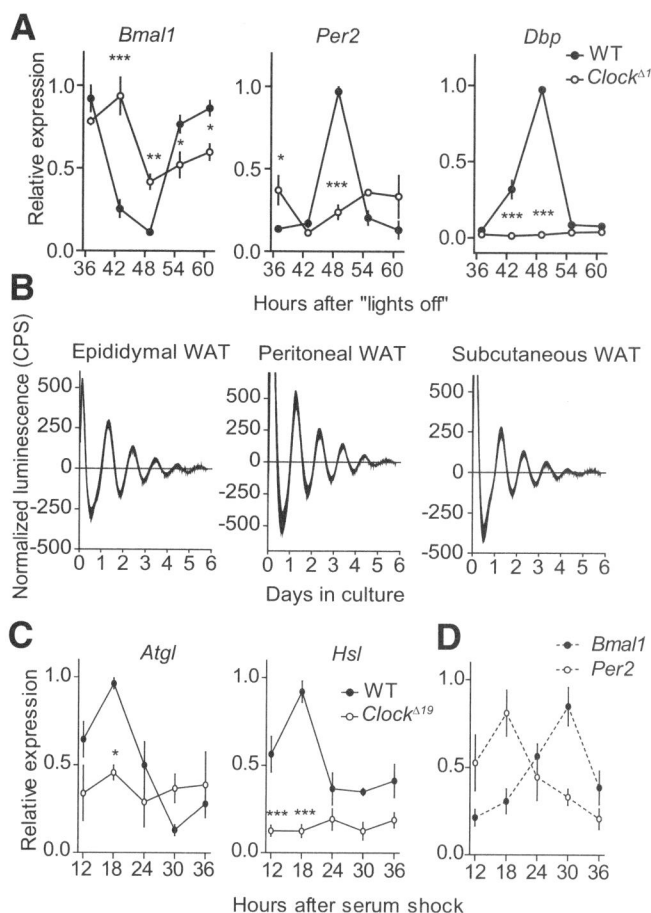

FIG. 5. Local WAT clocks regulate expression of *Atgl* and *Hsl*. *A*: Expression profiles of *Bmal1*, *Per2*, and *Dbp* mRNAs in WAT of wild-type (WT; closed circles) and *Clock$^{\Delta19}$* (open circles) mice in DD (*n* = 3/time point). *B*: Representative baseline-subtracted luminescence recordings from epididymal, peritoneal, and subcutaneous WAT explants of *PER2::LUCIFERASE* circadian reporter mice. *C*: Rhythmic expression of *Atgl* and *Hsl* transcripts in WT (closed circles), but not *Clock$^{\Delta19}$* (open circles), cultured fat-pad explants (*n* = 3/time point). *D*: Antiphasic expression of *Per2* (open circles) and *Bmal1* (closed circles) mRNAs in cultured WT fat-pad explants (*n* = 3/time point). All data are shown as means ± SEM. *$P < 0.05$; **$P < 0.01$; ***$P < 0.001$ by two-way ANOVA with Bonferroni posttest. CPS, counts per second.

with wild-type controls, implying decreased thermogenesis due to general energy shortage (Fig. 7*D*).

DISCUSSION

Circadian physiological rhythms are generated by interplay between systemic time cues (e.g., rhythmic hormones or metabolites) and the orchestration of transcriptional programs by local tissue oscillators. As a result many physiological parameters that exhibit diurnal variations are altered in mice with perturbed molecular clocks (5,6). In this article, we report that blood FFA and glycerol concentrations show strong variations across the day. This rhythm appears to not merely reflect rhythmic food intake and seems to critically depend on the presence of functional CLOCK/BMAL1. Moreover, in humans, it has been shown that FFA and glycerol are still rhythmic under constant routine conditions (25). During fasting conditions (e.g., during the daily rest phase), adipose-released FFAs become an important energy

source (26,27). Therefore, the mobilization of FFAs may be critically involved in the regulation of metabolic homeostasis.

In line with previous studies in rats (28,29), we showed circadian rhythms in baseline WAT lipolysis rates and FFA levels in the blood of wild-type mice. In *Clock$^{\Delta19}$* and *Bmal1$^{-/-}$* mutants, both rhythms were flattened and downregulated [our data and (30,31)], indicating defects in lipid mobilization. In agreement with this, it has previously been demonstrated that young *Bmal1$^{-/-}$* mice show increased adiposity (8,32,33), while C57BL/6 *Clock$^{\Delta19}$* animals are obese and are more sensitive to high-fat diet (4). Rhythmic clock gene expression has been detected in many tissues in rodents and humans including various adipose depots (10–12). Using *PER2::LUCIFERASE* fat-pad explants cultures, we showed that adipose clocks display similar endogenous rhythm sustainment as described for other peripheral oscillators. We identified *Atgl* and *Hsl*, which encode for two lipolysis pacemaker enzymes responsible for >95% of TG hydrolysis activity (34), as targets of the local WAT clock machinery. *Atgl/Hsl* transcriptional rhythms were accompanied by rhythmic lipolytic activity in explant cultures and rhythmic elevation of the lipolysis products FFAs and glycerol in the blood. Of note, increased *Atgl/Hsl* mRNA expression preceded the elevation of lipolytic products in the blood of wild-type animals by several hours, probably reflecting a delay between the initiation of the lipolytic response and the emergence of a measurable physiological effect. This delay results in high glycerol and FFA levels during the rest phase when both are used for energy production. *Hsl*-deficient mice show hypertrophic adipocytes, reduced lipolysis rates, and decreased FFA levels, though their body weight is normal (35). *Atgl* conventional and adipocyte-specific mutants display the same phenotype together with increased body weight (36–39). Although the precise mechanism by which impaired lipolysis contributes to the development of obesity is not well-understood, cell-based studies suggest that reduced expression of *Atgl* and *Hsl* leads to TG accumulation in lipid droplets in adipocytes (40,41). Consistent with this hypothesis, our data suggest that dampened circadian lipolysis rhythms, as seen in *Clock* and *Bmal1* mutant mice, may promote TG accumulation in WAT. Moreover, reduced availability of FFAs as peroxisome proliferator–activated receptor cofactors may disrupt oxidative metabolism in mitochondria in other organs (39,42). Of note, expression of both enzymes was reported to be decreased in adipose tissue in obesity, thus leaving a possibility that downregulation of *Atgl* and *Hsl* transcript levels in *Clock$^{\Delta19}$* and *Bmal1$^{-/-}$* animals might be rather the consequence than the cause of their adiposity. Our in vitro data suggest that *Atgl* and *Hsl* are direct targets of CLOCK/BMAL1, independent of metabolic state, but further studies are needed to clarify the impact of body weight and composition in this context (43,44). Moreover, we cannot exclude that disrupted feeding rhythms in *Clock$^{\Delta19}$* (Supplementary Fig. 2) mice may impinge on lipolysis rates via hormonal regulation (e.g., via leptin or insulin, which are known to induce and inhibit lipolysis, respectively) (45,46). However, circadian feeding profiles were not totally arrhythmic in *Clock* mutant mice, and *Atgl/Hsl* expression remained dampened in rhythmically fed *Clock* mutants. Further, reduced pancreatic secretion of insulin and hyperleptinemia have been reported in *Clock$^{\Delta19}$* mice (4,6), both of which appear insufficient to restore blood FFA and glycerol levels.

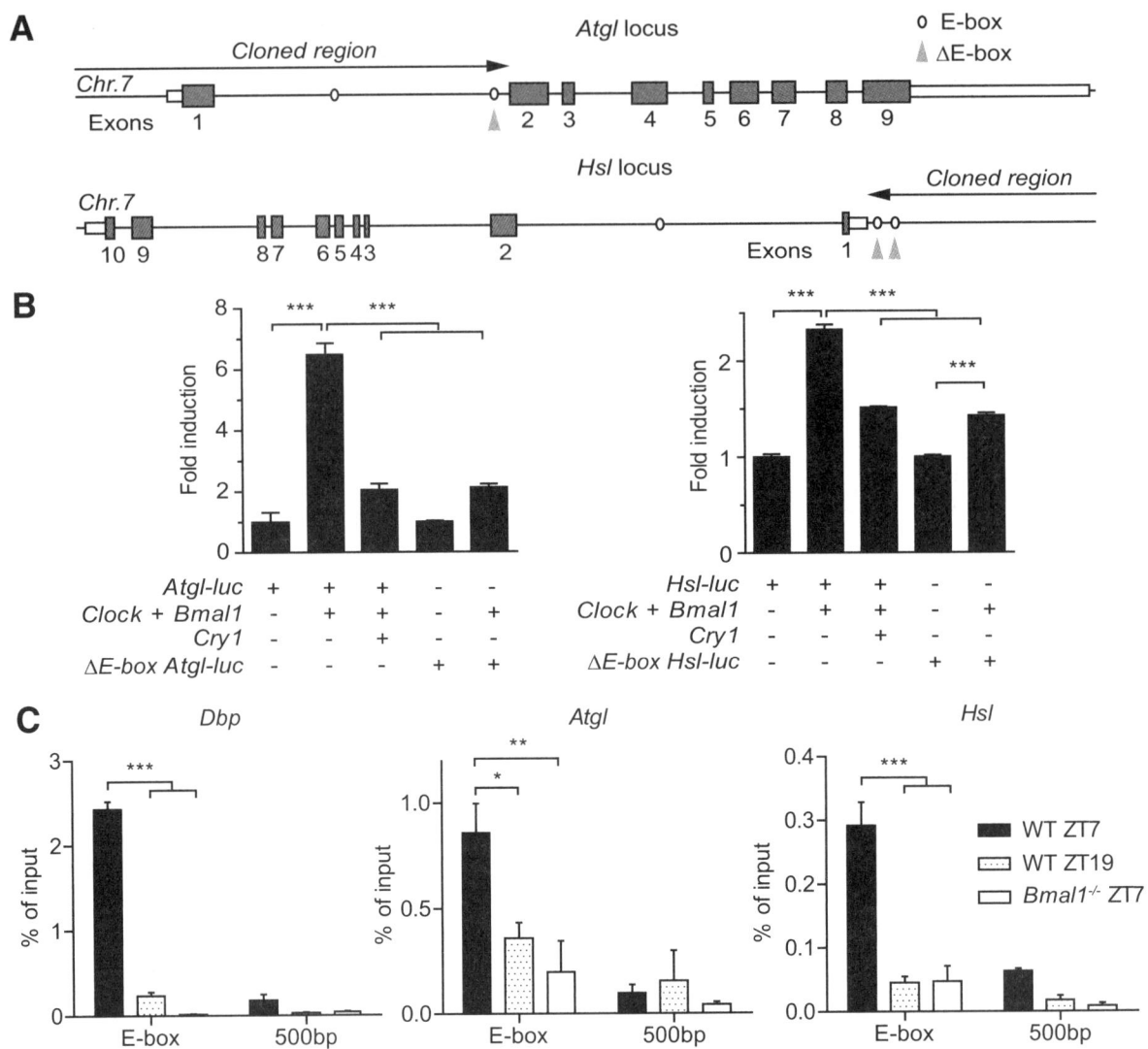

FIG. 6. CLOCK and BMAL1 drive rhythmic transcription of *Atgl* and *Hsl* via E-boxes. *A*: Maps of the 5′ regions of the genomic loci of murine *Atgl* (*top*) and *Hsl* (*bottom*) on chromosome 7 (*Chr.7*). Putative E-box enhancers are indicated by ovals. Black arrows depict the genomic sequences cloned for promoter studies. Mutated E-boxes are indicated by gray arrowheads. *B*: Luciferase reporter assays in HEK293 cells for wild-type (WT) and mutated *Atgl* (*left*) and *Hsl* (*right*) promoters in response to cotransfection with *Clock/Bmal1* and *Cry1* ($n = 3$; ***$P < 0.001$ by one-way ANOVA with Bonferroni posttest). *C*: Time-dependent BMAL1 binding to *Dbp*, *Atgl*, and *Hsl* E-boxes and 500-bp downstream regions as identified by ChIP in WAT ($n = 3$/time point [*$P < 0.05$; **$P < 0.01$; ***$P < 0.001$ by two-way ANOVA with Bonferroni posttest]). All data are shown as means ± SEM.

Instead, our results argue that rhythmic lipolysis is, at least in part, locally controlled by adipose circadian clocks. In line with this, oscillations of *Atgl* and *Hsl* mRNAs are sustained in fat pad explants ex vivo. Reporter gene and ChIP assays further indicate that CLOCK/BMAL1 directly and rhythmically bind to E-boxes in the promoters of *Atgl* and *Hsl*.

Mice with defective lipolysis exhibit impaired metabolic compensation during food deprivation (24). Consistently, our data reveal that *Clock*$^{\Delta19}$ mutants show aberrant fasting responses. Once external energy supplies are disrupted, glycogen stores become quickly depleted, while mice are unable to fully engage their lipid stores in WAT to deliver further energy for maintaining stable body temperature. Alternatively, the development of brown adipocytes may be affected in *Clock*$^{\Delta19}$ mice, or the *Clock*$^{\Delta19}$ mutation may directly impair brown adipose thermogenesis (11,39).

During the inactive phase, wild-type mice switch their energy substrate preference to lipids, which corresponds to a lower respiratory exchange ratio (47). *Hsl*- and *Atgl*-deficient animals, however, continue to primarily use carbohydrates during that time due to impaired FFA release into the blood (38). Remarkably, a similar respiratory exchange ratio phenotype was described for *Clock*$^{-/-}$ and *Bmal1*$^{-/-}$ mice (48,49), which, as our data suggest, could be explained by impaired lipid use. In contrast, animals lacking the transcriptional repressor and negative regulator of *Bmal1* REV-ERBα (NR1D1) show increased expression of both *Clock* and *Bmal1* and use lipids as the predominant energy source through their efficient FFA mobilization and membrane transport (50).

So far, the mechanistic link between circadian disruption and associated metabolic defects is not clearly understood. In this study, we show that adipose-tissue clocks may directly affect diurnal lipid homeostasis by

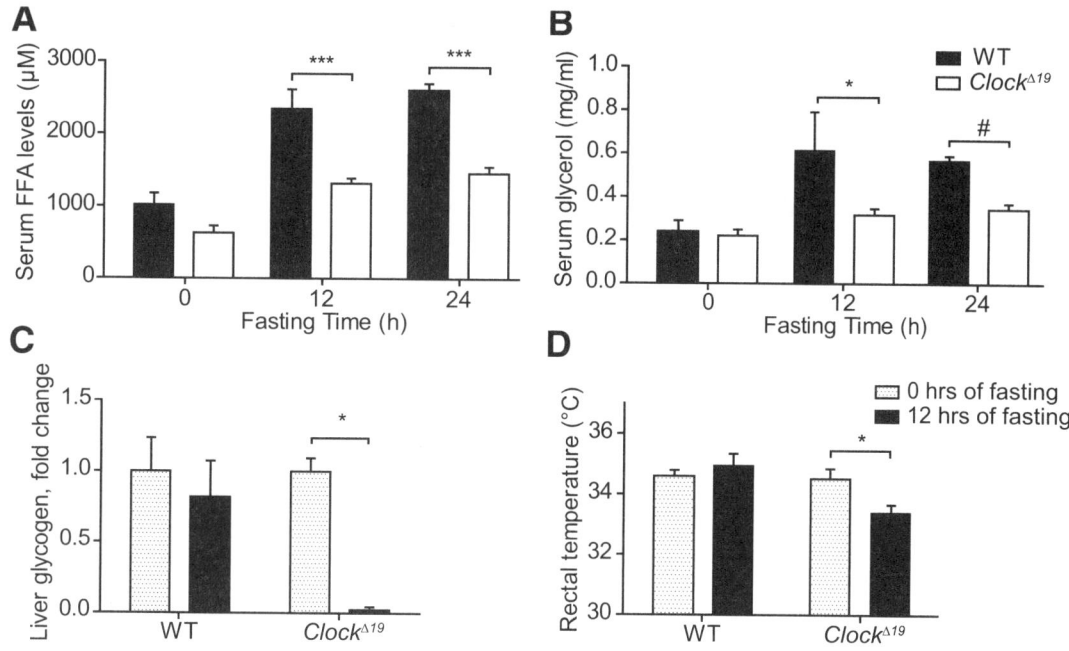

FIG. 7. Aberrant fasting responses in $Clock^{\Delta19}$ mice. Serum FFA (A) and glycerol (B) levels after 12 and 24 h of food deprivation in wild-type (WT; closed bars) and $Clock^{\Delta19}$ (open bars) mice (n = 3–5/time point). C: Normalized changes in liver glycogen content of WT and $Clock^{\Delta19}$ mice during 12-h fasting (n = 3 to 4). D: Rectal temperature in WT and $Clock^{\Delta19}$ animals during 12-h fasting (n = 6–12). All data are shown as means ± SEM. *P < 0.05; ***P < 0.001 by two-way ANOVA with Bonferroni posttest; #P < 0.001 by unpaired t test.

regulating FFA/glycerol mobilization from WAT stores via transcriptional regulation of the lipolytic machinery. By this, adipocyte clock function may directly impinge on energy homeostasis, thus representing a potential new target for pharmacological resetting of circadian physiology (51,52). Based on the evidence obtained from $Clock^{\Delta19}$ and $Bmal1^{-/-}$ mice, we suggest that impaired lipid mobilization may lead to an imbalance in energy homeostasis, promoting increased adiposity. It remains to be clarified, however, to which extent WAT lipolysis defects contribute to the obese phenotype seen in $Clock^{\Delta19}$ mutant mice since other alterations such as changed feeding patterns may further promote the development of obesity after circadian disruption (4,53,54).

ACKNOWLEDGMENTS

A.S. is supported by the Max Planck Society. H.O. is an Emmy Noether Fellow of the Deutsche Forschungsgemeinschaft and a Lichtenberg Fellow of the Volkswagen Foundation.

No potential conflicts of interest relevant to this article were reported.

A.S. and H.O. planned the study, researched data, and wrote the manuscript. J.M.-K. researched data. H.O. is the guarantor of this work and, as such, had full access to all the data in the study and takes responsibility for the integrity of the data and the accuracy of the data analysis.

The authors thank Dr. Ana Martinez Hernandez (Max-Planck-Institute for Biophysical Chemistry, Göttingen, Germany) for critical reading of the manuscript, and Dr. Moritz Rossner (Max-Planck-Institute for Experimental Medicine, Göttingen, Germany) and Dr. Steve A. Brown (University of Zürich, Zürich, Switzerland) for providing DNA constructs.

REFERENCES

1. Harmer SL, Panda S, Kay SA. Molecular bases of circadian rhythms. Annu Rev Cell Dev Biol 2001;17:215–253
2. Storch KF, Lipan O, Leykin I, et al. Extensive and divergent circadian gene expression in liver and heart. Nature 2002;417:78–83
3. Bray MS, Young ME. Circadian rhythms in the development of obesity: potential role for the circadian clock within the adipocyte. Obes Rev 2007; 8:169–181
4. Turek FW, Joshu C, Kohsaka A, et al. Obesity and metabolic syndrome in circadian Clock mutant mice. Science 2005;308:1043–1045
5. Rudic RD, McNamara P, Curtis AM, et al. BMAL1 and CLOCK, two essential components of the circadian clock, are involved in glucose homeostasis. PLoS Biol 2004;2:e377
6. Marcheva B, Ramsey KM, Buhr ED, et al. Disruption of the clock components CLOCK and BMAL1 leads to hypoinsulinaemia and diabetes. Nature 2010;466:627–631
7. Jeyaraj D, Haldar SM, Wan X, et al. Circadian rhythms govern cardiac repolarization and arrhythmogenesis. Nature 2012;483:96–99
8. Lamia KA, Storch KF, Weitz CJ. Physiological significance of a peripheral tissue circadian clock. Proc Natl Acad Sci USA 2008;105:15172–15177
9. Unger RH, Clark GO, Scherer PE, Orci L. Lipid homeostasis, lipotoxicity and the metabolic syndrome. Biochim Biophys Acta 2010;1801:209–214
10. Ando H, Yanagihara H, Hayashi Y, et al. Rhythmic messenger ribonucleic acid expression of clock genes and adipocytokines in mouse visceral adipose tissue. Endocrinology 2005;146:5631–5636
11. Zvonic S, Ptitsyn AA, Conrad SA, et al. Characterization of peripheral circadian clocks in adipose tissues. Diabetes 2006;55:962–970
12. Otway DT, Mäntele S, Bretschneider S, et al. Rhythmic diurnal gene expression in human adipose tissue from individuals who are lean, overweight, and type 2 diabetic. Diabetes 2011;60:1577–1581
13. Grimaldi B, Bellet MM, Katada S, et al. PER2 controls lipid metabolism by direct regulation of PPARγ. Cell Metab 2010;12:509–520
14. Shimba S, Ishii N, Ohta Y, et al. Brain and muscle Arnt-like protein-1 (BMAL1), a component of the molecular clock, regulates adipogenesis. Proc Natl Acad Sci USA 2005;102:12071–12076
15. Vitaterna MH, King DP, Chang AM, et al. Mutagenesis and mapping of a mouse gene, Clock, essential for circadian behavior. Science 1994;264:719–725
16. Bunger MK, Wilsbacher LD, Moran SM, et al. Mop3 is an essential component of the master circadian pacemaker in mammals. Cell 2000;103:1009–1017
17. Yoo SH, Yamazaki S, Lowrey PL, et al. PERIOD2:LUCIFERASE real-time reporting of circadian dynamics reveals persistent circadian

oscillations in mouse peripheral tissues. Proc Natl Acad Sci USA 2004; 101:5339–5346

18. Oster H, Damerow S, Kiessling S, et al. The circadian rhythm of glucocorticoids is regulated by a gating mechanism residing in the adrenal cortical clock. Cell Metab 2006;4:163–173

19. Brown SA, Ripperger J, Kadener S, et al. PERIOD1-associated proteins modulate the negative limb of the mammalian circadian oscillator. Science 2005;308:693–696

20. Oster H, Damerow S, Hut RA, Eichele G. Transcriptional profiling in the adrenal gland reveals circadian regulation of hormone biosynthesis genes and nucleosome assembly genes. J Biol Rhythms 2006;21:350–361

21. Panda S, Antoch MP, Miller BH, et al. Coordinated transcription of key pathways in the mouse by the circadian clock. Cell 2002;109:307–320

22. Pezuk P, Mohawk JA, Yoshikawa T, Sellix MT, Menaker M. Circadian organization is governed by extra-SCN pacemakers. J Biol Rhythms 2010;25: 432–441

23. Meng QJ, McMaster A, Beesley S, et al. Ligand modulation of REV-ER-Balpha function resets the peripheral circadian clock in a phasic manner. J Cell Sci 2008;121:3629–3635

24. Wu JW, Wang SP, Casavant S, Moreau A, Yang GS, Mitchell GA. Fasting energy homeostasis in mice with adipose deficiency of desnutrin/adipose triglyceride lipase. Endocrinology 2012;153:2198–2207

25. Dallmann R, Viola AU, Tarokh L, Cajochen C, Brown SA. The human circadian metabolome. Proc Natl Acad Sci USA 2012;109:2625–2629

26. Duncan RE, Ahmadian M, Jaworski K, Sarkadi-Nagy E, Sul HS. Regulation of lipolysis in adipocytes. Annu Rev Nutr 2007;27:79–101

27. Ahmadian M, Duncan RE, Sul HS. The skinny on fat: lipolysis and fatty acid utilization in adipocytes. Trends Endocrinol Metab 2009;20:424–428

28. Tsutsumi K, Inoue Y, Kondo Y. The relationship between lipoprotein lipase activity and respiratory quotient of rats in circadian rhythms. Biol Pharm Bull 2002;25:1360–1363

29. Benavides A, Siches M, Llobera M. Circadian rhythms of lipoprotein lipase and hepatic lipase activities in intermediate metabolism of adult rat. Am J Physiol 1998;275:R811–R817

30. Oishi K, Atsumi G, Sugiyama S, et al. Disrupted fat absorption attenuates obesity induced by a high-fat diet in Clock mutant mice. FEBS Lett 2006; 580:127–130

31. Kennaway DJ, Owens JA, Voultsios A, Boden MJ, Varcoe TJ. Metabolic homeostasis in mice with disrupted Clock gene expression in peripheral tissues. Am J Physiol Regul Integr Comp Physiol 2007;293:R1528–R1537

32. Guo B, Chatterjee S, Li L, et al. The clock gene, brain and muscle Arnt-like 1, regulates adipogenesis via Wnt signaling pathway. FASEB J 2012;26: 3453–3463

33. Hemmeryckx B, Himmelreich U, Hoylaerts MF, Lijnen HR. Impact of clock gene Bmal1 deficiency on nutritionally induced obesity in mice. Obesity (Silver Spring) 2011;19:659–661

34. Schweiger M, Schreiber R, Haemmerle G, et al. Adipose triglyceride lipase and hormone-sensitive lipase are the major enzymes in adipose tissue triacylglycerol catabolism. J Biol Chem 2006;281:40236–40241

35. Osuga J, Ishibashi S, Oka T, et al. Targeted disruption of hormone-sensitive lipase results in male sterility and adipocyte hypertrophy, but not in obesity. Proc Natl Acad Sci USA 2000;97:787–792

36. Haemmerle G, Lass A, Zimmermann R, et al. Defective lipolysis and altered energy metabolism in mice lacking adipose triglyceride lipase. Science 2006;312:734–737

37. Hoy AJ, Bruce CR, Turpin SM, Morris AJ, Febbraio MA, Watt MJ. Adipose triglyceride lipase-null mice are resistant to high-fat diet-induced insulin resistance despite reduced energy expenditure and ectopic lipid accumulation. Endocrinology 2011;152:48–58

38. Huijsman E, van de Par C, Economou C, et al. Adipose triacylglycerol lipase deletion alters whole body energy metabolism and impairs exercise performance in mice. Am J Physiol Endocrinol Metab 2009;297:E505–E513

39. Ahmadian M, Abbott MJ, Tang T, et al. Desnutrin/ATGL is regulated by AMPK and is required for a brown adipose phenotype. Cell Metab 2011;13: 739–748

40. Smirnova E, Goldberg EB, Makarova KS, Lin L, Brown WJ, Jackson CL. ATGL has a key role in lipid droplet/adiposome degradation in mammalian cells. EMBO Rep 2006;7:106–113

41. Zimmermann R, Strauss JG, Haemmerle G, et al. Fat mobilization in adipose tissue is promoted by adipose triglyceride lipase. Science 2004;306: 1383–1386

42. Haemmerle G, Moustafa T, Woelkart G, et al. ATGL-mediated fat catabolism regulates cardiac mitochondrial function via PPAR-α and PGC-1. Nat Med 2011;17:1076–1085

43. Oliver P, Caimari A, Díaz-Rúa R, Palou A. Diet-induced obesity affects expression of adiponutrin/PNPLA3 and adipose triglyceride lipase, two members of the same family. Int J Obes (Lond) 2012;36:225–232

44. Langin D, Dicker A, Tavernier G, et al. Adipocyte lipases and defect of lipolysis in human obesity. Diabetes 2005;54:3190–3197

45. Morimoto C, Tsujita T, Okuda H. Antilipolytic actions of insulin on basal and hormone-induced lipolysis in rat adipocytes. J Lipid Res 1998;39:957–962

46. Wang MY, Lee Y, Unger RH. Novel form of lipolysis induced by leptin. J Biol Chem 1999;274:17541–17544

47. Satoh Y, Kawai H, Kudo N, Kawashima Y, Mitsumoto A. Time-restricted feeding entrains daily rhythms of energy metabolism in mice. Am J Physiol Regul Integr Comp Physiol 2006;290:R1276–R1283

48. Eckel-Mahan KL, Patel VR, Mohney RP, Vignola KS, Baldi P, Sassone-Corsi P. Coordination of the transcriptome and metabolome by the circadian clock. Proc Natl Acad Sci USA 2012;109:5541–5546

49. Shimba S, Ogawa T, Hitosugi S, et al. Deficient of a clock gene, brain and muscle Arnt-like protein-1 (BMAL1), induces dyslipidemia and ectopic fat formation. PLoS ONE 2011;6:e25231

50. Delezie J, Dumont S, Dardente H, et al. The nuclear receptor REV-ERBα is required for the daily balance of carbohydrate and lipid metabolism. FASEB J 2012;26:3321–3335

51. Solt LA, Wang Y, Banerjee S, et al. Regulation of circadian behaviour and metabolism by synthetic REV-ERB agonists. Nature 2012;485:62–68

52. Hirota T, Lee JW, St John PC, et al. Identification of small molecule activators of cryptochrome. Science 2012;337:1094–1097

53. Hatori M, Vollmers C, Zarrinpar A, et al. Time-restricted feeding without reducing caloric intake prevents metabolic diseases in mice fed a high-fat diet. Cell Metab 2012;15:848–860

54. Barclay JL, Husse J, Bode B, et al. Circadian desynchrony promotes metabolic disruption in a mouse model of shiftwork. PLoS ONE 2012;7: e37150

Resistance to Aerobic Exercise Training Causes Metabolic Dysfunction and Reveals Novel Exercise-Regulated Signaling Networks

Sarah J. Lessard,[1] Donato A. Rivas,[2] Ana B. Alves-Wagner,[1] Michael F. Hirshman,[1] Iain J. Gallagher,[3] Dumitru Constantin-Teodosiu,[4] Ryan Atkins,[4] Paul L. Greenhaff,[4] Nathan R. Qi,[5] Thomas Gustafsson,[6] Roger A. Fielding,[2] James A. Timmons,[6,7] Steven L. Britton,[8] Lauren G. Koch,[8] and Laurie J. Goodyear[1]

Low aerobic exercise capacity is a risk factor for diabetes and a strong predictor of mortality, yet some individuals are "exercise-resistant" and unable to improve exercise capacity through exercise training. To test the hypothesis that resistance to aerobic exercise training underlies metabolic disease risk, we used selective breeding for 15 generations to develop rat models of low and high aerobic response to training. Before exercise training, rats selected as low and high responders had similar exercise capacities. However, after 8 weeks of treadmill training, low responders failed to improve their exercise capacity, whereas high responders improved by 54%. Remarkably, low responders to aerobic training exhibited pronounced metabolic dysfunction characterized by insulin resistance and increased adiposity, demonstrating that the exercise-resistant phenotype segregates with disease risk. Low responders had impaired exercise-induced angiogenesis in muscle; however, mitochondrial capacity was intact and increased normally with exercise training, demonstrating that mitochondria are not limiting for aerobic adaptation or responsible for metabolic dysfunction in low responders. Low responders had increased stress/inflammatory signaling and altered transforming growth factor-β signaling, characterized by hyperphosphorylation of a novel exercise-regulated phosphorylation site on SMAD2. Using this powerful biological model system, we have discovered key pathways for low exercise training response that may represent novel targets for the treatment of metabolic disease. *Diabetes* 62:2717–2727, 2013

C hronic complex diseases such as the metabolic syndrome and diabetes are tremendous burdens to our society, and regular physical activity (~150 min of aerobic training each week) is a primary recommendation for the prevention and treatment of these conditions (1–3). The potential for exercise to prevent chronic disease is exemplified by large-scale epidemiological studies demonstrating that cardiorespiratory fitness (i.e., aerobic exercise capacity) is one of the strongest predictors of health and longevity (4–6). For example, individuals with low aerobic exercise capacity have a more than four-fold higher risk of development of the metabolic syndrome and diabetes (7) and have up to five-fold higher all-cause mortality rates (8,9). The striking health risks associated with low aerobic exercise capacity are independent of other metabolic risk factors, including obesity and age (9–11), highlighting the importance of investigating the specific mechanisms that link exercise capacity to diabetes risk.

At present, the only clinically validated treatment for the improvement of exercise capacity is exercise training (12,13). However, significant variation exists in the ability to improve aerobic exercise capacity with exercise training in humans (14–16). In response to a standardized laboratory training protocol, changes in aerobic exercise capacity, as measured by $V_{O_{2max}}$, can range from negative or no gain in some individuals (nonresponders) to >100% improvement in others (high responders) (14,17). The fact that some individuals are completely unresponsive to aerobic improvements with exercise training infers the existence of "exercise resistance."

Considering the strong association between low aerobic exercise capacity and metabolic dysfunction (8), identifying mechanisms that contribute to the disparity in exercise training response may provide new targets for the treatment of chronic metabolic disease. However, the exercise capacity phenotype is determined by complex gene–environment interactions involving intrinsic factors (inborn) and those accrued in response to exercise training, making it challenging to isolate the critical mechanisms (17–20). Furthermore, animal models based on single-gene modifications (i.e., knockouts or transgenics) are inadequate to study the interaction between complex traits such as exercise capacity and metabolic disease. As such, we identified a need to develop genetically heterogeneous (noninbred) animal model systems that more closely embody human phenotypes and disease (19).

Here, we describe novel rat models of low aerobic response to training (LRT) and high aerobic response to training (HRT) that were created by divergent selective breeding to elucidate the mechanistic links between low aerobic adaptation to exercise training and disease risk. These models allowed us to directly test the hypothesis that nonresponders to exercise training have an increased risk for metabolic disease. Furthermore, because many of the health benefits attributed to exercise training stem from activation and remodeling of skeletal muscle, impaired adaptation in this tissue likely underlies the exercise-resistant phenotype. However, the multitude of concurrent

From the [1]Joslin Diabetes Center, Boston, Massachusetts; the [2]Jean Mayer United States Department of Agriculture Human Nutrition Research Center on Aging, Tufts University, Boston, Massachusetts; the [3]University of Stirling, Stirlingshire, Stirling, United Kingdom; the [4]University of Nottingham, University Park, Nottinghamshire, United Kingdom; the [5]Department of Internal Medicine, University of Michigan, Ann Arbor, Michigan; the [6]Karolinska Institutet, Huddinge, Sweden; the [7]Loughborough University, Leicestershire, United Kingdom; and the [8]Department of Anesthesiology, University of Michigan, Ann Arbor, Michigan.

Corresponding author: Laurie J. Goodyear, laurie.goodyear@joslin.harvard.edu.

Received 14 January 2013 and accepted 13 April 2013.

DOI: 10.2337/db13-0062

This article contains Supplementary Data online at http://diabetes.diabetesjournals.org/lookup/suppl/doi:10.2337/db13-0062/-/DC1.

transcriptional and signaling events that occur in skeletal muscle in response to exercise have made it difficult for previous research to establish which of these are essential for adaptive improvements to exercise capacity and health. Therefore, we used this contrasting animal model system to identify, using an unbiased approach, the molecular and morphological responses in skeletal muscle that are critical for improvements to exercise capacity and, potentially, metabolic health.

RESEARCH DESIGN AND METHODS

Artificial selection for LRT and HRT. To increase genetic heterogeneity, N:NIH out-crossed stock rats ($n = 152$) were used as the founder population (generation 0) rather than inbred strains. At ~10 weeks of age, the exercise capacity of each rat was measured using an incremental treadmill running test, which has been described previously (20). Each rat then underwent 24 sessions (3 days/week for 8 weeks) of treadmill running training using a protocol that increased in speed (from 10 to 20 m/min) and duration (from 20 to 30 min) each session. This moderate protocol was designed to ensure that all rats could complete the entire training schedule, regardless of their initial exercise capacity or relative change in capacity across training sessions (21). After completion of exercise training, the exercise capacity of each rat was measured (as described) and the training response was calculated as the change in exercise capacity as follows: posttraining exercise capacity − pretraining exercise capacity. Rats with the highest response to training were chosen for one line of selective breeding (HRT; 10 families/generation), and rats with the lowest response to training were chosen for an independent line (LRT; 10 families/generation). Approximately 100 offspring per line for each generation were assessed for training response and this selection process was repeated for 15 generations ($N = 3,114$ rats). Rats were fed rodent pellet diet (diet #5001; Purina Mills, Richmond, IN) and given free access to water. All procedures were performed in accordance with the University Committee on Use and Care of Animals at the University of Michigan.

Acute exercise bout. Forty female rats ($n = 20$ LRT and $n = 20$ HRT) from generation 12 were sent from University of Michigan to the Joslin Diabetes Center. After a 2-week acclimatization period, a subset of rats ($n = 13$/group) underwent an acute bout of exercise consisting of 25 min of treadmill running (15% incline) at a moderate speed (15 m/min). A second group of rats did not exercise and acted as sedentary controls ($n = 7$/group). Blood and tissue collection for the exercised rats occurred either immediately after the exercise bout ($n = 7$/group) or 3 h after the exercise bout ($n = 6$/group). All experiments were performed in accordance with the Institutional Animal Care and Use Committee of the Joslin Diabetes Center. The V_{O_2} and V_{CO_2} were measured using the Comprehensive Laboratory Monitoring System (Columbus Instruments).

Chronic exercise training. Forty female rats ($n = 20$ LRT and $n = 20$ HRT) from generation 15 underwent exercise capacity testing (as described) at 10–12 weeks of age. A subset of rats ($n = 10$/group) then underwent an 8-week exercise training protocol (as described). A second group of rats did not undergo exercise training and acted as sedentary controls. After the training period, all rats (exercise-trained and sedentary) underwent a second exercise capacity test for the calculation of exercise response as described. Blood and tissues were collected from exercise-trained rats 48 h after the last exercise bout to wash-out the potentially confounding effects of the last exercise bout.

Insulin and glucose tolerance tests. To assess glucose and insulin tolerance, sedentary rats were administered glucose (2 g/kg body weight) or insulin (0.75 units/kg body weight) by intraperitoneal injection, and blood glucose concentration was measured using a OneTouch Ultra (Lifescan) glucose monitoring system at specified time points after injection.

Blood metabolite and cytokine measurements. Plasma free fatty acid concentration was determined using an enzymatic colorimetric method (NEFA C; Wako Chemicals). Plasma interleukin-6, interleukin-1β, tumor necrosis factor (TNF)-α, and leptin concentrations were measured using a multiplex ELISA assay (Milliplex; Millipore). Plasma transforming growth factor (TGF)-β1 concentration was measured using an ELISA assay (MB100B; R&D Systems). Plasma triglycerides were measure using a colorimetric assay (Stanbio Laboratory 2200–430). Plasma glucose was measured using hexokinase reagent (Eagle Diagnostics #2821).

Citrate synthase activity. Whole-cell lysates from soleus and plantaris muscles were analyzed for citrate synthase activity as previously described (22).

Mitochondrial maximal ATP production rate. Twenty-four sedentary male rats ($n = 12$ LRT and $n = 12$ HRT) from generation 13 and 24 trained male rats ($n = 12$ LRT and $n = 12$ HRT) from generation 14 were sent from University of

Michigan to University of Nottingham. Mitochondria were isolated from freshly isolated soleus muscles ~1 week after completion of training and the rates of maximal ATP production in the presence of various substrates were determined using a luminescence technique as described previously (23). The substrate solutions tested were (final concentrations) as follows: glutamate 16.4 mmol/L and succinate 15 mmol/L; palmitoyl-L-carnitine and 5 μmol/L and malate 1.5 mmol/L (with human serum albumin 0.14 mg/mL); pyruvate 50 mmol/L and malate 22 mmol/L; succinate 2.5 mmol/L; and glutamate 32.75 mmol/L and malate 22 mmol/L.

Muscle glycogen content. An aliquot (~20 mg) of pulverized gastrocnemius muscle was hydrolyzed with HCl and neutralized with NaOH. The glucose concentration of the resulting lysate was analyzed using hexokinase reagent (Eagle Diagnostics #2821).

Liver triglyceride content. Triacylglycerol was extracted and saponified from an aliquot of liver (~25 mg) in ethanol/KOH at 55°C. Glycerol content was determined using a colorimetric assay (Sigma).

Western blotting. Gastrocnemius muscle lysates were solubilized in Laemmli buffer, separated by SDS-PAGE, and transferred to nitrocellulose membranes. The membranes were incubated with antibodies specific for the following: pERK 1/2 T202/Y204 (CST #4370); pSMAD4 T277 (Abgent AP7753); pSMAD3 S208 (Abgent AP9995); pSMAD2 S245/250/255 (CST #3104); pSMAD2 S465/467 (CST #3104); SMAD2 (CST #5339); pSMAD3 S423/425 (CST #9520); SMAD4 (CST #9515); active c-Jun N-terminal kinase (JNK; Promega V7931); JNK (CST #9252); pP38 mitogen-activated protein kinase (MAPK; CST #9211); P38 MAPK (CST #9212); pAkt (CST #9271); Akt (CST #9272); pAMPK (CST #2531); pACC (Millipore 07–303); ACC (Upstate); pTAK1 S412 (CST #9339); TGF-β–activated kinase (CST #4505); pCaMKII T286 (CST #3361); calcium/calmodulin-dependent protein kinase II (CaMKII; BD611292); CaMKK (BD); and AS160 (Upstate). The immunoreactive proteins were detected with enhanced chemiluminescence and quantified by densitometry.

Immunohistochemistry. Plantaris muscles from sedentary and exercise-trained rats were frozen in N_2-cooled isopentane and cut into 6-μm cross-sections. Sections were stained with antibodies against laminin (Sigma-Aldrich) and either myosin heavy chain I (4.951; DHSB) or myosin heavy chain IIA (SC-71; DHSB), or the endothelial marker CD31 (Serotec MCA1334EL), and visualized using fluorescent secondary antibodies under 100× magnification. Analysis of muscle capillary density (capillaries/mm^2) based on CD31 immunofluorescence was performed by OracleBio Limited using a customized vessel detection algorithm within Definiens Tissue Studio 3.5 image analysis software. Quantification of all images was performed in a blinded manner.

RNA isolation and microarray analysis. A portion of the soleus muscle taken from rats under resting conditions or 3 h after an acute bout of treadmill running exercise was preserved and frozen using RNAlater (Qiagen). RNA was extracted using QIAzol lysis reagent (Qiagen) and purified using RNeasy clean-up kit (Qiagen). RNA quality and integrity were assessed using an Agilent 2100 Bioanalyzer (Agilent Technologies). The Ambion WT Expression Kit (PN 4425209C) was used and labeling of cDNA was performed using the Affymetrix GeneChip WT Terminal Labeling Kit (PN 900671). Hybridization, washing, and staining were performed on Affymetrix GeneChip Rat Gene-ST 1.0 arrays. Low-level processing and significance analysis of microarrays analysis were undertaken as previously described (24,25) to generate a list of regulated genes. The gene list was then subject to ingenuity pathway analysis–based pathway analysis using the Upstream Analysis tool.

Statistical Analysis. Differences between groups were identified using a two-way ANOVA using phenotype and exercise as independent variables. When appropriate, Tukey post hoc testing was performed to assess differences between individual groups. Results are expressed as mean ± SEM and statistical significance was accepted at $P < 0.05$.

RESULTS

Selective breeding for LRT and HRT. Based on evidence that the ability to increase aerobic capacity with exercise training is determined by inherited factors (26), we aimed to create animal models of LRT and HRT via the process of selective breeding. Before selective breeding (generation 0), the average response of the rat population to this exercise training protocol resulted in 140 ± 15 m increase in exercise capacity. After 15 generations of selective breeding, rats bred as HRT improved endurance running capacity by 223 ± 20 m, whereas rats bred as LRT declined −65 ± 15 m in response to treadmill training. We closely evaluated 40 females (20 LRT and 20 HRT) by comparing groups that underwent

8 weeks of treadmill running exercise (exercise-trained) with untrained (sedentary) control groups. At 10 weeks of age, rats underwent exercise capacity testing, and it was determined that intrinsic exercise capacity (that which is present in the absence of training) was the same between LRT and HRT (Fig. 1A and B). After exercise training, exercise capacity was 67% higher in HRT compared with LRT (Fig. 1B). When the data were expressed as training response (Δ exercise capacity), LRT failed to improve exercise capacity and HRT had 54% increase in exercise capacity because of training (Fig. 1C; exercise-trained). Therefore, we have successfully created populations of nonresponders (LRT) and HRT through divergent selective breeding.

LRT display whole-body metabolic dysfunction. Clinical data demonstrate a strong correlation between low exercise capacity and metabolic disease (8). As such, we hypothesized that selection for LRT would segregate with higher metabolic disease risk. In support of this hypothesis, LRT displayed impaired whole-body insulin sensitivity (homeostasis model of insulin resistance; Fig. 2A) and higher circulating insulin concentrations under sedentary and exercise-trained conditions (Table 1). Consistent with training-independent insulin resistance, sedentary LRT had impaired glucose tolerance as assessed by the glucose area under the curve after intraperitoneal injection of 2 g/kg glucose (Fig. 2B) and blood glucose levels were higher in LRT 90 min after intraperitoneal injection of 0.75 units/kg insulin (Fig. 2C). LRT also had higher body (Fig. 2D) and gonadal fat pad (Fig. 2E) weights, higher plasma triglycerides (Fig. 2F), and higher circulating leptin (Table 1). Liver triglyceride content was 28% higher in LRT after exercise training (Fig. 2I), indicating metabolic dysfunction in this tissue. Notably, insulin resistance and adiposity in LRT were present in the absence of exercise training (sedentary condition), at a relatively young age (20 weeks), and under normal diet conditions (chow-fed, 13.5% calories from fat), demonstrating that primary metabolic defects co-selected with the genes that contribute to low aerobic training response.

Altered systemic inflammatory mediators are postulated to be contributing factors to the metabolic syndrome (27,28). Therefore, we measured the circulating levels of key inflammatory markers in LRT and HRT. Plasma cytokine levels were not different between untrained LRT and HRT rats (Fig. 2G and H, Table 1). However, after exercise training (samples taken 48 h after the last exercise bout), plasma concentrations of the inflammatory cytokine TNF-α were 85% higher in LRT (Fig. 2G), demonstrating that an altered inflammatory response to training accompanies the LRT phenotype. In contrast, plasma concentrations of the "anti-inflammatory" cytokine TGF-β were 50% lower in LRT compared with HRT after exercise training (Fig. 2H). Thus, TGF-β and TNF-α were divergently regulated by exercise training in LRT and HRT, indicating that these pleotropic cytokines may contribute to the training response phenotype.

LRT do not have impaired mitochondrial function in skeletal muscle. Although other organs (e.g., the heart) may contribute to the exercise capacity phenotypes in LRT and HRT, because of its significant contribution to total body mass, skeletal muscle has greater potential to influence both exercise capacity and whole-body metabolic health (29). Therefore, we measured several characteristics of skeletal muscle that have the potential to influence exercise capacity and metabolic health in LRT and HRT.

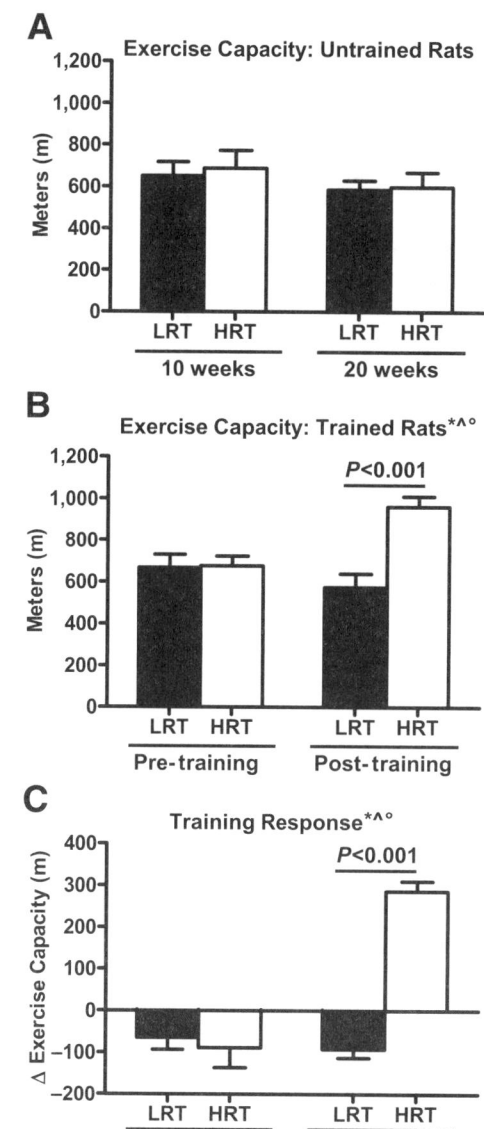

FIG. 1. Exercise capacity in rats bred for LRT and HRT. Exercise capacity (m) was measured using an incremental treadmill running test to exhaustion in (A) sedentary rats at 10 and 20 weeks of age and in (B) a separate group of age-matched trained rats before (pretraining) and after (posttraining) 8 weeks (3 days/week) of treadmill running exercise. C: Exercise response was calculated as the difference in exercise capacity before and after exercise training (exercise-trained) for each rat. The change in exercise capacity between 10 and 20 weeks of age is shown for animals in the control group (sedentary). *P < 0.05 for phenotype main effect; ^P < 0.05 for exercise main effect; °P < 0.05 for phenotype–exercise interaction by two-way ANOVA. P values obtained by Tukey post hoc testing are shown. n = 10–12/group.

Impaired mitochondrial capacity has been proposed as a mechanism contributing to the metabolic syndrome (30,31), and increased mitochondrial capacity contributes to improved aerobic exercise capacity with training (32). However, there was no difference in markers of mitochondrial density (citrate synthase activity in whole-muscle lysates) or mitochondrial function (maximal ATP production rates in isolated mitochondria) between LRT and HRT in the sedentary state (Table 2). Furthermore, LRT had normal increases in mitochondrial density and function in response to the moderate exercise training regimen (Table 2).

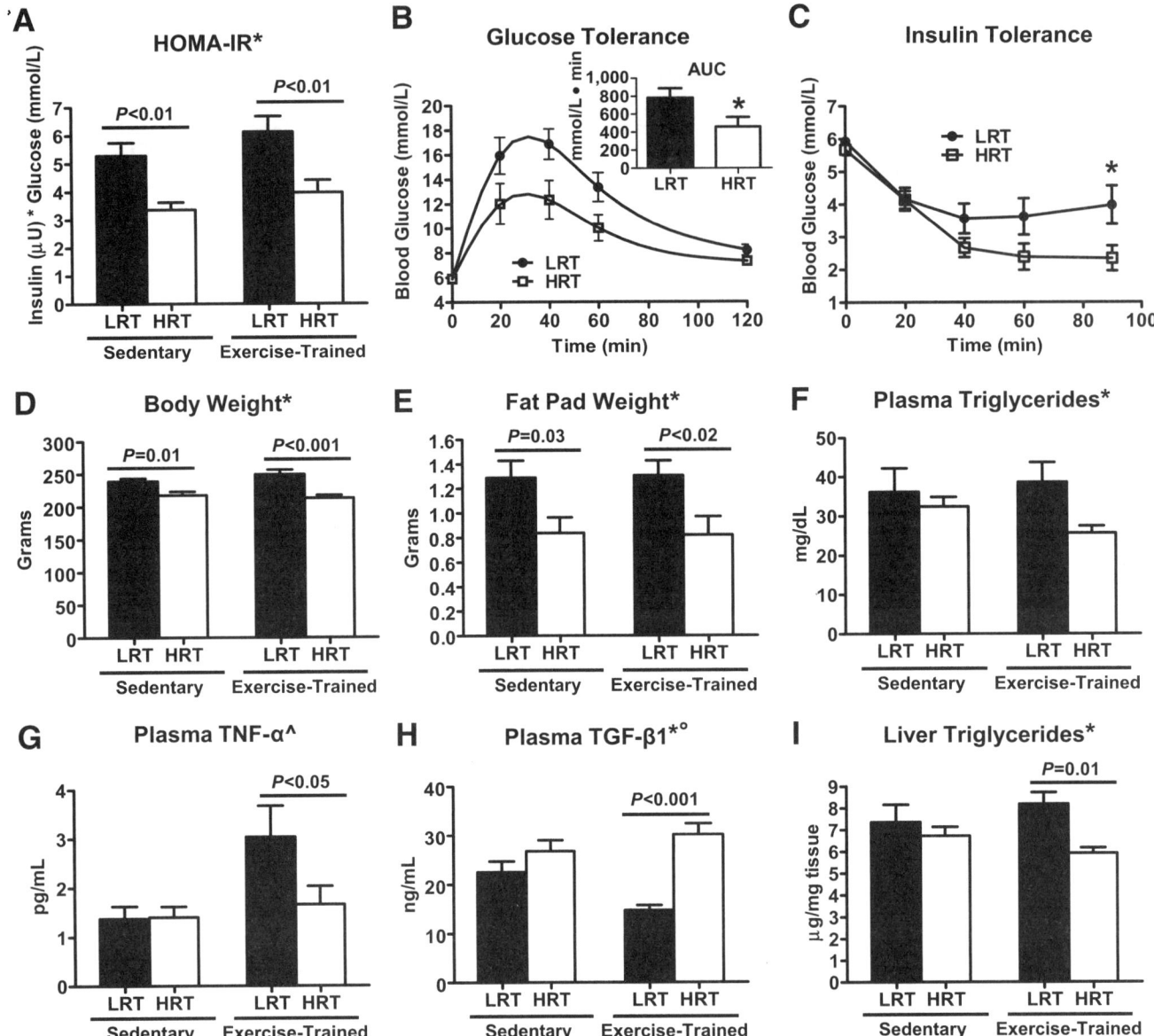

FIG. 2. Whole-body metabolic dysfunction in LRT. Fasting blood samples were collected from sedentary and exercise-trained LRT/HRT. *A*: Plasma glucose and insulin values were used to calculate the homeostasis model of insulin resistance (HOMA-IR). *B*: Glucose tolerance was assessed in sedentary rats after an intraperitoneal (IP) injection of 2 g/kg glucose and the area under curve (AUC) was calculated. *C*: Insulin tolerance was assessed after IP injection of 0.75 units/kg insulin. Body weight (*D*) and gonadal fat pad weight (*E*) were measured in sedentary and exercise-trained LRT and HRT. Plasma triglycerides (*F*), TNF-α (*G*), and TGF-β1 (*H*) concentrations were analyzed by ELISA. *I*: Liver triglycerides were estimated from total liver glycerol content. *$P < 0.05$ for phenotype main effect; ^$P < 0.05$ for exercise main effect; °$P < 0.05$ for phenotype–exercise interaction by two-way ANOVA. P values obtained by Tukey post hoc testing are displayed. $n = 10–12$/group.

Therefore, our results indicate that impaired mitochondrial function is not responsible for metabolic dysfunction or the failure to improve exercise capacity with training in LRT.

LRT have altered skeletal muscle fiber type. Endurance athletes often have a higher proportion of type I (oxidative) fibers in skeletal muscle (33), and low type I fiber content is associated with insulin resistance, obesity, and type 2 diabetes (34–36). Consistent with a proposed link between lower proportion of type I fibers and metabolic dysfunction, type I fibers accounted for ~7% of the total fibers in LRT compared with >20% in HRT (Fig. 3*A*). Therefore, higher type I fiber content may contribute to improved insulin sensitivity in HRT. However, fiber-type differences between LRT and HRT were independent of

exercise training and therefore cannot explain posttraining differences in exercise capacity. No differences were observed in type IIA (oxidative/glycolytic) fiber content (Supplementary Fig. 1).

LRT have impaired exercise-induced angiogenesis in skeletal muscle. Exercise training stimulates angiogenesis in skeletal muscle, and this may contribute to improved exercise capacity and metabolic health (10,37). Capillary density was similar in skeletal muscle from LRT and HRT under untrained conditions (Fig. 3*B*). In contrast, capillary density was 50% higher in HRT after exercise training (Fig. 3*B*). The failure of LRT to stimulate angiogenesis in response to training may contribute to divergent responses to training in these models. Overall, the skeletal muscle

TABLE 1
Plasma measurements taken from sedentary and exercise-trained LRT and HRT responders to exercise training

	LRT SED	LRT EXT	HRT SED	HRT EXT	Phenotype P	Exercise P
Insulin, ng/mL	1.04 ± 0.10	1.01 ± 0.10	0.69 ± 0.06*	0.78 ± 0.08*	0.002	0.75
Glucose, mmol/L	4.93 ± 0.10	4.94 ± 0.25	4.74 ± 0.16	4.89 ± 0.24	0.55	0.71
Leptin, pg/mL	5,760 ± 592	7,115 ± 734	3,725 ± 540*	4,058 ± 723*	<0.001	0.20
IL-1β, pg/mL	4.27 ± 0.79	3.32 ± 0.60	3.45 ± 0.85	3.49 ± 0.88	0.29	0.95
IL-6, pg/mL	17.77 ± 4.69	14.63 ± 2.37	29.60 ± 8.23	16.05 ± 2.40	0.2	0.11

n = 10/group. EXT, exercise-trained; IL, interleukin; SED, sedentary. *P < 0.05 vs. corresponding LRT value by Tukey post hoc testing.

characteristics of low type I fiber content in conjunction with impaired exercise-induced angiogenesis demonstrate a general alteration in muscle phenotype and impaired tissue remodeling in LRT.

Response to a single bout of treadmill running in LRT and HRT. It has been hypothesized that each single bout of exercise initiates signaling and transcriptional events that accumulate with repeated bouts to produce exercise training adaptations (38). However, a direct link between the acute molecular responses to exercise and the molecules that regulate long-term adaptation remains elusive (39) and our unique model affords an opportunity to provide new insight into this question. To determine differences in the molecular response to a single bout of exercise, LRT and HRT rats remained sedentary for 20 weeks after phenotyping to wash-out the effects of training. The detrained rats then performed a single bout of moderate-intensity treadmill running for 25 min at a speed of 15 m/min. Oxygen consumption, the respiratory exchange ratio, muscle glycogen concentrations, and serum free fatty acid concentrations were similarly altered by exercise in LRT and HRT, indicating that the intensity of the exercise bout was not different for the LRT and HRT rats (Supplementary Fig. 2). To test the hypothesis that LRT had altered exercised-induced signaling, we measured AMPK and Akt phosphorylation-molecular signals that have been proposed to be critical mediators of exercise training–induced adaptations in skeletal muscle (40,41). Exercise increased AMPK and Akt signaling in the muscle; however, there was no difference between LRT and HRT (Supplementary Fig. 3). These data suggest that as-yet-unidentified pathways mediate the adaptive response to exercise training.

Contrasting transcriptional responses to exercise in LRT and HRT. As a framework to identify the gene networks that regulate training response, a microarray

experiment was performed to establish the exercise-responsive networks that were differentially regulated in LRT and HRT. Microarray analysis of RNA extracted from soleus muscles in the basal state and 3 h after a single bout of exercise identified subsets of genes that were exclusively upregulated in response to exercise in LRT (n = 130 genes) and HRT (n = 59 genes; Supplementary Fig. 4), whereas 133 genes were downregulated in response to exercise exclusively in LRT (Supplementary Fig. 4). Analysis using ingenuity pathway analysis revealed that the LRT and HRT exercise-regulated transcriptomes shared no common ontological overlap, indicating a striking contrast in transcriptional responses to the same exercise bout in these models. Genes differentially regulated by exercise in LRT and HRT belonged to the functional categories of gene expression, development, cell-cycle regulation, cellular growth, proliferation, and movement (Supplementary Fig. 4D). This unbiased analysis of the global molecular responses to acute exercise demonstrates that inherent differences in the muscle remodeling response may contribute to the exercise adaptation phenotype.

SMAD3, CREB1, and histone deacetylase target genes are dysregulated in LRT. To identify the upstream processes underlying differential exercise induced gene network modulation between LRT and HRT, the ingenuity pathway analysis upstream analysis tool was used on their respective exercise-regulated transcriptomes. This analysis identified activation of SMAD3 and cAMP-responsive element–binding 1 (CREB1) target genes and inhibition of histone deacetylase (HDAC)-regulated genes after exercise in LRT (Fig. 4; $P < 1 \times 10^{-5}$). No such gene network nodes were found in the HRT exercise-regulated gene list, demonstrating that LRT activate a unique molecular response to exercise. Based on these data, we hypothesized that exercise-stimulated

TABLE 2
Skeletal muscle mitochondrial capacity is similar in LRT and HRT rats

	LRT SED	LRT EXT	HRT SED	HRT EXT	Phenotype P	Exercise P
Citrate synthase activity (nmol/min/mg muscle protein)						
Muscle						
Soleus	316.9 ± 3.8	343.5 ± 15.0	337.1 ± 18.1	368.7 ± 11.6	0.1	0.04
Maximal ATP production rate (nmol/min/min mitochondrial protein)						
Substrate						
Pyruvate/ malate	3.19 ± 0.55	5.26 ± 0.77*	3.29 ± 0.50	4.20 ± 0.84	0.49	0.03
Glutamate/ malate	3.84 ± 0.62	7.39 ± 1.22*	3.44 ± 0.67	5.65 ± 1.13	0.27	0.004
Glutamate/ succinate	6.01 ± 0.87	9.33 ± 1.45	5.56 ± 0.94	6.77 ± 1.40	0.22	0.06

Citrate synthase activity was measured in whole-muscle homogenates from SED and EXT rats (n = 6/group). Mitochondrial ATP production in response to various substrates was measured in mitochondria isolated from the soleus muscle of sedentary or exercise-trained rats (n = 12/group). EXT, exercise-trained; SED, sedentary. *P < 0.05 vs. corresponding SED value by Tukey post hoc testing.

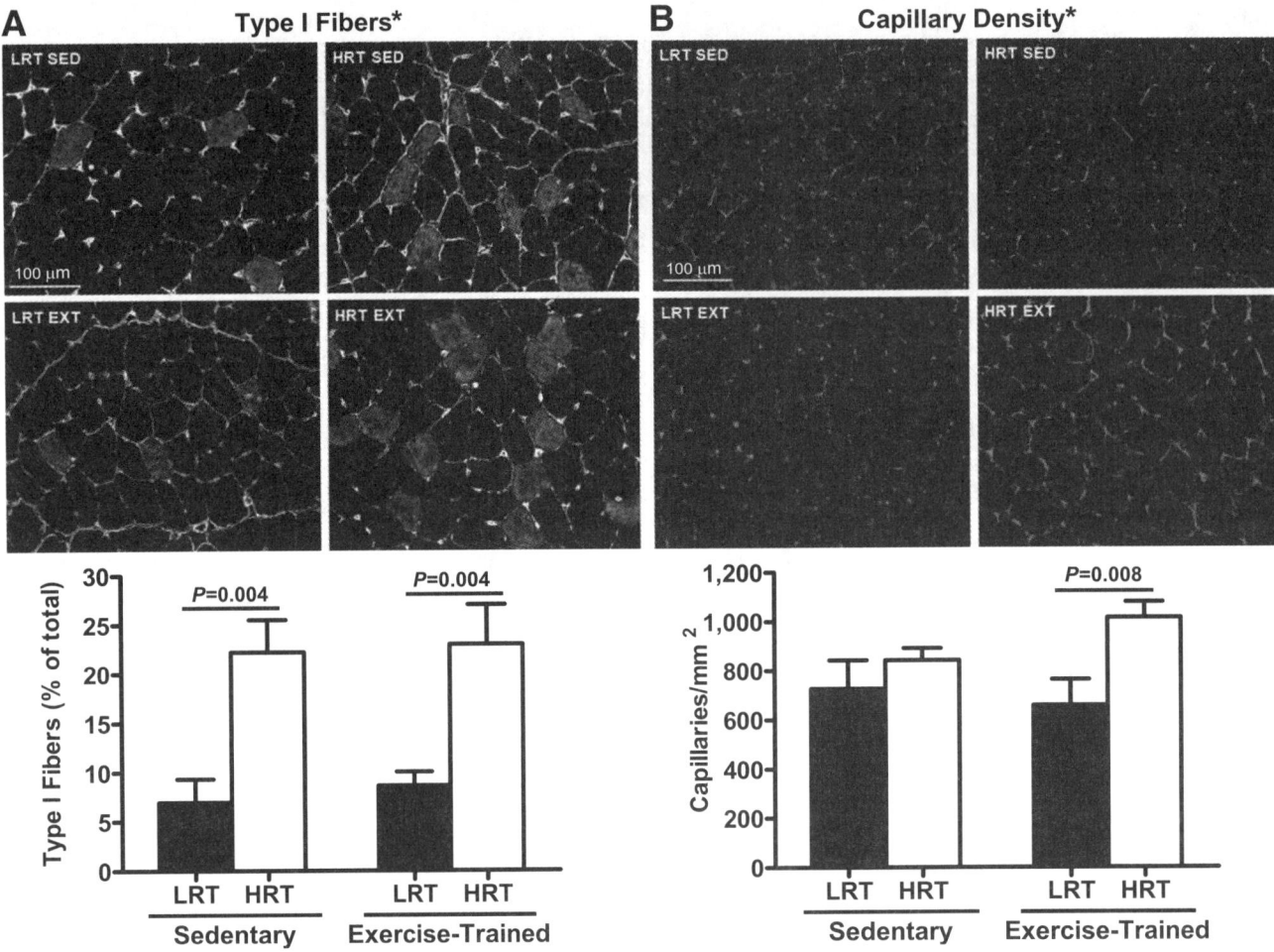

FIG. 3. HRT have fewer oxidative muscle fibers and impaired exercise-induced angiogenesis. Plantaris muscles from sedentary (SED) and exercise-trained (EXT) rats were frozen in N_2-cooled isopentane and cut into 6-μm cross-sections. *A*: Sections were stained with antibodies against laminin (white) and myosin heavy chain I (green) and visualized using fluorescent secondary antibodies under 100× magnification. Type I fiber content was expressed as % of total muscle fibers counted. *B*: Capillary density (capillaries/mm^2) was calculated in sections stained with an antibody against the endothelial marker CD31 (red). Nuclei were visualized with DAPI stain (blue). $n = 4$–5/group. *$P < 0.05$ for phenotype main effect by two-way ANOVA. *P* values obtained by Tukey post hoc testing are displayed.

protein signaling events that control SMAD, CREB, and HDAC transcription are dysregulated in LRT.

Muscle signal transduction is altered in LRT. CaMKII is an important mediator of intracellular calcium homeostasis and skeletal muscle plasticity (42,43), and is a key feature of the human exercise training transcriptome (44). CaMKII is a negative regulator of HDAC (43) that can mediate transcription via direct regulation of SMAD3 (45) and CREB1 (46), which were shown to contribute to the LRT exercise-responsive transcriptome, making altered CaMKII regulation a feasible mediator of dysregulated transcription in LRT. Phosphorylation of CaMKIIδγ at its autoregulatory site, Thr286, was higher in LRT, both in the basal state and after exercise, indicating constitutive activation of the enzyme (Fig. 5*B*). Constitutive activation of CaMKII in LRT was specific to the δγ isoforms of the enzyme (~55–60 kDa), because phosphorylation of the βm isoform (~70 kDa) was similar in LRT and HRT (Fig. 5*A*), which may reflect the different subcellular localization of these isoforms (47). Given the importance of CaMKII in many aspects of muscle signal transduction and remodeling processes (42,46), this chronic increase in CaMKII

activation likely contributes to altered transcription and impaired muscle plasticity in LRT.

SMAD3 is a primary mediator of TGF-β signaling and transcription in conjunction with its binding partner SMAD2 and molecular chaperone SMAD4 (48). To determine the mechanism behind altered exercise-induced SMAD3 transcription in LRT, we assessed canonical receptor-mediated TGF-β signaling by measuring the phosphorylation of SMAD2/3 at COOH terminal residues but found no phosphorylation of these sites in LRT and HRT skeletal muscle. Furthermore, exercise did not increase TGF-β–activated kinase phosphorylation in LRT or HRT (Fig. 5*A*), confirming that canonical TGF-β signaling is not activated by exercise. TGF-β–mediated transcription also can be regulated by an alternative pathway involving phosphorylation of SMADs in their linker region (49). Exercise had no effect on SMAD3 and SMAD4 linker phosphorylation in both phenotypes (Fig. 5*A*). In contrast, exercise robustly increased SMAD2 linker region phosphorylation (Ser245/250/255), an effect that was three-fold greater in LRT (Fig. 5*C*). Exercise-induced SMAD2 linker phosphorylation in skeletal muscle has not been previously reported; therefore, its functional role is

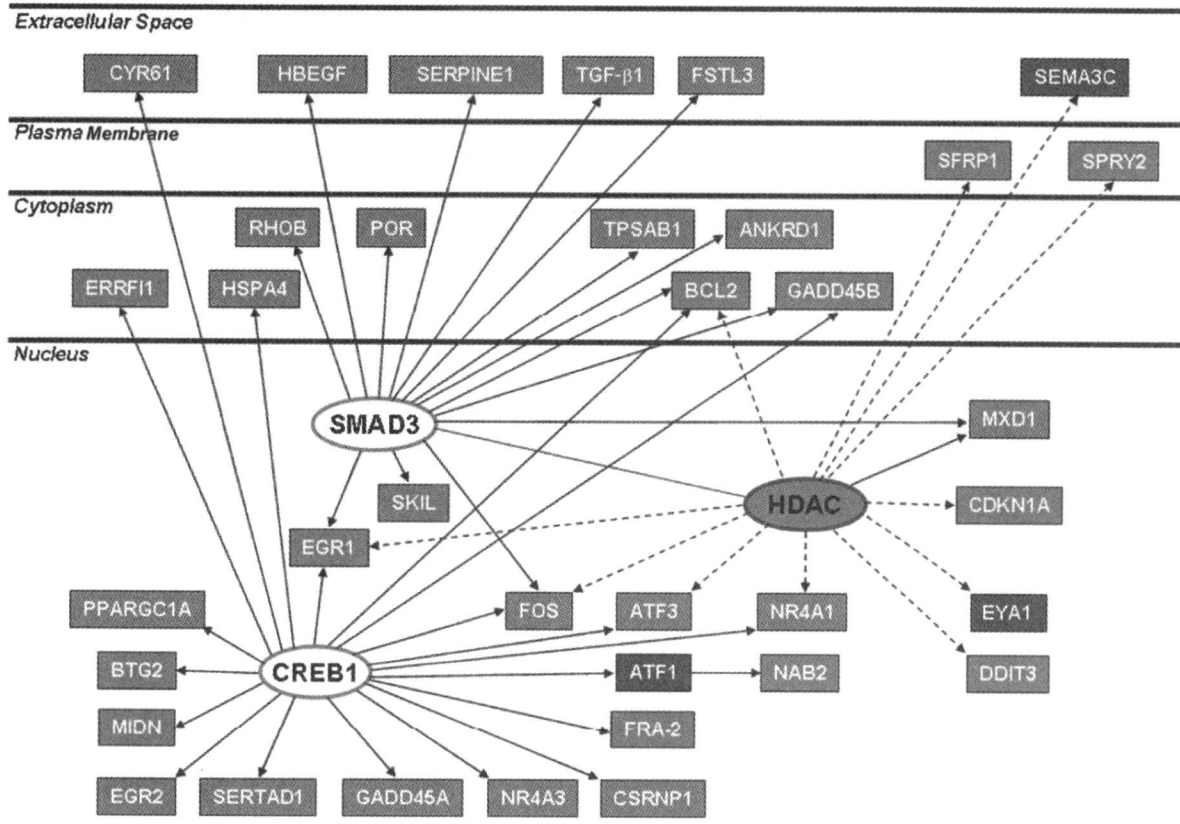

FIG. 4. Analysis of gene transcription in response to an acute bout of exercise identifies dysregulation of SMAD, CREB, and HDAC activity in LRT. RNA was extracted from the soleus muscles of rats under resting conditions or 3 h after an acute bout of treadmill running exercise. Genes that were significantly upregulated (red) or downregulated (blue) in response to exercise in LRT/HRT were identified using Affymetrix Rat ST 1.0 chips and analyzed using ingenuity pathway analysis (IPA; false discovery rate [FDR] = 5%, no fold-change filter). Transcription factor analysis in IPA clearly identified activation of SMAD3 (Z score = 2.3; $P = 1.1 \times 10^{-7}$) and CREB1 (Z score = 2.1; $P = 6.7 \times 10^{-6}$) target genes, whereas HDAC-regulated genes were inhibited (Z score = −2.8; $P = 1.1 \times 10^{-7}$) in response to exercise in LRT. Direct transcription factor/target gene relationships are indicated by solid arrows, and indirect relationships are indicated by broken arrows. No transcription factor enrichment was found in the HRT-regulated gene list, which was a set of entirely upregulated genes ($n = 156$, FDR = 5%, no fold-change filter) that bore no ontological or pathway overlap with the LRT dataset in IPA. $n = 5–6$ chips/group.

not yet understood. However, investigations of cultured fibroblasts indicate that phosphorylation of the SMAD linker region inhibits canonical TGF-β signaling (49) and may shift transcription toward target genes involved in extracellular matrix synthesis (50). Thus, we postulate that this novel phosphorylation site may contribute to impaired muscle remodeling in response to exercise in LRT.

Exercise increases JNK and p38 MAPK activity (51), and both JNK and p38 MAPK are upstream kinases for SMAD linker phosphorylation in vitro (50). Exercise increased JNK and p38 MAPK phosphorylation in both LRT and HRT; however, the increase was ~50% greater in LRT demonstrating hyperactivation of these signaling proteins (Fig. 5D and E). Based on our signal transduction and microarray analysis, we propose that the mechanism for the LRT phenotype involves the exercise-induced hyperactivation of JNK and p38 MAPK, leading to increased phosphorylation of their target, SMAD2, thereby resulting in increased transcription of SMAD3 target genes in LRT (Fig. 6).

DISCUSSION

We demonstrate that two-way selective breeding based on the aerobic response to exercise training generates rat models of LRT and HRT. Our results parallel clinical data in humans indicating that in response to standardized

aerobic exercise training, some individuals fail to improve their exercise capacity (nonresponders), whereas others achieve great gains (high responders) (14,15,52). The ability to enrich the trait of exercise response through selective breeding illustrates conclusively that inherited factors (genetic and epigenetic) determine this phenotype and validates our model for the study of this complex trait. Furthermore, despite strong clinical associations (8), previous research has not uncovered causative or mechanistic links between exercise training responsiveness and metabolic disease. We now demonstrate that selective breeding for the trait of LRT leads to whole-body metabolic dysfunction, including insulin resistance, increased adiposity, dyslipidemia, and inflammation. Remarkably, metabolic dysfunction in low-responders occurred even in the absence of training, suggesting an intrinsic metabolic defect segregates with the training response phenotype. These data are the first to establish a causative relationship between training response and metabolic disease risk, providing mechanistic validation for the numerous epidemiological studies that link aerobic exercise capacity and health.

To identify the molecular mechanisms that contribute to the LRT phenotype, we designed a novel multilevel approach using bioinformatic analysis of exercise-induced alterations in RNA networks to identify signal transduction

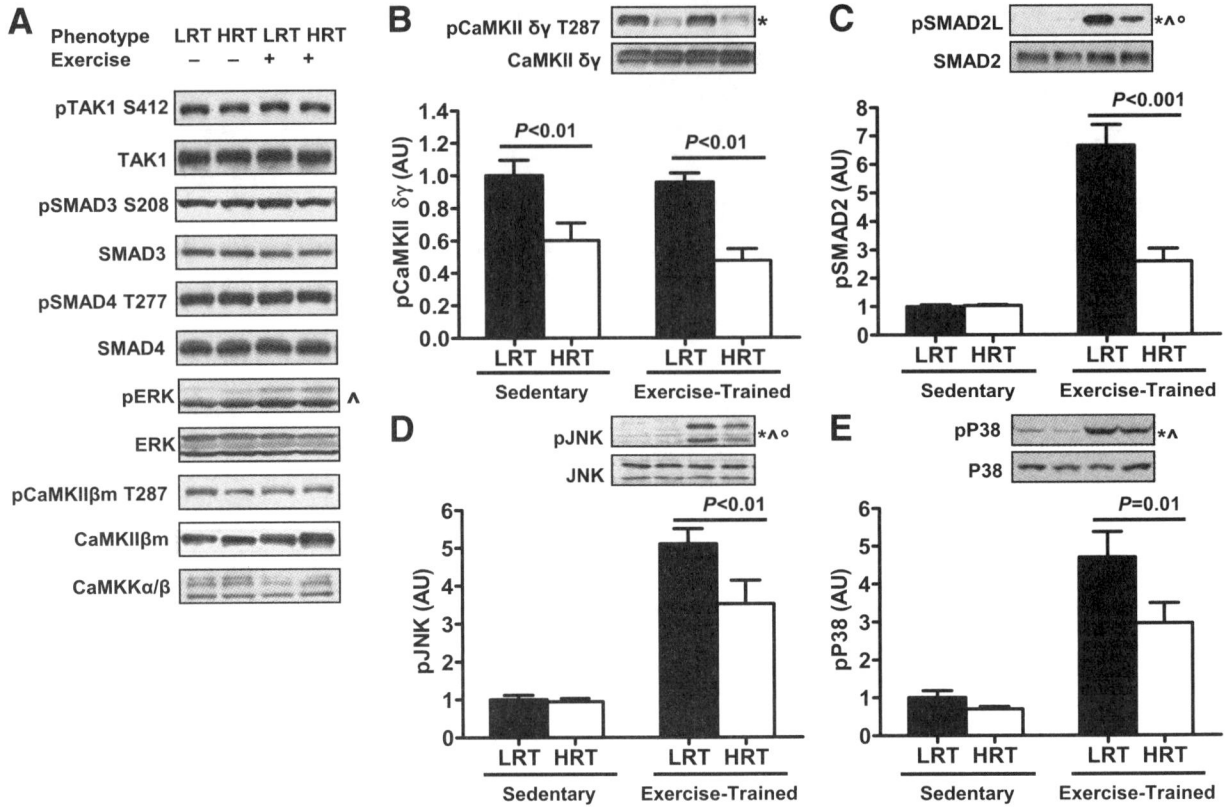

FIG. 5. Hyperphosphorylation of CaMKII, SMAD2, and MAPK in LRT. *A–E*: Phosphorylation of proteins involved in calcium, MAPK, and TGF-β MAPK signaling were measured by Western blotting in lysates from gastrocnemius muscle under resting conditions (basal) or immediately after an acute bout of exercise (exercise). ERK, extracellular signal–regulated kinase; P38, p38 mitogen-activated protein kinase; SMAD, mothers against decapentaplegic homolog. *n* = 6–7/group. *$P < 0.05$ for phenotype main effect; ^$P < 0.05$ for exercise main effect; °$P < 0.05$ for phenotype–exercise interaction by 2-way ANOVA. *P* values obtained by Tukey post hoc testing are displayed. AU, arbitrary units.

networks that regulate the molecular response to exercise. Our analysis revealed that gene networks involved in tissue remodeling are divergently regulated in LRT and HRT, a result that is consistent with analysis of gene networks regulated by exercise training in high-responding and low-responding humans (44,53). Specifically, we found that altered signaling via calcium, MAPK, and TGF-β pathways led to markedly different exercise-induced transcriptional networks in LRT. The involvement of multiple interacting pathways leading to hundreds of differentially regulated genes in LRT highlights the complexity of the exercise training response. The ability to study complex networks that more closely resemble human disease represents an advantage of using selective breeding as a tool over more traditional animal models based on single-gene modifications. Furthermore, our initial investigation examining the response to moderate aerobic training sets the stage for future studies using selective breeding models to investigate adaptations resulting from different exercise training modes (i.e., resistance vs. endurance) or intensities, which also have been associated with improved metabolic health.

Akt and AMPK, which represent signaling networks that have been extensively studied in the exercise and metabolism fields, were normally activated by exercise in LRT, suggesting they are insufficient to induce training adaptations. Therefore, using an unbiased approach based on bioinformatics analysis of skeletal muscle training response in humans (44,53) and the LRT/HRT models, we tested the hypothesis that TGF-β signaling regulates the training

response phenotype. The finding that exercise induces phosphorylation of SMAD2 in the linker region represents a novel exercise-regulated residue in skeletal muscle. Furthermore, exercise-induced SMAD2 linker phosphorylation was three-fold higher in LRT, suggesting altered TGF-β signaling contributes to the exercise-resistant phenotype. Because of its novelty, the role of SMAD2 linker phosphorylation in skeletal muscle is not known. However, investigations using cancer cell models demonstrate that SMAD linker region phosphorylation antagonizes canonical TGF-β signaling and may shift transcription of target genes toward those related to the extracellular matrix and tissue remodeling (49,50). At the whole-body level, LRT had two-fold lower levels of circulating TGF-β1 after exercise training compared with HRT, providing further evidence that altered TGF-β signaling is a key feature of the LRT phenotype. TGF-β is a potent stimulator of angiogenesis (54) and therefore represents a plausible mechanism for impaired skeletal muscle angiogenesis in LRT.

Dysregulated interactions between the MAPK and TGF-β signaling pathways are thought to be responsible for many disease states, including fibrosis and metastatic carcinoma (49,50). We now identify hyperactivation of JNK and P38 MAPK in response to exercise as a likely mechanism for enhanced SMAD2 linker phosphorylation in LRT (Fig. 6). MAPK activation is considered to be a normal response to acute exercise (51). However, chronic hyperactivation of JNK and P38 MAPK independent of exercise are

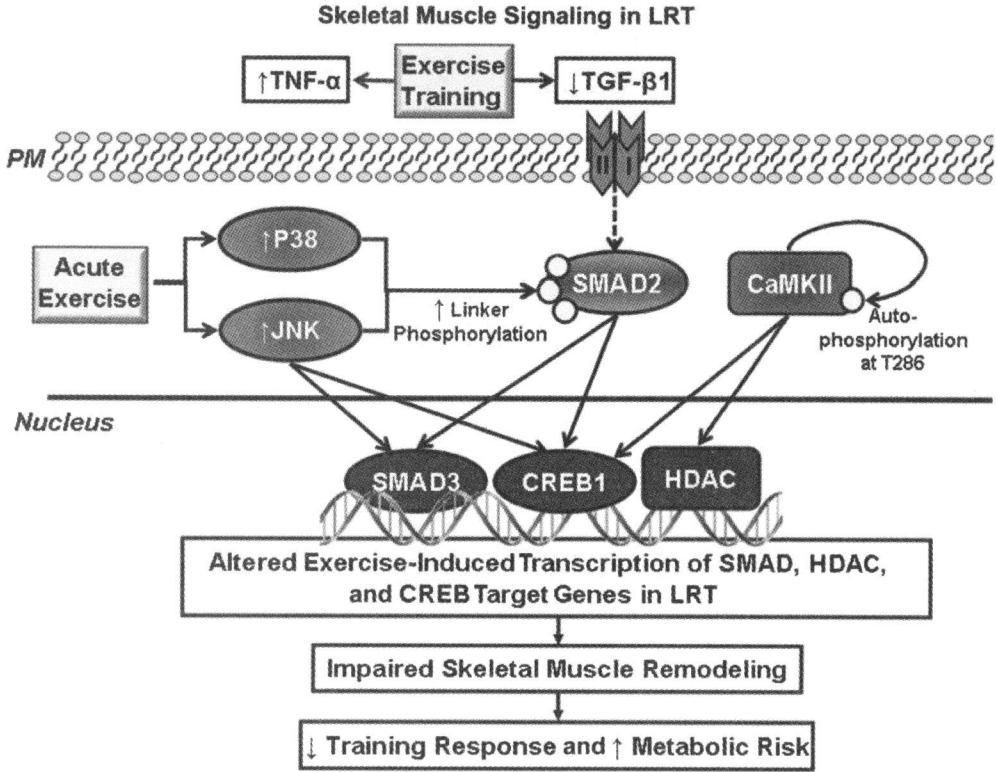

Skeletal Muscle Signaling in LRT

FIG. 6. Muscle signaling in LRT. A proposed sequence of signaling and transcriptional regulatory events that occurred in LRT was generated based on bioinformatic analysis of exercise-stimulated transcription and Western blotting analysis of skeletal muscle samples. In response to acute exercise, LRT have hyperactivation of JNK and P38 MAPK, leading to elevated phosphorylation of SMAD2 in its linker region at Ser245/250/255. Increased exercise-induced SMAD2 linker region phosphorylation results in altered gene expression by its binding partners SMAD3 and CREB1. Constitutive activation of CaMKII by phosphorylation of its autoregulatory site Thr286 also may contribute to altered transcription in LRT via its regulatory effects on HDAC and CREB1. Altered signal transduction and gene transcription likely lead to impaired remodeling of skeletal muscle in LRT, which, in turn, may contribute to decreased exercise capacity and whole-body metabolic dysfunction. ERK, extracellular signal–regulated kinase; P38, p38 mitogen-activated protein kinase; PM, plasma membrane; SMAD, mothers against decapentaplegic homolog.

associated with obesity, inflammation, and insulin resistance (28,55), all of which are consistent with the LRT disease risk phenotype. TNF-α was two-fold higher in LRT after exercise training and is a potent mediator of inflammation and a known activator of MAPK in muscle (27). Therefore, it is feasible that an exercise-induced inflammatory response interferes with TGF-β signaling and impairs muscle remodeling after exercise, contributing to the LRT phenotype. In line with this assertion, we found altered target gene expression of CREB1 and SMAD3 in response to acute exercise in LRT skeletal muscle, which are common mediators of the MAPK and TGF-β pathways (56,57).

In summary, using artificial selective breeding as a tool, we have generated animal models that establish physiological, tissue-specific, and molecular links between resistance to aerobic exercise training and metabolic disease. At the whole-body level, selective breeding for LRT caused significant metabolic dysfunction, including increased adiposity, insulin resistance, and inflammation. In skeletal muscle, LRT displayed impaired exercise-induced angiogenesis but a normal increase in mitochondrial capacity, indicating that the "supply" side, rather than the "demand" side, of aerobic energy transfer is limiting to exercise capacity. At the molecular level, increased stress and mitogenic signaling in response to acute exercise resulted in altered exercise-induced gene transcription in LRT. Furthermore, we identified a potentially novel role for TGF-β1 in exercise training adaptations and discovered that

SMAD2 linker phosphorylation is regulated by exercise and associated with the exercise-resistant phenotype of LRT. Using this powerful biological model system, we have discovered signaling networks that can be investigated as therapeutic targets for enhancing the improvement of aerobic capacity with exercise and thus the attenuation of metabolic disease in humans.

ACKNOWLEDGMENTS

This work was supported by National Institutes of Health grants RO1AR042238 and DK068626 (L.J.G.) and by Diabetes Research Center 5P30 DK 36836 (Joslin Diabetes Center) and DK089503 (University of Michigan). The HRT and LRT rat models are supported by the Department of Anesthesiology, University of Michigan Medical School, Michigan Diabetes Research and Training Center (NIH5P60 DK20572-P/FS; L.G.K.), National Center for Research Resources (R24 RR017718; L.G.K. and S.L.B.), and current support by Office of Research Infrastructure Programs/OD grant (ROD012098A) from the National Institutes of Health (L.G.K. and S.L.B.). This work also was supported by FP7 EU grant (J.A.T., T.G., and P.L.G.; METAPREDICT) and a grant from the Wallenberg Foundation, Sweden (T.G.).

S.L.B. was supported by National Institutes of Health grant RO1 DK077200. R.A.F. is supported by the United States Department of Agriculture under agreement 58-1950-0-014. D.A.R. is supported by the Boston Claude D. Pepper Older Americans Independence Center (1P30AG031679).

S.J.L. is supported by postdoctoral fellowships from the American Physiological Society (Physiological Genomics) and the Canadian Diabetes Association.

No potential conflicts of interest relevant to this article were reported.

S.J.L. designed experiments, performed experiments, analyzed the data, and wrote and edited the manuscript. D.A.R. performed experiments and analyzed the data. A.B.A.-W., M.F.H., I.J.G., R.A., N.R.Q., and T.G. performed experiments. D.C.-T. performed experiments and analyzed the data. P.L.G., R.A.F., S.L.B., L.G.K., and L.J.G. designed experiments. J.A.T. analyzed the data. L.G.K. designed experiments, analyzed the data, and wrote and edited the manuscript. L.J.G. designed experiments and wrote and edited the manuscript. L.J.G. is the guarantor of this work and, as such, had full access to all the data in the study and takes responsibility for the integrity of the data and the accuracy of the data analysis.

The authors acknowledge Animal Technicians Lori Gilligan and Molly Kalahar, University of Michigan, Ann Arbor, Michigan, for expert care and exercise training of the LRT and HRT rat colonies. The LRT and HRT models were created and are maintained at the University of Michigan and are available for collaborative study (contact: brittons@umich.edu or lgkoch@umich.edu).

REFERENCES

1. Hansen D, Dendale P, van Loon LJ, Meeusen R. The impact of training modalities on the clinical benefits of exercise intervention in patients with cardiovascular disease risk or type 2 diabetes mellitus. Sports Med 2010; 40:921–940
2. Sanz C, Gautier JF, Hanaire H. Physical exercise for the prevention and treatment of type 2 diabetes. Diabetes Metab 2010;36:346–351
3. Slentz CA, Houmard JA, Kraus WE. Exercise, abdominal obesity, skeletal muscle, and metabolic risk: evidence for a dose response. Obesity (Silver Spring) 2009;17(Suppl. 3):S27–S33
4. Blair SN, Kohl HW 3rd, Paffenbarger RS Jr, Clark DG, Cooper KH, Gibbons LW. Physical fitness and all-cause mortality. A prospective study of healthy men and women. JAMA 1989;262:2395–2401
5. Blair SN, Kampert JB, Kohl HW 3rd, et al. Influences of cardiorespiratory fitness and other precursors on cardiovascular disease and all-cause mortality in men and women. JAMA 1996;276:205–210
6. Kokkinos P, Myers J, Kokkinos JP, et al. Exercise capacity and mortality in black and white men. Circulation 2008;117:614–622
7. Grundy SM, Barlow CE, Farrell SW, Vega GL, Haskell WL. Cardiorespiratory fitness and metabolic risk. Am J Cardiol 2012;109:988–993
8. Church T. The low-fitness phenotype as a risk factor: more than just being sedentary? Obesity (Silver Spring) 2009;17(Suppl. 3):S39–S42
9. Church TS, Cheng YJ, Earnest CP, et al. Exercise capacity and body composition as predictors of mortality among men with diabetes. Diabetes Care 2004;27:83–88
10. Estacio RO, Regensteiner JG, Wolfel EE, Jeffers B, Dickenson M, Schrier RW. The association between diabetic complications and exercise capacity in NIDDM patients. Diabetes Care 1998;21:291–295
11. McAuley PA, Smith NS, Emerson BT, Myers JN. The obesity paradox and cardiorespiratory fitness. J Obes 2012;2012:951582
12. Goodyear LJ. The exercise pill—too good to be true? N Engl J Med 2008; 359:1842–1844
13. Hawley JA, Holloszy JO. Exercise: it's the real thing! Nutr Rev 2009;67: 172–178
14. Bouchard C, An P, Rice T, et al. Familial aggregation of VO(2max) response to exercise training: results from the HERITAGE Family Study. J Appl Physiol 1999;87:1003–1008
15. Kohrt WM, Malley MT, Coggan AR, et al. Effects of gender, age, and fitness level on response of VO2max to training in 60-71 yr olds. J Appl Physiol 1991;71:2004–2011
16. Lortie G, Simoneau JA, Hamel P, Boulay MR, Landry F, Bouchard C. Responses of maximal aerobic power and capacity to aerobic training. Int J Sports Med 1984;5:232–236
17. Timmons JA, Knudsen S, Rankinen T, et al. Using molecular classification to predict gains in maximal aerobic capacity following endurance exercise training in humans. J Appl Physiol 2010;108:1487–1496
18. Koch LG, Britton SL. Artificial selection for intrinsic aerobic endurance running capacity in rats. Physiol Genomics 2001;5:45–52
19. Koch LG, Britton SL. Development of animal models to test the fundamental basis of gene-environment interactions. Obesity (Silver Spring) 2008;16(Suppl. 3):S28–S32
20. Wisløff U, Najjar SM, Ellingsen O, et al. Cardiovascular risk factors emerge after artificial selection for low aerobic capacity. Science 2005;307:418–420
21. Koch LG, Green CL, Lee AD, Hornyak JE, Cicila GT, Britton SL. Test of the principle of initial value in rat genetic models of exercise capacity. Am J Physiol Regul Integr Comp Physiol 2005;288:R466–R472
22. Srere PA. Citrate synthase: [EC 4.1.3.7. Citrate oxaloacetate-lyase (CoA-acetylating)]. In Methods in Enzymology Citric Acid Cycle. John ML, Ed. New York, Academic Press, 1969, p. 3–11
23. Wibom R, Hagenfeldt L, von Döbeln U. Measurement of ATP production and respiratory chain enzyme activities in mitochondria isolated from small muscle biopsy samples. Anal Biochem 2002;311:139–151
24. Timmons JA, Wennmalm K, Larsson O, et al. Myogenic gene expression signature establishes that brown and white adipocytes originate from distinct cell lineages. Proc Natl Acad Sci USA 2007;104:4401–4406
25. Tusher VG, Tibshirani R, Chu G. Significance analysis of microarrays applied to the ionizing radiation response. Proc Natl Acad Sci USA 2001;98: 5116–5121
26. Prud'homme D, Bouchard C, Leblanc C, Landry F, Fontaine E. Sensitivity of maximal aerobic power to training is genotype-dependent. Med Sci Sports Exerc 1984;16:489–493
27. Nieto-Vazquez I, Fernández-Veledo S, Krämer DK, Vila-Bedmar R, Garcia-Guerra L, Lorenzo M. Insulin resistance associated to obesity: the link TNF-alpha. Arch Physiol Biochem 2008;114:183–194
28. Shoelson SE, Lee J, Goldfine AB. Inflammation and insulin resistance. J Clin Invest 2006;116:1793–1801
29. Dela F, Larsen JJ, Mikines KJ, Ploug T, Petersen LN, Galbo H. Insulin-stimulated muscle glucose clearance in patients with NIDDM. Effects of one-legged physical training. Diabetes 1995;44:1010–1020
30. Morino K, Petersen KF, Shulman GI. Molecular mechanisms of insulin resistance in humans and their potential links with mitochondrial dysfunction. Diabetes 2006;55(Suppl. 2):S9–S15
31. Szendroedi J, Phielix E, Roden M. The role of mitochondria in insulin resistance and type 2 diabetes mellitus. Nat Rev Endocrinol 2012;8:92–103
32. Holloszy JO. Regulation by exercise of skeletal muscle content of mitochondria and GLUT4. J Physiol Pharmacol 2008;59(Suppl. 7):5–18
33. Schiaffino S, Reggiani C. Fiber types in mammalian skeletal muscles. Physiol Rev 2011;91:1447–1531
34. Gaster M, Staehr P, Beck-Nielsen H, Schrøder HD, Handberg A. GLUT4 is reduced in slow muscle fibers of type 2 diabetic patients: is insulin resistance in type 2 diabetes a slow, type 1 fiber disease? Diabetes 2001;50: 1324–1329
35. Megeney LA, Neufer PD, Dohm GL, et al. Effects of muscle activity and fiber composition on glucose transport and GLUT-4. Am J Physiol 1993; 264:E583–E593
36. Tanner CJ, Barakat HA, Dohm GL, et al. Muscle fiber type is associated with obesity and weight loss. Am J Physiol Endocrinol Metab 2002;282: E1191–E1196
37. Gustafsson T, Kraus WE. Exercise-induced angiogenesis-related growth and transcription factors in skeletal muscle, and their modification in muscle pathology. Front Biosci 2001;6:D75–D89
38. Pilegaard H, Ordway GA, Saltin B, Neufer PD. Transcriptional regulation of gene expression in human skeletal muscle during recovery from exercise. Am J Physiol Endocrinol Metab 2000;279:E806–E814
39. Timmons JA. Variability in training-induced skeletal muscle adaptation. J Appl Physiol 2011;110:846–853
40. Baar K. Training for endurance and strength: lessons from cell signaling. Med Sci Sports Exerc 2006;38:1939–1944
41. Röckl KS, Witczak CA, Goodyear LJ. Signaling mechanisms in skeletal muscle: acute responses and chronic adaptations to exercise. IUBMB Life 2008;60:145–153
42. Chin ER. Intracellular Ca2+ signaling in skeletal muscle: decoding a complex message. Exerc Sport Sci Rev 2010;38:76–85
43. McGee SL, Hargreaves M. Histone modifications and exercise adaptations. J Appl Physiol 2011;110:258–263
44. Keller P, Vollaard NB, Gustafsson T, et al. A transcriptional map of the impact of endurance exercise training on skeletal muscle phenotype. J Appl Physiol 2011;110:46–59

45. Wicks SJ, Lui S, Abdel-Wahab N, Mason RM, Chantry A. Inactivation of smad-transforming growth factor beta signaling by Ca(2+)-calmodulin-dependent protein kinase II. Mol Cell Biol 2000;20:8103–8111

46. Singer HA. Ca2+/calmodulin-dependent protein kinase II function in vascular remodelling. J Physiol 2012;590:1349–1356

47. Griffith LC, Lu CS, Sun XX. CaMKII, an enzyme on the move: regulation of temporospatial localization. Mol Interv 2003;3:386–403

48. Shi Y, Massagué J. Mechanisms of TGF-beta signaling from cell membrane to the nucleus. Cell 2003;113:685–700

49. Matsuzaki K. Smad phosphoisoform signaling specificity: the right place at the right time. Carcinogenesis 2011;32:1578–1588

50. Burch ML, Zheng W, Little PJ. Smad linker region phosphorylation in the regulation of extracellular matrix synthesis. Cell Mol Life Sci 2011;68:97–107

51. Kramer HF, Goodyear LJ. Exercise, MAPK, and NF-kappaB signaling in skeletal muscle. J Appl Physiol 2007;103:388–395

52. Bouchard C, Rankinen T. Individual differences in response to regular physical activity. Med Sci Sports Exerc 2001;33(Suppl.):S446–S451; discussion S452–S453

53. Timmons JA, Jansson E, Fischer H, et al. Modulation of extracellular matrix genes reflects the magnitude of physiological adaptation to aerobic exercise training in humans. BMC Biol 2005;3:19

54. Orlova VV, Liu Z, Goumans MJ, ten Dijke P. Controlling angiogenesis by two unique TGF-β type I receptor signaling pathways. Histol Histopathol 2011;26:1219–1230

55. Gregor MF, Hotamisligil GS. Inflammatory mechanisms in obesity. Annu Rev Immunol 2011;29:415–445

56. Jang YS, Kim JH, Seo GY, Kim PH. TGF-β1 stimulates mouse macrophages to express APRIL through Smad and p38MAPK/CREB pathways. Mol Cells 2011;32:251–255

57. Newton K, Dixit VM. Signaling in innate immunity and inflammation. Cold Spring Harb Perspect Biol 2012;4:pii: a006049

Skeletal Muscle Triacylglycerol Hydrolysis Does Not Influence Metabolic Complications of Obesity

Mitch T. Sitnick,[1] Mahesh K. Basantani,[1] Lingzhi Cai,[1] Gabriele Schoiswohl,[1] Cynthia F. Yazbeck,[1] Giovanna Distefano,[1] Vladimir Ritov,[1] James P. DeLany,[1] Renate Schreiber,[2] Donna B. Stolz,[3] Noah P. Gardner,[4] Petra C. Kienesberger,[5] Thomas Pulinilkunnil,[5] Rudolf Zechner,[3] Bret H. Goodpaster,[1] Paul Coen,[1,6] and Erin E. Kershaw[1]

Intramyocellular triacylglycerol (IMTG) accumulation is highly associated with insulin resistance and metabolic complications of obesity (lipotoxicity), whereas comparable IMTG accumulation in endurance-trained athletes is associated with insulin sensitivity (the athlete's paradox). Despite these findings, it remains unclear whether changes in IMTG accumulation and metabolism per se influence muscle-specific and systemic metabolic homeostasis and insulin responsiveness. By mediating the rate-limiting step in triacylglycerol hydrolysis, adipose triglyceride lipase (ATGL) has been proposed to influence the storage/production of deleterious as well as essential lipid metabolites. However, the physiological relevance of ATGL-mediated triacylglycerol hydrolysis in skeletal muscle remains unknown. To determine the contribution of IMTG hydrolysis to tissue-specific and systemic metabolic phenotypes in the context of obesity, we generated mice with targeted deletion or transgenic overexpression of ATGL exclusively in skeletal muscle. Despite dramatic changes in IMTG content on both chow and high-fat diets, modulation of ATGL-mediated IMTG hydrolysis did not significantly influence systemic energy, lipid, or glucose homeostasis, nor did it influence insulin responsiveness or mitochondrial function. These data argue against a role for altered IMTG accumulation and lipolysis in muscle insulin resistance and metabolic complications of obesity. *Diabetes* 62:3350–3361, 2013

Obesity is a global public health problem and a major risk factor for insulin resistance and type 2 diabetes. These disorders are characterized by excess lipid accumulation in multiple tissues, primarily as triacylglycerols (TAGs). The lipotoxicity hypothesis suggests that this lipid excess promotes cellular dysfunction and cell death, which ultimately contribute to insulin resistance and metabolic disease (1). However, intracellular TAG accumulation is not always associated with adverse metabolic outcomes, suggesting that TAGs themselves are not pathogenic (2). In contrast, other non-TAG lipid metabolites such as fatty acids (FAs), diacylglycerols (DAGs), and ceramides have been shown to influence glucose homeostasis and insulin action by interfering with insulin signaling and glucose transport, promoting endoplasmic reticulum stress and mitochondrial dysfunction, and activating inflammatory and apoptotic pathways (reviewed in ref. 3). Nevertheless, the precise identities and sources of these bioactive lipid intermediates remain elusive (4,5). Furthermore, whether intracellular TAGs serve as a protective sink or a toxic source of deleterious lipid metabolites that contribute to insulin resistance remains unclear (6).

Since skeletal muscle is the major contributor to insulin-mediated glucose disposal, lipid excess in this tissue could have serious implications for systemic glucose homeostasis and insulin responsiveness (7). Indeed, numerous studies have demonstrated a strong association between intramyocellular triacylglycerol (IMTG) accumulation and insulin resistance (reviewed in ref. 8). In contrast, endurance exercise training is characterized by IMTG accumulation and insulin sensitivity (the athlete's paradox) (2). This variable association between IMTG accumulation and insulin responsiveness has largely been attributed to differences in the balance between lipid delivery and muscle oxidative capacity (8–10). Not surprisingly then, most studies have focused on the impact of muscle FA uptake and/or oxidation on glucose homeostasis and insulin action (11). However, experimental manipulations of these parameters cannot distinguish among the effects of IMTGs, IMTG metabolism, and other lipid intermediates. Furthermore, accumulating evidence suggests that muscle oxidative capacity cannot entirely explain differences in IMTGs or insulin responsiveness (12). These findings have led to speculation that dynamic IMTG metabolism (i.e., TAG synthesis or hydrolysis) may be critically involved in lipid-induced insulin resistance (6). However, few studies have specifically addressed the contribution of IMTG metabolism per se to this process.

The regulated storage and release of IMTGs remain poorly understood, but require the coordinated action of synthetic enzymes (i.e., diacylglycerol acyltransferases [DGATs]), hydrolytic enzymes (i.e., adipose triglyceride lipase [ATGL] and hormone sensitive lipase [HSL]), and other lipid droplet proteins (6). Specifically, modulating IMTG synthesis in murine skeletal muscle alters IMTG content and systemic glucose homeostasis, supporting a role for IMTG metabolism in metabolic disease (13–15). However, the metabolic impact of modulating IMTG hydrolysis in vivo remains unclear. Global deletion of either ATGL (16–19) or HSL (20) has produced variable results.

From the [1]Division of Endocrinology, Department of Medicine, University of Pittsburgh, Pittsburgh, Pennsylvania; the [2]Institute of Molecular Biosciences, University of Graz, Graz, Austria; the [3]Department of Cell Biology, University of Pittsburgh, Pittsburgh, Pennsylvania; the [4]Novartis Institute of Biomedical Research, Cambridge, Massachusetts; the [5]Department of Biochemistry and Molecular Biology, Dalhousie University, Dalhousie Medicine New Brunswick, Saint John, New Brunswick, Canada; and the [6]Department of Health and Physical Activity, University of Pittsburgh, Pittsburgh, Pennsylvania.

Received 4 April 2013 and accepted 10 June 2013.

DOI: 10.2337/db13-0500

This article contains Supplementary Data online at http://diabetes .diabetesjournals.org/lookup/suppl/doi:10.2337/db13-0500/-/DC1.

Corresponding author: Erin E. Kershaw, kershawe@pitt.edu.

M.T.S., M.K.B., and L.C. contributed equally to this work.

The former, but not the latter, results in massive IMTG accumulation with improvement in systemic glucose homeostasis, suggesting that inhibition of ATGL-mediated TAG hydrolysis protects against insulin resistance. In contrast, recent studies in cardiac muscle (21) and other tissues (22,23) indicate that ATGL-mediated TAG hydrolysis is required for mitochondrial function such that enhancing, rather than inhibiting, ATGL action may improve metabolic outcomes. Nevertheless, the autonomous role of skeletal muscle TAG catabolism in influencing muscle-specific and systemic metabolic phenotypes remains unknown.

The goal of the current study was to understand the contribution of IMTG hydrolysis to tissue-specific and systemic metabolic phenotypes, particularly glucose homeostasis and insulin action, in the context of obesity. We therefore generated animal models with decreased (skeletal muscle-specific ATGL knockout [SMAKO] mice) and increased (muscle creatine kinase [Ckm]-ATGL transgenic [Tg] mice) ATGL action exclusively in skeletal muscle, and assessed the metabolic consequences at baseline and in response to chronic high-fat feeding. Interestingly, modulation of IMTG hydrolysis via ATGL action did not significantly influence glucose homeostasis, insulin action, or other metabolic phenotypes in the context of obesity despite dramatic changes in IMTG content.

RESEARCH DESIGN AND METHODS

Animals. SMAKO mice were generated by crossing B6.129-Pnpla2^{tm1Eek} (ATGL-flox) mice with Myo-Cre mice (24). Ckm-ATGL Tg mice were generated by cloning murine ATGL in front of the Ckm promoter (25). B6.129-Pnpla2^{tm1Eek}, SMAKO, and Ckm-ATGL mice were generated as described in Figs. 2A and 5A and the Supplementary Data online. Male ATGL$^{flox/flox}$ Cre/+ mice were mated to female ATGL$^{flox/flox}$ +/+ mice to generate ATGL$^{flox/flox}$ Cre/+ (SMAKO) and ATGL$^{flox/flox}$ +/+ (control) mice. Male Ckm-ATGL Tg mice were mated to female wild-type (WT) mice to generate Tg and WT mice. Global ATGL knockout (ATGL$^{-/-}$ or GAKO) mice have been previously reported (16,17). Mice were housed under standard conditions (25°C, 14:10-h light/dark cycle) with ad libitum access to chow (Prolab Isopro RMH 3000; 14 kcal% fat) or high-fat diet (HFD; Research Diets D12451i, 45 kcal% fat). Body composition, energy expenditure, and metabolic parameters were performed as described (26). Experiments were approved by the University of Pittsburgh Institutional Animal Care and Use Committee and conducted in conformity with the Public Health Service Policy for Care and Use of Laboratory Animals.

Lipid analyses. DAGs (27), ceramides (27), and long-chain FA-CoAs (28) as well as TAG hydrolase activities (26) and radiolabeled palmitate oxidation (29) were determined in muscle homogenates and normalized to tissue wet weight or protein content.

Mitochondrial respiration. Respirometry was performed in permeabilized myofiber bundles using an Oxygraph-2K (Oroboros) (30). Assays were run at 37°C in oxygen-saturated (~150–220 μmol O$_2$) buffer (105 mmol K-MES, 30 mmol KCl, 10 mmol KH$_2$PO$_4$, 5 mmol MgCl$_2$, 5 mg/mL BSA, and 1 mmol EGTA [pH 7.4]) containing 25 μmol blebbistatin using the following titration protocol: 20 μmol palmitoylcarnitine, 2 mmol malate, 4 mmol ADP, 5 mmol glutamate, 10 mmol succinate, 10 μmol cytochrome c, 10 μg/mL oligomycin, and 2 μmol carbonylcyanide-p-trifluoromethoxyphenylhydrazone. Respiration rates were normalized to myofiber dry weight.

Insulin signaling and protein expression. Insulin signaling studies were performed (17) using the following primary antibodies: anti-pAkt (pT308) (4056S; Cell Signaling Technology), anti-pAkt (pS473), and anti-Akt (total) (05-736 and 07-416; EMD Millipore). For protein expression under non–insulin-stimulated conditions, the following antibodies were used: MitoProfile Antibody Cocktail (MS604; Mitosciences), anti-HSL (4017s; Cell Signaling Technology), anti-pHSL (S565 and S660) (4137S and 4126S; Cell Signaling Technology), antiperilipin (Plin)2 (20R-AP002; Fitzgerald Industries), anti-Plin5 (03-GP31; American Research Products), anti-ATGL (2439; Cell Signaling Technology), and anti-CGI58 (NB110-41576; Novus Biologicals). For loading controls, the following antibodies were used: anti-Ran GTPase (610340; BD Biosciences) or β-actin (4970; Cell Signaling Technology). Visualization was performed with Immun-Star WesternC Chemiluminescent Kit in a VersaDoc System and quantified using Quantity One 1-D software (Bio-Rad).

Tissue imaging. Muscles were frozen in isopentane in OCT and cut into 10-μm sections. For muscle morphology, sections were stained with hematoxylin and eosin (H&E). Alternatively, sections were processed for neutral lipid content (using Oil Red O [ORO]) and/or expression of specific proteins (using ATGL or other antibodies noted above) either alone or in combination with fiber type–specific antibodies from the Developmental Studies Hybridoma Bank (A4.840 [1], A4.74 [2A], 6H1 [2X], 10F5 [2B]) followed by secondary antibodies (A21044 and A10035; Invitrogen) (31). At least four random areas were visualized (DM4000B; Leica Microsystems), digitally captured (Retiga-2000R; QImaging), and quantified (Northern Eclipse; Empix Imaging). For transmission electron microscopy (TEM), muscles were fixed in 2.5% glutaraldehyde, postfixed in 1% osmium tetroxide, dehydrated, embedded in epon, and evaluated by TEM (JEM-1011; JEOL).

Gene expression. RNA extraction, reverse transcription, and gene expression analysis were performed using an Eppendorf Realplex System in accordance with Minimum Information for Publication of Quantitative Real-Time PCR Experiments (MIQE) guidelines (17,26).

Statistical analysis. Results are expressed as mean ± SEM. Comparisons were made by unpaired two-tailed Student t test or factorial ANOVA followed by determination of simple effects for pairwise comparisons. If indicated, comparisons were made by two-way ANOVA with repeated measures. For energy expenditure data, comparisons were made using generalized estimate equations. P values of <0.05 were considered statistically significant.

RESULTS

Endogenous ATGL expression in murine skeletal muscle is fiber type–specific and regulated by HFD feeding. Fiber type–specific quantitative immunofluorescence (IF) revealed that endogenous ATGL was predominantly expressed in type 2A and 2X fibers with lower expression in type 1 fibers and minimal expression in type 2B fibers (Fig. 1A and C and Supplementary Fig. 1A and B). Conversely, global deletion of ATGL resulted in fiber type–specific accumulation of IMTGs in types 2A, 2X, and 1 fibers (Fig. 1B and Supplementary Fig. 1C). The distribution of these fibers differs among murine muscles (Supplementary Fig. 1D). Endogenous ATGL protein directly correlated with IMTG content (Fig. 1E) and also increased in parallel with IMTGs following HFD feeding (Fig. 1C–E). Thus, endogenous ATGL is expressed and functional in type 2A > 2X > 1 murine muscle fibers and increases with diet-induced obesity.

Reducing IMTG hydrolysis via ATGL deletion increases IMTG content and subspecies of DAGs, but does not significantly influence other intramyocellular lipids or systemic lipid homeostasis. To reduce IMTG hydrolysis, SMAKO mice were generated by crossing ATGL-flox mice with Myo-Cre mice (24) (Fig. 2A). SMAKO mice had reduced ATGL mRNA (Fig. 2B) and protein (Fig. 2C) in skeletal but not cardiac muscle or other tissues. Accordingly, TAG hydrolase activity in skeletal muscle of SMAKO mice was dramatically reduced, could not be stimulated with the ATGL coactivator CGI-58, and was completely blunted in the presence of an HSL inhibitor (Fig. 2D). General muscle morphology did not differ between genotypes (Fig. 2E, top). Fiber type–specific quantitative IF of IMTG content, which is more sensitive and specific than whole-muscle biochemical IMTG analysis, revealed a dramatic fiber type–specific (2A > 2X > 1, but not 2B) increase in IMTGs in skeletal muscle of SMAKO mice that was comparable to GAKO mice (Fig. 2E and F). Cardiac muscle, in contrast, was unaffected (Supplementary Fig. 2). Lipidomic analysis of skeletal muscle (Fig. 2G) revealed no significant genotype effect on total DAGs, ceramides, or FA-CoAs. However, there was a trend toward increased total DAGs similar to GAKO mice (17). A detailed analysis of lipid classes in skeletal muscle revealed an effect of genotype on a few subspecies of DAGs (C14:0/C16:0-DAG, C14:0/C18:0-DAG, and C16:0/C18:0-DAG) and FA-CoAs (C14:0 and C16:0) (Supplementary Fig. 3). Finally, serum

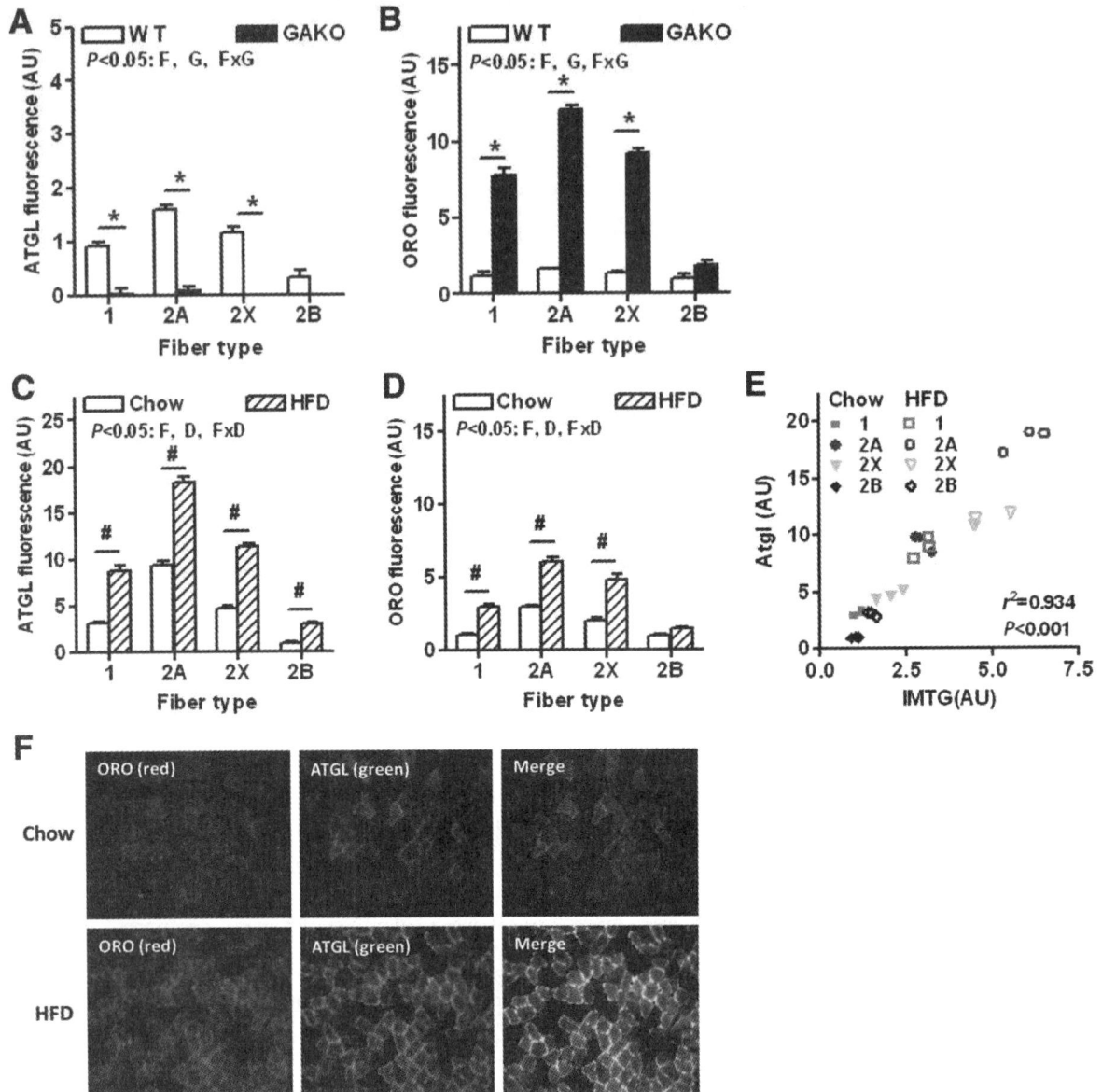

FIG. 1. Fiber type–specific expression of endogenous ATGL in murine skeletal muscle and regulation by HFD feeding. ATGL protein expression (ATGL IF in 2B fibers of GAKO mice set to 0) (*A*) and IMTG content by ORO staining (ORO IF of 2B fibers of WT mice set to 1) (*B*) in skeletal muscle fibers of chow-fed WT versus GAKO mice (♀, chow, 10 weeks, C57BL/6, gastrocnemius-plantaris-soleus [GPS] complex; *n* = 3 to 4/group). ATGL protein expression (ATGL IF in 2B fibers of WT-chow mice set to 1) (*C*) and IMTG content by ORO staining (ORO IF in 2B fibers of WT-chow mice set to 1) (*D*) in skeletal muscle fibers of chow- versus HFD-fed WT mice (♀, 22 weeks FVB, GPS complex; *n* = 3 to 4/group). *E*: Relationship between ATGL and IMTG (data from *C* and *D*). *F*: Representative images of ATGL and ORO IF in chow- and HFD-fed mice demonstrating overlap and enhanced staining with HFD. For overall effects having *P* < 0.05: D, diet; F, fiber type; G, genotype. For specific comparisons having *P* < 0.05: #for effect of diet; *for effect of genotype. AU, arbitrary units.

TAGs (Control-HFD 60 ± 5 vs. SMAKO-HFD 62 ± 5 mg/dL) and nonesterified FAs (Control-HFD 0.59 ± 0.05 vs. SMAKO-HFD 0.65 ± 0.06 mEq/L) did not differ between genotypes. Thus, decreasing IMTG hydrolysis via ATGL increases certain subspecies of DAGs and tends to increase total DAGs, but does not produce significant changes in other non-TAG intramyocellular lipids or systemic lipid homeostasis despite dramatic increases in IMTG content. **Reducing IMTG hydrolysis via ATGL deletion increases lipid droplet proteins but does not influence mitochondrial phenotypes.** Skeletal muscle FA oxidation increased with HFD feeding but was unaffected by genotype (Fig. 3*A*). Likewise, mitochondrial respiration in isolated

muscle fibers failed to identify any genotype effects in basal, substrate-stimulated, or uncoupled conditions (Fig. 3*B*). Consistent with these results, expression of mitochondrial oxidative phosphorylation proteins was not different between genotypes (Fig. 3*C*). Furthermore, imaging by TEM (Fig. 3*D*) and confocal microscopy (Supplementary Fig. 4) revealed no differences between genotypes for mitochondrial morphology or number, despite massive increases in lipid droplet size and number. Gene expression analysis revealed an increase in peroxisome proliferator–activated receptor (PPAR) α expression in chow- but not HFD-fed SMAKO mice (although threshold cycle was >35 using undiluted cDNA), but no effect of genotype on PPARδ, PPAR-γ

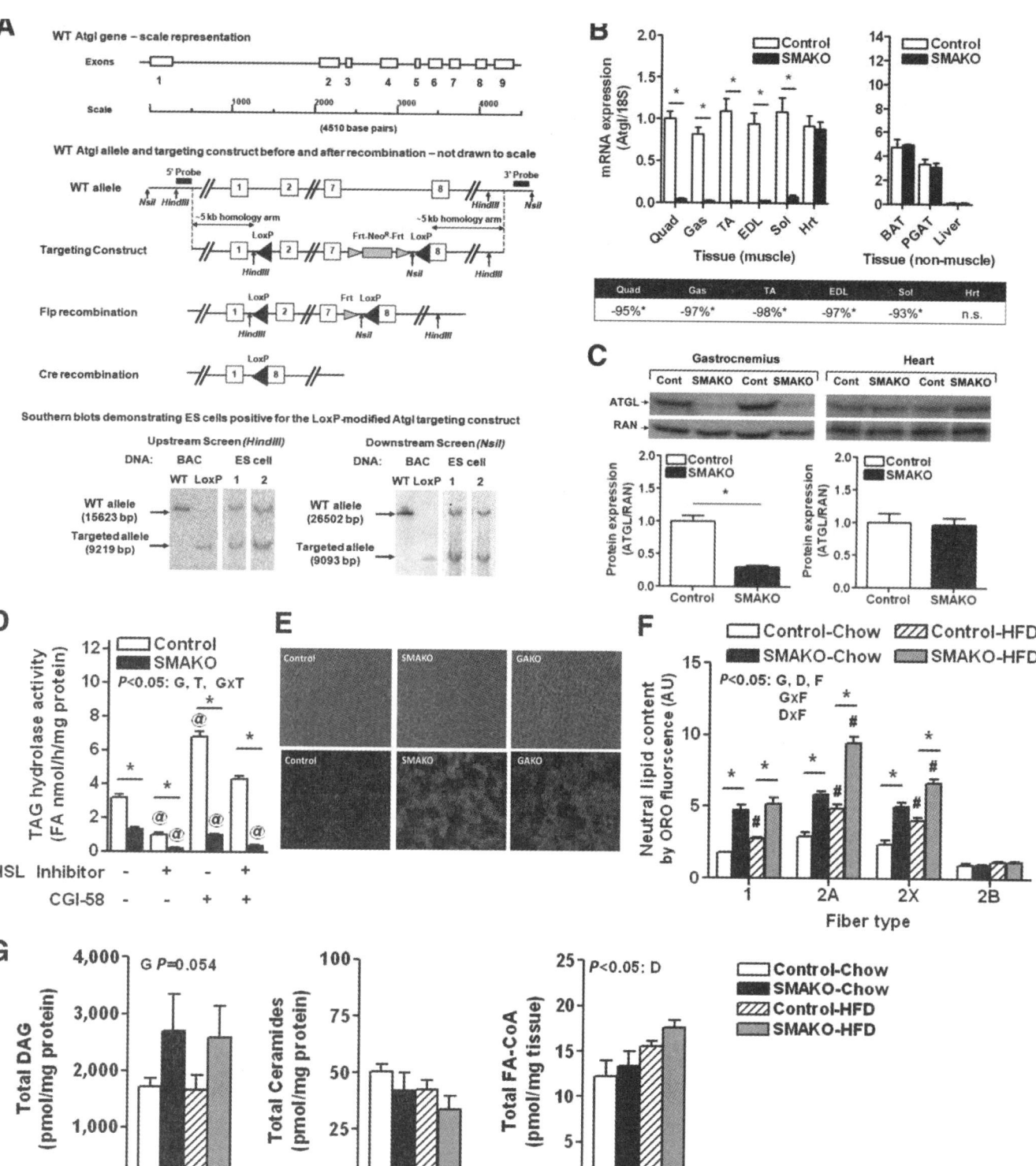

FIG. 2. Skeletal muscle–specific ATGL deletion and its impact on lipid homeostasis in SMAKO mice. *A*: The LoxP-modified ATGL construct. *B*: ATGL mRNA expression relative to 18S control gene by quantitative PCR in muscle and nonmuscle tissues with endogenous ATGL expression in quadriceps arbitrarily set to 1 (♀, 10 weeks, chow, fasted 12 h; *n* = 5 to 6/group). Percent decrease in ATGL mRNA expression in SMAKO relative to WT mice for select muscle tissues is shown in the table (*bottom*). *C*: ATGL protein expression relative to Ran GTPase (RAN) control in skeletal versus cardiac muscle (♀, 10 weeks, chow, fasted 12 h, gastrocnemius and heart; *n* = 5 to 6/group). *D*: TAG hydrolase activity at baseline and in the presence of the HSL-specific inhibitor 76-0079, the ATGL-specific activator CGI-58, or HSL inhibitor plus CGI-58 (♂, 28 weeks, chow, fasted 12 h, red gastrocnemius; *n* = 6/group). *E*: Skeletal muscle histology of control (*left*), SMAKO (*middle*), and GAKO (*right*) mice including general morphology by H&E staining (*top*) and IMTG content by ORO staining (*bottom*) (♂, 28 weeks, chow, fasted 12 h, gastrocnemius-plantaris-soleus [GPS] complex). *F*: IMTG content by ORO staining using quantitative IF (♂, 28 weeks, fasted 12 h, GPS complex, average of four muscle areas each; *n* = 4/group). Type 2B fibers of chow-fed WT mice are arbitrarily set to 1. *G*: Intramyocellular DAG, ceramide, and FA-CoA content using biochemical analysis of whole muscle (♂, 28 weeks, fasted 12 h, quadriceps; *n* = 3 to 4/group). For overall effects having *P* < 0.05: D, diet; F, fiber type; G, genotype; T, treatment (with HSL-inhibitor or CGI-58). For specific comparisons having *P* < 0.05: #for effect of diet; *for effect of genotype; and @for effect of treatment. AU, arbitrary units; BAC, bacterial artificial chromosome; BAT, brown adipose tissue; D, diet; EDL, extensor digitorum longus; ES, embryonic stem; Gas, gastrocnemius; Hrt, heart; PGAT, perigonadal adipose tissue; Quad, quadriceps; Sol, soleus; TA, tibialis anterior.

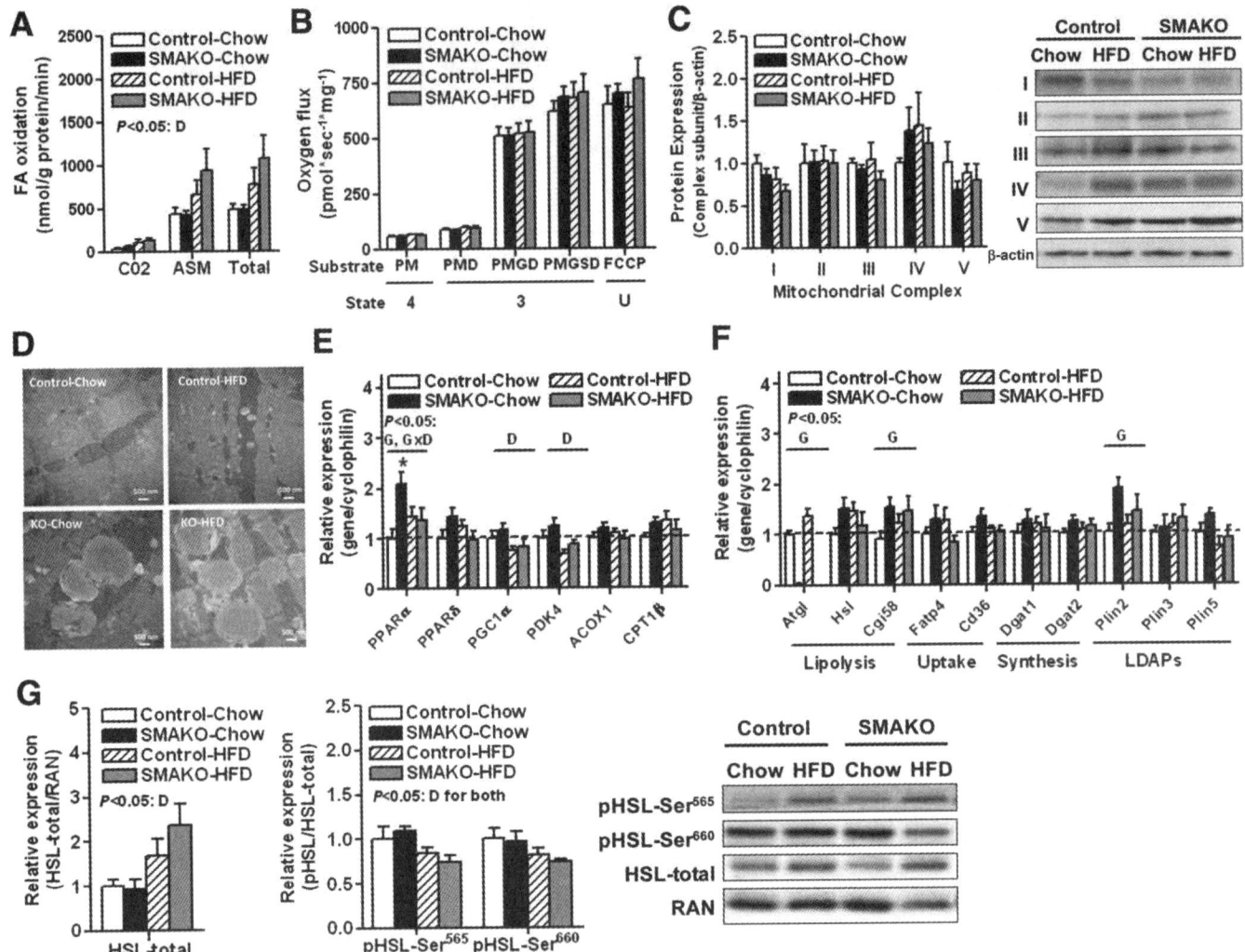

FIG. 3. Skeletal muscle mitochondrial function and expression of genes/proteins regulating lipid homeostasis in SMAKO mice. *A*: FA oxidation (♂, 28 weeks, fasted 12 h, red gastrocnemius; $n = 6$/group). ^{14}C-labeled incorporation into CO_2 and acid-soluble metabolites (ASMs) represent complete and incomplete oxidation, respectively. *B*: Mitochondrial respiration in permeabilized muscle fibers (♂, 28 weeks, fasted 12 h, soleus; $n = 6$/group). Oxygen consumption was measured following the sequential addition of the following substrates: palmitoylcarnitine (P), malate (M), ADP (D), glutamate (G), succinate (S), and cytochrome c, oligomycin, and carbonylcyanide-*p*-trifluoromethoxyphenylhydrazone (FCCP). The corresponding respiratory states are noted: ADP-driven respiration (state 3), respiration in the absence of ADP (state 4), and uncoupled respiration (state U). *C*: Expression of oxidative phosphorylation proteins in complexes I–V (NDUFB8 [complex I], SDHB [complex II], UQCRC2 [complex III], MTCO1 [complex IV], and ATP5A [complex V]) (♂, 28 weeks, fasted 12 h, tibialis anterior; $n = 6$/group). Data are normalized to protein expression of β-actin. *D*: TEM of skeletal muscle (♂, 28 weeks, fasted 12 h, red quadriceps, representative images). mRNA expression of PPARα/PGC1α and their target genes (*E*) and genes for lipid breakdown (lipolysis), uptake, and synthesis as well as lipid droplet–associated proteins (LDAPs) of the Plin family (*F*) relative to cyclophilin control with expression in WT-chow normalized to 1 (♂, 28 weeks, tibialis anterior; $n = 9$–13/group). *G*: Protein expression of total HSL normalized to Ran GTPase (RAN) control (*left*), phosphorylated HSL normalized to total HSL (*middle*), and representative immunoblots (*right*) (♂, 28 weeks, tibialis anterior; $n = 4$/group). For mRNA and protein expression, samples were confirmed to have low or no expression of Plin1, thereby confirming absence of significant fat contamination. For overall effects having $P < 0.05$: D, diet; G, genotype. Where an interaction was identified, specific comparisons having $P < 0.05$: *for effect of genotype.

coactivator (PGC) 1α, or PPAR target genes (Fig. 3*E*). ATGL mRNA expression was clearly decreased (>90%) in SMAKO muscle (Fig. 3*F*). However, expression of total HSL mRNA (Fig. 3*F*) and protein (Fig. 3*G*) as well as phosphorylation of HSL at Ser565 (AMPK target site, negative regulator of HSL action) and Ser660 (ERK target site, positive regulator of HSL action) (Fig. 3*G*) were unchanged. Likewise, no effects of genotype were identified on mRNA expression for genes involved in lipid uptake (FATP1 and CD36) or synthesis (DGAT1 and DGAT2). In contrast, CGI-58 and Plin2/Adrp mRNA (Fig. 3*F*) as well as CGI-58, Plin2/Adrp, and Plin5/Oxpat protein (Supplementary Fig. 5) were increased in SMAKO mice. However, these mechanisms were clearly

inadequate to compensate for loss of ATGL. Thus, reduced TAG hydrolysis in skeletal muscle does not influence lipid oxidation or mitochondrial phenotypes.

Reducing IMTG hydrolysis via ATGL deletion does not influence systemic energy homeostasis, glucose homeostasis, or insulin action. As expected, HFD feeding increased adiposity (Fig. 4*A* and *B*), altered energy substrate utilization (Fig. 4*E*), and impaired both glucose tolerance (Fig. 4*F*) and insulin sensitivity (Fig. 4*G*–*K*). In contrast, there were no effects of genotype on body weight (Fig. 4*A*), fat mass (Fig. 4*B*), lean mass (Fig. 4*C*), individual muscle weights (Fig. 4*D*), nonmuscle tissue weights (data not shown), or total energy intake and expenditure (data

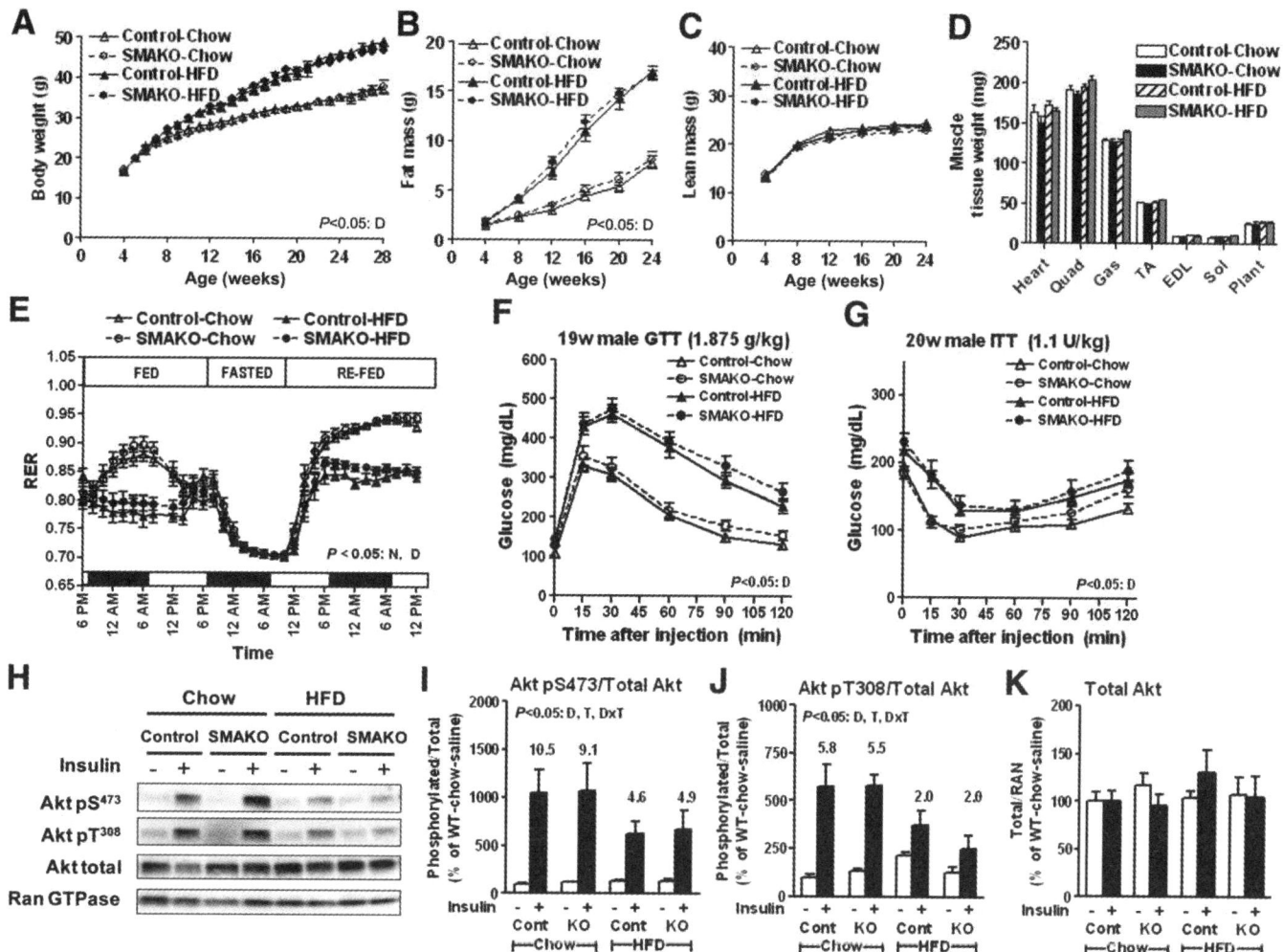

FIG. 4. Energy/glucose homeostasis and insulin action in SMAKO mice. Body weight (*A*), fat mass (*B*), and lean mass (*C*) (♂, 3–28 weeks; *n* ≥ 19/group). *D*: Muscle weights. With the exception of heart, data represent the average weight for both muscles from each mouse (♂, 28 weeks, fasted 12 h; *n* ≥ 19/group). EDL, extensor digitorum longus; Gas, gastrocnemius; Hrt, heart; Plant, plantaris; Quad, quadriceps; Sol, soleus; TA, tibialis anterior. *E*: RER using a Comprehensive Lab Animal Monitoring System (CLAMS) (♂, 11 weeks, weight-matched; *n* = 4/group). *F*: GTT at 19 weeks with 1.875 g/kg glucose i.p. (♂, fasted 12 h; *n* = 17–20/group). *G*: ITT at 20 weeks with 1.1 units/kg insulin i.p. (♂, fasted 4 h; *n* = 17–20/group). *H–K*: Insulin signaling studies: mice were fasted for 12 h, injected i.p. with saline or insulin at 10 units/kg body weight, and killed 10 min thereafter (♂, 28 weeks, tibialis anterior; *n* = 5–7/group). Representative immunoblots (*H*) and associated quantification of stoichiometric phosphorylation of Akt pS^{473}/Akt total (*I*), Akt pT^{308}/Akt total (*J*), and total Akt/Ran GTPase (RAN) control (*K*). Fold change in response to insulin treatment is indicated above the black bars. For overall effects having *P* < 0.05: D, diet; G, genotype; N, nutritional status (i.e., fasting/refeeding); T, treatment (i.e., with insulin). For clarity, only overall effects are shown.

not shown). Although alterations in IMTG metabolism could influence metabolic flexibility without affecting overall energy homeostasis, energy utilization (respiratory exchange ratio) during ad lib feeding, fasting, and refeeding transitions was likewise unchanged between genotypes (Fig. 4*E'*). In addition, no differences in serum glucose were identified between genotypes following a physiological (4-h) fast (Fig. 4*G*, time 0 of insulin tolerance test [ITT]), a prolonged (12-h) fast (Fig. 4*F*, time 0 of glucose tolerance test [GTT]), an intraperitoneal glucose challenge (Fig. 4*F*, GTT), or an intraperitoneal insulin challenge (Fig. 4*G*, ITT). Consistent with these findings, diet but not genotype effects were identified in skeletal muscle–specific insulin-stimulated phosphorylation of key proteins in the insulin signaling cascade including insulin receptor substrate 1 (data not shown) and Akt (Akt pS^{473} or Akt pT^{308}) (Fig. 4*H–K*). Thus, decreasing IMTG hydrolysis via ATGL deletion does not influence systemic energy homeostasis in the setting of acute or chronic nutritional challenges, nor does

it influence systemic or muscle-specific glucose homeostasis and insulin action.

Increasing IMTG hydrolysis via ATGL overexpression decreases IMTG content but does not change other intramyocellular lipids or systemic lipid homeostasis. To increase IMTG hydrolysis, we generated skeletal muscle–specific Ckm-ATGL Tg mice (Fig. 5*A*). Tg founder lines had increased ATGL mRNA (Fig. 5*B*) and protein (Fig. 5*C*) in skeletal but not cardiac muscle or other tissues. Notably, skeletal muscle ATGL mRNA expression in Tg mice was comparable to endogenous ATGL expression in adipose tissue (32). IF analysis confirmed an increase in ATGL protein expression within all skeletal muscle fiber types of Tg mice (Fig. 5*D* and *E*). Thus, ATGL transgene expression overlaps with endogenous ATGL expression. Tg muscle TAG hydrolase activity also increased in an ATGL-specific manner since it was increased in the presence of an HSL inhibitor (Fig. 5*F*). General muscle morphology did not differ between

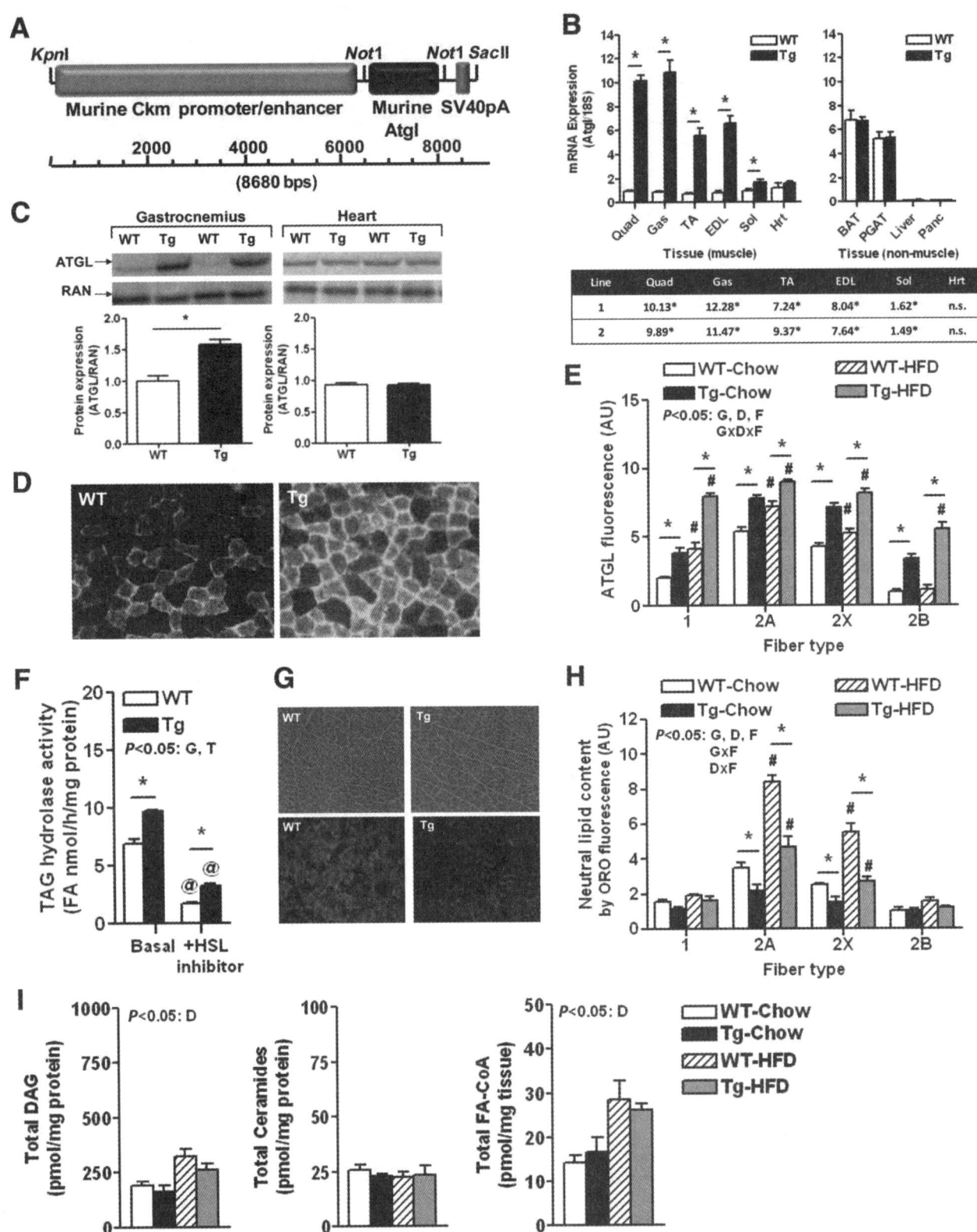

FIG. 5. Skeletal muscle–specific overexpression of ATGL and its impact on lipid homeostasis. *A*: The Ckm-ATGL transgene construct. *B*: ATGL mRNA expression relative to 18S control gene by quantitative PCR in muscle and nonmuscle tissues with endogenous ATGL expression in quadriceps arbitrarily set to 1 (Line 1, ♀, 8 weeks, chow, fasted 12 h; *n* = 4–5/group). The fold-increase in ATGL mRNA expression in Tg relative to WT mice for select muscle tissues in each of two founder lines is shown in the table (*bottom*). *C*: ATGL protein expression relative to Ran GTPase (RAN) control as determined by immunoblotting in skeletal versus cardiac muscle (Line 1, ♀, 17 weeks, chow, fasted 12 h, gastrocnemius and heart; *n* = 6/group). *D*: ATGL IF in skeletal muscle (Line 1, ♂, 17 weeks, chow, fasted 12 h, gastrocnemius). *E*: Quantitative fiber type–specific ATGL protein expression by IF (Line 1, ♂, 28 weeks, chow and HFD, fasted 12 h, gastrocnemius-plantaris-soleus [GPS] complex, average of four muscle areas each; *n* = 4/group). Type 2B fibers of chow-fed WT mice are arbitrarily set to 1. *F*: TAG hydrolase activity in the absence (basal) and presence of the HSL-specific inhibitor 76-0079 (Line 1, ♂, 12 weeks, chow, fasted 12 h, gastrocnemius; *n* = 3/group). *G*: Skeletal muscle histology of

genotypes (Fig. 5G, top). However, IMTGs were dramatically decreased in Tg mice with the greatest reduction in type 2A and 2X fibers (Fig. 5G and H). Lipidomic analysis of skeletal muscle (Fig. 5I) revealed no genotype effects on total DAGs, ceramides, or FA-CoAs. Furthermore, there was an effect of diet but not genotype on multiple subspecies of DAGs, ceramides, and FA-CoAs, with the only exceptions being reduced C16:0 ceramide and sphingosine (Supplementary Fig. 6). Furthermore, serum concentrations of TAGs (WT-HFD 122 ± 12 vs. Tg-HFD 126 ± 12 mg/dL) and nonesterified FAs (WT-HFD 0.62 ± 0.05 vs. Tg-HFD 0.59 ± 0.07 mEq/L) did not differ between genotypes. Thus, increasing IMTG hydrolysis via ATGL overexpression does not produce major changes in non-TAG intramyocellular lipids or systemic lipid homeostasis despite dramatic reductions in IMTG content.

Increasing IMTG hydrolysis via ATGL overexpression does not influence other pathways of lipid metabolism or mitochondrial phenotypes. As with SMAKO mice, FA oxidation was increased by HFD feeding but was unaffected by genotype (Fig. 6A). Likewise, mitochondrial respiration in isolated muscle fibers (Fig. 6B) and expression of mitochondrial proteins (Fig. 6C) did not differ between genotypes. Furthermore, TEM revealed no differences between genotypes for mitochondrial morphology or number, despite a clear reduction in lipid droplet size and number (Fig. 6D). Gene expression analysis revealed diet but not genotype effects on PPARα, PPARδ, PGC1α, and their target genes (Fig. 6E). ATGL mRNA expression was clearly increased (>12-fold) in skeletal muscle of Tg mice (Fig. 6F). However, expression of total HSL mRNA (Fig. 6F) and protein (Fig. 6G) as well as phosphorylation of HSL at Ser565 and Ser660 (Fig. 6G) were unchanged in Tg mice. Likewise, expression of other genes involved in lipid uptake, lipid synthesis, and/or modulation of ATGL action were not affected by genotype. Thus, in striking contrast to adipocyte specific overexpression of ATGL (23), increasing IMTG hydrolysis via ATGL overexpression has minimal to no effect on other lipid metabolic pathways or mitochondrial phenotypes.

Increasing IMTG hydrolysis via ATGL overexpression does not influence systemic energy homeostasis, glucose homeostasis, or insulin action. Again, the expected effects of HFD feeding were noted. However, there were no effects of genotype on body weight (Fig. 7A), fat mass (Fig. 7B), lean mass (Fig. 7C), individual muscle weights (Fig. 7D), nonmuscle tissue weights (data not shown), total energy intake and energy expenditure (data not shown), or respiratory exchange ratio (RER) during fed-fasted-refed conditions (metabolic flexibility) (Fig. 7E). In addition, no differences in serum glucose were identified between genotypes following a physiological (4-h) fast (Fig. 7G, time 0 of ITT), a prolonged (12-h) fast (Fig. 7F, time 0 of GTT), an intraperitoneal glucose challenge (Fig. 7F, GTT), or an intraperitoneal insulin challenge (Fig. 7G, ITT). Consistent with these findings, diet but not genotype effects were identified in skeletal muscle–specific

insulin-stimulated phosphorylation of key proteins in the insulin signaling cascade including insulin receptor substrate 1 (data not shown) and Akt (Akt pS473 or Akt pT308) (Fig. 7H–K). Thus, increasing IMTG hydrolysis via ATGL overexpression does not influence systemic energy homeostasis or either systemic or muscle-specific glucose homeostasis and insulin action.

DISCUSSION

The goal of the current study was to determine the role of IMTGs and IMTG hydrolysis in skeletal muscle and whole-body metabolism at baseline and in response to diet-induced obesity. Remarkably, we demonstrate that modulation of IMTG content and hydrolysis by altering ATGL action in skeletal muscle does not influence systemic energy, lipid, or glucose homeostasis, nor does it influence muscle-specific insulin action or mitochondrial function. The absence of profound metabolic phenotypes in skeletal muscle–specific ATGL mutant mice is striking considering the dramatic changes in IMTG hydrolysis and accumulation. These data provide compelling evidence that IMTG content, while often highly associated with insulin resistance and metabolic disease, is not causal in these disorders. These data further indicate that modulating IMTG hydrolysis neither promotes nor protects against deleterious metabolic consequences of obesity.

Although the effects of skeletal muscle lipid uptake and oxidation on glucose homeostasis and insulin action have been extensively studied (11), the metabolic consequences of IMTG metabolism itself remain less well-understood (6). With regards to IMTG synthesis, increasing muscle DGAT1 in vivo promotes insulin sensitivity (13,14), whereas increasing DGAT2 promotes insulin resistance (15). While both interventions similarly increase IMTG content, they differentially affect other non-TAG lipid metabolites (ceramides), suggesting that the latter rather than the former influences metabolic phenotypes. Thus, different proteins may have different metabolic effects, despite affecting similar metabolic pathways. With regards to IMTG hydrolysis, acutely modulating ATGL or HSL action in cultured human myotubes alters DAGs and disrupts glucose homeostasis and insulin action (33). However, the current study indicates that chronically modulating ATGL action in murine skeletal muscle in vivo fails to influence metabolic phenotypes. Several potential adaptations (i.e., increased CGI-58, Plin2, and Plin5 in SMAKO mice) may protect against lipid-induced insulin resistance but are clearly not sufficient to fully compensate for altered IMTG hydrolysis. These data indicate that changing IMTG content by altering IMTG hydrolysis is not pathogenic. The validity of these conclusions is supported by the finding that comparable changes in IMTG content by altering IMTG synthesis are sufficient to influence metabolic outcomes (13–15), whereas changes in IMTG hydrolysis are not.

Interestingly, enhancing IMTG hydrolysis in vivo has minimal effect on non-TAG lipid metabolites, and inhibiting

---

control (*left*) and Tg (*right*) mice including general morphology by H&E staining (*top*) and IMTG content by ORO staining (*bottom*) (Line 1, ♂, 12 weeks, HFD for 4 weeks, fasted 12 h, GPS complex). *H*: IMTG content by ORO staining using quantitative IF (Line 1, ♂, 28 weeks, chow and HFD, fasted 12 h, GPS complex, average of four muscle areas each; *n* = 4/group). Type 2B fibers of chow-fed WT mice are arbitrarily set to 1. *I*: Intramyocellular DAG, ceramide, and FA-CoA content using biochemical analysis of whole muscle (Line 1, ♂, 28 weeks, chow and HFD, fasted 12 h, quadriceps; *n* = 3/group). For overall effects having *P* < 0.05: D, diet; F, fiber type; G, genotype; T, treatment (with HSL-inhibitor). For specific comparisons having *P* < 0.05: #for effect of diet; *for effect of genotype; and @for effect of treatment. AU, arbitrary units; BAT, brown adipose tissue; EDL, extensor digitorum longus; Gas, gastrocnemius; Hrt, heart; Panc, pancreas; PGAT, perigonadal adipose tissue; Quad, quadriceps; Sol, soleus; TA, tibialis anterior.

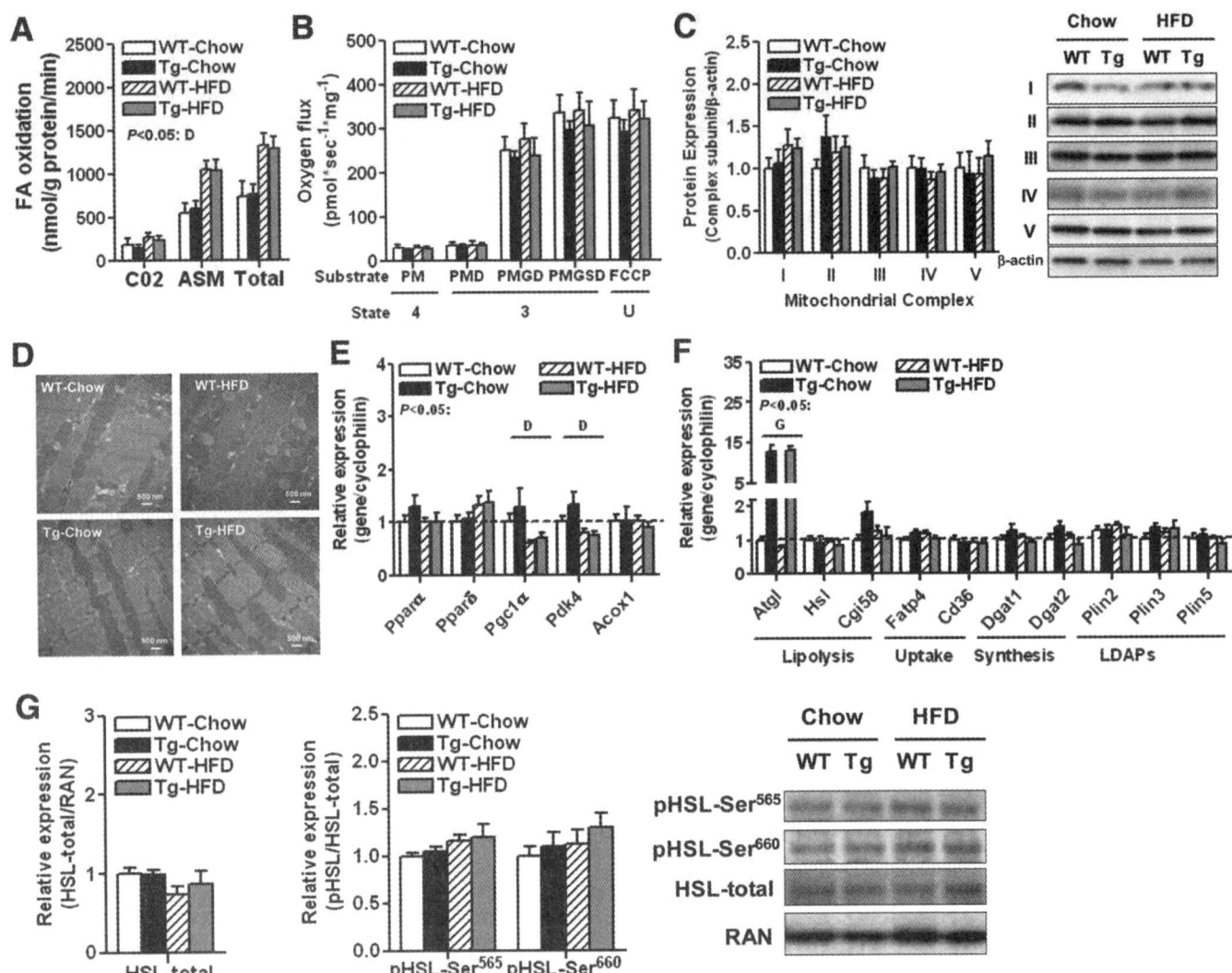

FIG. 6. Skeletal muscle mitochondrial function and expression of genes/proteins regulating lipid homeostasis in Ckm-ATGL mice. *A*: FA oxidation (♂, 28 weeks, fasted 12 h, red gastrocnemius; n = 5–8/group). *B*: Mitochondrial respiration in permeabilized muscle fibers (♂, 34 weeks, fasted 12 h, extensor digitorum longus; n = 3–6/group). *C*: Expression of oxidative phosphorylation proteins in complexes I–V (♂, 34 weeks, fasted 12 h, tibialis anterior; n = 4–7/group). Data are normalized to protein expression of β-actin. *D*: TEM of skeletal muscle (♂, 34 weeks, fasted 12 h, red quadriceps, representative images). mRNA expression of PPARα/PGC1α and their target genes (*E*) and genes for lipid breakdown (lipolysis), uptake, and synthesis as well as lipid droplet–associated proteins (LDAPs) of the Plin family (*F*) relative to cyclophilin control with expression in WT-chow normalized to 1 (♂, 34 weeks, tibialis anterior; n = 7–21/group). *G*: Protein expression of total HSL normalized to Ran GTPase (RAN) control (*left*), phosphorylated HSL normalized to total HSL (*middle*), and representative immunoblots (*right*) (♂, 34 weeks, tibialis anterior; n = 5–7/group). For mRNA and protein expression, samples were confirmed to have low or no expression of Plin1, thereby confirming absence of significant fat contamination. For overall effects having $P < 0.05$: D, diet; G, genotype.

IMTG hydrolysis increases certain subspecies of DAGs and tends to increase rather than decrease total DAGs. The lack of DAG accumulation with ATGL overexpression is likely due to sufficient residual capacity to further metabolize DAGs relative to the amount produced by IMTG hydrolysis. Furthermore, recent evidence suggests that the specific DAG species generated by ATGL cannot be directly used for phospholipid synthesis or activation of protein kinase C, mechanisms by which DAGs have been shown to influence glucose homoeostasis and insulin action (34). The reason why DAGs accumulate with ATGL deletion is less clear but also occurs in mice with global deletion of ATGL (17) and knockdown of the ATGL coactivator CGI-58 (35). Studies of the latter suggest that the increase in DAGs may result from compensatory increases in DAG synthesis without concomitant increases in TAG synthesis (35) and further suggests that the lack of

a physiological effect likely results from their subcellular localization to lipid droplets rather than membranes (35). Besides subcellular localization, the type of DAG stereoisomer (i.e., sn-1–2 vs. sn-1–3 vs. sni-2–3) and FA composition may also contribute to the dissociation between DAG concentrations and insulin responsiveness (5). Hence, modulating IMTG hydrolysis in vivo may not influence glucose homeostasis and insulin responsiveness because it does not produce physiologically relevant changes in the amount or cellular localization of specific bioactive non-TAG lipid metabolites.

In contrast, altering TAG hydrolysis could also affect metabolic phenotypes by influencing mitochondrial function via activation of PPAR nuclear transcription factors. A role for ATGL-mediated TAG hydrolysis in ligand-dependent (36) and ligand-independent (37,38) PPARα activation has been demonstrated in nonskeletal muscle

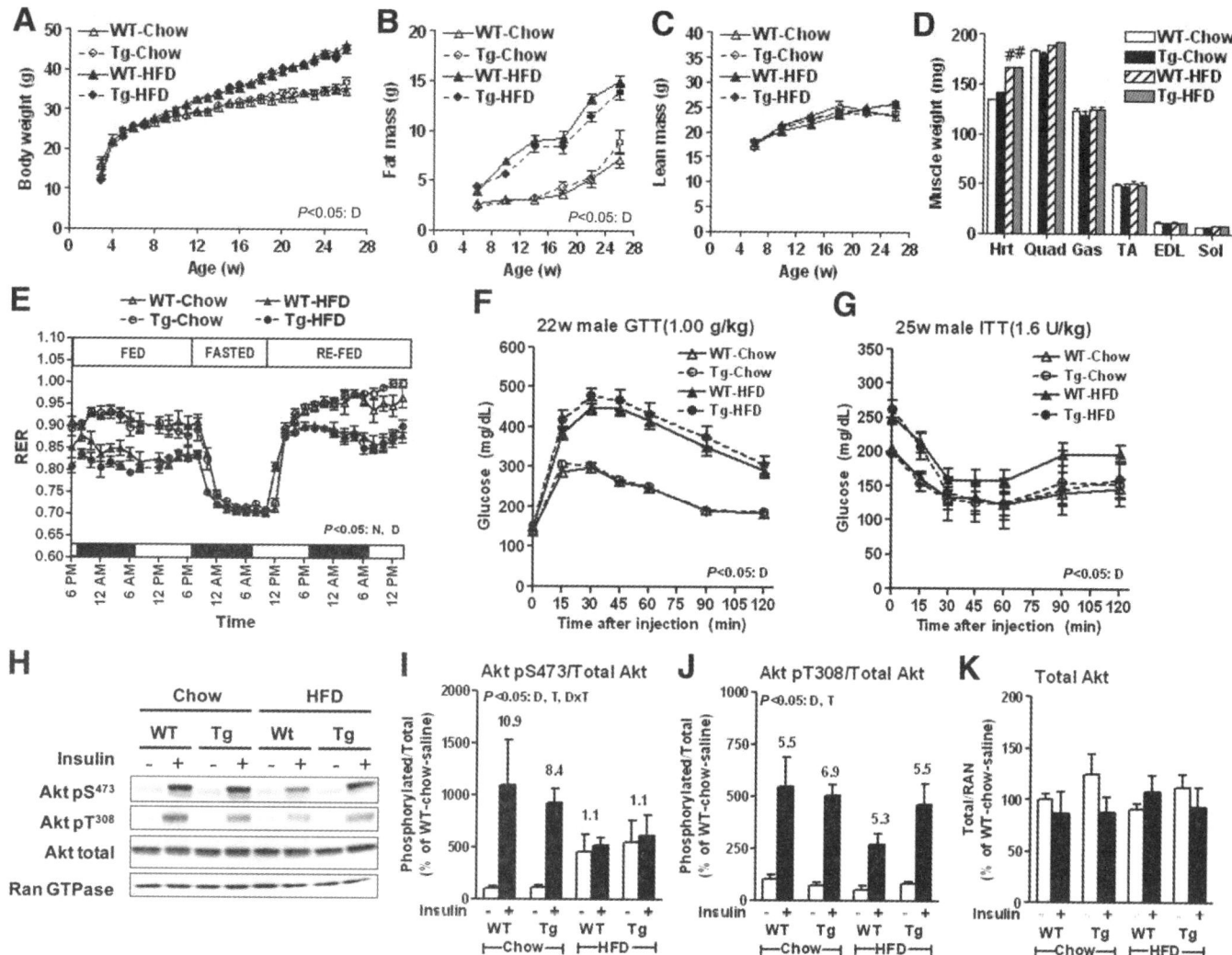

FIG. 7. Energy/glucose homeostasis and insulin action in Ckm-ATGL mice. Body weight (*A*), fat mass (*B*), and lean mass (*C*) (Line 1, ♂, 3–26 weeks; $n \geq 12$/group). *D*: Muscle weights (nonmuscle tissue weights also showed no genotype effects; data not shown). With the exception of heart, data represent the average weight for both muscles from each mouse (Line 1, ♂, 28 weeks, fasted 12 h; $n \geq 24$/group). EDL, extensor digitorum longus; Gas, gastrocnemius; Hrt, heart; Quad, quadriceps; Sol, soleus; TA, tibialis anterior. *E*: RER using a Comprehensive Lab Animal Monitoring System (CLAMS) (Line 1, ♂, 9 weeks, weight-matched; $n = 4$/group). *F*: GTT at 22 weeks with 1.0 g/kg glucose i.p. (♂, fasted 12 h; $n = 7$–22/group). *G*: ITT at 25 weeks with 1.6 units/kg insulin i.p. (Line 1, ♂, fasted 4 h; $n = 7$–22/group). *H–K*: Insulin signaling studies: Mice were fasted for 12 h, injected i.p. with saline or insulin at 10 units/kg body weight, and killed 10 min thereafter (♂, 34 weeks, tibialis anterior; $n = 5$–7/group). Representative immunoblots (*H*) and associated quantification of stoichiometric phosphorylation of Akt pS^{473}/Akt total (*I*), Akt pT^{308}/Akt total (*J*), and total Akt/Ran GTPase control (*K*). Fold change in response to insulin treatment is indicated above the black bars. For overall effects having $P < 0.05$: D, diet; N, nutritional status (i.e., fasting/refeeding); T, treatment (i.e., with insulin). For clarity, only overall effects are shown. For simple effects in *D*, #$P < 0.05$ for effect of diet.

cells. The physiological relevance of these findings has been corroborated in vivo in adipose tissue (23,39) and cardiac muscle (21). More recently, it has been shown that indirect modulation of ATGL action via its coactivator CGI-58 in human myotubes (40) or via Plin5 in rat muscle (41) influences PPAR target genes and mitochondrial function. Unexpectedly, changes in ATGL-mediated TAG hydrolysis in skeletal muscle in vivo do not significantly impact these parameters. These results are consistent with reports demonstrating IMTG accumulation but unaltered in vivo mitochondrial function in skeletal muscle of GAKO (42) and muscle-specific CGI-58 knockout mice (43). Thus, in striking contrast to cardiac muscle (21), in vivo modulation of TAG hydrolysis in skeletal muscle does not influence PPAR target genes or mitochondrial phenotypes.

The divergent consequences of altering IMTG hydrolysis in cardiac versus skeletal muscle may be due to differences in metabolic flux (10,44). In cardiac muscle (variable energy supply, chronically high energy demand), it has been proposed that FAs are preferentially directed to IMTG storage followed by coordinated ATGL-mediated release as energy substrates and PPAR ligands, thereby coupling hydrolysis to oxidation (21). In skeletal muscle (variable energy supply and demand), the above processes may only become physiologically relevant during functional but not nutritional stresses. Interestingly, enhancing TAG synthesis (via DGAT1) in rodent skeletal muscle (14,45) or TAG hydrolysis (via ATGL) in rodent adipose tissue are sufficient to drive FA oxidation (23) in the absence of functional stress, whereas enhancing TAG hydrolysis (via ATGL) in rodent skeletal muscle is not. While prior studies have suggested that ATGL-mediated TAG hydrolysis is important for working muscle (19,46), these studies were performed using GAKO mice, which have significant cardiac morbidity and defects in TAG catabolism in multiple tissues. Therefore, additional studies are required to determine the relative contribution of extra-versus intramyocellular TAG hydrolysis to skeletal muscle metabolism/function during functional stresses such as endurance or resistance exercise, which are believed to increase flux through the IMTG pool.

The regulated storage and release of both essential and deleterious lipid metabolites from intracellular TAG stores are among the most fundamental processes in metabolism. The complex relationship between intracellular TAGs and metabolic phenotypes is best exemplified in skeletal muscle, where IMTG accumulation is variably associated with insulin resistance (i.e., obesity) or insulin sensitivity (i.e., endurance exercise). The resolution of how IMTG metabolism contributes to these divergent phenotypes holds the key to understanding how these processes may be exploited for therapeutic benefit. Our study provides convincing evidence that IMTGs neither cause nor prevent insulin resistance and that manipulation of IMTG hydrolysis via altered ATGL action does not influence metabolic consequences of HFD-induced obesity. Additional functional studies will further enhance our understanding of TAG hydrolysis in muscle and whole-body physiology. Importantly, with few exceptions (21,47), tissue-specific modulation of ATGL-mediated TAG hydrolysis has largely produced beneficial effects (23,39,48–50). Thus, the lack of adverse metabolic consequences of altering ATGL action in skeletal muscle indicates that modulating TA hydrolysis may still be a viable therapeutic strategy for treating metabolic disorders. Additional studies in other metabolically relevant tissues are still required to more fully understand the health implications of TAG hydrolysis in normal physiology and disease.

ACKNOWLEDGMENTS

This work was supported by the following: National Institutes of Health grants R03-DK-077697 and R01-DK-090166 and a Howard Hughes Medical Institute Physician-Scientist Early Career Award (to E.E.K.); Claude D. Pepper Pilot Grant (to M.T.S.); Erwin Schrödinger Fellowship (to G.S.); and the Endocrine Fellows Foundation's Marilyn Fishman Grant for Diabetes Research (to C.F.Y.). Tissue lipid analysis was supported in part by the Lipidomics Shared Resource, Hollings Cancer Center, Medical University of South Carolina (P30-CA-138313); the Lipidomics Core in the SC Lipidomics and Pathobiology COBRE (P20-RR-017677); the National Center for Research Resources; and the Office of the Director of the National Institutes of Health (C06-RR-018823).

No potential conflicts of interest relevant to this article were reported.

M.T.S. and M.K.B. were project leaders for analysis of SMAKO and Ckm-ATGL mice, respectively. L.C. was the technical manager for all experiments and performed imaging analyses. G.S. and C.F.Y. performed experiments. G.D., B.H.G., and P.C. assessed mitochondrial respiration. V.R. and J.P.D. quantified FA-CoAs. R.S. and R.Z. performed TAG hydrolase activities. D.B.S. performed imaging analysis. N.P.G. helped generate and validate the mouse models. P.C.K. and T.P. contributed intellectual expertise and helped prepare the manuscript. E.E.K. generated mouse models, designed, executed, and analyzed experiments, and wrote the manuscript. All authors contributed intellectually to this work and reviewed and edited the manuscript. E.E.K. is the guarantor of this work and, as such, had full access to all the data in the study and takes responsibility for the integrity of the data and the accuracy of the data analysis.

Parts of this study were presented in poster form at the 73rd Scientific Sessions of the American Diabetes Association, Chicago, Illinois, 21–25 June 2013.

The authors thank the following for contributions: Jeffrey S. Flier, MD (Harvard Medical School) for mentoring and support; Eric Olson, PhD (University of Texas Southwestern) for providing Myo-Cre mice; C. Ronald Kahn, MD (Joslin Diabetes Center) for providing the Ckm promoter construct; Jacek Bielawski, PhD (Medical University of South Carolina) for expertise related to lipidomics; the University of Pittsburgh Center for Biological Imaging for equipment and expertise related to imaging; and the University of Pittsburgh Division of Endocrinology Metabolic Center for equipment and expertise related to metabolism.

REFERENCES

1. Schaffer JE. Lipotoxicity: when tissues overeat. Curr Opin Lipidol 2003;14:281–287
2. Goodpaster BH, He J, Watkins S, Kelley DE. Skeletal muscle lipid content and insulin resistance: evidence for a paradox in endurance-trained athletes. J Clin Endocrinol Metab 2001;86:5755–5761
3. Samuel VT, Shulman GI. Mechanisms for insulin resistance: common threads and missing links. Cell 2012;148:852–871
4. Cowart LA. Sphingolipids: players in the pathology of metabolic disease. Trends Endocrinol Metab 2009;20:34–42
5. Amati F. Revisiting the diacylglycerol-induced insulin resistance hypothesis. Obes Rev 2012;13(Suppl. 2):40–50
6. Bosma M, Kersten S, Hesselink MK, Schrauwen P. Re-evaluating lipotoxic triggers in skeletal muscle: relating intramyocellular lipid metabolism to insulin sensitivity. Prog Lipid Res 2012;51:36–49
7. Coen PM, Goodpaster BH. Role of intramyocelluar lipids in human health. Trends Endocrinol Metab 2012;23:391–398
8. van Loon LJ, Goodpaster BH. Increased intramuscular lipid storage in the insulin-resistant and endurance-trained state. Pflugers Arch 2006;451:606–616
9. Goodpaster BH. Mitochondrial deficiency is associated with insulin resistance. Diabetes 2013;62:1032–1035
10. Funai K, Semenkovich CF. Skeletal muscle lipid flux: running water carries no poison. Am J Physiol Endocrinol Metab 2011;301:E245–E251
11. Zhang L, Keung W, Samokhvalov V, Wang W, Lopaschuk GD. Role of fatty acid uptake and fatty acid beta-oxidation in mediating insulin resistance in heart and skeletal muscle. Biochim Biophys Acta 2010;1801:1–22
12. Holloszy JO. "Deficiency" of mitochondria in muscle does not cause insulin resistance. Diabetes 2013;62:1036–1040
13. Liu L, Zhang Y, Chen N, Shi X, Tsang B, Yu YH. Upregulation of myocellular DGAT1 augments triglyceride synthesis in skeletal muscle and protects against fat-induced insulin resistance. J Clin Invest 2007;117:1679–1689
14. Liu L, Shi X, Choi CS, et al. Paradoxical coupling of triglyceride synthesis and fatty acid oxidation in skeletal muscle overexpressing DGAT1. Diabetes 2009;58:2516–2524
15. Levin MC, Monetti M, Watt MJ, et al. Increased lipid accumulation and insulin resistance in transgenic mice expressing DGAT2 in glycolytic (type II) muscle. Am J Physiol Endocrinol Metab 2007;293:E1772–E1781
16. Haemmerle G, Lass A, Zimmermann R, et al. Defective lipolysis and altered energy metabolism in mice lacking adipose triglyceride lipase. Science 2006;312:734–737
17. Kienesberger PC, Lee D, Pulinilkunnil T, et al. Adipose triglyceride lipase deficiency causes tissue-specific changes in insulin signaling. J Biol Chem 2009;284:30218–30229
18. Hoy AJ, Bruce CR, Turpin SM, Morris AJ, Febbraio MA, Watt MJ. Adipose triglyceride lipase-null mice are resistant to high-fat diet-induced insulin resistance despite reduced energy expenditure and ectopic lipid accumulation. Endocrinology 2011;152:48–58
19. Huijsman E, van de Par C, Economou C, et al. Adipose triacylglycerol lipase deletion alters whole body energy metabolism and impairs exercise performance in mice. Am J Physiol Endocrinol Metab 2009;297:E505–E513
20. Kraemer FB, Shen WJ. Hormone-sensitive lipase knockouts. Nutr Metab (Lond) 2006;3:12

21. Haemmerle G, Moustafa T, Woelkart G, et al. ATGL-mediated fat catabolism regulates cardiac mitochondrial function via PPAR-α and PGC-1. Nat Med 2011;17:1076–1085

22. Reid BN, Ables GP, Otlivanchik OA, et al. Hepatic overexpression of hormone-sensitive lipase and adipose triglyceride lipase promotes fatty acid oxidation, stimulates direct release of free fatty acids, and ameliorates steatosis. J Biol Chem 2008;283:13087–13099

23. Ahmadian M, Duncan RE, Varady KA, et al. Adipose overexpression of desnutrin promotes fatty acid use and attenuates diet-induced obesity. Diabetes 2009;58:855–866

24. Li S, Czubryt MP, McAnally J, et al. Requirement for serum response factor for skeletal muscle growth and maturation revealed by tissue-specific gene deletion in mice. Proc Natl Acad Sci USA 2005;102:1082–1087

25. Brüning JC, Michael MD, Winnay JN, et al. A muscle-specific insulin receptor knockout exhibits features of the metabolic syndrome of NIDDM without altering glucose tolerance. Mol Cell 1998;2:559–569

26. Basantani MK, Sitnick MT, Cai L, et al. Pnpla3/Adiponutrin deficiency in mice does not contribute to fatty liver disease or metabolic syndrome. J Lipid Res 2011;52:318–329

27. Bielawski J, Szulc ZM, Hannun YA, Bielawska A. Simultaneous quantitative analysis of bioactive sphingolipids by high-performance liquid chromatography-tandem mass spectrometry. Methods 2006;39:82–91

28. Sun D, Cree MG, Wolfe RR. Quantification of the concentration and ^{13}C tracer enrichment of long-chain fatty acyl-coenzyme A in muscle by liquid chromatography/mass spectrometry. Anal Biochem 2006;349:87–95

29. Berggren JR, Boyle KE, Chapman WH, Houmard JA. Skeletal muscle lipid oxidation and obesity: influence of weight loss and exercise. Am J Physiol Endocrinol Metab 2008;294:E726–E732

30. Kuznetsov AV, Veksler V, Gellerich FN, Saks V, Margreiter R, Kunz WS. Analysis of mitochondrial function in situ in permeabilized muscle fibers, tissues and cells. Nat Protoc 2008;3:965–976

31. Koopman R, Schaart G, Hesselink MK. Optimisation of oil red O staining permits combination with immunofluorescence and automated quantification of lipids. Histochem Cell Biol 2001;116:63–68

32. Kershaw EE, Hamm JK, Verhagen LA, Peroni O, Katic M, Flier JS. Adipose triglyceride lipase: function, regulation by insulin, and comparison with adiponutrin. Diabetes 2006;55:148–157

33. Badin PM, Louche K, Mairal A, et al. Altered skeletal muscle lipase expression and activity contribute to insulin resistance in humans. Diabetes 2011;60:1734–1742

34. Eichmann TO, Kumari M, Haas JT, et al. Studies on the substrate and stereo/regioselectivity of adipose triglyceride lipase, hormone-sensitive lipase, and diacylglycerol-O-acyltransferases. J Biol Chem 2012;287:41446–41457

35. Cantley JL, Yoshimura T, Camporez JP, et al. CGI-58 knockdown sequesters diacylglycerols in lipid droplets/ER-preventing diacylglycerol-mediated hepatic insulin resistance. Proc Natl Acad Sci USA 2013;110:1869–1874

36. Mottillo EP, Bloch AE, Leff T, Granneman JG. Lipolytic products activate peroxisome proliferator-activated receptor (PPAR) α and δ in brown adipocytes to match fatty acid oxidation with supply. J Biol Chem 2012;287:25038–25048

37. Ong KT, Mashek MT, Bu SY, Greenberg AS, Mashek DG. Adipose triglyceride lipase is a major hepatic lipase that regulates triacylglycerol turnover and fatty acid signaling and partitioning. Hepatology 2011;53:116–126

38. Sapiro JM, Mashek MT, Greenberg AS, Mashek DG. Hepatic triacylglycerol hydrolysis regulates peroxisome proliferator-activated receptor alpha activity. J Lipid Res 2009;50:1621–1629

39. Ahmadian M, Abbott MJ, Tang T, et al. Desnutrin/ATGL is regulated by AMPK and is required for a brown adipose phenotype. Cell Metab 2011;13:739–748

40. Bosma M, Sparks LM, Hooiveld GJ, et al. Overexpression of PLIN5 in skeletal muscle promotes oxidative gene expression and intramyocellular lipid content without compromising insulin sensitivity. Biochim Biophys Acta 2013;1831:844–852

41. Badin PM, Loubière C, Coonen M, et al. Regulation of skeletal muscle lipolysis and oxidative metabolism by the co-lipase CGI-58. J Lipid Res 2012;53:839–848

42. Nunes PM, van de Weijer T, Veltien A, et al. Increased intramyocellular lipids but unaltered in vivo mitochondrial oxidative phosphorylation in skeletal muscle of adipose triglyceride lipase-deficient mice. Am J Physiol Endocrinol Metab 2012;303:E71–E81

43. Zierler KA, Jaeger D, Pollak NM, et al. Functional cardiac lipolysis in mice critically depends on comparative gene identification-58. J Biol Chem 2013;288:9892–9904

44. Muoio DM, Koves TR. Skeletal muscle adaptation to fatty acid depends on coordinated actions of the PPARs and PGC1 alpha: implications for metabolic disease. Appl Physiol Nutr Metab 2007;32:874–883

45. Timmers S, de Vogel-van den Bosch J, Hesselink MK, et al. Paradoxical increase in TAG and DAG content parallel the insulin sensitizing effect of unilateral DGAT1 overexpression in rat skeletal muscle. PLoS ONE 2011;6:e14503

46. Schoiswohl G, Schweiger M, Schreiber R, et al. Adipose triglyceride lipase plays a key role in the supply of the working muscle with fatty acids. J Lipid Res 2010;51:490–499

47. Wu JW, Wang SP, Alvarez F, et al. Deficiency of liver adipose triglyceride lipase in mice causes progressive hepatic steatosis. Hepatology 2011;54:122–132

48. Das SK, Eder S, Schauer S, et al. Adipose triglyceride lipase contributes to cancer-associated cachexia. Science 2011;333:233–238

49. Kienesberger PC, Pulinilkunnil T, Sung MM, et al. Myocardial ATGL overexpression decreases the reliance on fatty acid oxidation and protects against pressure overload-induced cardiac dysfunction. Mol Cell Biol 2012;32:740–750

50. Pulinilkunnil T, Kienesberger PC, Nagendran J, et al. Myocardial adipose triglyceride lipase overexpression protects diabetic mice from the development of lipotoxic cardiomyopathy. Diabetes 2013;62:1464–1477

Resveratrol Prevents β-Cell Dedifferentiation in Nonhuman Primates Given a High-Fat/High-Sugar Diet

Jennifer L. Fiori,[1] Yu-Kyong Shin,[1,2] Wook Kim,[1,3] Susan M. Krzysik-Walker,[1] Isabel González-Mariscal,[1] Olga D. Carlson,[1] Mitesh Sanghvi,[1] Ruin Moaddel,[1] Kathleen Farhang,[1] Shekhar K. Gadkaree,[1] Maire E. Doyle,[4] Kevin J. Pearson,[5,6] Julie A. Mattison,[5] Rafael de Cabo,[5] and Josephine M. Egan[1]

Eating a "Westernized" diet high in fat and sugar leads to weight gain and numerous health problems, including the development of type 2 diabetes mellitus (T2DM). Rodent studies have shown that resveratrol supplementation reduces blood glucose levels, preserves β-cells in islets of Langerhans, and improves insulin action. Although rodent models are helpful for understanding β-cell biology and certain aspects of T2DM pathology, they fail to reproduce the complexity of the human disease as well as that of nonhuman primates. Rhesus monkeys were fed a standard diet (SD), or a high-fat/high-sugar diet in combination with either placebo (HFS) or resveratrol (HFS+Resv) for 24 months, and pancreata were examined before overt dysglycemia occurred. Increased glucose-stimulated insulin secretion and insulin resistance occurred in both HFS and HFS+Resv diets compared with SD. Although islet size was unaffected, there was a significant decrease in β-cells and an increase in α-cells containing glucagon and glucagon-like peptide 1 with HFS diets. Islets from HFS+Resv monkeys were morphologically similar to SD. HFS diets also resulted in decreased expression of essential β-cell transcription factors forkhead box O1 (FOXO1), NKX6–1, NKX2–2, and *PDX1*, which did not occur with resveratrol supplementation. Similar changes were observed in human islets where the effects of resveratrol were mediated through Sirtuin 1. These findings have implications for the management of humans with insulin resistance, prediabetes, and diabetes. *Diabetes* 62:3500–3513, 2013

I n many developing countries, a rapid nutritional transition has occurred from a healthy diet, high in fiber and low in fat and calories, to calorie-dense meals, containing refined carbohydrates, red meats, sugary desserts and drinks, and high-fat foods (1). When "Westernized" diets are introduced, the population responds with weight gain leading to numerous health problems, including hypertension, coronary artery disease and strokes, respiratory effects, cancers, reproductive abnormalities, and type 2 diabetes mellitus (T2DM) (2). Obesity, a result of sedentary lifestyles and Westernized diets, has reached epidemic proportions and is the major risk factor for developing T2DM.

Currently 25.8 million Americans have adult-onset or T2DM and an additional 79 million exhibit a metabolic profile that is considered a precursor to T2DM (3). Several years ago, the Diabetes Prevention Program Trial (DPPT), targeting persons with prediabetes, found that the incidence of T2DM was reduced by 31% with metformin therapy and by 58% with lifestyle interventions, including exercise and weight reduction, over an average follow-up period of 2.8 years (4). However, in absolute terms, metformin had only a minor impact on the transition to diabetes, with diabetes developing in 13 of every 14 individuals receiving metformin. Although lifestyle intervention in a highly controlled setting faired twice as well, long-term modification of diet and activity patterns are very difficult for most adults to achieve. Further, despite the findings from the DPPT and recommendations for people with prediabetes to use metformin, lose weight, and start an exercise regimen, rates of diabetes continue to escalate. Therefore, it is extremely important to investigate the metabolic and physiologic alterations that occur in prediabetic states and elucidate the underlying etiopathology in order to develop effective strategies to prevent the transition to T2DM.

In the last several years, rodent studies and experiments in vitro have provided evidence that resveratrol, a naturally occurring phytoalexin found in numerous plant species, exerts beneficial effects in organisms and may be helpful in preventing some metabolic diseases, including diabetes (5). In animals given a high-fat diet, resveratrol has been shown to increase their survival and motor function (6), reduce visceral fat and liver mass indexes (7), and induce beneficial changes in lipid parameters (8). In addition, several different rodent models of diabetes have shown that resveratrol can reduce blood glucose levels (9), preserve β-cells (10), and improve insulin action (6). However, limited human data on metabolic effects of resveratrol are more controversial. A few studies have reported that resveratrol improves insulin sensitivity in adults who are obese (11), have T2DM (12), or have impaired glucose tolerance (13), whereas other studies have supported the idea that resveratrol supplementation does not improve metabolic function in nonobese women (14) or in obese men (15).

Although rodent models are helpful for understanding β-cell biology and some aspects of the pathogenesis of T2DM, they cannot reproduce the complexity of the human disease as well as that of nonhuman primates. T2DM

From the [1]Laboratory of Clinical Investigation, National Institute on Aging, National Institutes of Health, Baltimore, Maryland; the [2]Biochemistry Department, Boston University School of Medicine, Boston, Massachusetts; the [3]Department of Molecular Science and Technology, Ajou University, Suwon, Republic of Korea; the [4]Division of Endocrinology, Johns Hopkins Bayview Medical Center, Baltimore, Maryland; the [5]Translational Gerontology Branch, National Institute on Aging, National Institutes of Health, Baltimore, Maryland; and the [6]Graduate Center for Nutritional Sciences, University of Kentucky College of Medicine, Lexington, Kentucky.

Corresponding author: Josephine M. Egan, eganj@grc.nia.nih.gov.

Received 15 February 2013 and accepted 13 July 2013.

DOI: 10.2337/db13-0266

This article contains Supplementary Data online at http://diabetes .diabetesjournals.org/lookup/suppl/doi:10.2337/db13-0266/-/DC1.

occurs spontaneously in ad libitum–fed nonhuman primates (16). Also, monkey and human endocrine pancreata are similar with β- and α-cells interspersed, unlike rodent islets, and with similar islet size and cellular distribution of islet cell types (17). The metabolic and hormonal changes observed in humans with insulin resistance, prediabetes, and diabetes also occur in monkeys (18,19). Therefore, monkeys serve as ideal models for studying islets as they likely display evolving changes in response to increased insulin requirement. Additionally, these changes occur within a reasonable time frame of experimentation (18). We undertook a long-term study of monkeys given a high-fat/high-sugar diet to evaluate changes in islet function and morphology resulting from unremitting increased insulin requirement in the absence of dysglycemia and whether these changes were mitigated by resveratrol.

RESEARCH DESIGN AND METHODS

Animals. Twenty-four adult male rhesus monkeys (*Macaca mulatta*) were housed continuously at the National Institutes of Health (NIH) Animal Center (Poolesville, MD). The animal center is fully accredited by the American Association for Accreditation of Laboratory Animal Care, and all procedures were approved by the Animal Care and Use Committee of the National Institute on Aging Intramural Program.

Diet. During baseline assessments, all monkeys were maintained on standard NIH monkey chow (Purina Mills, St. Louis, MO). After baseline assessment, they were randomized into one of three groups: a healthy standard diet (SD; 4 monkeys) or a high-fat/high-sugar diet in combination with either placebo (HFS; 10 monkeys) or resveratrol (HFS+Resv; 10 monkeys). The SD was a purified diet consisting of 13% kcal in fat and <5% sucrose by weight. The HFS diet was a specially formulated purified ingredient diet with 42% kcal in fat and ~27% sucrose by weight (Teklad; Harlan, Indianapolis, IN). The monkeys were gradually switched to the HFS diet over a 3-week period. Monkeys received two meals per day at estimated ad libitum levels throughout the study, and water was always available. The average food consumption for weekly periods was the same for all three groups.

Resveratrol dosing. Resveratrol was supplied by DSM Nutritional Products North America (Parsippany, NJ). The dose for monkeys was derived from the protective dose reported in mice (22 mg/kg) (6) and was adjusted by allometric scaling to an average monkey body weight of 12.1 kg. The monkey equivalent dose was determined to be 40.7 mg. The resveratrol was used to formulate a flavored primate treat (Bio-Serv, Frenchtown, NJ) that was given to the monkeys prior to each meal. Thus, the monkeys received a total dose of 80 mg/day for the first year, and the resveratrol dose was increased to 240 mg twice a day during the second year. Monkeys in non-resveratrol groups received a cherry-flavored placebo treat (sugar pill) that was identical in looks and taste to the resveratrol treats.

Serum resveratrol levels. The extraction of resveratrol and its metabolites was performed with modifications of a previously published method (20). Briefly, 90 μL of methanol and 10 μL of hexestrol (internal standard) were added to 100 μL of serum, which was vortexed and centrifuged at 20,800 relative centrifugal force for 10 min at 4°C. The supernatant was transferred to an autosampler vial for further analysis. The chromatographic separation of resveratrol and its metabolites was carried out on a Shimadzu Prominence high-performance liquid chromatography system (Columbia, MD). The samples were introduced to the analytical column in 20-μL injections using a Shimadzu SIL 20A autosampler, which was maintained at 4°C. The separation of resveratrol, resveratrol-3-O-sulfate, resveratrol-3-O-glucuronide, and resveratrol-4′-O-glucuronide was accomplished using an Eclipse XDB-C18 guard column (4.6 × 12.5 mm) and a Discovery C18 column (150 × 4.6 mm; internal diameter 5 μm). The mobile phase consisted of water containing 0.1% acetic acid and 0.07% triethylamine as component A and acetonitrile as component B. A linear gradient was run as follows: 0–3 min, 20% B; 3–25 min, 20–60% B; 25–30 min, 60–20% B at a flow rate of 1.0 mL/min. Tandem mass spectrometry analysis was performed using the API4000 system with turbo ion spray (TIS) from Applied Biosystems (Foster City, CA). The data were acquired and analyzed using Analyst version 1.4.2. Negative electrospray ionization data were acquired using the following multiple reaction monitoring transitions: resveratrol (227–185); resveratrol–sulfate (307–227); resveratrol–glucuronide (403–227); and hexestrol (269–134). The TIS instrumental source settings for temperature (500°C), curtain gas (10 ψ), IS1 (60 ψ), IS2 (70 ψ), entrance potential (−10 V), and ion spray voltage (−4,500 V). The TIS compound parameter settings for declustering potential, collision energy,

and collision cell exit potential were −70, −25, and −7 V for resveratrol; −50, −28, and −9 V for resveratrol metabolites; and −82, −20, and −8 V for hexesterol.

Hormone assays. Intravenous glucose (IVG) challenge was performed with 300 mg/kg of 50% dextrose solution (Hospire, Inc., Lake Forest, IL). Blood samples were obtained by venipuncture of the femoral vein using a vacutainer and vacuum tubes. Glucose was measured in whole blood using the Ascensia Elite glucose meter (Bayer, Mishawaka, IN). Serum glucagon was measured by radioimmunoassay (Millipore, Billerica, MA), and serum insulin and media from human islets were measured by enzyme-linked immunosorbent assay (ELISA) (Mercodia, Uppsala, Sweden) according to the manufacturer's instructions. The insulin area under the curve (AUC) was determined using Prism (GraphPad, La Jolla, CA). The insulin sensitivity index (ISI) was calculated as previously described (21).

Immunofluorescence and densitometry. Dr. Frederic B. Askin from the Department of Pathology at The Johns Hopkins University School of Medicine (Baltimore, MD) provided anonymous human pancreas in paraffin blocks. Pancreata from two diabetic monkeys in a separate cohort were procured when animals were killed for medical reasons. Our monkeys were fasted overnight, and, after blood draw and euthanasia, the pancreata were excised. Human islets were provided by the National Institute of Diabetes and Digestive and Kidney Diseases–funded Integrated Islet Distribution Program at City of Hope and were embedded in Histogel (Thermo Scientific, Waltham, MA) after treatment. Both human islets and monkey pancreata were fixed in 4% paraformaldehyde, embedded in paraffin blocks, and sectioned (5 μm). After deparaffinization, sections were treated with antigen retrieval solution (BioGenex, Fremont, CA), washed, permeabilized, and blocked, and primary antibodies were added overnight at 4°C as follows: insulin (1:200; Millipore or Sigma, St. Louis, MO); glucagon (1:500; Millipore or Sigma); prohormone convertase (PC) 1/3 (1:200; provided by Dr. Donald Steiner, The University of Chicago, Chicago, IL); glucagon-like peptide 1 (GLP-1) (1:100; Sigma or US Biological, Swampscott, MA); Ki-67 (1:50; Dako, Carpinteria, CA); forkhead box O1 (FOXO1) (1:100; Cell Signaling Technology, Danvers, MA); pancreatic polypeptide (1:200; Millipore); somatostatin, phosphorylated insulin receptor (P-IR), and phosphorylated Bad (P-Bad; serine 136) (1:100; Santa Cruz Biotechnology, Santa Cruz, CA); and NKX2–2 and NKX6–1 (1:100; Novus Biologicals, Littleton, CO). After washing, sections were incubated with fluorescently labeled secondary antibodies (1:500; Rhodamine Red-X, FITC, Cy5; Jackson ImmunoResearch, West Grove, PA) with or without TO-PRO-3 (1:5,000; Molecular Probes, Grand Island, NY) for nuclear staining. Imaging was performed at 40× using a Zeiss (Jena, Germany) LSM-710 confocal microscope. Densitometry of staining was performed using ImageJ (NIH). Images were separated by color and inverted to black and white, and the integrated density was calculated for each stain using the tracing function.

Pancreatic islet size quantification. Multiple images (200 μm apart) from each monkey were assessed for signal intensity. Islet sizing was performed using the MATLAB (MathWorks, Natick, MA) Image Processing Toolbox. Each islet was carefully isolated using the roipoly tracing function. The various immunostains were separated by color into variables for processing. The resulting total islet, α-cell, and β-cell sizes were calculated based on total traced size, percentage of glucagon immunostain, and percentage of insulin immunostain, respectively. Somatostatin- and pancreatic polypeptide–positive cells were sized similarly. The percentage of cells per islet was determined by counting the number of insulin-, glucagon-, and TO-PRO-3–positive cells in each diet intervention.

Quantitative PCR. RNA was extracted using TRIzol (Invitrogen, Grand Island, NY) and an RNeasy Mini kit (Qiagen, Valencia, CA), and cDNA was synthesized using qScript cDNA Supermix (Quanta Biosciences, Gaithersburg, MD). Gene expression in monkey islets was quantified using SYBR green (Quanta Biosciences), and values were compared with standard curves and normalized to 18S (Ambion, Austin, TX). The monkey primers were: FOXO1 (forward: 5′-GGATGTGCATTCTATGGTGTACC-3′; and reverse: 5′-TTTCGGGATTGCTTA-TCTCAGAC-3′), NKX2–2 (forward: 5′-CCGGGCCGAGAAAGGTATG-3′; and reverse: 5′-GTTTGCCGTCCCTGACCAA-3′), NKX6–1 (forward: 5′-ATCTTCT-GGCCCGGAGTGA-3′; and reverse: 5′-CGCCAAGTATTTTGTTTGTTCG-3′), and PDX1 (forward: 5′-CGGAACTTTCTATTTAGGATGTGG-3′; and reverse: 5′-AAGATGTGAAGGTCATACTGGCTC-3′) (Integrated DNA Technologies, Coralville, IA). Gene expression in human islets was quantified using TaqMan Fast Advanced Master Mix (Invitrogen) and normalized to actin labeled with VIC. Human primers were labeled with FAM and purchased from Invitrogen (Taqman Gene Expression Assays). Quantitative PCR was performed on an ABI Prism 7300 (Applied Biosystems) detection system.

GLP-1 secretion assay. Human islets were incubated in Dulbecco's modified Eagle's medium (Gibco, Grand Island, NY) containing 5 mmol/L glucose (Sigma), 50 μmol/L dipeptidyl pepsidease-IV inhibitor (Millipore), and 3% bovine serum albumin at 37°C with 5% CO$_2$ overnight. Islets were then washed with medium, separated into several dishes containing 20 islets each, and

TABLE 1
Monkey characteristics and hormone levels at baseline (0 months) and after 24 months for indicated diets

Characteristics	SD (n = 4)		HFS (n = 10)		HFS+Resv (n = 10)	
	0 months	24 months	0 months	24 months	0 months	24 months
Age (years)	9.8 ± 0.8	12.8 ± 1.1	11.0 ± 0.6	13.8 ± 0.6	10.3 ± 0.5	13.1 ± 0.5
Weight (kg)	12.98 ± 1.21	13.49 ± 1.31	13.24 ± 1.21	16.69 ± 1.80*	12.82 ± 1.04	15.70 ± 1.12*
Fasting glucose (mg/dL)	58.77 ± 1.14	42.33 ± 2.31	60.07 ± 2.75	50.30 ± 1.47	61.24 ± 1.04	53.00 ± 2.88
Fasting insulin (μU/mL)	27.34 ± 6.61	89.15 ± 58.92	31.44 ± 16.04	63.48 ± 16.44	35.78 ± 13.24	94.22 ± 28.24
Insulin AUC after IVG challenge	6,254.00 ± 1,081.09	6,484.67 ± 1,851.36	5,710.90 ± 1,967.35	12,381.50 ± 2,732.90**	6,966.00 ± 1,683.51	14,836.00 ± 3,607.06*
ISI (10^{-3})	0.84 ± 0.17	0.82 ± 0.15	1.06 ± 0.18	0.36 ± 0.05*	1.03 ± 0.12	0.38 ± 0.07*
Fasting glucagon (pg/mL)	31.87 ± 5.59	46.33 ± 17.62	61.19 ± 14.91	45.3 ± 11.19	42.51 ± 3.80	55.80 ± 8.99

Data are shown as the mean ± SEM. *$P < 0.05$ and **$P < 0.01$, compared with baseline within each group.

placed in fresh medium. The islets were then incubated for 1 h at 37°C, after which medium was collected and secreted GLP-1 levels were measured by ELISA (Alpco Diagnostics, Salem, NH). Levels were normalized to total protein content as determined by a BCA Protein Assay (Pierce, Rockford, IL).

cAMP assay. Human islets were prepared as described above. Total protein was extracted using lysis buffer (0.01 mol/L TrisHcl, 1% Triton X-100, 0.15 mol/L NaCl, 0.5 mmol/L EDTA, and protease and phosphatase inhibitor cocktails). GLP-1 levels were measured by ELISA to determine the amount in total protein, and the islet extract was diluted to yield the different concentrations of GLP-1 (22). Chinese hamster ovary (CHO)/K1 cells were stably transfected with rat GLP-1 receptor (GLP-1R) as previously described (23). Both CHO/K1 and CHO/GLP-1R cells were treated with increasing concentrations (0–20 pmol/L) of full-length GLP-1 (Bachem, Torrance, CA) as well as GLP-1 islet extract for 30 min. After treatment, the cell supernatant was assayed using a Direct cAMP ELISA kit (Enzo Life Sciences, Farmingdale, NY) following the manufacturer's protocol.

Treatment of human islets. Human islets were prepared as described above 1 day prior to experimentation. Islets were then separated into several dishes containing 100 islets in fresh medium supplemented with 3% bovine serum albumin and 5 mmol/L glucose for the control condition or 13 mmol/L glucose and 500 μmol/L sodium palmitate (Sigma) for the HFS condition. Islets incubated under the HFS condition were also treated with 1 μmol/L EX-527 and/or 1 nmol/L resveratrol (TOCRIS Bioscience, Minneapolis, MN) for 24 h. Media were then collected for measuring insulin secretion, and islets were processed for quantitative PCR and immunofluorescence as described above.

Statistical analysis. Quantitative data are represented as the mean ± SEM. Differences between mean values were compared statistically by one-way ANOVA followed by Bonferroni post hoc comparison. A P value of <0.05 was considered statistically significant.

RESULTS

Monkey assessment and hormone levels. Adult male rhesus monkeys (average age at baseline 10.5 ± 0.4 years) were fed an SD, or an HFS or HFS+Resv diet for 24 months. Prior to euthanasia, the average serum concentrations of resveratrol and resveratrol-3-O-sulfate in HFS+Resv were 27.7 ± 8.6 and 239.1 ± 82.2 ng/mL, respectively, whereas the levels of resveratrol-4'-O-glucuronide and 3-O-glucuronide were below our quantitation limits; all were below detection levels in SD and HFS. SD monkeys gained very little weight, whereas HFS and HFS+Resv monkeys gained a significant amount over the 24-month period (Table 1). Based on fasting glucose and insulin levels at euthanasia, no metabolic dysregulation had occurred over 24 months within the feeding regimens (Table 1). All three groups had similar glucose levels after IVG challenge both at baseline and after 24 months (Fig. 1A). However, in both HFS and HFS+Resv monkeys, the serum insulin levels and the insulin AUC were significantly greater after IVG challenge compared with baseline levels, consistent with weight gain and insulin resistance (Fig. 1B and Table 1). The ISI of the SD animals was stable for the duration of the study, whereas both HFS and HFS+Resv animals exhibited decreased insulin sensitivity after 24 months on an HFS diet (Table 1). The fasting serum glucagon level was not significantly altered over 24 months in any group (Table 1). Within all of these parameters, there was a lot of heterogeneity in the monkeys in response to the diet intervention, both at 0 and 24 months (Supplementary Fig. 1).

An HFS diet resulted in morphological changes in islets that were prevented by resveratrol. On evaluating islet morphology, we found that although total islet size remained unchanged across the groups (Fig. 1D), α-cell mass was significantly increased with HFS at the expense of the β-cell mass compared with SD, with heterogeneity among the HFS islets in their numbers of α- and β-cells (Fig. 1E and F). This caused a significant alteration in the ratio of α-cell/β-cell mass (Fig. 1G). The total

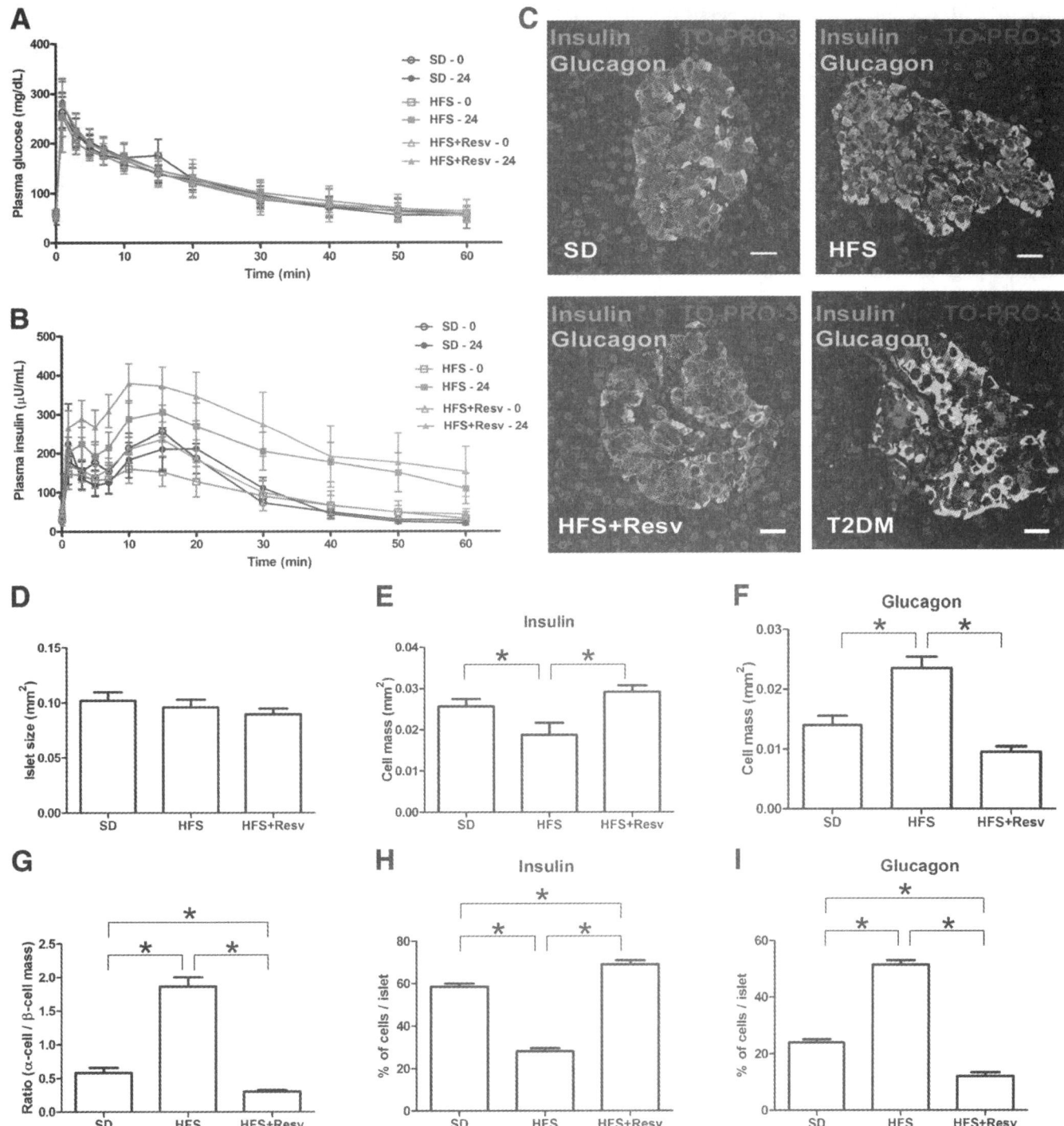

FIG. 1. HFS diet–induced morphological changes in pancreatic islets. *A* and *B*: Glucose (*A*) and insulin (*B*) levels at fasting and after IVG challenge (300 mg/kg) before (0, open bars) and after (24, closed bars) 24 months on SD (blue circle, $n = 4$), HFS diet (red square, $n = 10$), or HFS+Resv diet (green triangle, $n = 10$) interventions in adult rhesus monkeys. *C*: Representative images of immunostaining for insulin (red), glucagon (green), and TO-PRO-3 (blue) in islets of monkeys after 24 months on the indicated diet intervention, and in two nonstudy monkeys in which T2DM spontaneously developed. Scale bar = 20 μm. *D–F*: Quantification of total islet size (*D*), β-cell mass (insulin) (*E*), and α-cell mass (glucagon) (*F*). *G*: Ratio of α-cell mass to β-cell mass. *H* and *I*: The percentage of cells that were insulin-positive (*H*) and glucagon-positive (*I*) in each islet. Data are shown as the mean ± SEM. *$P < 0.05$.

number of α- and β-cells per islet was also counted and corroborated the α- and β-cell mass (Fig. 1*H* and *I*). The increase in α-cell mass did not occur with resveratrol treatment. HFS+Resv monkeys exhibited a significant decrease in α-cell mass and a lower ratio of α-cell/β-cell mass

compared with SD monkeys. The islet changes in HFS monkeys were similar to those of two nonstudy rhesus monkeys from our colony in which T2DM spontaneously developed, though the T2DM monkeys appeared to have even fewer β-cells (Fig. 1*C*, T2DM).

Lack of evidence for β-cell apoptosis or α-cell mitosis in islets from monkeys given an HFS diet. Because the change in the α-cell/β-cell ratio without dysglycemia was unexpected, we looked for β-cell apoptosis and α-cell mitosis. No detectable evidence of β-cell apoptosis was observed because we were unable to detect TUNEL-stained nuclei or cleaved caspase 1 or 3 in ~2,000 islets. Additionally, the expression of a prosurvival protein, P-Bad, was similar in all three groups (Fig. 2A). Despite the obvious increase in α-cell numbers with an HFS diet, no mitotic Ki-67–positive α-cells were found. Abundant Ki-67–positive cells were present in exocrine pancreas and small intestine (Fig. 2B). There were no differences in the numbers of somatostatin or pancreatic polypeptide islet cell types among diet interventions (Fig. 2C).

Resveratrol protected depletion of β-cell–specific transcription factors by an HFS diet. Next, we examined the effect of an HFS diet on insulin/IGF-I signaling and β-cell–specific transcription factors. HFS islets exhibited decreased numbers of tyrosine phosphorylated IR (activated insulin receptor), including within the remaining β-cells (Fig. 3A and B). P-IR in SD and HFS+Resv monkeys were similar, indicating that resveratrol was protective of P-IR in islets. Loss of β-cell P-IR in rodents causes profound defects in β-cell growth (24,25). Forkhead box protein O1 (FOXO1) is a downstream effector in β-cells of IR signaling, and total FOXO1 protein (Fig. 3C and D) and mRNA (Fig. 3E) levels were depleted in HFS islets. In β-cells of SD and HFS+Resv monkeys, total FOXO1 was similar. We next studied factors that are known to be affected by loss of FOXO1 and that are essential in maintaining β-cell phenotype (26). NKX6–1 is a transcriptional repressor that is tightly restricted to β-cell nuclei in adult islets and is known to suppress glucagon expression (27), and NKX2–2 is a transcriptional factor necessary for optimal insulin gene expression (28). Both NKX6–1 (Fig. 4A and B) and NKX2–2 (Fig. 4D and E) proteins and mRNA (Fig. 4C and F, respectively) were severely affected in HFS monkeys. Islets with the fewest number of β-cells had greatly diminished nuclear NKX6–1 expression, with a gradient of decreased expression of NKX6–1 in β-cells of different HFS monkeys (Fig. 4A, bottom panel). Similarly, the mRNA levels of PDX1, a transcription factor necessary for pancreatic development and β-cell maturation (29), were also significantly downregulated in HFS monkeys (Fig. 4G). Resveratrol appeared to protect β-cells from loss of P-IR, FOXO1, NKX6–1, NKX2–2, and PDX1, thereby preserving β-cell mass in HFS+Resv monkeys.

Resveratrol protected human islets from HFS-induced changes in morphology and loss of β-cell–specific transcription factors. Similar to observations in monkey islets after an HFS diet, when human islets were treated with high glucose and palmitate to mimic HFS conditions, the number of insulin-positive β-cells was decreased and the number of glucagon-positive α-cells was increased (Fig. 5A). No TUNEL- or Ki-67–positive nuclei were detected in the islets. Human islets that were incubated with HFS+Resv exhibited islet morphology similar to control islets. Insulin secretion was increased 2.6-fold with an HFS diet and 6.2-fold with an HFS+Resv diet, and treatment with EX-527, a selective Sirtuin 1 (SIRT1) inhibitor, significantly decreased insulin secretion (Fig. 5B). This indicates that the increase in insulin secretion observed with resveratrol treatment is mediated through SIRT1. Additionally, resveratrol treatment resulted in a significant increase in the mRNA expression of PDX1

(Fig. 5C), NKX6–1 (Fig. 5D), FOXO1 (Fig. 5E), and SIRT1 (Fig. 5F). When human islets were treated with EX-527, all of these transcription factors were expressed at levels similar to that of the control group, confirming that the effect of resveratrol in increasing β-cell–specific transcription factors in human islets is mediated, at least in part, through SIRT1.

Identification of PC1/3 and GLP-1 in α-cells. Because we observed a dramatic increase in α-cell numbers in HFS compared with SD monkeys, we closely examined the α-cell compartment. Glucagon, which functions to maintain fasting glucose levels by stimulating hepatic glucose production, is produced in α-cells resulting from the enzymatic cleavage of proglucagon by PC2 (30). The glucagon-positive cells in monkey islets costained with PC2, as expected (data not shown), and additionally expressed PC1/3 (Fig. 6A). Proglucagon is also produced in L-cells of the intestine and taste cells in taste buds, and the expression of PC1/3 in those cells leads to GLP-1 production (22,31). The α-cells in our monkeys expressed GLP-1 (Fig. 6B). There was a significant increase in the amount of GLP-1 staining with HFS because of the increased number of α-cells (Fig. 6C). Although PC1/3, as expected, was also present in some insulin-containing cells, GLP-1, similar to glucagon, never colocalized with insulin. The presence of PC1/3 and GLP-1 has been reported in human pancreatic islet cells, including those from T2DM patients (32). We also detected PC1/3 (Fig. 7A) and GLP-1 (Fig. 7B) immunostaining in α-cells of the human pancreas.

GLP-1 secreted from islets is biologically active. Because we did not have access to fresh monkey islets to ascertain whether the GLP-1 present in primate islets was biologically active, freshly isolated human islets were used. GLP-1 was detectably secreted into culture medium after 1 h from as little as 20 human islets (Fig. 7C). In order to determine whether the GLP-1 in islets was biologically active, we extracted total islet protein, measured GLP-1 by ELISA, and normalized it to protein content. The extract was then diluted to give the indicated concentrations of GLP-1 and added to CHO cells, and CHO cells were stably transfected with GLP-1R. Nontransfected CHO cells did not respond to GLP-1 treatment as measured by a direct cAMP assay (Fig. 7D). However, CHO cells stably transfected with GLP-1R responded to recombinant GLP-1 and islet extract GLP-1 in a dose-dependent manner. Islet-extracted GLP-1 actually resulted in a significant increase in cAMP levels (Fig. 7D), demonstrating that the GLP-1 present in human islets, and presumably monkey islets, is biologically active.

DISCUSSION

After 24 months on an HFS diet, monkeys had significant weight gain, increased serum insulin levels and insulin AUC after an IVG challenge, and decreased insulin sensitivity. Moreover, significant changes in islet morphology as a result of an HFS diet, independent of dysglycemia, were also present. Hyperglycemia or the diabetic state itself was not a secondary cause of these intraislet cellular changes. Most notably, the α-cell/β-cell ratio was significantly altered because of decreased numbers of insulin-containing cells and increased numbers of glucagon- and GLP-1–containing cells, whereas total islet size was unaltered. These morphological changes are similar to those observed in monkeys in which T2DM spontaneously developed (Fig. 1C), in vervet monkeys administered an 18-month

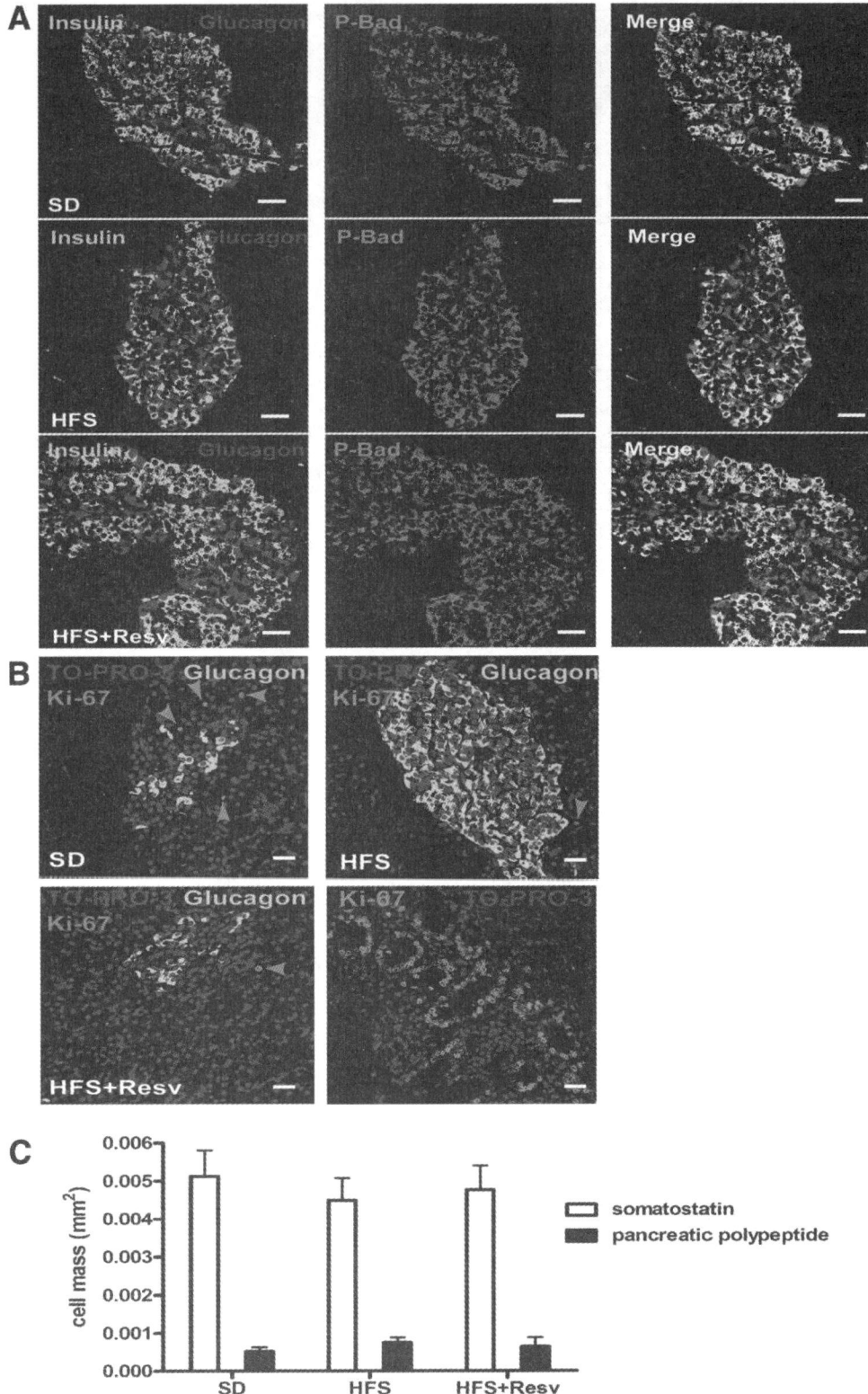

FIG. 2. Lack of apoptosis in β-cells, mitosis in α-cells, or changes in the number of other intraislet hormone cell types. *A*: Immunostaining for insulin (green), glucagon (blue), and P-Bad (red) in islets of monkeys after 24 months on SD (*top panel*), HFS diet (*middle panel*), or HFS+Resv diet (*bottom panel*). Scale bar = 20 μm. *B*: Ki-67 (red), glucagon (green), and TO-PRO-3 (blue) staining in islets of monkeys after 24 months on the indicated diets. Red arrows indicate Ki-67–positive cells that were detected in nonendocrine tissue. Ki-67 staining in the duodenum was used as a positive control. Scale bar = 20 μm. *C*: Quantification of somatostatin (white bars) and pancreatic polypeptide (black bars) cell mass in the different diet interventions. Data are shown as the mean ± SEM.

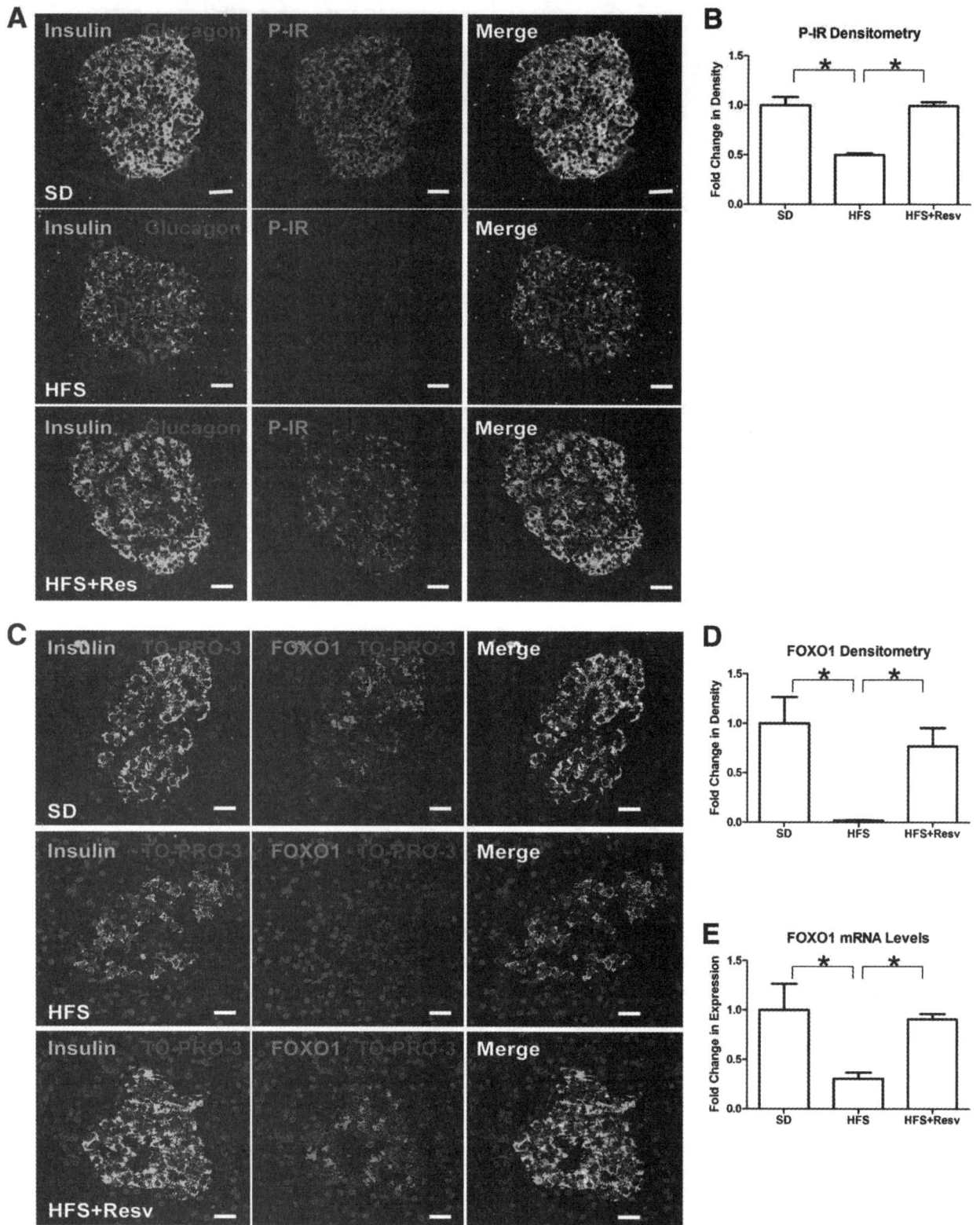

FIG. 3. Decreased P-IR and total FOXO1 levels in an HFS diet. *A*: Immunostaining for insulin (green), glucagon (blue), and tyrosine P-IR (red) in islets of monkeys after 24 months on SD (*top panel*), HFS diet (*middle panel*), or HFS+Resv diet (*bottom panel*). Scale bar = 20 μm. *B*: Quantitation of signal intensity for P-IR. Data are shown as the mean ± SEM. *P < 0.05. *C*: Immunostaining for insulin (green), TO-PRO-3 (blue), and total FOXO1 (red) in islets of monkeys after 24 months on SD (*top panel*), HFS (*middle panel*), or HFS+Resv (*bottom panel*) diets. Scale bar = 20 μm. *D* and *E*: Quantitation of signal intensity (*D*) and mRNA levels (*E*) for FOXO1. Data are shown as the mean ± SEM. *P < 0.05.

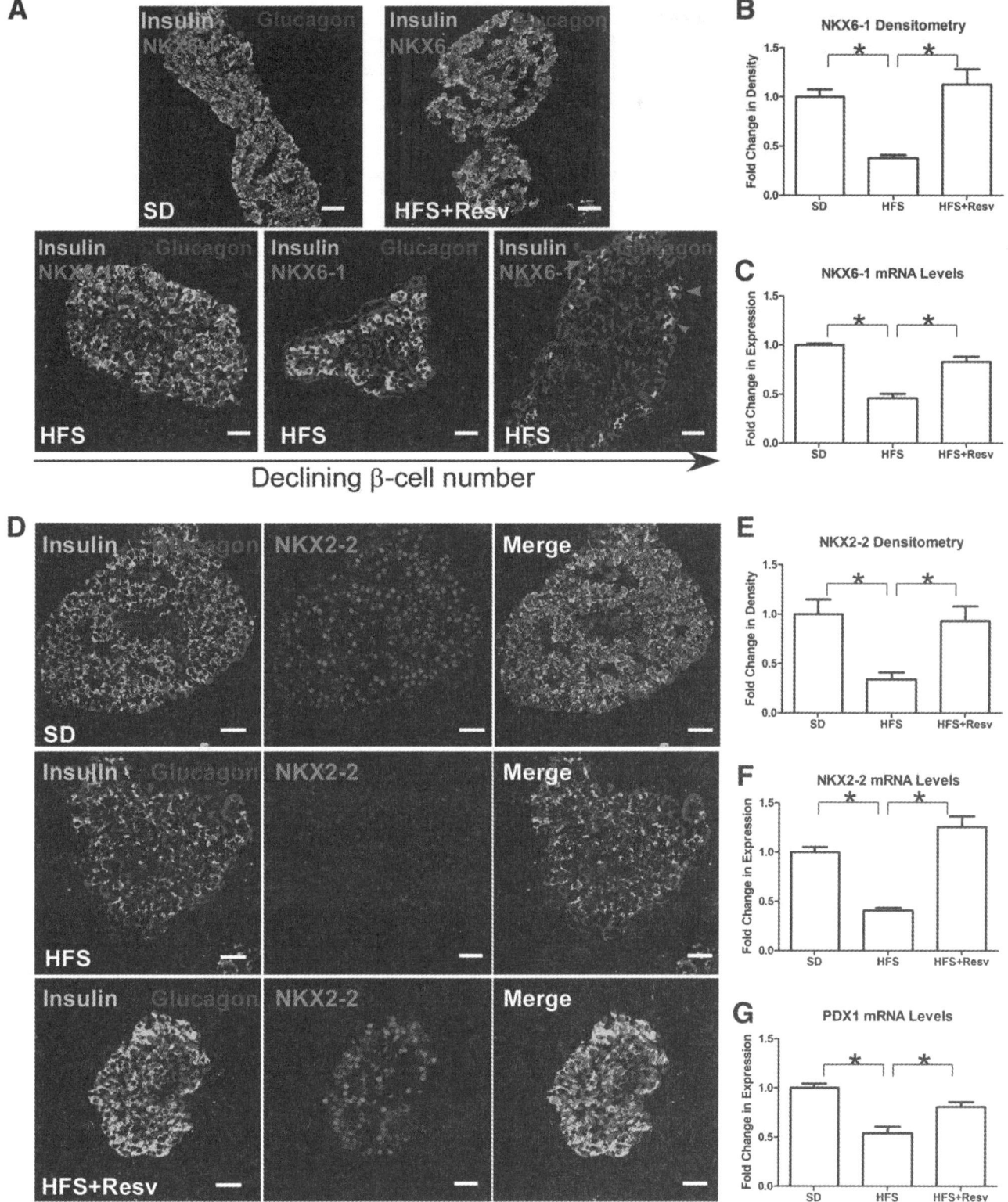

FIG. 4. Decreased nuclear expression of NKX6–1, NKX2–2, and PDX1 after an HFS diet. *A*: Immunostaining for insulin (green), glucagon (blue), and NKX6–1 (red) in monkeys after 24 months on the indicated diet. The islets from different HFS monkeys are shown in order of declining β-cell numbers (*bottom panel*); the red arrows indicate depletion of nuclear NKX6–1 in insulin-expressing cells. Scale bar = 20 μm. *B* and *C*: Quantitation of signal intensity (*B*) and mRNA levels (*C*) for NKX6–1. Data are shown as the mean ± SEM. *$P < 0.05$. *D*: Immunostaining for insulin (green), glucagon (blue), and NKX2–2 (red) in islets of monkeys after 24 months on SD (*top panel*), HFS diet (*middle panel*), or HFS+Resv diet (*bottom panel*). Scale bar = 20 μm. *E* and *F*: Quantitation of signal intensity (*E*) and mRNA levels (*F*) for NKX2–2. Data are shown as the mean ± SEM. *$P < 0.05$. *G*: Quantitation of mRNA levels for *PDX1*. Data are shown as the mean ± SEM. *$P < 0.05$.

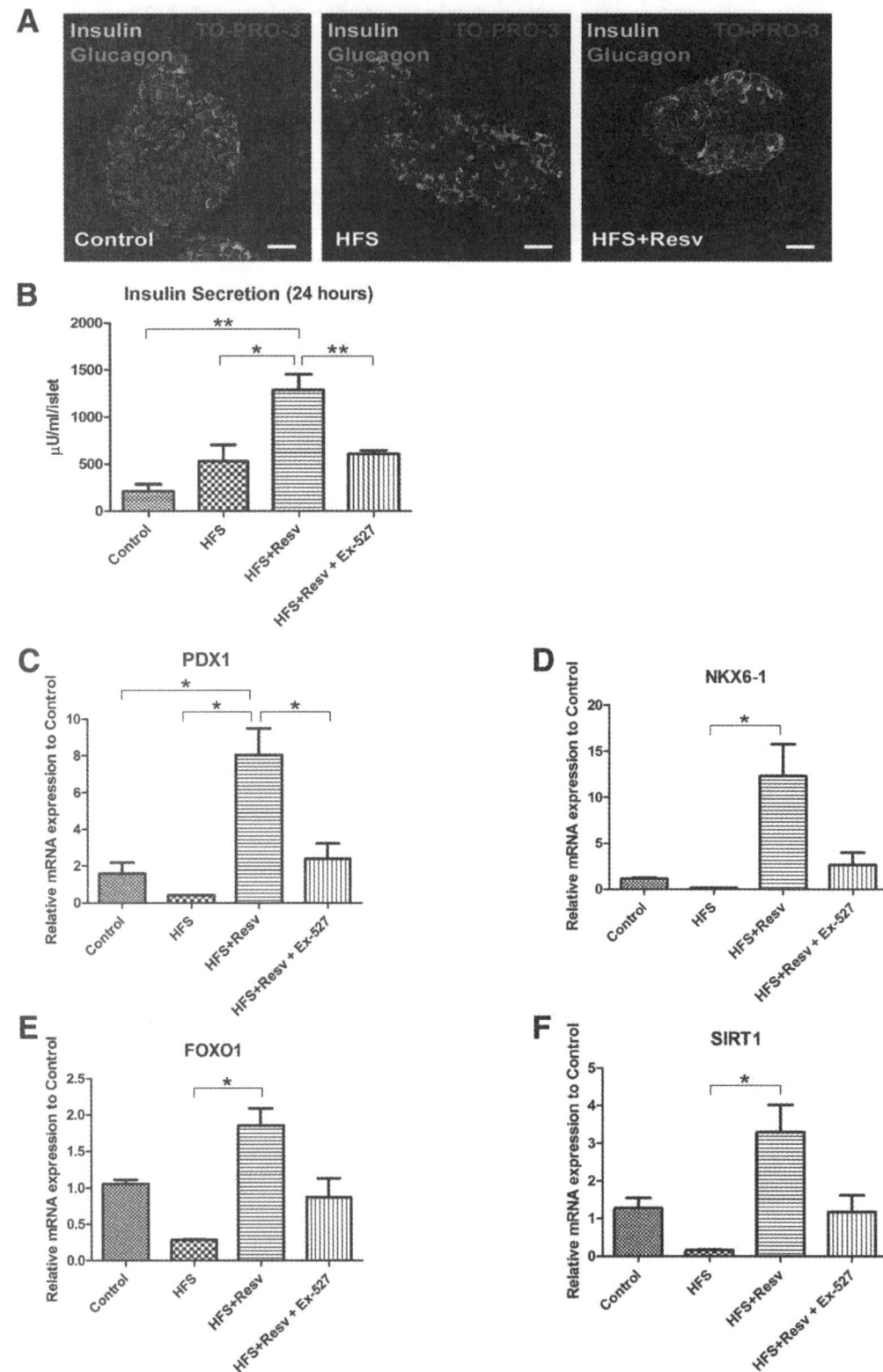

FIG. 5. Resveratrol protects islet morphology, increases insulin secretion, and increases mRNA expression of *PDX1*, *NKX6–1*, *FOXO1*, and *SIRT1* in human islets. *A*: Immunostaining for insulin (green), glucagon (red), and TO-PRO-3 (blue) in human islets. Scale bar = 20 μm. *B*: Insulin secretion per human islet after 24 h in low-glucose (Control), HFS, HFS+Resv, or HFS+Resv and a SIRT1 inhibitor (HFS+Resv + EX-527). *C–F*: Quantitation of mRNA levels for *PDX1* (*C*), *NKX6–1* (*D*), *FOXO1* (*E*), and *SIRT1* (*F*) in human islets after the indicated treatments. Data are shown as the mean ± SEM. *$P < 0.05$, **$P < 0.01$.

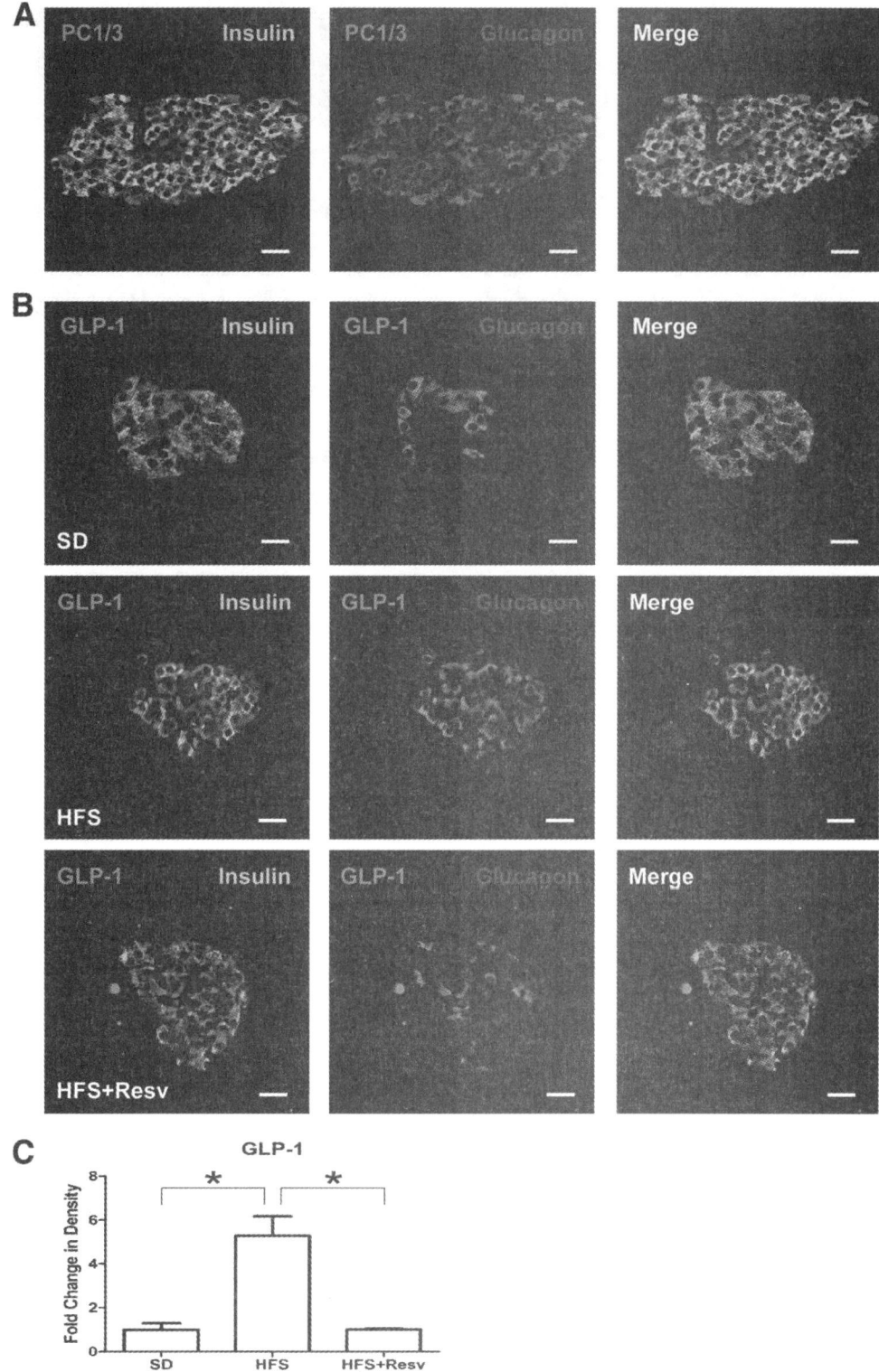

FIG. 6. Identification of PC1/3 and GLP-1 in monkey islets. *A*: Immunostaining for insulin (green), glucagon (blue), and PC1/3 (red) in SD monkey islets. *B*: Immunostaining for insulin (green), glucagon (blue), and GLP-1 (red) in islets of monkeys after 24 months on SD (*top panel*), HFS diet (*middle panel*), or HFS+Resv diet (*bottom panel*) interventions. Scale bar = 20 μm. *C*: Quantitation of signal intensity for GLP-1. Data are shown as the mean ± SEM. *$P < 0.05$.

atherogenic diet (33), and in the pathologies of diabetic human pancreata (34). Additionally, an HFS diet resulted in the depletion of β-cell–specific transcription factors FOXO1, NKX6–1, NKX2–2, and *PDX1*. Remarkably, monkeys given

resveratrol supplementation in addition to an HFS diet had islets that were similar in morphology to SD and maintained the critical transcription factors. The effect of resveratrol was independent of any effect it may have had on

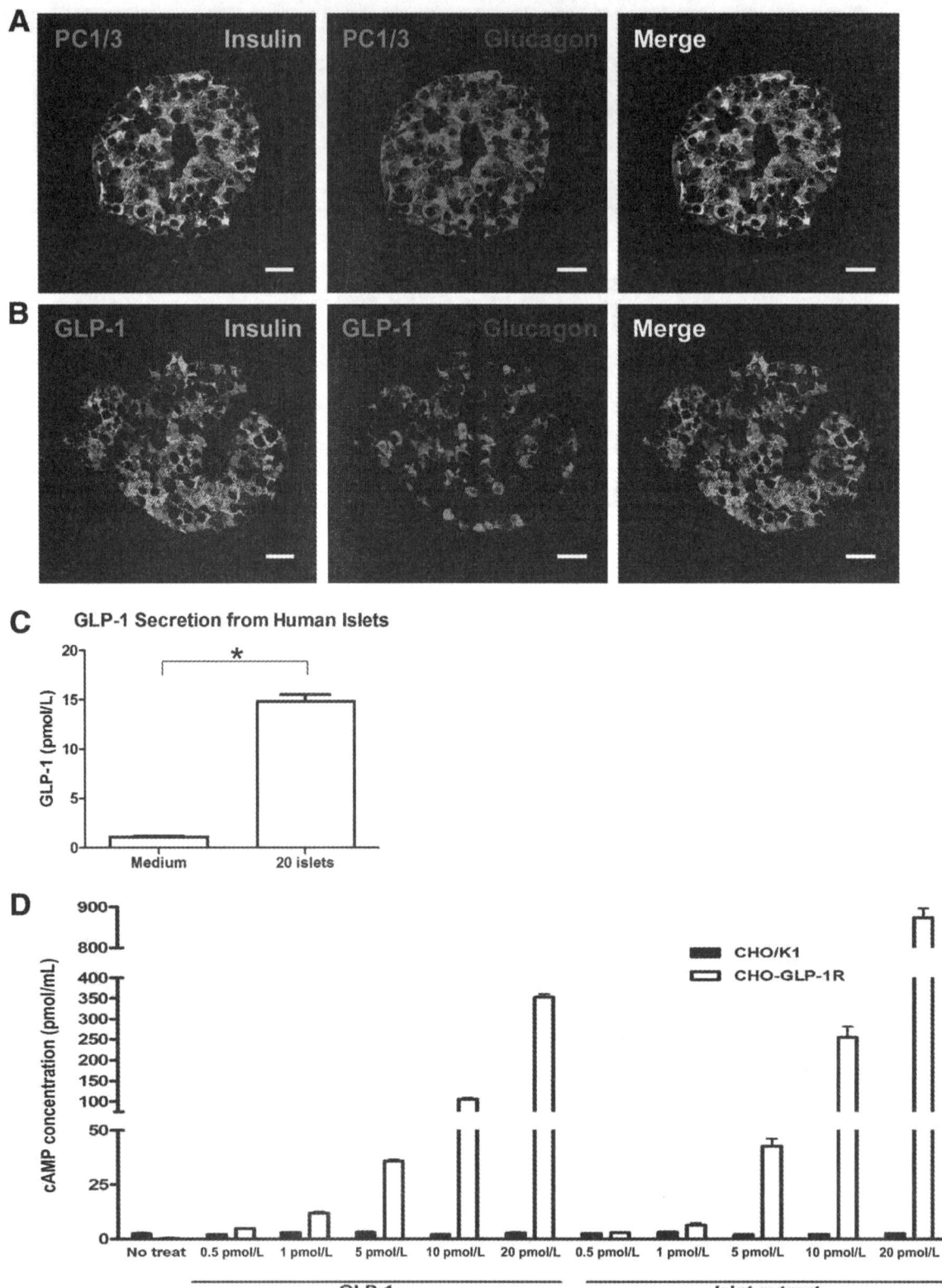

FIG. 7. Secretion of biologically active GLP-1 from human islets. *A* and *B*: Immunostaining for insulin (green) and glucagon (blue) along with PC1/3 (red) (*A*) or GLP-1 (red) (*B*) in human islets. Scale bar = 20 μm. *C*: Levels of secreted GLP-1 from medium alone or from 20 human islets into medium over 1 h as measured by ELISA. *D*: cAMP concentrations after treatment of CHO/K1 (black bars) and CHO-GLP-1R (white bars) cells with either increasing concentration of recombinant GLP-1 as a positive control or GLP-1 extracted from islets (Islet extract). Data are shown as the mean ± SEM from at least three independent experiments. *$P < 0.05$.

insulin-mediated glucose uptake (i.e., peripheral insulin sensitivity), because it did not prevent the decline in insulin sensitivity due to the HFS diet.

There are two possibilities for the increase in α-cell/β-cell ratio observed with HFS monkeys. The first is that β-cells underwent apoptosis and α-cells proliferated, but we did not capture either phenomenon because of the brevity of both. One possible signal for α-cell mitosis is that the neighboring β-cells act as brakes on α-cell turnover and this brake is lifted once a neighboring β-cell undergoes apoptosis. Additionally, apoptotic β-cells may shed microparticles/products that cause proliferation of neighboring α-cells. Indeed, apoptosis of β-cells in rodents stimulates proliferation of neighboring cells (35), and insulin itself is trophic in α-cell lines (36).

A decrease in β-cell mass has also been reported in humans with T2DM, and this was associated with an increase in islet amyloid deposition and β-cell apoptosis (37,38). Baboons, which serve as another model for T2DM (39), also exhibit severe islet amyloidosis, which is associated with increased β-cell apoptosis and decreased relative β-cell volume, as well as α-cell replication, hypertrophy, and increased relative volume (40). The increased α-cell proliferation correlated with hyperglucagonemia and hyperglycemia, neither of which was observed in our monkeys after 24 months on an HFS diet.

A second possibility for the islet findings in HFS monkeys is that β-cells dedifferentiated and became α-cells, thus explaining how islet size was unaltered. Our findings resemble the phenotype seen in FOXO1-null mice in that those mice, placed under metabolic stress, had reduced β-cell numbers due to dedifferentiation, not death, and some dedifferentiated cells became α-cells (26). We suggest that the loss of NKX6–1 and *PDX1* due to depletion of FOXO1 lifted the brake on the repression of glucagon transcription, and, as a consequence, β-cells, once dedifferentiated, became α cells. Single human β-cells normally express the glucagon gene, albeit at low levels compared with the insulin gene (41). In no instance did we find coexpression of insulin and glucagon or glucagon and NKX6–1, illustrating that regression of β-cells to a non–β-cell phenotype is necessary prior to conversion to α-cells. We conclude that unremitting hyperstimulation due to HFS food consumption, and not dysglycemia, is the so-called "metabolic stress" that causes depletion of FOXO1 and loss of β-cell phenotype. β-Cell loss of FOXO1, NKX6–2, and *PDX1* did not occur with HFS consumption when resveratrol was added to the diet. Similar effects have been described in vitro where resveratrol treatment of insulinoma INS-1E cells and human islets resulted in the upregulation of key genes for β-cell function, including *PDX1*, ultimately potentiating glucose-stimulated insulin secretion (42). We also found that resveratrol treatment resulted in a significant increase in *PDX1*, *NKX6–1*, and *FOXO1* mRNA expression in human islets incubated under HFS conditions. The increase in β-cell transcription factors was also associated with an increase in insulin secretion, as HFS+Resv-treated islets secreted insulin at levels 6.2-fold greater than control and 2.4-fold greater than HFS alone.

GLP-1 is a hormone with pleiotropic effects that helps to maintain blood glucose homeostasis. It is a powerful stimulant to insulin secretion in a glucose-dependent manner (43), increases proinsulin synthesis (44), modulates insulin sensitivity (45), and, in rodents, increases β-cell turnover (46). Additionally, glucagon secretion is inhibited by insulin (47) and by GLP-1 independently of insulin (48). We

suggest that increased α-cell–derived GLP-1 promoted enhanced glucose-mediated insulin secretion and contributed to the suppression of glucagon secretion in HFS monkeys. This allowed the remaining β-cells to secrete sufficient insulin to maintain euglycemia and suppress glucagon secretion. This mechanism would be successful as long as adequate numbers of β-cells remained. Eventually β-cell numbers would have declined to a limiting amount and circulating glucagon levels would rise because of lack of sufficient insulin for inhibition of secretion. At this time, dysglycemia would become evident.

Although nonhuman primate studies are crucial to more accurately elucidate the pathogenesis of T2DM in humans, several limitations are evident because of the nature of this model. In the current study, none of the monkeys in the HFS cohort developed overt diabetes, so islets from monkeys under metabolic stress were compared with those from monkeys in which diabetes spontaneously developed to show increasing progression of β-cell depletion. Additionally, we do not know whether the α-cell/β-cell ratio seen with HFS would revert to that of SD if the animals were returned to a healthy SD, so we cannot attest to the adaptability of α-cells once metabolic stress is alleviated. Finally, although we show that daily resveratrol supplementation prevented islet changes in the presence of an HFS diet, we were unable to show the biochemical pathways by which resveratrol was protective. Its effects may be through the activation of AMP-activated protein kinase or Sirtuins, and thus FOXO1 (49,50), through the inhibition of phosphodiesterases in β-cells (51), or through a combination of many pathways. In human islets, we were able to show that blocking SIRT1 prevented the resveratrol-induced increase in insulin secretion and upregulation of *PDX1*, *NKX6–1*, *FOXO1*, and *SIRT1* mRNA expression. This suggests that the positive effects of resveratrol on β-cell function in human islets are mediated through SIRT1.

This study was carried out in adult primates and has direct relevance to the human population that is currently facing a diabetic epidemic caused by obesity. Screening patients for early T2DM and prediabetes is a worthy goal in order to aggressively treat and preserve β-cell function (52,53). We submit, however, that islet changes occur before overt evidence of β-cell compromise and any dysglycemia are uncovered with usual testing, such as fasting glucose levels and hemoglobin A_{1c} measurements. Although lifestyle interventions and pharmacotherapy to maintain normal glucose homeostasis and prevent conversion of prediabetes to diabetes (54) are laudatory, they are expensive, require intense input from healthcare providers, and need to be persistent. They may also be too late because morphological changes causing predisposition to diabetes could have already occurred in islets. The addition of resveratrol and resveratrol-containing foods to one's daily diet may be a simple, inexpensive way to protect β-cells.

ACKNOWLEDGMENTS

This work was supported by the Intramural Research Program of the National Institute on Aging and by a grant from the Office of Dietary Supplements awarded to K.J.P. W.K. was supported by the Basic Science Research Program through the National Research Foundation of Korea (NRF) and funded by the Ministry of Science, ICT, and Future Planning (2012R1A1A1041352). M.E.D. was supported by the JDRF and The Sanford Project, Sioux Falls, SD.

No potential conflicts of interest relevant to this article were reported.

J.L.F. designed and performed experiments, analyzed data, and wrote the manuscript. Y.-K.S., W.K., S.M.K.-W., I.G.-M., and O.D.C. designed and performed experiments and analyzed data. M.S. and R.M. developed and performed the assays to determine serum resveratrol levels. K.F. and S.K.G. analyzed data. M.E.D. was responsible for procuring human islets from the Integrated Islet Distribution Program and for the treatment of human islets. K.J.P., J.A.M., and R.d.C. contributed to the design, execution, and analysis of experiments. J.M.E. contributed to the design of experiments, interpretation of data, and writing of the manuscript. All authors edited and reviewed the manuscript. J.M.E. is the guarantor of this work and, as such, had full access to all the data in the study and takes responsibility for the integrity of the data and the accuracy of the data analysis.

Parts of this study were presented at the 73rd Scientific Sessions of the American Diabetes Association, Chicago, Illinois, 21–25 June 2013.

The authors thank the animal care staff at the National Institutes of Health Animal Center: Edward Tilmont, Joanne Allard, Theresa Ward, Kaitlyn Lewis, Caitlin Younts, and veterinarian Dr. Rick Herbert. The authors also thank Hyekyung Yang for her assistance with processing human islets for staining. The authors are grateful to Fred E. Indig at the National Institute on Aging for his invaluable contributions with confocal imaging; and to DSM Nutritional Products for providing ResVida (resveratrol).

REFERENCES

1. Cordain L, Eaton SB, Sebastian A, et al. Origins and evolution of the Western diet: health implications for the 21st century. Am J Clin Nutr 2005; 81:341–354

2. Haslam DW, James WPT. Obesity. Lancet 2005;366:1197–1209

3. Centers for Disease Control and Prevention. *2011 National Diabetes Fact Sheet* [article online], 2011. Available from http://www.cdc.gov/diabetes/pubs/pdf/ndfs_2011.pdf. Accessed 15 February 2013

4. Knowler WC, Barrett-Connor E, Fowler SE, et al.; Diabetes Prevention Program Research Group. Reduction in the incidence of type 2 diabetes with lifestyle intervention or metformin. N Engl J Med 2002; 346:393–403

5. Szkudelska K, Szkudelski T. Resveratrol, obesity and diabetes. Eur J Pharmacol 2010;635:1–8

6. Baur JA, Pearson KJ, Price NL, et al. Resveratrol improves health and survival of mice on a high-calorie diet. Nature 2006;444:337–342

7. Shang J, Chen LL, Xiao FX, Sun H, Ding HC, Xiao H. Resveratrol improves non-alcoholic fatty liver disease by activating AMP-activated protein kinase. Acta Pharmacol Sin 2008;29:698–706

8. Rivera L, Morón R, Zarzuelo A, Galisteo M. Long-term resveratrol administration reduces metabolic disturbances and lowers blood pressure in obese Zucker rats. Biochem Pharmacol 2009;77:1053–1063

9. Su H-C, Hung L-M, Chen J-K. Resveratrol, a red wine antioxidant, possesses an insulin-like effect in streptozotocin-induced diabetic rats. Am J Physiol Endocrinol Metab 2006;290:E1339–E1346

10. Lee J-H, Song M-Y, Song E-K, et al. Overexpression of SIRT1 protects pancreatic beta-cells against cytokine toxicity by suppressing the nuclear factor-kappaB signaling pathway. Diabetes 2009;58:344–351

11. Timmers S, Konings E, Bilet L, et al. Calorie restriction-like effects of 30 days of resveratrol supplementation on energy metabolism and metabolic profile in obese humans. Cell Metab 2011;14:612–622

12. Brasnyó P, Molnár GA, Mohás M, et al. Resveratrol improves insulin sensitivity, reduces oxidative stress and activates the Akt pathway in type 2 diabetic patients. Br J Nutr 2011;106:383–389

13. Crandall JP, Oram V, Trandafirescu G, et al. Pilot study of resveratrol in older adults with impaired glucose tolerance. J Gerontol A Biol Sci Med Sci 2012;67:1307–1312

14. Yoshino J, Conte C, Fontana L, et al. Resveratrol supplementation does not improve metabolic function in nonobese women with normal glucose tolerance. Cell Metab 2012;16:658–664

15. Poulsen MM, Vestergaard PF, Clasen BF, et al. High-dose resveratrol supplementation in obese men: an investigator-initiated, randomized, placebo-controlled clinical trial of substrate metabolism, insulin sensitivity, and body composition. Diabetes 2013;62:1186–1195

16. Hansen BC. Investigation and treatment of type 2 diabetes in nonhuman primates. Methods Mol Biol 2012;933:177–185

17. Brissova M, Fowler MJ, Nicholson WE, et al. Assessment of human pancreatic islet architecture and composition by laser scanning confocal microscopy. J Histochem Cytochem 2005;53:1087–1097

18. Bremer AA, Stanhope KL, Graham JL, et al. Fructose-fed rhesus monkeys: a nonhuman primate model of insulin resistance, metabolic syndrome, and type 2 diabetes. Clin Transl Sci 2011;4:243–252

19. Ortmeyer HK, Sajan MP, Miura A, et al. Insulin signaling and insulin sensitizing in muscle and liver of obese monkeys: peroxisome proliferator-activated receptor gamma agonist improves defective activation of atypical protein kinase C. Antioxid Redox Signal 2011;14:207–219

20. Boocock DJ, Faust GES, Patel KR, et al. Phase I dose escalation pharmacokinetic study in healthy volunteers of resveratrol, a potential cancer chemopreventive agent. Cancer Epidemiol Biomarkers Prev 2007;16:1246–1252

21. Swarbrick MM, Havel PJ, Levin AA, et al. Inhibition of protein tyrosine phosphatase-1B with antisense oligonucleotides improves insulin sensitivity and increases adiponectin concentrations in monkeys. Endocrinology 2009;150:1670–1679

22. Shin Y-K, Martin B, Golden E, et al. Modulation of taste sensitivity by GLP-1 signaling. J Neurochem 2008;106:455–463

23. Montrose-Rafizadeh C, Wang Y, Janczewski AM, Henderson TE, Egan JM. Overexpression of glucagon-like peptide-1 receptor in an insulin-secreting cell line enhances glucose responsiveness. Mol Cell Endocrinol 1997;130: 109–117

24. Kulkarni RN, Brüning JC, Winnay JN, Postic C, Magnuson MA, Kahn CR. Tissue-specific knockout of the insulin receptor in pancreatic beta cells creates an insulin secretory defect similar to that in type 2 diabetes. Cell 1999;96:329–339

25. Ueki K, Okada T, Hu J, et al. Total insulin and IGF-I resistance in pancreatic beta cells causes overt diabetes. Nat Genet 2006;38:583–588

26. Talchai C, Xuan S, Lin HV, Sussel L, Accili D. Pancreatic β cell dedifferentiation as a mechanism of diabetic β cell failure. Cell 2012;150: 1223–1234

27. Watada H, Mirmira RG, Leung J, German MS. Transcriptional and translational regulation of beta-cell differentiation factor Nkx6.1. J Biol Chem 2000;275:34224–34230

28. Anderson KR, Torres CA, Solomon K, et al. Cooperative transcriptional regulation of the essential pancreatic islet gene NeuroD1 (beta2) by Nkx2.2 and neurogenin 3. J Biol Chem 2009;284:31236–31248

29. McKinnon CM, Docherty K. Pancreatic duodenal homeobox-1, PDX-1, a major regulator of beta cell identity and function. Diabetologia 2001;44: 1203–1214

30. Rouillé Y, Bianchi M, Irminger JC, Halban PA. Role of the prohormone convertase PC2 in the processing of proglucagon to glucagon. FEBS Lett 1997;413:119–123

31. Rouillé Y, Kantengwa S, Irminger JC, Halban PA. Role of the prohormone convertase PC3 in the processing of proglucagon to glucagon-like peptide 1. J Biol Chem 1997;272:32810–32816

32. Marchetti P, Lupi R, Bugliani M, et al. A local glucagon-like peptide 1 (GLP-1) system in human pancreatic islets. Diabetologia 2012;55:3262–3272

33. Louw J, Woodroof C, Seier J, Wolfe-Coote SA. The effect of diet on the Vervet monkey endocrine pancreas. J Med Primatol 1997;26:307–311

34. Folli F, Okada T, Perego C, et al. Altered insulin receptor signalling and β-cell cycle dynamics in type 2 diabetes mellitus. PLoS One 2011;6: e28050

35. Bonner C, Bacon S, Concannon CG, et al. INS-1 cells undergoing caspase-dependent apoptosis enhance the regenerative capacity of neighboring cells. Diabetes 2010;59:2799–2808

36. Liu Z, Kim W, Chen Z, et al. Insulin and glucagon regulate pancreatic α-cell proliferation. PLoS One 2011;6:e16096

37. Jurgens CA, Toukatly MN, Fligner CL, et al. β-cell loss and β-cell apoptosis in human type 2 diabetes are related to islet amyloid deposition. Am J Pathol 2011;178:2632–2640

38. Westermark P, Andersson A, Westermark GT. Islet amyloid polypeptide, islet amyloid, and diabetes mellitus. Physiol Rev 2011;91:795–826

39. Chavez AO, Lopez-Alvarenga JC, Tejero ME, et al. Physiological and molecular determinants of insulin action in the baboon. Diabetes 2008;57: 899–908

40. Guardado-Mendoza R, Davalli AM, Chavez AO, et al. Pancreatic islet amyloidosis, beta-cell apoptosis, and alpha-cell proliferation are determinants

of islet remodeling in type-2 diabetic baboons. Proc Natl Acad Sci USA 2009;106:13992–13997

41. Kirkpatrick CL, Marchetti P, Purrello F, et al. Type 2 diabetes susceptibility gene expression in normal or diabetic sorted human alpha and beta cells: correlations with age or BMI of islet donors. PLoS One 2010;5: e11053

42. Vetterli L, Brun T, Giovannoni L, Bosco D, Maechler P. Resveratrol potentiates glucose-stimulated insulin secretion in INS-1E beta-cells and human islets through a SIRT1-dependent mechanism. J Biol Chem 2011; 286:6049–6060

43. Nauck MA, Bartels E, Orskov C, Ebert RCW, Creutzfeldt W. Additive insulinotropic effects of exogenous synthetic human gastric inhibitory polypeptide and glucagon-like peptide-1-(7-36) amide infused at near-physiological insulinotropic hormone and glucose concentrations. J Clin Endocrinol Metab 1993;76:912–917

44. Alarcon C, Wicksteed B, Rhodes CJ. Exendin 4 controls insulin production in rat islet beta cells predominantly by potentiation of glucose-stimulated proinsulin biosynthesis at the translational level. Diabetologia 2006;49: 2920–2929

45. Zander M, Madsbad S, Madsen JL, Holst JJ. Effect of 6-week course of glucagon-like peptide 1 on glycaemic control, insulin sensitivity, and beta-cell function in type 2 diabetes: a parallel-group study. Lancet 2002; 359:824–830

46. Buteau J, Foisy S, Rhodes CJ, Carpenter L, Biden TJ, Prentki M. Protein kinase Czeta activation mediates glucagon-like peptide-1-induced pancreatic beta-cell proliferation. Diabetes 2001;50:2237–2243

47. Kaneko K, Shirotani T, Araki E, et al. Insulin inhibits glucagon secretion by the activation of PI3-kinase in In-R1-G9 cells. Diabetes Res Clin Pract 1999;44:83–92

48. Kawamori D, Akiyama M, Hu J, Hambro B, Kulkarni RN. Growth factor signalling in the regulation of α-cell fate. Diabetes Obes Metab 2011;13 (Suppl. 1):21–30

49. Brunet A, Sweeney LB, Sturgill JF, et al. Stress-dependent regulation of FOXO transcription factors by the SIRT1 deacetylase. Science 2004;303: 2011–2015

50. Wang A, Liu M, Liu X, et al. Up-regulation of adiponectin by resveratrol: the essential roles of the Akt/FOXO1 and AMP-activated protein kinase signaling pathways and DsbA-L. J Biol Chem 2011;286:60–66

51. Park S-J, Ahmad F, Philp A, et al. Resveratrol ameliorates aging-related metabolic phenotypes by inhibiting cAMP phosphodiesterases. Cell 2012; 148:421–433

52. Phillips LS, Olson DE. Diabetes: normal glucose levels should be the goal. Nat Rev Endocrinol 2012;8:510–512

53. Fradkin JE, Roberts BT, Rodgers GP. What's preventing us from preventing type 2 diabetes? N Engl J Med 2012;367:1177–1179

54. American Diabetes Association. Standards of medical care in diabetes—2012. Diabetes Care 2012;35(Suppl. 1):S11–S63

Sirt3 Regulates Metabolic Flexibility of Skeletal Muscle Through Reversible Enzymatic Deacetylation

Enxuan Jing,[1] Brian T. O'Neill,[1] Matthew J. Rardin,[2] André Kleinridders,[1] Olga R. Ilkeyeva,[3] Siegfried Ussar,[1] James R. Bain,[3] Kevin Y. Lee,[1] Eric M. Verdin,[4,5] Christopher B. Newgard,[3] Bradford W. Gibson,[2] and C. Ronald Kahn[1]

Sirt3 is an NAD^+-dependent deacetylase that regulates mitochondrial function by targeting metabolic enzymes and proteins. In fasting mice, Sirt3 expression is decreased in skeletal muscle resulting in increased mitochondrial protein acetylation. Deletion of Sirt3 led to impaired glucose oxidation in muscle, which was associated with decreased pyruvate dehydrogenase (PDH) activity, accumulation of pyruvate and lactate metabolites, and an inability of insulin to suppress fatty acid oxidation. Antibody-based acetyl-peptide enrichment and mass spectrometry of mitochondrial lysates from WT and Sirt3 KO skeletal muscle revealed that a major target of Sirt3 deacetylation is the E1α subunit of PDH (PDH E1α). Sirt3 knockout in vivo and Sirt3 knockdown in myoblasts in vitro induced hyperacetylation of the PDH E1α subunit, altering its phosphorylation leading to suppressed PDH enzymatic activity. The inhibition of PDH activity resulting from reduced levels of Sirt3 induces a switch of skeletal muscle substrate utilization from carbohydrate oxidation toward lactate production and fatty acid utilization even in the fed state, contributing to a loss of metabolic flexibility. Thus, Sirt3 plays an important role in skeletal muscle mitochondrial substrate choice and metabolic flexibility in part by regulating PDH function through deacetylation. *Diabetes* **62:3404–3417, 2013**

Skeletal muscle is the major oxidative tissue in mammals. Metabolic flexibility, i.e., the ability to switch between glucose and lipid oxidation, in muscle is essential to maintain normal energy metabolism and physiology. In the fed state, the main fuel source in muscle is insulin-induced glucose metabolism (1,2); during fasting, muscle switches its fuel utilization from glucose to lipid oxidation (3). Insulin resistance, type 2 diabetes, and obesity are strongly associated with impaired skeletal muscle substrate metabolism including decreased fasting lipid oxidation, impaired postprandial glucose oxidation, and reduced capacity for lipid oxidation during exercise (4,5). Thus, the flexibility and capacity of substrate metabolism are compromised in muscle in these states.

Recent reports have shown that mitochondrial dysfunction is a major contributor to the development of insulin resistance and diabetes (6,7). Transcription factors regulating mitochondrial function and biogenesis, such as peroxisome proliferator–activated receptor (PPAR)γ coactivator-1α, nuclear respiratory factor-1, and PPARα play critical roles in insulin sensitivity, glucose metabolism, and lipid metabolism in muscle (8–11). Mutations of key metabolic enzymes and subunits of the electron transporter chain can also lead to mitochondrial dysfunction and various degrees of myopathy and neuropathology. Among these, pyruvate dehydrogenase (PDH) complex deficiency due to mutations of the E1α subunit gene (PDHA1) that encodes the catalytic subunit of PDH is a genetic cause of mitochondrial dysfunction and inherited neurodegenerative disease in humans, implicating this subunit's critical role in metabolism (12,13).

The PDH complex catalyzes the rate-limiting step in aerobic carbohydrate metabolism and mediates the efficient conversion of pyruvate from glycolysis to energy in cells. The activity of this multienzyme complex is regulated, at least in part, by reversible phosphorylation of serine residues of the E1α subunit through PDH kinases (PDHKs) and PDH phosphatases whose enzymatic functions are regulated by cellular nutrient cues (14). Phosphorylation by PDHKs inhibits the E1α subunit, decreasing PDH activity; accordingly, inhibition of PDHKs is a potential therapeutic target for diabetes (15). Nutrient deprivation, such as starvation or diabetes, leads to increased NAD^+-to-NADH ratio and increases PDHK expression and activity, thereby inhibiting PDH in muscle; this is reversible with refeeding or insulin treatment (16). Besides phosphorylation, recent studies suggest that reversible acetylation/deacetylation may also regulate PDH catalytic subunit E1α (PDH E1α) function (17–19), although the pathways controlling this process have not been fully elucidated.

In recent years, NAD^+-dependent deacetylases called sirtuins (Sirt) have been shown to play important roles in metabolism (20,21). Among seven members of this protein family, Sirt3 is identified as the major mitochondrial deacetylase (22,23). Several recent studies have shown that Sirt3 regulates lipid metabolism, energy production, and stress response in different tissues through its deacetylase activity (24–26). In muscle, Sirt3 expression is regulated by nutrient signals and contractile activity and impacts downstream signaling events through AMP-activated protein kinase activation and PPARγ coactivator-1α expression (27,28). Sirt3 was implicated in the development of metabolic disease in humans when a commonly identified polymorphism that decreases Sirt3 activity was found to be associated with the development of metabolic syndrome (29). We previously demonstrated that skeletal muscle Sirt3 expression is downregulated in rodent models of diabetes

From the [1]Section on Integrative Physiology and Metabolism, Joslin Diabetes Center, Harvard Medical School, Boston, Massachusetts; the [2]Buck Institute for Research on Aging, Novato, California; the [3]Department of Medicine, Duke University Medical Center, Durham, North Carolina; the [4]Gladstone Institute of Virology and Immunology, San Francisco, California; and the [5]Department of Medicine, University of California, San Francisco, San Francisco, California.
Corresponding author: C. Ronald Kahn, c.ronald.kahn@joslin.harvard.edu.
Received 27 November 2012 and accepted 26 June 2013.
DOI: 10.2337/db12-1650
This article contains Supplementary Data online at http://diabetes .diabetesjournals.org/lookup/suppl/doi:10.2337/db12-1650/-/DC1.
E.J. and B.T.O. contributed equally to this study.

and upregulated by caloric restriction and that decreased Sirt3 expression induces oxidative stress and impairs insulin signaling in muscle (30). Sirt3 also regulates levels of reactive oxygen species (ROS) through deacetylation of SOD2 (26,31). In the current study, using a combination of proteomic, metabolomic, and functional approaches, we demonstrate that skeletal muscle Sirt3 regulates substrate metabolism by targeting mitochondrial PDH E1α subunit and PDH enzyme activity and thus optimizes the complex and intricate switch of substrate utilization between glucose and lipid oxidation and substrate flexibility.

RESEARCH DESIGN AND METHODS

Animal studies were performed according to protocols approved by the Institutional Animal Care and Use Committee. Male C57Bl/6 mice or *Sirt3⁻/⁻* and wild-type (WT) littermate controls backcrossed onto a C57Bl/6 background and maintained on a standard chow diet were used. Fed mice were allowed ad libitum access to food and killed at 9:00 A.M. For fasting studies, mice were transferred to a new cage without food for 24 h and then killed or refed for 4 or 16 h prior to sacrifice.

Insulin signaling in muscle strips. Extensor digitorum longus (EDL) or hemidiaphragms were dissected and incubated for 30 min in Krebs-Henseleit buffer (KHB) at 37°C and then transferred to KHB with or without 1 or 10 mU/mL insulin for 10 min. Muscle strips were blotted and snap frozen in liquid nitrogen.

Glycolysis, glycogen synthesis, glucose oxidation, and palmitate oxidation in muscle strips. Glycolysis, glycogen synthesis, glucose oxidation, and palmitate oxidation were measured in isolated muscle strips as previously described with the following modifications (32). Briefly, hemidiaphragms and EDL muscles were dissected and incubated for 30 min in KHB gassed with 95% O_2 and 5% CO_2. Muscle strips were transferred to gassed KHB containing 5 mmol/L glucose and 0.2 mmol/L palmitate bound to 3% fatty acid–free BSA, with or without 1 mU/mL insulin, and with radiolabeled tracers. For glycolysis, glycogen synthesis, and glucose oxidation, incubation buffer contained 20 μCi/mmol [U-¹⁴C]glucose and 80 μCi/mmol [5-³H]glucose, and muscles were incubated for 1 h with shaking at 37°C. Reactions were terminated by removal of the tissue from the incubation medium, followed by injection of 0.2 mL hyamine into the center wells and 0.1 mL 70% (w/v) $HClO_4$ into 1 mL of the contents of the flask. The rate of glucose oxidation was determined from the production of $^{14}CO_2$. Glycogen was purified by digestion of tissue in 1 mol/L NaOH and then precipitation in 66% ethanol with 100 mg unlabeled glycogen to determine the amount of glycogen synthesized from [U-¹⁴C]glucose and [5-³H]glucose incorporation. ³H₂O formation was measured by separating ³H₂O from 0.5 mL incubation buffer containing [5-³H]glucose on Poly-Prep Columns AG 1-X8-731-6212 (Bio-Rad) pretreated with 1 mol/L NaOH and then 0.3 mol/L Boric acid. The rate of glycolysis was determined from the difference between the rate of ³H₂O formed and the rate of substrate recycling determined from the difference between the rates of glycogen synthesis from [U-¹⁴C]glucose and [5-³H]glucose.

Cell culture maintenance. C2C12 cells (American Type Culture Collection, Manassas, VA) were maintained in high-glucose Dulbecco's modified Eagle's medium (DMEM) (Invitrogen) containing 10% FBS (Gemini Bioproducts) unless otherwise indicated. *Sirt3* short hairpin RNA (shRNA) and short hairpin green fluorescent protein (shGFP) control lentiviral constructs were purchased from Open Biosystems (Huntsville, AL). Stable Sirt3 knockdown and shGFP control cell lines were generated by viral transduction of C2C12 myoblasts and selection with puromycin. Wild-type PDH E1α cDNA lentiviral construct (Genecopeia) was used for site-directed mutagenesis (Stratagene) to generate K336Q and K336R mutations and further sequenced. WT, K336Q, and K336R overexpressing stable C2C12 cell lines were generated.

Proteomic analysis of acetylated skeletal muscle mitochondrial peptides. Mitochondria were isolated from hindlimb muscle of WT and SIRT3 KO mice as previously described (33) with the following adaptations: Muscle was homogenized with teflon-pestle in Medium 1 with deacetylase inhibitors (250 mmol/L sucrose, 1 mmol/L EDTA, and 10 mmol/L Tris-HCl, pH 7.4; protease and phosphatase inhibitors [PIs] [Sigma]; 10 mmol/L nicotinamide; and 1 μmol/L trichostatin A). Mitochondria were enriched by differential centrifugation and purified by centrifugation at 59,800g on 5–25% (w/v) linear Ficoll (Sigma) gradients. Purified mitochondria were lysed in radioimmunoprecipitation assay buffer containing protease, phosphatase, and deacetylase inhibitors. Approximately 1 mg total mitochondrial protein was digested with trypsin, and an acetylated peptide fraction was prepared using a combination of anti-AcK antibodies from ImmuneChem (cat. no. ICP0380-100) and Cell Signaling (cat. no. 9441) as previously described (34). Peptides were analyzed by

reversed-phase nano-high-performance liquid chromatography electrospray tandem mass spectrometry (HPLC-ESI-MS/MS) on a QSTAR Elite mass spectrometer. The resulting MS/MS datasets were analyzed using Mascot 2.3.2 (Matrix Sciences) and Protein Pilot 4.1 (AB Sciex, Foster City, CA) searched against the mouse SwissProt database (SwissProt 2011_04). Peptide scores outside of the 5% local false discovery rate were excluded. Skyline MS1 Filtering (34) was used to quantify changes in the MS1 ion abundances among acetylated peptides between WT and KO mice.

PDH activity assay. PDH activity was measured using two methods. The first used the Mitosciences Pyruvate Dehydrogenase Enzyme Activity Microplate Assay Kit (Abcam) in which PDH complexes from isolated mitochondria or cellular lysates are immunocaptured on a microplate. A reaction medium containing pyruvate and NAD⁺ is then added. The readout is the rate of production of NADH, which is coupled to a dye whose formation is monitored on a spectrophotometric plate reader, and activity is calculated from the rate of change in optical density at 410 nm. For in vivo experiments, muscle mitochondria were isolated as previously described (35), and equal amounts of mitochondrial protein were loaded into the immunocapture plate. For in vitro experiments, confluent myoblasts were treated as specified in the manufacturer's protocol. For specified experiments, PI cocktails 2 and 3 (Sigma) or 20 mmol/L dichloroacetate (DCA) was added to detergent-soluble fraction and buffer 1 prior to microplate incubation. Activity was normalized to protein content of the detergent-soluble fraction. For Western blots of extracts from PDH activity experiments, an aliquot of detergent soluble extracts was incubated at room temperature for 3 h to mimic microplate conditions and blotted using phospho-specific PDH E1α antibodies.

PDH activity was also measured in whole muscle homogenates based on the evolution of $^{14}CO_2$ from ¹⁴C-labeled pyruvate (36). Briefly, gastrocnemius muscle from randomly fed mice was snap frozen until use. Muscle homogenates (50 mg wet weight/mL) were incubated for 15 min at 37°C with either *1*) "inactivation" buffer containing 50 mmol/L NaF and 8 mmol/L ATP to prevent dephosphorylation of the PDH complex with or without the addition of deacetylase inhibitors (1 mmol/L nicotinamide and 1 μmol/L trichostatin A) or *2*) "activation" buffer containing 1 μg recombinant PDH phosphatase 1 (Abcam), 5 mmol/L DCA, 9 mmol/L $MgCl_2$, and 0.1 mmol/L $CaCl_2$ with or without deacetylase inhibitors. Activity was then measured in 20 μL homogenates diluted in reaction buffer for 10 min and terminated with 20% trichloroacetate and 30 mmol/L pyruvate as described in the protocol. Evolved $^{14}CO_2$ was collected in suspended center wells containing 1 mol/L hyamine hydroxide in methanol and counted in 4 mL Cytoscint scintillation fluid. Activity of homogenates treated with inactivating solution was termed "PDHa," as this likely represents the native activation of PDH in muscle. Activity of homogenates treated with activating solution was termed "PDHt," representing total activity of PDH present in muscle.

ATP and glycogen measurement. ATP levels were measured by an enzymatic coupled assay as previously described (37). Briefly, metabolites were isolated from pulverized muscle in 6% perchloric acid and neutralized with KOH and imidazole, and then ATP was measured as the change in optical density at 340 nm after addition of glucose, NADP⁺, glucose-6-phosphate dehydrogenase, and hexokinase. Glycogen content was measured as previously described (38).

Immunoprecipitation and Western analysis. Powdered muscle tissue, isolated muscle mitochondria, or confluent myoblasts were homogenized in radioimmunoprecipitation assay buffer (Millipore) with protease and PIs (Sigma) and deacetylase inhibitors (10 mmol/L nicotinamide/1 μmol/L trichostatin A). Lysates were subjected to SDS-PAGE and blotted using PDH E1α, PDHK4, LCAD, glyceraldehyde-3-phosphate dehydrogenase, insulin receptor β (Santa Cruz), phospho-IR/IGFR, phospho-Akt, phospho-ERK, Akt, extracellular signal–related kinase (ERK), VDAC, Sirt3, (Cell Signaling), or acetyl-lysine (Immunechem or Cell Signaling) antibodies. For immunoprecipitation assays, mitochondria were isolated in the presence of protease and deacetylase inhibitors as previously described (35), resuspended in IP lysis buffer (Pierce), and immunoprecipitated with anti–acetyl-lysine (AcK) agarose beads (Immunechem) with streptavidin beads (Pierce) as a control.

Oxygen consumption rate and extracellular acidification rate assays. Cellular oxygen consumption rate (OCR) was measured using a Seahorse Bioscience XF24 flux analyzer. Cells were seeded at 30,000 cells/well 24 h prior to the analysis in low-glucose (100 mg/dL) DMEM containing 10% FBS. Each experimental condition was analyzed using four to six biological replicates. For OCR experiments using palmitate, KHB buffer (pH 7.4) was added to each well and measurements were performed every 3 min with 2 min intermeasurement mixing. BSA-conjugated palmitate (final concentration 200 μmol/L) and etomoxir (final concentration 50 μmol/L) were injected sequentially. For extracellular acidification rate (ECAR) experiments with glucose as a substrate, sodium carbonate and glucose/pyruvate-free DMEM was used. Glucose and 2-deoxyglucose were injected sequentially to give final concentrations of 25 mmol/L.

Metabolomic assays for skeletal muscle amino acids, organic acids, and acylcarnitines. Amino acids, acylcarnitines, and organic acids were analyzed using stable isotope dilution techniques. Amino acids and acylcarnitine measurements were made by flow injection MS/MS using sample preparation methods described previously (39,40). The data were acquired using a Micromass Quattro MicroTM system equipped with a model 2777 autosampler, a model 1525 HPLC solvent delivery system, and a data system controlled by MassLynx 4.1 operating system (Waters, Millford, MA). Organic acids were quantified using methods described previously with Trace Ultra GC coupled to a Trace DSQ MS operating under Xcalibur 1.4 (Thermo Fisher Scientific, Austin, TX) (41).

Statistical analyses. All data are means ± SEM. Student t test was performed for comparison of two groups or ANOVA was performed for comparison of three or more groups to determine significance.

RESULTS

Sirt3 expression and mitochondrial acetylation is regulated by fasting. Quantitative real-time PCR using quadriceps (Quad), EDL, and soleus muscles from 8-week-old male WT C57Bl/6 mice revealed that 24 h of fasting suppressed Sirt3 mRNA expression in hindlimb muscles (Fig. 1A). All of these reductions returned to close to fed levels by 16 h of refeeding and the EDL muscle showed some recovery as early as 4 h after refeeding (Supplementary Fig. 1A). Western blotting analysis confirmed a parallel ~50% decrease of Sirt3 protein level in soleus and gastrocnemius muscle from fasted mice, which increased after refeeding to near-normal levels, as we have previously described in quadriceps (30) (Fig. 1B). There was some variability in the recovery of Sirt3 levels from experiment to experiment, but a decrease in Sirt3 levels in the fasted state was observed in all muscle groups tested (Supplementary Fig. 1A and C). In the fasted state, levels of expression also varied, with muscle fiber type being highest in red soleus and lower in white EDL muscle.

Western analysis of isolated mitochondria from skeletal muscle using an antibody against AcK revealed a general increase of mitochondrial protein acetylation after 24 h of fasting, coinciding with decreased Sirt3 levels. We observed a specific increase in acetylation of bands at 97, 72, and 47 kDa (Fig. 1C). The lower hyperacetylated band was in the migration position of PDH catalytic subunit E1α. We immunoprecipitated muscle mitochondrial lysates isolated from either fed or fasted mice using anti-AcK antibody and subjected the immunoprecipitates to Western blotting analysis with anti–PDH E1α antibody. The abundance of the PDH E1α protein from the immunoprecipitates represents its acetylation status. This analysis confirmed hyperacetylation of PDH E1α in fasted skeletal muscle (Fig. 1D).

Posttranslational modifications known to suppress PDH activity include PDH kinase–mediated phosphorylation targeting three serine residues of PDH E1α (S232, S293, and S300) (42). We tested serine phosphorylation of PDH E1α in muscle mitochondria using phospho-specific antibodies and found that S232 and S300 phosphorylation was increased during fasting coincident with the PDH E1α hyperacetylation (Fig. 1D). The changes in PDH E1α acetylation/phosphorylation after fasting were not explained by changes in PDH E1α total protein levels (Fig. 1D).

Sirt3 deletion induces a shift in substrate utilization away from glucose oxidation and increases PDH E1α phosphorylation suppressing PDH activity. We hypothesized that Sirt3 has its most prominent role in metabolic regulation in the fed state, when it is present at highest levels. To test this hypothesis, we assessed glucose and palmitate oxidation, as well as glycolysis and glycogen synthesis, in isolated muscle strips from fed WT and Sirt3

KO mice to fully characterize muscle substrate metabolism in the absence of Sirt3. Glucose oxidation in EDL muscles (composed primarily of glycolytic fibers) in the presence of 5 mmol/L glucose, 0.2 mmol/L palmitate, and 1 mU/mL insulin was significantly decreased in Sirt3 KO mice compared with controls (Fig. 2A). However, glycogen synthesis rates responded normally to insulin, and glycolytic rates were unchanged in Sirt3 KO, suggesting that glucose uptake was normal but that the end products of glycolysis were not fully oxidized in Sirt3 KO muscle generating lactate. Palmitate oxidation rate was quite low in EDL muscle and was unchanged between KO and WT. To determine whether these changes were due to insulin resistance, as we have observed in older 24-week animals (30), we measured insulin signaling in muscle strips from 8- to 16-week-old Sirt3 KO mice and controls. Interestingly, in this ex vivo experiment in EDL strips from younger mice in the fed or fasted state, we found no difference in insulin signaling between Sirt3 KO mice and controls (Fig. 2B). In hemidiaphragms (composed of more oxidative fibers) palmitate oxidation was increased in the presence of insulin, and glucose oxidation was not significantly changed in Sirt3 KO but tended to decrease (Fig. 2C). Again, there was no change in insulin signaling, glycolysis, or glycogen synthesis rates in hemidiaphragms from Sirt3 KO compared with WT controls (Supplementary Fig. 2A and B). These changes in substrate metabolism did not affect total glycogen content or ATP levels in tissues isolated in the fed or fasted states, and AMP-activated protein kinase phosphorylation was decreased in Sirt3 KO muscle upon fasting as previously described (Supplementary Fig. 2D and E) (27).

The decreased glucose oxidation rate in the insulin-stimulated state in muscle samples from Sirt3 KO mice indicated a potential regulatory role for Sirt3 on mitochondrial glucose oxidation. Since PDH E1α function can be regulated by phosphorylation on three serine residues (42), we assessed phosphorylation of PDH E1α in WT and Sirt3 KO skeletal muscle to determine whether deletion of Sirt3 mimics the effect of fasting on posttranslational modification of PDH E1α. Knockout of Sirt3 resulted in an increase in the phosphorylation of PDH E1α on S300 and tended to increase S232 (but not S293) in muscle of fed mice (Fig. 2D and Supplementary Fig. 2F), mimicking the increased phospho–PDH E1α observed in fasted WT mice. As observed in fasting, increased PDH E1α acetylation and phosphorylation in Sirt3 KO occurred without changes in the total level of PDH E1α or PDHK4 in either the fed or the fasted state (Fig. 2D and F).

Posttranslational modifications like phosphorylation of PDH E1α are known to have effects on PDH enzymatic activity (14,43); thus, we investigated whether the increased acetylation and phosphorylation of PDH E1α related to Sirt3 deletion would change catalytic activity of the PDH enzyme complex. Indeed, PDH activity measured by the immunocapture assay (see RESEARCH DESIGN AND METHODS) was significantly reduced in Sirt3 KO mitochondrial lysates compared with WT. Quantification of the slopes of the linear regressions demonstrated a >70% inhibition of PDH activity in KO mice (Fig. 2E). To further elucidate the possible regulatory role of acetylation on PDH activity, we determined active and total PDH activity in muscle homogenates from fed Sirt3 KO and WT mice as well as fasted C57Bl/6 mice by measurement of $^{14}CO_2$ production from ^{14}C-labeled pyruvate in the presence or absence of deacetylase inhibitors (see RESEARCH DESIGN AND METHODS). As in the mitochondrial isolates, PDHa activity

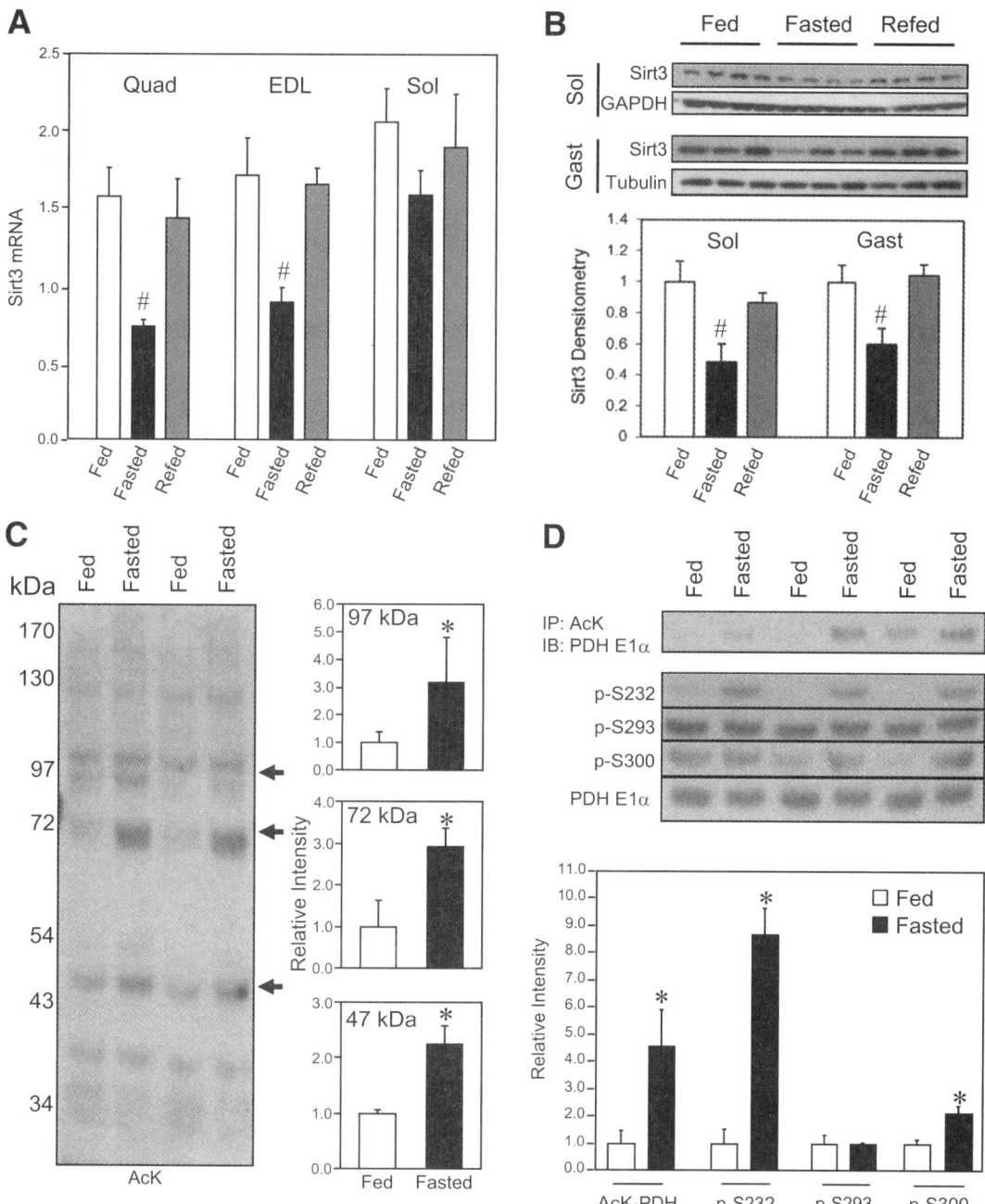

FIG. 1. Skeletal muscle Sirt3 expression and mitochondrial protein acetylation are regulated by fasting. Wild-type 8-week-old male C57Bl/6 mice were fed ad libitum, fasted for 24 h, or fasted and then refed for 16 h. After each treatment, RNA and protein were extracted and analyzed by real-time quantitative PCR (A) or Western blotting (B) for assessment of Sirt3 expression in quadriceps (Quad), EDL, soleus (Sol), and gastrocnemius (Gast) muscle groups ($n = 3–5$, #$P < 0.05$ vs. fed, ANOVA). C: Mixed hindlimb muscles (gastrocnemius and soleus) were collected from mice in the fed or fasted state. Muscle mitochondria were isolated in the presence of protease and deacetylase inhibitors as described in RESEARCH DESIGN AND METHODS. Mitochondrial protein lysates from each animal were subjected to SDS-PAGE and Western blotting using an antibody against AcK. The intensity of specified bands was quantified with ImageJ software ($n = 3$, *$P < 0.05$, Student t test). D: PDH E1α acetylation in muscle of fed or fasted mice was measured by immunoprecipitation (IP) of mitochondrial lysates using anti-AcK antibody. Immunoprecipitates were subjected to Western blotting analysis (IB) using anti–PDH E1α antibody. The same muscle mitochondrial lysates were directly subjected to SDS-PAGE electrophoresis and Western blotting using antibodies against phosphorylated serine sites p-232, p-293, and p-300 of the PDH E1α subunit and total protein of PDH E1α. Autoradiography of Western blots was quantified with ImageJ software ($n = 3$, *$P < 0.05$, Student t test). GAPDH, glyceraldehyde-3-phosphate dehydrogenase.

was significantly decreased in Sirt3 KO muscle to the level of fasted C57Bl/6 mice (Fig. 2G) without any changes in total PDH (Supplementary Fig. 2C). Remarkably, incubation of the muscle homogenates in the absence of deacetylase inhibitors, which likely allows other deacetylases outside the mitochondria but present in the tissue homogenate to

act on PDH, partially restored PDH activity from Sirt3 KO mice. Since inhibition of PDH activity in fasting muscle has profound effects on substrate metabolism, the observed reduction of PDH activity induced by Sirt3 deletion demonstrates that Sirt3 is an important regulator of the metabolic changes in fed skeletal muscle.

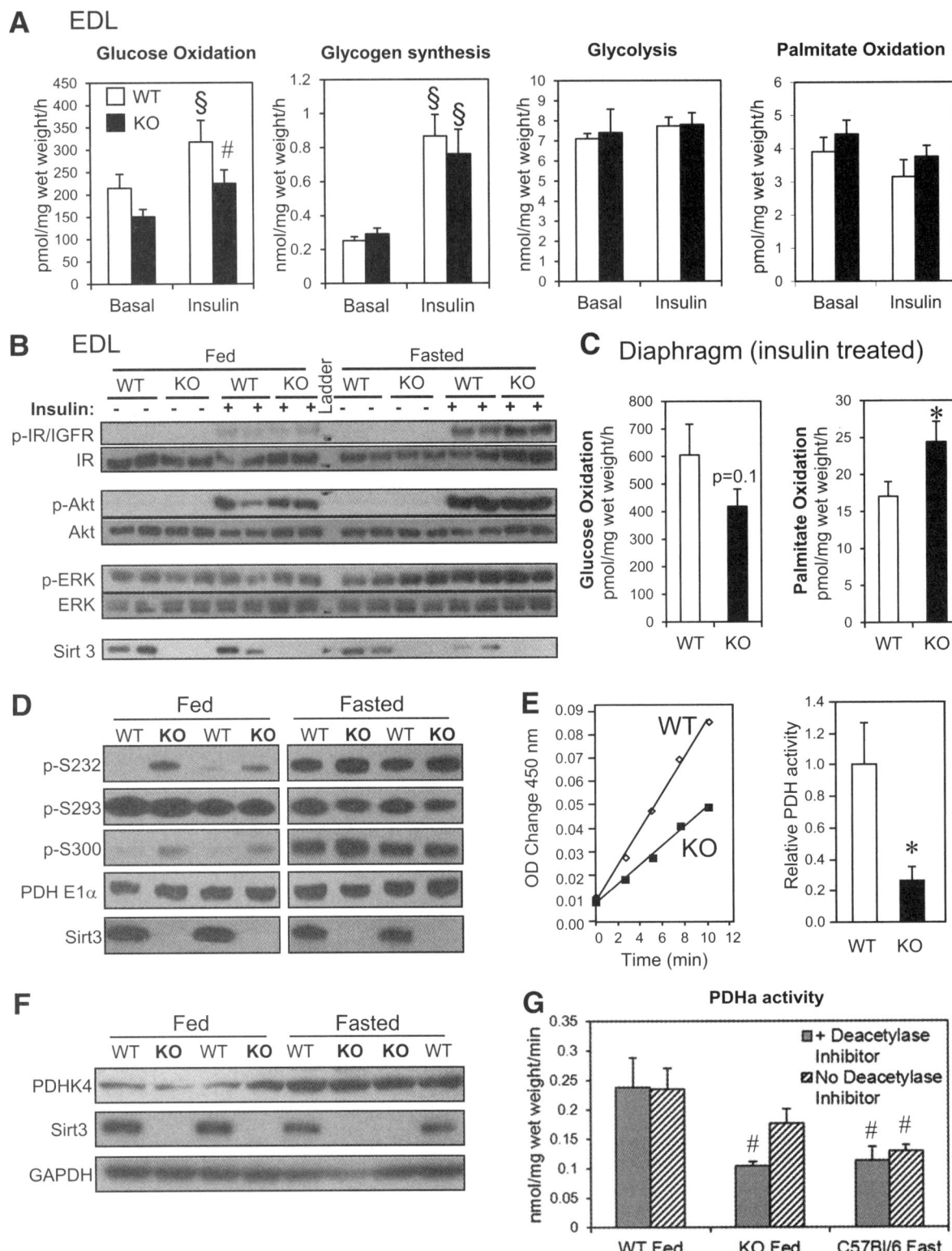

FIG. 2. Sirt3 deletion induces synergistic switch from glucose oxidation toward fatty acid oxidation and suppresses PDH activity by inducing PDH E1α hyperacetylation and hyperphosphorylation in fed Sirt3 KO skeletal muscle. *A*: Basal and insulin-stimulated (1 mU/mL) glucose oxidation, glycogen synthesis, glycolysis, and palmitate oxidation were measured in EDL muscles isolated from randomly fed 8- to 16-week-old WT and Sirt3 KO mice (*n* = 9; §*P* < 0.05 vs. basal, #*P* < 0.05 vs. WT, ANOVA). *B*: Basal and insulin-stimulated (10 mU/mL) phosphorylation of insulin/IGF-1 receptor, Akt, and ERK in tissue lysates of EDL muscles from fed and fasted 8- to 16-week-old WT and Sirt3 KO mice. *C*: Insulin-stimulated (1 mU/mL) glucose and palmitate oxidation were measured as described in RESEARCH DESIGN AND METHODS in diaphragms isolated from randomly fed 8- to 16-week-old WT and Sirt3 KO mice (*n* = 9; *P* < 0.05, Student *t* test). *D*: Mitochondrial lysates were subjected to Western blot analysis using antibodies against p-232, p-293, and p-300 serine phosphorylation sites on PDH E1α, total PDH E1α, and Sirt3 (densitometry in Supplementary Fig. 2*F*). *E*: PDH activity was measured in 20 mg mitochondrial lysate from hindlimb of fed WT and Sirt3 KO mice using a PDH activity microplate kit as described in RESEARCH DESIGN AND METHODS. The PDH activities were calculated by linear regression of the steady-state kinetics and quantified (*n* = 4–5,

PDH E1α subunit is a Sirt3 substrate. Using anti-AcK antibody to detect protein acetylation, we observed that Sirt3 KO muscle mitochondria displayed an elevation in acetylation similar to that seen in fasted WT mice (Fig. 3A), supporting the idea that Sirt3 is the primary mitochondrial deacetylase and consistent with our previous report in Sirt3 KO fed mice (23,30). To identify the potential Sirt3 targets in skeletal muscle during fasting (when Sirt3 levels are low) and in Sirt3 KO muscle, we performed a global acetyl-proteomic analysis (34). To this end, acetylated peptides were enriched from trypsinized mitochondrial protein lysates of WT and Sirt3 KO muscle using AcK antibody immunoprecipitation and subjected to mass spectrometry analysis. A total of 549 acetylated peptides were identified in the combined WT and KO muscle mitochondria. Among these, 299 acetylated peptides were present in both WT and KO samples, only 49 of which were detected exclusively in WT, whereas 201 acetylated peptides were exclusive to the Sirt3 KO, indicating increased acetylation induced by Sirt3 deletion (Fig. 3B). These 549 acetylated peptides corresponded to a total of 147 acetylated proteins, indicating that there were multiple acetylation sites for each protein (Fig. 3B). Our analysis revealed several lysine acetylation sites on PDH E1α (Fig. 3C). Among the peptides showing significantly increased acetylation in Sirt3 KO muscle mitochondria was one peptide representing acetylated lysine 336 (K336) of PDH E1α (Supplementary Fig. 3A). Quantitation of the MS1 precursor signals of this peptide between the four WT and four KO mice showed a threefold increase in acetylation at K336 in the Sirt3 KO animals (Fig. 3D), indicating that K336 is a substrate of Sirt3.

To confirm that Sirt3 directly acetylates PDH, we immunoprecipitated WT and Sirt3 KO muscle mitochondrial lysates from both fed and fasted mice using anti-AcK antibody and subjected the immunoprecipitates to Western blotting analysis with anti-PDH E1α antibody. This revealed that PDH E1α acetylation was increased significantly in Sirt3 KO muscle mitochondria (Fig. 3E), and this was specific, as no enrichment was observed using streptavidin beads as a control (Supplementary Fig. 3).

Sirt3 deletion in skeletal muscle induces an altered metabolic profile. To fully assess the metabolic effects of PDH E1α inhibition in Sirt3 KO skeletal muscle, we performed targeted gas chromatography/mass spectrometry and MS/MS metabolomic analysis on samples of skeletal muscle from fed WT and Sirt3 KO mice. We found significantly elevated levels of lactate, pyruvate, and α-ketoglutarate (α-KG) in Sirt3 KO skeletal muscle (Fig. 4A). The increase in lactate and pyruvate in Sirt3 KO muscles is consistent with suppression of PDH activity and decreased carbohydrate oxidation. We also observed a significant decrease in levels of acylcarnitines measured in Sirt3 KO muscle, suggestive of increased fatty acid use (Fig. 4B). Additionally, amino acids levels were decreased in Sirt3 KO muscle (Fig. 4C). Taken together, these metabolomic data indicate that Sirt3 deletion induces a metabolic derangement in skeletal muscle in which impaired PDH activity suppresses glucose oxidation and enhances lipid and amino acid catabolism.

Knockdown of Sirt3 in C2C12 myoblasts decreases PDH activity. To further elucidate the role of Sirt3 in PDH function, we determined PDH E1α acetylation and enzyme activity in C2C12 myoblasts in which Sirt3 was knocked down using shRNA (shSirt3). This resulted in a >90% decrease in Sirt3 protein by Western analysis (Fig. 5A, C, and D). Immunoprecipitation of mitochondrial lysates from shGFP control and shSirt3 myoblasts using anti-AcK antibody revealed significantly increased acetylated PDH E1α in knockdown cells (Fig. 5A). The increased acetylation of PDH E1α in vitro was associated with a 27% decrease in PDH activity in shSirt3 myoblasts measured by microplate immunocapture of PDH (Fig. 5B). However, in contrast to results in skeletal muscle in vivo from Sirt3 KO mice, shSirt3 myoblasts showed decreased phosphorylation at both S232 and S300 sites (Fig. 5C and D), suggesting that PDH E1α acetylation may inhibit PDH activity independent of phosphorylation.

Previous bioenergetic profiling using Seahorse XF flux analyzer with glucose and pyruvate as substrates showed that shSirt3 myoblasts had significantly lower uncoupled respiration (30). Since changes in the metabolomic profile suggested a switch in substrate utilization in Sirt3 KO muscles, we measured glucose and fatty acid oxidation occurred in a cell autonomous manner using shSirt3 knockdown myoblasts. Basal rates of lactate production, as indicated by ECAR, were similar in control and shSirt3 myoblasts. When given glucose as substrate, shSirt3 cells displayed a greater increase in ECAR compared with control (Fig. 5E). The area under the curve (AUC) quantification of ECAR was significantly higher in shSirt3 after glucose stimulation (Fig. 5F). As previously reported, OCRs were lower in shSirt3 myoblasts (Supplementary Fig. 4A and B) (30). OCR in the presence of 200 μmol/L palmitate was significantly higher in shSirt3 cells, and this was inhibited by addition of etomoxir, indicating higher rates of fatty acid β-oxidation in shSirt3 compared with control cells. AUC calculation after palmitate showed a ~35% increase in OCR in shSirt3 (Fig. 5G and H). Together, these data demonstrate that decreased Sirt3 expression induces a switch in muscle substrate utilization from glucose to fatty acid oxidation to compensate for decreased carbohydrate oxidation caused by inhibition of PDH activity.

Overexpression of K336Q or K336R mutants of PDH E1α decreases phosphorylation at S232 and S300 but does not affect PDH activity or substrate metabolism. To determine whether acetylation at lysine 336 of PDH E1α was sufficient to affect PDH activity, we created C2C12 myoblast cell lines with stable overexpression of WT PDH E1α or with either a K336Q or a K336R mutation. In some molecules, the lysine (K) to glutamine (Q) mutation can mimic the acetylated state, while the K to arginine (R) prevents acetylation and mimics the deacetylated state. Both K336Q and the K336R mutations caused a reduction in phosphorylation of S232 and S300 compared with overexpression of WT PDH E1α (Fig. 6A and B), indicating an important role of lysine 336 in control of serine phosphorylation. To dissect the effect of phosphorylation status versus K336 mutation on PDH activity, we determined PDH activity in the presence of PIs to promote phosphorylation

---

*P < 0.05, Student t test). F: Western blot analysis was performed on tissue lysates from gastrocnemius muscle from fed and fasted WT and Sirt3 KO for PDHK4, Sirt3, and glyceraldehyde-3-phosphate dehydrogenase. G: Native PDH activity (PDHa) was measured in gastrocnemius muscle homogenate from WT fed, Sirt3 KO fed, and fasted C57Bl/6 mice by collection of $^{14}CO_2$ release from ^{14}C-pyruvate. Prior to PDH assay, aliquots of homogenates were incubated in the presence of 50 mmol/L NaF with or without deacetylase inhibitors (1 mmol/L nicotinamide and 1 mol/L trichostatin A) as described in RESEARCH DESIGN AND METHODS (n = 6–7; #P < 0.05 vs. WT plus deacetylase inhibitors, ANOVA). OD, optical density.

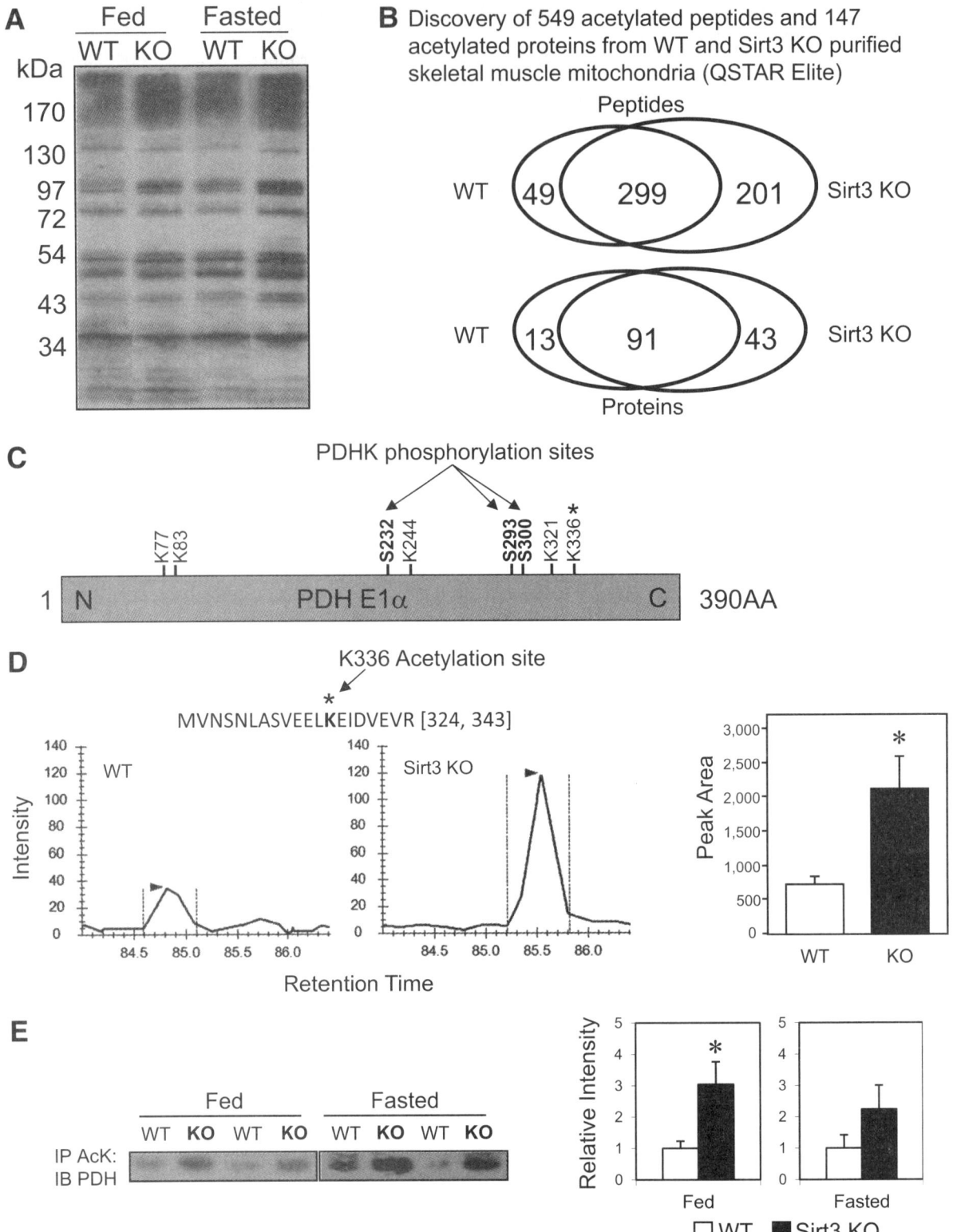

FIG. 3. Discovery of PDH E1α subunit as a target of Sirt3 in skeletal muscle. *A*: Muscle mitochondrial protein lysates from WT and Sirt3 KO mice in either the fed or fasted state were subjected to Western blotting analysis using anti-AcK antibody. *B*: Proteomic analysis using anti-AcK antibody–based acetylated peptide enrichment and mass spectrometry discovered a total of 549 acetylated peptides present in WT and Sirt3 KO skeletal muscle mitochondria. These peptides represented a total of 147 proteins. Venn diagrams show overlapping and distinctive patterns of distribution of acetylated peptides and proteins between WT and Sirt3 KO skeletal muscle. *C*: Schematic diagram of lysine acetylation sites and previously reported serine phosphorylation sites on PDH E1α. *D*: A representative MS1 chromatogram of the triply charged precursor peak at m/z 772.7303^{3+} (324-MVNSNLASVEELacKEIDVEVR-343) of PDH E1α was highly increased in Sirt3 KO skeletal muscle mitochondria compared with WT ($n = 4$; $P < 0.05$, Student t test). *E*: Skeletal muscle mitochondrial lysates from WT and Sirt3 KO mice in both fed and fasted states were immunoprecipitated (IP) with AcK antibody–bound beads. Immunoprecipitates of the mitochondrial lysate were subjected to Western blotting (IB) using an anti–PDH E1α antibody. Densitometry of either fed or fasted animals was calculated ($n = 4$; *$P < 0.05$, Student t test).

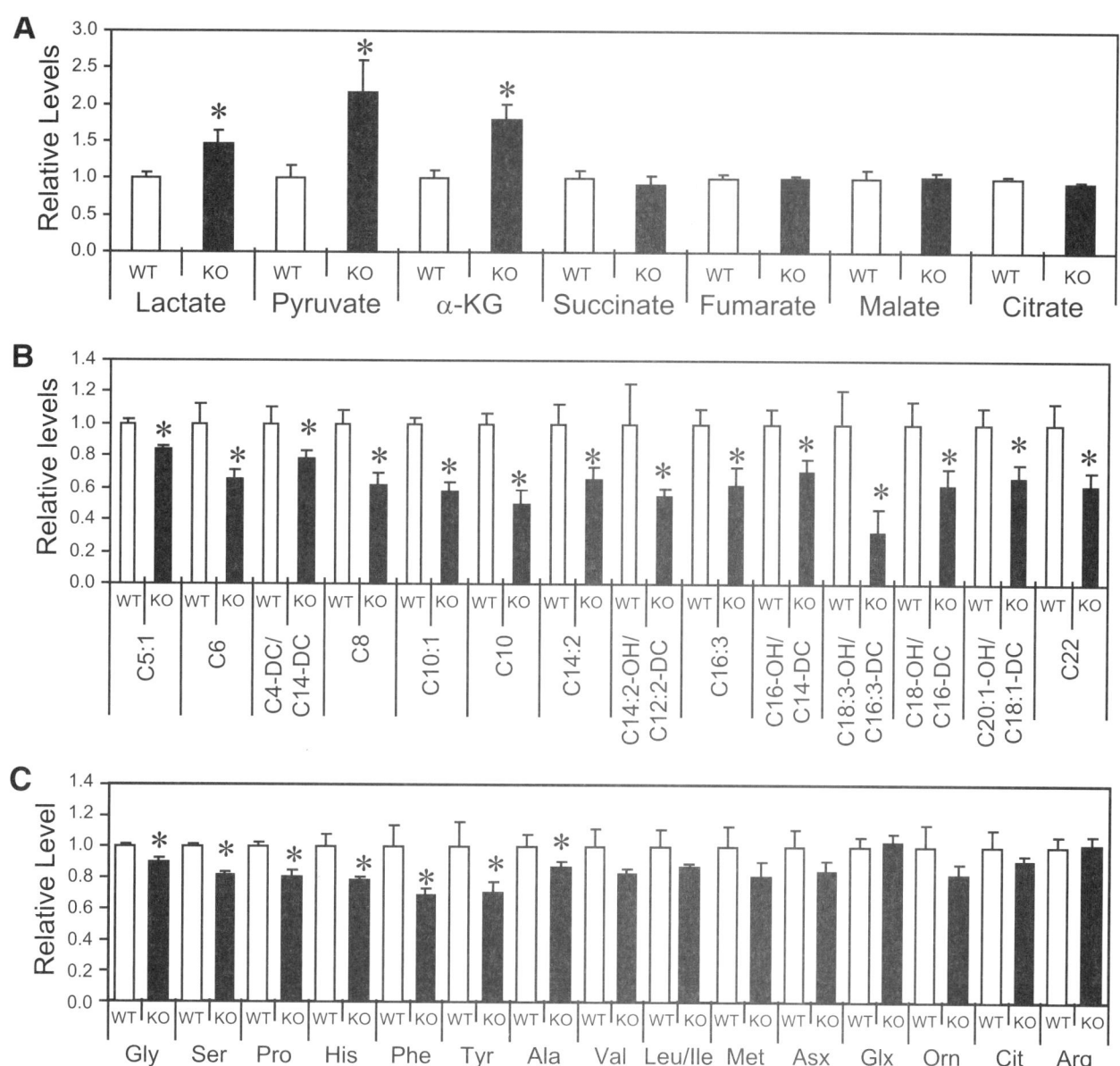

FIG. 4. Sirt3 deletion induces a substrate switch and derangement of metabolites in skeletal muscle. Quadriceps muscles from fed male WT and Sirt3 KO mice were collected and subjected to metabolomic analysis as described in RESEARCH DESIGN AND METHODS. Relative levels of organic acids and Kreb cycle intermediates are shown in *A*, levels of acylcarnitines in *B*, and amino acid levels in *C* (*n* = 4–5; *P < 0.05, Student *t* test). Asx, asparagine and aspartic acid; Cit, citrulline; Glx, glutamine and glutamic acid; Orn, ornithine.

or DCA, a PDH kinase specific inhibitor, to decrease phosphorylation of PDH E1α. PDH activity was unchanged in myoblasts harboring either of the K336Q or K336R mutations compared with WT controls (Fig. 6*C*) with or without addition of PI to preserve S293 and S300 phosphorylation or addition of DCA to maximally dephosphorylate PDH E1α (Fig. 6*D*).

To assess whether K336Q or K336R mutations could recapitulate the substrate switch observed in shSirt3 cells, we analyzed glucose-induced ECAR in WT, K336Q, or K336R myoblasts. No significant differences in glucose-stimulated ECAR were observed in the K336Q or K336R mutant cells compared with control (Fig. 6*E* and *F*). Thus, altering the ability of K336 to undergo acetylation did modify phosphorylation of PDH E1α but could not fully

recapitulate the effects of decreased Sirt3 expression on PDH complex activity and substrate metabolism.

DISCUSSION

Mitochondrial sirtuins are uniquely positioned to regulate energy metabolism via protein deacetylation. Although Sirt3, Sirt4, and Sirt5 have all been localized to mitochondria, previous reports have shown that only Sirt3 deletion induces mitochondrial protein hyperacetylation, suggesting that Sirt3 is the major mitochondrial protein deacetylase (23). Indeed, recent studies have shown that altered Sirt3 expression can have effects on lipid metabolism, ROS production, oxidative stress response, and cell survival (25,26,30,44,45).

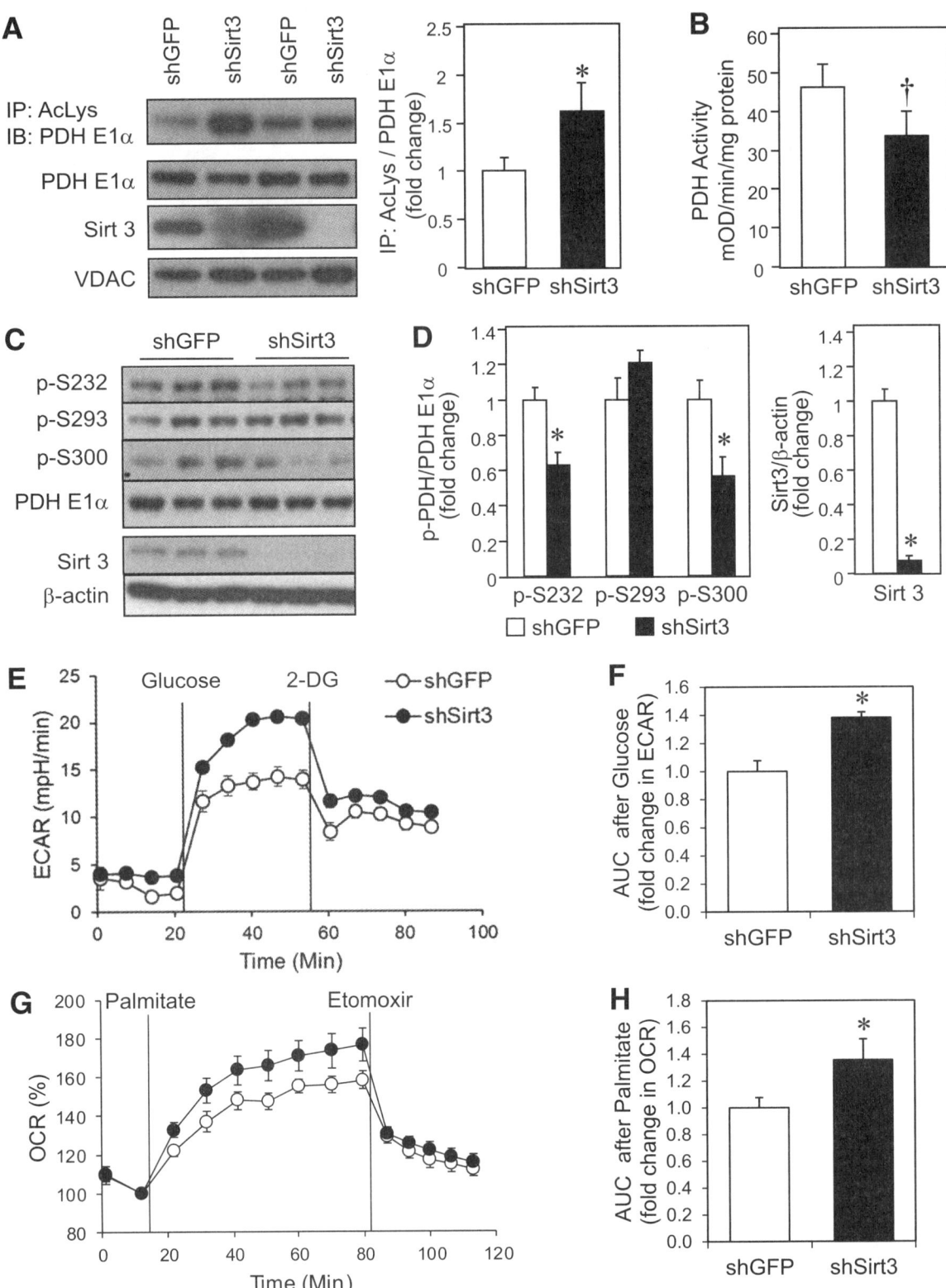

FIG. 5. Sirt3 knockdown in C2C12 myoblasts impairs PDH activity despite decreased phosphorylation of PDH E1α and leads to a substrate switch toward fatty acid utilization. A: Total mitochondrial protein lysates from shGFP control and shSirt3 myoblasts were immunoprecipitated (IP) with AcK (AcLys) antibody and subjected to Western blot analysis (IB) using an anti–PDH E1α antibody. The same mitochondrial lysates were directly subjected to Western blot analysis using antibodies against PDH E1α, Sirt3, and voltage-dependent anion channel (VDAC) as a mitochondrial loading control. Densitometry of PDH E1α from AcK immunoprecipitates was normalized to total PDH E1α (n = 4 separate experiments; *P < 0.05, Student t test). B: Total PDH activity was assessed in confluent control and shSirt3 myoblasts using PDH activity microplate assay kit and normalized to total protein from detergent extraction (n = 5 separate experiments; †P < 0.05, paired t test). C: Phosphorylation of PDH E1α and total Sirt3 levels were determined by Western blot analysis of whole cell lysates from confluent shGFP and shSirt3 C2C12 myoblasts. D: Densitometry of Western blots from C (n = 3 separate experiments, *P < 0.05, Student t test). E: ECAR was measured in shSirt3 and control myoblasts using a Seahorse flux analyzer after incubation in glucose-free Seahorse running media for 1 h at 37°C. A representative tracing of basal and

In the current study, we find that Sirt3 is an important mitochondrial factor in the regulation of skeletal muscle metabolic flexibility by targeting the enzymatic deacetylation of PDH E1α. Thus, when nutrients are abundant, Sirt3 deacetylation promotes PDH activity and postprandial glucose metabolism (Fig. 7A). During fasting, there is a decrease of Sirt3 in skeletal muscle, which leads to hyperacetylation of PDH E1α and promotes a metabolic switch from glucose to fatty acids as a predominant substrate (Fig. 7B). This can be mimicked by Sirt3 deletion, which results in decreased catalytic activity of PDH, decreased glucose oxidation, and an accumulation of pyruvate and lactate levels even in the fed state. Impaired glucose utilization in Sirt3 KO muscle induces a reliance on fatty acid β-oxidation for energy production. This results in increased breakdown of acylcarnitines and ROS generation and over time leads to insulin resistance (30).

Previous reports have suggested that 24 h of fasting increases Sirt3 levels in muscle (27), but in our hands, 24 h of fasting leads to a consistent decrease in Sirt3 in each muscle group tested. The difference between these two observations may be explained by the timing of the study (mice were killed at 6 P.M. in the former study and at 9 A.M. in our study) and the duration of fasting in the different fed and fasted groups. Peak feeding in mice occurs at the beginning of the nocturnal phase. Thus, fed mice killed at 9:00 A.M. are only a few hours after peak feeding time. On the other hand, when mice are killed at 6:00 P.M., even the "fed" mice are likely to have fasted or partially fasted for as many as 10–12 h prior to study, and the "24-h fasted" mice may have gone without food for as long as 36 h, resulting in dramatic wasting and changes in muscle protein composition (46). Alternatively, there may be circadian changes in expression of Sirt3 or some of its regulators, which is altered during prolonged periods of fasting.

Metabolic flexibility is the ability of an organism to adapt fuel oxidation in response to fuel availability (47). In both insulin resistance and type 2 diabetes, this metabolic flexibility is compromised in that skeletal muscle fails to switch substrate utilization from lipid metabolism to insulin-stimulated glucose oxidation (5,48). The current study demonstrates that mitochondrial Sirt3 can help optimize the switch of substrate oxidation toward glucose utilization by deacetylating PDH, a vital enzyme complex in glucose oxidation. Acute regulation of metabolic flexibility by Sirt3 upon refeeding is not due changes in Sirt3 levels, since 16 h of refeeding is required for full recovery of mRNA and protein levels. These acute changes in substrate flexibility going from the fed to the fasted state are more likely coordinated by a complex network of signaling cascades including insulin and nutrient-dependent phosphorylation events. This acute regulation may still be affected by Sirt3 intracellular partitioning or possible post-translational modification affecting its deacetylase activity. However, our data support the conclusion that Sirt3 plays an important role in regulating muscle metabolic flexibility upon refeeding by deacetylating PDH and, with dephosphorylation, allows for maximal enzyme activity for glucose oxidation.

Another interesting aspect of Sirt3 physiology is the differential regulation and physiological effects of this enzyme in different tissues. For example, during fasting Sirt3 expression is decreased in muscle but increased in liver (25,30). Mitochondrial protein acetylation patterns confirm that Sirt3 is more active in the fed state in skeletal muscle, whereas in liver Sirt3 is more active during fasting. Sirt3 also has different tissue-specific metabolic effects. Sirt3 deletion in liver suppresses lipid oxidation via suppression of LCAD activity (25), whereas deletion of Sirt3 in muscle decreases glucose oxidation and increases lipid oxidation, at least in part to compensate for PDH inhibition. This dichotomous role of Sirt3 in muscle versus liver may help to explain the report showing minimal changes in global metabolism when Sirt3 is deleted in a tissue-specific manor (49). Muscle-specific deletion of Sirt3 may lead to changes in mitochondrial substrate choice, which are compensated for by opposing Sirt3 action in liver, resulting in a balance at the whole-body level. Nonetheless, this differential regulation of Sirt3 expression and function in a tissue-dependent manner would allow Sirt3 to coordinately regulate divergent pathways of substrate utilization in different organs based on nutrient availability.

Reversible phosphorylation of PDH E1α by PDH kinases inhibits enzyme activity and, in starvation and diabetes, levels of PDH kinases increase in skeletal muscle (14,16,50). PDH kinases can be activated by a decrease in the NAD^+-to-NADH ratio, providing feedback inactivation of the PDH complex (51). Our studies demonstrate that increased acetylation of PDH E1α is associated with decreased PDH complex activity, leading us to speculate that PDH acetylation also regulates complex activity. Indeed, PDH activity was decreased in both Sirt3 KO muscle in vivo and Sirt3 knockdown myoblasts in vitro; the former was associated with increased phosphorylation of Ser^{232} and Ser^{300}, whereas the latter was associated with decreased serine phosphorylation. However, the degree of PDH activity decrease is different in the two models—55–70% in Sirt3 KO in vivo compared with 27% in shSirt3 in vitro—which could be related to phosphorylation status. Lastly, the observation that incubation of Sirt3 KO muscle homogenate in the absence of deacetylase inhibitors partially restored PDH activity supports the notion that acetylation of PDH inhibits its activity. Regulation of enzyme activity by acetylation may also help explain the observed accumulation of α-KG, as α-KG dehydrogenase is similar in structure and regulation to PDH, in that both use an E1 component that may be a target for acetylation and Sirt3-catalyzed deacetylation. Other mechanisms may also contribute to changes in PDH activity. For example, PDH and α-KG dehydrogenase contain many thiol groups, which are sensitive to ROS, and we have previously shown that deletion of Sirt3 causes increased ROS production in muscle from 24-week-old animals (30).

Mass spectrometry–based analysis revealed that PDH E1α is acetylated on multiple lysine residues. We focused our attention on lysine 336, since it exhibited one of the greatest levels of differential acetylation in Sirt3-depleted skeletal muscle. Our attempts to determine whether acetylation at

glucose-stimulated ECARs recorded before and after addition of 25 mmol/L glucose (final concentration) is shown. At the end of the glucose metabolism period, 2-deoxyglucose was injected to give a final concentration of 25 mmol/L. *F*: AUC calculation of glucose-stimulated ECAR from *E*. *G*: A representative tracing of palmitate OCR measured in control and Sirt3 knockdown cells after incubation with substrate-free buffer for 1 h at 37°C. Basal and palmitate-BSA–stimulated OCRs were recorded and plotted as a percentage over basal OCR. Finally, 50 μmol/L etomoxir was injected. *H*: AUC of palmitate-stimulated OCR from *G* ($n = 3$; *$P < 0.05$, Student *t* test). mOD, milli optical density.

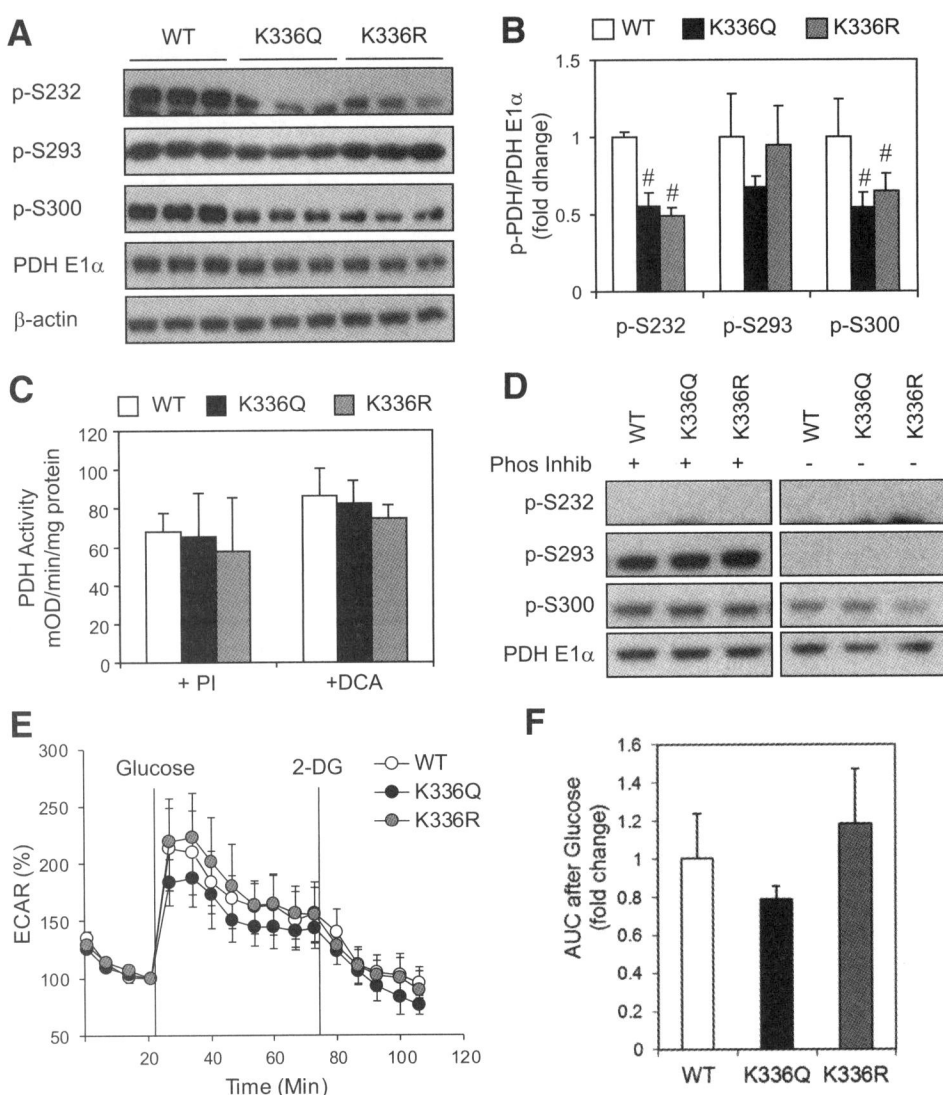

FIG. 6. Expression of a K336Q and K336R mutant of PDH E1α in C2C12 myoblasts decreases phosphorylation but does not affect PDH activity. *A*: Phosphorylation of PDH E1α levels determined by Western blot analysis of whole cell lysates from confluent C2C12 myoblasts expressing WT PDH E1α, K336Q, or K336R mutant of PDH E1α. *B*: Densitometry of Western blots from *A* ($n = 3$ separate experiments, #$P < 0.05$, ANOVA). *C*: Total PDH activity was assessed in confluent WT, K336Q, or K336R myoblasts using detergent extracts either with PIs 2 and 3 (Sigma) or 20 mmol/L DCA added to the PDH activity assay as described in RESEARCH DESIGN AND METHODS ($n = 2$–4 separate experiments). *D*: Western blot analysis of detergent extracts from *C* either with PI (Phos Inhib) or with DCA after 3 h incubation at room temperature in buffer 1 of the PDH activity assay kit. *E*: A representative example of Seahorse analysis of glucose-induced ECAR with PDH E1α WT, K336Q, and K336R mutants. *F*: AUC quantification after addition of glucose showed no statistical difference between mutants ($n = 4$ separate experiments). 2-DG, 2-deoxyglucose.

lysine 336 alone could alter PDH activity using the K336Q (which is regarded as an acetylation mimic) and K336R (which is regarded as a deacetylation mimic) mutations demonstrated that changing the ability of this lysine to become acetylated can cause alterations in phosphorylation of PDH E1α but did not change catalytic function or substrate metabolism in vitro. It is likely that acetylation of other lysine residues in the PDH complex contribute to the observed changes in PDH activity.

Identifying a role of Sirt3 in regulating metabolic flexibility and PDH activity in muscle may provide a new target for preventing and treating metabolic syndrome. Evidence for Sirt3 impacting human metabolic disease is accumulating. We have recently identified a single nucleotide polymorphism in the human Sirt3 gene that decreases its activity and is associated with metabolic syndrome (29). Indeed, targeting PDH activity in muscle for the treatment

of diabetes has been proposed as a way to increase glucose disposal, thereby decreasing circulating glucose levels (15). However, many of these treatments induce fasting hypoglycemia as a result of PDH activation during fasting. Since Sirt3 levels decrease in muscle with fasting, pharmacologic activation of Sirt3 in muscle should be beneficial, as it would have maximal effect in the fed state, when glucose levels are highest in diabetes.

In summary, our study demonstrates that Sirt3 plays an important role in control of substrate metabolism and adds another layer of regulation to the multiple pathways that control metabolic flexibility in skeletal muscle. In the fed state, Sirt3 expression/activity in muscle is high, resulting in deacetylation of many mitochondrial proteins, including PDH E1α. This enhances PDH complex activity and postprandial glucose metabolism. Thus, Sirt3 helps orchestrate the efficient use of available nutrients in skeletal muscle by

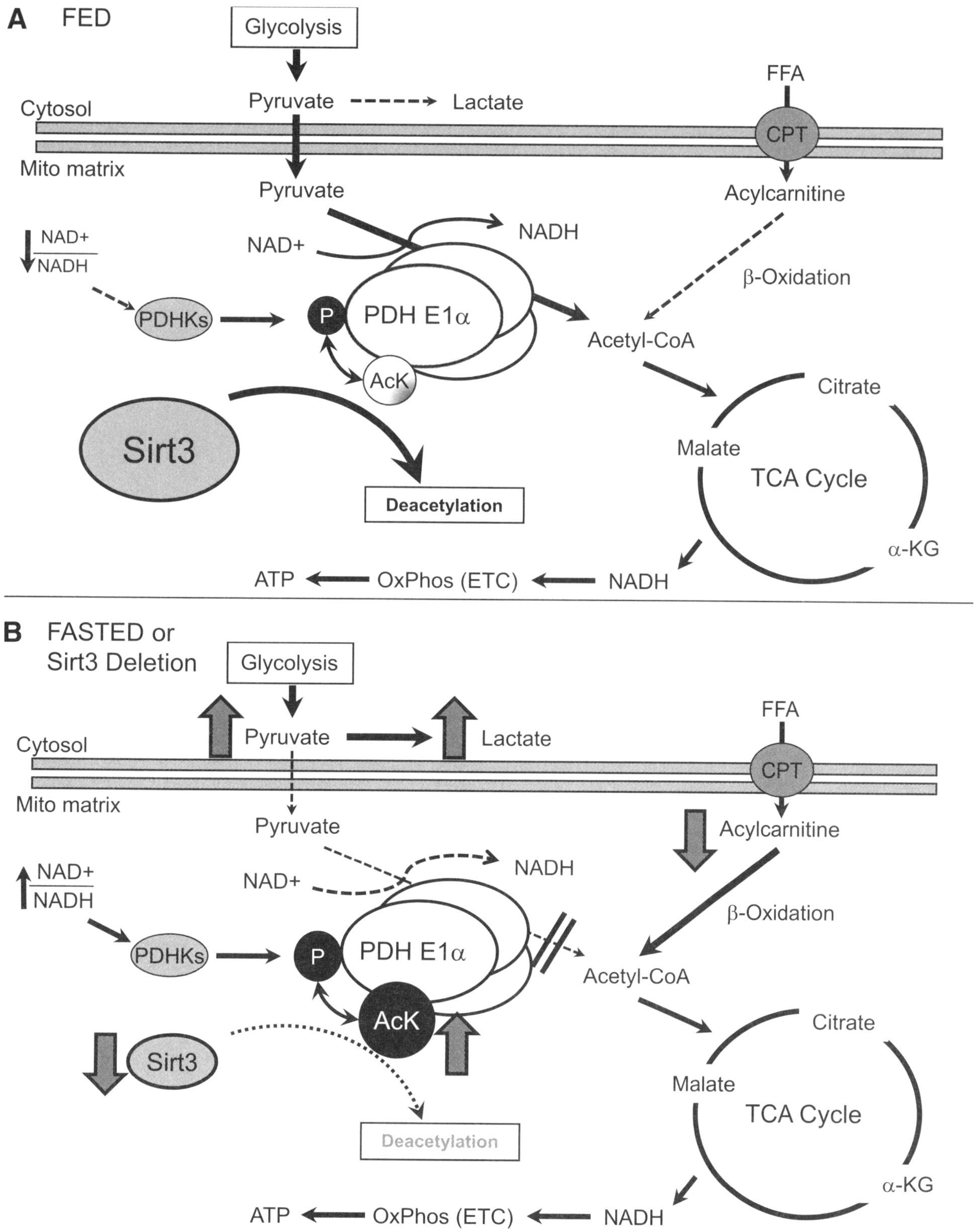

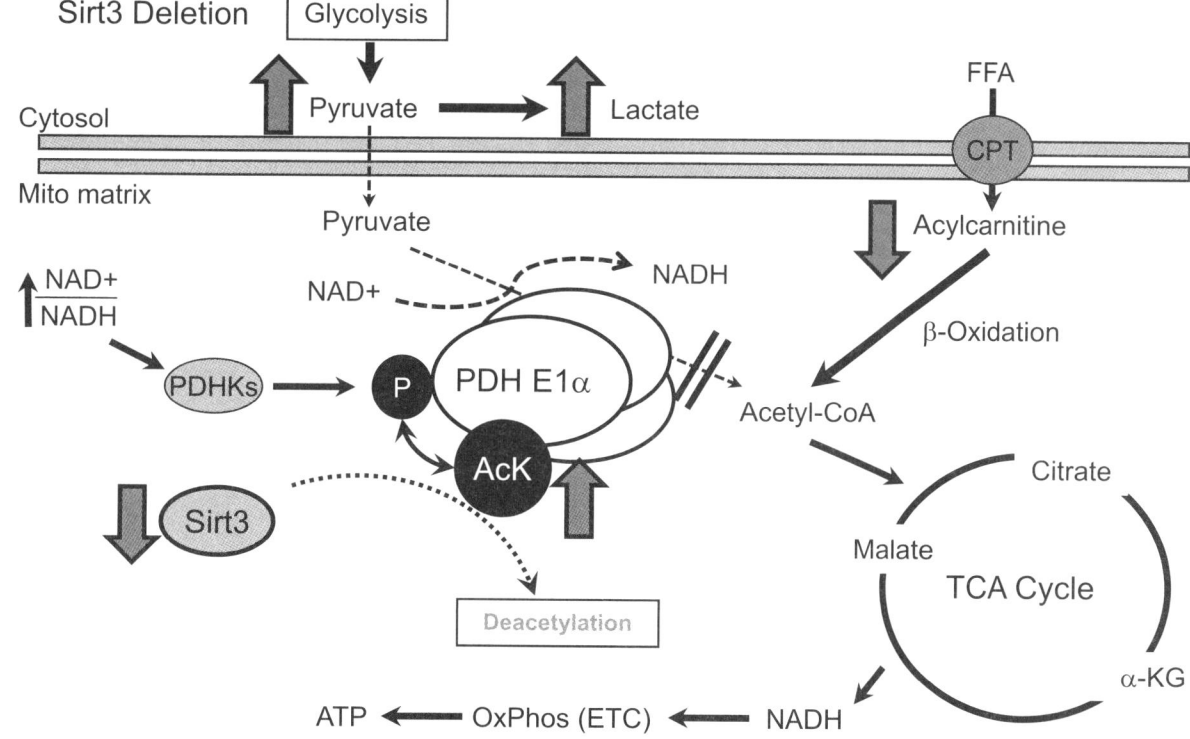

FIG. 7. Model for the role of Sirt3 in control of skeletal muscle substrate metabolism. Sirt3 regulates PDH E1α subunit deacetylation and activates PDH activity. *A:* In the fed state, Sirt3 skeletal muscle expression is abundant and leads to deacetylation of PDH E1α. This is associated with dephosphorylation of PDH allowing for maximal enzyme activation, enhanced glucose utilization, and increased flux of pyruvate to acetyl-CoA used by the tricarboxylic acid (TCA) cycle and electron transport chain (ETC) to generate ATP. *B:* In contrast, decreased Sirt3 expression in muscle by fasting or genetic deletion leads to PDH E1α hyperacetylation and decreased PDH complex activity, which is correlated with increased PDH E1α phosphorylation in vivo. The activity of PDH controls the substrate influx to the TCA cycle from glycolysis. In the case of Sirt3 deletion, inactivation of the PDH caused by hyperacetylation leads to metabolic inflexibility as evidenced by an inability to fully oxidize glucose, a shunt of excess pyruvate toward lactate production, and increased lipid oxidation even in the fed state. CPT, carnitine palmitoyl transferase; FFA, free fatty acid; Mito, mitochondrial; OxPhos, oxidative phosphorylation.

promoting metabolic flexibility through enzymatic deacetylation of PDH. Modulation of mitochondrial acetylation may offer a new therapeutic target for correcting some of the metabolic defects of obesity and type 2 diabetes.

ACKNOWLEDGMENTS

The primary funding for this project was National Institutes of Health Grant R24 DK085610. B.T.O. was funded by Joslin Training Grant T32DK007260. A.K. was funded by German Research Foundation project KL2399/1-1. S.U. was supported by a Human Frontier Science Program Long-Term fellowship. The authors acknowledge the support of National Center for Research Resources shared instrumentation grant S10 RR024615 (to B.W.G.) for the QSTAR Elite mass spectrometer used in these studies.

No potential conflicts of interest relevant to this article were reported.

E.J. and B.T.O. researched data and wrote the manuscript. M.J.R. researched data. A.K. contributed to discussion and researched data. O.R.I., S.U., J.R.B., and K.Y.L. researched data. E.M.V., C.B.N., and B.W.G. researched data and provided materials. C.R.K. oversaw the project, contributed to discussion, and helped write the manuscript. C.R.K. is the guarantor of this work and, as such, had full access to all the data in the study and takes responsibility for the integrity of the data and the accuracy of the data analysis.

REFERENCES

1. Kim JK, Zisman A, Fillmore JJ, et al. Glucose toxicity and the development of diabetes in mice with muscle-specific inactivation of GLUT4. J Clin Invest 2001;108:153–160
2. Fueger PT, Hess HS, Bracy DP, et al. Regulation of insulin-stimulated muscle glucose uptake in the conscious mouse: role of glucose transport is dependent on glucose phosphorylation capacity. Endocrinology 2004;145: 4912–4916
3. Storlien L, Oakes ND, Kelley DE. Metabolic flexibility. Proc Nutr Soc 2004; 63:363–368
4. van Loon LJ. Use of intramuscular triacylglycerol as a substrate source during exercise in humans. J Appl Physiol 2004;97:1170–1187
5. Befroy DE, Petersen KF, Dufour S, et al. Impaired mitochondrial substrate oxidation in muscle of insulin-resistant offspring of type 2 diabetic patients. Diabetes 2007;56:1376–1381
6. Leone TC, Lehman JJ, Finck BN, et al. PGC-1alpha deficiency causes multisystem energy metabolic derangements: muscle dysfunction, abnormal weight control and hepatic steatosis. PLoS Biol 2005;3:e101
7. Chow L, From A, Seaquist E. Skeletal muscle insulin resistance: the interplay of local lipid excess and mitochondrial dysfunction. Metabolism 2010;59:70–85
8. Espinoza DO, Boros LG, Crunkhorn S, Gami H, Patti ME. Dual modulation of both lipid oxidation and synthesis by peroxisome proliferator-activated receptor-gamma coactivator-1alpha and -1beta in cultured myotubes. FASEB J 2010;24:1003–1014
9. Finck BN, Bernal-Mizrachi C, Han DH, et al. A potential link between muscle peroxisome proliferator- activated receptor-alpha signaling and obesity-related diabetes. Cell Metab 2005;1:133–144
10. Summermatter S, Baum O, Santos G, Hoppeler H, Handschin C. Peroxisome proliferator-activated receptor gamma coactivator 1alpha (PGC-1alpha) promotes skeletal muscle lipid refueling in vivo by activating de novo lipogenesis and the pentose phosphate pathway. J Biol Chem 2010;285:32793–32800
11. Baar K, Song Z, Semenkovich CF, et al. Skeletal muscle overexpression of nuclear respiratory factor 1 increases glucose transport capacity. FASEB J 2003;17:1666–1673
12. Rahman S, Blok RB, Dahl HH, et al. Leigh syndrome: clinical features and biochemical and DNA abnormalities. Ann Neurol 1996;39:343–351
13. Cameron JM, Levandovskiy V, Mackay N, Tein I, Robinson BH. Deficiency of pyruvate dehydrogenase caused by novel and known mutations in the E1alpha subunit. Am J Med Genet A 2004;131:59–66
14. Bowker-Kinley MM, Davis WI, Wu P, Harris RA, Popov KM. Evidence for existence of tissue-specific regulation of the mammalian pyruvate dehydrogenase complex. Biochem J 1998;329:191–196
15. Mayers RM, Leighton B, Kilgour E. PDH kinase inhibitors: a novel therapy for Type II diabetes? Biochem Soc Trans 2005;33:367–370
16. Wu P, Inskeep K, Bowker-Kinley MM, Popov KM, Harris RA. Mechanism responsible for inactivation of skeletal muscle pyruvate dehydrogenase complex in starvation and diabetes. Diabetes 1999;48:1593–1599
17. Zhao S, Xu W, Jiang W, et al. Regulation of cellular metabolism by protein lysine acetylation. Science 2010;327:1000–1004
18. Choudhary C, Kumar C, Gnad F, et al. Lysine acetylation targets protein complexes and co-regulates major cellular functions. Science 2009;325:834–840
19. Schwer B, Eckersdorff M, Li Y, et al. Calorie restriction alters mitochondrial protein acetylation. Aging Cell 2009;8:604–606
20. Michan S, Sinclair D. Sirtuins in mammals: insights into their biological function. Biochem J 2007;404:1–13
21. Milne JC, Denu JM. The Sirtuin family: therapeutic targets to treat diseases of aging. Curr Opin Chem Biol 2008;12:11–17
22. Cooper HM, Spelbrink JN. The human SIRT3 protein deacetylase is exclusively mitochondrial. Biochem J 2008;411:279–285
23. Lombard DB, Alt FW, Cheng HL, et al. Mammalian Sir2 homolog SIRT3 regulates global mitochondrial lysine acetylation. Mol Cell Biol 2007;27: 8807–8814
24. Ahn BH, Kim HS, Song S, et al. A role for the mitochondrial deacetylase Sirt3 in regulating energy homeostasis. Proc Natl Acad Sci USA 2008;105: 14447–14452
25. Hirschey MD, Shimazu T, Goetzman E, et al. SIRT3 regulates mitochondrial fatty-acid oxidation by reversible enzyme deacetylation. Nature 2010; 464:121–125
26. Qiu X, Brown K, Hirschey MD, Verdin E, Chen D. Calorie restriction reduces oxidative stress by SIRT3-mediated SOD2 activation. Cell Metab 2010;12:662–667
27. Palacios OM, Carmona JJ, Michan S, et al. Diet and exercise signals regulate SIRT3 and activate AMPK and PGC-1alpha in skeletal muscle. Aging (Albany, NY Online) 2009;1:771–783
28. Hokari F, Kawasaki E, Sakai A, Koshinaka K, Sakuma K, Kawanaka K. Muscle contractile activity regulates Sirt3 protein expression in rat skeletal muscles. J Appl Physiol 2010;109:332–340
29. Hirschey MD, Shimazu T, Jing E, et al. SIRT3 deficiency and mitochondrial protein hyperacetylation accelerate the development of the metabolic syndrome. Mol Cell 2011;44:177–190
30. Jing E, Emanuelli B, Hirschey MD, et al. Sirtuin-3 (Sirt3) regulates skeletal muscle metabolism and insulin signaling via altered mitochondrial oxidation and reactive oxygen species production. Proc Natl Acad Sci USA 2011; 108:14608–14613
31. Chen Y, Zhang J, Lin Y, et al. Tumour suppressor SIRT3 deacetylates and activates manganese superoxide dismutase to scavenge ROS. EMBO Rep 2011;12:534–541
32. Jeoung NH, Wu P, Joshi MA, et al. Role of pyruvate dehydrogenase kinase isoenzyme 4 (PDHK4) in glucose homoeostasis during starvation. Biochem J 2006;397:417–425
33. McKeel DW, Jarett L. Preparation and characterization of a plasma membrane fraction from isolated fat cells. J Cell Biol 1970;44:417–432
34. Schilling B, Rardin MJ, MacLean BX, et al. Platform-independent and label-free quantitation of proteomic data using MS1 extracted ion chromatograms in skyline: application to protein acetylation and phosphorylation. Mol Cell Proteomics 2012;11:202–214
35. Frezza C, Cipolat S, Scorrano L. Organelle isolation: functional mitochondria from mouse liver, muscle and cultured fibroblasts. Nat Protoc 2007;2:287–295
36. Kerr D, Grahame G, Nakouzi G. Assays of pyruvate dehydrogenase complex and pyruvate carboxylase activity. Methods Mol Biol 2012;837:93–119
37. Goodyear LJ, Giorgino F, Balon TW, Condorelli G, Smith RJ. Effects of contractile activity on tyrosine phosphoproteins and PI 3-kinase activity in rat skeletal muscle. Am J Physiol 1995;268:E987–E995
38. Bouskila M, Hirshman MF, Jensen J, Goodyear LJ, Sakamoto K. Insulin promotes glycogen synthesis in the absence of GSK3 phosphorylation in skeletal muscle. Am J Physiol Endocrinol Metab 2008;294:E28–E35
39. An J, Muoio DM, Shiota M, et al. Hepatic expression of malonyl-CoA decarboxylase reverses muscle, liver and whole-animal insulin resistance. Nat Med 2004;10:268–274
40. Wu JY, Kao HJ, Li SC, et al. ENU mutagenesis identifies mice with mitochondrial branched-chain aminotransferase deficiency resembling human maple syrup urine disease. J Clin Invest 2004;113:434–440
41. Jensen MV, Joseph JW, Ilkayeva O, et al. Compensatory responses to pyruvate carboxylase suppression in islet beta-cells. Preservation of glucose-stimulated insulin secretion. J Biol Chem 2006;281:22342–22351

42. Rardin MJ, Wiley SE, Naviaux RK, Murphy AN, Dixon JE. Monitoring phosphorylation of the pyruvate dehydrogenase complex. Anal Biochem 2009;389:157–164

43. Akhmedov D, De Marchi U, Wollheim CB, Wiederkehr A. Pyruvate dehydrogenase E1α phosphorylation is induced by glucose but does not control metabolism-secretion coupling in INS-1E clonal β-cells. Biochim Biophys Acta 2012;1823:1815–1824

44. Bell EL, Emerling BM, Ricoult SJ, Guarente L. SirT3 suppresses hypoxia inducible factor 1α and tumor growth by inhibiting mitochondrial ROS production. Oncogene 2011;30:2986–2996

45. Yang H, Yang T, Baur JA, et al. Nutrient-sensitive mitochondrial NAD+ levels dictate cell survival. Cell 2007;130:1095–1107

46. Jagoe RT, Lecker SH, Gomes M, Goldberg AL. Patterns of gene expression in atrophying skeletal muscles: response to food deprivation. FASEB J 2002;16:1697–1712

47. Galgani JE, Moro C, Ravussin E. Metabolic flexibility and insulin resistance. Am J Physiol Endocrinol Metab 2008;295:E1009–E1017

48. DeFronzo RA, Tripathy D. Skeletal muscle insulin resistance is the primary defect in type 2 diabetes. Diabetes Care 2009;32(Suppl. 2):S157–S163

49. Fernandez-Marcos PJ, Jeninga EH, Canto C, et al. Muscle or liver-specific Sirt3 deficiency induces hyperacetylation of mitochondrial proteins without affecting global metabolic homeostasis. Sci Rep 2012;2:425

50. Linn TC, Pettit FH, Reed LJ. Alpha-keto acid dehydrogenase complexes. X. Regulation of the activity of the pyruvate dehydrogenase complex from beef kidney mitochondria by phosphorylation and dephosphorylation. Proc Natl Acad Sci USA 1969;62:234–241

51. Harris RA, Bowker-Kinley MM, Huang B, Wu P. Regulation of the activity of the pyruvate dehydrogenase complex. Adv Enzyme Regul 2002;42:249–259

Glucokinase Activation Ameliorates ER Stress–Induced Apoptosis in Pancreatic β-Cells

Jun Shirakawa,[1] Yu Togashi,[1] Eri Sakamoto,[1] Mitsuyo Kaji,[1] Kazuki Tajima,[1] Kazuki Orime,[1] Hideaki Inoue,[1] Naoto Kubota,[2] Takashi Kadowaki,[2] and Yasuo Terauchi[1]

The derangement of endoplasmic reticulum (ER) homeostasis triggers β-cell apoptosis, leading to diabetes. Glucokinase upregulates insulin receptor substrate 2 (IRS-2) expression in β-cells, but the role of glucokinase and IRS-2 in ER stress has been unclear. In this study, we investigated the impact of glucokinase activation by glucokinase activator (GKA) on ER stress in β-cells. GKA administration improved β-cell apoptosis in Akita mice, a model of ER stress–mediated diabetes. GKA increased the expression of IRS-2 in β-cells, even under ER stress. Both glucokinase-deficient Akita mice and IRS-2–deficient Akita mice exhibited an increase in β-cell apoptosis, compared with Akita mice. β-cell–specific IRS-2–overexpressing (βIRS-2-Tg) Akita mice showed less β-cell apoptosis than Akita mice. IRS-2–deficient islets were vulnerable, but βIRS-2-Tg islets were resistant to ER stress–induced apoptosis. Meanwhile, GKA regulated the expressions of C/EBP homologous protein (CHOP) and other ER stress–related genes in an IRS-2–independent fashion in islets. GKA suppressed the expressions of CHOP and Bcl2-associated X protein (Bax) and protected against β-cell apoptosis under ER stress in an ERK1/2-dependent, IRS-2–independent manner. Taken together, GKA ameliorated ER stress–mediated apoptosis by harmonizing IRS-2 upregulation and the IRS-2–independent control of apoptosis in β-cells. *Diabetes* **62:3448–3458, 2013**

T he decline in β-cell mass as a result of increased apoptosis is an important property of type 2 diabetes (1,2). Endoplasmic reticulum (ER) stress is a key mediator of β-cell apoptosis (3,4). Hence, the development of therapeutic strategies to safeguard residual β-cells against ER stress–induced apoptosis is needed for the adequate care and cure of type 2 diabetes.

Glucokinase, a member of the hexokinase family, is mainly expressed in hepatocytes, pancreatic β-cells, and certain subgroups of hypothalamic neurons, forming a key component of the main glucose sensor in β-cells (5–8). Glucokinase also mediates the glucose signal–induced upregulation of insulin receptor substrate 2 (IRS-2) expression in β-cells through calcineurin or CREB (9–12). IRS-2 is required for the maintenance of the β-cell mass and plays an important role in compensatory β-cell expansion against peripheral insulin resistance and in β-cell survival, preventing diabetes (9,13–15). Mice that were heterozygous for β-cell glucokinase (βGck[+/−]) and that were fed a diet rich in linoleic acid and sucrose exhibited increased ER stress and apoptosis in β-cells, compared with wild-type (WT) mice (16). Consequently, we speculated that glucokinase is also involved in the regulation of ER stress–induced apoptosis in β-cells.

Glucokinase activators (GKAs) have been shown to reduce blood glucose levels in several diabetic animal models and type 2 diabetic patients (10,11,17–19). GKAs promote β-cell proliferation, which is driven by the increased expression of IRS-2 and the activation of its downstream signaling pathway (11,20,21). However, the physiological advantage of GKA-mediated signaling during β-cell apoptosis has been obscure (22,23), and the effect of GKAs on ER stress in β-cells remains unknown.

These conditions inspired us to undertake a detailed investigation of the impact of GKA on ER stress and apoptosis in β-cells. Here, we report the protective effects of GKA against ER stress–induced apoptosis in β-cells, the nature of this mechanism, and the significance of glucokinase and IRS-2 in the regulation of ER stress in β-cells.

RESEARCH DESIGN AND METHODS

Animals and animal care. Akita mice with a C57BL/6J background were obtained from Japan SLC. We backcrossed βGck[+/−] (7), IRS-2[−/−] (15), or β-cell–specific IRS-2–overexpressing (βIRS-2-Tg) mice (9) with C57BL/6J mice >10 times. Akita mice were crossed with βGck[+/−], IRS-2[−/−], or βIRS-2-Tg mice to obtain βGck[+/−];Akita, IRS-2[−/−];Akita, or βIRS-2-Tg;Akita offspring. *db/db* (Lepr[+/−]) mice were also obtained from CLEA Japan. High fat–fed WT and βGck[+/−] mice were generated as described previously (9). All the experiments were conducted on male littermates. All the animal procedures were performed in accordance with the institutional animal care guidelines and the guidelines of the Animal Care Committee of the Yokohama City University. The animal housing rooms were maintained at a constant room temperature (25°C) and on a 12-h light (7:00 A.M.)/dark (7:00 P.M.) cycle.

Drugs. GKA Cpd A [2-amino-5-(4-methyl-4H-(1,2,4)-triazole-3-yl-sulfanyl)-N-(4-methyl-thiazole-2-yl)benzamide] (24), was purchased from Calbiochem, Ro-28-1675 [(R)-3-cyclopentyl-2-(4-methanesulfonyl-phenyl)-N-thiazol-2-yl-propionamide] (17) was purchased from Axon Medchem, and Cpd B (3-[(1S)-2-hydroxy-1-methylethoxy]-5-[4-(methylsulfonyl)phenoxy]-N-1,3-thiazol-2-ylbenzamide) (25) was provided by Merck Sharp & Dohme. The neonatal WT and Akita mice were weaned at 19 days after birth and were fed a standard diet (MF; Oriental Yeast, Tokyo, Japan) or a standard diet containing 0.01% GKA Cpd A (Calbiochem), 0.4% sitagliptin (STG) (Januvia; Suzuken Co., Nagoya, Japan), or 0.5% phloridzin (PHZ) (Sigma-Aldrich). βGck[+/−];Akita and IRS-2[−/−];Akita mice were fed a standard diet or a standard diet containing 0.01% GKA until 33 days of age or 0.5% PHZ until 8 weeks of age.

Biochemical parameters and glucose tolerance test. The plasma glucose levels, blood insulin levels, and glycogen content in the liver were determined using a Glutest Neo Super (Sanwa Chemical Co.), an insulin kit (Morinaga), and a Determiner-GL-E Kit (Wako Pure Chemical Industries), respectively. The plasma alanine aminotransferase, free fatty acid, total cholesterol, and triglyceride levels were assayed using enzymatic methods (Wako Pure Chemical Industries). All the mice were denied access to food for 20–24 h before the oral glucose tolerance test (OGTT) and then were orally loaded with glucose at 1.5 mg/g body weight. For single administration experiments, 33-day-old mice received either the vehicle (Solutol HS-15; BASF) or GKA (30 mg/kg orally) before oral glucose loading (1.5 mg/g).

From the [1]Department of Endocrinology and Metabolism, Graduate School of Medicine, Yokohama City University, Yokohama, Japan; and the [2]Department of Diabetes and Metabolic Diseases, Graduate School of Medicine, University of Tokyo, Tokyo, Japan.

Corresponding author: Yasuo Terauchi, terauchi-tky@umin.ac.jp.

Received 12 January 2013 and accepted 14 June 2013.

DOI: 10.2337/db13-0052

This article contains Supplementary Data online at http://diabetes .diabetesjournals.org/lookup/suppl/doi:10.2337/db13-0052/-/DC1.

Histological analysis. More than five pancreatic tissue sections from each animal were analyzed after fixation and paraffin embedding. The sections were immunostained with antibodies to insulin (Santa Cruz Biotechnology) or glucagon (Abcam). Biotinylated secondary antibodies, a VECTASTAIN Elite ABC Kit, and a DAB Substrate Kit (Vector Laboratories) were used to examine the sections using bright-field microscopy to determine the β-cell mass, and Alexa Fluor 488–, 555–, and 647–conjugated secondary antibodies (Invitrogen) were used for fluorescence microscopy. All the images were acquired using a BZ-9000 microscope (Keyence) or FluoView FV1000-D confocal laser scanning microscope (Olympus). The proportion of the area of pancreatic tissue occupied by the β-cells was calculated using BIOREVO software (Keyence), as described previously (16). TUNEL staining was performed in vivo or in vitro using the ApopTag In Situ Detection Kit (Chemicon). For TUNEL staining, at least 100 islets per mouse (in vivo) or 30 islets per isolated islet group (in vitro) attached to poly-L-lysine–coated coverslips (Falcon) were analyzed using the FluoView FV1000-D confocal laser scanning microscope to assess the proportion of immunostained nuclei among the insulin-positive cells.

Islet culture. Islets were isolated from mice as described elsewhere (16). Isolated islets were cultured overnight in RPMI 1640 medium (Wako Pure Chemical Industries) containing 2.8, 5.6, 11.1, or 22.2 mmol/L glucose supplemented with 10% FCS, 100 units/mL penicillin, and 100 μg/mL streptomycin. Islets were treated with 1 μmol/L thapsigargin, 10 μmol/L tunicamycin, 50 μmol/L nifedipine, 10 μmol/L FK506, 20 μmol/L U0126, 10 μmol/L UK14304 (Sigma-Aldrich), 30 μmol/L GKA Cpd A, 0.5 μmol/L GSK-3 inhibitor (BIO), 10 μmol/L Akti-1/2 (Calbiochem), 10 mmol/L D-mannoheptulose (Toronto Research Chemicals), 200 μmol/L diazoxide (Wako Pure Chemical Industries), 200 nmol/L OSI-906 (Selleck Chemicals), 10 μmol/L GKA Ro-28-1675 (Axon Medchem), or 2 μmol/L GKA Cpd B (provided by Merck Sharp & Dohme). All the reagents were added concomitantly to the medium in each experiment.

Real-time PCR. Total RNA was isolated from pancreatic islets using an RNase-free DNase and RNeasy Kit (Qiagen, Valencia, CA). cDNA was prepared using the High Capacity cDNA Reverse Transcription Kits (Applied Biosystems) and was subjected to quantitative PCR using TaqMan Gene Expression Assays (7900 Real-Time PCR System; Applied Biosystems) with THUNDERBIRD qPCR Master Mix (TOYOBO). All the probes were purchased from Applied Biosystems. Each quantitative reaction was performed in duplicate. Data were normalized according to the β-actin level.

Immunoblotting. For immunoblotting, >100 isolated islets were lysed in ice-cold RIPA buffer (Cell Signaling Technology) with complete protease inhibitor cocktail (Roche Diagnostics). After centrifugation, the extracts were subjected to immunoblotting with antibodies to C/EBP homologous protein (CHOP) (GADD153), ATF4, GRP78, phosphor-eIF-2α, ATF3, Bcl2-associated X protein (Bax), X-box binding protein 1 (XBP1), ATF6α (Santa Cruz Biotechnology), GSK-3β, phospho-GSK-3β (Ser9), extracellular signal–related kinase 1/2 (ERK1/2), phospho-ERK1/2 (Thr202/Tyr204), IRS-2, phospho-eIF2α (Ser51), eIF2α, IRE1α, phospho-PERK, PERK (Cell Signaling Technology), glyceraldehyde-3-phosphate dehydrogenase (GAPDH), phospho-IRE1 (Ser724) (Abcam), and β-actin (Sigma-Aldrich). Densitometry was performed using Image J software.

cDNA microarray analysis. Islets were isolated from mice as described elsewhere (16). Islets of 8-week-old C57BL/6J mice were treated for 24 h with 30 μmol/L GKA (Cpd A) or vehicle (DMSO) at 5.6 mmol/L glucose RPMI-1640 medium containing 5.6 mmol/L glucose supplemented with 10% FCS. The cDNA microarray analysis was performed using the Agilent-026655 whole mouse genome array (GPL10333) (Agilent). Replicate (n = 2) microarray studies were performed for each treatment. The data were analyzed using Genespring GX software (Agilent). The data were normalized in a per-chip and per-spot intensity-dependent manner. The data files have been deposited in the NCBI GEO database GSE41248 (http://www.ncbi.nlm.nih.gov/geo/query/acc.cgi?acc=GSE41248).

Flow cytometry. To assay apoptosis based on cleaved caspase-3 expression, the islets were fixed with 2% formaldehyde, perforated with 0.01% Triton X-100, stained with phycoerythrin-conjugated anticleaved caspase-3 antibody (Asp175; Cell Signaling Technology), and analyzed using a FACS Canto II (BD Biosciences). The mean fluorescence of normal-sized (small populations of forward scatter were excluded) and propidium iodide-negative survival cell fractions was calculated using FACS Diva software (BD Biosciences).

Statistical analyses. All the data were reported as the means ± SE and were analyzed using the Student t test or ANOVA. Differences were considered significant if the P value was <0.05 (*) or <0.01 (**).

RESULTS

GKA ameliorated β-cell apoptosis in Akita mice. To address whether GKA ameliorates ER stress and apoptosis in β-cells, we used Akita mice, which carry a heterozygous conformation-altering mutation (Cys96Tyr) in the *Ins2* gene and manifest enhanced ER stress and the apoptosis

of β-cells (26,27). WT or Akita mice were fed a standard diet or a diet containing GKA, the DPP-4 inhibitor STG, or the SGLT1 and SGLT2 inhibitor PHZ (Supplementary Fig. 1A). Because DPP-4 inhibitor reportedly protected β-cell ER stress and apoptosis in diabetic mice and PHZ could lower blood glucose levels via a reduction of renal glucose transport, we assessed the impacts of these drugs on β-cell apoptosis as controls (16). Prior to the administration of these diets, the Akita mice already exhibited impaired glucose tolerance and deteriorated insulin secretion after glucose loading but retained similar body weights, fed blood glucose levels, β-cell areas, islet diameters, and β-cell proportions, compared with the WT mice (Supplementary Fig. 1B–H). Body weight gain and serum lipid profiles were not significantly different among the five groups (Fig. 1A and Supplementary Fig. 2A). GKA and PHZ, but not STG, improved the plasma glucose levels in Akita mice (Fig. 1B). The OGTT after a 20–24-h fast revealed that Akita mice had abnormal glucose tolerance and severely exacerbated insulin secretion, compared with WT mice (Supplementary Fig. 2B and C). Of note, GKA, STG, and PHZ did not restore insulin secretion during the OGTT, suggesting that these agents were insufficient to improve β-cell function in Akita mice (Supplementary Fig. 2B and C).

Subsequently, Akita and WT mice were treated with GKA or a vehicle 30 min before an OGTT. GKA significantly reduced the blood glucose levels before and after glucose administration in both WT and Akita mice (Supplementary Fig. 2D). GKA facilitated insulin secretion in WT mice, but it failed to improve impaired insulin secretion in Akita mice (Supplementary Fig. 2E). On the other hand, in Akita mice, the liver glycogen content was increased by GKA (Supplementary Fig. 2F). Accordingly, the glucose-lowering effect of GKA in Akita mice was partly attributed to the facilitation of glucose utilization in the liver.

In Akita mice, the β-cell mass and the β-cell ratio in the islets were significantly decreased, the islet morphology was abnormal, and the number of TUNEL-positive apoptotic β-cells was significantly greater than that in WT mice (Fig. 1C–E). GKA and STG, but not PHZ, restored the β-cell mass, normalized the islet morphology, and significantly decreased the number of TUNEL-positive apoptotic β-cells in Akita mice (Fig. 1C–E and Supplementary Fig. 2G). GKA significantly decreased the mRNA expression of CHOP, CEBP-β, and Bax, and it significantly increased the mRNA expression of IRS-2 in islets, compared with the expression levels in untreated Akita mice (Fig. 1F).

Role of glucokinase in ER stress–induced β-cell apoptosis. To assess the role of glucokinase in ER stress, we generated Akita mice with the β-cell–specific heterozygous ablation of glucokinase (βGck$^{+/-}$;Akita). The βGck$^{+/-}$;Akita mice exhibited an equivalent body weight gain and lipid levels but had aggravated blood glucose levels and glucose tolerance (Fig. 2A–D and Supplementary Fig. 3A–D). However, glucokinase deficiency no longer produced any impairment in insulin secretion in insulin-defective Akita mice (Fig. 2D and Supplementary Fig. 3C). Although the βGck$^{+/-}$;Akita mice depicted a similar β-cell mass (Fig. 2E), the number of TUNEL-positive β-cells was significantly higher in the βGck$^{+/-}$;Akita mice than in WT mice (Fig. 2F and Supplementary Fig. 3E). Of note, the reversal of hyperglycemia by PHZ in βGck$^{+/-}$;Akita mice did not improve β-cell apoptosis (Supplementary Fig. 3F–J). A gene expression analysis of

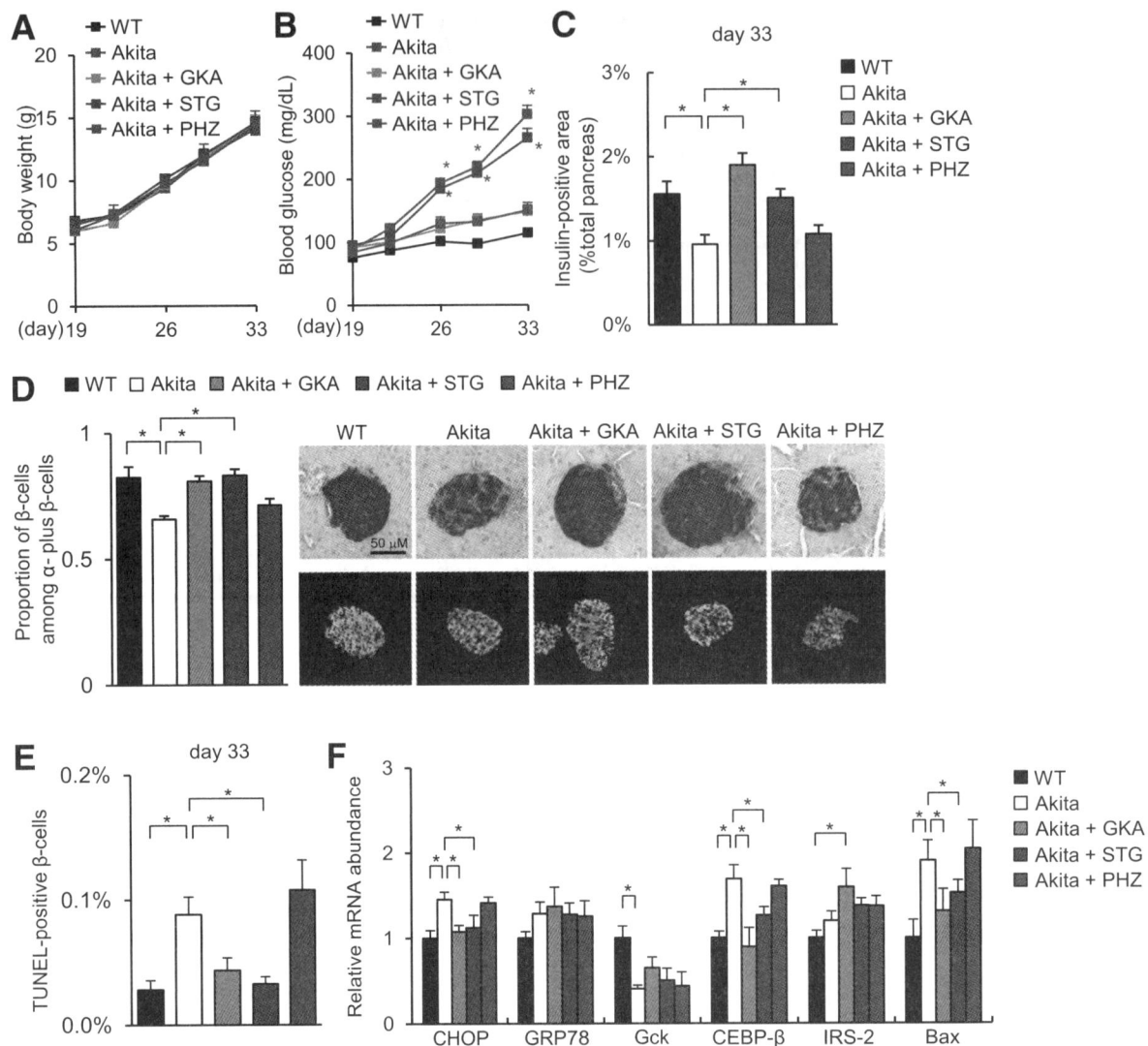

FIG. 1. GKA ameliorated β-cell apoptosis in Akita mice. The experiments were performed in Akita mice after 14 days on a standard diet or a diet containing 0.01% GKA, 0.4% STG, or 0.5% PHZ. Details are described in Supplementary Fig. 1A. A: Body weight gain ($n = 8$). B: Fed blood glucose levels ($n = 8$). *$P < 0.05$ vs. WT mice. C: β-cell mass ($n = 6$–8). The β-cell area is shown as a proportion of the area of the entire pancreas (aged 33 days). D, left: Quantification of β-cell mass as a proportion of the total α-cell plus β-cell mass in the islet (aged 33 days, $n = 6$). D, right: Pancreatic sections were stained with antibodies to insulin (green) and glucagon (red). The scale bar represents 50 μm. E: The proportion of TUNEL-positive cells is shown as a percentage of the total number of insulin-positive cells in the sections (aged 33 days, $n = 6$). F: The mRNA expression levels of the molecules indicated in the islets (aged 33 days, $n = 5$). *$P < 0.05$.

isolated islets demonstrated a decreased expression of IRS-2 and an increased expression of Bax in βGck$^{+/-}$; Akita mice, compared with Akita mice (Fig. 2G). These results suggested that the insufficiency of glucokinase in β-cells was vulnerable to ER stress by the absence of the induced expression of IRS-2.

Role of IRS-2 in ER stress–induced β-cell apoptosis.
Next, we generated IRS-2–deficient Akita (IRS-2$^{+/-}$;Akita and IRS-2$^{-/-}$;Akita) mice. IRS-2$^{+/-}$;Akita mice exhibited a modest decrease in body weight gain and deterioration in their blood glucose levels, compared with Akita mice (Fig. 3A and B). As we reported (11), IRS-2$^{-/-}$ mice remained euglycemic with normal β-cell mass in the C57BL/6J background, while these mice demonstrated diabetes and decreased β-cell mass in other genetic backgrounds. IRS-2$^{-/-}$;Akita mice showed a more severe impairment of body weight gain, overt hyperglycemia, increased mortality, a further decrease in β-cell mass, and the enhancement

of β-cell apoptosis compared with Akita mice (Fig. 3A–D and Supplementary Fig. 4A and B). The serum lipid levels in the IRS-2$^{-/-}$;Akita mice were similar to those in the Akita mice (Supplementary Fig. 4C). The administration of PHZ partly reduced the blood glucose levels and lethality but did not affect the β-cell mass or β-cell apoptosis in IRS-2$^{-/-}$;Akita mice (data not shown).

We investigated changes in gene expressions in isolated islets of IRS-2–deficient (IRS-2$^{-/-}$) mice under ER stress induced by treatment with thapsigargin. The expression levels of CHOP or Bax were increased in IRS-2$^{-/-}$ islets under ER stress, compared with WT islets, at 5.6 or 11.1 mmol/L glucose but not at 2.8 mmol/L glucose (Fig. 3E). Under basal unstimulated conditions, elevated expression levels of GPR78, ATF6α, PERK, eIF2α, and IRE1α were observed in IRS-2$^{-/-}$ islets (Fig. 3F and Supplementary Fig. 4D). IRS-2$^{-/-}$ islets also showed reduced phosphorylation levels of GSK-3β (Fig. 3F), increased expression of

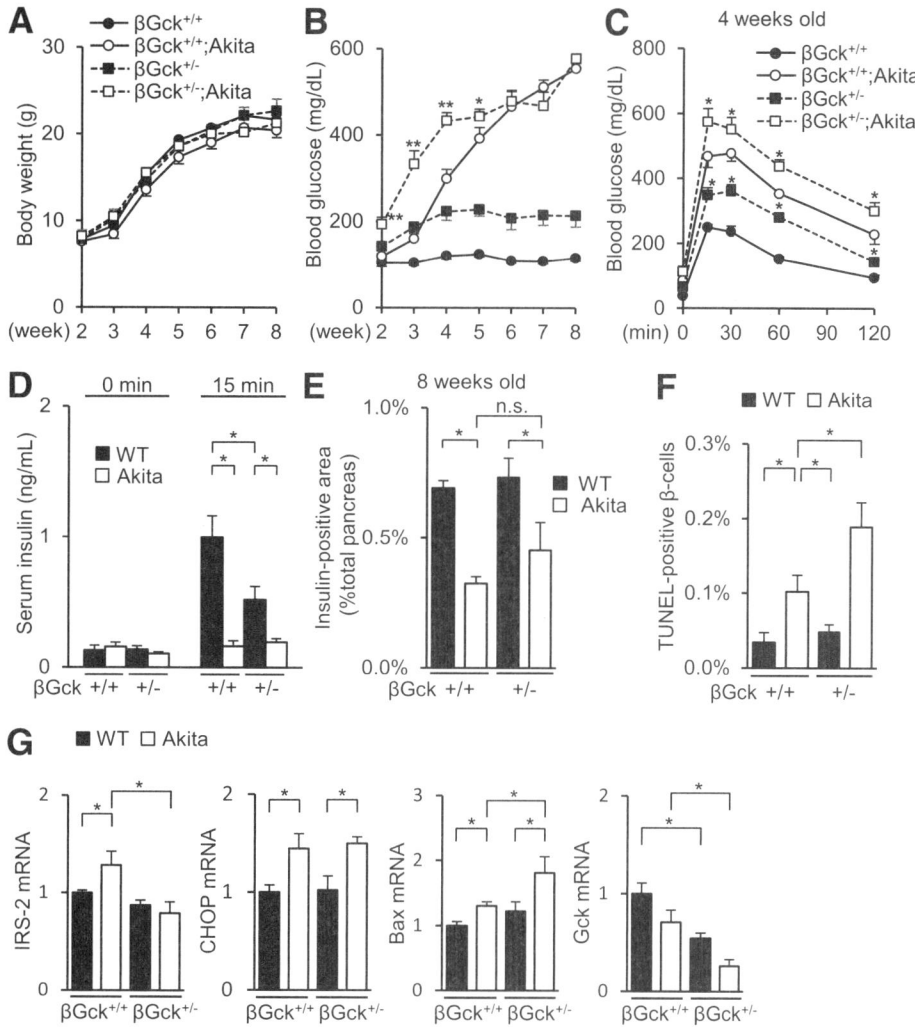

FIG. 2. β-Cell–specific heterozygous ablation of glucokinase (βGck^+/−) worsened β-cell apoptosis in Akita mice. *A:* Body weight gain (*n* = 8–14). *B:* Fed blood glucose levels (*n* = 8–14). *P < 0.05 and **P < 0.01 vs. Akita mice. *C* and *D:* Glucose tolerance test (aged 4 weeks, *n* = 6–8). *C:* Plasma glucose levels. *P < 0.05 vs. Akita mice. *D:* Serum insulin levels. *E:* β-Cell mass (*n* = 6). The β-cell area is shown as a proportion of the area of the entire pancreas (aged 8 weeks). *F:* The proportion of TUNEL-positive cells is shown as a percentage of the total number of insulin-positive cells in the sections (aged 8 weeks, *n* = 6). *G:* The mRNA expression levels of the molecules indicated in the islets (aged 8 weeks, *n* = 6). *P < 0.05. n.s., not significant.

cleaved caspase-3 (Fig. 3*G*), and augmentation of β-cell apoptosis (Fig. 3*H* and Supplementary Fig. 4*E*) in the presence of ER stress at 5.6 mmol/L glucose. Correspondingly, a GSK-3 inhibitor (BIO) recuperated this apoptosis in IRS-2^−/− islets (Fig. 3*H*).

Akita mice with the β-cell–specific transgenic overexpression of IRS-2 (βIRS-2-Tg;Akita) were also generated. Although the body weight gain and β-cell mass showed no significant changes, βIRS-2-Tg;Akita mice exhibited an improved glucose tolerance, enhanced glucose-induced insulin secretion, and the amelioration of β-cell apoptosis, compared with Akita mice (Fig. 4*A–F* and Supplementary Fig. 5*A–C*). The β-cell mass of βIRS-2-Tg;Akita mice tended to be higher than that of Akita mice, with a value similar to that in WT mice (Fig. 4*E*). Consistent with the results of the apoptotic analysis (Fig. 4*F*), the expression level of Bax in islets was significantly lower in the βIRS-2-Tg;Akita mice than in Akita mice (Fig. 4*G*). Isolated βIRS-2-Tg islets also showed reduced expression levels of Bax (Fig. 4*H*) and the restoration of β-cell apoptosis (Fig. 4*I* and Supplementary Fig. 5*D*) in the presence of ER stress.

IRS-2–independent regulation of ER stress–related genes by GKA. We compared the gene expression profiles between GKA-treated and vehicle-treated isolated islets to identify the target genes of GKA. Genes for which the expression levels were increased by greater than twofold or reduced by <0.5-fold by GKA treatment, relative to the expression levels in control islets, were identified (NCBI GEO database GSE41248) (Supplementary Table 1). We confirmed that insulin gene and insulin signal molecules, such as IRS-2, PDX-1, and PIK3R1, were upregulated by GKA (Fig. 5*A*). Interestingly, GKA decreased the expression of CHOP and increased the expression of *Stc2, Ero-1β, Sdf2l1,* and *Edem-2,* which are reportedly ER stress–related genes (Fig. 5*A*). However, the expressions of the other ER stress–related genes, such as *Bip, IRE-1α, PERK, ATF6, Xbp1, ATF3, ATF4,* or *4EBP1,* were unaffected by GKA (data not shown). High glucose evoked identical changes in the gene expressions of ER stress–related genes (Supplementary Fig. 6*A*), and mannoheptulose, a glucokinase inhibitor, completely abolished these changes (Supplementary Fig. 6*B*). In the presence of diazoxide,

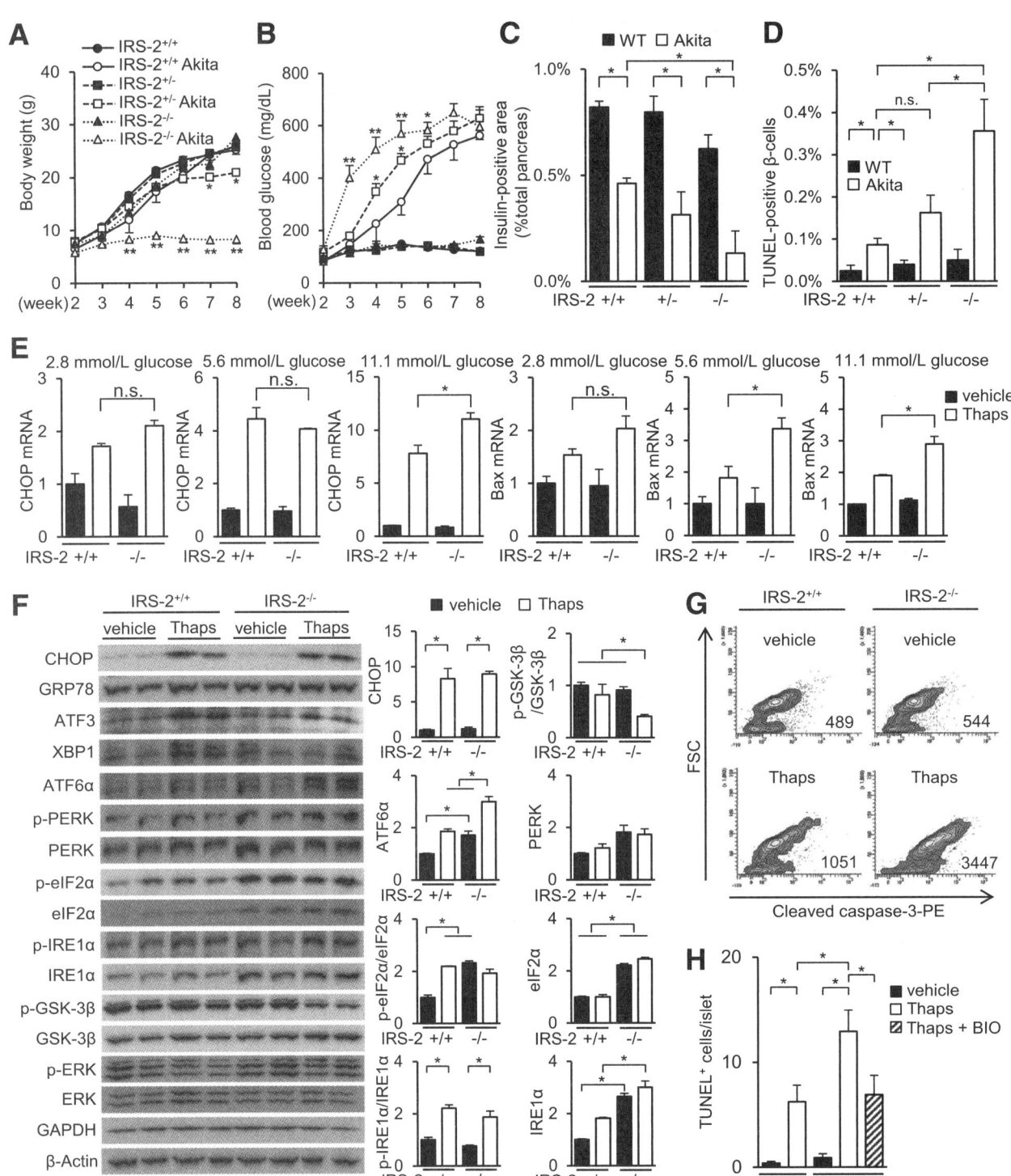

FIG. 3. IRS-2–deficient Akita (IRS-2$^{-/-}$;Akita) mice demonstrated a decreased β-cell mass and the enhancement of β-cell apoptosis. *A*: Body weight gain ($n = 8$–18). *$P < 0.05$ vs. Akita mice. *B*: Fed blood glucose levels ($n = 8$–18). *$P < 0.05$ and **$P < 0.01$ vs. Akita mice. *C*: β-Cell mass ($n = 8$). The β-cell area is shown as a proportion of the area of the entire pancreas (aged 8 weeks). *D*: The proportion of TUNEL-positive cells is shown as a percentage of the total number of insulin-positive cells in the sections (aged 8 weeks, $n = 8$). *E–H*: Isolated islets of WT (IRS-2$^{+/+}$) or IRS-2$^{-/-}$ mice were incubated with 1 μmol/L thapsigargin (Thaps) or vehicle for 24 h at 2.8, 5.6, or 11.1 mmol/L glucose (*E*) or at 5.6 mmol/L glucose (*F–H*). *E*: mRNA expression levels in the islets ($n = 8$). *F, left*: The total cell extracts from the islets were subjected to immunoblotting as indicated. *F, right*: Intensity of the signals quantified by densitometry ($n = 4$). *G*: Flow-cytometric analysis of cleaved caspase-3 levels in islets. Values shown represent the mean fluorescence of normal-sized cells (upper populations of forward scatter [FSC], i.e., viable cells) in the indicated population. The results of one of three independent experiments are shown. *H*: Number of TUNEL-positive β-cells in the islets (at least 30 islets per indicated group). A GSK-3 inhibitor, 0.5 μmol/L BIO, was added concomitantly with thapsigargin. *$P < 0.05$. n.s., not significant.

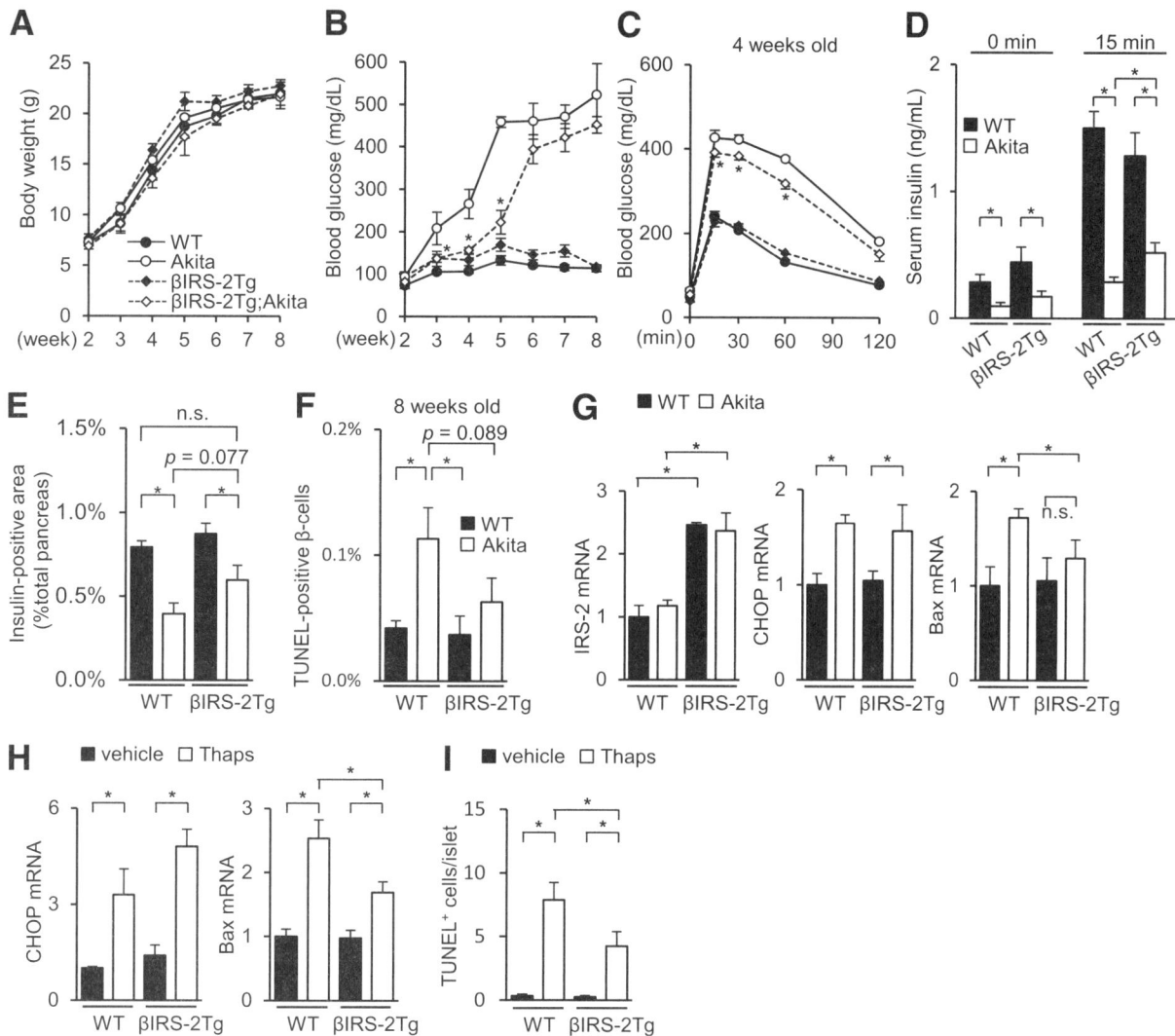

FIG. 4. Akita mice with β-cell–specific transgenic overexpression of IRS-2 (βIRS-2-Tg;Akita) were resistant to ER stress–induced apoptosis. *A*: Body weight gain (*n* = 10–14). *B*: Fed blood glucose levels (*n* = 10–14). *P < 0.05 vs. Akita mice. *C* and *D*: Glucose tolerance test (aged 4 weeks, *n* = 7–9). *C*: Plasma glucose levels. *P < 0.05 vs. Akita mice. *D*: Serum insulin levels. *E*: β-Cell mass (*n* = 7). The β-cell area is shown as a proportion of the area of the entire pancreas (aged 8 weeks). *F*: The proportion of TUNEL-positive cells is shown as a percentage of the total number of insulin-positive cells in the pancreas sections (aged 8 weeks, *n* = 6). *G*: mRNA expression levels in the islets (aged 8 weeks, *n* = 6). *H* and *I*: Isolated islets of WT or βIRS-2-Tg mice were incubated with 1 μmol/L thapsigargin (Thaps) or vehicle for 24 h at 5.6 mmol/L glucose. *H*: mRNA expression levels in the islets (*n* = 6). *I*: Number of TUNEL-positive β-cells in the islets (at least 30 islets per indicated group). *P < 0.05. n.s., not significant.

a K_{ATP} channel opener, the changes in IRS-2, Stc2, and Sdf2l1 were abrogated (Supplementary Fig. 6*C*). Treatment with the IGF-1R/insulin receptor inhibitor OSI-906 did not affect GKA-induced changes in ER stress–related gene expressions (Supplementary Fig. 6*D*). GKA decreased the expression of CHOP also in MIN6 cells (Supplementary Fig. 6*H*).

Because ER stress in β-cells reportedly occurs in *db/db* mice, the effects of GKA on ER stress–related genes were assessed in islets from 9-week-old *db/db* mice. Interestingly, the upregulation of IRS-2, PDX1, Stc2, Sdf2l1, and Ero1-β was attenuated, but the induction of Edem-2 was retained in *db/db* islets after GKA treatment (Supplementary Fig. 6*E*). βGck$^{+/-}$ mice failed to exhibit an elevated expression of IRS-2 in a diet-induced obesity (DIO) model (9). Although the upregulation of IRS-2 by GKA was greater in islets from DIO mice than from lean mice with a βGck$^{+/+}$ background, the βGck$^{+/-}$ islets from the DIO and

lean mice exhibited similar IRS-2 expression levels (Supplementary Figure 6*F*). βGck$^{+/-}$ islets also exhibited the increased expression of CHOP under unstimulated conditions and a reduction in Stc2 induction after GKA treatment (Supplementary Figure 6*F*).

Whether IRS-2 is required for the regulation of ER stress–related genes by GKA is uncertain. Accordingly, we used IRS-2$^{-/-}$ islets to address this question. In IRS-2$^{-/-}$ islets, the GKA-induced changes in the expression levels of genes related to ER stress were essentially preserved, not impaired (Fig. 5*B*). Hence, GKA regulates the expressions of ER stress–related genes, regardless of IRS-2 deficiency. Blocking L-type Ca^{2+} channels with nifedipine or calcineurin with FK506 (tacrolimus) prevented the GKA-induced increase in the expression of IRS-2 but had little effect on the regulation of ER stress–related gene expressions by GKA (Fig. 5*C*). In contrast, the changes in CHOP, Stc2, and Sdf2l1 expressions by GKA were completely blunted by the

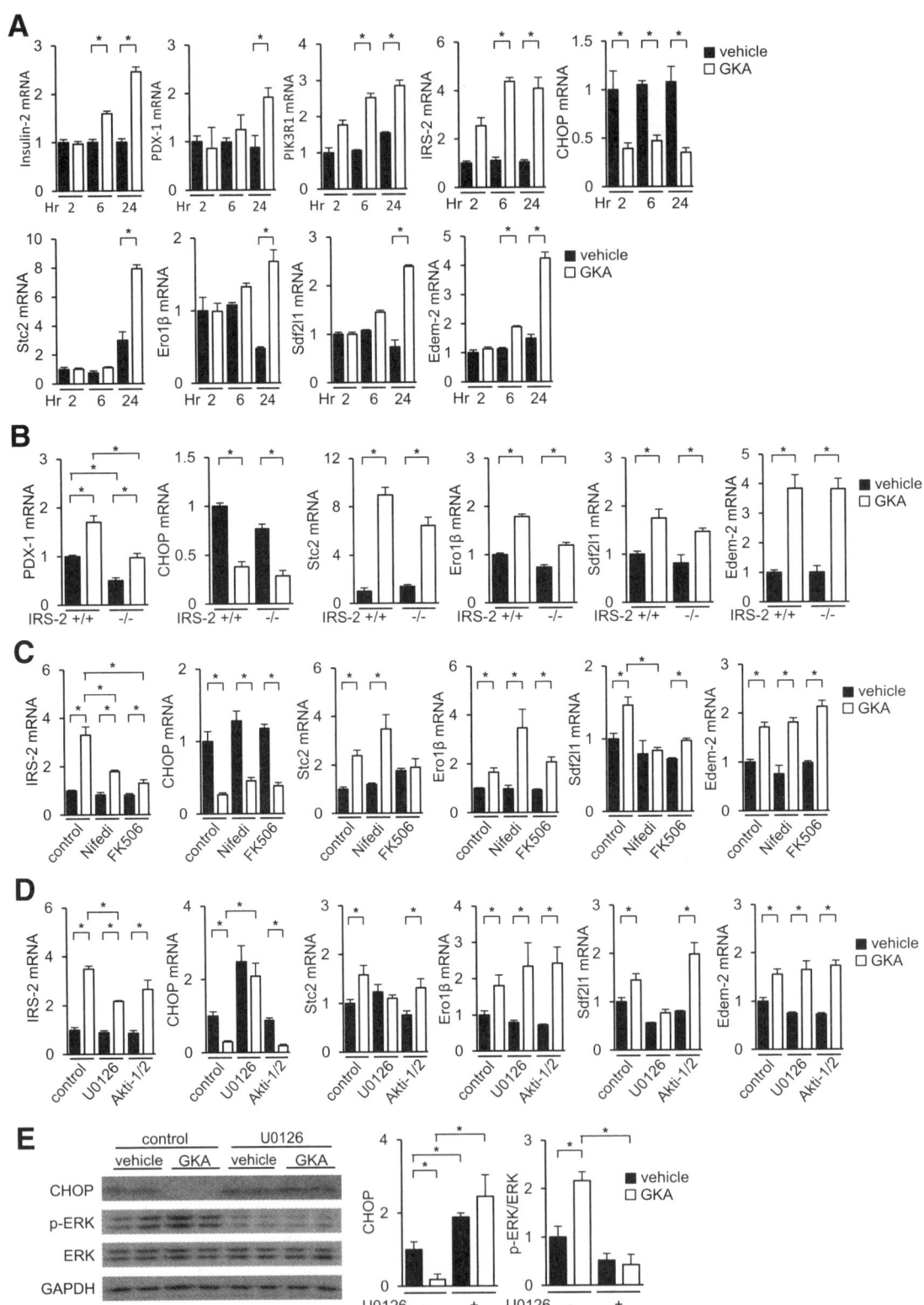

FIG. 5. IRS-2–independent and ERK-dependent regulation of ER stress–related genes by GKA in islets. *A–D*: The mRNA expression levels in the islets (aged 8 weeks, *n* = 6). *A*: Islets of C57BL/6J mice were incubated with 30 μmol/L GKA (Cpd A) at 5.6 mmol/L glucose. *B*: Islets of WT (IRS-2$^{+/+}$) or IRS-2$^{-/-}$ mice were incubated with 30 μmol/L GKA at 5.6 mmol/L glucose for 24 h. *C*: Islets of C57BL/6J mice were incubated with 30 μmol/L GKA at 5.6 mmol/L glucose for 24 h, in the presence of 50 μmol/L nifedipine (Nifedi, calcium channel blocker) or 10 μmol/L FK506 (tacrolimus, calcineurin inhibitor). *D*: Islets of C57BL/6J mice were incubated with 30 μmol/L GKA at 5.6 mmol/L glucose for 24 h, in the presence of 20 μmol/L U0126 (MEK inhibitor) or 10 μmol/L Akti-1/2 (Akt/PKB inhibitor). *E*: Islets of C57BL/6J mice were incubated with 30 μmol/L GKA at 5.6 mmol/L glucose for 24 h in the presence of 20 μmol/L U0126. *E, left*: Total cell extracts from islets were subjected to immunoblotting as indicated. *E, right*: Intensity of the signals quantified by densitometry (ImageJ) (*n* = 4). *P < 0.05.

blockade of MEK1/2 with U0126 but not by the Akt inhibitor (Akti-1/2) (Fig. 5D). The upregulation of IRS-2 by GKA was retained despite its significant attenuation by U0126 (Fig. 5D). GKA phosphorylated ERK1/2 and reduced CHOP protein in islets, and these actions induced by GKA were restricted in the presence of U0126 (Fig. 5E). The selective α2-adrenergic agonist UK14304 reduced glucose-stimulated ERK1/2 activation (28). UK14304 suppressed the GKA-mediated modifications in the expression levels of IRS-2, CHOP, Stc2, and Sdf2l1 (Supplementary Fig. 6G). Thus, the regulation of CHOP and other ER stress–related genes by GKA was IRS-2 independent and partly ERK1/2 dependent.

IRS-2–independent amelioration of ER stress–induced apoptosis by GKA.

CHOP triggers ER stress–induced apoptosis in β-cells in several diabetic mouse models (27,29). Since GKA reduced the expression of CHOP via an ERK-dependent, IRS-2–independent manner, we assessed the effects of GKA on isolated islets under ER stress. GKA increased the gene expression of IRS-2 and decreased the expressions of CHOP and Bax in WT islets under ER stress induced by thapsigargin, an inhibitor of sarco/endoplasmic reticulum Ca^{2+} ATPase (Fig. 6A). Interestingly, a transient increase in IRS-2 expression was observed in islets and MIN6 insulinoma cells after treatment with either

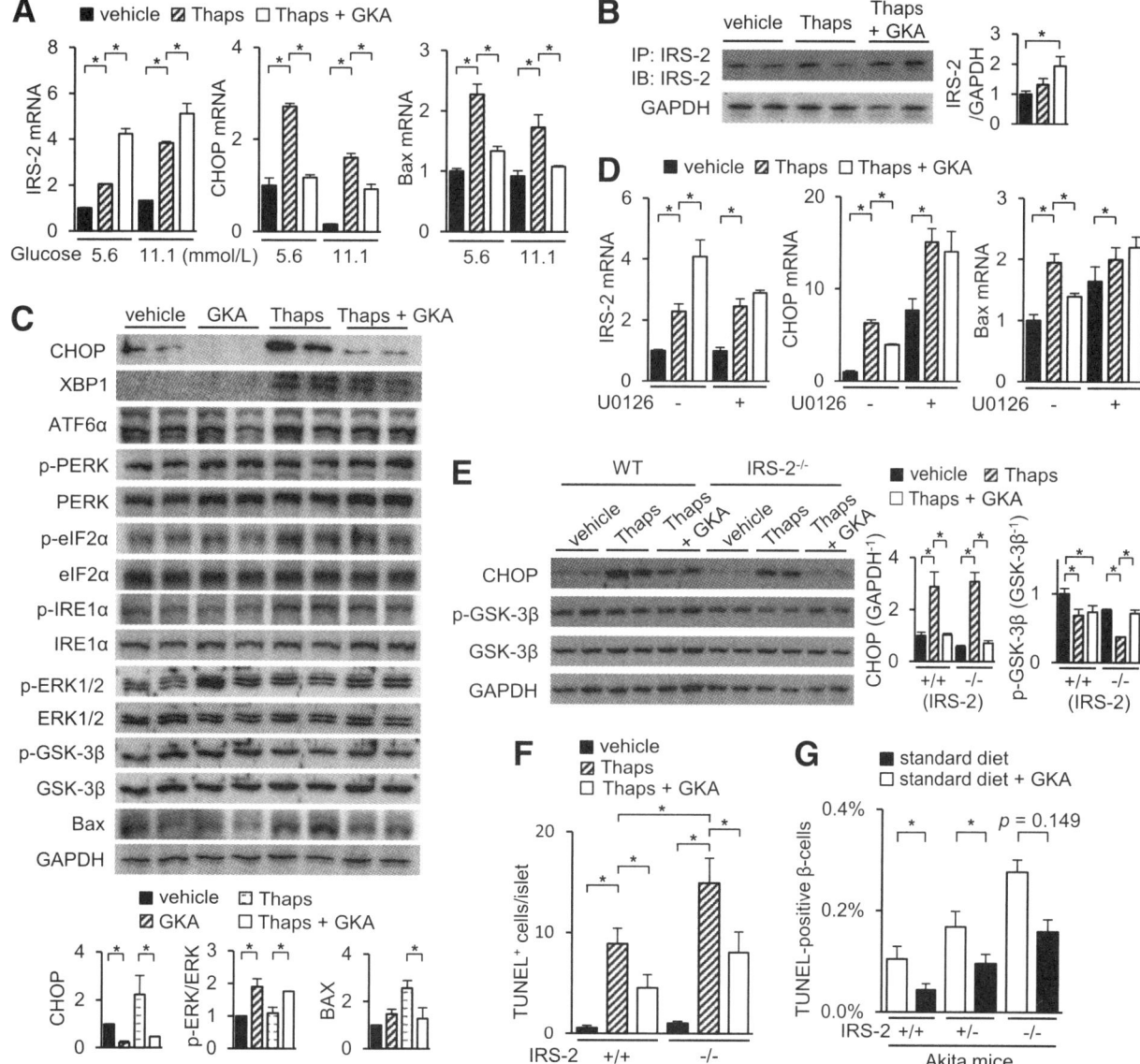

FIG. 6. GKA ameliorates ER stress–induced apoptosis via IRS-2–independent pathway. Islets from C57BL/6J mice (aged 8 weeks) were incubated with 1 μmol/L thapsigargin (Thaps) and 30 μmol/L GKA (Cpd A) at 5.6 (A–C) or 11.1 mmol/L (A) glucose for 24 h. A: mRNA expression levels in the islets (n = 6). B, left: The immunoprecipitated or total cell extracts from the islets were subjected to immunoblotting as indicated. B, right: Intensity of the signals quantified by densitometry (n = 4). C, top: The total cell extracts from the islets were subjected to immunoblotting as indicated. C, bottom: Intensity of the signals quantified by densitometry (n = 4). D: Islets of C57BL/6J mice (aged 8 weeks) were incubated with 30 μmol/L GKA and 1 μmol/L Thaps at 5.6 mmol/L glucose for 24 h in the presence of 20 μmol/L U0126 (MEK inhibitor). The mRNA expression levels (n = 6). E and F: Islets of WT (IRS-2^{+/+}) or IRS-2^{−/−} mice were incubated with 1 μmol/L Thaps and 30 μmol/L GKA for 24 h at 5.6 mmol/L glucose. E: mRNA expression levels in the islets (n = 6). F: Number of TUNEL-positive β-cells in the islets (at least 30 islets per indicated group). G: IRS-2^{+/+};Akita, IRS-2^{+/−};Akita, or IRS-2^{−/−}; Akita mice were fed standard diet containing GKA from day 19 to 33 after birth. The proportion of TUNEL-positive cells is shown as a percentage of the total number of insulin-positive cells in the pancreas sections (aged 33 days, n = 4–7). *P < 0.05. IB, immunoblotting; IP, immunoprecipitation.

thapsigargin or tunicamycin, a blocker of the synthesis of all N-linked glycoproteins (N-glycans) (Fig. 6A and Supplementary Fig. 7I). This transient IRS-2 induction is also displayed in Akita mice in vivo (Supplementary Fig. 2H). The protein level of IRS-2 was increased by GKA but not by thapsigargin alone (Fig. 6B). The expressions of ATF3 and ATF4 were not affected by GKA (Supplementary Fig. 7A). GKA induced a similar outcome in WT islets under both palmitate-induced ER stress (Supplementary Fig. 7B) and tunicamycin-induced ER stress (data not shown). Two other classes of GKAs, Ro-28-1675 and Cpd-B, also produced parallel changes in gene expression in the islets (Supplementary Fig. 7C). In islets under ER stress, GKA significantly increased the phosphorylation level of ERK and decreased the protein levels of CHOP and Bax (Fig. 6C). But GKA did not influence the protein levels of XBP1, ATF6α, PERK, eIF2α, and IRE1α and those phosphorylation levels (Fig. 6C and Supplementary Fig. 7D). In the presence of the MEK inhibitor U0126 or selective α2-adrenergic agonist UK14304, the GKA-induced suppression of CHOP and Bax under ER stress was inhibited (Fig. 6D and Supplementary Fig. 7E and F), but OSI906 had no effect on them (Supplementary Fig. 7G). A high glucose level also increased IRS-2 and decreased CHOP expression but did not affect Bax levels under ER stress (Supplementary Fig. 7H). GKA reduced the expression of cleaved caspase-3 in β-cells (Supplementary Fig. 7J) and TUNEL-positive β-cells (Fig. 6F) under ER stress. Thus, GKA directly protected ER stress–induced apoptosis in islets. In accordance with the IRS-2–independent regulation of ER stress–related genes by GKA, GKA suppressed the expressions of CHOP and Bax even in IRS-2$^{-/-}$ islets under ER stress (Fig. 6E). Furthermore, GKA increased the phosphorylation level of GSK-3β, decreased the CHOP protein level, and protected against β-cell apoptosis in IRS-2$^{-/-}$ islets under ER stress (Fig. 6E and F and Supplementary Fig. 7K). To assess this IRS-2–independent potency of GKA in vivo, we fed IRS-2$^{+/-}$;Akita and IRS-2$^{-/-}$;Akita mice diets containing GKA for 14 days and evaluated the levels of β-cell apoptosis. GKA partially reversed the increase in β-cell apoptosis in IRS-2$^{+/-}$;Akita and IRS-2$^{-/-}$;Akita mice (Fig. 6G and Supplementary Fig. 7L).

DISCUSSION

The present report describes a previously unidentified function of the activation of glucokinase in governing ER stress–induced β-cell apoptosis (Fig. 7). Consistent with the established antiapoptotic effects of IRS-2–mediated signaling in β-cells (13), genetic modification of this signaling pathway altered the levels of β-cell apoptosis induced by ER stress in Akita mice. Notably, GKA reduced the expression of CHOP and Bax and directly ameliorated ER stress–induced apoptosis in β-cells through an ERK-dependent, IRS-2–independent pathway.

In Akita mice, GKA improved β-cell apoptosis in a glycemic control–independent manner, since the improvement of hyperglycemia by PHZ did not affect β-cell apoptosis. The antihyperglycemic action of PHZ was thought to be caused by the inhibition of intestinal glucose uptake and renal glucose reabsorption, but these mechanisms might not be sufficient for the preservation of β-cell mass in Akita mice. This concept was also supported by the results that the increase in β-cell apoptosis in βGck$^{+/-}$;Akita mice was not reversed by glycemic control with PHZ. GKA retained the normoglycemia in Akita mice, possibly by safeguarding the β-cell mass.

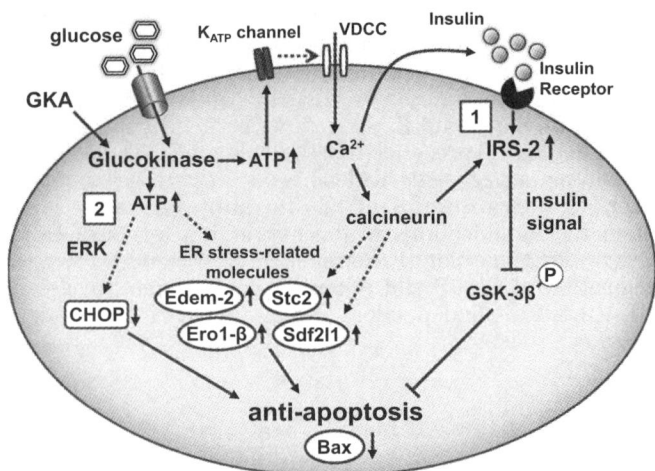

FIG. 7. An illustrative model of amelioration of ER stress–induced β-cell apoptosis by GKA. Activation of glucokinase in β-cells induces insulin secretion and the upregulation of IRS-2, which results in the activation of insulin signaling and β-cell proliferation. Under ER stress, GKA correspondingly increases IRS-2 and inactivates GSK-3β by its phosphorylation (1). GKA also decreases CHOP expression via ERK-dependent pathway and increases the expression of ER stress–related molecules, such as Stc2, Ero-1, Sdf2l1, and Edem-2 (2). These multiple pathways in β-cells coordinately suppress the proapoptotic gene *Bax*, allowing adaptation and survival against ER stress. VDCC, voltage-dependent Ca^{2+} channel; K$_{ATP}$ channel, ATP-sensitive potassium channel.

Since ER stress led to the reactive induction of IRS-2 expression in β-cells, we hypothesized that a reduction in IRS-2 expression would lead to an increase in β-cell apoptosis in βGck$^{+/-}$;Akita mice. Predictably, the loss of IRS-2 aggravated glycemic control and β-cell apoptosis in Akita mice. IRS-2 deficiency in islets also caused a reduction in the inhibition of GSK-3β by its phosphorylation under ER stress, and an inhibitor of GSK-3 restored ER stress–induced apoptosis in IRS-2$^{-/-}$ islets. Thus, the glucokinase/IRS-2/Akt/GSK-3β signaling pathway is thought to be involved in the antiapoptotic effect of GKA against ER stress. Our results are consistent with previous observations that GSK-3β haploinsufficiency corrected β-cell apoptosis in IRS-2$^{-/-}$ mice (30), and the attenuation of the regulation of GSK-3β by insulin signaling partly caused ER stress–induced apoptosis (31). Considering the report that PDX1 deficiency induced β-cell susceptibility to ER stress (32), the GKA-induced upregulation of PDX1 expression might be somewhat associated with the regulation of apoptosis.

A major question to be addressed in future studies is the pathophysiological significance of the modulation of ER stress–related genes, such as the downregulation of CHOP and the upregulation of Stc2, Ero-1β, Sdf2l1, or Edem-2 that are triggered by GKA. The suppression of CHOP evidently averts apoptosis induced by ER stress (27,29,33). The overexpression of Stc2 also reduces pancreatic tissue apoptosis in cerulein-induced pancreatitis model mice through the alteration of PERK signaling (34). Ero-1β, an oxidoreductase, plays a role in the efficient oxidative maturation of proinsulin and glycemic control in mice (35). Edem-2 assists folding-incompetent glycoprotein degradation from the ER via ER-associated degradation (36). Thus, increases in the expressions of Stc2, Ero-1β, and Edem-2 in response to GKA make physiological sense with respect to the prevention of ER stress–induced apoptosis. *Sdf2l1* is also known to be an ER stress–inducible gene (37), but its function in ER stress remains obscure.

Some studies have shown that CREB or the Ca^{2+}/calcineurin signal mediates the glucose signal–induced augmentation of IRS-2 expression in β-cells (9,12,38), and ATF3 evokes the repression of IRS-2 expression, resulting in β-cell apoptosis (39). We demonstrated that GKA upregulated IRS-2 via Ca^{2+}-calcineurin but did not affect ATF3 levels in β-cells. The insulin receptor plays a crucial role in β-cell proliferation in response to insulin resistance (40). However, we noted that even if signals from insulin and IGF-1 receptors were canceled by OSI-906, GKA satisfactorily increased IRS-2 and regulated ER stress–related genes. Meanwhile, ERK1/2 mediated the modification of ER stress–related gene expressions by GKA. As the suppression of CHOP by glucose signals has been implicated in ERK1/2 and MafA (41), MafA might influence other GKA-induced ER stress regulators. The cooperative nature of insulin signaling and ERK for cell survival against ER stress has been previously reported (42). We advocate this concept as being a valid model for β-cells.

Numerous studies have shown that chronic exposure to high glucose induces β-cell ER stress and reactive oxygen species production, resulting in cell death (43,44). Does this mean that the hyperactivation of glucokinase in response to GKA is toxic to β-cells? Some reports had suggested that β-cell apoptosis induced by exposure to chronic high glucose levels arises from a reduction in glucokinase expression and a reduction in the interactions between glucokinase and mitochondria (45–47). Furthermore, the glucokinase-binding domain of BAD controls insulin secretion and β-cell apoptosis at the mitochondria (48). Glucose signaling may have two-sided effects, providing crucial tasks for β-cell adaptation or apoptosis depending on the unique metabolic niche. Therefore, a balance between β-cell adaptation and β-cell apoptosis is presumably scheduled by the combination of diversity, magnitude, and timing of glucose signaling. Based on our results, glucokinase activation could provide plural points for the regulation of ER stress–induced apoptosis in β-cells (Fig. 7). These multiple pathways in β-cells may allow a timely adaptation and survival against ER stress. In this study, successful treatment was portrayed by early intervention with GKA. One proposal is that glucokinase activation should be promoted during the early stage of diabetes or prediabetes, but not in overt diabetes, since we and others have previously reported that GKA failed to restore serious β-cell damage under oxidative stress (11,49).

In this study, ER stresses were assessed in insulin gene–mutated Akita mice and were induced by chemicals such as thapsigargin. Under conditions related to obesity and type 2 diabetes, ER stress is activated in various tissues such as hypothalamus, liver, muscle, adipose tissue, and β-cells in both human and mouse (50,51). In the context of insulin resistance, ER stress in liver serves as a key homeostatic regulator of protein, lipid, and glucose metabolism (52,53). Therefore, more physiological or pathophysiological models ought to be examined for possible effects of GKA on ER stress. Lastly, but perhaps most importantly, further analyses of the efficacy and feasibility of glucokinase activation in the clinical management of diabetes are needed to open new avenues for β-cell–protective interventions.

ACKNOWLEDGMENTS

This work was supported in part by Grants-in-Aid for Scientific Research (B) 21390282 and (B) 24390235 from the Ministry of Education, Culture, Sports, Science and Technology of Japan, a Medical Award from the Japan Medical Association, a Grant-in-Aid from the Japan Diabetes Foundation, a Grant-in-Aid from the Uehara Memorial Foundation, a Grant-in-Aid from the Naito Foundation, a Grant-in-Aid from the Takeda Life Foundation (to Y.Te.), a Grant-in-Aid for JSPS fellows, a Grant-in-Aid from Yokohama General Promotion Foundation, a Grant-in-Aid from the Novo Nordisk Insulin Research Foundation, a Grant-in-Aid from Japan Foundation for Applied Enzymology, a Grant-in-Aid from Kanae Memorial Foundation, and a Grant-in-Aid from Banyu Life Science Foundation International (to J.S.). No other potential conflicts of interest relevant to this article were reported.

J.S. designed and performed experiments, analyzed the data, and wrote the manuscript. Y.To., K.T., K.O., and H.I. contributed to discussions. E.S. and M.K. performed experiments. N.K. and T.K. provided mice for this study, contributed to discussions, and reviewed the manuscript. Y.Te. wrote the manuscript, reviewed and edited the manuscript, and contributed to discussions. Y.Te. is the guarantor of this work and, as such, had full access to all the data in the study and takes responsibility for the integrity of the data and the accuracy of the data analysis.

Parts of this study were presented in abstract form at the 71st Scientific Sessions of the American Diabetes Association, San Diego, California, 24–28 June 2011, and the 72nd Scientific Sessions of the American Diabetes Association, Philadelphia, Pennsylvania, 8–12 June 2012.

The authors thank Misa Katayama (Yokohama City University) for secretarial assistance.

REFERENCES

1. Donath MY, Halban PA. Decreased beta-cell mass in diabetes: significance, mechanisms and therapeutic implications. Diabetologia 2004;47:581–589
2. Butler AE, Janson J, Bonner-Weir S, Ritzel R, Rizza RA, Butler PC. Beta-cell deficit and increased beta-cell apoptosis in humans with type 2 diabetes. Diabetes 2003;52:102–110
3. Eizirik DL, Cardozo AK, Cnop M. The role for endoplasmic reticulum stress in diabetes mellitus. Endocr Rev 2008;29:42–61
4. Laybutt DR, Preston AM, Akerfeldt MC, et al. Endoplasmic reticulum stress contributes to beta cell apoptosis in type 2 diabetes. Diabetologia 2007;50:752–763
5. Matschinsky F, Liang Y, Kesavan P, et al. Glucokinase as pancreatic beta cell glucose sensor and diabetes gene. J Clin Invest 1993;92:2092–2098
6. Grupe A, Hultgren B, Ryan A, Ma YH, Bauer M, Stewart TA. Transgenic knockouts reveal a critical requirement for pancreatic beta cell glucokinase in maintaining glucose homeostasis. Cell 1995;83:69–78
7. Terauchi Y, Sakura H, Yasuda K, et al. Pancreatic beta-cell-specific targeted disruption of glucokinase gene. Diabetes mellitus due to defective insulin secretion to glucose. J Biol Chem 1995;270:30253–30256
8. Shirakawa J, Tanami R, Togashi Y, et al. Effects of liraglutide on β-cell-specific glucokinase-deficient neonatal mice. Endocrinology 2012;153:3066–3075
9. Terauchi Y, Takamoto I, Kubota N, et al. Glucokinase and IRS-2 are required for compensatory beta cell hyperplasia in response to high-fat diet-induced insulin resistance. J Clin Invest 2007;117:246–257
10. Nakamura A, Terauchi Y, Ohyama S, et al. Impact of small-molecule glucokinase activator on glucose metabolism and beta-cell mass. Endocrinology 2009;150:1147–1154
11. Nakamura A, Togashi Y, Orime K, et al. Control of beta cell function and proliferation in mice stimulated by small-molecule glucokinase activator under various conditions. Diabetologia 2012;55:1745–1754
12. Demozay D, Tsunekawa S, Briaud I, Shah R, Rhodes CJ. Specific glucose-induced control of insulin receptor substrate-2 expression is mediated via $Ca2+$-dependent calcineurin/NFAT signaling in primary pancreatic islet β-cells. Diabetes 2011;60:2892–2902
13. Hennige AM, Burks DJ, Ozcan U, et al. Upregulation of insulin receptor substrate-2 in pancreatic beta cells prevents diabetes. J Clin Invest 2003;112:1521–1532

14. Withers DJ, Burks DJ, Towery HH, Altamuro SL, Flint CL, White MF. Irs-2 coordinates Igf-1 receptor-mediated beta-cell development and peripheral insulin signalling. Nat Genet 1999;23:32–40

15. Kubota N, Tobe K, Terauchi Y, et al. Disruption of insulin receptor substrate 2 causes type 2 diabetes because of liver insulin resistance and lack of compensatory beta-cell hyperplasia. Diabetes 2000;49:1880–1889

16. Shirakawa J, Amo K, Ohminami H, et al. Protective effects of dipeptidyl peptidase-4 (DPP-4) inhibitor against increased β cell apoptosis induced by dietary sucrose and linoleic acid in mice with diabetes. J Biol Chem 2011;286:25467–25476

17. Grimsby J, Sarabu R, Corbett WL, et al. Allosteric activators of glucokinase: potential role in diabetes therapy. Science 2003;301:370–373

18. Efanov AM, Barrett DG, Brenner MB, et al. A novel glucokinase activator modulates pancreatic islet and hepatocyte function. Endocrinology 2005;146:3696–3701

19. Matschinsky FM. Assessing the potential of glucokinase activators in diabetes therapy. Nat Rev Drug Discov 2009;8:399–416

20. Salpeter SJ, Klein AM, Huangfu D, Grimsby J, Dor Y. Glucose and aging control the quiescence period that follows pancreatic beta cell replication. Development 2010;137:3205–3213

21. Porat S, Weinberg-Corem N, Tornovsky-Babaey S, et al. Control of pancreatic β cell regeneration by glucose metabolism. Cell Metab 2011;13:440–449

22. Futamura M, Yao J, Li X, et al. Chronic treatment with a glucokinase activator delays the onset of hyperglycaemia and preserves beta cell mass in the Zucker diabetic fatty rat. Diabetologia 2012;55:1071–1080

23. Wei P, Shi M, Barnum S, Cho H, Carlson T, Fraser JD. Effects of glucokinase activators GKA50 and LY2121260 on proliferation and apoptosis in pancreatic INS-1 beta cells. Diabetologia 2009;52:2142–2150

24. Futamura M, Hosaka H, Kadotani A, et al. An allosteric activator of glucokinase impairs the interaction of glucokinase and glucokinase regulatory protein and regulates glucose metabolism. J Biol Chem 2006;281:37668–37674

25. Iino T, Hashimoto N, Sasaki K, et al. Structure-activity relationships of 3,5-disubstituted benzamides as glucokinase activators with potent in vivo efficacy. Bioorg Med Chem 2009;17:3800–3809

26. Wang J, Takeuchi T, Tanaka S, et al. A mutation in the insulin 2 gene induces diabetes with severe pancreatic beta-cell dysfunction in the Mody mouse. J Clin Invest 1999;103:27–37

27. Oyadomari S, Koizumi A, Takeda K, et al. Targeted disruption of the Chop gene delays endoplasmic reticulum stress-mediated diabetes. J Clin Invest 2002;109:525–532

28. Gibson TB, Lawrence MC, Gibson CJ, et al. Inhibition of glucose-stimulated activation of extracellular signal-regulated protein kinases 1 and 2 by epinephrine in pancreatic beta-cells. Diabetes 2006;55:1066–1073

29. Song B, Scheuner D, Ron D, Pennathur S, Kaufman RJ. Chop deletion reduces oxidative stress, improves beta cell function, and promotes cell survival in multiple mouse models of diabetes. J Clin Invest 2008;118:3378–3389

30. Tanabe K, Liu Z, Patel S, et al. Genetic deficiency of glycogen synthase kinase-3beta corrects diabetes in mouse models of insulin resistance. PLoS Biol 2008;6:e37

31. Srinivasan S, Ohsugi M, Liu Z, Fatrai S, Bernal-Mizrachi E, Permutt MA. Endoplasmic reticulum stress-induced apoptosis is partly mediated by reduced insulin signaling through phosphatidylinositol 3-kinase/Akt and increased glycogen synthase kinase-3beta in mouse insulinoma cells. Diabetes 2005;54:968–975

32. Sachdeva MM, Claiborn KC, Khoo C, et al. Pdx1 (MODY4) regulates pancreatic beta cell susceptibility to ER stress. Proc Natl Acad Sci USA 2009;106:19090–19095

33. Marciniak SJ, Yun CY, Oyadomari S, et al. CHOP induces death by promoting protein synthesis and oxidation in the stressed endoplasmic reticulum. Genes Dev 2004;18:3066–3077

34. Fazio EN, Dimattia GE, Chadi SA, Kernohan KD, Pin CL. Stanniocalcin 2 alters PERK signalling and reduces cellular injury during cerulein induced pancreatitis in mice. BMC Cell Biol 2011;12:17

35. Zito E, Chin KT, Blais J, Harding HP, Ron D. ERO1-beta, a pancreas-specific disulfide oxidase, promotes insulin biogenesis and glucose homeostasis. J Cell Biol 2010;188:821–832

36. Olivari S, Molinari M. Glycoprotein folding and the role of EDEM1, EDEM2 and EDEM3 in degradation of folding-defective glycoproteins. FEBS Lett 2007;581:3658–3664

37. Fukuda S, Sumii M, Masuda Y, et al. Murine and human SDF2L1 is an endoplasmic reticulum stress-inducible gene and encodes a new member of the Pmt/rt protein family. Biochem Biophys Res Commun 2001;280:407–414

38. Jhala US, Canettieri G, Screaton RA, et al. cAMP promotes pancreatic beta-cell survival via CREB-mediated induction of IRS2. Genes Dev 2003;17:1575–1580

39. Li D, Yin X, Zmuda EJ, et al. The repression of IRS2 gene by ATF3, a stress-inducible gene, contributes to pancreatic beta-cell apoptosis. Diabetes 2008;57:635–644

40. Okada T, Liew CW, Hu J, et al. Insulin receptors in beta-cells are critical for islet compensatory growth response to insulin resistance. Proc Natl Acad Sci USA 2007;104:8977–8982

41. Lawrence MC, McGlynn K, Naziruddin B, Levy MF, Cobb MH. Differential regulation of CHOP-10/GADD153 gene expression by MAPK signaling in pancreatic beta-cells. Proc Natl Acad Sci USA 2007;104:11518–11525

42. Hu P, Han Z, Couvillon AD, Exton JH. Critical role of endogenous Akt/IAPs and MEK1/ERK pathways in counteracting endoplasmic reticulum stress-induced cell death. J Biol Chem 2004;279:49420–49429

43. Back SH, Kaufman RJ. Endoplasmic reticulum stress and type 2 diabetes. Annu Rev Biochem 2012;81:767–793

44. Tang C, Han P, Oprescu AI, et al. Evidence for a role of superoxide generation in glucose-induced beta-cell dysfunction in vivo. Diabetes 2007;56:2722–2731

45. Kooptiwut S, Kebede M, Zraika S, et al. High glucose-induced impairment in insulin secretion is associated with reduction in islet glucokinase in a mouse model of susceptibility to islet dysfunction. J Mol Endocrinol 2005;35:39–48

46. Kim WH, Lee JW, Suh YH, et al. Exposure to chronic high glucose induces beta-cell apoptosis through decreased interaction of glucokinase with mitochondria: downregulation of glucokinase in pancreatic beta-cells. Diabetes 2005;54:2602–2611

47. Joe MK, Lee HJ, Suh YH, et al. Crucial roles of neuronatin in insulin secretion and high glucose-induced apoptosis in pancreatic beta-cells. Cell Signal 2008;20:907–915

48. Danial NN, Walensky LD, Zhang CY, et al. Dual role of proapoptotic BAD in insulin secretion and beta cell survival. Nat Med 2008;14:144–153

49. Meininger GE, Scott R, Alba M, et al. Effects of MK-0941, a novel glucokinase activator, on glycemic control in insulin-treated patients with type 2 diabetes. Diabetes Care 2011;34:2560–2566

50. Flamment M, Hajduch E, Ferré P, Foufelle F. New insights into ER stress-induced insulin resistance. Trends Endocrinol Metab 2012;23:381–390

51. Cnop M, Foufelle F, Velloso LA. Endoplasmic reticulum stress, obesity and diabetes. Trends Mol Med 2012;18:59–68

52. Fu S, Watkins SM, Hotamisligil GS. The role of endoplasmic reticulum in hepatic lipid homeostasis and stress signaling. Cell Metab 2012;15:623–634

53. Bechmann LP, Hannivoort RA, Gerken G, Hotamisligil GS, Trauner M, Canbay A. The interaction of hepatic lipid and glucose metabolism in liver diseases. J Hepatol 2012;56:952–964

Blunted Refeeding Response and Increased Locomotor Activity in Mice Lacking FoxO1 in Synapsin-Cre-Expressing Neurons

Hongxia Ren,[1,2] Leona Plum-Morschel,[1,2] Roger Gutierrez-Juarez,[3] Taylor Y. Lu,[1,2] Ja Young Kim-Muller,[1,2] Garrett Heinrich,[1,2] Sharon L. Wardlaw,[1,2] Rae Silver,[4] and Domenico Accili[1,2]

Successful development of antiobesity agents requires detailed knowledge of neural pathways controlling body weight, eating behavior, and peripheral metabolism. Genetic ablation of FoxO1 in selected hypothalamic neurons decreases food intake, increases energy expenditure, and improves glucose homeostasis, highlighting the role of this gene in insulin and leptin signaling. However, little is known about potential effects of FoxO1 in other neurons. To address this question, we executed a broad-based neuronal ablation of FoxO1 using *Synapsin* promoter–driven Cre to delete floxed *Foxo1* alleles. Lineage-tracing experiments showed that NPY/AgRP and POMC neurons were minimally affected by the knockout. Nonetheless, *Syn-Cre-Foxo1* knockouts demonstrated a catabolic energy homeostatic phenotype with a blunted refeeding response, increased sensitivity to leptin and amino acid signaling, and increased locomotor activity, likely attributable to increased melanocortinergic tone. We confirmed these data in mice lacking the three *Foxo* genes. The effects on locomotor activity could be reversed by direct delivery of constitutively active FoxO1 to the mediobasal hypothalamus, but not to the suprachiasmatic nucleus. The data reveal that the integrative function of FoxO1 extends beyond the arcuate nucleus, suggesting that central nervous system inhibition of FoxO1 function can be leveraged to promote hormone sensitivity and prevent a positive energy balance. *Diabetes* 62:3373–3383, 2013

The alarming increase in the prevalence of obesity and the advances in the ability to genetically map and modify biochemical pathways of hormone action and nutrient sensing have rekindled interest in understanding how the central nervous system (CNS) regulates energy homeostasis and metabolism (1). CNS integration of feeding behavior and nutrient turnover reveals a complex anatomic and functional architecture, with redundant control mechanisms and shared functions that have thus far thwarted attempts at identifying specific networks that can be pharmacologically engaged to control body weight.

Key to solving the stalemate is refinement of our knowledge of the integrated circuitry of CNS metabolic functions. For example, leptin—the main appetite-suppressing hormone—acts at multiple CNS sites in qualitatively different fashions, affecting not only neurohormonal aspects but also reward aspects of feeding (2). Likewise, characterization of specific neuronal populations in areas traditionally linked to food intake, such as the mediobasal hypothalamus (MBH), has revealed a complex pattern of neuronal populations regulating this process as well as interdependent signaling pathways that regulate the activity of these neurons (3,4).

FoxO1 has emerged during the past decade as a critical node in relaying the hormonal status and nutritional status of the organism, allowing target cells to implement transcriptional programs that reflect energy conservation or dispersal. Among its protean functions are the regulation of hepatic glucose production (5,6) and bile acid synthesis (7), the integration of different aspects of pancreatic endocrine function (8), and developmental functions in the differentiation of adipose, muscle, and enteroendocrine progenitor cells (9–11). In the CNS, we and others (12–16) previously have shown that FoxO1 lies astride of insulin and leptin signaling in neuropeptide-producing cells of the arcuate nucleus, orchestrating a complex transcriptional program that includes melanocortin signaling (17) and orphan G-protein-coupled receptors, and whose ultimate outcome is to promote food intake and reduce energy expenditure (18).

The purpose of the current study was to extend our knowledge of the actions of neural FoxO1 beyond the narrow confines of the arcuate nucleus. Impetus for these experiments was provided by the realization that therapeutic modalities based on FoxO1 loss-of-function may be desirable for weight-control purposes. However, to implement such approaches, one needs to map the gamut of pathophysiologic FoxO1 actions in the CNS as a way to ascertain potential liabilities. The studies described in this article were designed to fill this gap.

RESEARCH DESIGN AND METHODS

Experimental animals. The Columbia University Animal Care and Utilization Committee approved all procedures. Normal chow diet included 62.1% of calories from carbohydrates, 24.6% of calories from protein, and 13.2% of calories from fat (PicoLab rodent diet 20, 5053; Purina Mills); high-fat diet (HFD) included 20% of calories from carbohydrates, 20% of calories from protein, and 60% of calories from fat (D12492; Research Diets). We measured weight and length to calculate BMI, and we estimated body composition by nuclear magnetic resonance (Bruker Optics). We generated *Syn*-specific *FoxO* single or triple knockouts by mating *Syn-Cre* transgenic mice with *Foxo1*$^{flox/flox}$ mice or *Foxo1*$^{flox/flox}$*3a*$^{flox/flox}$*4*$^{flox/flox}$ mice (19) and genotyped them as previously described (18). We excluded from analyses knockout mice that showed widespread recombination because of stochastic embryonic expression of *Syn-Cre*. We used cohorts of adult male mice, with 6–8 mice per genotype in most experiments (unless otherwise noted). We used the Rosa-Gfp reporter mice (B6;129-Gt(ROSA)26Sor^{tm2sho}/J; JAX Stock Number 004077) for lineage-tracing experiments.

From the [1]Berrie Diabetes Center, New York, New York; the [2]Department of Medicine, Columbia University, New York, New York; the [3]Diabetes Research and Training Center, Albert Einstein College of Medicine, Bronx, New York; and the [4]Department of Psychology, Columbia University, New York, New York.

Corresponding author: Domenico Accili, da230@columbia.edu.

Received 15 April 2013 and accepted 20 June 2013.

DOI: 10.2337/db13-0597

H.R. and L.P.-M. contributed equally to this work.

Metabolic analyses. We measured food intake with feeding racks (Firma Wenzel). For refeeding experiments, we habituated mice to feeding racks for 3 days, fasted them for 18 h, placed feeding racks 2 h after the start of the light phase, and measured food intake thereafter. We used a TSE Labmaster Platform (TSE Systems) for indirect calorimetry and activity measurements (17). For mice receiving adenovirus injection, we measured the wheel-running activity after the established protocol (20). Briefly, wheel-running activity was monitored remotely by Vitalview (Minimitter, Bend, OR), with counts collected in 10-min bins, and visualized using double-plotted actograms. We measured blood glucose by the One-Touch Ultra meter (LifeScan, Milpitas, CA), insulin and leptin were measured by ELISA, glucagon was measured by radioimmunoassay (Linco Research, St. Charles, MO), plasma free fatty acids and cholesterol were measured by nonesterified fatty acid hazard ratio and cholesterol-E test reagents, respectively (Wako Chemicals, Richmond, VA), and triglycerides were measured by serum triglyceride determination kit (Sigma-Aldrich, St. Louis, MO). Body composition was determined using Bruker Minispec nuclear magnetic resonance (Bruker Optics, Billerica, MA). We performed euglycemic-hyperinsulinemic clamps as previously described (21).

Immunostaining. We perfused mice with saline and then with 4% paraformaldehyde. We froze brains in Tissue-Tek O.C.T. Compound (Sakura) and cut 30-μm–thick coronal sections for green fluorescent protein (GFP)-specific immunohistochemistry (Molecular Probes/Invitrogen). We acquired images with a Nikon eclipse microscope.

RNA procedures. We extracted RNA with Trizol (Invitrogen) and performed quantitative PCR using SYBR Green I (Roche). Primer sequences are available on request. We used equal amounts of total RNA for reverse transcription and measured threshold cycle for each gene. β-Actin was used as an internal control. Data were quantified by standard delta ratio threshold cycle method.

Hypothalamic neuropeptide assays. We extracted MBH in 0.1 N HCl. We measured β-endorphin and α-melanocyte–stimulating hormone (MSH) by radioimmunoassay (17).

Statistical analyses. We analyzed data with Student t test, one-way ANOVA, or two-way ANOVA. $P < 0.05$ was considered statistically significant (*$P < 0.05$; **$P < 0.01$; ***$P < 0.001$).

RESULTS

Generation and analysis of neuronal FoxO1 knockout mice.

To generate neuron-specific FoxO1 knockout mice, we crossed *Foxo1^{lox/lox}* and *Syn-Cre* mice. Cre-mediated deletion of the loxP-flanked *Foxo1* exon 2 resulted in null

Foxo1 alleles in Synapsin-expressing neurons (hereafter called *Syn-Foxo1*). To assess the distribution of *Foxo1* ablation in the CNS, we introduced a reporter allele that encodes GFP as a marker of Cre-mediated recombination. GFP immunohistochemistry revealed Cre-mediated recombination across the brain, including cortex, hippocampus, and multiple hypothalamic nuclei. The frequency of *Syn-Cre*–mediated recombination varied in different brain regions. Hippocampus and dorsal medial nucleus showed the highest fractions of recombined cells, whereas cortex, ventral medial nucleus, and paraventricular hypothalamic nucleus had fewer GFP⁺ cells. The arcuate nucleus showed limited recombination, and the suprachiasmatic nucleus (SCN) showed little if any recombination (Fig. 1A). To provide a quantitative assessment of *Foxo1* deletion, we assayed recombination using genomic DNA extracted from various brain regions. These data are consistent with the immunohistochemistry and also show extensive recombination in the brain stem, but not in peripheral tissues (Fig. 1B).

Limited *Syn-Cre*–mediated recombination in NPY/AgRP and POMC neurons.

FoxO1 ablation in MBH AgRP/NPY and POMC neurons has striking effects on energy homeostasis and peripheral metabolism (17,18). To assess potential contributions of FoxO1 ablation in these neurons to the overall phenotype of *Syn-Foxo1* mice, we determined the extent of *Syn-Cre*–mediated recombination in these two neuronal populations. To this end, we generated double-transgenic mice in which neurons undergoing *Syn-Cre*–mediated recombination was labeled red by a *Rosa-Tomato* allele (*Syn-Tom*) (22), whereas NPY/AgRP or POMC neurons were labeled green by *Npy-Gfp* or *Pomc-Gfp* transgenes, i.e., *Syn-Tom;Npy-Gfp* (Fig. 2A–E) and *Syn-Tom;Pomc-Gfp* (Fig. 2F–J), respectively. Double fluorescence demonstrated that *Npy*-labeled or *Pomc-Gpf*–labeled neurons had minimal overlap with *Syn-Tom* neurons (Fig. 2A, B, F, and G). We quantified the

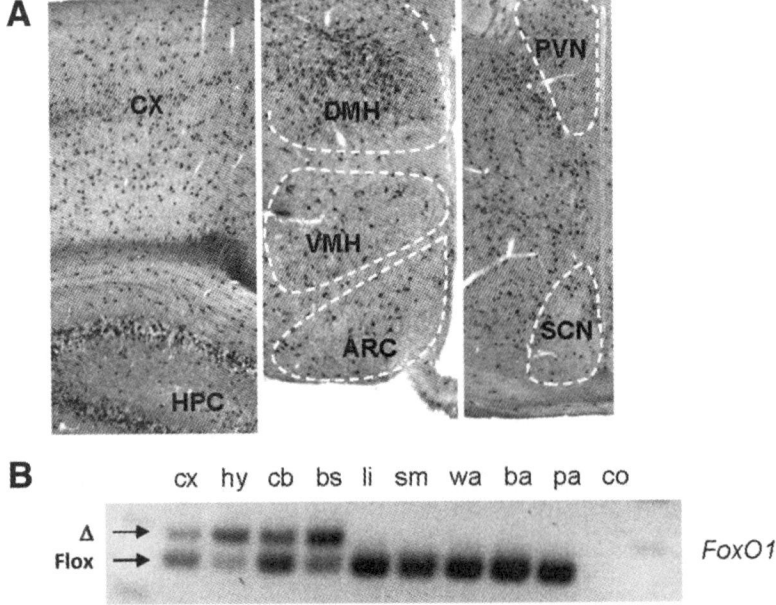

FIG. 1. Generation of *Syn-Foxo1*⁻/⁻ mice. *A*: GFP immunohistochemistry in the hypothalamus of *Syn-Gfp* mice as a reporter of Cre-mediated recombination (black) in cortex (CX), hippocampus (HPC), and various hypothalamic nuclei (dorsal medial nucleus [DMH], ventral medial nucleus [VMH], arcuate nucleus [ARC], paraventricular hypothalamic nucleus [PVN], and SCN). *B*: Detection of recombined *Foxo1* allele in brain, including cortex (cx), hypothalamus (hy), cerebellum (cb), and brain stem (bs), but not in other tissues, including liver (li), skeletal muscle (sm), white adipose tissue (wa), brown adipose tissue (ba), and pancreas (pa), or in wild-type control (co).

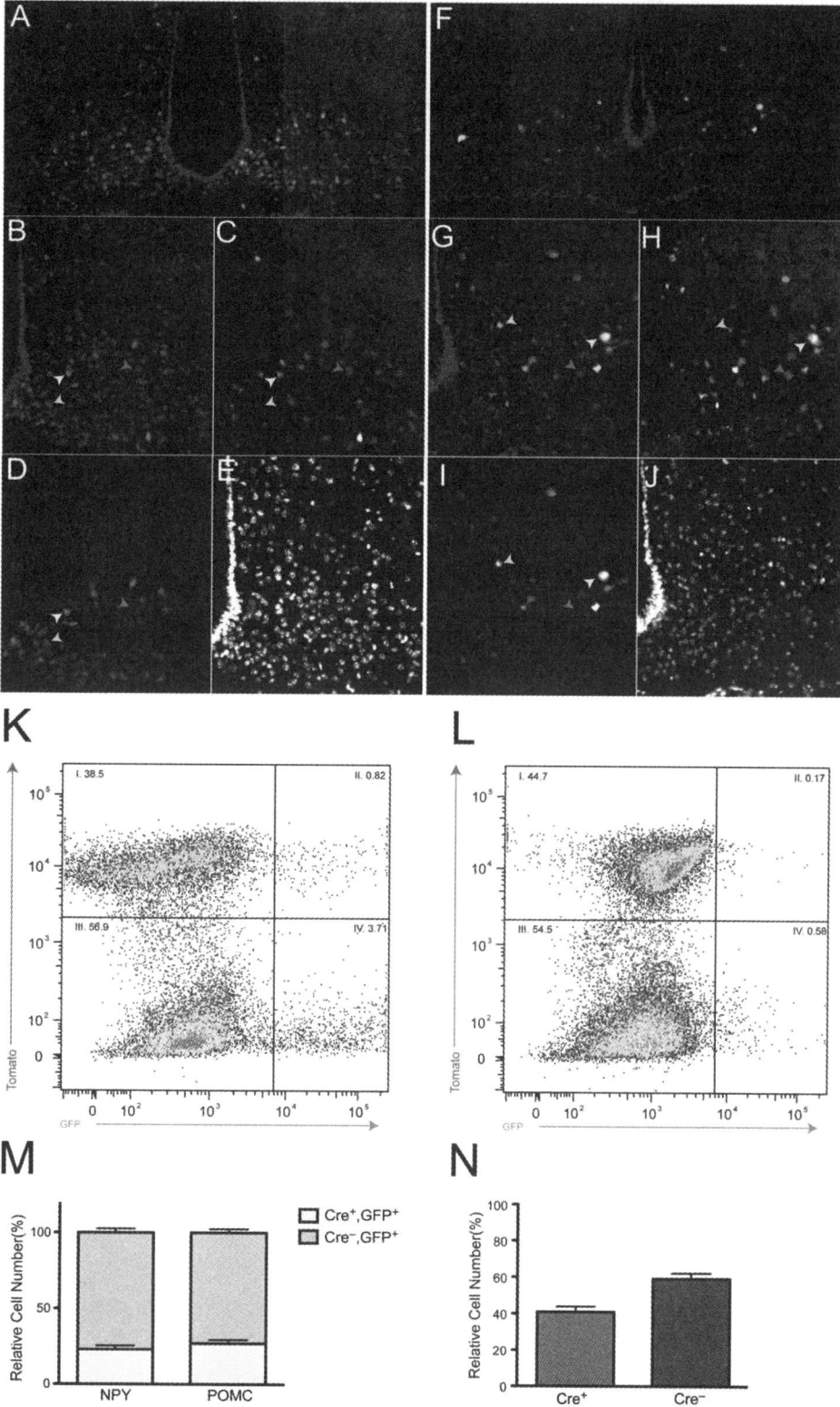

FIG. 2. Limited *Syn-Cre*–mediated recombination in NPY-AgRP and POMC neurons. *A–J*: Fluorescence microscopy of arcuate nucleus from *Syn-Cre;Rosa-Tomato* mice carrying *Npy-Gfp* (*A–E*) or *Pomc-Gfp* (*F–J*) transgene. Neurons exhibiting *Syn-Cre*–mediated recombination are labeled red and those expressing *Npy-Gfp* (*A*) or *Pomc-Gfp* (*F*) are green. Double-positive neurons are yellow. Magnified merged views (*B*, *G*) showing limited overlapping and individual channels for *Tomato* (*C*, *H*), *Npy-Gfp* (*D*), *Pomc-Gfp* (*I*), and DAPI (*E*, *J*). *K* and *L*: Representative fluorescence-activated cell sorting analysis of dissociated hypothalamic neurons of *Syn-Cre;Rosa-Tomato;Npy-Gfp* mice (*B*) and *Syn-Cre;Rosa-Tomato;Pomc-Gfp* mice (*C*). The percentage of each quadrant over the total sorted cells is listed. *M*: Quantification of the percentage of NPY or POMC neurons with active *Syn-Cre* by fluorescence-activated cell sorting analysis (*n* = 3). *N*: Quantification of the percentage of *Syn-Cre*–recombined neurons in the hypothalamus by fluorescence-activated cell sorting analysis (*n* = 6).

findings using fluorescence-activated cell sorting in which double-labeled neurons were distinct from single-labeled neurons (Fig. 2K and L, *upper* and *lower right quadrants*, respectively). *Syn-Tom* neurons accounted for ~20% of NPY neurons, ~20% of POMC neurons (Fig. 2M), and ~40% of hypothalamic neurons (Fig. 2N). We estimated that NPY and POMC neurons combined constitute <5% of total sorted MBH neurons. Thus, we conclude that *Syn-Cre* primarily targets neurons other than NPY and POMC in the hypothalamus.

Increased central hormonal and nutrient sensitivity in *Syn-Foxo1* mice. We evaluated *Syn-Foxo1* mice by measuring plasma metabolites and energy expenditure with different diets. In chow-fed animals, we did not detect differences in body weight and composition, or in plasma triglycerides (Table 1). Measurements of respiratory exchanges failed to reveal alterations of V_{O_2} and V_{CO_2}, indicating that basal energy homeostasis was unaltered (data not shown).

However, when we measured the response to fasting and refeeding, we found that *Syn-Foxo1* mice fed significantly less after an overnight fast (Fig. 3A). Specifically, during the 6-h refeeding, wild-type and knockout mice consumed 0.3831 and 0.2921 kcal/g body weight (calories normalized by body weight), respectively. To explain this observation, we measured hormonal sensitivity. Serum leptin levels were significantly decreased in fasted and ad libitum–fed *Syn-Foxo1* mice (Fig. 3B). We examined leptin signaling by immunohistochemistry with antiphospho-Stat3 (pStat3) antibody in refed mice. The number of cells displaying pStat3 immunoreactivity and the intensity of the signal increased nearly two-fold in *Syn-Foxo1* mice (Fig. 3C). Next, we examined whether the increase in leptin signaling was cell-autonomous. To this end, we generated *Syn-Foxo1* mice bearing a *Rosa-Tom* allele and measured pStat3 immunoreactivity in response to refeeding after an overnight fast. The expectation of this experiment was that if the decreased rebound food intake was attributable to increased leptin sensitivity in FoxO1-deficient neurons, then knockout mice should show increased pStat3 signal (green fluorescence) in neurons that were marked by FoxO1 ablation (red fluorescence), giving rise to yellow fluorescence. We observed that most of the pStat3 signal colocalized with recombined neurons, indicating that FoxO1 ablation increases leptin-induced pStat3 generation in a cell-autonomous manner (Fig. 3D).

Hypothalamic amino acid signaling regulates satiety and feeding behaviors (23). We measured amino acid sensitivity by immunostaining with antibody to the mTOR substrate, phospho-ribosomal protein S6 (pS6). *Syn-Foxo1* mice had increased pS6, predominantly in dorsal medial nucleus (Fig. 3E), a site of *Syn-Cre*–dependent recombination (Fig. 1A). Using *Syn-Tom* to label recombined neurons, we sought to determine whether the increase of pS6 was caused by FoxO1 deletion in a cell-autonomous or cell-nonautonomous manner. We saw that increased pS6 staining occurred equally in FoxO1-deleted and FoxO1-intact dorsal medial nucleus neurons, indicating that the effect of FoxO1 ablation is at least partly cell-nonautonomous (Fig. 3F).

Altered insulin secretion in *Syn-Foxo1* mice. The CNS further regulates pancreatic hormone secretion, especially through the adrenosympathetic system (24). We therefore measured insulin secretion induced by the β3-adrenergic receptor agonist, CL-316243. Activating β3-adrenergic receptor quickly increases insulin secretion by pancreatic β-cells and free fatty acid release by adipocytes. After CL-316243 injection, *Syn-Foxo1* mice showed consistently lower glucose (Fig. 4A), secondary to increased insulin release (Fig. 4B). Serum free fatty acid levels were comparable with those of controls (Fig. 4C), indicating that the effect of the *Foxo1* mutation on insulin release is not secondary to increased lipolysis with β3-adrenergic receptor agonist stimulation. Next, we examined insulin secretion in static incubations of purified pancreatic islets and found small but significant increases induced by low (5 mmol/L) and high (25 mmol/L) glucose concentrations (Fig. 4D). Total insulin content and secretion in response to KCl-induced depolarization were comparable (Fig. 4D). Islet size tended to be larger in *Syn-Foxo1* animals, but not significantly larger (Fig. 4E). These data indicate that FoxO1 ablation in *Syn-Cre* neurons increased sympathoadrenal responses. Using the *Syn-Tom* reporter, we found no evidence of Cre-mediated recombination in the pancreas of *Syn-Foxo1* animals (data not shown), effectively ruling out a direct effect of FoxO1 ablation in β-cells (25). The increased insulin secretion from β-cells in response to adrenosympathetic stimuli did not alter fasted and fed glucagon levels (Fig. 4F). However, *Syn-Foxo1* mice exhibited significantly lower circulating insulin levels (Table 1), indicating increased insulin sensitivity.

TABLE 1
Metabolic measurements

		WT	*Syn-Foxo1*	P
Weight, g		28.64 ± 1.27	27.77 ± 0.77	NS
Body composition, %	Fat mass	12.9 ± 2.5	14.3 ± 1.1	NS
	Lean mass	73.2 ± 1.5	73 ± 1	NS
Glucose, mg/dL	Ad libitum	136 ± 10	124 ± 3	NS
	Fasted	66 ± 3	66 ± 4	NS
	Refed	174 ± 14	159 ± 5	NS
	Fasted (HFD)	87 ± 7	68 ± 4	<0.05
Insulin, ng/mL	Ad libitum	3.3 ± 0.4	1.8 ± 0.4	<0.03
	Fasted	0.6 ± 0.1	0.5 ± 0.1	NS
	Refed	7.7 ± 1.1	4.7 ± 0.7	<0.05
Triglyceride, mg/dL	Ad libitum	117 ± 20	165 ± 14	NS

Fasting measurements were performed after an overnight fast. Refed measurements were performed 4–6 h after refeeding. Ad libitum samples were collected 2–3 h after lights-on for 13- to 16-week-old male knockout mice and control littermates fed chow diet unless otherwise indicated. Data are means ± SEM. N = 8–10 for each genotype and measurement. WT, wild-type; NS, not significant.

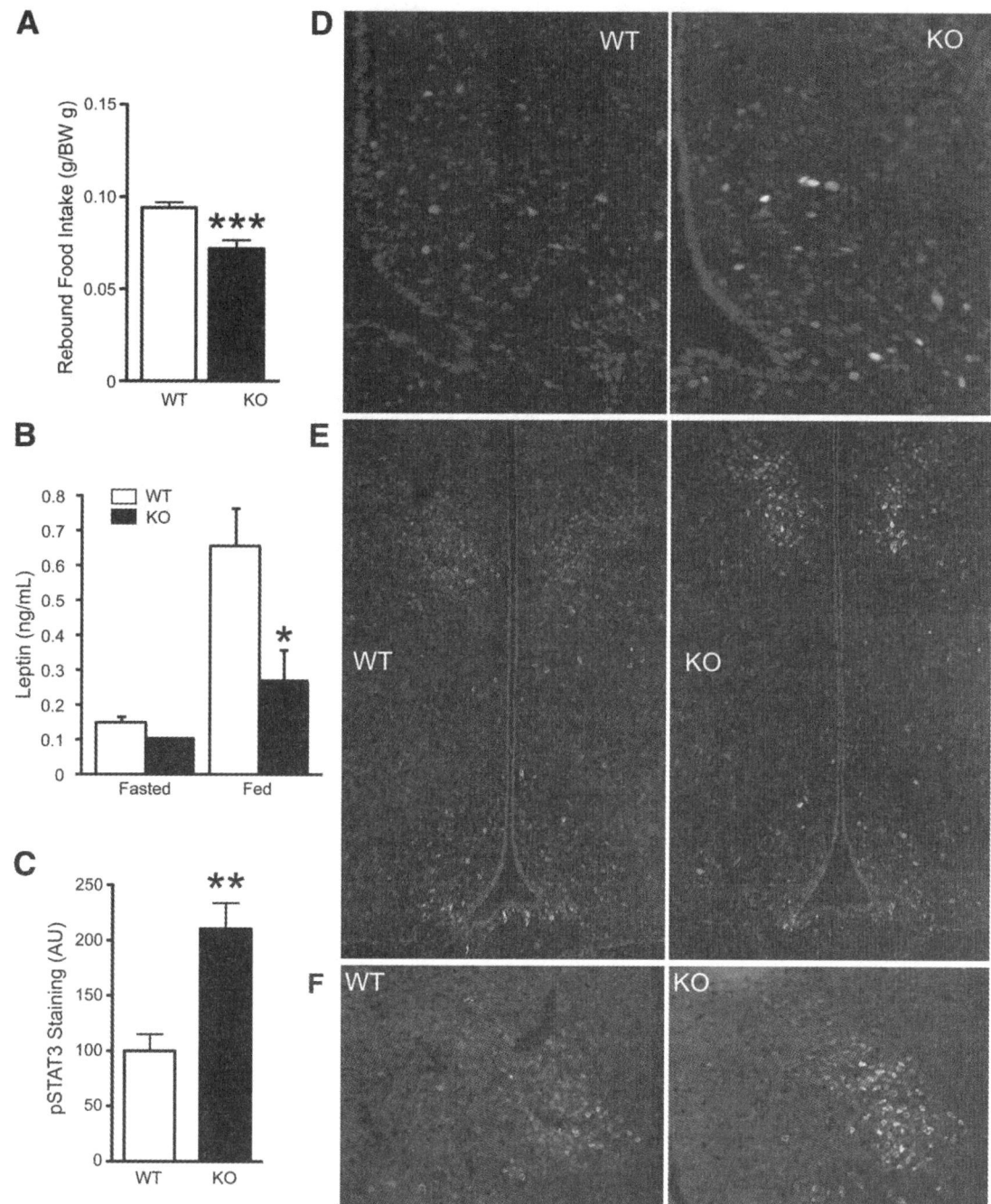

FIG. 3. Increased central hormonal and nutrient sensitivity in *Syn-Foxo1* mice. *A*: Rebound food intake after an overnight fast (*n* = 6 for each genotype). *B*: Serum leptin measured after overnight fasting or refeeding (*n* = 6–8 for each genotype). *C*: Quantification of the integrated intensity of pSTAT3 staining in the arcuate nucleus from refed wild-type and *Syn-Foxo1$^{-/-}$* mice (*n* = 6). *D*: pStat3 staining (green) in the arcuate nucleus from refed wild-type (*Syn-Foxo1$^{+/+}$;Rosa-Tomato*) and knockout (*Syn-Foxo1$^{-/-}$;Rosa-Tomato*) mice. *Syn-Cre* neurons are labeled in red. Nuclei are staining with DAPI (blue). *E*: Increased pS6 staining (green) in the hypothalamus from *Syn-Foxo1;Rosa-Tomato* mice. *Syn-Cre*–recombined neurons are labeled in red. Nuclei are staining with DAPI (blue). *F*: pS6 staining (green) in dorsal medial nucleus of the hypothalamus from *Syn-Foxo1;Rosa-Tomato* and control mice. AU, arbitrary units; BW, body weight; KO, knockout; WT, wild-type. *P < 0.05; **P < 0.01; ***P < 0.001.

Increased locomotor activity and melanocortin signaling in *Syn-Foxo1* mice. Male *Syn-Foxo1* mice had increased locomotor activity during the dark phase of the light cycle (Fig. 5*A*). Previous studies have shown that FoxO1 ablation in POMC neurons increased locomotor activity because of increased α-MSH processing and melanocortin signaling (17). Given that only a minority of POMC neurons were targeted in *Syn-Foxo1* mice (Fig. 2),

the cause of increased locomotion in *Syn-Foxo1* mice is likely different from that for *Pomc-Foxo1* knockout mice. In fact, α-MSH and β-endorphin levels in the MBH were comparable between wild-type and *Syn-Foxo1* mice (Fig. 5*B* and *C*), indicating that processing of POMC-derived hormones occurs normally in the knockout mice. The α-MSH is rapidly metabolized in vivo by prolyl-carboxypeptidase (Prcp) (26). The ratio of α-MSH to β-endorphins in *Syn-Foxo1*

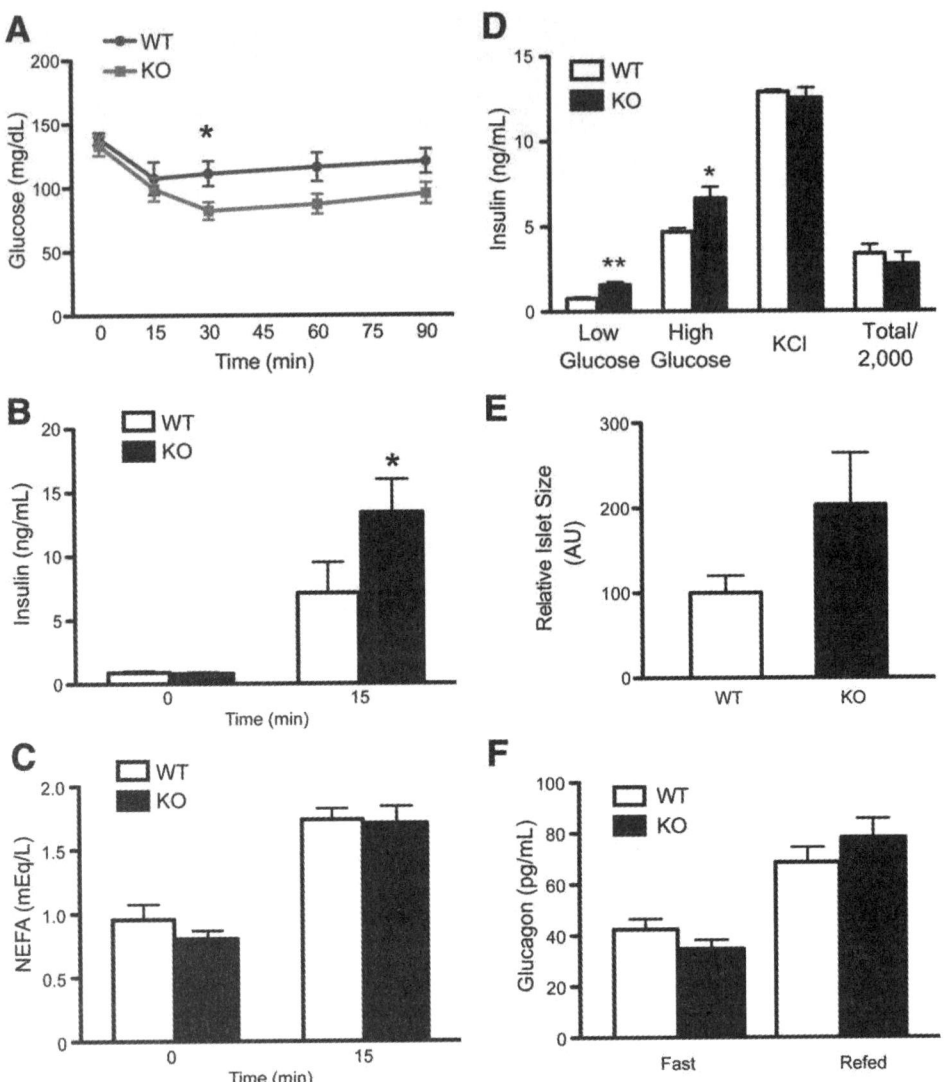

FIG. 4. Altered brain–pancreas axis in *Syn-Foxo1*$^{-/-}$ mice. Glucose (*A*), insulin (*B*), and nonesterified fatty acid (*C*) levels after β3-adrenergic receptor agonist injection (*n* = 7 for each genotype). *D*: Insulin secretion from islets isolated from *Syn-Foxo1* and wild-type mice (*n* = 8 for each genotype). Total/2,000: 1:2,000 dilution of islet insulin content obtained by acid extraction. *E*: Islet size quantification by morphometry (*n* = 6–8 for each genotype). *F*: Fasted and fed glucagon levels (*n* = 6–8 for each genotype). AU, arbitrary units; KO, knockout; NEFA, nonesterified fatty acid; WT, wild-type. *P < 0.05; **P < 0.01.

mice was slightly higher compared with that of wild-type mice (0.471 ± 0.025 vs. 0.419 ± 0.014, respectively; P = not significant), consistent with the possibility that slower inactivation of α-MSH may contribute to increased melanocortinergic tone. α-MSH signaling exerts negative feedback regulation on its peptide processing, reducing Pcsk1 expression (17). *Pcsk1* and *Prcp* expression were significantly reduced in the hypothalamus of *Syn-Foxo1* mice during the phase of increased locomotor activity (Fig. 5*E* and *F*). These data suggest that increased melanocortin signaling in *Foxo1* knockout mice contributes to the increased locomotor activity.

We tested this hypothesis by a gain-of-function approach. We reasoned that if FoxO1 loss-of-function increased locomotor activity, then a gain-of-function mutant should reverse this phenotype. We injected adenovirus encoding the constitutively active FoxO1-ADA mutant (9) into the MBH. After this manipulation, we observed increased hypothalamic *Foxo1* when compared with mice

that received control GFP adenovirus (Fig. 5*G*). After recovery, we individually housed mice in activity hotels provided with a running wheel and monitored wheel rotations to assess locomotor activity during the 24-h light–dark cycle. Mice injected with FoxO1-ADA showed less locomotor activity during the dark phase (Fig. 5*H*). Of note, as a negative control, mice with FoxO1-ADA injection into the SCN—a site spared by *Syn-Cre* recombination—demonstrated no change in activity patterns (data not shown). The SCN is the site of the master clock of the brain, and it known for its role in controlling daily rest–activity rhythms. This result indicates that the activity phenotype is not caused by changes in SCN.

Single and triple FoxO ablation in neurons protect equally from HFD-induced weight gain. We next investigated whether the comparatively mild phenotype seen in *Syn-Foxo1* mice could be explained by compensatory actions of the two closely related isoforms, FoxO3 and FoxO4 (19). To this end, we generated triple-knockout

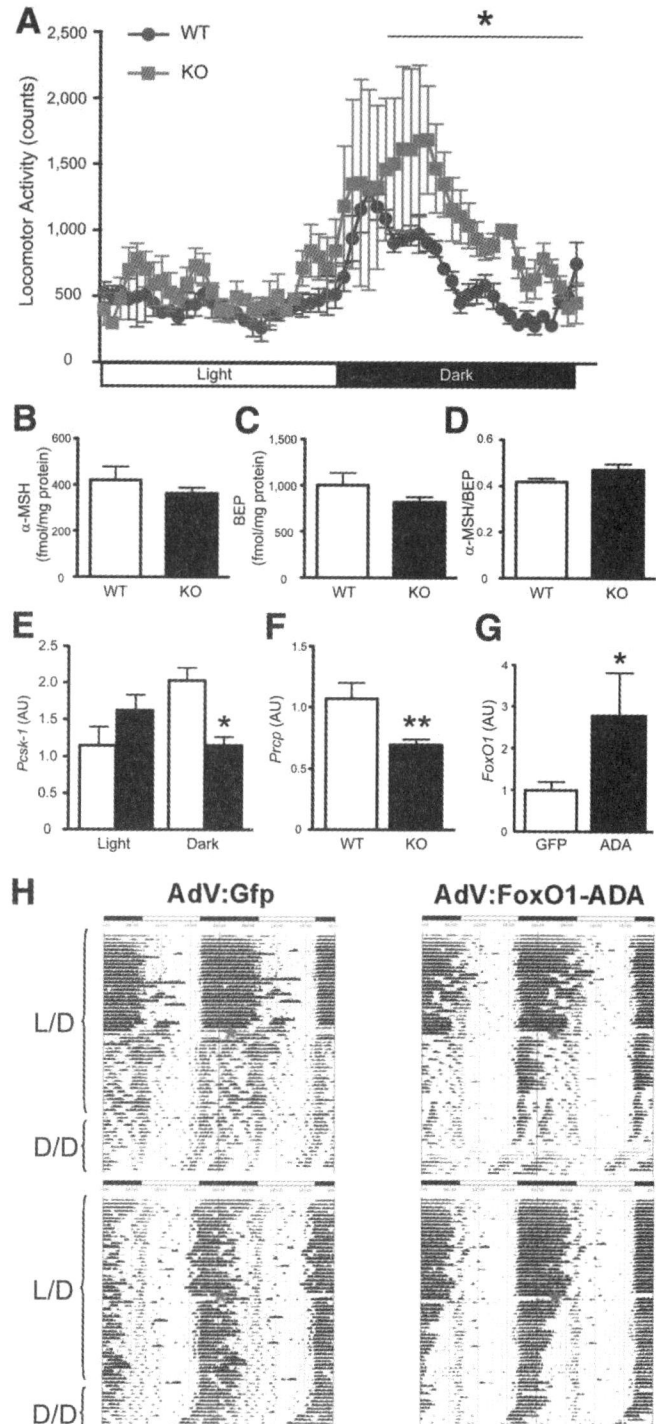

mice using *Syn-Cre* (*Syn-Foxo1,3,4*). mRNA measurements in hypothalamus and hippocampus from wild-type and *Syn-Foxo1,3,4* mice revealed significant reductions of *Foxo1* and *Foxo3*, whereas *Foxo4* was undetectable (Fig. 6*A*). *Syn-Foxo1,3,4* and wild-type mice showed comparable body weight when fed the normal chow diet (Fig. 6*B*). When fed HFD after weaning, triple-knockout mice gained less weight compared with wild-type mice (Fig. 6*C*), likely because of reduced fat accumulation, as indicated by body composition studies (Fig. 6*D*).

Next, we determined whether the knockout protected from weight gain induced by HFD feeding. We used mice backcrossed onto B6 background to minimize individual variation. Wild-type mice rapidly gained weight when fed HFD, whereas knockout mice consistently maintained a significantly lower body weight (Fig. 6*E*). We analyzed body composition after 4 months of HFD feeding and found that knockout mice had significantly less fat mass compared with wild-type mice (Fig. 6*F*). We compared these mice with triple *Syn-Foxo1,3,4* mice, and we found that the extent of protection from HFD-induced fat accumulation was the same. The triple-knockout mice fed HFD had lower body weight than wild-type mice (33.8 ± 0.8 g; knockout mice: 31.3 ± 0.7 g; $P = 0.035$). Then, we analyzed energy balance in this cohort by indirect calorimetry. Interestingly, knockout mice had significantly increased V_{O_2} (Fig. 6*G*), locomotor activity, and energy expenditure during both light and dark phases (Fig. 6*H* and *I*). Knockout mice had respiratory quotients comparable with those of wild-type mice (Fig. 6*J*). In conclusion, FoxO1 ablation in *Syn-Cre*–expressing neurons increased energy expenditure in HFD-fed animals and partly offset diet-induced weight gain.

Distinct energy balance and glucose homeostasis phenotypes of *Pomc;Agrp-Foxo1* mice. POMC and AgRP neurons in the arcuate nucleus are critical CNS components for controlling metabolic homeostasis. We have reported that knocking out FoxO1 in either POMC or AgRP neurons improves energy and glucose homeostasis (17,18). Curiously, we found that only few POMC and AgRP neurons undergo *Syn-Cre*–mediated recombination (Fig. 2), yet *Syn-Foxo1* mice have an improved metabolic profile (Fig. 3). To distinguish the collective contribution of POMC and AgRP neurons from that of other CNS neurons, we characterized the phenotype of mice with combined FoxO1 knockout in both POMC and AgRP neurons. In contrast to *Syn-Foxo1* mice, *Pomc;Agrp-Foxo1* mice fed normal chow exhibited a lean phenotype, with lower body weight (Fig. 7*A*), decreased fat mass (Fig. 7*B*), and increased lean mass (Fig. 7*C*). Furthermore, during the 24-h light cycle *Pomc; Agrp-Foxo1* mice showed significantly reduced V_{O_2} (Fig. 7*D*) and elevated respiratory quotient but unaltered locomotor activity (Fig. 7*E*) compared with wild-type mice.

Considering this energy partitioning phenotype, we analyzed hepatic glucose production in *Pomc;Agrp-Foxo1* mice by euglycemic-hyperinsulinemic clamp studies. Glucose infusion rates trended higher in *Pomc;Agrp-Foxo1* mice (Fig. 7*G*), likely because of increased rates of glucose disposal (Fig. 7*H*), but neither difference reached statistical significance. Interestingly, hepatic glucose production

FIG. 5. Locomotor activity and melanocortin signaling in single and triple *Syn-Foxo* knockout mice. *A*: Locomotor activity during the 24-h light-dark cycle in *Syn-Foxo1,3,4* and control wild-type mice (*n* = 8 for each genotype). We measured activity by beam breaks in metabolic chambers used for indirect calorimetry studies. The α-MSH (*B*), β-endorphin (*C*), and α-MSH:BEP ratios (*D*) in *Syn-Foxo1* and control wild-type mice (*n* = 8–9 for each genotype) are shown. *Pcsk1* (*E*) and *Prcp* (*F*) mRNA levels during the dark phase of the light cycle (*n* = 6–8 for each genotype). *G*: *Foxo1* mRNA in the MBH after delivery of FoxO1-ADA or GFP adenovirus (*n* = 6 for each genotype). Data are expressed as fold-change compared with control (normalized to 1). *H*: Locomotor activity after delivery of FoxO1-ADA or GFP adenovirus. Activity was measured by wheel rotations for each individually housed mouse with a running wheel during 12-h light/12-h dark cycle or continuous 24-h dark cycle. We show two representative continuous activity recordings

over 48 h for each genotype. Red asterisk depicts the time of viral injection. AU, arbitrary units; BEP, β-endorphin; D/D, 24-h dark cycle; KO, knockout; L/D, 12-h light/12-h dark cycle; WT, wild-type. *$P < 0.05$; **$P < 0.01$.

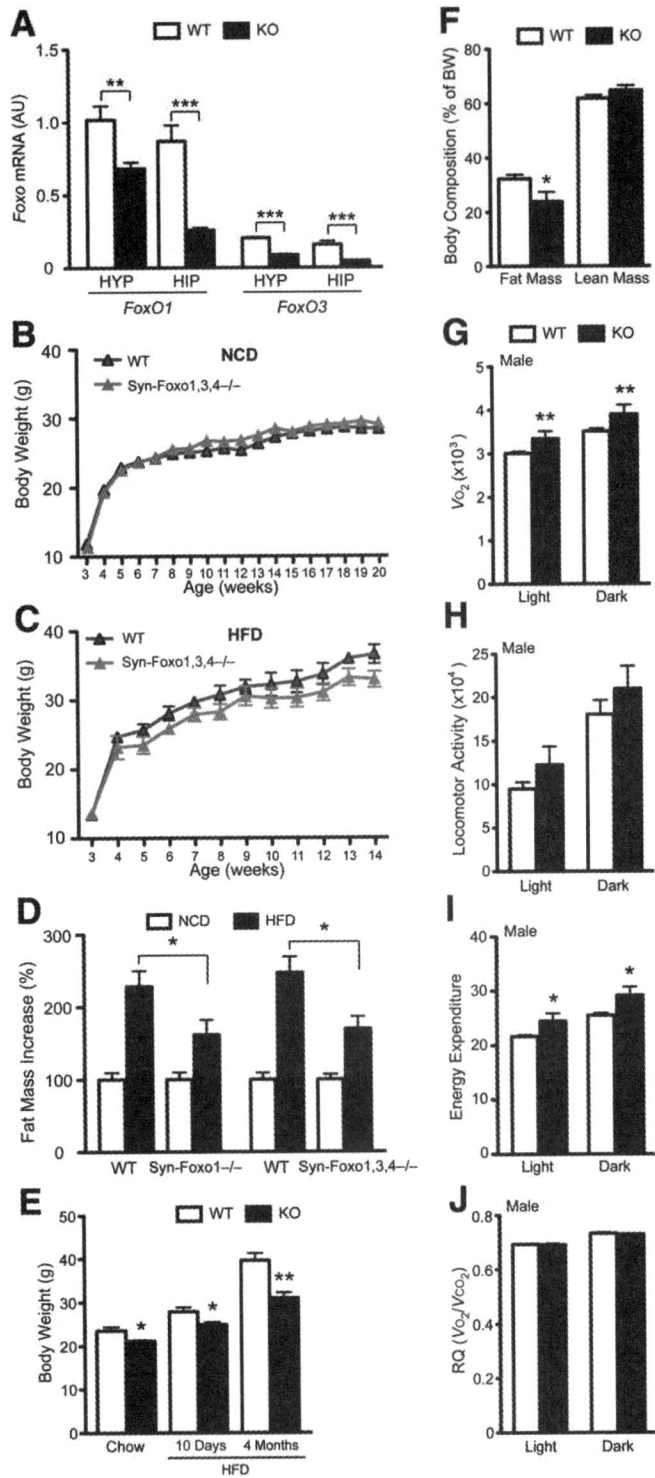

FIG. 6. FoxO ablation in neurons protects from HFD-induced weight gain. *A: Foxo* mRNA levels in the hypothalamus and hippocampus (*n* = 6–8 for each genotype). *B* and *C*: Growth curve of *Syn-Foxo1,3,4* and wild-type mice fed chow (*n* = 32–35 for each genotype; *B*) or HFD (*n* = 6 for each genotype; *C*). *D*: Body composition of mice fed HFD (*n* = 6–10 for each genotype). Body weight (*E*) and body composition (*F*) of *Syn-Foxo1* and wild-type mice fed HFD at 11 weeks of age (*n* = 5–6 for each genotype). *G–J*: Indirect calorimetry measurements. Oxygen consumption (mL/h/kg) (*G*), locomotor activity (counts) (*H*), energy expenditure (W/kg) (*I*), and respiratory quotient (*J*) of male mice fed HFD (*n* = 8 for each genotype). AU, arbitrary units; BW, body weight; HIP, hippocampus; HYP, hypothalamus; KO, knockout; NCD, normal chow diet; RQ, respiratory quotients; WT, wild-type. **P < 0.05; **P < 0.01; ***P < 0.001.

was unchanged (Fig. 7*I*), unlike in *Agrp-Foxo1* mice (18). Based on these results, we conclude that FoxO1 function in POMC and AgRP has concordant effects to increase energy expenditure but has opposing actions on hepatic glucose production, as intimated by a previous study (21). The metabolic functions of FoxO1 in *Syn-Cre*–expressing neurons appear to be distinct from those in AgRP and POMC neurons.

DISCUSSION

In this work, we describe the metabolic and energy balance phenotypes associated with deletion of transcription factor FoxO1, a key metabolic sensor, in *Syn-Cre*–expressing neurons that are found scattered in the cortex, hippocampus, hypothalamus, and brain stem. *Syn-Foxo1* mice display a catabolic energy balance phenotype associated with increased sensitivity to hormone and nutrient signaling within the CNS and increased locomotor activity, possibly attributable to low α-MSH turnover leading to enhanced melanocortin signaling. The heterogeneity of *Syn-Cre*–mediated recombination, as assessed by lineage tracing, limits our ability to assign the observed phenotype to a specific neuronal subtype. Nonetheless, we used three alternative approaches to begin to map the functional neuroanatomy of FoxO functions in the CNS. First, lineage-tracing approaches show that only ~20% of NPY/AgRP and POMC neurons display *Syn-Cre*–dependent recombination, effectively ruling a major contribution of these key neuronal populations to the energy balance and metabolic phenotypes of *Syn-Foxo1* mice. We supported this conclusion by analyzing mice with combined ablations of FoxO1 in AgRP and POMC neurons, and by showing that the phenotypes differ. Second, concurrent ablation in *Syn-Cre* neurons of the three insulin-regulated FoxO isoforms, FoxO1, FoxO3, and FoxO4, also conferred a catabolic energy expenditure phenotype, with improved glucose metabolism and resistance to HFD, demonstrating that FoxO functions likely overlap, similar to previous observations (6,27). Third, we used a gain-of-function approach to map the increased activity phenotype to the MBH. We conclude that in addition to their established role in neuropeptide synthesis and processing, FoxO1, FoxO3, and FoxO4 have anabolic functions in other areas of the CNS.

A new finding of the present work is the increase in insulin secretion observed in response to a β3-AR agonist. This likely reflects an effect of FoxO1 on sympathetic activity, possibly because of loss of FoxO1 function in the brain stem (28,29). Our conclusion is that the integrative neuronal function of FoxO1 extends beyond the arcuate nucleus, suggesting that broad-based inhibition of FoxO1 function in the CNS can promote hormone sensitivity and prevent metabolic disease.

Key components of insulin and leptin signaling pathways have been studied using pan-neuronal ablation approaches (30). Our data emphasize that there is no such thing as a truly pan-neuronal knockout, and that caution should be exerted in comparing knockouts performed with different Cre drivers. Mice with *Nestin-Cre*–driven insulin receptor knockout (31) develop diet-induced obesity with increases in body fat, mild insulin resistance, increased plasma leptin, and hypertriglyceridemia, demonstrating that neuronal insulin receptor function affects energy balance. With the caveats stated, it is reassuring that the overall direction of the metabolic changes is consistent with the opposing cellular actions of insulin receptor and FoxO (5), especially

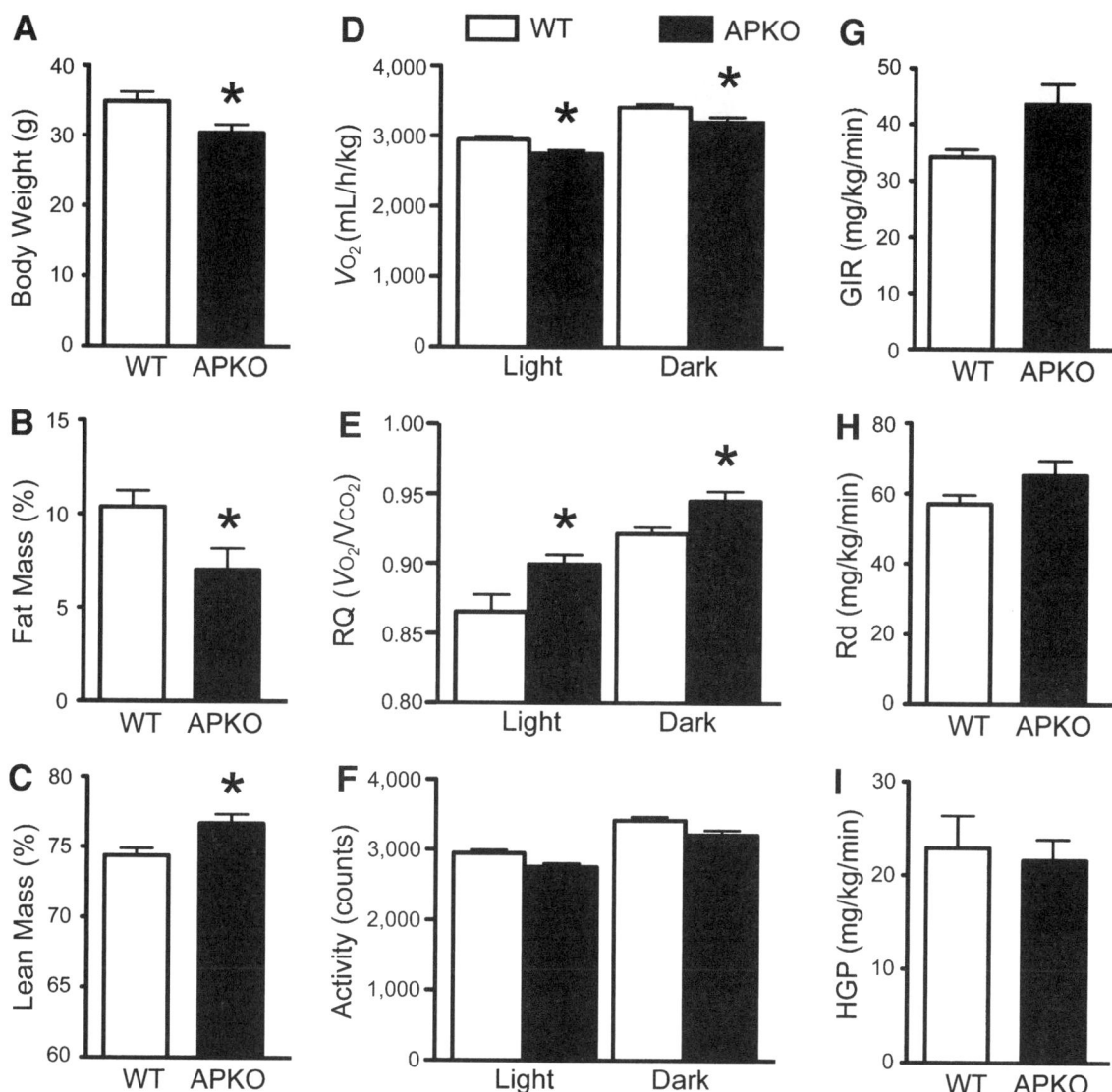

FIG. 7. Distinct energy balance and glucose homeostasis phenotypes of *Pomc;Agrp-Foxo1*$^{-/-}$ mice. Body weight (*A*), fat content (*B*), and lean mass (*C*) (*n* = 8–9 for each genotype). Oxygen consumption (*D*), respiratory quotient (*E*), and locomotor activity (*F*) (*n* = 9 for each genotype). Glucose infusion (*G*), glucose disposal (*H*), and hepatic glucose production (*I*) during euglycemic-hyperinsulinemic clamps (*n* = 4–6 for each genotype). APKO, *Pomc;Agrp-Foxo1*$^{-/-}$; GIR, glucose infusion rate; HGP, hepatic glucose production; Rd, glucose disposal; RQ, respiratory quotient; WT, wild-type. *$P < 0.05$.

because the latter acts as a relay node for multiple extra-cellular signals (32). Similarly, *Syn-Cre* neuron–specific leptin receptor deletion gave rise to obesity associated with increased plasma glucose, insulin, and leptin in a manner that was directly related to the extent of hypo-thalamic leptin receptor ablation (33). These data lend support to previous work indicating that FoxOs act to in-tegrate insulin with leptin signaling by virtue of their ability to antagonize STAT3 signaling in response to decreasing levels of phospho-Akt (13). Conversely, neuron-specific knockout or knockdown of protein tyrosine phosphatase-1b, a negative regulator of insulin and leptin signaling, improves insulin and leptin sensitivity and protects from diet-induced obesity (34,35). Nonetheless, there are telling differences between the phenotypes resulting from protein tyrosine phosphatase-1b and FoxO ablation, for example, with regard to peripheral metabolism and locomotor activity. These data indicate that FoxO relays multiple pathways

acting not only through Akt but also possibly through other kinases. The nature of these kinases and their target sites on FoxO1, as well as the physiologic consequences of their activation on FoxO1 function, represent important areas for further research. In addition to insulin and leptin, FoxO1 mediates the effects of other key hormones on metabolism, such as ghrelin (36). We found in our studies that the diverse, if internally consistent, effects of FoxO ablation on energy homeostasis impinge equally on insulin and leptin signaling, sensitizing the body to both. More challenging is the question of which cellular mechanisms and neuronal relay systems are used to effect these actions.

In this study, we found that mice with FoxO1 knockout in *Syn-Cre*–expressing neurons have increased melano-cortin signaling tone, manifested as increased locomotor activity. The finding that constitutively active FoxO1 ex-pression in MBH, but not in SCN, reduces locomotor ac-tivity highlights the physiological importance of FoxO1 function in MBH. MBH includes several neuronal populations that are critical for metabolic regulation. For example, FoxO1 activation in POMC and AgRP neurons results in anabolic function, but the underlying effectors and molecular mechanisms are starkly different (12–15,17,18). In POMC neurons, FoxO1 knockout promotes leanness, decreases food intake, increases leptin sensitivity, and increases melanocortin signaling. We have proposed that the key effector of these actions is carboxypeptidase, the protease responsible for cleaving POMC to α-MSH and β-endorphin, which are normally suppressed by FoxO1 (17). In AgRP neurons, FoxO1 regulates expression of AgRP itself (13) and also of the orphan G-protein-coupled receptor Gpr17, whose pharmacological modulation affects food intake and, hence, shows promise as a target of antiobesity drugs (18). Unlike ablation in POMC neurons, ablation in AgRP neurons also had a substantial effect on hepatic glucose production, adding one important potential therapeutic benefit to CNS-targeted FoxO inhibition (18). The ventral medial nucleus is also a site of FoxO1 action (16). Mice lacking FoxO1 in ventral medial nucleus steroidogenic factor-1–expressing neurons are lean because of increased energy expenditure and have increased insulin sensitivity, suggesting that the overarching role of FoxO as a mediator of energy balance extends to multiple CNS sites.

The adult mammalian brain also contains neural stem cells that can give rise to neurons, astrocytes, and oligodendrocytes (37). FoxO1, FoxO3, and FoxO4 cooperatively regulate neural stem cell homeostasis and play important roles in neural stem cell proliferation and renewal, possibly through their regulation of cellular metabolism (27).

FoxO isoforms include FoxO1, FoxO3, and FoxO4. Based on estimates from quantitative PCR analysis, FoxO1 is the major isoform expressed in the brain. FoxO3 is expressed at lower levels, whereas FoxO4 expression is virtually undetectable. These different FoxO isoforms could have functional redundancy, and other isoforms may compensate for the loss of one isoform. For example, this is the case in the liver, where triple ablation of *Foxo* genes causes more pronounced effects than the single FoxO1 knockout with fasting hypoglycemia, increased glucose tolerance and insulin sensitivity, and decreased plasma insulin levels (6). This paradigm appears to hold true in the brain, because our data show that triple FoxO knockouts in the brain are better protected from weight gain induced by HFD, indicating potentially redundant contributions of other FoxO genes to CNS regulation of energy balance.

Understanding the integrative function of FoxO1 in the CNS is crucial for harnessing its therapeutic potential for metabolic diseases. The data presented in this study are reassuring in this regard because we observed no untoward effect of single or triple FoxO ablation. Further, we saw that the effects linked to *Syn-Cre* ablation are qualitatively similar to those observed in more restricted knockouts (16–18), allaying fears that broad-based FoxO inhibition might adversely affect cellular survival, behavior, and overall energy homeostasis.

ACKNOWLEDGMENTS

This study was supported by National Institutes of Health grants DK58282 and DK63608 (Columbia Diabetes Research Center), American Diabetes Association mentor-based fellowship, and Berrie Fellowship Award (H.R.).

No potential conflicts of interest relevant to this article were reported.

H.R. designed and conducted experiments, analyzed data, and wrote the manuscript. L.P.-M. designed and conducted experiments, analyzed data, and wrote the manuscript. R.G.-J. conducted glucose clamp experiments. T.Y.L. and J.Y.K.-M. conducted experiments. G.H. analyzed data. S.L.W. and R.S. designed experiments and analyzed data. D.A. designed experiments, analyzed data, and wrote the manuscript. D.A. is the guarantor of this work and, as such, had full access to all the data in the study and takes responsibility for the integrity of the data and the accuracy of the data analysis.

The authors thank members of the Accili laboratory for insightful data sessions and for critical reading of the manuscript. The authors thank Thomas K. Kolar and Ana M. Flete Castro (Department of Medicine, Columbia University) for excellent technical support. The authors thank Dr. Matthew Butler (Department of Psychology, Columbia University) for helping with wheel-running experiments.

REFERENCES

1. Morton GJ, Schwartz MW. Leptin and the central nervous system control of glucose metabolism. Physiol Rev 2011;91:389–411
2. Gautron L, Elmquist JK. Sixteen years and counting: an update on leptin in energy balance. J Clin Invest 2011;121:2087–2093
3. Suzuki K, Jayasena CN, Bloom SR: Obesity and appetite control. Exp Diabetes Res 2012;2012:824305
4. Varela L, Horvath TL. Leptin and insulin pathways in POMC and AgRP neurons that modulate energy balance and glucose homeostasis. EMBO Rep 2012;13:1079–1086
5. Matsumoto M, Pocai A, Rossetti L, Depinho RA, Accili D. Impaired regulation of hepatic glucose production in mice lacking the forkhead transcription factor Foxo1 in liver. Cell Metab 2007;6:208–216
6. Haeusler RA, Kaestner KH, Accili D. FoxOs function synergistically to promote glucose production. J Biol Chem 2010;285:35245–35248
7. Haeusler RA, Pratt-Hyatt M, Welch CL, Klaassen CD, Accili D. Impaired generation of 12-hydroxylated bile acids links hepatic insulin signaling with dyslipidemia. Cell Metab 2012;15:65–74
8. Talchai C, Xuan S, Lin HV, Sussel L, Accili D. Pancreatic beta cell dedifferentiation as mechanism of beta cell failure in diabetes. Cell 2012;150:1223–1234
9. Nakae J, Kitamura T, Kitamura Y, Biggs WH 3rd, Arden KC, Accili D. The forkhead transcription factor Foxo1 regulates adipocyte differentiation. Dev Cell 2003;4:119–129
10. Kitamura T, Kitamura YI, Funahashi Y, et al. A Foxo/Notch pathway controls myogenic differentiation and fiber type specification. J Clin Invest 2007;117:2477–2485
11. Talchai C, Xuan S, Kitamura T, DePinho RA, Accili D. Generation of functional insulin-producing cells in the gut by Foxo1 ablation. Nat Genet 2012;44:406–412, S1
12. Kim MS, Pak YK, Jang PG, et al. Role of hypothalamic Foxo1 in the regulation of food intake and energy homeostasis. Nat Neurosci 2006;9:901–906
13. Kitamura T, Feng Y, Kitamura YI, et al. Forkhead protein FoxO1 mediates Agrp-dependent effects of leptin on food intake. Nat Med 2006;12:534–540
14. Iskandar K, Cao Y, Hayashi Y, et al. PDK-1/FoxO1 pathway in POMC neurons regulates Pomc expression and food intake. Am J Physiol Endocrinol Metab 2010;298:E787–E798
15. Kim HJ, Kobayashi M, Sasaki T, et al. Overexpression of FoxO1 in the hypothalamus and pancreas causes obesity and glucose intolerance. Endocrinology 2012;153:659–671
16. Kim KW, Donato J Jr, Berglund ED, et al. FOXO1 in the ventromedial hypothalamus regulates energy balance. J Clin Invest 2012;122:2578–2589
17. Plum L, Lin HV, Dutia R, et al. The obesity susceptibility gene Cpe links FoxO1 signaling in hypothalamic pro-opiomelanocortin neurons with regulation of food intake. Nat Med 2009;15:1195–1201
18. Ren H, Orozco IJ, Su Y, et al. FoxO1 target Gpr17 activates AgRP neurons to regulate food intake. Cell 2012;149:1314–1326
19. Paik JH, Kollipara R, Chu G, et al. FoxOs are lineage-restricted redundant tumor suppressors and regulate endothelial cell homeostasis. Cell 2007;128:309–323
20. Butler MP, Karatsoreos IN, LeSauter J, Silver R. Dose-dependent effects of androgens on the circadian timing system and its response to light. Endocrinology 2012;153:2344–2352

21. Lin HV, Plum L, Ono H, et al. Divergent regulation of energy expenditure and hepatic glucose production by insulin receptor in agouti-related protein and POMC neurons. Diabetes 2010;59:337–346

22. Madisen L, Zwingman TA, Sunkin SM, et al. A robust and high-throughput Cre reporting and characterization system for the whole mouse brain. Nat Neurosci 2010;13:133–140

23. Stefater MA, Seeley RJ. Central nervous system nutrient signaling: the regulation of energy balance and the future of dietary therapies. Annu Rev Nutr 2010;30:219–235

24. Thorens B. Sensing of glucose in the brain. Handbook Exp Pharmacol 2012;209:277–294

25. Buteau J, Accili D. Regulation of pancreatic beta-cell function by the forkhead protein FoxO1. Diabetes Obes Metab 2007;9(Suppl. 2):140–146

26. Diano S. New aspects of melanocortin signaling: a role for PRCP in α-MSH degradation. Front Neuroendocrinol 2011;32:70–83

27. Paik JH, Ding Z, Narurkar R, et al. FoxOs cooperatively regulate diverse pathways governing neural stem cell homeostasis. Cell Stem Cell 2009;5:540–553

28. Luiten PG, ter Horst GJ, Buijs RM, Steffens AB. Autonomic innervation of the pancreas in diabetic and non-diabetic rats. A new view on intramural sympathetic structural organization. J Auton Nerv Syst 1986;15:33–44

29. Kreier F, Kap YS, Mettenleiter TC, et al. Tracing from fat tissue, liver, and pancreas: a neuroanatomical framework for the role of the brain in type 2 diabetes. Endocrinology 2006;147:1140–1147

30. Plum L, Belgardt BF, Brüning JC. Central insulin action in energy and glucose homeostasis. J Clin Invest 2006;116:1761–1766

31. Brüning JC, Gautam D, Burks DJ, et al. Role of brain insulin receptor in control of body weight and reproduction. Science 2000;289:2122–2125

32. Eijkelenboom A, Burgering BM. FOXOs: signalling integrators for homeostasis maintenance. Nat Rev Mol Cell Biol 2013;14:83–97

33. Cohen P, Zhao C, Cai X, et al. Selective deletion of leptin receptor in neurons leads to obesity. J Clin Invest 2001;108:1113–1121

34. Bence KK, Delibegovic M, Xue B, et al. Neuronal PTP1B regulates body weight, adiposity and leptin action. Nat Med 2006;12:917–924

35. Picardi PK, Calegari VC, Prada PO, et al. Reduction of hypothalamic protein tyrosine phosphatase improves insulin and leptin resistance in diet-induced obese rats [corrected in Endocriology 2013;154:1667]. Endocrinology 2008;149:3870–3880

36. Varela L, Vázquez MJ, Cordido F, et al. Ghrelin and lipid metabolism: key partners in energy balance. J Mol Endocrinol 2011;46:R43–R63

37. Rafalski VA, Brunet A. Energy metabolism in adult neural stem cell fate. Prog Neurobiol 2011;93:182–203

Mitochondrial Substrate Availability and Its Role in Lipid-Induced Insulin Resistance and Proinflammatory Signaling in Skeletal Muscle

Christopher Lipina,[1] Katherine Macrae,[1] Tamara Suhm,[2] Cora Weigert,[2,3] Agnieszka Blachnio-Zabielska,[4] Marcin Baranowski,[4] Jan Gorski,[4] Karl Burgess,[5] and Harinder S. Hundal[1]

The relationship between glucose and lipid metabolism has been of significant interest in understanding the pathogenesis of obesity-induced insulin resistance. To gain insight into this metabolic paradigm, we explored the potential interplay between cellular glucose flux and lipid-induced metabolic dysfunction within skeletal muscle. Here, we show that palmitate (PA)-induced insulin resistance and proinflammation in muscle cells, which is associated with reduced mitochondrial integrity and oxidative capacity, can be attenuated under conditions of glucose withdrawal or glycolytic inhibition using 2-deoxyglucose (2DG). Importantly, these glucopenic-driven improvements coincide with the preservation of mitochondrial function and are dependent on PA oxidation, which becomes markedly enhanced in the absence of glucose. Intriguingly, despite its ability to upregulate mitochondrial PA oxidation, glucose withdrawal did not attenuate PA-induced increases in total intramyocellular diacylglycerol and ceramide. Furthermore, consistent with our findings in cultured muscle cells, we also report enhanced insulin sensitivity and reduced proinflammatory tone in soleus muscle from obese Zucker rats fed a 2DG-supplemented diet. Notably, this improved metabolic status after 2DG dietary intervention is associated with markedly reduced plasma free fatty acids. Collectively, our data highlight the key role that mitochondrial substrate availability plays in lipid-induced metabolic dysregulation both in vitro and in vivo. *Diabetes* 62:3426–3436, 2013

There is significant evidence in the literature linking elevation in free fatty acid (FFA) levels with development of peripheral insulin resistance and its associated metabolic perturbations, including impaired glucose uptake (1). However, as yet, there is no unified view that adequately explains how these pathophysiological events develop. Randle et al. (2) first postulated that increased mitochondrial fatty acid oxidation (associated with FFA oversupply) may impair glucose uptake and utilization via metabolite-induced allosteric inhibition of key glycolytic enzymes. Specifically, inhibition of pyruvate dehydrogenase and phosphofructokinase by acetyl CoA and citrate generated from excessive FFA oxidation would culminate in accumulation of glucose-6-phosphate (G6P) that, in turn, would promote allosteric inhibition of hexokinase with a concomitant reduction in glucose uptake. However, the concept that suppressed glycolytic flux underlies lipid-induced metabolic dysfunction has been challenged by an alternative school of thought implicating ectopic accumulation of lipids as the primary cause of insulin resistance in skeletal muscle (3,4). In particular, lipid oversupply in the form of excess saturated fatty acids including palmitate (PA) (C16:0) promotes intramyocellular accumulation of bioactive lipids such as diacylglycerol (DAG) and ceramide. These lipids have been implicated strongly in the development of insulin resistance via their inhibitory effects on proximal insulin signaling, and as such, their effects may depend or be further accentuated by glucose overloading (i.e., glucolipotoxicity). Notably, activated DAG-sensitive protein kinase C (PKC) isoforms suppress insulin action via elevated serine phosphorylation of insulin receptor substrates, such as insulin receptor substrate (IRS)-1 (5,6), whereas ceramide induces a targeted loss in activation of the serine/threonine kinase, Akt, by insulin (7). Both IRS and Akt serve as critical components of the insulin signaling cascade, and so their dysregulation impairs key processes under the control of insulin, including glucose uptake and glycogen synthesis.

In accordance with evidence supporting a role for lipotoxic intermediates in the pathogenesis of insulin resistance, a number of studies have also explored the relationship between insulin sensitivity and mitochondrial function. Importantly, various indicators of impaired mitochondrial capacity have been reported in skeletal muscle from insulin-resistant or obese human subjects including, for example, a reduction in the activity or expression of carnitine palmitoyltransferase-1, which mediates mitochondrial fatty acid uptake, and that of various oxidative enzymes and respiratory chain components coinciding with suppressed ATP synthesis (8–13). Furthermore, obesity-induced reductions in peroxisome proliferator–activated receptor γ coactivator (PGC)-1α, a key transcriptional coordinator of mitochondrial biogenesis, and elevated expression of muscle nuclear factor κB (NF-κB)-dependent proinflammatory genes (e.g., interleukin-6 [IL-6], tumor necrosis factor-α), may contribute significantly to FFA-induced mitochondrial dysfunction and insulin resistance (12,14–18). Collectively, these observations support the idea that mitochondrial dysfunction (associated with lipid oversupply) may restrict FFA oxidation and promote their greater partitioning into bioactive lipid intermediates, such as ceramide and DAG, that negatively regulate insulin action.

From the [1]Division of Cell Signalling and Immunology, Sir James Black Centre, College of Life Sciences, University of Dundee, Dundee, U.K.; the [2]Division of Endocrinology, Diabetology, Angiology, Nephrology, Pathobiochemistry and Clinical Chemistry, Department of Internal Medicine, University of Tübingen, Tübingen, Germany; the [3]Institute for Diabetes Research and Metabolic Diseases of the Helmholtz Centre Munich at the University of Tübingen, Tübingen, Germany (Paul Langerhans Institute Tübingen), Member of the German Centre for Diabetes Research; the [4]Department of Physiology, Medical University of Bialystok, Bialystok, Poland; and the [5]Glasgow Polyomics Metabolomics Facility, University of Glasgow, Glasgow, U.K.

Corresponding author: Harinder S. Hundal, h.s.hundal@dundee.ac.uk.

Received 15 February 2013 and accepted 29 May 2013.

DOI: 10.2337/db13-0264

This article contains Supplementary Data online at http://diabetes .diabetesjournals.org/lookup/suppl/doi:10.2337/db13-0264/-/DC1.

Herein, given the current focus on fuel substrate–derived metabolites, lipotoxic intermediates, and mitochondrial energetics, we sought to explore their interrelationship and involvement in obesity and FFA-induced metabolic dysregulation by assessing the effects of restricting glucose utilization both in vitro and in vivo. Together, our data underscore the important role that mitochondrial substrate overload, in particular with respect to glucose and fatty acid provision, plays in the development of lipid-mediated insulin resistance and associated proinflammatory cytokine production in skeletal muscle.

RESEARCH DESIGN AND METHODS

Ten-week-old male obese (*fa/fa*) and lean (*Fa/fa*) Zucker rats obtained from Harlan UK (Oxon, U.K.) were maintained on a 12-h light/dark cycle and fed ad libitum a standard or 2-deoxyglucose (2DG) (0.4% w/w) supplemented chow diet for 28 days. The 2DG diet was prepared by pulverizing standard chow pellets and reconstituting with 2DG powder. Body weights and food intake were monitored twice weekly. After the 28-day dietary regimen, animals were fasted overnight (16 h) and subsequently anesthetized by injection of sodium pentobarbitone (60 mg/kg i.p.). Blood sampling, careful excision, and rapid freezing in liquid nitrogen of soleus from one hindlimb were then performed prior to administration of insulin (10 units/kg i.v., Actrapid; Novo Nordisk, Bagsværd, Denmark). Five minutes post–insulin administration, soleus muscle from the contralateral hindlimb was removed and immediately frozen in liquid nitrogen for storage at −80°C. All animal procedures complied with the U.K. Animal Scientific Procedures Act.

Muscle cell culture, cell treatments, and analysis. Methods used for culturing and treating rat (L6) and primary human myotubes with PA and their preparation for immunoblotting, RNA extraction, conventional RT-PCR and real-time quantitative (qPCR) analysis, PA oxidation, and whole-cell oxygen consumption and analysis of intramyocellular DAG and ceramide have previously been described (19–22) or are described in the Supplementary Data.

Measurement of intracellular metabolites. L6 myotubes were incubated with 0.5 mmol/L PA in the absence or presence of 5 mmol/L glucose as indicated in the appropriate figure legends. After treatment, cells were lysed in ice-cold chloroform/methanol/water (1:3:1) and resulting samples analyzed by liquid chromatography–mass spectrometry (LCMS) as previously described (23). Analysis of LCMS data was performed using MzMatch (24) and IDEOM (23) software, with metabolites confirmed by mass and retention time analysis being matched against authentic standards or classified as putative, based on mass, predicted retention time, and biochemical reference (23).

Determination of blood and tissue biochemistry. Plasma FFA concentration was measured using the EnzyChrom Free Fatty Acid Assay Kit from BioAssay Systems (Hayward, CA). Triglyceride concentration in blood plasma was determined using the Triglyceride Assay kit from Cayman Chemical (Ann Arbor, MI). Circulating blood glucose levels were measured using an Alpha-TRAK Blood Glucose Monitoring System (Abbott Laboratories).

Statistical analyses. For multiple comparisons, statistical analysis was performed using one-way ANOVA or a *t* test where appropriate. Data analysis was performed using GraphPad Prism software and considered statistically significant at P values <0.05.

RESULTS

Effects of PA and glucose availability on Akt-directed insulin signaling. Sustained (16 h) PA overprovision caused a substantial reduction in the insulin-dependent phosphorylation/activation of Akt and that of forkhead box O3 (FOXO3a) and glycogen synthase kinase-3 α/β; both established Akt targets in L6 myotubes (Fig. 1*A*). To determine whether this reduced insulin signaling capacity was a consequence of substrate competition, we investigated the effects of incubating myotubes with PA for 16 h in *1*) glucose-free media, *2*) glucose-free media to which 2DG (a nonmetabolizable glucose analog and glycolytic inhibitor) was added as a glucose substitute, or *3*) glucose-containing media to which 2DG was added as a competitive glucose supplement. This strategy revealed that while Akt phosphorylation by insulin was severely blunted by PA when glucose was present (Fig. 1*B* [compare

lanes 1 and *2*]), this inhibition was not detected in myotubes incubated with PA in the absence of glucose or when glucose had been substituted or media cosupplemented with 2DG (Fig. 1*B* [compare *lanes 4* and *8* with *2*]). In line with the ability to restrain the insulin-desensitizing effect of PA upon glucose withdrawal or 2DG provision, phosphorylation of FOXO3a and glycogen synthase kinase-3 α/β was also enhanced (Fig. 1*B*). This enhancement was not just restricted to proximal insulin signaling events but was also evident by changes in hexokinase II gene expression, which represents a more distal insulin-regulated response (Fig. 1*C*). Since the insulin-desensitizing effects of PA on Akt-directed insulin signaling were potently repressed in the absence of glucose, we assessed whether we could define a threshold glucose concentration at which glucolipotoxicity was no longer evident. Figure 1*D* shows that 0.5 mmol/L PA induced a significant reduction in insulin-dependent Akt phosphorylation when cells were incubated in the presence of glucose at concentrations >0.2 mmol/L.

To exclude the possibility that the insulin-sensitizing effect conferred by limiting glucose availability/metabolism may be a phenomenon restricted to rat skeletal muscle cells, Fig. 1*E* shows that primary human skeletal myotubes exposed to PA also exhibit significant reduction in Akt phosphorylation, which was antagonized by glucose deprivation.

It is important to stress that the reduction in Akt phosphorylation that we observe in muscle cells after incubation with PA (Fig. 1) is not restricted to this fatty acid alone. Indeed, exposure of L6 myotubes to stearate (a C18:0 saturated fatty acid) or to a fatty acid mixture comprising PA, stearate, oleate, and palmitoleate (at concentrations found in plasma of obese, insulin resistant rodents) promotes a loss in insulin-dependent Akt phosphorylation, which, in both instances, can be attenuated if muscle cells are held in glucose-free or 2DG-supplemented media (Supplementary Fig. 1).

Effect of PA and glucose availability on proinflammatory signaling. Sustained myotube exposure to PA also stimulates NF-κB signaling, which depends critically upon upstream activation of the mitogen-activated protein kinase (extracellular signal–related kinase [ERK]) pathway (19). Figure 2*A* shows that PA induces a dose-dependent activation of ERK1/2 and IκB kinase (IKK) α/β with concomitant loss of inhibitor of κB (IκB) α. However, this PA-induced activation of ERK and IκBα loss were attenuated in myotubes maintained in glucose-free media (Fig. 2*B* and *C*) or when either glucose was substituted with 2DG or this glycolytic inhibitor was added to glucose-containing media (Fig. 2*C* [compare *lanes 6* and *8* with lane *2*]). However, unlike Akt activation (Fig. 1*C*), the loss of this protein in response to PA was only abrogated when glucose was completely absent from the media. Consistent with the stimulation that PA promotes in NF-κB signaling when glucose is available, PA induced robust increases in the expression of two NF-κB target genes: IL-6 and cytokine-induced neutrophil chemoattractant-1 (CINC-1) (the rat homolog of IL-8), which was not seen in myotubes deprived of glucose (Fig. 2*E* and *F*). These findings were replicated in primary human myotubes (Fig. 2*G*).

Effects of PA and glucose availability upon intramyocellular DAG and ceramides. PA-induced increases in intramyocellular DAG and ceramide have been shown to impair IRS-1 and Akt activation (6,25,26). The ability to restrain the insulin-desensitizing effect of PA when glucose is limiting may be linked to a reduction in PA-driven

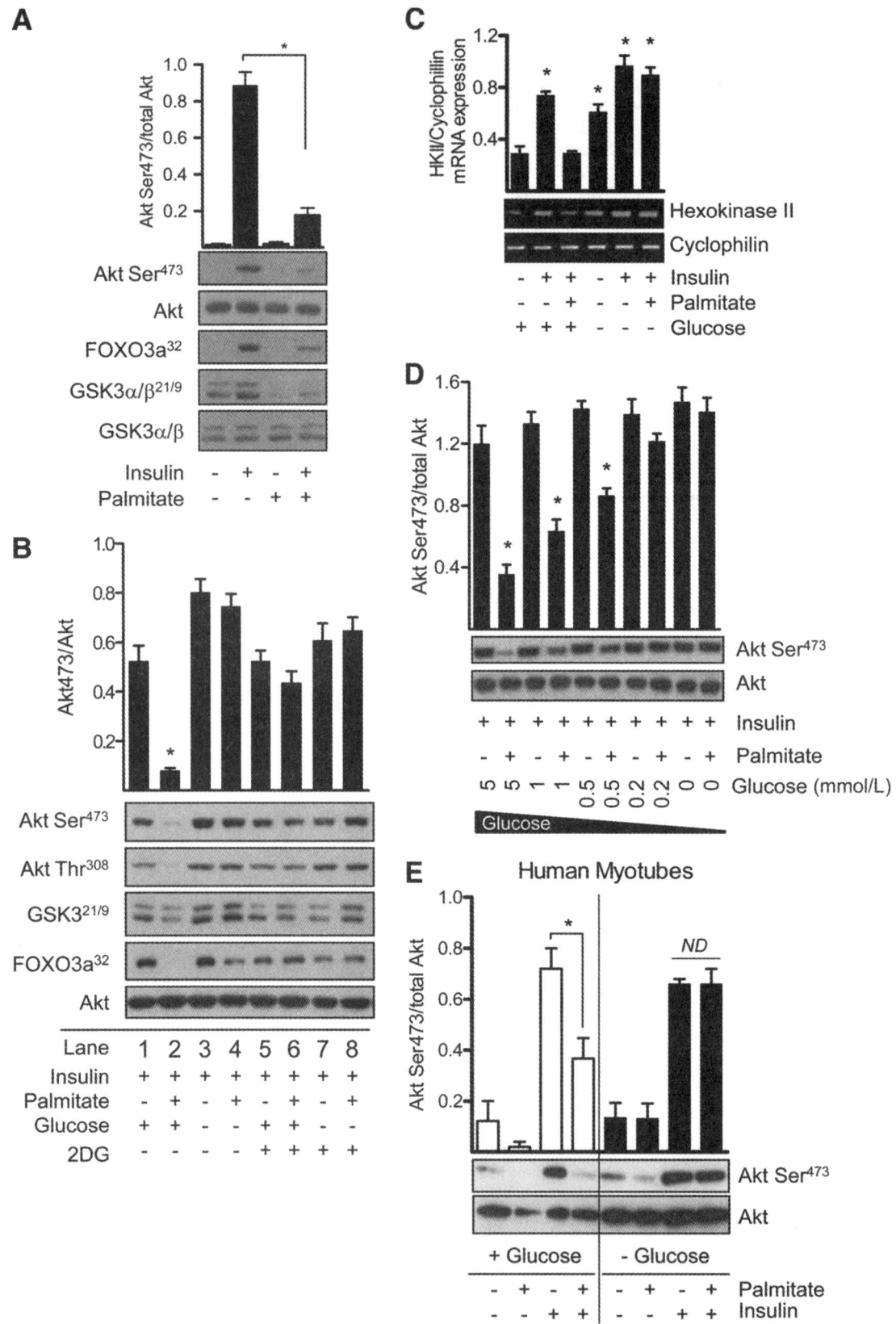

FIG. 1. Limiting glucose availability or its metabolism antagonizes PA-induced insulin resistance in L6 myotubes. *A* and *B*: L6 myotubes were treated with 0.5 mmol/L PA for 16 h in the absence or presence of 5 mmol/L D-glucose with or without 5 mmol/L 2DG as indicated prior to stimulation with insulin (20 nmol/L for 10 min). Resulting cell lysates were analyzed by immunoblotting using the antibodies indicated. *$P < 0.05$ between bars indicated or vs. non–PA treated. Data values presented as mean ± SEM, $n = 3$. *C*: L6 myotubes were incubated with 0.5 mmol/L PA in the absence or presence of 5 mmol/L glucose for a total of 16 h. For the final 4 h, cells were treated with 100 nmol/L insulin or vehicle control prior to extraction of total cellular RNA. Hexokinase II (HKII) mRNA expression relative to the internal control cyclophilin was subsequently

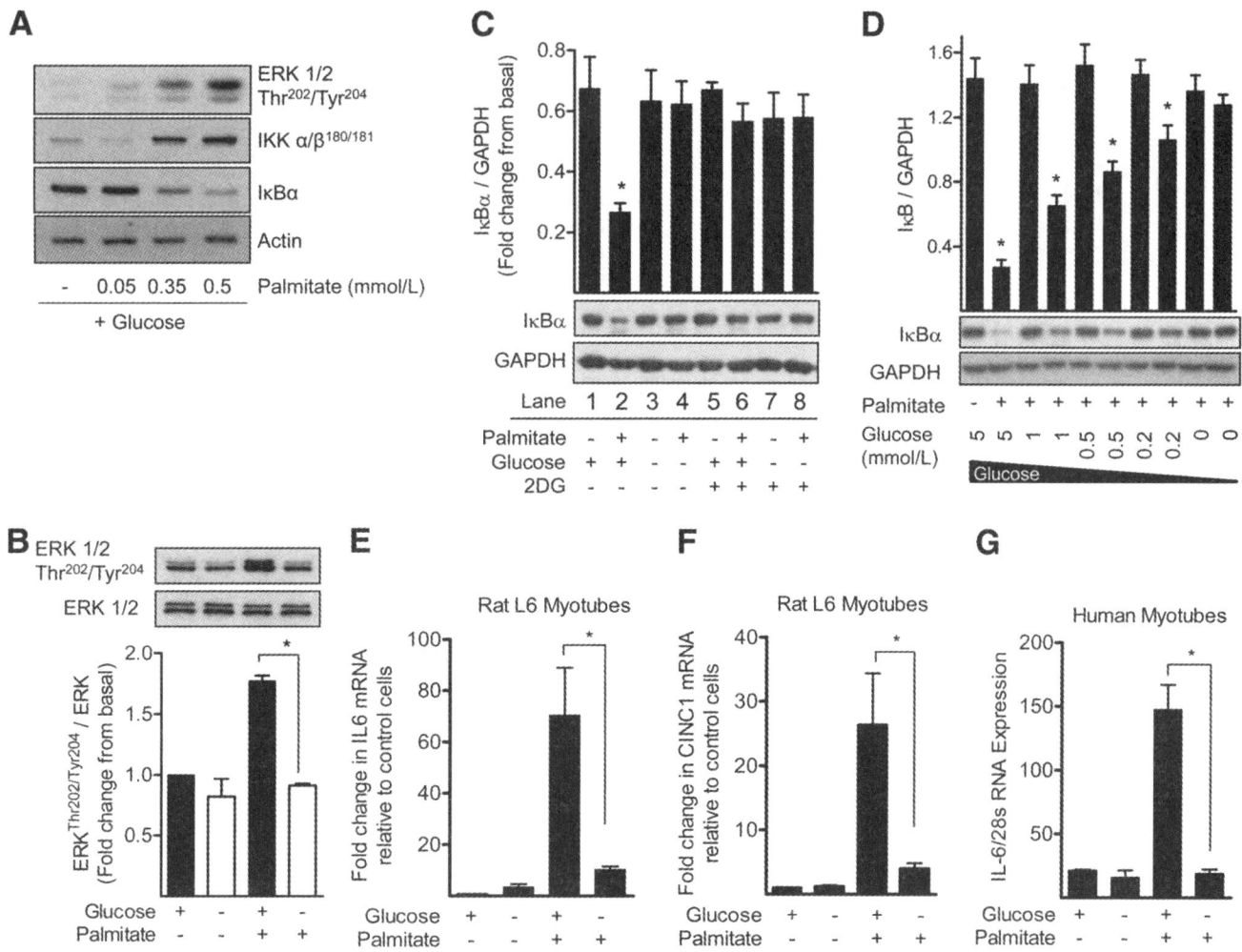

FIG. 2. Limiting glucose availability or its utilization antagonizes PA-induced inflammation in L6 myotubes. *A–C*: L6 myotubes were treated with different concentrations of PA (*A*) or 0.5 mmol/L PA (*B* and *C*) for 16 h in media containing or lacking either 5 mmol/L D-glucose or 5 mmol/L 2DG as indicated. Resulting cell lysates were immunoblotted using the antibodies indicated. *D*: L6 myotubes were incubated with 0.5 mmol/L PA for 16 h in the presence of different concentrations of glucose as indicated. Resulting cell lysates were immunoblotted using the antibodies shown. Relative band intensity values presented are the mean ± SEM from three independent experiments. *Significant change (*P* < 0.05) from the untreated control (*lane 1*). *E–G*: L6 myotubes (*E* and *F*) and human primary skeletal muscle myotubes (*G*) were treated with 0.5 mmol/L (for 16 h) or 0.25 mmol/L (for 22 h) PA, respectively, in the absence or presence of 5 mmol/L D-glucose. After cell treatments, total RNA was extracted and used to determine relative mRNA expression of IL-6 and CINC-1 to glyceraldehyde-3-phosphate dehydrogenase (GAPDH) or 28S rRNA by qPCR as indicated. Data values presented are mean ± SEM (*n* = 3 for L6 myotubes; *n* = 4 for human primary skeletal muscle myotubes). *P* < 0.05 between the indicated bars.

accumulation of DAG and ceramides. However, Fig. 3*A* and *B* shows that while DAG and ceramides were increased by more than twofold when myotubes were incubated with PA in glucose-containing media, glucose withdrawal or its substitution with 2DG had no impact on the accumulation of either lipid. Our liquid chromatography–mass spectrometry analysis permits quantification of multiple DAGs and ceramides and reveals that while most are elevated in response to PA, glucose withdrawal or glycolytic inhibition with 2-DG only affected accumulation of a few select DAG and ceramide species (Supplementary Fig. 2 [DAGs:

C18:0/C18:0, C18:1/C81:1] and Supplementary Fig. 3 [ceramide: C14:0, C18:1]). It is possible that under these circumstances, the lipotoxic effects associated with DAG and ceramide are negated by their generation in membrane compartments spatially segregated from those in which insulin signaling is initiated. To test this possibility, we incubated myotubes with increasing concentrations of C2 ceramide, a cell-permeable ceramide analog whose cellular distribution is unlikely to be constrained to specific membrane pools. Figure 3*C* shows that regardless of glucose availability, Akt activation by insulin was inhibited by C2 ceramide.

determined by RT-PCR analysis. Relative band intensity values presented are the mean ± SEM from three independent experiments. *Significant change (*P* < 0.05) from the untreated control (*lane 1*). *D*: L6 myotubes were incubated with 0.5 mmol/L PA for 16 h in the presence of different concentrations of glucose as indicated prior to stimulation with insulin (20 nmol/L for 10 min). Resulting cell lysates were immunoblotted using the antibodies shown. Relative band intensity values presented are the mean ± SEM from three independent experiments. *Significant change (*P* < 0.05) from the insulin/5 mmol/L glucose bar value (*lane 1*). *E*: Representative immunoblot for total and phosphorylated Ser[473] Akt in primary human skeletal muscle myotubes treated with 0.25 mmol/L PA for 22 h in media containing or lacking 5 mmol/L D-glucose prior to stimulation with insulin (100 nmol/L for 10 min). Data values presented as mean ± SEM, *n* = 4. (*P* < 0.05 between the indicated bars.) ND, no difference.

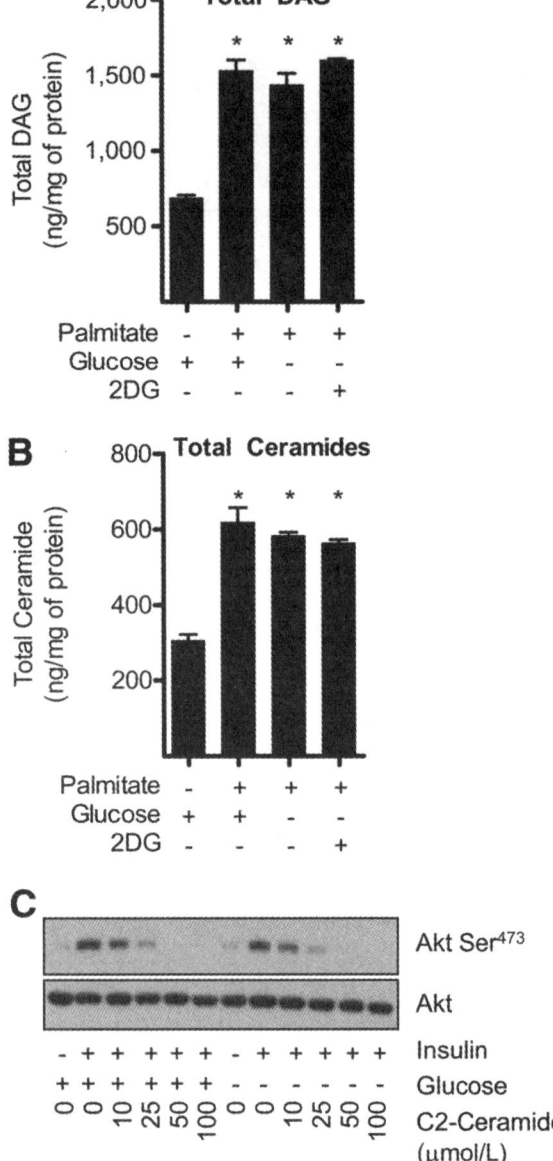

FIG. 3. Limiting glucose availability does not prevent PA-induced ceramide and DAG accumulation in L6 myotubes. *A* and *B*: Total cellular DAG (*A*) and ceramide (*B*) content in L6 myotubes after treatment with 0.5 mmol/L PA (or vehicle control) for 16 h in the absence or presence of 5 mmol/L D-glucose or 5 mmol/L 2DG as indicated. *C*: L6 myotubes were treated with different concentrations of C2 ceramide for 2 h in serum-free media containing or lacking 5 mmol/L D-glucose prior to insulin stimulation (20 nmol/L for 10 min). Resulting cell lysates were immunoblotted for total and phosphorylated Ser[473] Akt. Data are presented as mean ± SEM from three independent experiments.

Effects of substrate availability on mitochondrial function. Insulin resistance and heightened proinflammatory signaling may be a consequence of mitochondrial dysfunction induced by substrate overload. Figure 4*A* shows that cellular respiration fell significantly (~50%) when myotubes were incubated with PA and glucose. This reduced aerobic capacity was not observed when cells were exposed to PA alone or when glucose was substituted with 2DG. In line with these observations, analysis of ATP and ADP revealed that the ATP-to-ADP ratio fell significantly from 16.2 ± 1.2 to 8.1 ± 1.0 in myotubes incubated with

PA and glucose, whereas this ratio was unaltered in cells exposed to PA alone (not shown). The ability to maintain cellular respiration in myotubes treated with just PA implies that cells may oxidize PA more efficiently. Indeed, PA oxidation was approximately threefold greater than in myotubes incubated with PA and glucose together (Fig. 4*B*). This increase in PA oxidation was sensitive to 2-bromopalmitate and etomoxir, two carnitine palmitoyltransferase-1 inhibitors (27). To assess whether the reduced respiratory rate associated with PA and glucose overload is a consequence of impaired mitochondrial integrity/function, we monitored the abundance of PGC-1α, cytochrome c oxidase subunit IV (COXIV), and succinate dehydrogenase (SDHA). These proteins were reduced substantially in cells treated with PA and glucose but maintained when either nutrient was present alone or when glucose metabolism was inhibited by 2DG (Fig. 4*C*).

Consistent with the reduction in SDHA associated with glucose/PA overload (Fig. 4*C*), we observed a significant decline in fumarate, the product of succinate oxidation by SDHA, and malate, which is generated from hydration of fumarate. Intriguingly, both metabolites were significantly elevated in myotubes incubated with PA alone, most likely due to increased anaplerotic flux via reactions contributing to their maintenance. Since glucose withdrawal or glycolytic inhibition is protective against the insulin-desensitizing and proinflammatory effects of PA, we hypothesized that this may depend on using PA as fuel when glucose supply is restricted. Indeed, inhibiting mitochondrial PA uptake using 2-bromopalmitate induced a dose-dependent reduction in insulin-stimulated Akt phosphorylation and IκBα loss in response to PA despite the absence of glucose (Fig. 4*E*).

The ability to sustain PA oxidation in the absence of glucose requires maintaining levels of key tricarboxylic acid (TCA) cycle metabolites such as oxaloacetate (OAA) via anaplerotic reactions like that catalyzed by pyruvate carboxylase. As anticipated, cells incubated with PA alone exhibit a dramatic reduction in glycolytic intermediates, such as G6P and glyceraldehyde 3-phosphate (Fig. 5*A*). Intriguingly, however, despite withdrawing glucose the abundance of pyruvate (the end product of glycolysis) was maintained in myotubes treated with PA alone (Fig. 5*B*). We postulated that irreversible carboxylation of pyruvate by pyruvate carboxylase may help sustain mitochondrial anaplerosis. To test this hypothesis, the effect of phenylacetic acid (PAC), a pyruvate carboxylase inhibitor, was assessed in myotubes treated with PA in the absence and presence of glucose. Figure 5*C* and *D* show that while the insulin-desensitizing and proinflammatory effect of PA is attenuated by glucose withdrawal, this protective effect was progressively eroded by PAC in a dose-dependent manner.

Since pyruvate would normally be generated via glycolysis, it is likely that in the absence of glucose it is generated by transamination of alanine prior to being channeled into mitochondria for OAA synthesis by pyruvate carboxylase. Figure 5*E* and *F* shows that aminooxyacetate, a transaminase inhibitor (28), antagonized the protective effect conferred by glucose withdrawal upon Akt phosphorylation and IκBα.

Effects of 2DG on metabolic homeostasis in obese Zucker (*fa/fa*) rats. To validate whether restricting skeletal muscle glucose utilization confers similar insulin-sensitizing and anti-inflammatory effects in vivo, the effect of a glucopenic dietary intervention in an appropriate animal model was investigated. Obese male Zucker (*fa/fa*) rats and their lean littermates were placed on either a

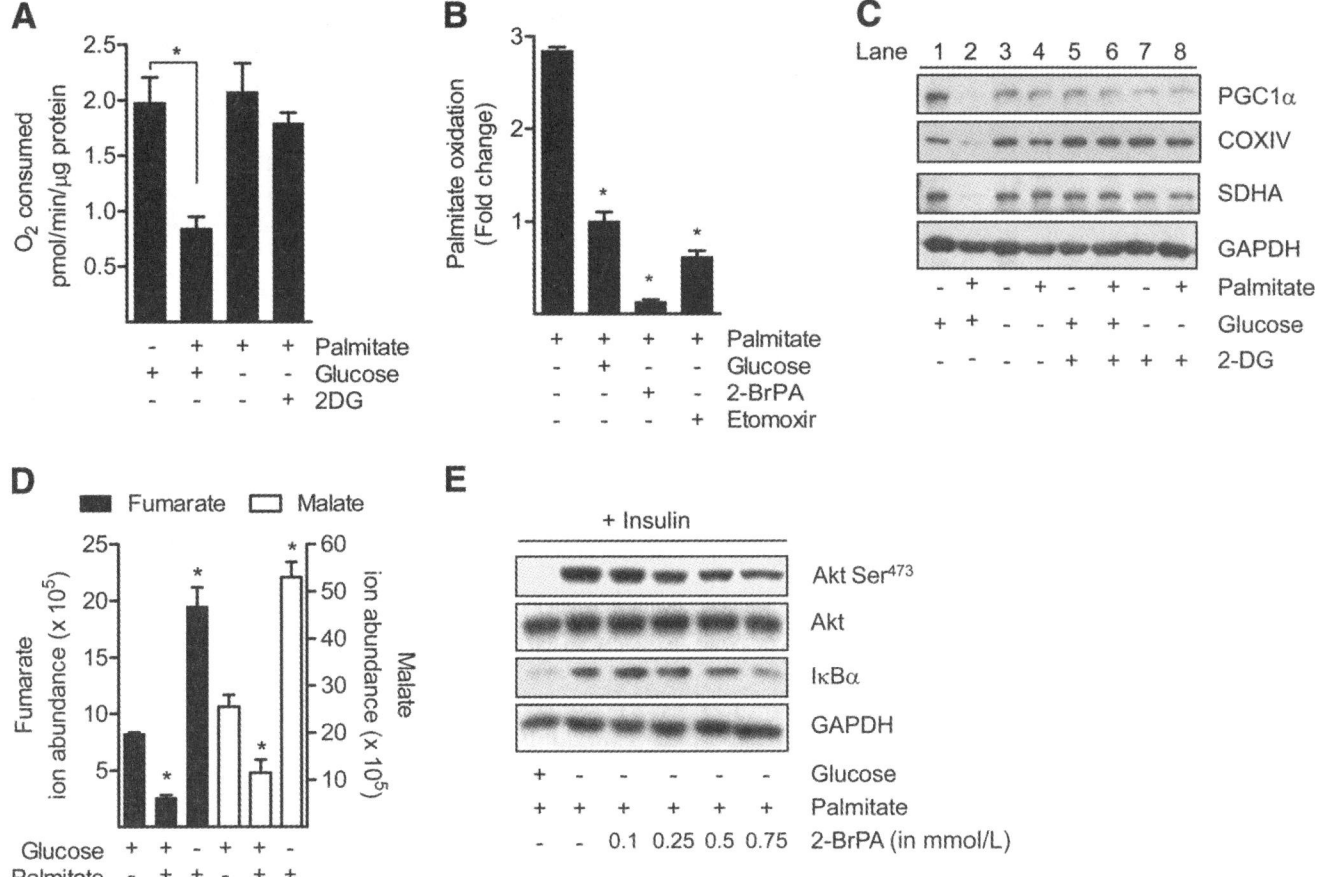

FIG. 4. Improvements in mitochondrial function in response to restricted glucose availability or its utilization contributes to enhanced insulin sensitivity and reduced proinflammatory signaling. *A*: L6 myotubes were incubated with 0.5 mmol/L PA (or vehicle control) for 16 h in media supplemented with or without 5 mmol/L D-glucose or 5 mmol/L 2DG as shown. Oxygen consumption rates were subsequently measured as described in Supplementary Data. *$P < 0.05$ vs. non–PA treated. *B*: L6 myotubes were incubated in the absence or presence of 5 mmol/L D-glucose for 3 h in the absence or presence of 2-bromopalmitate (2-BrPA) (100 µmol/L) or etomoxir (100 µmol/L), as indicated, prior to determining the rate of [3H]PA oxidation. *$P < 0.05$ compared with glucose-containing treatment. *C*: Representative immunoblot for PGC-1α, COXIV, SDHA, and glyceraldehyde-3-phosphate dehydrogenase (GAPDH) in L6 myotubes treated with 0.5 mmol/L PA (or vehicle control) for 16 h in the absence or presence of 5 mmol/L D-glucose or 5 mmol/L 2DG. *D*: Fumarate and malate content in L6 myotubes after treatment with 0.5 mmol/L PA (or vehicle control) for 16 h in the absence or presence of 5 mmol/L D-glucose. *$P < 0.05$ vs. non–PA treated. *E*: L6 myotubes were incubated with 0.5 mmol/L PA (or vehicle control) for 16 h in media containing or lacking 5 mmol/L D-glucose in the presence of different concentrations of 2-bromopalmitate as indicated. Cells were then stimulated with insulin (20 nmol/L for 10 min) and resulting cell lysates used to immunoblot for native and phosphorylated Ser473 Akt, IκBα, and glyceraldehyde-3-phosphate dehydrogenase. All data are presented as mean ± SEM from three independent experiments.

normal chow diet or one supplemented with 2DG for 28 days. Figure 6*A* shows that lean and obese rats on the 2DG diet gain considerably less weight than their respective counterparts fed the normal chow diet, although the effect was far greater (approximately threefold) in obese than lean animals (Supplementary Table 1). Although weight gain in the lean animals on the 2DG diet was consistently lower at each measurement point over the 28-day period compared with lean controls fed the standard diet, the difference between these groups (unlike the obese animals) fell short of being significant. Despite no enforced restriction on how much food animals could eat, obese rats consumed marginally less on the 2DG diet, whereas no differences were observed in food intake in lean animals (Fig. 6*B*).

Effects of 2DG upon plasma glucose, FFAs, triglyceride, epididymal fat pad, and soleus mass. Figure 6*C* shows that fasting plasma glucose remained significantly higher in obese compared with lean animals reflecting the fact that the obese animals used in our study are severely glucose intolerant and insulin resistant. Intake of 2DG induced a

modest reduction in circulating glucose in both lean and obese rats (by ~18%). This finding is consistent with the known glucopenic effect induced by 2DG consumption (29). Obese Zucker rats are characteristically hyperlipidemic. In line with this, plasma triglyceride was elevated by ~11-fold and FFAs by ~2.5-fold compared with their lean littermates (Fig. 6*D* and *E*). Although 2DG intake induced a slight reduction in plasma triglyceride in obese animals, this was not significant (Fig. 6*D*). In contrast, 2DG consumption induced a profound reduction in plasma FFAs in obese rats (Fig. 6*E*), which occurs alongside a modest but significant fall in epididymal fat mass (Fig. 6*F*). Similar reductions were not apparent in lean animals fed 2DG. No notable changes in soleus mass between animals fed the standard chow or 2DG diets were observed (data not shown).

2DG intake improves insulin signaling and reduces inflammatory tone in muscle of obese rats. Figure 7*A* shows that there were no detectable differences in the insulin-dependent phosphorylation of Akt in solei from three lean animals fed either the standard or the 2DG diet.

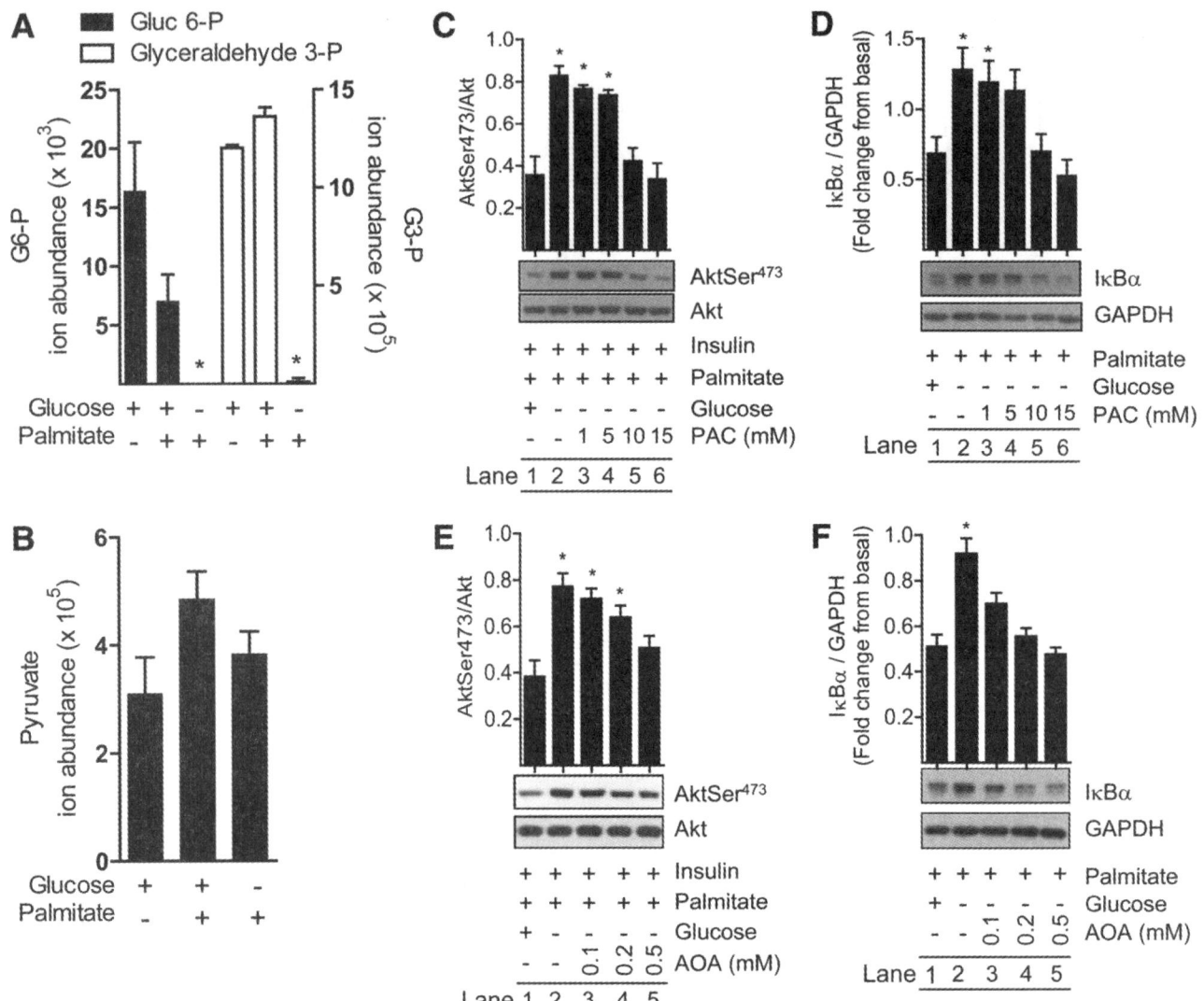

FIG. 5. Mitochondrial anaplerosis via sustained cellular pyruvate underpins the beneficial metabolic effects of glucose withdrawal. *A* and *B*: Intracellular levels of G6P (Gluc 6-P) and glyceraldehyde 3-phosphate (glyceraldehyde 3-P) (*A*) and pyruvate (*B*) in L6 myotubes treated with 0.5 mmol/L PA (or vehicle control) for 16 h in the absence or presence of 5 mmol/L D-glucose as determined by LCMS analysis. *C–F*: L6 myotubes were incubated with 0.5 mmol/L PA (or vehicle control) for 16 h in the absence or presence of 5 mmol/L D-glucose and different concentrations of PAC (*C* and *D*) or aminooxyacetic acid (AOA) (*E* and *F*) as shown. After treatments, resulting cell lysates were subjected to SDS-PAGE and immunoblotted for total and phosphorylated Ser[473] Akt, IκBα, and GAPDH as indicated. All data are presented as mean ± SEM (*n* = 3). *P < 0.05 vs. cells treated with D-glucose alone (*A*). *P < 0.05 vs. PA-treated cells in the presence of 5 mmol/L D-glucose (*C–F*). GAPDH, glyceraldehyde-3-phosphate dehydrogenase.

In contrast, a similar analysis from five obese animals on the standard diet revealed that muscle Akt phosphorylation in response to insulin was severely blunted, consistent with the significant insulin resistance exhibited by these animals (Fig. 7*B*). Strikingly, solei from five separate obese animals fed 2DG all exhibited a significant increase in Akt phosphorylation (Fig. 7*B*). Analysis of IκBα abundance revealed a significant fall in soleus of obese animals on the normal diet compared with those fed 2DG (Fig. 7*C*). In line with this, the relative expression of muscle IL-6 and CINC-1 mRNA was significantly lower in animals fed the 2DG-supplemented diet (Fig. 7*D*).

DISCUSSION

A central tenet of the Randle hypothesis is that increased provision and oxidation of FFAs in skeletal muscle suppresses uptake and utilization of glucose as a consequence of an increase in G6P that results in allosteric inhibition of key glycolytic enzymes (2). Our findings do not support this premise, given that we observed a modest reduction in the steady-state abundance of G6P when muscle cells were rendered insulin resistant by PA in the presence of glucose (Fig. 5*A*). Lipid infusion and clamp studies also show that while raising plasma FFAs in healthy individuals impairs glucose handling in skeletal muscle, such disturbances are preceded by a fall rather than an increase in intramuscular G6P as originally hypothesized by Randle (30). Together, these observations suggest that mechanisms other than a reduction in glycolytic drive are likely to play a more prominent role in fatty acid–induced insulin resistance in skeletal muscle.

Numerous studies suggest that accumulation of fatty acid–derived DAG and ceramide are better predictors of

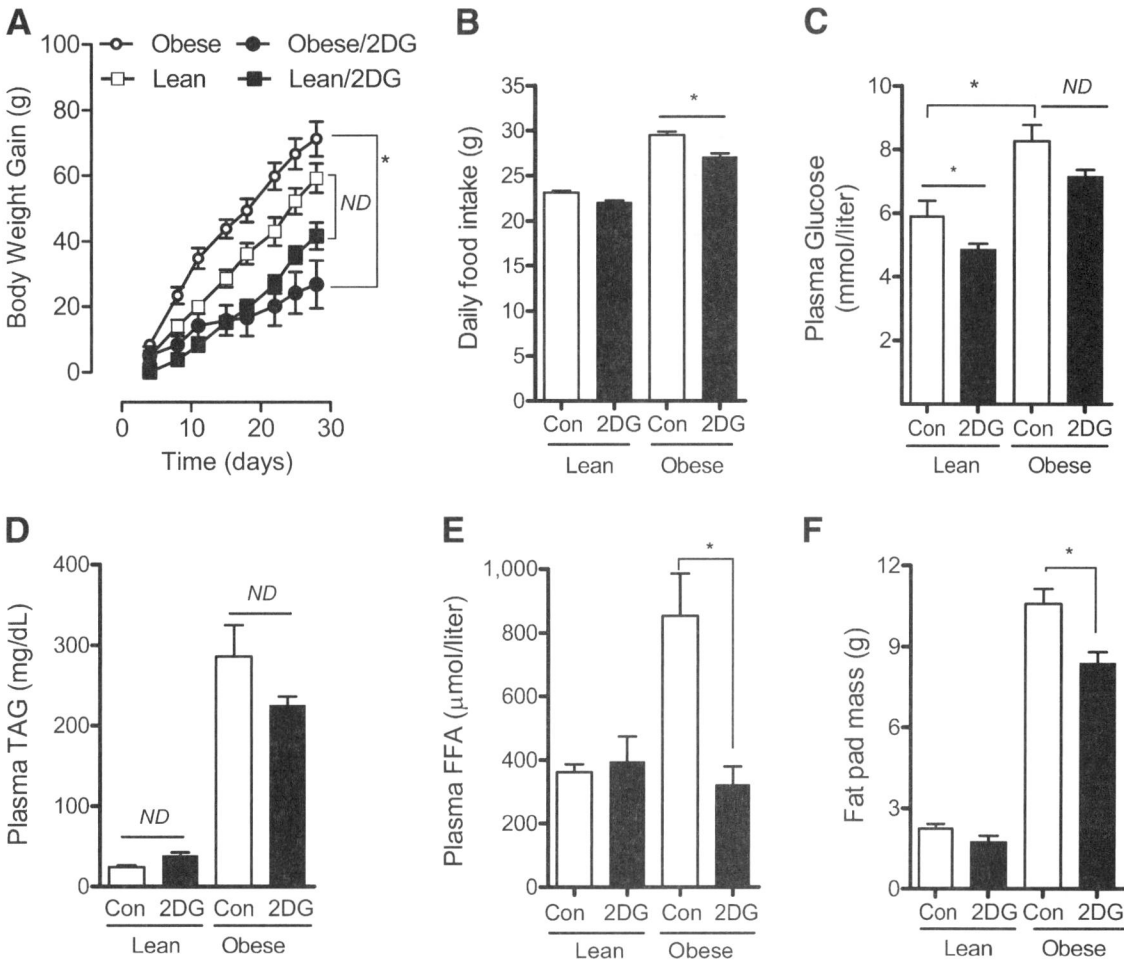

FIG. 6. Obese *fa/fa* Zucker rats maintained on a 2DG-supplemented diet gain less body weight and exhibit reduced plasma FFAs. Ten-week-old male lean *Fa/fa* and obese *fa/fa* Zucker rats were maintained on an ad libitum standard chow diet (Con) or one supplemented with (0.4% w/w) 2DG for 28 days. Corresponding changes in body weight gain (*A*) and mean daily food intake (*B*) for each animal genotype/diet group were monitored twice weekly and daily, respectively. Plasma glucose (*C*), triacylglycerol (TAG) (*D*), and total FFAs (*E*) were measured using blood specimens from anesthetized rats after an overnight fast as described in RESEARCH DESIGN AND METHODS. Average epididymal fat pad weights from each animal genotype/diet group are presented (*F*). All data are expressed as mean ± SEM (*n* = 5/group). *$P < 0.05$, obese 2DG vs. obese control. ND, no difference.

reduced insulin sensitivity (reviewed in 3,4). Indeed, studies in rodents and cultured myotubes have demonstrated that inhibiting enzymes involved in endogenous ceramide synthesis (e.g., dihydroceramide desaturase-1 and serine palmitoyl transferase) not only improves glucose homeostasis but also restrains the insulin-desensitizing effects of PA (6,31). Intriguingly, while suppressing de novo ceramide synthesis from PA is insulin sensitizing in the short term, sustained loss of serine palmitoyl transferase activity in myotubes induces greater partitioning of PA toward DAG biosynthesis, which then promotes insulin resistance via PKC-mediated serine phosphorylation of IRS-1 (6). These observations support a significant role for DAG and ceramides in fatty acid–induced insulin resistance. However, the current findings demonstrate that muscle cells held in glucose-free media are protected against the deleterious effects of PA despite increases in intramyocellular DAG and ceramide. These findings imply that the lipotoxic effect of these lipids can be muted under certain circumstances and add to the current debate as to whether their accumulation is inextricably linked to development of tissue insulin resistance (32–34). Our studies indicate that glucose or its metabolites may play a permissive role in the

pathogenic action of DAG and ceramide. Glucose availability/metabolism may not only influence accumulation of select DAG/ceramide species but also result in these lipids or their signaling effectors being spatially segregated from molecules mediating insulin and proinflammatory signaling. The finding that cell-permeable ceramide impairs Akt activation, irrespective of whether myotubes are held in media containing glucose, supports the "segregation" hypothesis. Moreover, we have previously demonstrated that a critical feature underpinning inhibition of Akt in response to ceramide is recruitment and retention of the kinase within caveolin-enriched microdomains (CEMs) (35). This targeting to CEMs is, in turn, dependent upon caveolar recruitment of atypical PKCs, which are potently activated by ceramide and which physically interact with Akt and caveolin. Intriguingly, we find that while PA induces recruitment of atypical PKCs to CEMs in muscle cells, this recruitment is substantially reduced in PA-treated muscle cells that have be coincubated with 2DG (Supplementary Fig. 4). It is currently unclear how 2DG restrains PA-induced caveolar targeting of PKCs, but the observation implies that the inability to relocalize atypical PKCs to CEMs under glucopenic conditions may,

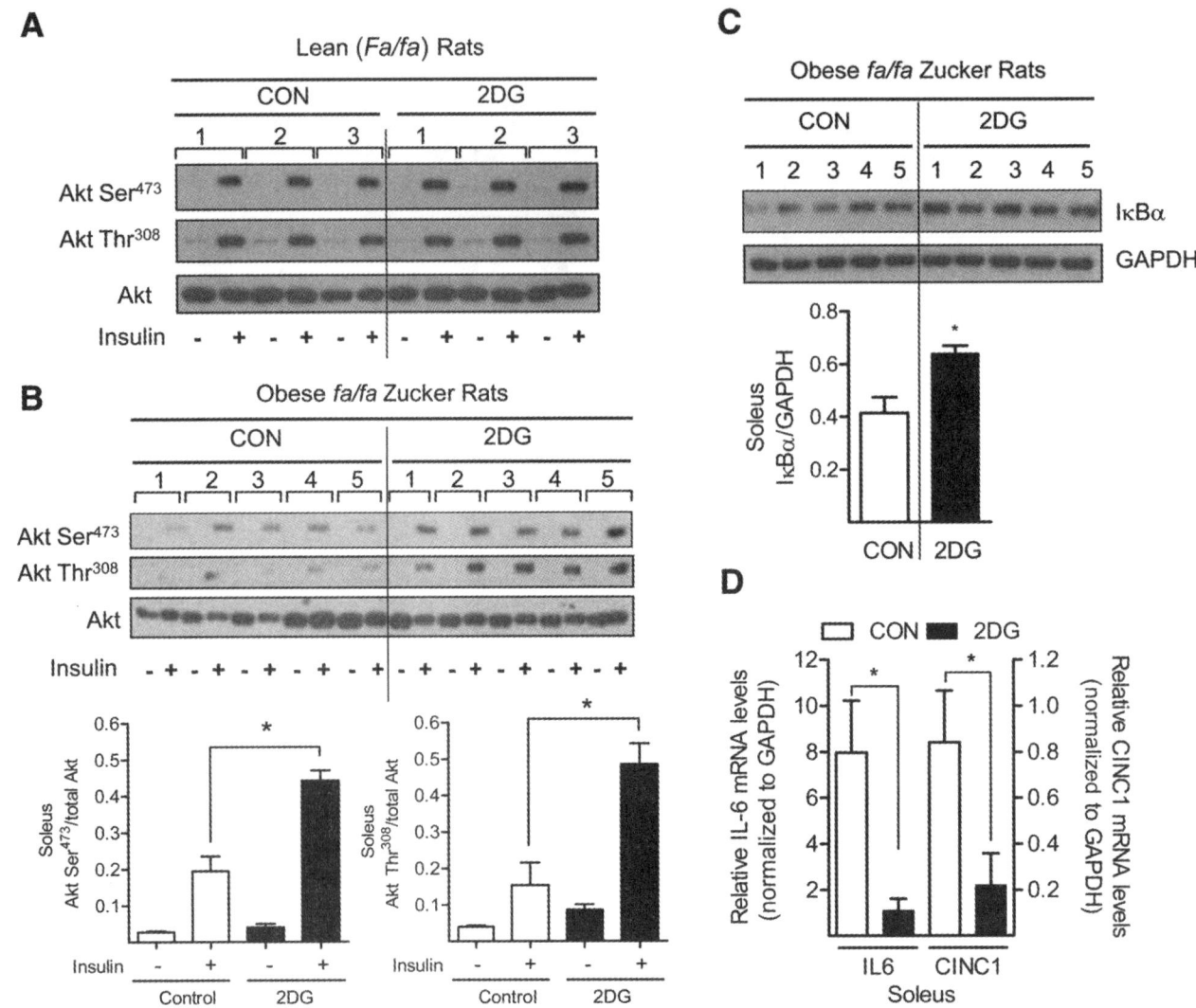

FIG. 7. Obese Zucker rats maintained on a 2DG-supplemented diet exhibit improved skeletal muscle insulin sensitivity and reduced cytokine expression. Ten-week-old lean (*Fa/fa*) and obese *fa/fa* Zucker rats were maintained on an ad libitum standard chow diet (CON) or one supplemented with 2DG (0.4% w/w) for 28 days. After overnight starvation, rats were anesthetized immediately prior to receiving an intravenous injection of insulin (10 units/kg) for 5 min. Solei were isolated from each animal as described in RESEARCH DESIGN AND METHODS. Insulin signaling (total Akt, phosphorylated Ser473Akt, and phosphorylated Thr308 Akt) was measured using lysates prepared from solei isolated 5 min after insulin injection. (*A*: Lean animals, *n* = 3/group. *B*: Obese animals, *n* = 5/group.) For each animal, the phosphorylated Akt signal in each lane was normalized to total Akt in that lane. These normalized values were then averaged from the 5 animals in each group to compare insulin-induced phosphorylation of Akt (Ser473 and Thr308) in muscle of obese animals on the control diet versus that of obese animals on the 2DG diet (*B*, *lower panel*). *C*: Lysates from non–insulin-stimulated solei from obese animals were used for immunoblot analysis of proinflammatory signaling (IκBα, glyceraldehyde-3-phosphate dehydrogenase [GAPDH]) (*B*) (*n* = 5/group). Total RNA extracted from non–insulin-stimulated solei was used to determine IL-6 and CINC-1 (*D*) relative to GAPDH mRNA expression by qPCR analysis (*C*) (*n* = 5/group). All values are presented as mean ± SEM. *P < 0.05, obese 2DG vs. obese control (corresponding insulin treatment in *B*) or between indicated bar values.

in part, explain how the inhibitory effects of PA on Akt signaling are attenuated despite a prevailing intramyocellular increase in PA-derived ceramide.

It is plausible that the protective effect conferred by glucose withdrawal/2DG supplementation against the proinflammatory potential of PA may be linked to suppressing effects that the fatty acid may have upon either reactive oxygen species formation or signaling initiated via Toll-like receptor 4 (TLR4). However, we are able to discount the notion that reactive oxygen species may be involved given that application of antioxidants (N-acetylcysteine and vitamin C) did not curtail PA-induced activation of the ERK-IKK signaling axis (Supplementary Fig. 5). The involvement of TLR4 in our cells can also be excluded, given that while LPS (a TLR4 ligand) induced IKK-directed signaling in bone marrow

dendritic cells, it had no observable effect on proinflammtory NF-κB signaling in our muscle cells (Supplementary Fig. 6).

Mitochondrial dysfunction associated with FFA overload has been implicated in the pathogenesis of skeletal muscle insulin resistance (36,37). Koves et al. (38) demonstrated that increasing FFA oxidation by chronic high-fat feeding or genetic obesity in mice imposes a major substrate load on muscle's oxidative machinery that eventually surpasses the respiratory drive for ATP synthesis. Under these circumstances, FFAs undergo incomplete oxidation resulting in accumulation of acylcarnitines, which then promote insulin resistance by mechanisms that currently remain unclear (38). Accumulation of acylcarnitines is, nonetheless, likely to be a secondary consequence of reduced mitochondrial respiratory drive brought about by the impact that sustained fatty acid overload has upon production of reactive oxygen species (39,40) and genes encoding PGC-1α and respiratory chain components that, together, will reduce the abundance, function, and integrity of mitochondria (12,13,16). Consistent with previous studies, we observe a significant decline in PGC-1α expression and mitochondrial respiration but, importantly, demonstrate that these are a likely consequence of being unable to deal with not only the carbon load born from PA but also that originating from glucose. Moreover, the improved insulin sensitivity and reduced proinflammatory drive conferred by glucose withdrawal/glycolytic inhibition requires PA oxidation, since the metabolic benefits associated with glucose restriction are antagonized by inhibiting mitochondrial PA uptake. Equally, it is noteworthy that inhibiting fatty acid entry (and, hence, influx of fatty acid–derived carbon) into mitochondria when glucose is available averts the insulin-desensitizing effect associated with fatty acid overprovision (38). Together, these observations imply that, irrespective of which metabolic fuel is available, as long as the total or combined fuel load does not exceed mitochondrial oxidative capacity and respiratory drive is maintained within a normal threshold, the fidelity with which insulin activates molecules such as Akt is likely to be upheld.

Our work demonstrates that the ability to sustain PA oxidation and preserve insulin sensitivity when glucose availability is restricted depends on maintaining mitochondrial anaplerosis. Inhibiting transaminases and pyruvate carboxylase, which support anaplerotic generation of OAA, would ultimately "run down" the TCA cycle with a concomitant decline in respiratory activity and energy balance. The failure to oxidize PA would then reinstate the insulin-desensitizing and proinflammatory potential of PA. Since inhibiting mitochondrial anaplerosis will promote incomplete fatty acid oxidation, we cannot exclude the possibility that impaired insulin signaling seen under these conditions is attributable to intramitochondrial acylcarnitine accumulation (38).

Reduced calorie intake has been shown to increase PGC-1α expression, mitochondrial density, oxygen consumption, and ATP production (41,42). These beneficial gains have been linked to sirtuin 1 (SIRT1), which deacetylates PGC-1α, thereby enhancing transcription of mitochondrial oxidative genes (43). AMP kinase (AMPK) has been implicated as a SIRT1 activator (44), and very recent work indicates that mice lacking AMPKα2 in skeletal muscle lose the insulin-sensitizing effect associated with calorie restriction (45). Since glucose withdrawal and 2DG supplementation are known to stimulate AMPK and the activated kinase supports mitochondrial fatty acid uptake by reducing cytosolic levels of malonyl CoA (via phosphorylation/inhibition of acetyl CoA carboxylase), it is plausible that the insulin-sensitizing and anti-inflammatory effect associated with glucose withdrawal may involve AMPK. In line with this possibility, we find that muscle cells in which AMPK expression/activity has been stably silenced by ~90% (46) exhibit a compromised response to glucose withdrawal in terms of repressing the PA effect upon Akt activation and IκBα loss (Supplementary Fig. 7). It is conceivable that because myotubes still express some residual, albeit small (~10%), measure of AMPK activity or SIRT1 is activated via AMPK-independent mechanisms that this may account for some of the salutary effects of glucose withdrawal that remain in the AMPK-silenced myotubes. However, while activation of SIRT1 by such mechanisms cannot be excluded, two different deacetylase inhibitors

failed to suppress the protective effect conferred by glucose withdrawal upon Akt and IκBα when myotubes were overloaded with PA (Supplementary Fig. 8).

Since calorie restriction preserves mitochondrial function and tissue sensitivity to insulin, the development of calorie restriction mimetics may offer an effective approach for combating insulin resistance and tissue inflammation in conditions such as diabetes and obesity. In accord with our cell-based observations and carbohydrate-restriction studies (47), we demonstrate that dietary supplementation of 2DG as a calorie restriction mimetic (48) in an obese rodent model induces a dramatic reduction in circulating FFAs that is associated with improved insulin-dependent Akt phosphorylation and reduced inflammatory tone in skeletal muscle. While we cannot exclude the possibility that the reduction in plasma FFAs may be a consequence of reduced lipolysis, the finding that epididymal fat pad mass was reduced significantly in 2DG-fed obese animals implies that the fall in circulating FFAs may be linked to their greater oxidation in tissues such as muscle. Whether these 2DG-driven responses in vivo are a direct consequence of enhanced mitochondrial function via, for example, the AMPK–PGC-1α axis is currently unclear, but testing this possibility more thoroughly is a major goal of future work.

In summary, our report reveals that chronic overprovision of PA induces a marked reduction in insulin action and heightened proinflammatory signaling in skeletal muscle. These responses are associated with mitochondrial dysfunction that most likely stems from an inability to match oxidative capacity to excess fuel supply. Importantly, reducing the carbon load on mitochondria by glucose withdrawal or glycolytic inhibition helps preserve the ability to oxidize PA and restrains its insulin-desensitizing and proinflammatory potential in muscle cells. In support of this concept, a glucopenic diet proffered to obese insulin-resistant animals induces beneficial gains in skeletal muscle insulin action and inflammatory status. Together, these observations indicate that strategies that maintain/improve mitochondrial oxidative capacity may help limit metabolic dysfunction associated with fatty acid overload in skeletal muscle.

ACKNOWLEDGMENTS

This work was supported by grants from the Biotechnology and Biological Sciences Research Council and Diabetes UK to H.S.H.; and, in part, by funds from the German Research foundation to C.W. (GRK 1302/2) and from the German Federal Ministry of Education and Research (BMBF) to the German Centre for Diabetes Research (DZD e.V.).

No potential conflicts of interest relevant to this article were reported.

C.L., K.M., and T.S. participated in the design, execution, and analysis of experimental work and data. C.W. was involved in conceiving the experimental/research program, data interpretation, and manuscript preparation and editing. A.B.-Z. and M.B. participated in the design, execution, and analysis of experimental work and data. J.G. was involved in conceiving the experimental/research program, data interpretation, and manuscript preparation and editing. K.B. participated in the design, execution, and analysis of experimental work and data. H.S.H. was involved in conceiving the experimental/research program, data interpretation, and manuscript preparation and editing. H.S.H. is the guarantor of this work and, as such, had full access to all the data in the study and takes responsibility for the integrity of the data and the accuracy of the data analysis.

The authors thank Heike Runge (University of Tübingen) for excellent technical assistance and Dr. Clare Stretton (University of Dundee) for useful discussions.

REFERENCES

1. Boden G. Obesity, insulin resistance and free fatty acids. Curr Opin Endocrinol Diabetes Obes 2011;18:139–143
2. Randle PJ, Garland PB, Hales CN, Newsholme EA. The glucose fatty-acid cycle. Its role in insulin sensitivity and the metabolic disturbances of diabetes mellitus. Lancet 1963;1:785–789
3. Erion DM, Shulman GI. Diacylglycerol-mediated insulin resistance. Nat Med 2010;16:400–402
4. Chavez JA, Summers SA. A ceramide-centric view of insulin resistance. Cell Metab 2012;15:585–594
5. Yu C, Chen Y, Cline GW, et al. Mechanism by which fatty acids inhibit insulin activation of insulin receptor substrate-1 (IRS-1)-associated phosphatidylinositol 3-kinase activity in muscle. J Biol Chem 2002;277:50230–50236
6. Watson ML, Coghlan M, Hundal HS. Modulating serine palmitoyl transferase (SPT) expression and activity unveils a crucial role in lipid-induced insulin resistance in rat skeletal muscle cells. Biochem J 2009;417:791–801
7. Lipina C, Hundal HS. Sphingolipids: agents provocateurs in the pathogenesis of insulin resistance. Diabetologia 2011;54:1596–1607
8. Kim JY, Hickner RC, Cortright RL, Dohm GL, Houmard JA. Lipid oxidation is reduced in obese human skeletal muscle. Am J Physiol Endocrinol Metab 2000;279:E1039–E1044
9. Kelley DE, He J, Menshikova EV, Ritov VB. Dysfunction of mitochondria in human skeletal muscle in type 2 diabetes. Diabetes 2002;51:2944–2950
10. Petersen KF, Befroy D, Dufour S, et al. Mitochondrial dysfunction in the elderly: possible role in insulin resistance. Science 2003;300:1140–1142
11. Ritov VB, Menshikova EV, He J, Ferrell RE, Goodpaster BH, Kelley DE. Deficiency of subsarcolemmal mitochondria in obesity and type 2 diabetes. Diabetes 2005;54:8–14
12. Sparks LM, Xie H, Koza RA, et al. A high-fat diet coordinately downregulates genes required for mitochondrial oxidative phosphorylation in skeletal muscle. Diabetes 2005;54:1926–1933
13. Heilbronn LK, Gan SK, Turner N, Campbell LV, Chisholm DJ. Markers of mitochondrial biogenesis and metabolism are lower in overweight and obese insulin-resistant subjects. J Clin Endocrinol Metab 2007;92:1467–1473
14. Gao Z, Hwang D, Bataille F, et al. Serine phosphorylation of insulin receptor substrate 1 by inhibitor kappa B kinase complex. J Biol Chem 2002;277:48115–48121
15. Sinha S, Perdomo G, Brown NF, O'Doherty RM. Fatty acid-induced insulin resistance in L6 myotubes is prevented by inhibition of activation and nuclear localization of nuclear factor kappa B. J Biol Chem 2004;279:41294–41301
16. Petersen KF, Dufour S, Befroy D, Garcia R, Shulman GI. Impaired mitochondrial activity in the insulin-resistant offspring of patients with type 2 diabetes. N Engl J Med 2004;350:664–671
17. Chen XH, Zhao YP, Xue M, et al. TNF-alpha induces mitochondrial dysfunction in 3T3-L1 adipocytes. Mol Cell Endocrinol 2010;328:63–69
18. Zhang J, Gao Z, Yin J, Quon MJ, Ye J. S6K directly phosphorylates IRS-1 on Ser-270 to promote insulin resistance in response to TNF-(alpha) signaling through IKK2. J Biol Chem 2008;283:35375–35382
19. Green CJ, Macrae K, Fogarty S, Hardie DG, Sakamoto K, Hundal HS. Counter-modulation of fatty acid-induced pro-inflammatory nuclear factor κB signalling in rat skeletal muscle cells by AMP-activated protein kinase. Biochem J 2011;435:463–474
20. Weigert C, Brodbeck K, Staiger H, et al. Palmitate, but not unsaturated fatty acids, induces the expression of interleukin-6 in human myotubes through proteasome-dependent activation of nuclear factor-kappaB. J Biol Chem 2004;279:23942–23952
21. Blachnio-Zabielska AU, Persson XM, Koutsari C, Zabielski P, Jensen MD. A liquid chromatography/tandem mass spectrometry method for measuring the in vivo incorporation of plasma free fatty acids into intramyocellular ceramides in humans. Rapid Commun Mass Spectrom 2012;26:1134–1140
22. Dimopoulos N, Watson M, Sakamoto K, Hundal HS. Differential effects of palmitate and palmitoleate on insulin action and glucose utilization in rat L6 skeletal muscle cells. Biochem J 2006;399:473–481
23. Creek DJ, Jankevics A, Breitling R, Watson DG, Barrett MP, Burgess KE. Toward global metabolomics analysis with hydrophilic interaction liquid chromatography-mass spectrometry: improved metabolite identification by retention time prediction. Anal Chem 2011;83:8703–8710
24. Scheltema RA, Jankevics A, Jansen RC, Swertz MA, Breitling R. PeakML/mzMatch: a file format, Java library, R library, and tool-chain for mass spectrometry data analysis. Anal Chem 2011;83:2786–2793
25. Powell DJ, Turban S, Gray A, Hajduch E, Hundal HS. Intracellular ceramide synthesis and protein kinase Czeta activation play an essential role in palmitate-induced insulin resistance in rat L6 skeletal muscle cells. Biochem J 2004;382:619–629
26. Lee JS, Pinnamaneni SK, Eo SJ, et al. Saturated, but not n-6 polyunsaturated, fatty acids induce insulin resistance: role of intramuscular accumulation of lipid metabolites. J Appl Physiol 2006;100:1467–1474
27. Ruddock MW, Stein A, Landaker E, et al. Saturated fatty acids inhibit hepatic insulin action by modulating insulin receptor expression and postreceptor signalling. J Biochem 2008;144:599–607
28. McKenna MC, Tildon JT, Stevenson JH, Boatright R, Huang S. Regulation of energy metabolism in synaptic terminals and cultured rat brain astrocytes: differences revealed using aminooxyacetate. Dev Neurosci 1993;15:320–329
29. Wan R, Camandola S, Mattson MP. Intermittent fasting and dietary supplementation with 2-deoxy-D-glucose improve functional and metabolic cardiovascular risk factors in rats. FASEB J 2003;17:1133–1134
30. Roden M, Price TB, Perseghin G, et al. Mechanism of free fatty acid-induced insulin resistance in humans. J Clin Invest 1996;97:2859–2865
31. Holland WL, Brozinick JT, Wang LP, et al. Inhibition of ceramide synthesis ameliorates glucocorticoid-, saturated-fat-, and obesity-induced insulin resistance. Cell Metab 2007;5:167–179
32. Farese RV Jr, Zechner R, Newgard CB, Walther TC. The problem of establishing relationships between hepatic steatosis and hepatic insulin resistance. Cell Metab 2012;15:570–573
33. Amati F. Revisiting the diacylglycerol-induced insulin resistance hypothesis. Obes Rev 2012;13(Suppl. 2):40–50
34. Timmers S, Nabben M, Bosma M, et al. Augmenting muscle diacylglycerol and triacylglycerol content by blocking fatty acid oxidation does not impede insulin sensitivity. Proc Natl Acad Sci USA 2012;109:11711–11716
35. Hajduch E, Turban S, Le Liepvre X, et al. Targeting of PKCzeta and PKB to caveolin-enriched microdomains represents a crucial step underpinning the disruption in PKB-directed signalling by ceramide. Biochem J 2008;410:369–379
36. Turner N, Heilbronn LK. Is mitochondrial dysfunction a cause of insulin resistance? Trends Endocrinol Metab 2008;19:324–330
37. Muoio DM, Neufer PD. Lipid-induced mitochondrial stress and insulin action in muscle. Cell Metab 2012;15:595–605
38. Koves TR, Ussher JR, Noland RC, et al. Mitochondrial overload and incomplete fatty acid oxidation contribute to skeletal muscle insulin resistance. Cell Metab 2008;7:45–56
39. Bonnard C, Durand A, Peyrol S, et al. Mitochondrial dysfunction results from oxidative stress in the skeletal muscle of diet-induced insulin-resistant mice. J Clin Invest 2008;118:789–800
40. Yuzefovych L, Wilson G, Rachek L. Different effects of oleate vs. palmitate on mitochondrial function, apoptosis, and insulin signaling in L6 skeletal muscle cells: role of oxidative stress. Am J Physiol Endocrinol Metab 2010;299:E1096–E1105
41. Nisoli E, Tonello C, Cardile A, et al. Calorie restriction promotes mitochondrial biogenesis by inducing the expression of eNOS. Science 2005;310:314–317
42. Civitarese AE, Carling S, Heilbronn LK, et al.; CALERIE Pennington Team. Calorie restriction increases muscle mitochondrial biogenesis in healthy humans. PLoS Med 2007;4:e76
43. Gerhart-Hines Z, Rodgers JT, Bare O, et al. Metabolic control of muscle mitochondrial function and fatty acid oxidation through SIRT1/PGC-1alpha. EMBO J 2007;26:1913–1923
44. Cantó C, Gerhart-Hines Z, Feige JN, et al. AMPK regulates energy expenditure by modulating NAD+ metabolism and SIRT1 activity. Nature 2009;458:1056–1060
45. Wang P, Zhang RY, Song J, et al. Loss of AMP-activated protein kinase-α2 impairs the insulin-sensitizing effect of calorie restriction in skeletal muscle. Diabetes 2012;61:1051–1061
46. Turban S, Stretton C, Drouin O, et al. Defining the contribution of AMP-activated protein kinase (AMPK) and protein kinase C (PKC) in regulation of glucose uptake by metformin in skeletal muscle cells. J Biol Chem 2012;287:20088–20099
47. Kirk E, Reeds DN, Finck BN, Mayurranjan SM, Patterson BW, Klein S. Dietary fat and carbohydrates differentially alter insulin sensitivity during caloric restriction. Gastroenterology 2009;136:1552–1560
48. Ingram DK, Roth GS. Glycolytic inhibition as a strategy for developing calorie restriction mimetics. Exp Gerontol 2011;46:148–154

Disordered Control of Intestinal Sweet Taste Receptor Expression and Glucose Absorption in Type 2 Diabetes

Richard L. Young,[1,2,3,4] Bridgette Chia,[1,4] Nicole J. Isaacs,[2] Jing Ma,[2,5] Joan Khoo,[2,6] Tongzhi Wu,[2,3] Michael Horowitz,[2,3] and Christopher K. Rayner[2,3,4]

We previously established that the intestinal sweet taste receptors (STRs), T1R2 and T1R3, were expressed in distinct epithelial cells in the human proximal intestine and that their transcript levels varied with glycemic status in patients with type 2 diabetes. Here we determined whether STR expression was *1*) acutely regulated by changes in luminal and systemic glucose levels, *2*) disordered in type 2 diabetes, and *3*) linked to glucose absorption. Fourteen healthy subjects and 13 patients with type 2 diabetes were studied twice, at euglycemia (5.2 ± 0.2 mmol/L) or hyperglycemia (12.3 ± 0.2 mmol/L). Endoscopic biopsy specimens were collected from the duodenum at baseline and after a 30-min intraduodenal glucose infusion of 30 g/150 mL water plus 3 g 3-O-methylglucose (3-OMG). STR transcripts were quantified by RT-PCR, and plasma was assayed for 3-OMG concentration. Intestinal STR transcript levels at baseline were unaffected by acute variations in glycemia in healthy subjects and in type 2 diabetic patients. T1R2 transcript levels increased after luminal glucose infusion in both groups during euglycemia ($+5.8 \times 10^4$ and $+5.8 \times 10^4$ copies, respectively) but decreased in healthy subjects during hyperglycemia (-1.4×10^4 copies). T1R2 levels increased significantly in type 2 diabetic patients under the same conditions ($+6.9 \times 10^5$ copies). Plasma 3-OMG concentrations were significantly higher in type 2 diabetic patients than in healthy control subjects during acute hyperglycemia. Intestinal T1R2 expression is reciprocally regulated by luminal glucose in health according to glycemic status but is disordered in type 2 diabetes during acute hyperglycemia. This defect may enhance glucose absorption in type 2 diabetic patients and exacerbate postprandial hyperglycemia. *Diabetes* **62:3532–3541, 2013**

Glucose in the small intestinal lumen induces feedback that regulates gastric emptying, absorptive function, and energy intake (1–3), mediated both by vagal nerve pathways and secretion of gut peptides (4), including glucose-dependent insulinotropic polypeptide (GIP) from enteroendocrine K cells and glucagon-like peptide 1 (GLP-1) from L cells. These "incretins" substantially augment insulin secretion when glucose is given orally compared with an isoglycemic intravenous infusion (5). The rate of gastric emptying and the secretion and action of the incretin hormones are both key determinants of postprandial glycemia. However, the precise mechanism of glucose detection in the small intestine remains unclear.

Lingual sweet taste cells possess two G-protein–coupled receptors, T1R2 and T1R3, which form a heterodimeric sweet taste receptor (STR) for sugars, D-amino acids, sweet proteins, and artificial sweeteners (6,7). T1R2/R3 activation liberates the α-subunit of the G-protein gustducin (α-gustducin), leading to intracellular Ca^{2+} release, gating of a taste-specific transient receptor potential ion channel TRPM5 (8), cellular depolarization, and release of mediators that activate lingual afferent nerves.

We, and others, have shown that STRs, α-gustducin, and TRPM5 are also expressed with cellular and regional specificity in the animal and human intestine, where they may serve as glucose sensors (4,9–13). In addition to expression in intestinal sweet taste cells, some of these taste components are also expressed in separate intestinal cell populations that detect umami (T1R3, α-gustducin, TRPM5), bitter, and fats (α-gustducin, TRPM5) (4). STR activation may be linked to gut hormone secretion, because mice deficient in T1R3 or α-gustducin exhibit defective glucose-induced GLP-1 release (14), whereas the STR blocker, lactisole, decreases GLP-1 secretion and increases glycemic excursions after intragastric or intraduodenal glucose infusion in humans (15,16). Animal studies also indicate that STR activation increases the availability and function of the primary intestinal glucose transporter, sodium-glucose cotransporter-1 (SGLT-1) (17,18), although this link has not been assessed directly in humans.

Patients with type 2 diabetes frequently demonstrate disordered gastrointestinal responses to nutrients, with delayed gastric emptying in up to 30–50%, abnormally rapid emptying in a few (19,20), and a high prevalence of gastrointestinal symptoms (21). GLP-1 and GIP secretion has been inconsistently reported to be diminished in patients with type 2 diabetes (22,23), whereas intestinal levels of SGLT-1 and the capacity for glucose absorption may be increased (24). Any of these abnormalities could potentially relate to disordered intestinal sensing of glucose. We previously reported that duodenal expression of STRs during fasting was comparable in unselected patients with type 2 diabetes and nondiabetic control subjects but was inversely related to the blood glucose concentration at the time of biopsy in type 2 diabetic patients (13). In rodents, we, and others, have also shown that intestinal STR transcript and protein levels are rapidly downregulated upon acute luminal exposure to glucose or artificial sweeteners (13,25). Our current aims were, therefore, to evaluate the modulation of duodenal STR expression in response to acute changes in luminal and systemic glucose exposure in healthy humans and to determine whether

From the [1]Nerve-Gut Research Laboratory, University of Adelaide, Adelaide, South Australia, Australia; the [2]Discipline of Medicine, University of Adelaide, Adelaide, South Australia, Australia; the [3]Centre of Research Excellence in Translating Nutritional Science to Good Health, University of Adelaide, Adelaide, South Australia, Australia; the [4]Department of Gastroenterology and Hepatology, Royal Adelaide Hospital, Adelaide, South Australia, Australia; the [5]Department of Endocrinology and Metabolism, Shanghai Renji Hospital, Shanghai Jiaotong University, Shanghai, China; and the [6]Department of Endocrinology, Changi General Hospital, Singapore.
Corresponding author: Richard L. Young, richard.young@adelaide.edu.au.
Received 11 April 2013 and accepted 5 June 2013.
DOI: 10.2337/db13-0581
See accompanying commentary, p. 3336.

STR regulation is disordered in type 2 diabetes and related to changes in glucose absorption and/or gut hormone secretion.

RESEARCH DESIGN AND METHODS

Subjects. Fourteen healthy subjects and 13 patients with type 2 diabetes were studied in randomized, crossover fashion. The mean duration of known diabetes in the latter group was 5 ± 1 years, HbA$_{1c}$ was $6.3 \pm 0.2\%$ (45 ± 2 mmol/mol), and all were free of significant comorbidities and managed by diet alone. The protocol was approved by the Human Research Ethics Committee of the Royal Adelaide Hospital and conducted in accordance with the Declaration of Helsinki as revised in 2000. Each subject provided written informed consent.

Screening visit. Each subject attended the laboratory at 0830 h after an overnight fast of 12 h for solids and 10 h for liquids. An intravenous cannula was inserted for blood sampling, and subjects consumed a glucose drink (75 g glucose dissolved in water to 300 mL, labeled with 150 mg ^{13}C acetate) within 5 min ($T = -5$ to 0 min). Blood was sampled at $T = -5$, 30, 60, 120, and 180 min to measure blood glucose by a glucometer (Medisense Precision QID; Abbott Laboratories, Bedford, MA). Breath samples were collected before and every 5 min after oral glucose during the first hour, and every 15 min for a further 2 h to measure $^{13}CO_2$ concentrations by isotope ratio mass spectrometer (ABCA 2020; Europa Scientific, Crewe, U.K.). The gastric half-emptying time was calculated using the formula of Ghoos et al. (26). Gastrointestinal symptoms were assessed by a standard questionnaire (maximum score, 27), as previously described (27). Autonomic nerve function was assessed in the type 2 diabetes patients using standardized cardiovascular reflex tests, with a score ≥ 3 (of a maximum of 6) indicating autonomic dysfunction (28).

Endoscopy protocol. After the screening visit, each subject was studied twice, separated by at least a week, with female subjects studied exclusively during the follicular phrase of the menstrual cycle to limit variations in gut hormone concentrations (29). Subjects attended the laboratory at 0830 h after an overnight fast, and an insulin/glucose clamp was established to achieve euglycemia (~5 mmol/L) or hyperglycemia (~12 mmol/L) (30). A 50-mL intravenous bolus of 25% glucose (Baxter Healthcare, Old Toongabbie, NSW, Australia) was administered on the hyperglycemic day, and 0.9% saline (Baxter Healthcare) on the euglycemic day, over 1 min each, followed by continuous infusion of the same solution starting at 150 mL/h and adjusted according to blood glucose measurements every 5 min on the hyperglycemic day or remaining at 150 mL/h on the euglycemic day. On the euglycemic day, 25% dextrose was infused intravenously if the blood glucose concentration fell below 5 mmol/L. In addition, 100 IU of insulin (Actrapid; Novo Nordisk, Baulkham Hills, NSW, Australia), in 500 mL 4% succinylated gelatin solution (Gelofusine; B. Braun Australia, Bella Vista, NSW, Australia), was infused intravenously at a variable rate to maintain euglycemia. Once blood glucose concentrations were stable for 30 min (12.3 ± 0.2 mmol/L on the hyperglycemic day or 5.2 ± 0.2 mmol/L on the euglycemic day), a small diameter video endoscope (GIF-XP160; Olympus, Tokyo, Japan) was passed via an anesthetized nostril into the second part of the duodenum, from which mucosal biopsy specimens were collected using standard biopsy forceps and placed into RNAlater (Qiagen, Sydney, NSW, Australia) or 4% paraformaldehyde for 2 h. At $T = 0$ an intraduodenal infusion containing 30 g glucose and 3 g glucose absorption marker 3-O-methyglucose (3-OMG; Sigma-Aldrich, St. Louis, MO) was commenced via the biopsy channel of the endoscope, and continued for 30 min (1 g/min; 4 kcal/min). At $T = 10$ and $T = 30$ min, additional biopsy specimens were collected. Blood samples (20 mL) were taken every 10 min over 1 h to determine concentrations of 3-OMG, C-peptide, GLP-1, and GIP.

Assays. Plasma total GLP-1 concentrations were measured by radioimmunoassay (GLPIT-36HK; Millipore, Billerica, MA) with sensitivity of 3 pmol/L and intra- and interassay coefficients of variation (CV) of 4.2% and 10.5%. Total plasma GIP was measured by radioimmunoassay as previously reported, with sensitivity of 2 pmol/L and intra- and interassay CV of 6.1% and 15.4%, respectively (31). Plasma C-peptide concentrations were measured by ELISA (10-1136-01; Mercodia, Uppsala, Sweden), with sensitivity of 15 pmol/L and intra- and interassay CV of 3.6% and 3.3%. Serum 3-OMG concentrations were measured by liquid chromatography and mass spectrometry, with sensitivity of 10 pmol/L (32).

Quantification of gene expression by real-time RT-PCR. RNA was extracted from tissues using an RNeasy Mini kit (Qiagen), following the manufacturer's instructions, and RNA yield and quality were determined using a NanoDrop (NanoDrop Technologies, Wilmington, DE). Quantitative real-time RT-PCR was then used to determine the absolute expression of sweet taste molecules. Validated human primers for T1R2, α-gustducin, and TRPM5 were used as primer assays (QuantiTect, Qiagen). T1R3 primers were designed using Primer 3.0 software (Applied Biosystems, Foster City, CA) based on target sequences obtained from the National Center for Biotechnology Information nucleotide database (Table 1). Absolute standard curves were generated by including known copy number standards in RT-PCR for each target (Table 2), as described (13). RT-PCR was performed on a Chromo4 (MJ Research, Waltham, MA) real-time instrument attached to a PTC-200 Peltierthermal cycler (MJ Research) using a QuantiTect SYBR Green one-step RT-PCR kit (Qiagen) according to the manufacturer's specifications, as previously described (13). Each assay was performed in triplicate and included internal no-template and no-RT controls. All replicates were averaged for final mRNA copy number, which was expressed as copies/50 ng of total RNA.

Immunohistochemistry. Fixed tissues were cryoprotected (30% sucrose in PBS), embedded in cryomolds, and frozen before sectioning at 6–10 μm (Cryocut 1800; Leica Biosystems, Nussloch, Germany) and thaw mounting onto gelatin-coated slides. Immunoreactivity was detected using rabbit T1R2 primary (H90, 1:400, SC-50305; Santa Cruz Biotechnology, Santa Cruz, CA), goat GLP-1 primary (1:400, SC-7782; Santa Cruz Biotechnology), monoclonal 5-hydroxytryptamine (5-HT; 1:1000, M0758; Dako Australia, Victoria, Australia), and GIP primary antibodies (1:800, AB30679; Abcam). All were visualized using species-specific secondary antibodies conjugated to Alexa Fluor dyes (1:200 in PBS-Tween 20) as previously described (12,13). Antigen retrieval (S1700; Dako) was performed for T1R2 according to the manufacturer's instructions. Nucleated epithelial cells immunopositive for individual targets were counted per square millimeter of high-power field and averaged over at least 10 intact transverse sections per subject.

Data analysis. The incremental area under the curve (iAUC) for 3-OMG, GLP-1, and GIP concentrations was calculated using the trapezoidal rule (33) and analyzed by one-factor ANOVA using Prism software (version 6.0; GraphPad Software Inc., La Jolla, CA). These variables were also assessed using repeated-measures ANOVA, with treatment and time as factors. Post hoc comparisons, adjusted for multiple comparisons by Holm-Sidak's correction, were performed if ANOVAs showed significant effects. One-way ANOVA, with Holm-Sidak's post hoc test, was used to compare differences in duodenal levels of STR transcripts between healthy subjects and type 2 diabetic patients. Relationships between transcript expression and other factors were evaluated by the Pearson correlation coefficient (r). We calculated that 12 subjects had 80% power to detect a one-third difference in duodenal T1R2 expression in paired studies ($\alpha = 0.05$), compared with control (13). P values ≤ 0.05 were considered statistically significant. Data are expressed as mean $\pm$ SEM.

RESULTS

All subjects tolerated the study well. The patients with type 2 diabetes were older than the healthy subjects, but

TABLE 1
Human primers used for absolute quantification of target genes in RT-PCR

Gene	Accession no.	Primer information	Amplicon length (bp)
T1R2 (TASR2)	NM_152232	QT01026508	94
T1R3 (TASR3)	NM_152228	Forward (5' to 3'): CAAAACCCAGACGACATCG Reverse (5' to 3'): CATGCCAGGAACCGAGAC	101
Gα$_{gust}$ (GNAT3)	XM_001129050	QT00049784	111
TRPM5	NM_014555	QT00034734	115

QT, QuantiTect primer assay (Qiagen).

TABLE 2

Human primers used to generate RT-PCR product containing target amplicon to create absolute standard curves

Gene	Forward primer (5'–3')	Reverse primer (5'–3')	Amplicon length (bp)
T1R2	TACCTGCCTGGGGATTAC	AAATAGGGAGAGGAAGTTGG	390
T1R3	AGGGCTAAATCACCACCAGA	CCAGGTACCAGGTGCACAGT	953
$G\alpha_{gust}$	GAGGACCAACGACAACTTTA	ACAATGGAGGTTGTTGAAAA	491
TRPM5	CTTGCTGCCCTAGTGAAC	CTGCAGGAAGTCCTTGAGTA	639

gastrointestinal symptom scores, BMI, and gastric emptying of glucose did not differ (Table 3). Five type 2 diabetic patients had autonomic dysfunction, but none had evidence of peripheral neuropathy, nephropathy, retinopathy, or macrovascular complications. As expected, blood glucose concentrations were higher in type 2 diabetic patients during fasting and after oral glucose ($P < 0.05$; Fig. 1A).

Baseline STR expression. Transcripts for T1R2, T1R3, α-gustducin, and TRPM5 were readily detected in duodenal biopsy specimens by quantitative RT-PCR. TRPM5 was the most abundant STR transcript in all subjects, with lower levels of α-gustducin and much lower levels of T1R2 and T1R3; T1R2 was the least expressed transcript (Fig. 2A). TRPM5 transcript levels in healthy subjects during euglycemia were 34 ± 8-fold higher than those of T1R2 ($P < 0.001$), whereas α-gustducin levels were 22 ± 7-fold higher ($P < 0.05$) and T1R3 levels were 12 ± 5-fold higher.

Effects of acute changes in glycemia on STR expression. Fasting expression of STR transcripts was unaffected by the glycemic state in health or type 2 diabetes and did not differ between the groups (Fig. 2B–E).

Effects of luminal glucose on duodenal STR expression. Owing to intersubject variability in STR expression, responses to luminal glucose were evaluated as changes from baseline. During euglycemia, T1R2 transcript levels increased in response to duodenal glucose infusion in health and in type 2 diabetes after 30 min ($+5.9 \times 10^4$ and $+5.8 \times 10^4$ copies; Fig. 3A). During hyperglycemia, T1R2 transcript levels decreased in healthy subjects after 30 min (-1.4×10^4 copies) but increased in type 2 diabetic patients ($+6.9 \times 10^5$ copies), so that levels in health were lower at 30 min during hyperglycemia than euglycemia and lower than in type 2 diabetic patients during either glycemic state (subject × time interactions $P < 0.01$ for each). Levels of T1R3, α-gustducin, and

TRPM5 transcript, in contrast, did not significantly change in response to luminal glucose under either glycemic condition (Fig. 3B–D).

Plasma hormone concentrations. Fasting plasma GLP-1 concentrations did not differ between health and type 2 diabetes and were not acutely affected by the glycemic state. Plasma GLP-1 increased in response to duodenal glucose infusion in all groups ($P < 0.001$; Fig. 1C), with higher concentrations evident in type 2 diabetic patients at 40 min irrespective of glycemic status (subject × time interactions $P < 0.01$) and at 50 min during euglycemia compared with healthy subjects (subject × time interactions $P < 0.05$). The iAUC for GLP-1 was higher in type 2 diabetic patients during euglycemia and hyperglycemia compared with healthy subjects ($P < 0.05$ each; Table 4).

Fasting plasma GIP concentrations did not differ between healthy subjects and type 2 diabetic patients and were not acutely affected by the glycemic state. Plasma GIP increased in response to duodenal glucose infusion in both groups ($P < 0.001$; Fig. 1D), with higher GIP concentrations evident in type 2 diabetic patients at 40 min irrespective of glycemic status and higher concentrations during euglycemia at 20 and 50 min compared with healthy subjects (subject × time interaction $P < 0.05$). The iAUC was higher in type 2 diabetic patients during euglycemia compared with healthy subjects ($P < 0.05$; Table 4).

Fasting C-peptide concentrations were higher during hyperglycemia than during euglycemia in healthy subjects ($P < 0.001$; Fig. 1E) but not in type 2 diabetic patients. C-peptide concentrations increased in response to duodenal glucose infusion in both groups during hyperglycemia (subject × time interaction $P < 0.05$; iAUC $P < 0.001$) but not during euglycemia (Fig. 1E and Table 4). C-peptide concentrations during hyperglycemia were higher in healthy subjects than in type 2 diabetic patients throughout the

TABLE 3

Demographic, anthropometric, metabolic, and gastrointestinal parameters of the study participants

	Healthy subjects $n = 14$	Type 2 diabetic patients $n = 13$	P value
Sex			
Male	9	4	
Female	5	9	
Age (years)	31 ± 3	66 ± 2	<0.001
BMI (kg/m^2)	25 ± 1	27 ± 1	NS
HbA$_{1c}$ (%)		6.3 ± 0.2	
Duration of known diabetes (years)		5.0 ± 0.9	
Fasting blood glucose at screening (mmol/L)	5.9 ± 0.2	7.4 ± 0.4	<0.01
2-h blood glucose after oral load (mmol/L)	6.3 ± 0.4	12.3 ± 1.1	<0.001
Gastrointestinal symptom score (maximum, 27)	1.9 ± 0.6	1.2 ± 0.3	NS
Autonomic function score (maximum, 6)		2.6 ± 0.5	
Gastric half-emptying (min)	123 ± 8	130 ± 12	NS

Data are number or mean $\pm$ SEM. NS, not significant.

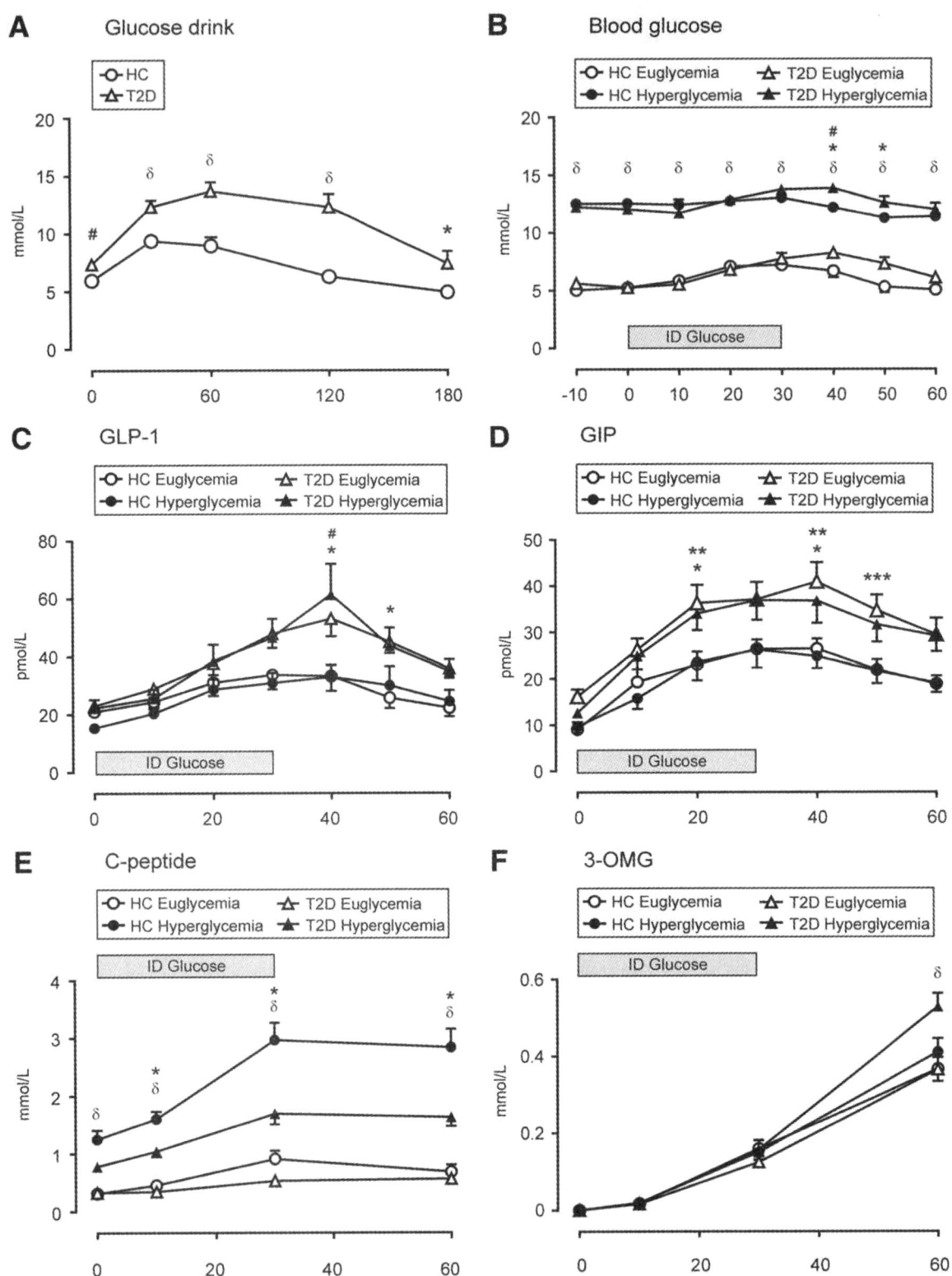

FIG. 1. Effects of oral glucose or intraduodenal (ID) glucose infusion on blood glucose levels and plasma levels of hormones and the glucose absorption marker 3-OMG in healthy control (HC) subjects and type 2 diabetic (T2D) patients during euglycemia or hyperglycemia. (A) Blood glucose levels after a glucose drink in HC subjects and T2D patients. *$P < 0.05$, #$P < 0.01$, δ$P < 0.001$ T2D compared with HC. (B) Blood glucose levels after ID glucose infusion during glycemic clamp. δ$P < 0.001$ HC euglycemic compared with hyperglycemic groups and T2D euglycemic compared with T2D hyperglycemic; *$P < 0.05$ T2D euglycemic compared with HC euglycemic; #$P < 0.05$ T2D hyperglycemic compared with HC hyperglycemic. (C) Plasma GLP-1. *$P < 0.05$ T2D groups compared with HC euglycemic; #$P < 0.01$ T2D groups compared with HC hyperglycemic. (D) Plasma GIP. *$P < 0.05$ T2D groups compared with HC euglycemic; **$P < 0.05$ T2D groups compared with HC hyperglycemic; ***$P < 0.05$ T2D euglycemic compared with HC groups. (E) C-peptide. δ$P < 0.001$ HC hyperglycemic compared with euglycemic groups; *$P < 0.05$ T2D hyperglycemic compared with other groups. (F) 3-OMG. δ$P < 0.001$ T2D hyperglycemic compared with other groups. Data are mean ± SEM; significance represents treatment × time interactions.

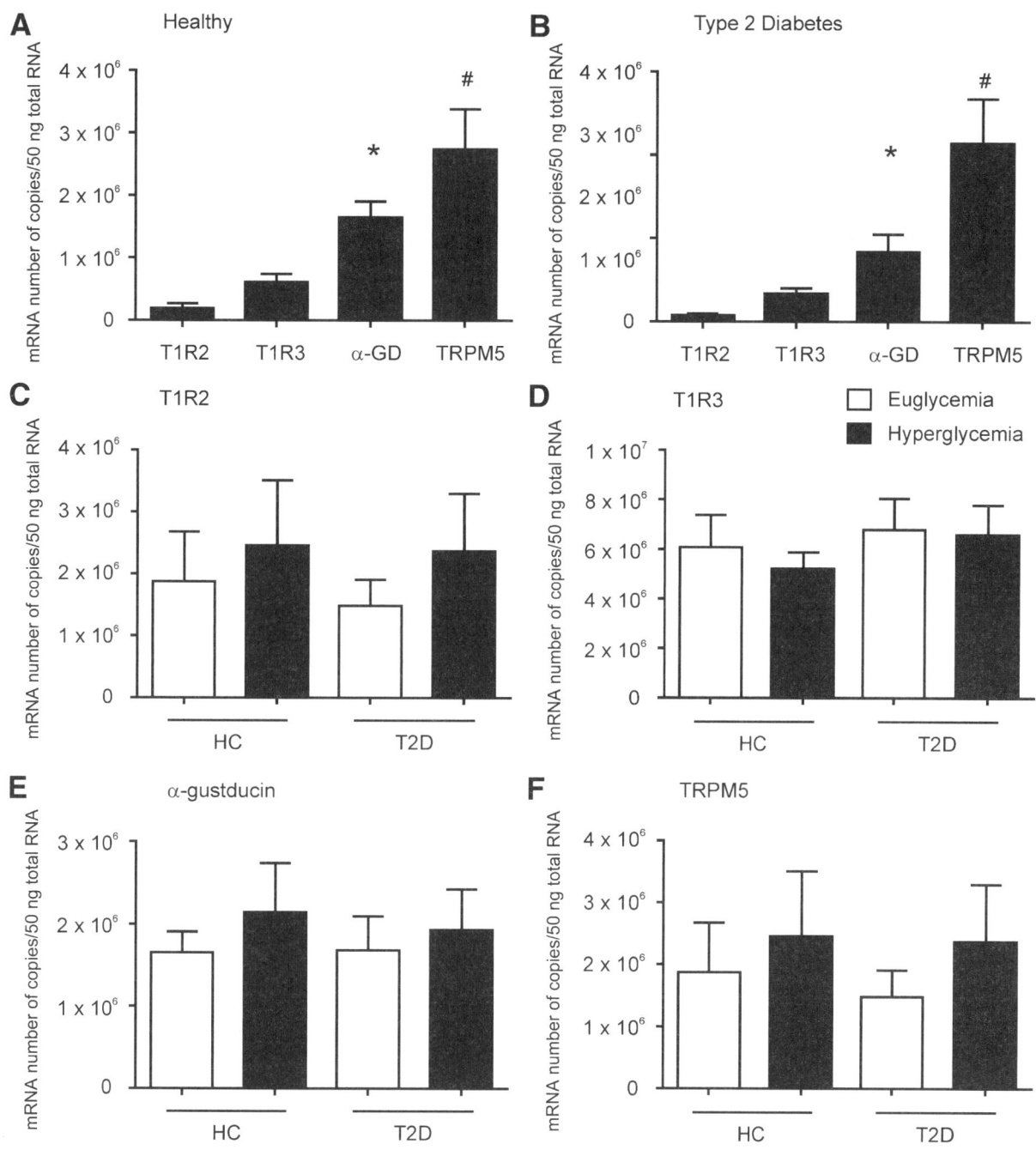

FIG. 2. Absolute transcript levels of STR in the duodenum of healthy subjects and type 2 diabetic patients at stable euglycemia and hyperglycemia. Absolute expression (copy number) of STR transcripts at baseline in the duodenum of healthy subjects (*A*) or patients with type 2 diabetes (*B*). (*A*) TRPM5 levels were 15-fold higher, α-gustducin 9-fold higher, and T1R3 3-fold higher than T1R2 levels in healthy subjects. (*B*) TRPM5 levels were 29-fold higher, α-gustducin 11-fold higher, and T1R3 5-fold higher than T1R2 levels in patients with type 2 diabetes. *$P < 0.05$ and #$P < 0.01$ compared with T1R2. Duodenal levels of T1R2 (*C*), T1R3 (*D*), α-gustducin (*E*), and TRPM5 (*F*) transcript in healthy control (HC) subjects and type 2 diabetic (T2D) patients at stable euglycemia or hyperglycemia. No significant differences in transcript levels were detected at stable baseline. Data are mean ± SEM. α-GD, α-gustducin

glucose infusion (subject × time interaction $P < 0.05$; iAUC $P < 0.001$).

Serum 3-OMG concentrations. Serum 3-OMG concentrations increased over time in all groups but were higher at 60 min in type 2 diabetic patients during hyperglycemia than in any other group (subject × time interaction $P < 0.001$; Fig. 1*F*). The iAUC for 3-OMG was higher in type 2 diabetic patients and in healthy subjects during hyperglycemia than during euglycemia ($P < 0.05$; Table 4).

Phenotype of human intestinal sweet taste cells. Immunolabeling for T1R2 was evident in single cells dispersed throughout the mucosal epithelium in healthy subjects and type 2 diabetic patients (Fig. 4). Immunopositive cells showed a homogenous distribution of the label throughout the cytoplasm, were largely open or "flask-shaped," and were found with equal frequency within villi or crypts. In dual-labeling experiments in healthy subjects, 19 ± 11% of T1R2-labeled duodenal cells

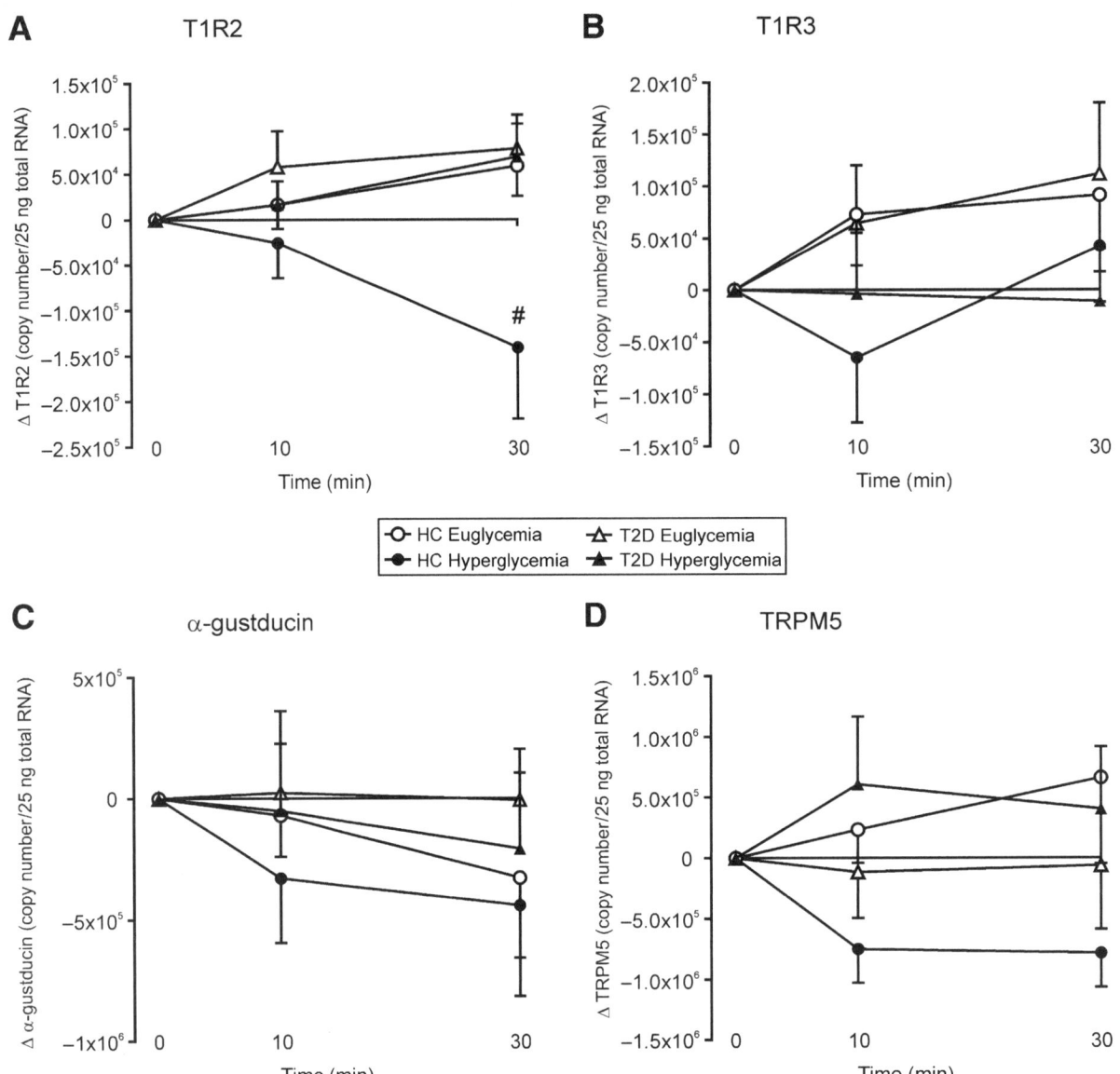

FIG. 3. Effects of intraduodenal glucose infusion on sweet taste molecule transcript levels in healthy control (HC) subjects and type 2 diabetic (T2D) patients during euglycemia or hyperglycemia. (A) Change in absolute expression of T1R2 in human duodenum during intraduodenal glucose infusion under euglycemic or hyperglycemic clamp. #$P < 0.01$ HC hyperglycemic compared with all other groups. T1R3 (B), α-gustducin (C), and TRPM5 (D). Data are mean ± SEM.

coexpressed GLP-1, whereas 13 ± 8% of L cells coexpressed T1R2 (Fig. 4A). In a similar manner, 15 ± 10% of T1R2-labeled duodenal cells coexpressed GIP, whereas 12 ± 8% of K cells coexpressed T1R2 (Fig. 4B). Separate populations of T1R2-labeled cells coexpressed 5-HT (31 ± 6%),

whereas 5 ± 1% of enterochromaffin (EC) cells coexpressed T1R2 in healthy subjects (Fig. 4C). During fasting, an equivalent number of T1R2 immunopositive cells were evident in healthy subjects and in type 2 diabetic patients, under euglycemia or hyperglycemia, and the

TABLE 4
iAUC for GLP-1, GIP, C-peptide, and 3-OMG in healthy subjects and type 2 diabetic patients

iAUC$_{60}$ (pmol/L/min)	Healthy subjects		Type 2 diabetic patients		P value (one-factor ANOVA)
	Euglycemia	Hyperglycemia	Euglycemia	Hyperglycemia	
GLP-1	1,530 ± 152	1,403 ± 122	2,373 ± 219[a,b]	2,446 ± 354[a,b]	<0.05[a,b]
GIP	1,308 ± 126	1,261 ± 160	1,978 ± 181[a,b]	1,849 ± 197	<0.05[a,b]
C-peptide	2,028 ± 178	7,796 ± 715[a]	1,599 ± 184[b]	4,756 ± 405[a,b,c]	<0.001[a,b,c]
3-OMG	542 ± 45	747 ± 55[a]	565 ± 48[b]	715 ± 37[a,c]	<0.05[a,b,c]

iAUC$_{60}$, incremental area under the curve at 60 min. Data are mean ± SEM. Significantly different from [a]healthy euglycemia, [b]healthy hyperglycemia, and [c]type 2 diabetes euglycemia.

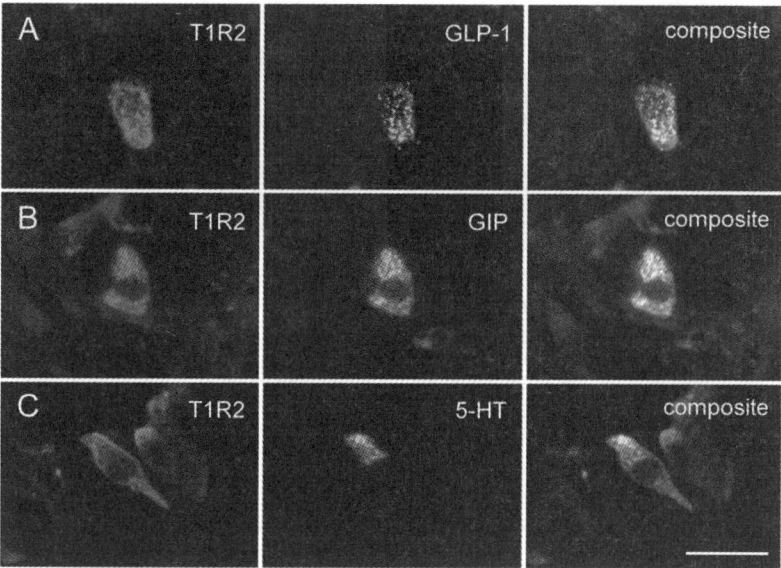

FIG. 4. Subsets of L cells, K cells, and EC cells express STR in healthy human duodenum. (*A*) Immunolabeling for GLP-1 was present in 19 ± 11% of T1R2-labeled duodenal cells in healthy control subjects at euglycemia, whereas 13 ± 8% of L cells coexpressed T1R2. (*B*) GIP was present in 15 ± 10% of T1R2-labeled cells in healthy control subjects at euglycemia, whereas 12 ± 8% of K cells coexpressed T1R2. (*C*) In a similar manner, separate populations of T1R2-labeled cells coexpressed 5-HT (31 ± 6%), whereas 5 ± 1% of EC cells coexpressed T1R2. (*A–C*) Scale bar = 20 μm.

number did not change during the duodenal glucose infusion. Similarly, the proportion of cells immunopositive for GLP-1, GIP, and 5-HT did not differ between healthy subjects and type 2 diabetic patients or with glycemic state or exposure to luminal glucose, although a trend for increased L cells in fasting type 2 diabetic patients was evident (data not shown; $P = 0.07$).

Relationships between variables. Absolute copy numbers of STR transcripts during fasting and after the 30-min glucose infusion did not correlate with age, sex, BMI, symptom score, or gastric half-emptying time in either group, and in type 2 diabetic patients, they were not related to duration of diabetes, HbA_{1c}, autonomic dysfunction, or symptom score. In contrast, the change in T1R2 transcript level after luminal glucose exposure correlated with the iAUC for 3-OMG in healthy subjects during euglycemia ($r = 0.73$, $P < 0.05$), and the change in TRPM5 transcript level with plasma GLP-1 concentrations at 30 min ($r = 0.62$, $P < 0.05$) in the same group. Changes in T1R2 ($r = 0.78$, $P < 0.01$) and T1R3 transcript levels ($r = 0.59$, $P < 0.05$) in type 2 diabetic patients during hyperglycemia also correlated with plasma GIP concentrations at 30 min, and the change in T1R2 correlated with the iAUC for GIP ($r = 0.69$, $P < 0.05$).

DISCUSSION

This study is the first to define changes in expression of intestinal STR transcripts in healthy humans and patients with type 2 diabetes in response to acute changes in systemic and luminal glucose. We have shown that absolute levels of STR transcripts are unaffected by acute variations in glycemia during fasting in either group but that T1R2 expression increases upon exposure to luminal glucose during euglycemia. In contrast, T1R2 expression decreases markedly in response to luminal glucose during hyperglycemia in health but increases under the same conditions in type 2 diabetes. Type 2 diabetic patients also exhibit increased glucose absorption during acute hyperglycemia

compared with healthy subjects, suggesting that dysregulated expression of intestinal STRs can perpetuate postprandial hyperglycemia in this group.

We confirmed our previous observation that fasting STR transcript levels are similar in health and in type 2 diabetes irrespective of age, sex, or BMI (13). Although we previously observed that levels of STR transcript were inversely related to fasting blood glucose concentrations in unselected type 2 diabetic patients presenting for endoscopy, we have now established unequivocally that acute changes in glycemia do not influence fasting intestinal STR expression in health or in "well-controlled" type 2 diabetes. The apparent discrepancy in these observations may reflect the effects of more longstanding hyperglycemia or differences in the duration of fasting in the earlier cross-sectional study. We have now shown that the intestinal STR system is, in contrast, highly responsive to the presence of luminal glucose, with rapid and reciprocal regulation of T1R2 transcripts in health, depending on the prevailing blood glucose concentration. Comparable changes were evident in T1R3 and TRPM5 transcript levels, although these were not statistically significant. Increased intersubject variability seen for T1R3 and TRPM5 transcript levels may be due to their expression in additional populations of intestinal cells tuned to detect other taste modalities and, therefore, unresponsive to luminal and/or systemic glucose.

Healthy subjects who displayed the largest glucose-induced increase in duodenal T1R2 transcript levels during euglycemia had the highest plasma concentrations of the glucose absorption marker 3-OMG. Because SGLT-1 is responsible for the active transport of luminal 3-OMG, our findings support a role of intestinal T1R2 signals in the regulation of glucose absorption via SGLT-1. Indeed, intestinal STR activation has been shown to upregulate SGLT-1 transcript, apical protein, and function in a number of species (17,18). Accordingly, reciprocal regulation of T1R2 in human health may increase SGLT-1 function at euglycemia to facilitate glucose absorption and reduce

SGLT-1 function during hyperglycemia to limit postprandial glycemic excursion. However, despite a reduction in T1R2 transcript after luminal glucose exposure during hyperglycemia, our healthy subjects still displayed greater rates of glucose absorption than during euglycemia, which might be accounted for by changes in SGLT-1 lagging behind those in T1R2. Our finding that plasma 3-OMG concentrations were elevated in type 2 diabetic patients during hyperglycemia is in keeping with the concept that SGLT-1 transporter capacity was maintained, or increased, in the presence of luminal glucose under these conditions. In fact, even small changes in SGLT-1 may increase this risk, because type 2 diabetic patients are reported to have up to fourfold higher levels of transcript, protein, and function of this transporter at baseline compared with healthy control subjects (24). We note that an increased level of facilitated glucose transport via the basolateral glucose transporter GLUT2 may have contributed to plasma levels of 3-OMG in the current study; however, the role of STR signals to direct the apical insertion of GLUT2 in enterocytes appears to be limited to rodents (25,34).

The link between STR stimulation and incretin hormone release in healthy humans is not clear. Most in vivo studies indicate that acute administration of nonnutritive sweeteners does not trigger incretin secretion in humans or rodents (35–37). Nonetheless, we observed that subsets of duodenal L cells, K cells, and EC cells were immunopositive for T1R2, in accord with previous reports (4,12,14). Together with positive associations between luminal glucose-induced changes in some STR transcripts and measures of GLP-1 and GIP secretion in the current study, it remains possible that STRs do have a regulatory role in gut hormone release. The inhibition of glucose-induced GLP-1 secretion in healthy humans by the STR blocker, lactisole (15), supports this concept. We also recognize that STR signals may serve autocrine and/or paracrine functions within the intestinal mucosa that are not reflected in circulating gut hormone concentrations; the latter appear to be a blunt marker for local concentrations of GLP-1 (38). There is also a large body of evidence indicating that the intestinotrophic gut peptide, glucagon-like peptide 2 (GLP-2), coreleased from L cells with GLP-1, is a powerful local stimulus to increase intestinal glucose transport via SGLT-1 and GLUT2 in rodents and in patients with short bowel syndrome (39–41). Importantly, GLP-2 release has recently been revealed as STR-dependent in animals and in a human enteroendocrine cell line (42,43), highlighting an important link between STRs and GLP-2 in the regulation of intestinal glucose transport.

Reports concerning postprandial incretin hormone release in patients with type 2 diabetes have been inconsistent, with plasma GLP-1 concentrations after a mixed meal being either reduced (22) or intact (44), although such studies are potentially confounded by failure to control for differences in the rate of gastric emptying, which is frequently delayed in longstanding diabetes or during acute hyperglycemia (20). Our observation that GLP-1 and GIP responses to a standardized rate of duodenal glucose infusion were maintained, and indeed increased, in type 2 diabetic patients, supports our previous findings (45) and is in keeping with the trend for increased L-cell density in these patients in the current study and a report of an increased density of L cells and mixed L/K cells in the duodenum of well-controlled type 2 diabetic patients (46). There is now strong evidence that SGLT-1

transport is a key stimulus for release of GLP-1 and GIP, which occurs even after exposure to nonmetabolized SGLT-1 substrates and is inhibited by pharmacological blockade or genetic ablation of SGLT-1 in rodents (47–49). Therefore, increased SGLT-1 capacity could explain enhanced glucose-induced GLP-1 and GIP responses in our type 2 diabetic patients. Any deficiency in the incretin effect in type 2 diabetes is likely to be explained by impaired β-cell function rather than by deficient incretin hormone secretion (45,50), and indeed, defective C-peptide responses in our type 2 diabetic patients during hyperglycemia support this assertion. Acute hyperglycemia had no effect on GLP-1 or GIP secretion, as noted previously (51,52). Although SGLT-1 transport appears a major determinant of GLP-1 and GIP release, other transporters (49,53) or signaling pathways (54) may also be involved, so increased glucose absorptive capacity during hyperglycemia may not necessarily result in enhanced GLP-1 or GIP concentrations.

Our study had a number of limitations. Transcriptional regulation of intestinal T1R2 occurred rapidly in humans, but we did not quantify changes in STR protein in parallel due to ethical considerations on the additional biopsy specimens required. However, similarly rapid changes in these proteins after glucose or sucralose exposure are known to occur in apical membrane vesicles of rat jejunum (25). We did not assess effects on SGLT-1 transcript or protein here, although measures of glucose absorption with 3-OMG reflect, in large part, SGLT-1 function as the primary intestinal glucose transporter in humans. There was considerable interindividual variability in baseline expression of intestinal STR transcripts, so that our study was insufficiently powered to detect relationships between absolute transcript levels and concentrations of gut hormones and 3-OMG. Our 3-OMG measurements were limited to 60 min, and differences between groups or glycemic states might have become more marked after this point. The duodenal glucose infusion was also relatively brief, being limited by the tolerability of unsedated endoscopy. Our type 2 diabetic patients had relatively good glycemic control, and more marked differences from health might be observed in patients with a higher HbA$_{1c}$. The type 2 diabetic patients were older than the healthy control subjects, although we have not previously shown any age-related differences in postprandial GLP-1 responses (55).

In conclusion, we have shown that the intestinal STR system is reciprocally regulated in the presence of luminal glucose according to glycemic status in health but not in type 2 diabetes. In the latter, T1R2 dysregulation potentially increases the risk of postprandial hyperglycemia, but the intestinal STR system appears unlikely to be a major determinant of circulating GLP-1 or GIP concentrations in humans.

ACKNOWLEDGMENTS

This study was supported by grants awarded to R.L.Y. by the National Health and Medical Research Council (NHMRC) of Australia (grant no. 627127) and to R.L.Y., M.H., and C.K.R. from Diabetes Australia. T.W. was supported by an NHMRC Overseas Clinical Postdoctoral Training Fellowship (grant no. 519349)

No potential conflicts of interest relevant to this article were reported.

R.L.Y. and C.K.R. conceived, designed, and supervised the study, obtained funding, acquired data, undertook statistical analyses and interpreted data, and drafted and critically reviewed the manuscript. B.C. and N.J.I. acquired data and provided technical support. J.M., J.K., and T.W. assisted in study design, acquired data, and critically reviewed the manuscript. M.H. designed the study, interpreted data, and critically reviewed the manuscript. R.L.Y. and C.K.R. are the guarantors of this work and, as such, had full access to all the data in the study and take responsibility for the integrity of the data and the accuracy of the data analysis.

The authors thank the Endoscopy Unit staff, Department of Gastroenterology and Hepatology, Royal Adelaide Hospital, for their assistance with the study; Dr. Kate Sutherland, University of Sydney, for contributing to the molecular assays in this study; and Kylie Lange, National Health and NHMRC Centre of Research Excellence in Translating Nutritional Science to Good Health, University of Adelaide, for professional biostatistical support.

Preliminary accounts of this study were presented at the Digestive Disease Week meeting of the American Gastroenterological Association, Chicago, IL, 7–11 May 2011; and at the Joint International Neurogastroenterology & Motility Meeting, Bologna, Italy, 6–8 September 2012.

REFERENCES

1. Raybould HE, Hölzer H. Dual capsaicin-sensitive afferent pathways mediate inhibition of gastric emptying in rat induced by intestinal carbohydrate. Neurosci Lett 1992;141:236–238
2. Horowitz M, Edelbroek MA, Wishart JM, Straathof JW. Relationship between oral glucose tolerance and gastric emptying in normal healthy subjects. Diabetologia 1993;36:857–862
3. Pilichiewicz AN, Chaikomin R, Brennan IM, et al. Load-dependent effects of duodenal glucose on glycemia, gastrointestinal hormones, antropyloroduodenal motility, and energy intake in healthy men. Am J Physiol Endocrinol Metab 2007;293:E743–E753
4. Young RL. Sensing via intestinal sweet taste pathways. Front Neurosci 2011;5:23
5. Holst JJ, Gromada J. Role of incretin hormones in the regulation of insulin secretion in diabetic and nondiabetic humans. Am J Physiol Endocrinol Metab 2004;287:E199–E206
6. Nelson G, Hoon MA, Chandrashekar J, Zhang Y, Ryba NJ, Zuker CS. Mammalian sweet taste receptors. Cell 2001;106:381–390
7. Li X, Staszewski L, Xu H, Durick K, Zoller M, Adler E. Human receptors for sweet and umami taste. Proc Natl Acad Sci U S A 2002;99:4692–4696
8. Pérez CA, Huang L, Rong M, et al. A transient receptor potential channel expressed in taste receptor cells. Nat Neurosci 2002;5:1169–1176
9. Höfer D, Püschel B, Drenckhahn D. Taste receptor-like cells in the rat gut identified by expression of alpha-gustducin. Proc Natl Acad Sci U S A 1996;93:6631–6634
10. Dyer J, Salmon KS, Zibrik L, Shirazi-Beechey SP. Expression of sweet taste receptors of the T1R family in the intestinal tract and enteroendocrine cells. Biochem Soc Trans 2005;33:302–305
11. Bezençon C, le Coutre J, Damak S. Taste-signaling proteins are coexpressed in solitary intestinal epithelial cells. Chem Senses 2007;32:41–49
12. Sutherland K, Young RL, Cooper NJ, Horowitz M, Blackshaw LA. Phenotypic characterization of taste cells of the mouse small intestine. Am J Physiol Gastrointest Liver Physiol 2007;292:G1420–G1428
13. Young RL, Sutherland K, Pezos N, et al. Expression of taste molecules in the upper gastrointestinal tract in humans with and without type 2 diabetes. Gut 2009;58:337–346
14. Jang HJ, Kokrashvili Z, Theodorakis MJ, et al. Gut-expressed gustducin and taste receptors regulate secretion of glucagon-like peptide-1. Proc Natl Acad Sci U S A 2007;104:15069–15074
15. Steinert RE, Gerspach AC, Gutmann H, Asarian L, Drewe J, Beglinger C. The functional involvement of gut-expressed sweet taste receptors in glucose-stimulated secretion of glucagon-like peptide-1 (GLP-1) and peptide YY (PYY). Clin Nutr 2011;30:524–532
16. Gerspach AC, Steinert RE, Schönenberger L, Graber-Maier A, Beglinger C. The role of the gut sweet taste receptor in regulating GLP-1, PYY, and CCK release in humans. Am J Physiol Endocrinol Metab 2011;301:E317–E325
17. Margolskee RF, Dyer J, Kokrashvili Z, et al. T1R3 and gustducin in gut sense sugars to regulate expression of Na+-glucose cotransporter 1. Proc Natl Acad Sci U S A 2007;104:15075–15080
18. Stearns AT, Balakrishnan A, Rhoads DB, Tavakkolizadeh A. Rapid upregulation of sodium-glucose transporter SGLT1 in response to intestinal sweet taste stimulation. Ann Surg 2010;251:865–871
19. Rayner CK, Schwartz MP, van Dam PS, et al. Small intestinal glucose absorption and duodenal motility in type 1 diabetes mellitus. Am J Gastroenterol 2002;97:3123–3130
20. Horowitz M, O'Donovan D, Jones KL, Feinle C, Rayner CK, Samsom M. Gastric emptying in diabetes: clinical significance and treatment. Diabet Med 2002;19:177–194
21. Bytzer P, Talley NJ, Leemon M, Young LJ, Jones MP, Horowitz M. Prevalence of gastrointestinal symptoms associated with diabetes mellitus: a population-based survey of 15,000 adults. Arch Intern Med 2001;161:1989–1996
22. Toft-Nielsen MB, Damholt MB, Madsbad S, et al. Determinants of the impaired secretion of glucagon-like peptide-1 in type 2 diabetic patients. J Clin Endocrinol Metab 2001;86:3717–3723
23. Vilsbøll T, Krarup T, Deacon CF, Madsbad S, Holst JJ. Reduced postprandial concentrations of intact biologically active glucagon-like peptide 1 in type 2 diabetic patients. Diabetes 2001;50:609–613
24. Dyer J, Wood IS, Palejwala A, Ellis A, Shirazi-Beechey SP. Expression of monosaccharide transporters in intestine of diabetic humans. Am J Physiol Gastrointest Liver Physiol 2002;282:G241–G248
25. Mace OJ, Affleck J, Patel N, Kellett GL. Sweet taste receptors in rat small intestine stimulate glucose absorption through apical GLUT2. J Physiol 2007;582:379–392
26. Ghoos YF, Maes BD, Geypens BJ, et al. Measurement of gastric emptying rate of solids by means of a carbon-labeled octanoic acid breath test. Gastroenterology 1993;104:1640–1647
27. Horowitz M, Maddox AF, Wishart JM, Harding PE, Chatterton BE, Shearman DJ. Relationships between oesophageal transit and solid and liquid gastric emptying in diabetes mellitus. Eur J Nucl Med 1991;18:229–234
28. Ewing DJ, Clarke BF. Diagnosis and management of diabetic autonomic neuropathy. Br Med J (Clin Res Ed) 1982;285:916–918
29. Brennan IM, Feltrin KL, Nair NS, et al. Effects of the phases of the menstrual cycle on gastric emptying, glycemia, plasma GLP-1 and insulin, and energy intake in healthy lean women. Am J Physiol Gastrointest Liver Physiol 2009;297:G602–G610
30. Rayner CK, Verhagen MA, Hebbard GS, DiMatteo AC, Doran SM, Horowitz M. Proximal gastric compliance and perception of distension in type 1 diabetes mellitus: effects of hyperglycemia. Am J Gastroenterol 2000;95:1175–1183
31. Vanis L, Gentilcore D, Rayner CK, et al. Effects of small intestinal glucose load on blood pressure, splanchnic blood flow, glycemia, and GLP-1 release in healthy older subjects. Am J Physiol Regul Integr Comp Physiol 2011;300:R1524–R1531
32. Deane AM, Summers MJ, Zaknic AV, et al. Glucose absorption and small intestinal transit in critical illness. Crit Care Med 2011;39:1282–1288
33. Wolever TM. Effect of blood sampling schedule and method of calculating the area under the curve on validity and precision of glycaemic index values. Br J Nutr 2004;91:295–301
34. Shirazi-Beechey SP, Moran AW, Batchelor DJ, Daly K, Al-Rammahi M. Glucose sensing and signalling; regulation of intestinal glucose transport. Proc Nutr Soc 2011;70:185–193
35. Ma J, Bellon M, Wishart JM, et al. Effect of the artificial sweetener, sucralose, on gastric emptying and incretin hormone release in healthy subjects. Am J Physiol Gastrointest Liver Physiol 2009;296:G735–G739
36. Wu T, Zhao BR, Bound MJ, et al. Effects of different sweet preloads on incretin hormone secretion, gastric emptying, and postprandial glycemia in healthy humans. Am J Clin Nutr 2012;95:78–83
37. Brown RJ, Walter M, Rother KI. Ingestion of diet soda before a glucose load augments glucagon-like peptide-1 secretion. Diabetes Care 2009;32:2184–2186
38. D'Alessio D, Lu WJ, Sun W, et al. Fasting and postprandial concentrations of GLP-1 in intestinal lymph and portal plasma: evidence for selective release of GLP-1 in the lymph system. Am J Physiol Regul Integr Comp Physiol 2007;293:R2163–R2169
39. Cheeseman CI. Upregulation of SGLT-1 transport activity in rat jejunum induced by GLP-2 infusion in vivo. Am J Physiol 1997;273:R1965–R1971
40. Au A, Gupta A, Schembri P, Cheeseman CI. Rapid insertion of GLUT2 into the rat jejunal brush-border membrane promoted by glucagon-like peptide 2. Biochem J 2002;367:247–254

41. Jeppesen PB, Hartmann B, Thulesen J, et al. Glucagon-like peptide 2 improves nutrient absorption and nutritional status in short-bowel patients with no colon. Gastroenterology 2001;120:806–815

42. Daly K, Al-Rammahi M, Arora DK, et al. Expression of sweet receptor components in equine small intestine: relevance to intestinal glucose transport. Am J Physiol Regul Integr Comp Physiol 2012;303:R199–R208

43. Sato S, Hokari R, Kurihara C, et al. Dietary lipids and sweeteners regulate glucagon-like peptide-2 secretion. Am J Physiol Gastrointest Liver Physiol 2013;304:G708–G714

44. Vollmer K, Holst JJ, Baller B, et al. Predictors of incretin concentrations in subjects with normal, impaired, and diabetic glucose tolerance. Diabetes 2008;57:678–687

45. Ma J, Pilichiewicz AN, Feinle-Bisset C, et al. Effects of variations in duodenal glucose load on glycaemic, insulin, and incretin responses in type 2 diabetes. Diabet Med 2012;29:604–608

46. Theodorakis MJ, Carlson O, Michopoulos S, et al. Human duodenal enteroendocrine cells: source of both incretin peptides, GLP-1 and GIP. Am J Physiol Endocrinol Metab 2006;290:E550–E559

47. Gorboulev V, Schürmann A, Vallon V, et al. Na(+)-D-glucose cotransporter SGLT1 is pivotal for intestinal glucose absorption and glucose-dependent incretin secretion. Diabetes 2012;61:187–196

48. Parker HE, Reimann F, Gribble FM. Molecular mechanisms underlying nutrient-stimulated incretin secretion. Expert Rev Mol Med 2010;12:e1

49. Parker HE, Adriaenssens A, Rogers G, et al. Predominant role of active versus facilitative glucose transport for glucagon-like peptide-1 secretion. Diabetologia 2012;55:2445–2455

50. Woerle HJ, Carneiro L, Derani A, Göke B, Schirra J. The role of endogenous incretin secretion as amplifier of glucose-stimulated insulin secretion in healthy subjects and patients with type 2 diabetes. Diabetes 2012;61: 2349–2358

51. Vilsbøll T, Krarup T, Sonne J, et al. Incretin secretion in relation to meal size and body weight in healthy subjects and people with type 1 and type 2 diabetes mellitus. J Clin Endocrinol Metab 2003;88:2706–2713

52. Kuo P, Wishart JM, Bellon M, et al. Effects of physiological hyperglycemia on duodenal motility and flow events, glucose absorption, and incretin secretion in healthy humans. J Clin Endocrinol Metab 2010;95:3893–3900

53. Cani PD, Holst JJ, Drucker DJ, et al. GLUT2 and the incretin receptors are involved in glucose-induced incretin secretion. Mol Cell Endocrinol 2007; 276:18–23

54. Reimann F, Habib AM, Tolhurst G, Parker HE, Rogers GJ, Gribble FM. Glucose sensing in L cells: a primary cell study. Cell Metab 2008;8:532–539

55. Trahair LG, Horowitz M, Rayner CK, et al. Comparative effects of variations in duodenal glucose load on glycemic, insulinemic, and incretin responses in healthy young and older subjects. J Clin Endocrinol Metab 2012;97:844–851

Teplizumab (Anti-CD3 mAb) Treatment Preserves C-Peptide Responses in Patients With New-Onset Type 1 Diabetes in a Randomized Controlled Trial

Metabolic and Immunologic Features at Baseline Identify a Subgroup of Responders

Kevan C. Herold,[1] Stephen E. Gitelman,[2] Mario R. Ehlers,[3] Peter A. Gottlieb,[4] Carla J. Greenbaum,[5] William Hagopian,[6] Karen D. Boyle,[7] Lynette Keyes-Elstein,[7] Sudeepta Aggarwal,[8] Deborah Phippard,[8] Peter H. Sayre,[3] James McNamara,[9] Jeffrey A. Bluestone,[2] and the AbATE Study Team*

Trials of immune therapies in new-onset type 1 diabetes (T1D) have shown success, but not all subjects respond, and the duration of response is limited. Our aim was to determine whether two courses of teplizumab, an Fc receptor–nonbinding anti-CD3 monoclonal antibody, reduces the decline in C-peptide levels in patients with T1D 2 years after disease onset. We also set out to identify characteristics of responders. We treated 52 subjects with new-onset T1D with teplizumab for 2 weeks at diagnosis and after 1 year in an open-label, randomized, controlled trial. In the intent to treat analysis of the primary end point, patients treated with teplizumab had a reduced decline in C-peptide at 2 years (mean −0.28 nmol/L [95% CI −0.36 to −0.20]) versus control (mean −0.46 nmol/L [95% CI −0.57 to −0.35]; $P = 0.002$), a 75% improvement. The most common adverse events were rash, transient upper respiratory infections, headache, and nausea. In a post hoc analysis we characterized clinical responders and found that metabolic (HbA$_{1c}$ and insulin use) and immunologic features distinguished this group from those who did not respond to teplizumab. We conclude that teplizumab treatment preserves insulin production and reduces the use of exogenous insulin in some patients with new-onset T1D. Metabolic and immunologic features at baseline can identify a subgroup with robust responses to immune therapy. *Diabetes* 62:3766–3774, 2013

From the [1]Department of Immunobiology and Internal Medicine, Yale University, New Haven, Connecticut; the [2]Department of Pediatrics, University of California, San Francisco, California; the [3]Immune Tolerance Network, San Francisco, California; the [4]Department of Pediatrics and Medicine, Barbara Davis Center, University of Colorado, Aurora, Colorado; the [5]Benaroya Research Institute, Seattle, Washington; the [6]Pacific Northwest Diabetes Research Institute, Seattle, Washington; the [7]Rho Federal Systems Division, Chapel Hill, North Carolina; the [8]Immune Tolerance Network, Bethesda, Maryland; and the [9]National Institute of Allergy and Infectious Diseases, Bethesda, Maryland.
Corresponding author: Kevan C. Herold, kevan.herold@yale.edu.
Received 4 March 2013 and accepted 26 June 2013.
DOI: 10.2337/db13-0345. Clinical trial reg. no. NCT00129259, clinicaltrials.gov.
This article contains Supplementary Data online at http://diabetes.diabetesjournals.org/lookup/suppl/doi:10.2337/db13-0345/-/DC1.
*A list of other members of the AbATE Study Team can be found in the APPENDIX.
See accompanying commentary, p. 3656.

A number of trials have shown that the progression of type 1 diabetes (T1D) can be modulated by immune therapies. Cyclosporin A, azathioprine plus prednisone, and, more recently, CTLA4Ig, rituximab, and Fc receptor (FcR)–nonbinding anti-CD3 monoclonal antibody (mAb) treatments have reduced the fall in C-peptide responses that occurs in the first 2 years after disease onset (1–5). While the effects of therapy are not permanent, there is evidence that in at least some individuals, responses to immune therapy may persist for as long as 3 years after diagnosis, whereas in others there is no response to drug treatment (6,7). The reasons why immune therapies have not induced lasting remissions of the disease and why some individuals are more responsive to treatment than others are not known. One factor may involve the pharmacokinetics of the immune therapy in individual subjects (8). However, even drugs that have been given continuously, such as CTLA4Ig or cyclosporin A, have diminishing effects over time (3,9). Alternatively, there may be individual factors that affect escape from the effects of immune therapy, such as immune receptor signaling pathways or inflammatory mediators (10,11). Finally, there may be factors that affect β-cells, such as inflammatory cytokines (12). Glucose toxicity itself has been thought to affect these responses. In the Diabetes Control and Complications Trial (DCCT), individuals in the intensive control group showed less decline in stimulated C-peptide levels than those in the conventional control group (13).

Identifying individuals who are likely to respond to drug therapy would be valuable for the selection of patients for treatment. In previous studies, we and others showed that a single course of FcR-nonbinding anti-CD3 mAb given soon after the diagnosis of T1D improved C-peptide responses for 1 year after diagnosis, but the responses waned after that time (1,2,5). Therefore, we conducted a prospective, randomized, controlled trial of teplizumab in patients with new-onset T1D to test the effects of two courses of the drug, 1 year apart, on C-peptide responses 2 years after diagnosis. Using post hoc analyses, we also sought to identify the clinical and immunologic features of subjects who showed clinical responses to the drug. Our data show that treatment with an FcR-nonbinding anti-CD3 mAb can preserve insulin secretion in patients with new-onset T1D. Metabolic control and insulin use at the time of study enrollment were the strongest predictors of response as well as immunologic features. The lasting effect of metabolic features on responses to immune therapy has not been previously appreciated and deserves further study.

RESEARCH DESIGN AND METHODS

Study design and patients. This was a randomized, open-label study performed at six medical centers conducted between 2005 and 2011. Eligible individuals were between 8 and 30 years of age, diagnosed with T1D within 8 weeks of study enrollment, and positive for anti-GAD65, anti-ICA512, or ICA. Written consent was obtained from all participants. The study was approved by the institutional review boards at each institution. A data and safety monitoring board reviewed safety data at least yearly. This study is registered with clinicaltrials.gov (NCT00129259). The complete protocol is available at www.immunetolerance.org.

Randomization and masking. Subjects were randomized to drug treatment or a control group in a 2:1 ratio within randomly ordered blocks of six or three. The study was open label, but core laboratory personnel were masked to the treatment assignments.

Treatment and assessments. The drug treatment group received a 14-day course of teplizumab (day 1, 51 $\mu g/m^2$; day 2, 103 $\mu g/m^2$; day 3, 206 $\mu g/m^2$; day 4, 413 $\mu g/m^2$; days 5–14, 826 $\mu g/m^2$; median cumulative dose 11.6 mg; interquartile range 5.7 mg) diluted in normal saline solution and administered intravenously (14). The control group did not receive a placebo infusion. Subjects received ibuprofen, diphenhydramine, acetaminophen, or all three for infusion-related reactions. Drug treatment was discontinued during a treatment cycle if thrombocytopenia ($<140,000/mm^3$ on day 1 or $<100,000/mm^3$ on other days), anemia, neutropenia, fever (grade 3 or higher), liver function abnormalities (of two to three times the upper limit of the reference interval), hyperbilirubinemia, international normalized ratio >1.3, or other adverse events (AEs) grade 3 or higher occurred. Participants were not permitted to receive the second treatment cycle if they had an acute febrile illness within 4 weeks or developed anti-idiotype antibodies of $>1:1000$ titer or IgE isotype. Both groups were seen at regular intervals and received contact by a certified diabetes educator (CDE) every 2 weeks with a target treatment goal of a HbA_{1c} $<7.5\%$ (58 mmol/mol).

Subjects in both groups underwent a 4-h mixed-meal tolerance test (MMTT) every 6 months for 2 years, as described previously (2). After 1 year, subjects in the drug treatment group who had detectable C-peptide responses from MMTTs at all time points and who had not met stopping criteria for drug administration received a second course of teplizumab ($n = 40$) (median cumulative dose 12.4 mg, interquartile range 5.08 mg). A temporary hold in the protocol because of a drug manufacturing and safety review caused four of the first five subjects to receive their second course of drug later than the prescribed 1 year time point. These subjects had MMTTs within 100 days of 24 months after study entry. Insulin use was determined from patient logs and calculated as the average units per kilogram per day over the 3 days before the study visit.

Laboratory tests. Autoantibodies were measured by radioimmunoassay at the Barbara Davis Center (Aurora, CO) and immunofluorescence was tested at the University of Florida. C-peptide and HbA_{1c} levels were measured by two-site immunoenzymometric assay (Tosoh, San Francisco, CA) and ion exchange high-performance liquid chromatography (Bio-Rad Diagnostics) at the Northwest Lipid Research Laboratory (Seattle, WA) (3,15). The lower limit of detection in the C-peptide assay was 0.05 nmol/L. Serum teplizumab levels were measured in a subset (6) of drug-treated subjects using a previously defined flow cytometry–based assay (2). The peak teplizumab levels (mean ± SD) in serum collected before the last infusion of the first (day 13) and second cycles were 1095 ± 329 ($n = 4$) and 1097 ± 851 ng/ml ($n = 2$), respectively. The trough levels, calculated as the median of the values 1 and 6 h after the last infusion (where available), were 412 ± 215 and 514 ± 399 ng/ml, respectively.

Flow cytometry. Peripheral mononuclear blood cells were isolated from whole blood at study entry and frozen at a core facility. Thawed cells were stained with 10-color panels, which included mAbs to CD2, CD4, CD8, CCR4, CCR5, CCR6, CCR7, CXCR3, CXCR5, CD25, CD28, CD38, CD39, CD45RA, CD45RO, CD127, Helios, Foxp3, TNFR2, PD-1, NKG2A (BD Pharmingen, San Jose, CA) and analyzed by flow cytometry on an LSRII cytometer. For intracellular cytokine staining, cells were stimulated for 6 h with or without phorbol myristic acid (500 ng/ml) and ionomycin (500 pg/ml) and stained with mAbs to interferon (IFN)-γ, tumor necrosis factor, interleukin (IL)-13, IL-17, and IL-10 (BD Pharmingen) and analyzed by flow cytometry.

Statistical analyses. The 4-h C-peptide area under the curve (AUC) was calculated using the trapezoidal rule over the 4-h period (0–240 min). For this computation, the "time 0" C-peptide value was taken as the average of C-peptide values measured at time points -10 and 0 min. The AUC calculation was based on the time points available from the MMTT. Results reported as less than the lower limit of detection were imputed as zero for the MMTT at that time point. The primary end point was predefined as a comparison of the change in the mean 4-h C-peptide AUC from baseline, adjusted for the baseline C-peptide response, in the drug versus control groups at 24 months. Treated subjects who completed the MMTT at baseline and received at least 1 dose of study drug ($n = 52$) and subjects randomized to the control group with a baseline MMTT ($n = 25$) were used in the intent to treat (ITT) analysis. Seven subjects in the ITT population did not have an MMTT at month 24 (four in the control group, three in the teplizumab group). For the ITT analysis of the primary end point missing month 24 values were imputed using an algorithm designed to underestimate the true difference between arms. If the last available AUC value was zero, the missing month 24 AUC was imputed as zero. If the last observed AUC value was more than zero, the month 24 AUC values among subjects in the same arm were regressed on AUC values from the prior time point to yield a regression line and 95% CIs. Missing month 24 AUC values were imputed as predicted values from the upper 95% confidence band for control subjects and from the lower 95% confidence band for subjects in the teplizumab arm. A sensitivity analysis was conducted using the t statistic derived from the model with imputed data but reducing the degrees of freedom to account for the seven imputed values. The P values from both the primary and sensitivity analyses agreed to the fourth decimal place for the test of the treatment effect.

For group comparisons, C-peptide AUC values were transformed to ln(AUC + 1) values. An F test derived from an ANCOVA with baseline ln(AUC + 1) value as a covariate was used to compare treatment groups. Means and 95% CIs are presented on the untransformed scale. Percentage improvement was calculated as:

$$100\% \times (Least\ squares\ [LS]\ mean\ for\ treated - LS\ mean\ for\ controls)/$$
$$LS\ mean\ for\ controls.$$

Similar methods, using a repeated measures analysis with baseline response as a covariate, were used for secondary clinical and mechanistic end points and for exploratory analyses using groups defined by responder status. Longitudinal analyses also were applied to test trends over time. For secondary and exploratory analyses, corrections were not made for multiple comparisons.

Baseline differences between treatment groups were evaluated using P values as descriptive measures of the strength of association; Mann-Whitney U tests and χ^2 tests were used for continuous assessments and categorical characteristics, respectively. SAS software version 9.2 was used.

The sample size was based on a group comparison of ln(AUC + 1) after adjusting for baseline differences. On the basis of data from a prior study (1), we assumed that the ln(AUC + 1) after adjusting for baseline would be 0.309 in the teplizumab group. The current study was powered to detect a 50% worsening in adjusted 24-month C-peptide AUC in the control group compared with the treated group (i.e., assume mean AUC = $[\exp(0.31) - 1] = 0.36$ for the teplizumab group compared with 0.181 for the control group). With 2:1 randomization and a two-sided test of significance at $\alpha = 0.05$, 72 subjects were needed for 92% power. The study accrued 77 subjects in the ITT population.

RESULTS

Recruitment and treatment of patients with new-onset T1D. We screened 125 subjects <8 weeks from diagnosis of T1D and enrolled 83 (Fig. 1). Six subjects left the study before the first MMTT and are not included in the ITT analysis ($n = 77$). Fifty-two of the subjects randomized to drug treatment received all or part of the first drug course and are included in the ITT analysis; 15 discontinued teplizumab treatment after receiving some of cycle 1 or 2 (Supplementary Table 1). Twelve of the 15 subjects developed laboratory abnormalities or experienced AEs, leading to drug discontinuation. There were no significant differences between the study groups at entry (Table 1). The majority of subjects (94%) were <18 years old; 64% were ≤12 years old.

Effects of teplizumab treatment on C-peptide and clinical responses. Teplizumab treatment significantly

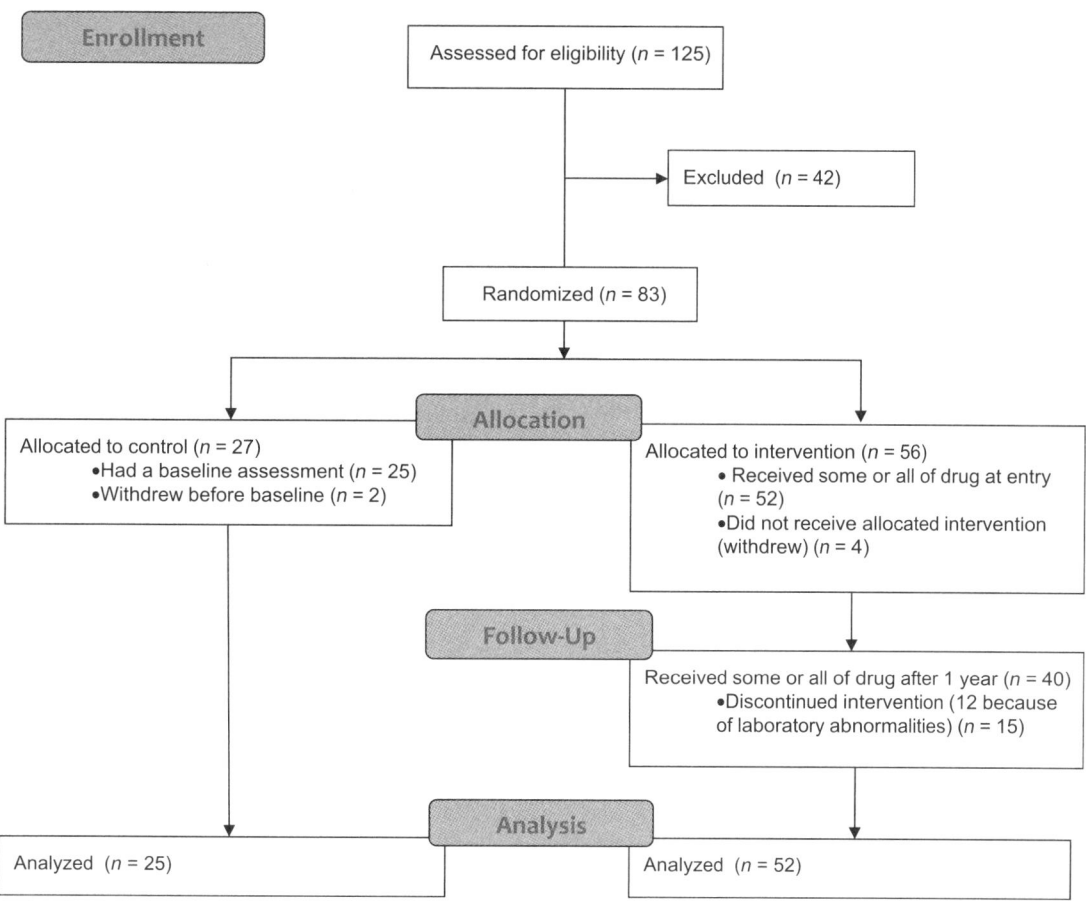

FIG. 1. Enrollment, randomization, and participation. Subjects ($n = 125$) were screened and 83 were eligible for enrollment. The majority of subjects who were excluded failed to meet entry criteria. Of 83 subjects randomized, 25 in the control group and 52 in the teplizumab group underwent an MMTT at baseline, received the first dose of study drug (teplizumab group), and are included in the ITT analysis. Of the subjects randomized to the teplizumab group, 12 did not receive the second course of drug because of AEs leading to discontinuation during cycle 1 ($n = 6$), had predefined laboratory abnormalities that precluded readministration ($n = 4$), or were withdrawn ($n = 2$). In addition, 3 of 40 subjects who started cycle 2 discontinued treatment because of AEs. The reasons for drug discontinuation are listed in Supplementary Table 1.

reduced the loss of C-peptide 2 years after study entry ($P = 0.002$; Table 2, Fig. 2A). After adjusting for the baseline imbalance, the mean C-peptide AUC level at year 2 was 75% higher in the teplizumab arm compared with controls. Likewise, the drop in C-peptide AUC from baseline to year 2, adjusting for baseline C-peptide AUC, was on average smaller in patients treated with teplizumab compared with the untreated controls as an absolute ($P = 0.002$) or percentage change ($P < 0.001$) from baseline (Table 2). Treated subjects were estimated to reach 6-month control group values 15.9 months later than the control group (i.e., month 21.9) (Fig. 2B). At the month 24 visit, more subjects treated with teplizumab had detectable levels of C-peptide compared with control subjects ($P = 0.002$; Fig. 2C).

Intensive diabetes care with contact with a CDE was provided to all subjects to "treat to target" of <7.5% (58 mmol/mol). There was not a significant difference in the HbA$_{1c}$ levels in the drug and control groups ($P = 0.093$) over the 24-month study, although at 9 and 15 months the change from baseline HbA$_{1c}$ levels were significantly higher in the control group ($P = 0.035$ and 0.011, respectively; Fig. 3A). The drug-treated group used significantly less insulin to achieve this level of glycemic control ($P = 0.036$; Fig. 3B).

Adverse events. Drug-related events were transient and resolved (Supplementary Table 2–5). There were a total of

11 serious AEs (SAEs) in 10 drug-treated subjects and 2 SAEs in 1 control subject (Supplementary Table 2). The AEs and those occurring in >15% of all subjects are shown in Supplementary Tables 3–5. Cytokine release syndrome was identified in five treated subjects. The rates of severe hypoglycemia were similar in the drug and control groups.

Of the patients in the drug-treated group who were seropositive for Epstein-Barr virus (EBV) ($n = 21$) and cytomegalovirus ($n = 16$), nine and two patients, respectively, had a transient increase in the viral load detected by PCR 1 month after the first course of drug treatment, and three and one, respectively, had an increase after the second course of the drug (range 100–5,500 copies/ml; median 200). Five subjects with an increase in EBV viral load had possible symptoms of transient EBV infection. In all subjects the viral loads were undetectable 2 months after treatment.

Effects of teplizumab treatment on autoantibodies. The titers of biochemical autoantibodies were similar in the treatment groups at baseline. There was a significant reduction in the titer of anti–zinc transporter 8 antibodies but not the other biochemical autoantibodies in the drug-treated group at the end of year 1 ($P < 0.05$). The differences at 2 years were not statistically significant (Supplementary Fig. 1).

TABLE 1
Baseline characteristics

	Teplizumab group ($n = 52$)	Control group ($n = 25$)	P value*
Age (years)	12.7 (4.9)	12.3 (4.1)	0.86
8–12 (%)	65.4	60.0	0.67
13–17 (%)	26.9	36.0	—
18–30 (%)	7.7	4.0	—
Male (%)	53.8	64.0	0.47
Hispanic (%)	3.8	8.0	0.59
African American (%)	3.8	4.0	0.81
BMI (kg/m^2)	19.5 (3.77)	20.1 (4.15)	0.41
Time since diagnosis (days)	40.4 (8.3)	37.6 (9.0)	0.14
Insulin use (units/kg/day)	0.39 (0.26)	0.39 (0.17)	0.75
HbA$_{1c}$ % [mmol/mol]	7.43 (0.99) [57.7 (10.9)]	7.70 (1.23) [60.7 (13.5)]	0.40
C-peptide AUC (nmol/L)	0.72 (0.29)	0.67 (0.28)	0.41
GAD65 (% positive)	76.5	95.7	0.05
IA.2ic (% positive)	98.0	95.7	0.53
MIAA (% positive)	70.6	73.9	0.99
ZnT8 (% positive)	86.3	65.2	0.06

Data are mean (SD) unless otherwise indicated. *P values for continuous variables are from the t test, and P values for categorical variables are from χ^2 or Fisher exact test.

Identification of responders. The C-peptide responses varied widely among drug-treated subjects, suggesting there was a spectrum of responses. In a post hoc analysis we sought to identify clinical and immunologic features that differentiated those individuals who did and did not show a response to teplizumab treatment. For the purpose of generating a hypothesis, we differentiated the responses of the drug-treated subjects based on changes in C-peptide secretion in the untreated control group at 24 months (Fig. 4A). All of the 25 control subjects lost ≥40% of the baseline C-peptide response by 24 months, and 27 of 49 drug-treated subjects showed a similar loss of ≥40%. Conversely, 22 of 49 of the drug-treated subjects (45%) lost <40% of baseline C-peptide; we refer to them as "responders." The three subjects with missing month 24 C-peptide results were not evaluated for responder status.

Our analysis of the percentage loss of C-peptide, shown in Fig. 4A, did not indicate whether the pattern of the response

to drug treatment reflected a true qualitative difference, in which the curves describing the change in the C-peptide responses were different from the untreated controls, or a quantitative difference, in which the curves describing the change in C-peptide responses were similar to the untreated control group but shifted over time, as suggested by our ITT analysis of all of the drug-treated subjects (Fig. 2A). Therefore, we compared the C-peptide AUC over time in the responders, nonresponders, and control subjects (Fig. 4B). This analysis suggested that the responders showed both quantitative and qualitative differences in their response to teplizumab. Even after 18 months, the average C-peptide level for responders was 113% of the baseline response and decreased from baseline by an average of only 6% at month 24. After adjusting for baseline differences, the C-peptide levels were nearly threefold (on average, 199%) higher among responders versus control subjects at month 24 but were not different in the nonresponders versus controls.

TABLE 2
Primary end point analysis of MMTT-stimulated 4-h C-peptide AUC (nanomoles per liter)

	Drug-treated group	Control group	P value*
ITT	$n = 52$	$n = 25$	
BL (nmol/L)†	0.72 (0.64–0.80)	0.67 (0.55–0.78)	
24 months (nmol/L)†	0.44 (0.32–0.56)	0.21 (0.11–0.30)	
24 months, adjusted for BL (nmol/L)‡	0.42 (0.35–0.5)	0.24 (0.13–0.35)	
Change from BL to 24 months, adjusted for BL (nmol/L)‡	−0.28 (−0.36 to −0.20)	−0.46 (−0.57 to −0.35)	0.002
Mean percentage change from BL to 24 months, adjusted for BL (%)‡	−45.1 (−53.35 to −36.86)	−72.2 (−84.10 to −60.27)	<0.001
Per protocol§	$n = 35$	$n = 21$	
BL (nmol/L)†	0.67 (0.58–0.76)	0.66 (0.53–0.78)	
24 months (nmol/L)†	0.39 (0.29–0.49)	0.18 (0.08–0.28)	
24 months, adjusted for BL (nmol/L)‡	0.38 (0.32–0.45)	0.19 (0.11–0.27)	
Change from BL to 24 months, adjusted for BL (nmol/L)‡	−0.28 (−0.34 to −0.22)	−0.48 (−0.56 to −0.39)	<0.001
Mean percentage change from BL to 24 months, adjusted for BL (%)‡	−45.6 (−55.02 to −36.15)	−76.3 (−88.50 to −64.13)	<0.001

*The P value for the group comparison of change is for the F test derived from an ANCOVA for change in ln(AUC + 1) from BL to 24 months that includes BL ln(AUC + 1) value as a covariate. The P value for the group comparison of "mean percentage change" is for the F test derived from the ANCOVA for percentage change from BL to 24 months that includes BL AUC value as a covariate. †Means and 95% CIs are on the untransformed scale. ‡Means and 95% CIs are on the untransformed scale and corrected for the BL imbalance in AUC using an ANCOVA model. The mean AUC across groups is 0.7038 and 0.6640 for ITT and per protocol analyses, respectively. §Missing month 24 AUCs are imputed for the ITT analysis but are excluded for the per protocol results. BL, baseline.

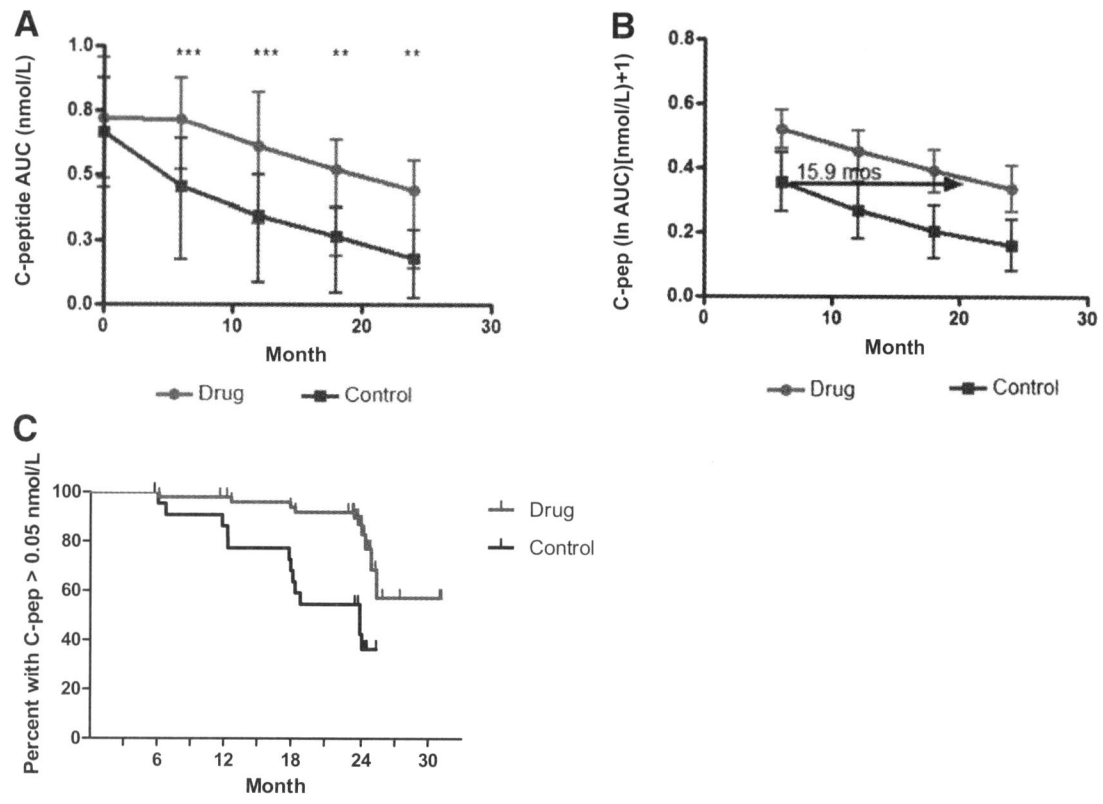

FIG. 2. C-peptide (C-pep) responses in drug-treated and control subjects. *A*: The mean ± 25th and 75th percentiles of the C-pep AUC (nanomoles per liter) are shown for the drug and control groups (***$P = 0.002$; **$P < 0.02$, ANCOVA for each time point). *B*: Estimates and 95% CIs from a mixed effects model, with fixed effects for treatment group and linear and quadratic trends over time and random subject-level effects for intercepts and linear trends over time. Drug-treated subjects are estimated to have a delay of decline in C-pep by 15.9 months (i.e., would reach control 6-month values 21.9 months after study entry). *C*: Proportion of subjects with detectable C-pep (i.e., >0.05 nmol/L). The actual study dates when the MMTTs were performed are shown. There was a significantly greater loss of detectable C-pep secretion in the control group at month 24 ($P = 0.002$, χ^2 test).

Metabolic and immunologic features of responders at baseline.

The patients' age, sex, BMI, duration of disease, and baseline autoantibody titers were not predictors of the response to teplizumab treatment (Fig. 5*A*). The responders and nonresponders did not receive significantly different amounts of drug. However, clinical responders had lower HbA$_{1c}$ levels (mean 7.05% [95% CI 6.689–7.411%] vs. 7.78% [7.360–8.203%]; mean 53.54 mmol/mol [95% CI 49.59–57.49 mmol/mol] vs. 61.54 mmol/mol [56.93–66.14 mmol/mol]; $P = 0.011$) and used less insulin (mean 0.28 units/kg/day [95% CI 0.204–0.357 units/kg/day] vs. 0.49 units/kg/day [0.376–0.606 units/kg/day]; $P = 0.004$) at baseline (Fig. 5*B*) even after correcting for baseline C-peptide AUC ($P = 0.018$ and 0.008, respectively). The baseline C-peptide AUC responses in the responders (mean 0.78 nmol/L [95% CI 0.65–0.91 nmol/L]) and nonresponders (0.68 pmolM/L [0.56–0.79 pmolM/L]) were not significantly different ($P = 0.245$).

There was a lower frequency of CD4+CCR4+ memory and naïve T cells ($P = 0.027$ and 0.047), CD4+CCR6+ naïve CD4+ T cells ($P = 0.044$), naïve CCR4+ CD8+ T cells ($P = 0.029$), and IFN-γ-producing CD8+ T cells ($P = 0.03$) at baseline. There was a higher number of activated CD8+ terminally differentiated effector and CD8+ effector memory T cells ($P = 0.011$ and 0.017) in responders versus nonresponders (Table 3).

DISCUSSION

In this randomized controlled trial we show that two courses of treatment with FcR-nonbinding anti-CD3 mAb (teplizumab) reduced the loss of C-peptide 2 years after the first treatment in patients with new-onset T1D. Fewer drug-treated subjects lost detectable insulin production. Less exogenous insulin was needed to maintain equivalent or lower levels of HbA$_{1c}$ (3,4). However, the responses to the drug varied and, therefore, in a post hoc analysis, we sought to identify individuals who were clinical responders and distinct from the nonresponders and to compare the immunologic and metabolic features of these subgroups. The strongest differences were in metabolic features: responders had lower levels of HbA$_{1c}$ and insulin use at baseline. In addition, responders had reduced numbers of Th1-like cells and other differences in T-cell subsets. These findings suggest lasting effects of metabolic control before treatment on responses to immune therapy since the end point of the study was 2 years after enrollment and the glucose control during the study period was not significantly different.

The results of this trial suggest a more robust effect on the course of T1D (75% higher C-peptide responses vs. control) than was recently reported by the Protégé Study, a phase III trial that also used teplizumab (approximately 33% higher C-peptide responses vs. placebo) (14). A number of design differences in these two trials may account for this. Although the control arm did not receive placebo, subjects were randomized to treatment arms and balanced at baseline, and there were few dropouts. Our study was restricted to North American sites where the diagnosis of disease was made relatively early, there were fewer insulin

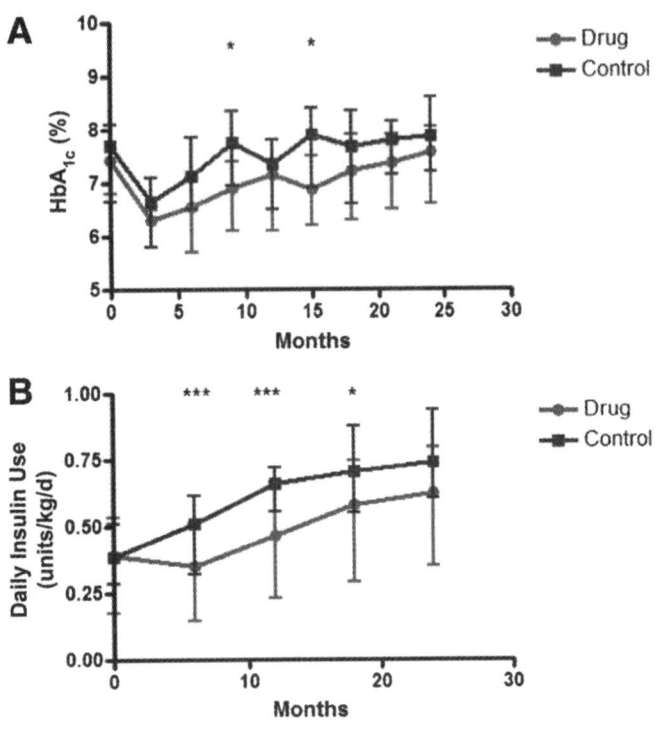

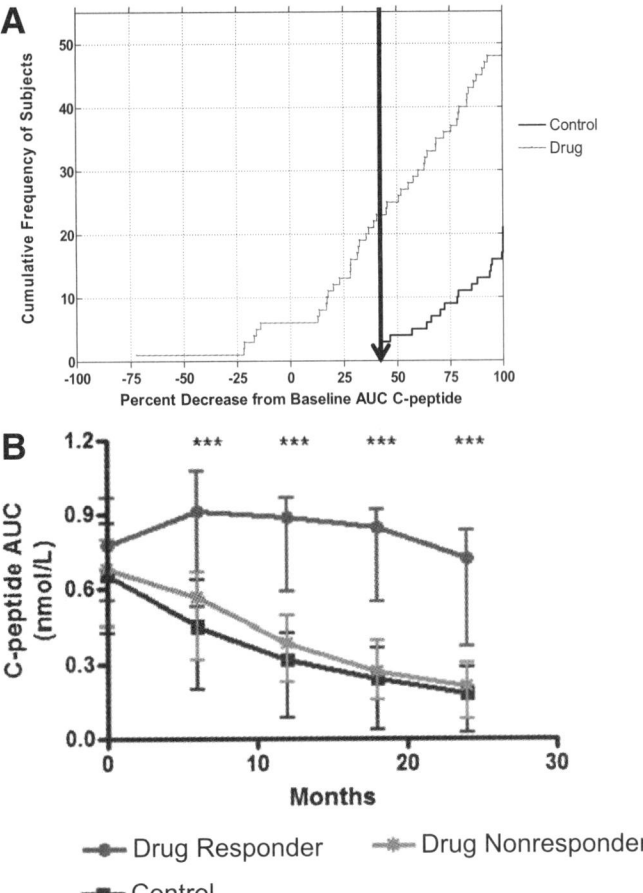

FIG. 3. Insulin use and HbA₁c in drug and control groups. *A*: HbA₁c levels in the drug and control groups (means ± 25th and 75th percentiles are shown; *P < 0.05). *B*: Average insulin use in the 3 days before the visit was calculated (group means ± 25th and 75th percentiles; *P < 0.05, ***P < 0.005; P < 0.001 for overall trend at month 12, and P = 0.022 at month 18 using ANCOVA).

FIG. 4. Identification of clinical responders to teplizumab. *A*: The cumulative frequency of subjects and distribution of percentage decrease from baseline C-peptide AUC at month 24. The arrow shows the smallest percentage loss of C-peptide AUC in the control group. *B*: The C-peptide AUC at each time point (means ± 25th and 75th percentiles) is shown for the responders (red line) and nonresponders (green line) in the drug-treated group and for the control subjects (blue line). ***P < 0.001 between responders and nonresponders at each time point based on ANCOVAs.

requirements and lower HbA₁c levels, and the frequency of diabetic ketoacidosis was low. Although we did not find a significant effect of age on treatment efficacy, unlike the Protégé trial, our subjects were younger, and the rate of decline in C-peptide responses is greater in younger subjects (16).

The differences in the rates of AEs and SAEs were greater in the drug-treated versus the control group in this trial. In addition to teplizumab-associated events, the drug-treated group was seen more frequently, which may have contributed to further imbalance in reporting AEs. The SAE most closely related to the study drug, cytokine release syndrome, was transient. Of the 52 subjects randomized to drug treatment, 12 were unable to receive the second course of the drug because of protocol-defined rules for stopping treatment. The rules were based on prior experience to prevent more significant AEs with continued drug administration (6), but the AEs were generally of low grade at the time of discontinuation.

We used a definition for responders based on the characteristics of the randomized control group in this study. Previous studies used definitions of responders based on the absence of a decline in C-peptide or features of the C-peptide assay (1,17), which, when applied to our dataset, identified a smaller subgroup. It is important to note that our designation of drug-treated subjects as responders and nonresponders did not reflect a clear bimodal division but rather was based on overall changes in the C-peptide responses in the drug-treated group that were different from the untreated controls, all of whom had levels at least 40% less than the baseline responses. Nevertheless, when analyzed in this way the responders and nonresponders

had quantitatively and qualitatively different responses, which did not simply reflect a delay in the decline in the C-peptide response, as suggested by our ITT analysis, or as reported with other successful immune therapies such as abatacept or rituximab (3,4). Instead, in the responder group the effects of teplizumab were robust and durable, with C-peptide values above the baseline level for at least 18 months on average and a C-peptide response of almost three times that of the untreated group after 2 years, whereas in the nonresponders even the initial effect was modest. Within the responder group identified in this way, we did not find a clear bimodal distribution; there were subjects in whom the C-peptide response did not change or even increased after 2 years and others in whom the decline in C-peptide responses were slightly less than 40% of the baseline response. Our original objective in this trial was to test whether a second course of drug treatment at 1 year would improve the clinical responses that appeared to wane during the second year after a single course of teplizumab. The second course of teplizumab did not seem to have an effect on the drug-treated group as a whole, but the robust pattern of response in the responders raises the

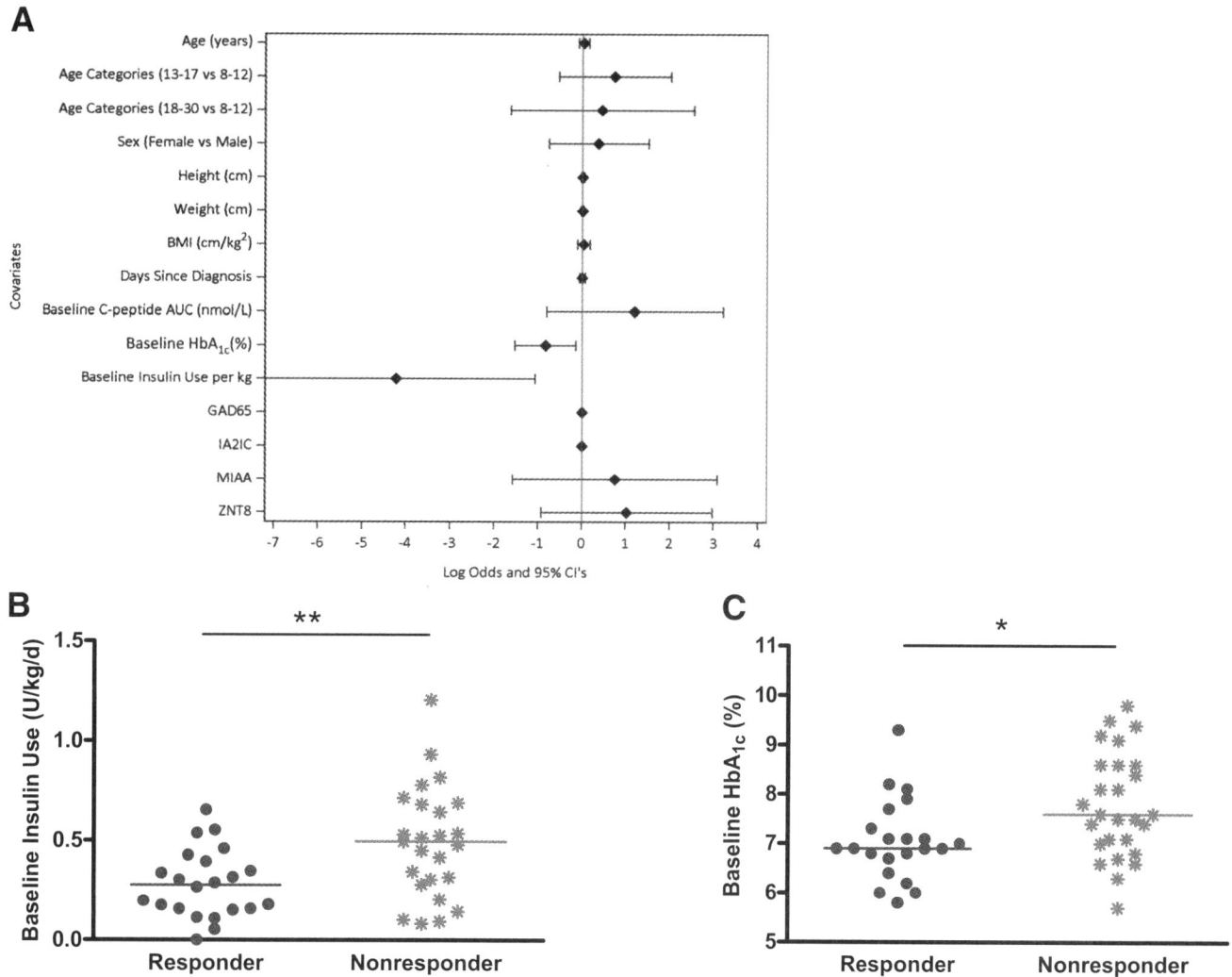

FIG. 5. Baseline clinical characteristics in responders versus nonresponders. *A*: Ladder plot of covariates and clinical response. The effects of the indicated covariates on the ratio of log odds of responder status and 95% CIs are shown. The baseline HbA$_{1c}$ (P = 0.011) and insulin use (P = 0.004) were inversely associated with response. Baseline insulin use (*B*) and HbA$_{1c}$ (*C*) in the drug-treated responders (red) and nonresponders (green) (**P = 0.004, *P = 0.011).

possibility that the second course was effective in maintaining C-peptide levels in this subset. However, we cannot directly assess this since we did not have a comparison group receiving a single treatment course.

A surprising finding was the differences in metabolic and immunologic features of the drug-treated responder group compared with the drug-treated nonresponders. HbA$_{1c}$ and insulin use at the time of study enrollment were

TABLE 3
Immunologic features of responders at baseline

Cell population	Responder (n = 18*)	Nonresponder (n = 21 or 22*)	P value
CCR4+ naïve CD4 T cells	12.6 (7.24)	17.5 (6.24)	0.047
CCR6+ naïve CD4 T cells	6.8 (5.85)	9.8 (5.12)	0.044
CCR4+ naïve CD8 T cells	14.4 (6.96)	19.4 (5.70)	0.029
CCR4+ memory CD4 T cells	29.7 (7.56)	34.6 (7.95)	0.027
CD8 effector memory T cells	6.5 (2.45)	4.8 (2.93)	0.017
CD38+ terminally differentiated CD8 effector T cells	82.7 (8.88)	76.5 (8.80)	0.011
CD8+ IFN-γ+	8.9 (6.53)	14.7 (10.29)	0.033

Data are mean (SD). Peripheral blood mononuclear cells from baseline visits were thawed and stained for viability and a combination of 25 markers, divided in panels of 6, for a 10-color flow experiment. FlowJo software (TreeStar, Inc.) was used to sequentially gate the cell populations. The percentages of cells that were positive in their respective parent population (CD2+CD4+ or CD2+CD8+) are shown. Cell populations that were significantly different between drug-treated responders and nonresponders are listed. *Samples were unavailable for subjects who did not meet minimal body weight for sampling for mechanistic studies.

significantly lower among responders compared with nonresponders. These parameters are thought to reflect endogenous β-cell function, yet baseline C-peptide AUC measurements were not significantly different between the groups. An effect of tight glucose control on preservation of C-peptide responses was shown in the DCCT, and for that reason all subjects kept in close contact with a CDE with the intent to maintain HbA_{1c} ≤7.5% (58 mmol/mol) (13). The mechanisms whereby glucose control and insulin sensitivity might lead to improved responses are unknown. Metabolic pathways can affect effector and memory T-cell differentiation and function (18,19). Glucose can stimulate IL-1β production by β-cells, which may impair the effects of the FcR-nonbinding anti-CD3 mAb (20,21). Chronic exposure to elevated glucose causes a deterioration of β-cell function as a consequence of oxidative stress (22). The damage inflicted on β-cells before the immune therapy may render the cells incapable of recovery and repair. However, even more striking was the difference in insulin use between responders and nonresponders. Since we did not find a significant difference in C-peptide responses between the responders and nonresponders, this finding suggests differences in insulin sensitivity: chronic insulin resistance may cause metabolic stress of residual β-cells, rendering them susceptible to immune-mediated damage. The contribution of metabolic factors to immune therapeutic responses has not been reported within the drug-treatment groups in earlier immune therapy trials, but we observed an interesting similar trend in an analysis of two previous trials of teplizumab that we conducted (data not reported) (1,15). Although a trend for lower HbA_{1c} (<6.0%), but not lower insulin usage, favoring response to abatacept, was suggested previously (3), that analysis compared drug- and placebo-treated subjects, whereas our analysis involved only subjects within the drug-treated group.

In addition, we found differences in immune parameters in the responder versus nonresponder groups. The decreased IFN-γ–producing CD8+ and CCR4+CD4+ T cells at baseline in responders suggest a lower frequency of Th1-like T cells, which may be contributory since a Th1 phenotype has been associated with pathogenic T cells (23–25). In this exploratory analysis we did not correct for multiple comparisons; in addition, longitudinal studies of these subsets and others that have been implicated as mediators of the effects of teplizumab will be necessary to understand the role of cellular responses in the clinical response (26–31).

In summary, we found a robust effect of an FcR-nonbinding anti-CD3 mAb in a subset of patients with new-onset T1D. Within this subgroup, we found differences in metabolic and immunologic parameters, suggesting that both contribute to the efficacy that we observed. Our studies support the potential value of this immunotherapeutic approach. The results highlight the interactions between host factors and drug action, which ultimately determine the clinical value of treatment.

ACKNOWLEDGMENTS

This research was performed as a project of the Immune Tolerance Network (National Institutes of Health contract no. N01 AI15416), an international clinical research consortium headquartered at the Benaroya Research Institute and supported by the National Institute of Allergy and Infectious Diseases and the Juvenile Diabetes Research Foundation. The work also was supported by grants UL1 RR024131 from the National Center for Research Resources and UL1 RR024139 from the National Center for Advancing Translational Science.

MacroGenics provided teplizumab. LifeScan Division of Johnson & Johnson provided blood glucose monitoring meters and strips to participants.

K.C.H. has received grant support from MacroGenics, Inc. J.A.B. has a patent on the teplizumab molecule. No other potential conflicts of interest relevant to this article were reported.

The sponsor (Immune Tolerance Network and the National Institute of Allergy and Infectious Diseases) participated in study design, analysis, and writing of the manuscript.

K.C.H., S.E.G., M.R.E., P.A.G., C.J.G., and W.H. carried out the clinical trial and wrote the manuscript. K.D.B. and L.K.-E. performed statistical analysis and wrote the manuscript. S.A., D.P., and J.A.B. analyzed mechanistic data and wrote the manuscript. P.H.S. served as clinical monitor, designed the protocol, and wrote the manuscript. J.M. designed the protocol, analyzed the data, and wrote the manuscript. K.C.H. is the guarantor of this work and, as such, had full access to all the data in the study and takes responsibility for the integrity of the data and the accuracy of the data analysis.

Special thanks is given to Margaret Lund Fitzgibbon, RN (National Institute of Allergy and Infectious Diseases).

APPENDIX

Other members of the AbATE Study Team include Melissa Johnson, Preeti Chugha, PhD, and Tracia Debnam (Immune Tolerance Network); Jennifer Sherr, MD, Frank Waldron-Lynch, MD, PhD, Linda Rink, RN, Kimberly Kunze, and Anna Wurtz (Yale University); Jennifer Bollyky, MD, Deborah Hefty, RN, CDE, Marli McCulloch-Olson, and Srinath Sanda, MD (Benaroya Research Institute); Stephen Rosenthal, MD, Saleh Adi, MD, Christine Torok, RN, and Rebecca Wesch (University of California, San Francisco); Jenna Lungaro, Allison Proto, RN, Amy Wallace, and Kimber Westbrook (Barbara Davis Center); and Rachel Hervey (Pacific Northwest Research Institute).

REFERENCES

1. Herold KC, Gitelman SE, Masharani U, et al. A single course of anti-CD3 monoclonal antibody hOKT3gamma1(Ala-Ala) results in improvement in C-peptide responses and clinical parameters for at least 2 years after onset of type 1 diabetes. Diabetes 2005;54:1763–1769
2. Herold KC, Hagopian W, Auger JA, et al. Anti-CD3 monoclonal antibody in new-onset type 1 diabetes mellitus. N Engl J Med 2002;346:1692–1698
3. Orban T, Bundy B, Becker DJ, et al.; Type 1 Diabetes TrialNet Abatacept Study Group. Co-stimulation modulation with abatacept in patients with recent-onset type 1 diabetes: a randomised, double-blind, placebo-controlled trial. Lancet 2011;378:412–419
4. Pescovitz MD, Greenbaum CJ, Krause-Steinrauf H, et al.; Type 1 Diabetes TrialNet Anti-CD20 Study Group. Rituximab, B-lymphocyte depletion, and preservation of beta-cell function. N Engl J Med 2009;361:2143–2152
5. Keymeulen B, Vandemeulebroucke E, Ziegler AG, et al. Insulin needs after CD3-antibody therapy in new-onset type 1 diabetes. N Engl J Med 2005;352:2598–2608
6. Herold KC, Gitelman S, Greenbaum C, et al.; Immune Tolerance Network ITN007AI Study Group. Treatment of patients with new onset type 1 diabetes with a single course of anti-CD3 mAb Teplizumab preserves insulin production for up to 5 years. Clin Immunol 2009;132:166–173
7. Keymeulen B, Walter M, Mathieu C, et al. Four-year metabolic outcome of a randomised controlled CD3-antibody trial in recent-onset type 1 diabetic

patients depends on their age and baseline residual beta cell mass. Diabetologia 2010;53:614–623

8. Press RR, de Fijter JW, Guchelaar HJ. Individualizing calcineurin inhibitor therapy in renal transplantation—current limitations and perspectives. Curr Pharm Des 2010;16:176–186

9. Bougnères PF, Landais P, Boisson C, et al. Limited duration of remission of insulin dependency in children with recent overt type I diabetes treated with low-dose cyclosporin. Diabetes 1990;39:1264–1272

10. Bertin-Maghit S, Pang D, O'Sullivan B, et al. Interleukin-1β produced in response to islet autoantigen presentation differentiates T-helper 17 cells at the expense of regulatory T-cells: Implications for the timing of tolerizing immunotherapy. Diabetes 2011;60:248–257

11. Yang XO, Nurieva R, Martinez GJ, et al. Molecular antagonism and plasticity of regulatory and inflammatory T cell programs. Immunity 2008;29:44–56

12. Larsen CM, Faulenbach M, Vaag A, et al. Interleukin-1-receptor antagonist in type 2 diabetes mellitus. N Engl J Med 2007;356:1517–1526

13. Effect of intensive therapy on residual beta-cell function in patients with type 1 diabetes in the diabetes control and complications trial. A randomized, controlled trial. The Diabetes Control and Complications Trial Research Group. Ann Intern Med 1998;128:517–523

14. Sherry N, Hagopian W, Ludvigsson J, et al.; Protégé Trial Investigators. Teplizumab for treatment of type 1 diabetes (Protégé study): 1-year results from a randomised, placebo-controlled trial. Lancet 2011;378:487–497

15. Herold KC, Gitelman SE, Willi SM, et al. Teplizumab treatment may improve C-peptide responses in participants with type 1 diabetes after the new-onset period: a randomised controlled trial. Diabetologia 2013;56:391–400

16. Greenbaum CJ, Beam CA, Boulware D, et al.; Type 1 Diabetes TrialNet Study Group. Fall in C-peptide during first 2 years from diagnosis: evidence of at least two distinct phases from composite Type 1 Diabetes TrialNet data. Diabetes 2012;61:2066–2073

17. Herold KC, Pescovitz MD, McGee P, et al.; Type 1 Diabetes TrialNet Anti-CD20 Study Group. Increased T cell proliferative responses to islet antigens identify clinical responders to anti-CD20 monoclonal antibody (rituximab) therapy in type 1 diabetes. J Immunol 2011;187:1998–2005

18. Gerriets VA, Rathmell JC. Metabolic pathways in T cell fate and function. Trends Immunol 2012;33:168–173

19. Cham CM, Gajewski TF. Glucose availability regulates IFN-gamma production and p70S6 kinase activation in CD8+ effector T cells. J Immunol 2005;174:4670–4677

20. Mandrup-Poulsen T, Spinas GA, Prowse SJ, et al. Islet cytotoxicity of interleukin 1. Influence of culture conditions and islet donor characteristics. Diabetes 1987;36:641–647

21. Maedler K, Sergeev P, Ris F, et al. Glucose-induced beta cell production of IL-1beta contributes to glucotoxicity in human pancreatic islets. J Clin Invest 2002;110:851–860

22. Robertson RP, Harmon J, Tran PO, Tanaka Y, Takahashi H. Glucose toxicity in beta-cells: type 2 diabetes, good radicals gone bad, and the glutathione connection. Diabetes 2003;52:581–587

23. Antonelli A, Fallahi P, Ferrari SM, et al. Serum Th1 (CXCL10) and Th2 (CCL2) chemokine levels in children with newly diagnosed type 1 diabetes: a longitudinal study. Diabet Med 2008;25:1349–1353

24. Coppieters KT, Dotta F, Amirian N, et al. Demonstration of islet-autoreactive CD8 T cells in insulitic lesions from recent onset and long-term type 1 diabetes patients. J Exp Med 2012;209:51–60

25. Itoh N, Hanafusa T, Miyazaki A, et al. Mononuclear cell infiltration and its relation to the expression of major histocompatibility complex antigens and adhesion molecules in pancreas biopsy specimens from newly diagnosed insulin-dependent diabetes mellitus patients. J Clin Invest 1993; 92:2313–2322

26. Ablamunits V, Bisikirska B, Herold KC. Acquisition of regulatory function by human CD8(+) T cells treated with anti-CD3 antibody requires TNF. Eur J Immunol 2010;40:2891–2901

27. Ablamunits V, Henegariu O, Preston-Hurlburt P, Herold KC. NKG2A is a marker for acquisition of regulatory function by human CD8+ T cells activated with anti-CD3 antibody. Eur J Immunol 2011;41:1832–1842

28. Bisikirska B, Colgan J, Luban J, Bluestone JA, Herold KC. TCR stimulation with modified anti-CD3 mAb expands CD8+ T cell population and induces CD8+CD25+ Tregs. J Clin Invest 2005;115:2904–2913

29. Belghith M, Bluestone JA, Barriot S, Mégret J, Bach JF, Chatenoud L. TGF-beta-dependent mechanisms mediate restoration of self-tolerance induced by antibodies to CD3 in overt autoimmune diabetes. Nat Med 2003; 9:1202–1208

30. You S, Leforban B, Garcia C, Bach JF, Bluestone JA, Chatenoud L. Adaptive TGF-beta-dependent regulatory T cells control autoimmune diabetes and are a privileged target of anti-CD3 antibody treatment. Proc Natl Acad Sci U S A 2007;104:6335–6340

31. Waldron-Lynch F, Henegariu O, Deng S, Preston-Hurlburt P, Tooley J, Flavell R, Herold KC. Teplizumab induces human gut-tropic regulatory cells in humanized mice and patients. Sci Transl Med 2012;4:118ra112

PREVENTION & TREATMENT

Personalized Genetic Risk Counseling to Motivate Diabetes Prevention

A randomized trial

RICHARD W. GRANT, MD, MPH[1]
KELSEY E. O'BRIEN, BA[2]
JESSICA L. WAXLER, CGC[3]
JASON L. VASSY, MD, MPH, SM[2,4]
LINDA M. DELAHANTY, MS, RD[4,5]
LAURIE G. BISSETT, MS[5]

ROBERT C. GREEN, MD, MPH[4,6,7]
KATHERINE G. STEMBER, BA[2]
CANDACE GUIDUCCI, BS[8]
ELYSE R. PARK, PHD, MPH[4,9]
JOSE C. FLOREZ, MD, PHD[4,5,8,10]
JAMES B. MEIGS, MD, MPH[2,4]

OBJECTIVE—To examine whether diabetes genetic risk testing and counseling can improve diabetes prevention behaviors.

RESEARCH DESIGN AND METHODS—We conducted a randomized trial of diabetes genetic risk counseling among overweight patients at increased phenotypic risk for type 2 diabetes. Participants were randomly allocated to genetic testing versus no testing. Genetic risk was calculated by summing 36 single nucleotide polymorphisms associated with type 2 diabetes. Participants in the top and bottom score quartiles received individual genetic counseling before being enrolled with untested control participants in a 12-week, validated, diabetes prevention program. Middle-risk quartile participants were not studied further. We examined the effect of this genetic counseling intervention on patient self-reported attitudes, program attendance, and weight loss, separately comparing higher-risk and lower-risk result recipients with control participants.

RESULTS—The 108 participants enrolled in the diabetes prevention program included 42 participants at higher diabetes genetic risk, 32 at lower diabetes genetic risk, and 34 untested control subjects. Mean age was 57.9 ± 10.6 years, 61% were men, and average BMI was 34.8 kg/m^2, with no differences among randomization groups. Participants attended 6.8 ± 4.3 group sessions and lost 8.5 ± 10.1 pounds, with 33 of 108 (30.6%) losing $\geq$5% body weight. There were few statistically significant differences in self-reported motivation, program attendance, or mean weight loss when higher-risk recipients and lower-risk recipients were compared with control subjects ($P > 0.05$ for all but one comparison).

CONCLUSIONS—Diabetes genetic risk counseling with currently available variants does not significantly alter self-reported motivation or prevention program adherence for overweight individuals at risk for diabetes.

Diabetes Care 36:13–19, 2013

Nearly 80 million Americans are currently at increased risk for diabetes, with worldwide diabetes prevalence projected to reach 440 million by 2030 (1,2). Robust clinical trial evidence has demonstrated that lifestyle changes leading to increased exercise and weight loss can substantially reduce the risk for diabetes (3–5). Despite the relative cost-effectiveness of nonpharmacologic approaches to diabetes prevention (6,7), efforts to translate the intensive behavioral change interventions of clinical trials into the community setting have had only modest success (8–11).

New approaches to conveying personal risk, such as individualized diabetes genetic risk testing, may enable more effective diabetes prevention (12). One promise of genome-based "personalized medicine" has been the potential to motivate individuals to make lifestyle changes that ameliorate their disease risk (13,14). Type 2 diabetes is an ideal clinical paradigm for testing this assumption given the high prevalence of an easily identified pre-disease phenotype, the strong evidence linking behavior change to risk reduction, suboptimal translation of proven behavioral change interventions into clinical practice, and recent rapid progress in diabetes genetic epidemiology.

Patients and providers have both indicated that learning about higher genetic risk results would likely motivate individuals to change their behavior to prevent diabetes (15,16). This prediction has not yet been convincingly demonstrated in controlled trials (17). In addition, genetic testing that reveals a decreased genetic risk could provide false reassurance to individuals with a high phenotypic risk (18). This concern has also not yet been rigorously examined. Therefore, we conducted a randomized, controlled trial to test the hypothesis that diabetes genetic risk testing and counseling can motivate the behavior changes necessary to prevent diabetes. Given the potential for false reassurance with lower-risk results, we separately investigated the effect of disclosing increased or decreased diabetes genetic risk compared with untested control participants.

RESEARCH DESIGN AND METHODS

Study design

The Genetic Counseling/Lifestyle Change for Diabetes Prevention (GC/LC) Study was a prospective, three-arm parallel

From the [1]Division of Research, Kaiser Permanente Northern California, Oakland, California; the [2]Division of General Medicine, Massachusetts General Hospital, Boston, Massachusetts; the [3]Department of Pediatrics, Massachusetts General Hospital, Boston, Massachusetts; the [4]Harvard Medical School, Boston, Massachusetts; the [5]Diabetes Center, Massachusetts General Hospital, Boston, Massachusetts; the [6]Partners Center for Personalized Genetic Medicine, Boston, Massachusetts; the [7]Division of Genetics, Brigham and Women's Hospital, Boston, Massachusetts; the [8]Program in Medical and Population Genetics, Broad Institute, Cambridge, Massachusetts; the [9]Mongan Institute for Health Policy, Massachusetts General Hospital, Boston, Massachusetts; and the [10]Center for Human Genetic Research, Massachusetts General Hospital, Boston, Massachusetts.
Corresponding author: Richard W. Grant, richard.w.grant@kp.org.
Received 7 May 2012 and accepted 28 June 2012.
DOI: 10.2337/dc12-0884. Clinical trial reg. no. NCT01034319, clinicaltrials.gov.
This article contains Supplementary Data online at http://care.diabetesjournals.org/lookup/suppl/doi:10.2337/dc12-0884/-/DC1.

group, randomized, controlled clinical trial conducted among individuals at increased phenotypic risk for type 2 diabetes that tested two hypotheses: 1) receiving a higher diabetes genetic risk result would improve motivation and participation in a 12-session weekly diabetes prevention program compared with untested control subjects; and 2) receiving a lower diabetes genetic risk result would decrease motivation and participation compared with untested control subjects. This study was investigator-initiated, funded by the National Institute of Diabetes and Digestive and Kidney Diseases, and conducted at Massachusetts General Hospital in Boston.

Details of the study design have been published previously (19). Briefly, eligible individuals were randomly allocated using random numbers in concealed envelopes in a four-to-one ratio to diabetes genetic risk testing versus no testing. Investigators implemented the random allocation, enrollment, and assignment. Participants with top and bottom quartile of diabetes genetic risk were enrolled with untested control subjects into a 12-week group-based Lifestyle Balance diabetes prevention program modeled after the Diabetes Prevention Program protocol and previously validated in patients with metabolic syndrome (9). Participants determined to have average diabetes genetic risk received their results but were not studied further. This study was approved by the Partners Human Research Committee Institutional Review Board. All participants provided written informed consent before enrollment.

Study participants

Participants were recruited from primary care practices within our institution, with the permission of their primary care physicians, between January 2010 and March 2011. Patients were eligible to participate in the study if they were aged 21 years or older, overweight (defined as BMI ≥ 29.1 kg/m^2 in men, ≥ 27.2 kg/m^2 in women), met one other criterion for metabolic syndrome without an existing diagnosis of type 2 diabetes (20), and were physically able and willing to participate in a 12-week group session program designed to achieve weight loss through dietary change and increased physical activity.

Blood samples for individuals randomized to genetic testing were drawn for diabetes genetic risk assessment and genotyped at the Broad Institute (Cambridge, MA) using the Sequenom MassARRAY iPLEXGold platform (Sequenom, Inc.,

San Diego, CA). A summary genetic risk score was calculated from 36 successfully genotyped risk alleles previously associated with type 2 diabetes (21).

Calculation of relative and absolute diabetes genetic risk

Individualized genetic risk assessment was performed by multiplying the relative genetic risk, as determined using diabetes incidence data from the Framingham Offspring Study (FOS) (22), by the absolute phenotypic risk of the study population. In FOS, 17.9% patients in the top quartile of genetic risk score distribution (>38) developed diabetes (46% relative increase compared with middle two average quartiles), whereas 9.9% in the bottom quartile (scores <34) developed diabetes (18% relative decrease compared with "average" risk). We estimated the absolute diabetes incidence for participants meeting our study eligibility criteria as ~11% over 3 years using previously published data from within our hospital network (23). Multiplying relative genetic risk by this absolute phenotypic-based risk resulted in posttest absolute 3-year risk estimates of 17% (higher genetic risk recipients), 11% (untested control subjects), and 9% (lower genetic risk recipients) for type 2 diabetes.

Intervention implementation

Participants with results showing higher and lower diabetes genetic risk each received a 15-min structured, individual genetic counseling session conducted by a certified genetic counselor. Details of the session have published previously (24). Each participant received a detailed diabetes genetic risk report listing results for each successfully tested single nucleotide polymorphisms and the individual's overall diabetes genetic risk category (Supplementary Data). The one-on-one genetic counseling sessions explained the genetic test results, discussed the relative contributions of genetic versus lifestyle factors to the development of diabetes, and placed the recipient's genetic risk results within the context of his or her overall risk for diabetes. A primary goal of the counseling session was to use the genetic test result as an opportunity to encourage overall diabetes risk reduction through behavioral changes.

Counseled intervention participants and untested control subjects participated in a 12-week diabetes prevention program conducted by an experienced dietitian from our institution's Diabetes

Center who was masked to the genetic results. The diabetes prevention groups combined intervention and control participants to eliminate any group-based intervention effects. Participants were asked to refrain from discussing their genetic testing status and results. Masking was well preserved, with the correct prediction of participant testing status by the dietitian after completion of the 12-week program no better than chance (33.2%).

Outcome measures

We posited a causal pathway for diabetes prevention by which changes in patient motivation would lead to changes in the health-related behaviors that in turn would induce the physiologic changes necessary to prevent diabetes. To capture changes in motivation, we assessed self-reported confidence and motivation to make diabetes-related lifestyle changes (exercise, weight loss, and adoption of a low-fat diet) and stage of change for achieving these behaviors (25–27). To assess behavioral changes, we measured number of sessions attended for the 12-week Lifestyle Balance program because prior research has demonstrated a positive dose–response relationship between attendance and diabetes prevention (28). Finally, we also assessed weight change from baseline to program completion.

Statistical analyses

For our primary analyses, we examined changes in self-reported responses from baseline to study end, separately comparing higher-risk and lower-risk recipients with untested control participants. The study was designed to have sufficient power for assessing 1) the difference between comparison arms from baseline to study completion in self-reported stages of change, and 2) differences in program attendance. We estimated that with 30 intervention participants in each arm and 30 control participants, we had 97% power to detect a 90% increase in higher-risk intervention patients versus a 50% increase in control participants regarding stage of change at 0.05 two-sided significance and 78% power to show a 21% decrease in motivation comparing lower-risk intervention patients with control participants. For attendance, we estimated that the study sample size would provide 96% power to detect a 20% difference in number of diabetes prevention sessions attended (i.e., difference of 1.7 visits assuming that control participants attended 8.5 of 12 visits).

For stages of change, we dichotomized the results into percentage of participants who improved or increased versus all others. Changes from baseline in 10-point scales for motivation and confidence were analyzed as continuous data using t tests and dichotomized data (increase vs. no increase) using χ^2 tests. Program attendance was analyzed as a continuous variable (using t tests and Wilcoxon rank sum to compare means and medians) and also dichotomized as proportion of participants attending at least seven sessions (a threshold consistent with the Centers for Disease Control and Prevention's attendance criteria for diabetes prevention recognition programs) (29) as the goal for group-based diabetes prevention programs. All analyses were intention-to-treat.

In a planned secondary analysis, we also compared the relative effect and durability of the genetic counseling intervention between higher- versus lower-risk intervention recipients after completion of the 12-week program.

RESULTS

Study participants
We contacted 687 potentially eligible participants by telephone. After excluding ineligible 83 individuals, 177 of 604 participants (29.3%) consented to participate. Study allocation arms were well balanced (Table 1). All participants reported high motivation (9.4 on a scale of 0–10) to prevent diabetes, although motivation and confidence for making specific changes involving weight loss, diet, and increasing exercise were lower, ranging from 6.8 to 8.4.

Changes in self-reported attitudes
Enrollment in the 12-week diabetes prevention program led to small, generally favorable changes in risk perception, motivation (with the exception of exercise), and confidence that were not statistically different comparing higher- or lower-risk result recipients with control participants (Table 2). There was some evidence that lower-risk result recipients had less intent to exercise, with 37.5% of these participants increasing their stage of change for exercise compared with 64.7% of control participants ($P = 0.03$).

Differences in program attendance and weight loss
Study participants attended a mean of 6.8 ± 4.3 of 12 diabetes prevention group sessions. The 12-week Lifestyle Change program had a beneficial overall effect, with enrollees losing a mean of 8.5 ± 10.1

Table 1—*Baseline characteristics of the 116 participants by intervention allocation*

	Control subjects $n = 38$	Higher genetic risk $n = 44$	P	Lower genetic risk $n = 34$	P
Age (years), mean ± SD	59.6 ± 10.8	56.2 ± 8.9	0.12	61.0 ± 12.0	0.61
Male sex, n (%)	25 (65.8)	25 (56.8)	0.41	19 (55.9)	0.39
Race, n (%)					
Black	1 (2.6)	3 (6.8)	0.63	0	1.0
White	32 (84.2)	33 (75.0)		30 (88.2)	
Other	5 (13.2)	8 (18.2)		4 (11.8)	
BMI (kg/m^2), mean ± SD	34.7 ± 3.6	34.8 ± 5.5	0.96	36.1 ± 6.2	0.27
Annual household income, n (%)					
<$50,000	13 (36.1)	12 (27.9)	0.55	12 (37.5)	0.39
$50,000–99,000	9 (25.0)	9 (20.9)		12 (37.5)	
>$100,000	14 (38.9)	22 (51.2)		8 (25.0)	
Education, n (%)					
≤12th grade or General Educational Development test	4 (10.5)	8 (18.2)	0.5	12 (35.3)	0.05
1–3 years of college	13 (34.2)	11 (25.0)		9 (26.5)	
≥ 4 years of college	21 (55.3)	25 (56.8)		13 (38.2)	
Family history of diabetes, n (%)	19 (50.0)	25 (56.8)	0.54	21 (61.8)	0.32
Current health, n (%)					
Poor	0	0	0.73	1 (2.9)	0.72
Fairly poor	4 (10.5)	3 (6.8)		4 (11.8)	
Average	14 (36.8)	16 (36.4)		9 (26.5)	
Good	14 (36.8)	14 (31.8)		16 (47.1)	
Very good	6 (15.8)	11 (25.0)		4 (11.8)	
Diabetes risk perception (% reporting "moderate/high" risk)	73.5	65.6*	0.47	68.8	0.69
Motivation (10-point scale) for					
Weight loss	8.0	8.3	0.44	8.1	0.80
Dietary change	7.8	8.3	0.16	8.1	0.38
Exercise increase	8.2	8.4	0.54	8.0	0.70
Diabetes prevention	9.4	9.5	0.84	9.5	0.85
Confidence (10-point scale) for					
Weight loss	7.0	7.6	0.19	6.8	0.69
Dietary change	7.3	8.0	0.15	7.0	0.58
Exercise increase	7.8	7.9	0.74	7.0	0.13
Diabetes prevention	8.2	8.1	0.86	7.7	0.33
Stage of change (% in action/maintenance)					
Weight loss	12 (35.2)	15 (35.7)	0.97	9 (28.1)	0.53
Diet	5 (15.2)	10 (23.8)*	0.35	4 (12.5)*	0.76
Exercise	8 (23.5)	13 (31.0)	0.47	5 (15.6)	0.41

P values compare higher-risk recipients vs. control participants and lower-risk recipients vs. control participants. Race, income, education, and family history of diabetes are self-reported. Motivation and confidence questions are based on 10-point Likert scales ranging from 0 (not at all) to 10 (highest motivation/very confident). Prochaska stages of change progress from precontemplative to contemplative, preparation, action, and maintenance (25–27). *One missing response.

pounds ($P < 0.001$) and 33 of 108 participants (30.6%) losing ≥5% body weight. However, despite clear room for improvement in program attendance and goal weight achievement, receipt of personal genetic risk information and counseling had no statistically significant effect on measured behaviors compared with untested control participants (Table 3 and Fig. 1). Recipients

of higher-risk results attended 0.4 more sessions (95% CI −1.6 to 2.5; $P = 0.67$) and lost more weight (BMI difference −0.2 kg/m^2 [−0.5 to 0.9]; $P = 0.52$) compared with control participants. Lower-risk recipients attended 0.3 fewer sessions (−1.9 to 2.4; $P = 0.82$) and also lost more weight (BMI difference −0.3 kg/m^2 [−0.5 to 1.1]; $P = 0.48$) compared with control participants.

Table 2—*Changes from baseline in self-reported measures of risk perception, motivation, confidence, and stage of change for diabetes prevention behaviors, comparing recipients of higher and lower genetic risk results with untested control subjects*

	Control n = 34	Higher n = 42	P	Lower n = 32	P
Increased diabetes risk perception	4 (11.8)	9 (22.0)*	0.25	1 (3.1)	0.18
Increased motivation					
Weight loss	17 (50.0)	12 (28.6)	0.056	13 (40.6)	0.44
Dietary change	15 (44.1)	16 (38.1)	0.60	12 (37.5)	0.58
Exercise increase	11 (32.4)	10 (23.8)	0.41	8 (25.0)	0.51
Diabetes prevention	3 (8.8)	7 (16.7)	0.31	5 (15.6)	0.40
Increased confidence					
Weight loss	18 (52.9)	15 (35.7)	0.13	18 (52.9)	0.21
Dietary change	16 (47.1)	20 (47.6)	0.96	11 (35.5)*	0.34
Exercise increase	14 (41.2)	17 (40.5)	0.95	11 (34.4)	0.57
Diabetes prevention	11 (32.4)	17 (40.5)	0.47	13 (41.9)*	0.42
Increased in stage of change					
Weight loss	20 (58.8)	22 (53.7)	0.65	19 (59.4)	0.96
Diet	17 (51.5)	21 (50.0)	0.90	12 (40.0)	0.36
Exercise	22 (64.7)	19 (45.2)	0.09	12 (37.5)	0.03

Data are shown as *n* (%). *P* values compare higher-risk recipients vs. control participants and lower-risk recipients vs. control participants. Number (%) with increased motivation and confidence based on improvement from baseline in response to 10-point Likert scale ranging from 0 (not at all) to 10 (very confident/highest motivation). Prochaska stages of change progress from precontemplative to contemplative, preparation, action, and maintenance (25–27). *One missing response.

Secondary analysis of higher- versus lower-risk intervention arms

After completing the 12-week prevention program, 74 intervention participants (96%) recalled their diabetes genetic risk status (e.g., "higher" or "lower"), although only 2 (3%) could accurately recall their numeric genetic risk score. In an exploratory analysis, we found that higher-risk result recipients more often reported that the initial genetic counseling intervention had made them "much more/somewhat more" motivated to participate in the 12-week program (78.6% vs. 43.8% for lower-risk participants, *P* = 0.003) and to make lifestyle changes to prevent diabetes (85.7% vs. 56.3% for lower-risk

participants, *P* = 0.008). A significant proportion of lower-risk result recipients reported that they had not thought about their genetic risk results in the prior 3 months (43.8% vs. 16.7% of higher result recipients, *P* = 0.02). Despite these self-reported differences, program attendance and weight loss were not statistically different when the two intervention arms were compared (*P* > 0.05).

CONCLUSIONS—Among overweight primary care patients at increased phenotypic risk for type 2 diabetes, receiving a higher genetic risk result and counseling did not significantly improve motivation

to adopt diabetes prevention behaviors or significantly increase program attendance or weight loss compared with untested control patients. Conversely, receiving a lower genetic risk result did not appear to significantly detract from motivation or attendance.

The GC/LC Study is one of the first rigorous, controlled trials to directly address the effect of diabetes genetic risk information on patient behavior. Our study has several important strengths. We designed our genetic counseling intervention to be intensive yet relatively brief to maximize the translatability to the real-world clinical setting. Delivered by an experienced genetic counselor, the counseling intervention was designed to educate recipients about the relative contributions of both genetic and behavioral risk and to emphasize that changing their behavior could reduce their overall diabetes risk. This approach received positive preliminary feedback by study participants for its effect on perceived control and general satisfaction with the genetic counseling process (24). Crucially, all study participants were then enrolled in an evidence-based and validated diabetes prevention program designed to provide them with the tools and skills necessary to achieve the required behavior changes for diabetes prevention. We believe that using the genetic test disclosure as a "teachable moment" to engage patients in risk-reducing behavior change represents a powerful model for how genetic testing for common chronic diseases can be implemented into primary care practice. By coupling information (genetic test results and counseling) to a mechanism for participants to act on the information (diabetes prevention program), the GC/LC Study created an ideal context for genetic testing to succeed as a motivator.

Our study was also designed to directly address the potential for false reassurance from receiving results showing a lower genetic risk, particularly among patients with increased risk based on family history or validated phenotypic measures. We did not uncover a strong negative influence of receiving a "lower" risk result, with the possible exception of one exercise measure. From our exit surveys, it appears that many lower-risk recipients underemphasized their genetic test results. We suspect that most of the genetically tested patients with average results would have had a similar response, indicating that diabetes genetic risk

Table 3—*Differences in program attendance and weight loss, comparing recipients of higher and lower genetic risk results with untested control subjects*

	Control n = 34	Higher n = 42	P	Lower n = 32	P
Classes attended of 12 scheduled					
Mean ± SD	6.6 ± 4.7	7.0 ± 4.0	0.67	6.8 ± 4.2	0.82
Median (interquartile range)	9 (1–11)	8 (3–11)	0.84	8 (3.5–10)	0.97
Attended ≥7 classes, *n* (%)	20 (58.8)	26 (61.9)	0.78	20 (62.5)	0.76
Weigh loss (pounds), mean ± SD	7.52 ± 9.59	8.74 ± 9.60	0.58	9.18 ± 11.6	0.53
BMI reduction (kg/m²), mean ± SD	1.02 ± 1.45	1.23 ± 1.47	0.52	1.30 ± 1.80	0.48
Lost 7% body weight, *n* (%)	6 (17.7)	10 (23.8)	0.51	6 (18.8)	0.91

P values compare higher-risk recipients vs. control subjects and lower-risk recipients vs. control subjects.

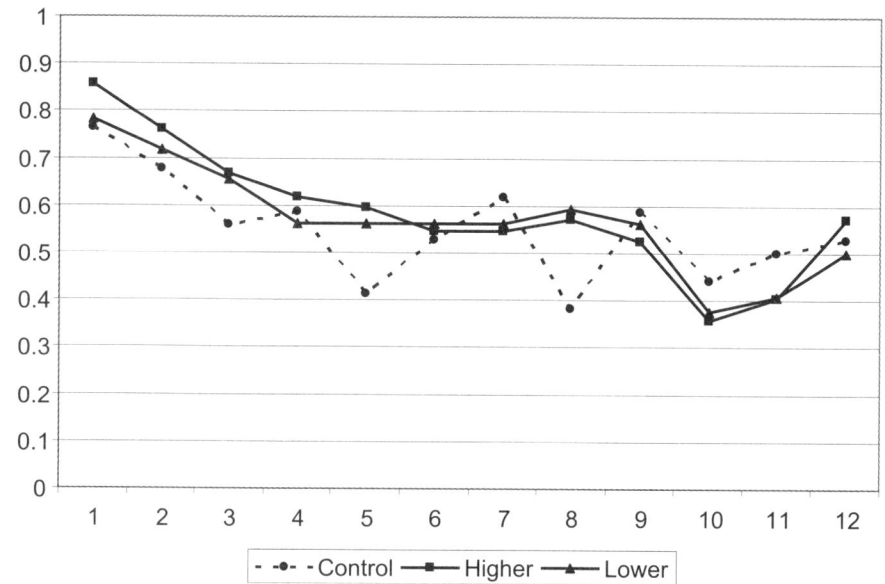

Figure 1—*Proportion of participants attending each week of the 12-week Diabetes Prevention Program.*

testing and counseling, even if it ultimately provides greater predictive power, will likely have little benefit but will do little harm for most tested patients who do not have higher results.

Despite these study strengths, several limitations must be considered. Perhaps foremost of these is the limited predictive value of current diabetes genetic risk testing, which required us to focus on the highest-risk patients to maximize the resulting contrast between tested and untested participants. Even in this group, with an estimated 3-year risk for diabetes of 11%, the recalculated risk based on relative genetic risk results resulted in only modest changes. Thus, we do not know whether greater genetic predictive ability in the future will have a bigger impact on changing behavior. However, given that 96% of our intervention patients remembered their qualitative genetic risk (i.e., "higher" or "lower") but not their quantitative risk score (provided as a hand-out during the counseling session), we suspect that marginal improvements in risk prediction will not lead to substantially greater impact on patient behavior.

Another limitation of current genetic knowledge is that results do not alter the actual behavioral intervention; thus, although the risk information is personalized, the intervention itself is not. The Diabetes Prevention Program recently showed that an intensive lifestyle intervention benefits participants regardless of overall genetic risk (30), but future research

focused on unique gene-environment interactions may help to further tailor interventions (e.g., some patients may benefit preferentially from caloric restriction or certain dietary plans, others from aerobic exercise or resistance training) (31) and therefore lead to truly personalized behavioral treatments. Finally, although we cannot exclude small differences in self-reported measures that did not reach statistical significance, we have good confidence that any difference in self-reported measures did not translate into significant changes in attendance behavior.

Our results must be considered within the context of the study design. We randomized in two stages to provide a clinically relevant test of genetic testing versus no testing on preventive behavior, while also efficiently focusing on the genetic risk extremes among tested participants. For the second-stage allocation of intervention participants, we relied on the concept of Mendelian randomization (e.g., the random allocation of parental alleles during gametogenesis) to identify top and bottom quartiles of genetic risk score distribution (32). A strategy of using the lowest quartile of score as "normal" would have increased the effect size in the highest quartile and would have eliminated the problem of presenting "lower" genetic risk results to otherwise phenotypically high-risk individuals. However, it seemed unethical to portray low-score outliers as normal given the population

distribution in which the vast majority of individuals fall within a relatively narrow middle range. In addition, creating more extreme cut points, such as the top decile of risk, would have resulted in higher relative risk differences at the expense of identifying an increasingly smaller number of participants, which would have diminished the clinical relevance of our results.

Focusing as we did on phenotypically high-risk participants might have limited the effect of the genetic risk results because these participants might already have been maximally motivated. The paradox of this limitation is that less motivated individuals are also less likely to be interested in genetic testing. Given the modest success rate among control participants in our study and among other community-based programs described in the literature (8–11), new tools to achieve enduring behavior change are clearly needed. One challenge for the future is to identify the subset of patients for whom genetic test results represent the tipping point from inaction to action.

Our findings build on an emerging literature in translational genomics and health outcomes (33–35) and have implications for current direct-to-consumer home genetic testing (36). Such tests may benefit self-selected individuals but may also have negative consequences in patient-borne costs and the potential for triggering expensive diagnostic cascades (37). Without further evidence of efficacy from controlled clinical trials, such testing cannot yet be recommended in routine clinical care for diabetes prevention. Other important applications of personalized genetic testing deserve further study, including clinically applied pharmacogenomic profiling (38) and evaluation of phenotypically lower-risk younger patients who have yet to manifest diabetes-related phenotypic traits.

In summary, a diabetes genetic risk assessment and counseling intervention for overweight individuals based on 36 single nucleotide polymorphisms neither improved nor substantially detracted from an evidence-based behavioral intervention to prevent diabetes.

Acknowledgments—This study received funding support from National Institute of Diabetes and Digestive and Kidney Diseases Grants R21-DK84527 and K24-DK080140. No potential conflicts of interest relevant to this article were reported.

R.W.G. obtained funding, oversaw the clinical trial, researched data, and wrote the manuscript. K.E.O., J.L.W., and K.G.S. contributed to the conduct of the clinical trial, researched data, and reviewed and edited the manuscript. J.L.V. researched data and reviewed and edited the manuscript. L.M.D., L.G.B., R.C.G., C.G., E.R.P., J.C.F., and J.B.M. contributed to the conduct of the clinical trial and reviewed and edited the manuscript. R.W.G. is the guarantor of this work and, as such, had full access to all the data in the study and takes responsibility for the integrity of the data and the accuracy of the data analysis.

The results of this study, titled "Can Genetic Testing Motivate Behavior Change and Weight Loss?" were presented at the "New Frontiers in Weight Management" symposium at the 72nd Scientific Sessions of the American Diabetes Association, Philadelphia, Pennsylvania, 8–12 June 2012.

The authors acknowledge the Diabetes Prevention Support Center of the University of Pittsburgh for providing the written materials for the Group Lifestyle Balance program.

References

1. Flegal KM, Carroll MD, Ogden CL, Curtin LR. Prevalence and trends in obesity among US adults, 1999-2008. JAMA 2010;303: 235–241
2. Wild S, Roglic G, Green A, Sicree R, King H. Global prevalence of diabetes: estimates for the year 2000 and projections for 2030. Diabetes Care 2004;27:1047–1053
3. Knowler WC, Barrett-Connor E, Fowler SE, et al.; Diabetes Prevention Program Research Group. Reduction in the incidence of type 2 diabetes with lifestyle intervention or metformin. N Engl J Med 2002;346: 393–403
4. Tuomilehto J, Lindström J, Eriksson JG, et al.; Finnish Diabetes Prevention Study Group. Prevention of type 2 diabetes mellitus by changes in lifestyle among subjects with impaired glucose tolerance. N Engl J Med 2001;344:1343–1350
5. Pan XR, Li GW, Hu YH, et al. Effects of diet and exercise in preventing NIDDM in people with impaired glucose tolerance. The Da Qing IGT and Diabetes Study. Diabetes Care 1997;20:537–544
6. Jacobs-van der Bruggen MA, van Baal PH, Hoogenveen RT, et al. Cost-effectiveness of lifestyle modification in diabetic patients. Diabetes Care 2009;32:1453–1458
7. Herman WH, Hoerger TJ, Brandle M, et al.; Diabetes Prevention Program Research Group. The cost-effectiveness of lifestyle modification or metformin in preventing type 2 diabetes in adults with impaired glucose tolerance. Ann Intern Med 2005; 142:323–332
8. Ackermann RT, Finch EA, Brizendine E, Zhou H, Marrero DG. Translating the diabetes prevention program into the community. The DEPLOY pilot study. Am J Prev Med 2008;35:357–363
9. Seidel MC, Powell RO, Zgibor JC, Siminerio LM, Piatt GA. Translating the Diabetes Prevention Program into an urban medically underserved community: a nonrandomized prospective intervention study. Diabetes Care 2008;31:684–689
10. Absetz P, Oldenburg B, Hankonen N, et al. Type 2 diabetes prevention in the real world: three-year results of the GOAL Lifestyle Implementation Trial. Diabetes Care 2009;32:1418–1420
11. Kramer MK, Kriska AM, Venditti EM, et al. Translating the Diabetes Prevention Program: a comprehensive model for prevention training and program delivery. Am J Prev Med 2009;37:505–511
12. McBride CM, Bowen D, Brody LC, et al. Future health applications of genomics: priorities for communication, behavioral, and social sciences research. Am J Prev Med 2010;38:556–565
13. Hamburg MA, Collins FS. The path to personalized medicine. N Engl J Med 2010;363:301–304
14. McBride CM, Koehly LM, Sanderson SC, Kaphingst KA. The behavioral response to personalized genetic information: will genetic risk profiles motivate individuals and families to choose more healthful behaviors? Annu Rev Public Health 2010; 31:89–103
15. Grant RW, Hivert M, Pandiscio JC, Florez JC, Nathan DM, Meigs JB. The clinical application of genetic testing in type 2 diabetes: a patient and physician survey. Diabetologia 2009;52:2299–2305
16. Markowitz SM, Park ER, Delahanty LM, O'Brien KE, Grant RW. Perceived impact of diabetes genetic risk testing among patients at high phenotypic risk for type 2 diabetes. Diabetes Care 2011;34:568–573
17. Marteau TM, French DP, Griffin SJ, et al. Effects of communicating DNA-based disease risk estimates on risk-reducing behaviours. Cochrane Database Syst Rev 2010:CD007275
18. Evans JP, Meslin EM, Marteau TM, Caulfield T. Genomics. Deflating the genomic bubble. Science 2011;331:861–862
19. Grant RW, Meigs JB, Florez JC, et al. Design of a randomized trial of diabetes genetic risk testing to motivate behavior change: the Genetic Counseling/Lifestyle Change (GC/LC) Study for Diabetes Prevention. Clin Trials 2011;8: 609–615
20. Grundy SM, Cleeman JI, Daniels SR, et al.; American Heart Association; National Heart, Lung, and Blood Institute. Diagnosis and management of the metabolic syndrome: an American Heart Association/National Heart, Lung, and Blood Institute Scientific Statement. Circulation 2005;112:2735–2752
21. de Miguel-Yanes JM, Shrader P, Pencina MJ, et al.; MAGIC Investigators; DIAGRAM + Investigators. Genetic risk reclassification for type 2 diabetes by age below or above 50 years using 40 type 2 diabetes risk single nucleotide polymorphisms. Diabetes Care 2011;34:121–125
22. Meigs JB, Shrader P, Sullivan LM, et al. Genotype score in addition to common risk factors for prediction of type 2 diabetes. N Engl J Med 2008;359:2208–2219
23. Hivert MF, Grant RW, Shrader P, Meigs JB. Identifying primary care patients at risk for future diabetes and cardiovascular disease using electronic health records. BMC Health Serv Res 2009;9:170
24. Waxler JL, O'Brien KE, Delahanty LM, et al. Genetic counseling as a tool for type 2 diabetes prevention: a new genetic counseling framework for common polygenetic disorders. J Genet Couns 2012 Feb 3 [Epub ahead of print]
25. Greene GW, Rossi SR, Reed GR, Willey C, Prochaska JO. Stages of change for reducing dietary fat to 30% of energy or less. J Am Diet Assoc 1994;94:1105–1110; quiz 1111–1112
26. Marcus BH, Selby VC, Niaura RS, Rossi JS. Self-efficacy and the stages of exercise behavior change. Res Q Exerc Sport 1992; 63:60–66
27. O'Connell D, Velicer WF. A decisional balance measure and the stages of change model for weight loss. Int J Addict 1988; 23:729–750
28. Lindström J, Ilanne-Parikka P, Peltonen M, et al.; Finnish Diabetes Prevention Study Group. Sustained reduction in the incidence of type 2 diabetes by lifestyle intervention: follow-up of the Finnish Diabetes Prevention Study. Lancet 2006; 368:1673–1679
29. Williamson DF, Marrero DG. Scaling up type 2 diabetes prevention programs for high risk persons: progress and challenges in the United States. In *Diabetes Prevention in Practice*. Schwarz P, Reddy P, Greaves C, Dunbar JA, Schwarz J, Eds. Dresden, TUMAINI Institute for Prevention Management, 2010, p. 69–82
30. Hivert MF, Jablonski KA, Perreault L, et al.; DIAGRAM Consortium; Diabetes Prevention Program Research Group. Updated genetic score based on 34 confirmed type 2 diabetes loci is associated with diabetes incidence and regression to normoglycemia in the Diabetes Prevention Program. Diabetes 2011;60: 1340–1348
31. Rosado EL, Bressan J, Martins MF, Cecon PR, Martínez JA. Polymorphism in the PPARgamma2 and beta2-adrenergic genes and diet lipid effects on body composition, energy expenditure and eating behavior of obese women. Appetite 2007; 49:635–643

32. Thanassoulis G, O'Donnell CJ. Mendelian randomization: nature's randomized trial in the post-genome era. JAMA 2009;301: 2386–2388

33. Collins F. Has the revolution arrived? Nature 2010;464:674–675

34. Green RC, Roberts JS, Cupples LA, et al.; REVEAL Study Group. Disclosure of APOE genotype for risk of Alzheimer's disease. N Engl J Med 2009;361:245–254

35. Scheuner MT, Sieverding P, Shekelle PG. Delivery of genomic medicine for common chronic adult diseases: a systematic review. JAMA 2008;299:1320–1334

36. Bloss CS, Schork NJ, Topol EJ. Effect of direct-to-consumer genomewide profiling to assess disease risk. N Engl J Med 2011; 364:524–534

37. Verrilli DW, Welch HG. The impact of diagnostic testing on therapeutic interventions. JAMA 1996;275:1189–1191

38. Wang L, McLeod HL, Weinshilboum RM. Genomics and drug response. N Engl J Med 2011;364:1144–1153

Divide and Conquer: The Multidisciplinary Approach to Achieving Significant Long-Term Weight Loss and Improved Glycemic Control in Obese Patients With Type 2 Diabetes

Ramy H. Bishay, BSc, MSc, MBBS, Abdullah Omari, MBBS, DDU, MMED, FRACP, PhD, Johnson Zang, BMedSc, MBBS, Anna Lih, MBBS, PhD, FRACP, and Nic Kormas, MBBS, FRACP

Type 2 diabetes has become a worldwide epidemic, estimated to affect 1 in 14 adults, or 380 million people, globally by 2025.[1,2] The problem is particularly acute in Australia, where the prevalence of diagnosed diabetes more than doubled between 1989 and 2005, amounting to 3 million people affected by the disease.[3,4] Diabetes is the most common reason for renal dialysis, blindness in people < 60 years of age, nontraumatic lower-limb amputation, and cardiovascular disease and is the sixth-highest cause of death by disease in Australia.[3,5]

First-line best-practice management includes brief counseling to promote lifestyle changes in diet, exercise, and education, with the aim to improve insulin resistance, reduce hypertension, correct dyslipidemia, and achieve weight reduction.[6] Patients at high risk of developing type 2 diabetes and who are refractory to lifestyle intervention may be treated with pharmacological agents and insulin, many of which contribute to further weight gain.[7,8]

According to several recent studies, a large proportion of newly diagnosed cases are potentially preventable or could at least be delayed through lifestyle and behavioral modification.[9–11] Data from 20 longitudinal cohort studies illustrate consistently that regular physical activity substantially reduces the risk of developing type 2 diabetes by 20–30%, with the greatest benefits obtained in obese patients with impaired glucose regulation undergoing moderate- or vigorous-intensity exercise.[11,12] One recent study validated a rigorous lifestyle intervention program with counseling for physical activity, nutrition, and weight loss, resulting in a risk reduction of 40–60% in adults with impaired glucose tolerance.[12]

Recent research supports the potential benefit of significant weight loss leading to diabetes "remission" (i.e., consistent normalization of blood glucose levels and A1C). In a pivotal study by Dixon et al.,[13] 73% of patients who were randomized to laparoscopic gastric banding achieved remission of their diabetes compared to 13% in the conventional therapy group, and the relative risk of remission for the surgical group was 5.5. The surgical group also had 20.0% body weight loss, representing 62.5% excess body weight (vs. 1.4% body weight loss or 4.3% excess body weight loss in standard group) at 2 years. Furthermore, remission was related to weight loss ($R^2 = 0.46$) and lower baseline A1C levels (combined $R^2 = 0.52$).

Nonsurgical metabolic rehabilitation poses several theoretical and logistical problems, and there is no currently advocated model. Previously reported strategies have included telephone-derived interventions,[2] 1-day outpatient motivational workshops,[14] general recommendation-based lifestyle programs,[15] a supervised resistance training program,[16] a supervised program of combined resistance and aerobic training,[17] and a home-based walking and resistance program.[18] These studies have all shown modest, short-term amelioration of cardiometabolic risk factors, but with various degrees of efficacy. In general, an absolute reduction of 0.4–0.5% in A1C can be achieved, with varying degrees of weight loss and modest improvement in lipid profiles. Nonetheless, these studies point to weight loss as the most important determinant in improving health outcomes in high-risk and diagnosed type 2 diabetes patients with cardiovascular risk factors.

With some exceptions,[19–24] data are lacking with respect to ameliorating health risks in obese patients with established type 2 diabetes. We have established a multidisciplinary, nonsurgical metabolic rehabilitation program (MRP) with a mandatory exercise component and weight loss as the primary intervention. This study followed a small population of obese patients with type 2 diabetes presenting to the MRP, an outpatient program established at a tertiary teaching hospital in Sydney, Australia. We hypothesized that an intensive exercise program with multidisciplinary support could achieve significant improvement in cardiometabolic risk factors and that these results could be sustained in the long term.

Methods

This was a retrospective study from 2004 to 2007 of patients enrolled in the MRP. Participants were required to fulfill three criteria: *1*) have a BMI > 30 kg/m², *2*) have established type 2 diabetes, and *3*) have a referral from their general practitioner or treating endocrinologist. Patients with cardiac or other conditions that precluded undertaking intensive exercise sessions or having a body weight > 150 kg were excluded. The minimum commitment was 1 year plus 80% attendance at all sessions. No exclusions were made related to duration of diabetes, primary or secondary causes of diabetes, or other comorbidities.

Design

The program consisted of clinical consultations and supervised exercise classes. It included *1*) appointments with an endocrinologist specializing in obesity and diabetes management conducted monthly for the first 6 months and then every 2–3 months thereafter; *2*) dietitian appointments, including an initial consultation, a follow-up visit at 6 weeks, an annual visit, and eight group sessions conducted throughout the duration of the program to help patients with a healthy eating plan and meal replacement (e.g., Optifast); *3*) appointments with diabetes educators, including an initial visit and every 6 months thereafter if needed to provide monitoring of blood glucose levels and advice on administering medication; *4*) psychologist appointments, including

an initial visit and four group sessions conducted throughout the duration of the program to detect and treat psychosocial barriers to healthy eating and exercise; *5*) physiotherapists available on request to treat physical factors limiting patients' ability to exercise; and *6*) exercise physiologists available daily for 6 days/week to help assess, prescribe, and supervise exercise.

The Bodylines program, a validated educational weight loss program developed at the Royal Prince Alfred Hospital in Sydney, New South Wales, Australia, was delivered in modules and integrated in the group sessions conducted by the dietitians and psychologists.

Exercise sessions were held in the early mornings and late afternoons each day to facilitate participation. The minimum level of participation was attendance at three exercise sessions per week, for a total of 180 minutes of supervised exercise in the hospital gymnasium. Patients were also prescribed 120 minutes (2 × 60 minutes) of exercise routines for off-clinic days to achieve an overall cumulative amount of 300 minutes/week of exercise, inclusive of the supervised exercise sessions. Off-clinic exercise routines could include walking, swimming, or whatever exercise was conducive to the patient's environment.

The supervised exercise sessions included a combination of resistance and aerobic exercises. The aerobic component lasted a total of 20–30 minutes using a variety of methods including treadmills, bikes, rowers, steppers, mini-trampolines, rebounders, step-up boxes, and lap-walking with light hand weights. Intensity levels were based on achievement of a heart rate (HR) response of 60–80% of predicted maximal HR (average range 110–140 beats per minute), taking into account age, fitness level, risk of injury, and cardiorespiratory

risk factors. For patients who were on negatively chronotropic medications (e.g., beta-blockers), rate of perceived exertion of the individual patient was used instead, aiming for 5–8 out of a maximum 10 as a subjective scale of exertion as a guide.

The resistance component usually consisted of 20–30 minutes, with the remaining 5–10 minutes for cooling down, stretches, and abdominal exercises. It included mostly pin-loaded machines and free weights (e.g., dumbbells), with patients given appropriate exercises taking into account their tolerance range and fitness, physical limitations, past injuries, age, medications, comorbidities, cardiac risk factors, and exercise history. Generally, the appropriate weight was a load that could be completed in 8–15 repetitions. This was repeated for up to three sets during the session, with the exercise routine designed to include a balance of opposing muscle groups (e.g., chest and upper back, quads and hamstring, etc.) with alternating upper-body and lower-body exercises to ensure maximum recovery between exercises. The emphasis was on resistance, not on body-building or heavy weight lifting, so as to minimize the risk of injury.

Physiological parameters were collected before enrollment and every 6 months for 30 months or until voluntary discharge from the program. The physical parameters collected included weight, waist circumference, BMI, A1C, systolic and diastolic blood pressure, and HDL cholesterol, LDL cholesterol, and triglyceride levels.

All contact and patient details were stored confidentially by the study coordinator in a private database file and de-identified. The local human research ethics committee approved the study.

All data are expressed as mean ± standard error of mean (SEM). Percentage change was calculated as a percentage difference from baseline. Excess body weight (EBW) was defined as current weight (kg) minus $25 \times$ height $(m)^2$. Statistical significance was determined using a repeated-measures, one-way analysis of variance. Pair-wise comparisons between different time points were calculated using the Holm-Sidak method. All statistical analyses were performed with SigmaStat (Systat Software Inc., Chicago, Ill.). Probability values < 0.05 were considered statistically significant.

Results

Of 62 participants enrolled, 15 were excluded from analysis because they participated for < 1 year. Forty-seven patients continued to 18 months; 44 participated for 24 months; and 41 participated for the full 30 months of the study period.

Baseline data are summarized in Table 1. There were approximately equal numbers of male (45%) and female (55%) participants. Ethnicity was divided as follows: 72% Caucasian, 21% Mediterranean, and the remainder divided among Hispanic, Asian, and Indian backgrounds (7%). Given the small cohort studied, subanalyses taking into account sex and ethnic differences were not analyzed.

The average age was 59.1 ± 9.4 years (range 33–72 years), and the mean weight was 104.7 ± 19.9 kg, representing a baseline EBW of 35.0 ± 16.6 kg. Baseline BMI (37.6 ± 5.7 kg/m²) fell within the World Health Organization obese class II.[25] Waist circumference at enrollment was 113.4 ± 12.6 cm, reflecting the substantially increased risk of cardiometabolic complications in this patient cohort.[25]

Patients had suboptimal glycemic control, with an average A1C of

Table 1. Baseline Data of Participants in the MRP	
Baseline Parameters	**Mean ± SEM**
Sex (*n* [%]) Male Female	 21 (45) 26 (55)
Duration of diagnosis (years)	10.5 ± 7.2 (range 1–34)
Weight (kg)	104.7 ± 19.9
Height (m)	1.67 ± 0.1
BMI (kg/m²)	37.6 ± 5.7
Waist circumference (cm)	113.4 ± 12.6
EBW	35.0 ± 16.6
A1C (%)	8.2 ± 1.6
Systolic blood pressure (mmHg)	137.0 ± 18.6
Diastolic blood pressure (mmHg)	79 ± 9.1
HDL cholesterol (mg/dl)	48.7 ± 24.7
LDL cholesterol (mg/dl)	97.8 ± 34.8
Triglycerides (mg/dl)	183.2 ± 88.5
Patients taking anti-lipid medications (*n* [%])	31 (66)
Patients taking antihypertensive medications (*n* [%])	35 (74)
Patients taking oral hypoglycemic medications (*n* [%])	38 (81)
Patients taking insulin ± oral agents (*n* [%])	12 (25)
Patients with metabolic syndrome	47 (100)

8.2 + 1.6%, despite the fact that the majority were on conventional treatment with oral hypoglycemic agents (81%) or insulin plus oral agent therapy (25%). Although 74% were taking antihypertensive medications, patients were clinically defined as hypertensive (systolic blood pressure of 137.0 ± 18.6 mmHg and diastolic blood pressure of 79 ± 9.1 mmHg). Sixty-six percent of patients were taking anti-lipid therapy. Baseline HDL cholesterol (48.7 ± 24.7 mg/dl), LDL cholesterol (97.8 ± 34.8 mg/dl), and triglyceride levels (183.2 ± 88.5 mg/dl) were suboptimal according to

the recommended target ranges for adults with type 2 diabetes.[26]

The average duration of diabetes was 10.5 ± 7.2 years (range 1–34 years). All patients were treated in a diabetes clinic or in a private practice by an endocrinologist, and 67% were referred to the MRP by their treating endocrinologist.

The average number of exercise sessions attended per week was 4.1 ± 0.9, with 94% of patients attending an average of at least two sessions per week and 87% of patients attending an average of at least three sessions per week.

Significant reductions were achieved in all parameters (Figure 1*A–H*) as early as 6 months (6-month values vs. baseline, *P* < 0.001, are marked with α). Continued reductions were seen at 12 months (all values vs. 6-month values, *P* < 0.001, marked with asterisks) in weight (8.4 ± 0.9 kg), weight loss (7.9 ± 0.8%), EBW (26.8 ± 2.3 kg), EBW loss (25.3 ± 2.8%), reduction in BMI (8.4 ± 1.1%), reduction in waist circumference (6.5 ± 0.9%), percentage reduction in A1C (11.4 ± 2.1%), and absolute reduction in A1C (1.1 ± 0.2 percentage points).

All parameters were maintained for as long as 30 months: weight (10.8 ± 1.7 kg), weight loss 9.8 ± 1.4%, EBW (25.2 ± 2.3 kg), BW loss (29.5 ± 4.1%), reduction of BMI (10.0 ± 1.5%), reduction of waist circumference (6.3 ± 1.3%), percentage of A1C reduction (9.7 ± 2.5%), and absolute reduction in A1C (0.9 ± 0.2 percentage points).

Significant reductions in systolic blood pressure (6.4 ± 1.99%, *P* = 0.015) and diastolic blood pressure (6.6 ± 2.0%, *P* = 0.008) were observed at 1 year. Insulin dosage was halved at 30 months (from 93.8 ± 6.3 IU to 46.0 ± 5.0 IU, *P* < 0.01).

A significant increase in HDL cholesterol was observed at 24 months (10.6 ± 4.3%, *P* = 0.049 [from 50.3 ± 31 mg/dl to 58.0 ± 15.5 mg/dl, *P* = 0.018]). Despite a general observable decrease at 30 months, LDL cholesterol and triglyceride levels (10.0 ± 7.3 and 12.9 ± 6.6%, respectively) were not significantly different from baseline at 30 months.

Discussion

This study demonstrated that obese diabetes patients with suboptimal control of cardiometabolic risk factors despite standard best care can achieve significant improvements in weight, waist circumference, physical activity, and glycemic control in an

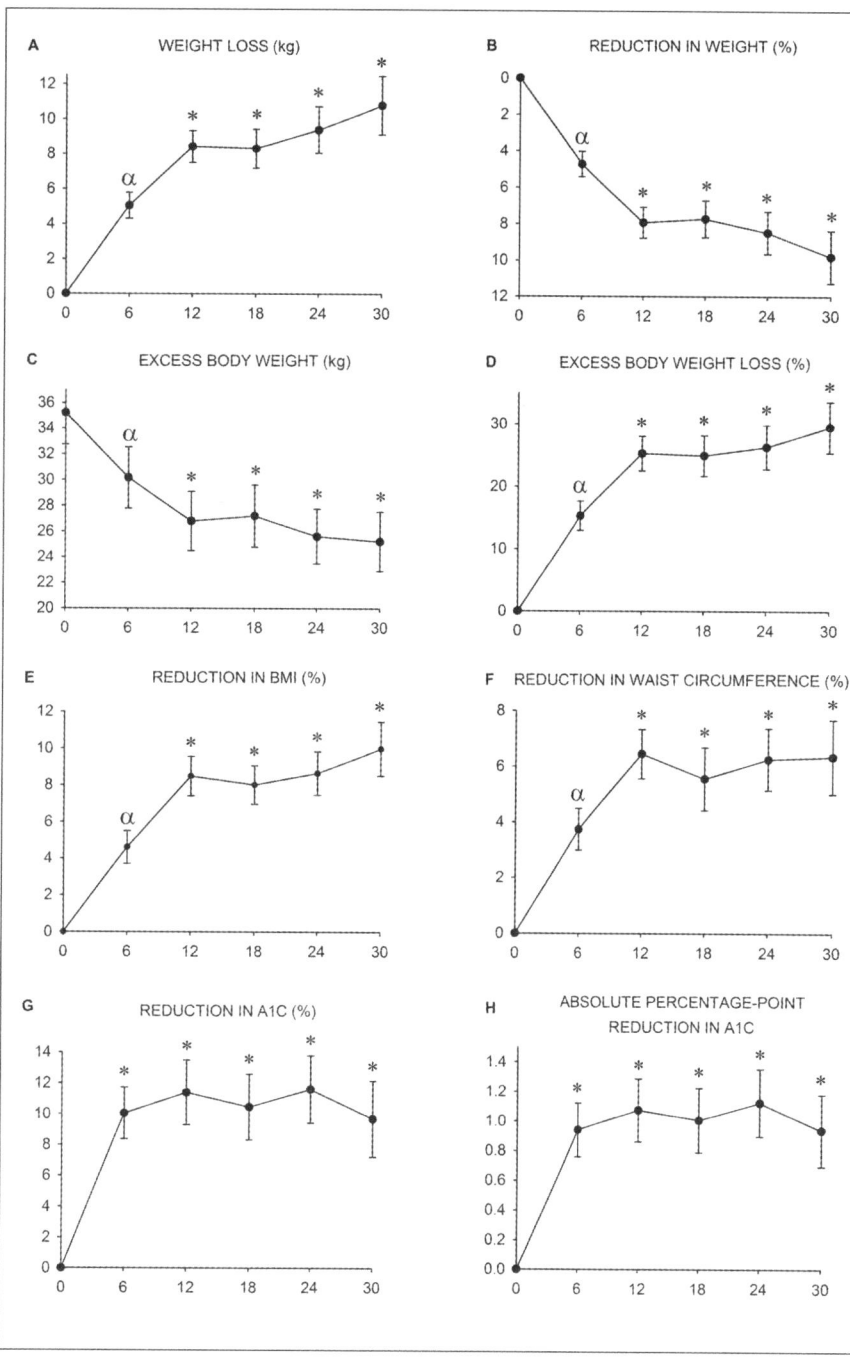

Figure 1. Significant reduction in cardiometabolic parameters maintained for 30 months in obese diabetes patients with multidisciplinary metabolic rehabilitation. A: *Weight loss (kg);* B: *weight reduction (%);* C: *EBW (kg);* D: *reduction in EBW (%);* E: *reduction in BMI (%);* F: *reduction in waist circumference (%);* G: *reduction in A1C (%); and* H: *absolute reduction in A1C (%). Significant differences versus baseline are indicated with* α *(P < 0.001) and significant differences versus 6-month values are indicated with asterisks (P < 0.001). All data are expressed as mean ± SEM.*

intensive, nonsurgical interventional program focused on weight reduction, increased physical activity, dietary modification, and psychosocial support at 30 months.

Numerous randomized, controlled studies illustrate a beneficial effect on several metabolic parameters achieved through intensive interventional programs,[15,27–31] but these programs often offer limited information because the time period is typically ≤ 1 year. Our program, which employed dietitians, clinical nurse educators in obesity and diabetes, physiotherapists, exercise physiologists, personal trainers, a psychologist, and an endocrinologist, achieved consistent long-term results.

Similarly, the Finnish Diabetes Prevention Study [20] showed favorable long-term results using multidisciplinary approaches in a randomized, controlled study involving patients with prediabetes (i.e., impaired glucose tolerance), in which patients were allocated to either a usual-care control group (dietary and exercise advice plus annual specialist visits) or an intensive lifestyle intervention group (dietary and exercise counseling plus circuit-type resistance training sessions). The intervention group lost 4.5 and 3.5 kg, whereas the control group lost 1.0 and 0.9 kg after 1 and 3 years, respectively. The gains, although modest, were sustained over the long term at 3 years' follow-up. This may reflect the necessity of a more intensive intervention to achieve meaningful outcomes in a high-risk population, whether for patients with prediabetes or established diabetes.

To date, the most comprehensive comparison between intensive lifestyle intervention and standard care is the Look AHEAD trial.[21–23] Although baseline characteristics with respect to average age, BMI, weight, and waist circumference

were not significantly different in our study compared to the Look AHEAD trial, our participants were more complex at baseline, with a minimum BMI ≥ 30 kg/m² (vs. 25 kg/m²), poorer glycemic control (A1C 8.2 vs. 7.3%) and more hypertension (systolic blood pressure 137 vs. 128 mmHg, diastolic blood pressure 79 vs. 69 mmHg). Furthermore, 100% of our participants had a diagnosis of metabolic syndrome, and 24% were using insulin, versus 93 and 14.8%, respectively in the Look AHEAD trial.[22] Our patients also had an appreciable mean time from diagnosis of type 2 diabetes of 10.5 years.

At 1 year, the Look AHEAD study achieved 8.6% weight loss in the intervention group versus 7.9% in our study.[21] By 3 years, modest results were sustained for weight loss (5.5%), although our cohort lost more weight (9.8%), possibly because of the nearly doubled prescribed exercise requirement in our study (300 vs. 175 minutes per week), of which 180 minutes was supervised in our gymnasium. This finding substantiates the superiority of supervised exercise in achieving better outcomes.[16]

We also achieved a reduction in A1C of 11.4 versus 6.3% at 1 year and 9.7 versus 3.2% at 30 months.[23] This reflects the likely benefit of our increased exercise requirements and the favorable effects of a combination of aerobic and resistance training on glycemic control.[17,24] The reduction in A1C in our study is significant considering that the U.K. Prospective Diabetes Study[32] demonstrated that for each 1% reduction in A1C, there were reductions of 21% in deaths related to diabetes, 14% in the incidence of myocardial infarction, and 37% in microvascular complications.[32]

Modest reductions in systolic blood pressure were reflected simi-

larly in the Look AHEAD trial and in our study (6.8 and 6.4%, respectively), although our study achieved a greater reduction in diastolic blood pressure at 1 year (6.6 vs. 3.0%) and increased HDL cholesterol at 2 years (10.6 vs. 9.6%). Blood pressure continued to decrease for 30 months, although this change was statistically nonsignificant.

Although there is a clear, short-term association between blood pressure reduction and weight loss and caloric restriction,[33] previous studies observed a rebound of blood pressure over the long term despite maintained weight loss.[34] A recent review by Aucott et al.[35] of nine clinical trials and eight cohort studies found that reductions in systolic blood pressure (but less reliably in diastolic blood pressure) of 1 mmHg to each 1 kg of weight loss may be expected, but only for short follow-up periods of 2–3 years, possibly because of the secondary effects of medications, diet, and pre-study blood pressure levels.

Studies have shown the rates of comorbid mental health problems to be substantially higher in diabetic patients than in the general population, with associated poorer functional status and clinical outcomes, more complications, and increased mortality.[36] Our program employed an onsite psychologist with inclusion of individual and group sessions to counsel patients about psychosocial barriers to achieving better emotional and psychological well-being, as well as to empower patients to become active participants in their own diabetes management. These strategies, which generally included assisting patients with decision-making and problem-solving skills, augmenting their confidence, supporting their goals, and promoting self-efficacy, have been shown to lead to better glycemic control and encourage positive behavior change in type 2 diabetes patients.[37–39] These approaches are also consistent with the recently revised American Diabetes Association standards of practice guidelines, which promote a more patient-centered model incorporating group sessions, ongoing support, and behavioral goal-setting as crucial aspects of diabetes self-management education.[40]

Conclusion

In summary, cardiometabolic improvements were maintained over the long term in obese adults with complex type 2 diabetes using intensive multidisciplinary metabolic rehabilitation. Limitations of this study included its retrospective design and small number of subjects, which likely precluded reaching an appreciable statistical power to show long-term significant changes in lipid profiles and possibly blood pressure. The aim, however, was to establish improvements in health outcomes in high-risk obese patients with type 2 diabetes before larger-scale studies are implemented.

The effect of pharmacological unloading, particularly on lipid profiles and blood pressure, may also partially explain the lack of long-term significance in these parameters, as many patients reached clinical targets and ceased medications. Future studies involving larger numbers of patients with randomization to either usual "best-practice" clinics or the MRP are needed to evaluate long-term health outcomes.

ACKNOWLEDGMENTS

Author contributions to this article were as follows: R.H.B. researched and analyzed the data, participated in the conceptual design, and prepared the manuscript. A.O. supplied a significant portion of the data at 12 months and reviewed and edited the manuscript. J.Z. collected data from months 12–30. A.L. provided further review and editing of the manuscript. N.K. critiqued the data, manuscript, and access to the patient cohort for study. An abstract based on this study was accepted for presentation at the Australian Diabetes Society annual scientific meeting in 2011. The authors thank Professor Markus Seibel, head of the Department of Endocrinology and Metabolism, Concord Repatriation General Hospital, in Concord, New South Wales, Australia, for encouraging the organization of this study and Karen Evans for her assistance with the manuscript, particularly the exercise component.

REFERENCES

[1]Iqbal N: The burden of type 2 diabetes: strategies to prevent or delay onset. *Vasc Health Risk Manag* 3:511–520, 2007

[2]Eakin EG, Reeves MM, Lawler SP, Oldenburg B, Del Mar C, Wilkie K, Spencer A, Battistutta D, Graves N: The Logan Healthy Living Program: a cluster randomized trial of a telephone-delivered physical activity and dietary behavior intervention for primary care patients with type 2 diabetes or hypertension from a socially disadvantaged community: rationale, design and recruitment. *Contemp Clin Trials* 29:439–454, 2008

[3] Australian Institute of Health and Welfare: Diabetes: Australian facts 2008. Diabetes series no. 8. Cat. no. CVD 40. Canberra, Australian Institute of Health and Welfare. Available from www.aihw.gov.au. Accessed 12 November 2012

[4]Mbanya JC, Gan D, Allgot B, Bakker K, Brown JB, Ramachandran A, Roglic G, Shaw J, Silink M, Siminerio L, Soltesz G, Williams R, Zimmet P: *Diabetes Atlas*. 3rd ed. Brussels, Belgium, International Diabetes Federation, 2006

[5]Barr ELM, Marliano DJ, Zimmet PZ, Polkinghorne KR, Atkins RC, Dunstan DW, Murray SG, Je S; The Australian Diabetes, Obesity and Lifestyle Study (AusDiab) 2005: Tracking the Accelerating Epidemic: Its Causes and Outcomes. Melbourne, Australia, International Diabetes Institute, 2006. Available from http://www.bakeridi.edu.au/Assets/Files/AUSDIAB_Report_2005.pdf. Accessed 12 November 2012

[6]Arroyo BJ, Caixas PA, Pi-Sunyer FX: Treatment of type 2 diabetes: revision of current therapeutical options and priorities. *Med Clin (Barc)* 129:746–757, 2007

[7]Rosenstock J, Hassman DR, Madder RD, Brazinsky SA, Farrell J, Khutoryansky N, Hale PM, for the Repaglinide Versus Nateglinide Comparison Study Group: Repaglinide versus nateglinide monotherapy: a randomized, multicenter study. *Diabetes Care* 27:1265–1270, 2004

[8]McFarlane SI: Antidiabetic medications and weight gain: implications for the practicing physician. *Curr Diabetes Rep* 9:249–254, 2009

[9]Jakicic JM, Jaramillo SA, Balasubramanyam A, Bancroft B, Curtis JM, Mathews A, Pereira M, Regensteiner JG, Ribisl PM: Effect of a lifestyle intervention on change in cardiorespiratory fitness in adults with type 2 diabetes: results from the Look AHEAD study. *Int J Obes (Lond)* 33:305–316, 2009

[10]O'Gorman DJ, Krook A: Exercise and the treatment of diabetes and obesity. *Endocrinol Metab Clin North Am* 37:887–903, 2008

[11]Gill JM, Cooper AR: Physical activity and prevention of type 2 diabetes mellitus. *Sports Med* 38:807–824, 2008

[12]Qi L, Hu FB, Hu G: Genes, environment, and interactions in prevention of type 2 diabetes: a focus on physical activity and lifestyle changes. *Curr Mol Med* 8:519–532, 2008

[13]Dixon JB, O'Brien PE, Playfair J, Chapman L, Schachter LM, Skinner S, Proietto J, Bailey M, Anderson M: Adjustable gastric banding and conventional therapy for type 2 diabetes: a randomized controlled trial. *JAMA* 299:316–323, 2008

[14]Amati F, Barthassat V, Miganne G, Hausman I, Monnin DG, Costanza MC, Golay A: Enhancing regular physical activity and relapse prevention through a 1-day therapeutic patient education workshop: a pilot study. *Patient Educ Couns* 68:70–78, 2007

[15]Bo S, Ciccone G, Baldi C, Benini L, Dusio F, Forastiere G, Lucia C, Nuti C, Durazzo M, Cassader M, Gentile L, Pagano G: Effectiveness of a lifestyle intervention on metabolic syndrome: a randomized controlled trial. *J Gen Intern Med* 22:1695–1703, 2007

[16]Dunstan DW, Vulikh E, Owen N, Jolley D, Shaw J, Zimmet P: Community center-based resistance training for the maintenance of glycemic control in adults with type 2 diabetes. *Diabetes Care* 29:2586–2591, 2006

[17]Sigal RJ, Kenny GP, Boule NG, Wells GA, Prud'homme D, Fortier M, Reid RD, Tulloch H, Coyle D, Phillips P, Jennings A, Jaffey J: Effects of aerobic training, resistance training, or both on glycemic control in type 2 diabetes: a randomized trial. *Ann Intern Med* 147:357–369, 2007

[18]Aylin K, Arzu D, Sabri S, Handan TE, Ridvan A: The effect of combined resistance and home-based walking exercise in type 2 diabetes patients. *Int J Diabetes Dev Ctries* 29:159–165, 2009

[19]Wadden TA, West DS, Delahanty L, Jakicic J, Rejeski J, Williamson D, Berkowitz RI, Kelley DE, Tomchee C, Hill JO, Kumanyika S: The Look AHEAD study: a description of the lifestyle intervention and the evidence supporting it. *Obesity (Silver Spring)* 14:737–752, 2006

[20]Lindstrom J, Louheranta A, Mannelin M, Rastas M, Salminen V, Eriksson J, Uusitupa M, Tuomilehto J: The Finnish Diabetes Prevention Study (DPS): lifestyle intervention and 3-year results on diet and physical activity. *Diabetes Care* 26:3230–3236, 2003

[21]Pi-Sunyer X, Blackburn G, Brancati FL, Bray GA, Bright R, Clark JM, Curtis JM, Espeland MA, Foreyt JP, Graves K, Haffner SM, Harrison B, Hill JO, Horton ES, Jakicic J, Jeffery RW, Johnson KC, Kahn S, Kelley DE, Kitabchi AE, Knowler WC, Lewis CE, Maschak-Carey BJ, Montgomery B, Nathan DM, Patricio J, Peters A, Redmon JB, Reeves RS, Ryan DH, Safford M, Van Dorsten B, Wadden TA, Wagenknecht L, Wesche-Thobaben J, Wing RR, Yanovski SZ: Reduction in weight and cardiovascular disease risk factors in individuals with type 2 diabetes: one-year results of the look AHEAD trial. *Diabetes Care* 30:1374–1383, 2007

[22]Wing RR, Jakicic J, Neiberg R, Lang W, Blair SN, Cooper L, Hill JO, Johnson KC, Lewis CE: Fitness, fatness, and cardiovascular risk factors in type 2 diabetes: Look AHEAD study. *Med Sci Sports Exerc* 39:2107–2116, 2007

[23]Wing RR: Long-term effects of a lifestyle intervention on weight and cardiovascular risk factors in individuals with type 2 diabetes mellitus: four-year results of the Look AHEAD trial. *Arch Intern Med* 170:1566–1575, 2010

[24]Vadstrup ES, Frolich A, Perrild H, Borg E, Roder M: Lifestyle intervention for type 2 diabetes patients: trial protocol of the Copenhagen Type 2 Diabetes Rehabilitation Project [article online]. *BMC Public Health* 9:166, 2009 (doi: 10.1186/1471-2458-9-166)

[25]World health Organization: Obesity: preventing and managing the global epidemic: report of a WHO Consultation. Geneva, Swizerland, World Health Organization, 2000

[26]American Diabetes Association: Position statement: Management of dyslipidemia in adults with diabetes. *Diabetes Care* 23(Suppl. 1):S57–S60, 2000

[27]Corpeleijn E, Feskens EJ, Jansen EH, Mensink M, Saris WH, de Bruin TW, Blaak EE: Improvements in glucose tolerance and insulin sensitivity after lifestyle intervention are related to changes in serum fatty acid profile and desaturase activities: the SLIM study. *Diabetologia* 49:2392–2401, 2006

[28]Dreimane D, Safani D, MacKenzie M, Halvorson M, Braun S, Conrad B, Kaufman F: Feasibility of a hospital-based, family-centered intervention to reduce weight gain in overweight children and adolescents. *Diabetes Res Clin Pract* 75:159–168, 2007

[29]Bronner Y, Boyington JE: Developing weight loss interventions for African-American women: elements of successful models. *J Natl Med Assoc* 94:224–235, 2002

[30]Eriksson KM, Westborg CJ, Eliasson MC: A randomized trial of lifestyle intervention in primary healthcare for the modification of cardiovascular risk factors. *Scand J Public Health* 34:453–461, 2006

[31]Whittemore R, Melkus G, Wagner J, Dziura J, Northrup V, Grey M: Translating the Diabetes Prevention Program to primary care: a pilot study. *Nurs Res* 58:2–12, 2009

[32]Stratton IM, Adler AI, Neil HA, Matthews DR, Manley SE, Cull CA, Hadden D, Turner RC, Holman RR: Association of glycaemia with macrovascular and microvascular complications of type 2 diabetes (UKPDS 35): prospective observational study. *BMJ* 321:405–412, 2000

[33]Brinkworth GD, Wycherley TP, Noakes M, Clifton PM: Reductions in blood pressure following energy restriction for weight loss do not rebound after re-establishment of energy balance in overweight and obese subjects. *Clin Exp Hypertens* 30:385–396, 2008

[34]Sjostrom CD, Peltonen M, Wedel H, Sjostrom L: Differentiated long-term effects of intentional weight loss on diabetes and hypertension. *Hypertension* 36:20–25, 2000

[35]Aucott L, Rothnie H, McIntyre L, Thapa M, Waweru C, Gray D: Long-term weight loss from lifestyle intervention benefits blood pressure: a systematic review. *Hypertension* 54:756–762, 2009

[36]de Groot M, Pinkerman B, Wagner J, Hockman E: Depression treatment and satisfaction in a multicultural sample of type 1 and type 2 diabetic patients. *Diabetes Care* 29:549–553, 2006

[37]Anderson RM, Funnell MM, Fitzgerald JT, Marrero DG: The Diabetes Empowerment Scale: a measure of psychosocial self-efficacy. *Diabetes Care* 23:739–743, 2000

[38]Krichbaum K, Aarestad V, Buethe M: Exploring the connection between self-efficacy and effective diabetes self-management. *Diabetes Educ* 29:653–662, 2003

[39]Trento M, Passera P, Borgo E, Tomalino M, Bajardi M, Cavallo F, Porta M: A 5-year randomized controlled study of learning, problem solving ability, and quality of life modifications in people with type 2 diabetes managed by group care. *Diabetes Care* 27:670–675, 2004

[40]Inzucchi SE, Bergenstal RM, Buse JB, Diamant M, Ferrannini E, Nauck M, Peters AL, Tsapas A, Wender R, Matthews DR: Management of hyperglycemia in type 2 diabetes: a patient-centered approach: position statement of the American Diabetes Association (ADA) and the European Association for the Study of Diabetes (EASD). *Diabetes Care* 35:1364–1379, 2012

All of the authors are based in Sydney, New South Wales, Australia. Rami H. Bishay, BSc, MSc, MBBS, and Johnson Zang, BMedSc, MBBS, were medical students at the Sydney Medical School of the University of Sydney and undertook clerkships at the Department of Endocrinology and Metabolism at the Concord Repatriation General Hospital, during which the study was performed. Dr. Bishay is now a senior resident in internal medicine (medical registrar) at St. George Hospital, and Dr. Zang is now a senior medical resident at Bankstown Hospital. Abdullah Omari, MBBS, DDU, MMED, FRACP, PhD, is a consultant physician (specialist) in vascular medicine and head of the Department of Vascular Medicine at St. Vincent's General Hospital and a conjoint lecturer at the University of New South Wales. Anna Lih, MBBS, PhD, FRACP, is a consultant physician (specialist) in endocrinology and metabolism at the Department of Endocrinology and Metabolism at Concord Repatriation General Hospital and the Sydney Medical School of the University of Sydney. Nic Kormas, MBBS, FRACP, is a consultant physician (specialist) in endocrinology and metabolism at the Department of Endocrinology and Metabolism, Concord Repatriation General Hospital, and the Royal Prince Alfred Hospital. He is also founder and director of the metabolic rehabilitation program at Concord Repatriation General Hospital and its satellite branch, the University Medical Clinics of Camden and Campbelltown Hospitals.

Diabetes and Depression in the Hispanic/Latino Community

Eduardo Colon, MD, Aida Giachello, PhD, LaShawn McIver, MD, MPH, Guadalupe Pacheco, MSW, and Leonel Vela, MD, MPH

Editor's note: *The terms "Hispanic" and "Latino" are used interchangeably to refer to people who were born in or descended from those born in Mexico, Puerto Rico, Cuba, Central or South America, or any other Caribbean island. In this article, the term "Hispanic" is used throughout.*

Nearly 12% of all Hispanics have diabetes, compared to 7.1% of non-Hispanic whites. The prevalence of diagnosed diabetes is not homogenous within subgroups of the Hispanic population, but instead ranges from as low as 7.6% for Cubans to as high as 13.3 and 13.8% for Puerto Rican and Mexican Americans, respectively.[1] Disparities in some diabetes-related complications are also higher among Hispanics compared to non-Hispanic whites.[2,3]

The prevalence rates for depression are significantly higher among adults with diabetes than among those without diabetes.[4] People with type 1 or type 2 diabetes are twice as likely to experience depression.[4] Comorbid depression affects 15–30% of all adults with diabetes and is associated with more diabetes-related symptoms, worse glycemic control, poorer self-management (worse adherence to dietary and medication recommendations, less physical activity, and less frequent glucose monitoring and foot care),[5] higher prevalence of complications, reduced quality of life, and increased mortality.[6–10] Despite that, fewer than 25% of people with diabetes

and depression are adequately treated.[6,11,12]

Limited data exist about the prevalence of comorbid depression among Hispanics. Current research shows that Hispanics with diabetes are less likely to be diagnosed with comorbid depression,[13] despite prevalence rates equal to or higher than rates among non-Hispanic whites,[14] and they are half as likely to receive treatment.[15] This article briefly describes depression in the Hispanic community; the relationship between diabetes, depression, and culture; and how advocacy can play a role in addressing this problem.

Depression, Diabetes, and Culture: The Combined Effect

Studies of Hispanic culture and health often describe Hispanics as having a set of health beliefs and behaviors and definitions of health and illness, including perceived causes of illnesses. Hispanics also stress the role of the family, religion, and other traditional practices depending on their years in the United States and their levels of acculturation and assimilation to the U.S. mainstream society.

Cherrington et al.[6] found that Hispanics with diabetes, when talking about depression, describe depressive symptoms and emotional distress. They use terms such as sadness, apathy, and loss of pleasure and describe more somatic complaints. They also describe lack of motivation to interact with family

members, get out of bed, go to work, and engage in self-care behaviors.[6]

The lack of validated assessment tools for depression in Hispanics may explain why they are least likely to be diagnosed and treated for depression. Hispanics also tend to attribute symptoms of fatigue, low energy, and dizziness to having both diabetes and depression.[6]

Cherrington et al.[6] found that Hispanics who were diagnosed with diabetes had feelings of hopelessness and were upset about the potential consequences of developing complications and that Hispanics who were experiencing difficulties in diabetes management became anxious and depressed. These researchers argue that there is a bi-directional relationship between emotional health and diabetes.

The prevalence of depression varies by age and sex. A study by Liang et al.[16] found higher levels of depressive symptoms (regardless of diabetes) among middle-aged and older Hispanics and blacks than among white Americans of the same age-groups. Compared to white non-Hispanics and African-American woman, Hispanic women have more severe chronic depression. Some studies argue that, in Hispanic women, there is a correlation between depression and exposure to a number of psychosocial and environmental stressors, including poverty, stress associated with single parenting, gender roles, low educational achievement, social isolation, language barriers, migration, and the processes associated with acculturation and adaptation.[16]

Hispanics are frequently described as having strong family ties (a concept expressed as familialismo)[6,17] that protect them from depression and other mental health conditions. For example, there is evidence that the risk of depression is reduced with increasing level of familial support among foreign-born Mexicans.[18] Some studies indicate that the family plays both a positive and a negative role in diabetes; it can be a source of support and a source of stress.[6] The emotional impact of family as social support varies depending on the extent to which individuals feel supported or understood by family members.[6] Men generally report significant family support for their illness (particularly from wives), whereas women often feel unsupported.

Hispanic health research literature also documents a belief in a strong connection between powerful emotions and diabetes, leading some Hispanics to believe that diabetes is the result of a traumatic event (e.g., a car accident or the death of close relative), which is often described as a susto (fright). This is based on the culturally bound belief that strong emotions can lead to bodily changes.[6] This perceived connection persists beyond onset and diagnosis of diabetes and into disease management.[6]

In terms of diabetes treatment, some Hispanics seek medical care from traditional healers (curanderos) or employ home remedies or over-the-counter medications, particularly when they experience financial or cultural and linguistic barriers to accessing the health and mental health system.[19,20] Finally, the stigma associated with mental illnesses, including depression, affects whether they seek mental health services

such as counseling and whether they start and adhere to antidepressant medications.[21] One study looked at the rates of adherence to psychotropic medications for patients at a community mental health center. Even after controlling for confounders such as age and social support, the adherence rates for monolingual Hispanics were significantly less than for white non-Hispanics.[22]

The Role of Advocacy

Diabetes is a serious and growing epidemic in the Hispanic community. Understanding depression and diabetes in disparately affected populations is important, not only for providers, but also for policymakers who work to construct health policies addressing the needs of people with diabetes. There is an ongoing need for more studies on comorbid depression and diabetes; for affordable and culturally linguistic assessment, educational, and treatment tools, including the integration of depression education into diabetes management and control; for increased community awareness of the relationship between diabetes and depression; and for a larger bilingual and bicultural diabetes and mental health workforce.

The goal of the American Diabetes Association (ADA) Diabetes Advocates program is to bring attention to issues affecting people living with diabetes and to advocate for public policy solutions. ADA leads this charge for people with diabetes. The ADA's efforts to address the disparate impact of diabetes on Hispanic populations through public policy change is led by its Latino Diabetes Action Council (LDAC). Composed of a cross-section of leaders from the Hispanic community, LDAC provides leadership on numerous legislative efforts, develops public policy strategies, and provides a strong voice for the ADA's focus on

health disparities in its 2012–2015 strategic plan.[23]

How can health professionals get involved and help advocate for patients with diabetes? As demonstrated in this article, we know it is important for people with diabetes and depression to receive proper care so that their depression does not impair their ability to carry out diabetes care tasks and therefore compromise their health status. ADA Diabetes Advocates can influence policies to address these and other issues faced by people with diabetes.

Diabetes Advocates fought for the passage of the Patient Protection and Affordable Care Act (ACA), which includes many new tools in the fight to stop diabetes in the disparately affected populations who represent a disproportionate number of the uninsured or underinsured in the United States. For example, under the ACA, screening for depression is now a preventive service covered at no cost for adults. This means that people with diabetes who may have undiagnosed depression can be screened without having to pay a copayment, have co-insurance, or meet an insurance deductible. Once the law is fully implemented, people with diabetes and depression will no longer be legally denied insurance or forced to pay a higher premium because of a preexisting condition. These and other efforts are crucial to addressing the needs of people in Hispanic communities living with diabetes.

Health care providers play a key role in combating the disparate impact of diabetes and depression on Hispanic populations. Become a champion for all patients by joining ADA's Diabetes Advocates. Information about how to become an advocate is available online at www.diabetes.org/advocate.

REFERENCES

[1]Centers for Disease Control and Prevention: National diabetes fact sheet: national estimates and general information on diabetes and prediabetes in the United States, 2011. Atlanta, Ga., U.S. Department of Health and Human Services, Centers for Disease Control and Prevention, 2011

[2]Harris MI, Klein R, Cowie CC, Rowland M, Byrd-Holt DD: Is the risk of diabetic retinopathy greater in non-Hispanic blacks and Mexican Americans than in non-Hispanic whites with type 2 diabetes? A U.S. population study. *Diabetes Care* 121:1230–1235, 1998

[3]Young BA, Maynard C, Boyko EJ: Racial differences in diabetic nephropathy, cardiovascular disease, and mortality in a national population of veterans. *Diabetes Care* 26:2392–2399, 2003

[4]Anderson RJ, Freedland K, Clouuse RE, Lustman PJ: The prevalence of comorbid depression in adults with diabetes: a meta-analysis. *Diabetes Care* 24:1069–1078, 2001

[5]Gonzalez JS, Safren SA, Cagliero E, Wexler DJ, Delahanty L, Wittenberg E, Blais MA, Meigs JB, Grant RW: Depression, self-care, and medication adherence in type 2 diabetes. *Diabetes Care* 30:2222–2227, 2007

[6]Cherrington A, Guadalupe X, Ayala BS, Corbie-Smith G: Examining knowledge, attitudes, and beliefs about depression among Latino adults with type 2 diabetes. *Diabetes Educ* 32:603–611, 2006

[7]de Groot M, Anderson R, Freedland KE, Clouse RE, Lustman PJ: Association of depression and diabetes complications: a meta-analysis. *Psychosom Med* 63:619–630, 2001

[8]Hanninen JA, Taka JK, Keinanen-Kiukannanniemi SM: Depression in subjects with type 2 diabetes: predictive factors and relation to quality of life. *Diabetes Care* 22:997–998, 1999

[9]Sullivan MD, O'Connor P, Feeney P, Hire D, Simmons DL, Raisch DW, Fine LJ, Narayan KMV, Ali MK, Katon WJ: Depression predicts all-cause mortality. *Diabetes Care* 35:1708–1715, 2012

[10]Katon WJ, Rutter C, Simon G, Lin EH, Ludman E, Ciechanowski P, Kinder L, Von Korff M: The association of comorbid depression with mortality in patients with type 2 diabetes. *Diabetes Care* 28:2668–2672, 2005

[11]Rubin RR, Ciechanowski P, Egede LE, Lin EH, Lustman PJ: Recognizing and treating depression in patients with diabetes. *Curr Diab Rep* 4:119–125, 2004

[12]Rubin RR, Knowler WC, Ma Y, Marrero DG, Edelstein SL, Walker EA, Garfield SA, Fisher EB, Diabetes Prevention Program Research Group: Depression symptoms and antidepressant medicine use in Diabetes Prevention Program participants. *Diabetes Care* 15:685–690, 2005

[13]Shah ZC, Huffman FG: Depression among Hispanic women with type 2 diabetes. *Ethn Dis* 15:685–690, 2005

[14]Black SA, Markides KS: Depressive symptoms and mortality in older Mexican Americans. *Ann Epidemiol* 9:45–52, 1999

[15]Gross R, Olfson M, Gameroff MJ, Carasquillo O, Shea S, Feder A, Landtigua R, Weissman MM: Depression and glycemic control in Hispanic primary care patients with diabetes. *J Gen Intern Med* 20:460–466, 2005

[16]Liang J, Xu X, Quiñones AR, Bennett JM, Ye W: Multiple trajectories of depressive symptoms in middle and late life: racial/ethnic variations. *Psychol Aging* 26:761–777, 2011

[17]Lipton RB, Losey LM, Giachello AL, Mendez J, Girotti MH: Attitudes and issues in treating Latino patients with type 2 diabetes: views of healthcare providers. *Diabetes Educ* 24:67–71, 1998

[18]Almeida J, Subramanian SV, Kawachi I, Molnar BE: Is blood thicker than water? Social support, depression and the modifying role of ethnicity/nativity status. *J Epidemiol Community Health* 65:51–56, 2011

[19]Lipton R, Losey L, Giachello AL, Corral M, Girotti MH, Mendez JJ: Factors affecting diabetes treatment and patient education among Latinos: results of a preliminary study in Chicago. *J Med Syst* 20:267–276, 1996

[20]Giachello AL: Issues of access and use. In *Latino Health in the U.S.: A Growing Challenge.* Molina CW, Aguirre-Molina M, Eds. Washington, D.C., American Public Health Association, 1994, p. 83–111

[21]Cabassa LJ, Hansen MC, Palinkas LA, Ell K: Azucar y nervios: explanatory models and treatment experiences of Hispanics with diabetes and depression. *Soc Sci Med* 66:2413–2424, 2008

[22]Diaz E, Woods SW, Rosenheck RA: Effects of ethnicity on psychotropic medications adherence. *Community Ment Health J* 41:521–537, 2005

[23]American Diabetes Association: Annual report and strategic plan. Available from http://www.diabetes.org/about-us/annual-report-and-strategic-plan.html. Accessed 6 November 2012

Eduardo Colon, MD, is a member of the ADA LDAC and a psychiatrist in the Department of Psychology at Hennepin County Medical Center in Minneapolis, Minn. Aida Giachello, PhD, is a member of the ADA LDAC and a professor in the Department of Preventive Medicine at the Feinberg School of Medicine at Northwestern University in Chicago. LaShawn McIver, MD, MPH, is the ADA national director of public policy and strategic alliances in Alexandria, Va. Guadalupe Pacheco, MSW, is a member of the ADA LDAC and the senior health advisor to the director at the Office of Minority Health in the U.S. Department of Health and Human Services in Rockville, Md. Leonel Vela, MD, is a member of the ADA LDAC and the regional dean and a professor at the University of Texas Health Science Center in San Antonio.

Depression as a Predictor of Weight Regain Among Successful Weight Losers in the Diabetes Prevention Program

David W. Price, MD[1,2]
Yong Ma, PhD[3]
Richard R. Rubin, PhD[4,5]
Leigh Perreault, MD[6]
George A. Bray, MD[7]
David Marrero, PhD[8]

William C. Knowler, MD, DRPH[9]
Elizabeth Barrett-Connor, MD[10]
D. Yvette LaCoursiere, MD[11]
for the Diabetes Prevention Program
   Research Group*

OBJECTIVE—To determine whether depression symptoms or antidepressant medication use predicts weight regain in overweight individuals with impaired glucose tolerance (IGT) who are successful with initial weight loss.

RESEARCH DESIGN AND METHODS—A total of 1,442 participants who successfully lost at least 3% of their baseline body weight after 12 months of participation in the randomized controlled Diabetes Prevention Program (DPP) continued in their assigned treatment group (metformin, intensive lifestyle, or placebo) and were followed into the Diabetes Prevention Program Outcome Study (DPPOS). Weight regain was defined as a return to baseline DPP body weight. Participant weight and antidepressant medication use were assessed every 6 months. Depression symptoms (Beck Depression Inventory [BDI] score ≥11) were assessed every 12 months.

RESULTS—Only 2.7% of the overall cohort had moderate to severe depression symptoms at baseline; most of the participants with BDI score ≥11 had only mild symptoms during the period of observation. In unadjusted analyses, both depression symptoms (hazard ratio 1.31 [95% CI 1.03–1.67], $P = 0.03$) and antidepressant medication use at either the previous visit (1.72 [1.37–2.15], $P < 0.0001$) or cumulatively as percent of visits (1.005 [1.002–1.008], $P = 0.0003$) were predictors of subsequent weight regain. After adjustment for multiple covariates, antidepressant use remained a significant predictor of weight regain ($P < 0.0001$ for the previous study visit; $P = 0.0005$ for the cumulative measure), while depression symptoms did not.

CONCLUSIONS—In individuals with IGT who do not have severe depression and who initially lose weight, antidepressant use may increase the risk of weight regain.

Diabetes Care 36:216–221, 2013

• •

From the [1]Institute for Health Research, Kaiser Permanente Colorado, Denver, Colorado; the [2]Department of Family Medicine, University of Colorado Anschutz Medical Campus, Aurora, Colorado; the [3]Biostatistics Center, George Washington University, Rockville, Maryland; the [4]Department of Medicine, Johns Hopkins University School of Medicine, Baltimore, Maryland; the [5]Department of Pediatrics, Johns Hopkins University School of Medicine, Baltimore, Maryland; the [6]Department of Endocrinology, University of Colorado University of Colorado Anschutz Medical Campus, Aurora, Colorado; [7]Pennington Biomedical Research Center, Baton Rouge, Louisiana; the [8]Department of Medicine, Indiana University School of Medicine, Indianapolis, Indiana; the [9]National Institute of Diabetes and Digestive and Kidney Diseases, Phoenix, Arizona; the [10]Department of Family and Preventative Medicine, University of California, San Diego, La Jolla, California; and the [11]Department of Reproductive Medicine, University of California, San Diego, La Jolla, California.

Corresponding author: David W. Price, dppmail@biostat.bsc.gwu.edu, david.price@ucdenver.edu, or david .price@kp.org.

Received 10 February 2012 and accepted 24 July 2012.

DOI: 10.2337/dc12-0293. Clinical trial reg. nos. NCT00004992 and NCT00038727, clinicaltrials.gov.

This article contains Supplementary Data online at http://care.diabetesjournals.org/lookup/suppl/doi:10 .2337/dc12-0293/-/DC1.

*A full list of investigators can be found in the Supplementary Data online.

The opinions expressed are those of the investigators and do not necessarily reflect the views of the funding agencies.

Depression is common in obese individuals (1–4) and is 50–100% more prevalent in those with diabetes than in the general population (3,4). Depression symptoms are associated with an increased risk of type 2 diabetes (5,6), and antidepressant medication use may also be associated with the development of diabetes in high-risk individuals (7–9). Both depression symptoms and antidepressant medications have been associated with overweight/obesity in individuals with or at increased risk of type 2 diabetes (7,10).

Depression is known to impair adherence to treatment recommendations in several chronic illnesses, including diabetes (11,12). This raises the possibility that problems with motivation and concentration, two cardinal symptoms of depression, could interfere with adherence to weight-loss efforts such as those shown to reduce the risk of developing type 2 diabetes in the Diabetes Prevention Program (DPP) (13) and the Finnish Diabetes Prevention Study (14). An analysis of a subset of DPP participants showed that higher baseline levels of depression symptoms were associated with lower levels of baseline physical activity (15). Another analysis from the original DPP cohort suggested that baseline depression symptoms did not adversely impact the chances of successful initial weight loss among participants randomized to the intensive lifestyle arm (16). It is not known whether depression symptoms at baseline affected weight in the metformin or placebo arms of the DPP clinical trial.

Weight regain is common after successful weight loss. To our knowledge, no studies have examined mood or antidepressant use as predictors of weight regain in individuals with prediabetes or diabetes who were previously successful in losing weight. In this study, we explored the association between weight gain and depression symptoms or antidepressant use in participants who successfully lost at least 3% of their baseline body weight after 1 year of the DPP. We examined the associations between depression symptoms or antidepressant use and weight regain 6 months subsequently. We also examined the associations between cumulative depression symptoms or antidepressant use over the course of the DPPOS and weight regain. Our hypotheses were that depression symptoms would predict weight regain and that antidepressant use would predict weight regain. These associations would suggest the importance of regular monitoring for depression in successful weight loss participants in order to intervene early to decrease the risk of weight regain and for close follow-up for weight regain in individuals taking antidepressants.

RESEARCH DESIGN AND

METHODS—The DPP was a randomized controlled clinical trial designed to compare the effects of lifestyle modification (achievement of $\geq$150 min of exercise per week and 7% weight loss) or metformin on delaying the onset of type 2 diabetes in overweight or obese adults who had impaired glucose tolerance and impaired fasting glucose (17,18). Participants with major psychiatric disorders and those taking greater than moderate doses of antidepressants were excluded (19). The first phase of the DPP study concluded after a mean 2.8 years of follow-up, with the finding that both lifestyle and metformin treatment resulted in significantly reduced risk of progression to type 2 diabetes compared with placebo (13). The study then continued in 2001 as the Diabetes Prevention Program Outcomes Study (DPPOS), designed to assess the effects of lifestyle or metformin on preventing long term macro- and microvascular complications of diabetes. In the DPPOS, participants continued in their assigned DPP treatment group: metformin, intensive lifestyle modification, or placebo. While weight loss per se was not a goal for participants in the metformin or placebo groups, all three treatment groups received exercise and weight loss advice in DPPOS and were eligible to attend quarterly lifestyle education sessions. Lifestyle intervention participants were also offered additional semiannual weight loss–specific campaigns. While the mechanism of weight loss in the metformin group may differ than other groups, all three treatment groups were included in this analysis because the objective was to see what the presence of depression symptoms did to the risk of weight regain among those who successfully lost weight regardless of the intervention or mechanism.

Data were collected longitudinally throughout the DPP/DPPOS. Participants' weight was collected every 6 months during both DPP and DPPOS through October 2008. As the weight regain event happened throughout the course of the study, the weight regain outcome was defined as a time-to-event variable at the subject level. Concurrent medication data were collected every 6 months in DPP/DPPOS. Nutrition data were collected at DPP baseline and year 1 and DPPOS years 1, 2, and year 5. Psychological and behavioral questionnaires were administrated annually in both DPP and DPPOS (17,18). Analyses in this paper are limited to successful weight losers, defined as participants randomized to the lifestyle, metformin, or placebo arms who achieved at least the median or greater weight loss (3% of baseline body weight) at the 12-month visit after randomization. The primary outcome of this analysis was weight regain (i.e., failure to maintain weight loss), defined as time to the first measured occurrence of a regain to the DPP baseline weight. We took a participant-centric perspective in selecting return to baseline weight, rather than a set kilogram definition, of weight regain, as we believe the former approach more closely mirrors concerns regarding how those who attempt weight loss and clinicians gauge the success of their efforts in real-world settings.

Data collection in this analysis, spanning the DPP and DPPOS, continued for a mean of 10 years. Participant data were censored at the point of weight regain. Cox proportional hazard models were used to examine the association between the key predictors (depression symptoms and antidepressant use) and the main outcome of weight regain. We hypothesized that both variables would predict weight regain. "Depression symptoms" was defined categorically as a Beck Depression Inventory (BDI) score $\geq$11. The BDI is a 21-item questionnaire, widely used clinically and in research, that has been shown to reliably detect mild, moderate, and severe levels of depression; the cut point of $\geq$11 indicates at least mild depression symptoms (19). Presence or absence of antidepressant use (selective serotonin uptake inhibitors, tricyclic antidepressants, serotonin/norepinephrine reuptake inhibitors, and dopamine agonists) was derived from concurrent medication data.

Because depression symptoms and antidepressant use were measured repeatedly

throughout the study, we used time-dependent covariate analyses to model the relationship between depression and weight regain. Predictors in the models included depression symptoms 6 months prior to assessment of weight regain, percent of time having depression symptoms at previous DPP/DPPOS visits, taking an antidepressant 6 months earlier, and percent of time taking an antidepressant at previous DPP/DPPOS visits. For variables measured only at annual visits, such as depression scores, missing values at the semiannual visits were imputed using the previous annual visit data. Other nonstructural missing values were very sporadic and imputed using the last-value-carried-forward approach. Again using time-to-event analyses, we then sequentially assessed for the effect of several covariates potentially related to weight gain, including 1) baseline treatment group (lifestyle, metformin, and placebo); 2) age, sex, and ethnicity; 3) marital status, income level, and education level; 4) BMI at randomization and percent weight loss at the 12-month DPP visit; 5) baseline activity and nutrient intake at DPP entry and at entry into the analysis and time-dependent leisure activity; 6) medical comorbidity (assessed by number of chronic medications at the visit before weight regain), total number of serious adverse events before weight regain, incident diagnosis of diabetes, and initiation of diabetes medications other than metformin during follow-up; 7) diabetes status plus antiglycemic medication use; 8) average leisure activity throughout the study period; and 9) DPP baseline participant self-rating of general health using the General and Physical Functioning questions of the SF-36 and mild or greater levels of anxiety. (Serious adverse medical events include conditions resulting in hospitalization for >24 hours, prolongation of a current hospitalization, permanent or severe disability, death, or congenital abnormality in pregnancy; are life threatening; or are involved in an accidental or intentional medication overdose.) Anxiety was assessed with the Beck Anxiety Inventory, a 21-item self-administered questionnaire shown to reliably detect mild levels of anxiety at a score $\geq$8 (20). Participants were not asked the indication (depression vs. anxiety) for antidepressant use at DPPOS visits; however, only 16% of participants had mild or greater levels of anxiety, and depression and anxiety symptoms are often comorbid (21). To examine the possibility that the association between depression symptoms or antidepressant use and weight regain varied by the degree of initial weight loss, we examined the interaction between percentage of initial weight loss (3–7%, or approximately 7–15 pounds, versus ≥ 7%) and the depression variables. The SAS system was used for all analyses (version 9.3; SAS Institute, Cary, NC).

RESULTS—Baseline characteristics of DPP participants who lost ≥3% of their baseline body weight as of the 12-month DPP visit and those who did not are shown in Table 1. Of the original 3,234 DPP enrollees, 1,452 (44.9%) had lost at least 3% of their baseline body weight at the time of the 12-month DPP visit, which was the point of maximum weight loss for

most participants. Seventy-one percent of DPP lifestyle participants achieved ≥3% weight loss compared with 42% of participants randomized to metformin and 21% of participants randomized to placebo ($P < 0.001$). Participants who lost ≥3% weight were older at DPP baseline (50.9 compared with 49.1 years of age, $P < 0.0001$) and had a lower baseline BMI (32.4 vs. 33.2 kg/m^2, $P = 0.0028$). Non-Hispanic white participants were somewhat more successful losing 3% of baseline weight compared with participants in other ethnic groups ($P < 0.01$), and married participants were slightly more successful compared with those who were not married ($P < 0.05$). Baseline antidepressant use, depression symptoms, anxiety symptoms, caloric intake,

and leisure activity did not differ between participants losing weight and those not losing weight. Ten participants had no subsequent visits and were excluded from further analysis. Therefore, 1,442 participants are included in this analysis: 762 (52.8%) of successful weight losers were lifestyle participants, 452 (31.4%) were metformin participants, and 228 (15.8%) participated in the placebo arm. The median weight loss in the three groups was 8.5% (25th–75th percentile 6.1–12.0), 6.0% (4.3–8.9), and 5.7% (4.1–8.1), respectively. Among the 1,442 study participants who lost ≥3% of their baseline body weight as of the 12-month DPP visit, 826 (57%) regained their baseline weight, which occurred, on average, after 5.1 years of follow-up. Weight regain occurred in 124 (55.6%) lifestyle participants, 245 (54.2%) metformin participants, and 157 (68.9%) placebo participants. The crude incidence rate of weight regain to baseline in the three groups was 10.3 per 100 person-years for lifestyle, 10.3 for metformin, and 17.9 for the placebo group ($P < 0.0001$). As shown in Fig. 1, the difference between placebo and the other two groups was significant ($P < 0.0001$) beginning at the 6-month visit after the start of this analysis. Treatment group and weight loss at year one were independently associated with weight regain (data not shown).

Overall, 25.6% of the cohort in this analysis experienced elevated depression symptoms and 23.4% reported antidepressant use at least once during the assessment period. The majority of depressed participants had mild symptoms (BDI 11–15); only 36% of participants with depression symptoms (2.7% of the overall cohort) had more severe depression symptoms (BDI score of ≥16), limiting our power to conduct subset analyses on the most severely depressed (likely major depressive disorder) participants. The percentage of participants with categorically defined depression symptoms at a given study assessment point fluctuated throughout the study, while the percentage of participants taking antidepressant medication at a study assessment point trended upward toward 11–12% (Fig. 2)—a finding consistent with secular prevalence and trends (22). Less than 7.4% of participants simultaneously reported both depression symptoms and antidepressant use at any visit during the assessment period.

In unadjusted models, both depression symptoms (hazard ratio 1.31 [95%

Table 1—*Comparison of participants who lost ≥3% baseline weight vs. those who did not*

Characteristics at DPP baseline	Weight loss at DPP year 1 visit	
	<3% ($n = 1,782$)	≥3% ($n = 1,452$)
Treatment groups*		
Intensive lifestyle	312 (28.9)	767 (71.1)
Metformin	618 (57.6)	455 (42.4)
Placebo	852 (78.7)	230 (21.3)
Age at randomization (years)*	49.1 (42.5–56.7)	50.9 (43.8–59.0)
Sex		
Female	1,219 (55.6)	972 (44.4)
Male	563 (54.0)	480 (46.0)
Race/ethnicity&		
Caucasian	930 (52.6)	838 (47.4)
African American	392 (60.8)	253 (39.2)
Hispanic	282 (55.5)	226 (44.5)
American Indian	98 (57.3)	73 (42.7)
Asian	80 (56.3)	62 (43.7)
Married#		
Yes	1,138 (53.6)	986 (46.4)
No	644 (58.0)	466 (42.0)
Education (years)		
≤12	468 (56.1)	366 (43.9)
13–16	833 (53.5)	723 (46.5)
≥17	481 (57.0)	363 (43.0)
BMI (kg/m^2)&	33.2 (29.1–37.9)	32.4 (28.8–36.7)
Leisure activity (MET h/week)	10.0 (4.1–20.5)	9.6 (3.7–20.7)
Calorie intake (kcal)	1,904 (1,470–2,576)	1,886 (1,436–2,522)
Depression symptoms (BDI ≥11)		
Yes	186 (56.7)	142 (43.3)
No	1,563 (54.7)	1,296 (45.3)
Anxiety symptom (BAI ≥8)		
Yes	286 (55.2)	232 (44.8)
No	1,463 (54.8)	1,206 (45.2)
Antidepressant use		
Yes	92 (56.8)	70 (43.2)
No	1,690 (55.0)	1,382 (45.0)

Data are n (%) or median (interquartile range). BAI, Beck Anxiety Inventory. *$P < 0.0001$. &$P < 0.01$. #$P < 0.05$.

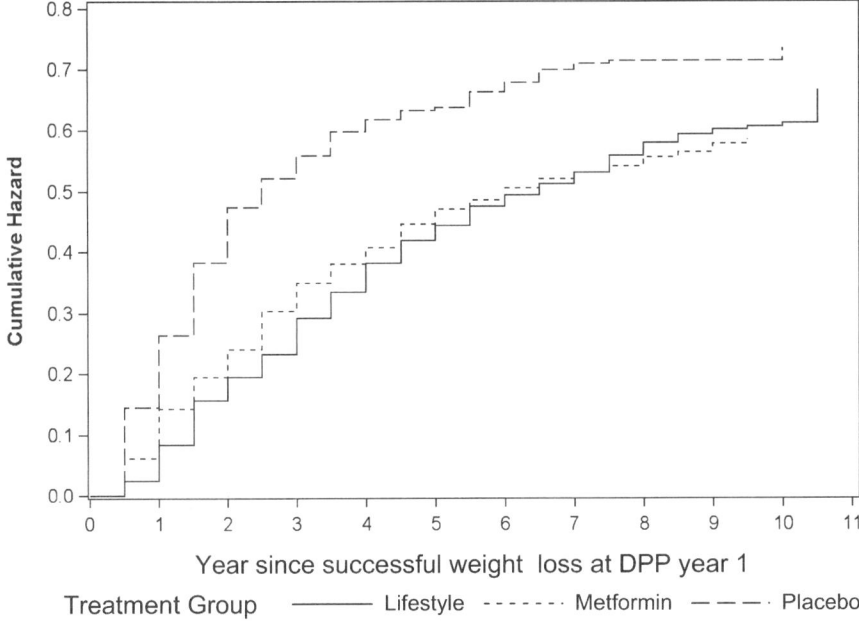

Figure 1—*Cumulative incidence of weight regain by DPP treatment group.*

significant interactions between depression symptoms and treatment group. After adjustment for all covariates, depression symptoms at the previous visit no longer predicted weight regain; however, use of antidepressant medication at either the previous visit (1.735 [1.338–2.250], $P < 0.0001$) or any prior study visits as a percent (1.006 [1.002–1.009], $P = 0.0005$) remained a significant predictor for weight regain. The association of antidepressant use and subsequent weight regain was also noted in the subgroup of selective serotonin reuptake inhibitor (SSRI) participants (1.92 [1.43–2.58], $P < 0.0001$ for the previous visit; 1.006 [1.003–1.01] for any prior study visit, adjusted for the same covariates as in the antidepressant model). In fact, the antidepressant effect is mostly driven by the SSRI users. To determine whether the association between depression symptoms or antidepressant use and weight regain might be different in moderate and substantial initial weight losers, we performed a sensitivity analysis to look for a significant interaction between the weight loss categorical variable (3–7 vs. ≥7% weight loss) and the four depression measures. Because no significant interaction was found, we did not conduct further subgroup analyses.

CI 1.03–1.67], $P = 0.03$) and antidepressant use noted at the study visit 6 months previously (1.72 [1.37–2.15], $P < 0.0001$) were predictors of weight regain. Cumulative antidepressant use calculated as a percentage of all prior visits was also

noted to predict weight regain (1.005 [1.002–1.008], $P = 0.0003$), while cumulative depression symptoms calculated as a percentage of all prior study visits was not predictive (1.003 [1.000–1.006], $P = 0.09$). There were no

CONCLUSIONS—Fifty-seven percent of successful weight losers (≥3% from baseline after 1 year of the DPP) regained their initially lost weight after an average of 5.1 years; 43% of successful weight losers were able to maintain some amount of weight loss. These findings are not surprising, given the results of other studies that substantiate the difficulties of sustaining initial weight loss over the long term (23). Participants in the active DPP treatment arms (lifestyle and metformin) were somewhat more successful in maintaining weight loss than placebo group participants (with differences becoming evident early in the follow-up period), yet many active group participants also regained weight. The weight regain similarities between the metformin and lifestyle groups in this analysis parallel those seen in the entire DPPOS cohort and in part reflect the fact that some lifestyle components were offered to metformin group participants, and the lifestyle group intervention became somewhat less intense after the completion of the initial DPP study (24).

In unadjusted models, both depression symptoms and antidepressant use

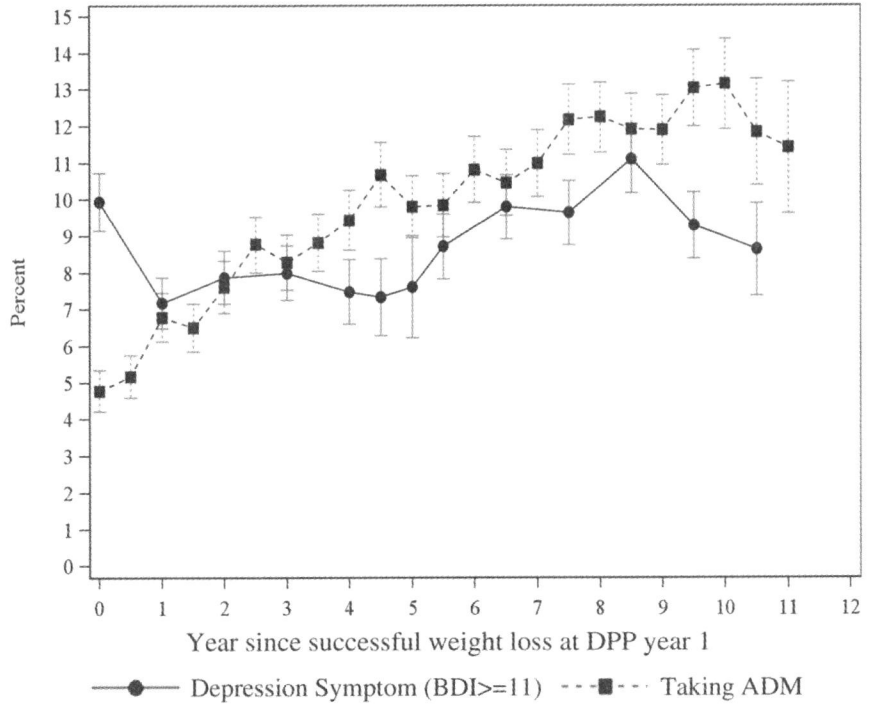

Figure 2—*Depression symptoms and antidepressant medication use over time among participants who achieved at least 3% weight loss.*

at either the previous DPP visit or their cumulative measures were associated with weight regain. After adjustment for multiple factors potentially related to weight gain, antidepressant use, but not depression symptoms, remained associated with a risk of weight regain in these participants. The risk of weight regain was 72% higher for participants using antidepressants at the visit 6 months prior compared with non–antidepressant users. This association remained when the analysis was restricted to SSRI antidepressant users.

SSRIs were the most frequently used (78%) antidepressants among DPP participants (25). Even though SSRIs are traditionally thought to be associated with less weight gain than are many older antidepressants, recent examinations (26) have suggested the tendency for some SSRI users to gain weight over time—a finding consistent with other DPP analyses (7). It is therefore possible that the weight regain seen in our participants is due to antidepressant side effects. The small number of participants using non-SSRI antidepressants precluded a comparison of risk of weight regain by antidepressant class.

There are several possible explanations for the failure of depression symptoms in predicting weight gain in our cohort. While weight gain is a feature of some forms of depression, it is not as prevalent as weight loss (27). Other investigators have found that the prevalence of obesity is related to depression severity (1,2). Individuals with more severe depression were excluded from DPP—only 2.7% had moderate or greater levels of depression at the time of initial enrollment (18)—and most of the participants with BDI score ≥11 during the period of observation had only mild symptoms. Therefore, it is possible that more severe, but not milder, depression symptoms would be related to weight regain, but we did not have enough power to detect this association. This would not discount the association between antidepressant medication use and weight regain, however.

Depression symptoms were assessed annually during our period of observation, while antidepressant medication use was assessed every 6 months. Thus, it is possible that, similar to the initial DPP cohort, depression symptoms in our participants were of short duration and may have resolved by the time of follow-up assessment (25). The frequent attention DPP participants received throughout the study may have helped lead to symptom resolution in some participants with

milder depression symptoms. It is also possible that antidepressants were effective in treating the mild depression symptoms in our population, leading to symptom resolution while antidepressant use continued. While the DPP and DPPOS were not designed to ascertain this, a recent analysis (26) noting marginal differences between antidepressants and placebo for participants with mild depression symptoms lessens this possibility. We therefore cannot differentiate between spontaneous, antidepressant-aided, and psychosocial support–assisted resolution of depression symptoms in our cohort. All of these possibilities would lead to a failure to detect an association between depression symptoms as a predictor of weight regain.

Our analysis was also limited by the small number of participants (7.4%) reporting both depression symptoms and antidepressant use. The lower-than-expected prevalence of depression in our sample may be the result of DPP study selection criteria (individuals taking higher than the normal starting antidepressant dose were excluded) and recruitment bias (depressed individuals may have been less likely to volunteer for a long intensive study). The vast majority of participants in our cohort had mild depression symptoms that did not likely meet the threshold for major depressive disorder, which may explain why many participants with depression symptoms did not report taking antidepressants. We therefore could not test for differences between participants with both depression symptoms and antidepressant use compared with participants with only depression symptoms or only antidepressant use. Furthermore, the mild nature of depression symptoms in our cohort may limit the generalizability of our findings to other populations of individuals at risk for diabetes with more severe depression.

In our study of successful initial weight losers, after adjustment for multiple relevant covariates, antidepressant use at the previous (6 month) DPPOS visit was predictive of weight regain on follow-up. This suggests that overweight individuals with impaired glucose intolerance who successfully lose weight and who are recent antidepressant medication users may be at higher risk for regaining weight than non–antidepressant users with impaired glucose tolerance. Maintaining initially successful weight loss strategies over time can be difficult (23). These at-risk individuals may benefit from ongoing support via regularly structured coaching

and reinforcement to help them maintain their successful weight loss strategies and refine them for new or unexpected challenges to maintaining behavior change. Early detection of weight regain could lead to intensification of weight loss strategies or the addition of new strategies to minimize regained weight. Future studies could design and elucidate practical, effective strategies for real-world settings to help these at-risk individuals maintain successful weight loss.

Acknowledgments—During the DPPOS, the National Institute of Diabetes and Digestive and Kidney Diseases (NIDDK) of the National Institutes of Health provided funding to the clinical centers and the coordinating center for the design and conduct of the study and collection, management, analysis, and interpretation of the data. The Southwestern American Indian Centers were supported directly by the NIDDK, including its Intramural Research Program, and the Indian Health Service. The General Clinical Research Center Program, National Center for Research Resources, supported data collection at many of the clinical centers. Funding was also provided by the National Institute of Child Health and Human Development, the National Institute on Aging, the National Eye Institute, the National Heart, Lung and Blood Institute, the Office of Research on Women's Health, the National Institute on Minority Health and Health Disparities, the Centers for Disease Control and Prevention, and the American Diabetes Association.

Bristol-Myers Squibb and Parke-Davis provided additional funding and material support during the DPP. Lipha (Merck-Sante) provided medication, and LifeScan Inc. donated materials during the DPP and DPPOS. No other potential conflicts of interest relevant to this article were reported.

D.W.P. researched data, contributed to discussion, wrote the manuscript, and edited the manuscript. Y.M. researched data, contributed to discussion, wrote the manuscript, and edited the manuscript. R.R.R. and L.P. contributed to discussion and edited the manuscript. G.A.B., D.M., and W.C.K. researched data, contributed to the discussion, and reviewed and edited the manuscript. E.B.-C. wrote the manuscript. D.Y.L. contributed to discussion and edited the manuscript. D.W.P. is the guarantor of this work and, as such, had full access to all the data in the study and takes responsibility for the integrity of the data and the accuracy of the data analysis.

The research group gratefully acknowledges the commitment and dedication of the participants of the DPP and DPPOS. The writing group thanks Nicole Butler, George Washington University Biostatistics Center, for her assistance with manuscript preparation. A complete list of centers, investigators, and staff can be found in the Supplementary Data online.

References

1. Strine TW, Mokdad AH, Dube SR, et al. The association of depression and anxiety with obesity and unhealthy behaviors among community-dwelling US adults. Gen Hosp Psychiatry 2008;30:127–137
2. Simon GE, Ludman EJ, Linde JA, et al. Association between obesity and depression in middle-aged women. Gen Hosp Psychiatry 2008;30:32–39
3. Everson SA, Maty SC, Lynch JW, Kaplan GA. Epidemiologic evidence for the relation between socioeconomic status and depression, obesity, and diabetes. J Psychosom Res 2002;53:891–895
4. Blazer DG, Moody-Ayers S, Craft-Morgan J, Burchett B. Depression in diabetes and obesity: racial/ethnic/gender issues in older adults. J Psychosom Res 2002;53:913–916
5. Mezuk B, Eaton WW, Albrecht S, Golden SH. Depression and type 2 diabetes over the lifespan: a meta-analysis. Diabetes Care 2008;31:2383–2390
6. Knol MJ, Twisk JWR, Beekman ATF, Heine RJ, Snoek FJ, Pouwer F. Depression as a risk factor for the onset of type 2 diabetes mellitus. A meta-analysis. Diabetologia 2006;49:837–845
7. Rubin RR, Ma Y, Marrero DG, et al.; Diabetes Prevention Program Research Group. Elevated depression symptoms, antidepressant medicine use, and risk of developing diabetes during the diabetes prevention program. Diabetes Care 2008;31:420–426
8. Kivimäki M, Tabák AG, Lawlor DA, et al. Antidepressant use before and after the diagnosis of type 2 diabetes: a longitudinal modeling study. Diabetes Care 2010;33:1471–1476
9. Rubin RR, Ma Y, Peyrot M, et al.; Diabetes Prevention Program Research Group. Antidepressant medicine use and risk of developing diabetes during the diabetes prevention program and diabetes prevention program outcomes study. Diabetes Care 2010;33:2549–2551
10. Rubin RR, Gaussoin SA, Peyrot M, et al. Knowler WC for the Look AHEAD Research Group. Cardiovascular disease risk factors, depression symptoms and antidepressant medicine use in the Look AHEAD (Action for Health in Diabetes) clinical trial of weight loss in diabetes. Diabetologia 2010;55:1581–1589
11. Lin EH, Katon W, Von Korff M, et al. Relationship of depression and diabetes self-care, medication adherence, and preventive care. Diabetes Care 2004;27:2154–2160
12. Ciechanowski PS, Katon WJ, Russo JE, Hirsch IB. The relationship of depressive symptoms to symptom reporting, self-care and glucose control in diabetes. Gen Hosp Psychiatry 2003;25:246–252
13. Knowler WC, Barrett-Connor E, Fowler SE, et al.; Diabetes Prevention Program Research Group. Reduction in the incidence of type 2 diabetes with lifestyle intervention or metformin. N Engl J Med 2002;346:393–403
14. Tuomilehto J, Lindström J, Eriksson JG, et al.; Finnish Diabetes Prevention Study Group. Prevention of type 2 diabetes mellitus by changes in lifestyle among subjects with impaired glucose tolerance. N Engl J Med 2001;344:1343–1350
15. Delahanty LM, Conroy MB, Nathan DM; Diabetes Prevention Program Research Group. Psychological predictors of physical activity in the diabetes prevention program. J Am Diet Assoc 2006;106:698–705
16. Wing RR, Hamman RF, Bray GA, et al.; Diabetes Prevention Program Research Group. Achieving weight and activity goals among diabetes prevention program lifestyle participants. Obes Res 2004;12:1426–1434
17. The Diabetes Prevention Program Research Group. The Diabetes Prevention Program. Design and methods for a clinical trial in the prevention of type 2 diabetes. Diabetes Care 1999;22:623–634
18. Rubin RR, Fujimoto WY, Marrero DG, et al.; DPP Research Group. The Diabetes Prevention Program: recruitment methods and results. Control Clin Trials 2002;23:157–171
19. Beck AT, Steers RA. *Manual of the Beck Depression Inventory*. San Antonio, TX, Psychological Corp., 1993
20. Beck AT, Epstein N, Brown G, Steer RA. An inventory for measuring clinical anxiety: psychometric properties. J Consult Clin Psychol 1988;56:893–897
21. Gaynes BN, Rush AJ, Trivedi MH, Wisniewski SR, Balasubramani GK, Spencer DC. Major depression symptoms in primary care and psychiatric care settings: a cross-sectional analysis. Ann Fam Med 2007;5:126–134
22. Pratt LA, Brody DJ, Gu Q. Antidepressant use in persons aged 12 and over: United States. 2005–2008. NCHS data brief, no. 76. Hyattsville, MD, National Center for Health Statistics, 2011
23. Turk MW, Yang K, Hravnak M, Sereika SM, Ewing LJ, Burke LE. Randomized clinical trials of weight loss maintenance: a review. J Cardiovasc Nurs 2009;24:58–80
24. Knowler WC, Fowler SE, Hamman RF, et al.; Diabetes Prevention Program Research Group. 10-year follow-up of diabetes incidence and weight loss in the Diabetes Prevention Program Outcomes Study. Lancet 2009;374:1677–1686
25. Rubin RR, Knowler WC, Ma Y, et al.; Diabetes Prevention Program Research Group. Depression symptoms and antidepressant medicine use in Diabetes Prevention Program participants. Diabetes Care 2005;28:830–837
26. Gartlehner G, Hansen RA, Thieda P, et al. Comparative effectiveness of second-generation antidepressants in the pharmacologic treatment of adult depression. Comparative effectiveness rev. no. 7 [article online], 2007. Rockville, MD, Agency for Healthcare Research and Quality. Available from www.effectivehealthcare.ahrq.gov/reports/final.cfm. Accessed on 27 December 2010
27. Thase ME. Recognition and diagnosis of atypical depression. J Clin Psychiatry 2007;68(Suppl. 8):11–16

Association Among Depression, Physical Functioning, and Hearing and Vision Impairment in Adults With Diabetes

Paul D. Loprinzi, PhD, Ellen Smit, PhD, and Gina Pariser, PT, PhD

Abstract

Objective. Individuals with diabetes may be at an increased risk for depression given the potential diabetes-induced link between sensory impairment, physical functioning, and depression. As a result, the purposes of this study were *1)* to examine the association between sensory impairment and depression among adults of all ages with diabetes, *2)* to examine whether dual sensory impairment and physical functioning are independently associated with depression, and *3)* to examine the association between physical functioning and sensory impairment.

Design and Methods. Data from the 2005–2006 National Health and Nutrition Examination Survey were used in the present study and, after exclusions, 567 participants (18–85 years of age) with evidence of diabetes constituted the analytic sample. Sensory impairment (vision and hearing), physical functioning, and depression were reported from questionnaires.

Results. After controlling for age, sex, race/ethnicity, comorbidity index, smoking, BMI, physical activity, and glycemic control, dual sensory impairment (odds ratio [OR] 7.48, 95% CI 2.09–26.71) and physical dysfunction (unable to perform activities; OR 3.21, 95% CI 1.28–8.08) were associated with increased depression symptoms. After adjustments, participants who were unable to perform activities had a 1.73 (95% CI 0.94–3.19, *P* = 0.07), 2.78 (0.78–9.87, *P* = 0.11), and 2.21 (0.50–9.68, *P* = 0.29) nonsignificant greater odds, respectively, of having hearing, vision, and dual sensory impairment than participants who were able to perform activities.

Conclusion. Adults with diabetes who have dual sensory impairment and physical functioning limitations are more likely to report depression symptoms. This highlights the importance of preventing and improving sensory impairments, physical functioning, and depression among adults with diabetes.

Address correspondence to Paul Loprinzi, PhD, Bellarmine University Department of Exercise Science, Donna & Allan Lansing School of Nursing & Health Sciences, Louisville, KY 40205.

Diabetes is associated with sensory impairment, including both vision and hearing impairment,[1,2] with the underlying mechanisms occurring through unfavorable glucose-induced changes in inflammation, microvasculature, and sensory nerves.[3,4] Studies also have shown that individuals with diabetes are at an increased risk for depression,[5] which is not surprising given the psychological and emotional problems linked with sensory impairment and diabetes.[6,7] Notably, diabetes may also be linked with depression through other mechanisms such as elevated inflammation[8] or through lifestyle factors such as physical activity and smoking.[9]

The majority of studies examining the association between sensory impairment and depression have examined this relationship for single-sensory impairment alone (i.e., hearing or vision impairment).[10,11] Fewer studies have examined the association between dual sensory impairment (i.e., having both hearing and vision impairment) and depression.[10,11] Those that have usually restricted the sample to older adults (despite the fact that sensory impairment does not always start during the late adult years)[12,13] and did not always employ multivariate analyses to control for potential confounding variables.[11] Furthermore, we have a limited understanding of the association between dual sensory impairment and depression among adults with diabetes.

In addition to the link between sensory impairment and diabetes, individuals with diabetes may have considerable functional impairment, through changes in health status and mobility.[14] Although sensory impairment may influence depression, physical functioning has also been linked to depression symptoms.[15] We currently have a dearth of studies examining the concurrent independent effects of dual sensory impairment and physical functioning on depression symptoms.

Providing some insight into this, McDonnall[16] employed a longitudinal study to examine the association between physical status and depression among older adults with and without dual sensory loss. Physical status was assessed using three measures, including physical activity, physical condition, and BMI. All three physical status measures were associated with depression symptoms for individuals who had or who developed dual sensory loss.

The primary aims of this study were to increase our knowledge base in this area of research by 1) examining the association between single and dual sensory impairment and depression among adults of all ages with diabetes while controlling for potential confounding variables and 2) examining whether dual sensory impairment and physical functioning are independently associated with depression. A secondary purpose of this study was to examine the association between physical functioning and sensory impairment because, in the general population, studies have shown that those with sensory impairment have less functional independence.[17-19]

Study Methods

Design and participants

For this study, we used data from the 2005–2006 National Health and Nutrition Examination Survey (NHANES).[20] Briefly, NHANES employs a representative sample of noninstitutionalized U.S. civilians selected by a complex, multistage probability design. Participants were interviewed in their homes and subsequently examined in mobile examination centers (MECs) across numerous U.S. geographical locations. The study was approved by the National Center for Health Statistics ethics review board, with informed consent obtained from all participants before data collection. The final sample for the present study included 567 adult NHANES participants between 18 and 85 years of age after excluding participants who did not have diabetes or had missing data for the study variables.

Assessment of diabetes status

Administered in participants' homes, the NHANES included several questions related to diabetes. Participants were asked if they had ever been told by a doctor or health professional that they had or have diabetes or sugar diabetes and if they are now taking insulin. A subsample of NHANES participants was examined in a morning fasting session. Fasting glucose was measured from a blood sample, and participants with a fasting glucose level ≥ 126 mg/dl were considered to have diabetes. Finally, participants were also considered to have evidence of diabetes if they had an A1C value ≥ 6.5%.

Measurement of depression status

At the MECs, participants completed the Patient Health Questionnaire-9 (PHQ-9)[21] during the computer-assisted personal interview. The PHQ-9 depression scale consists of the nine diagnostic criteria for depressive disorders as listed in the fourth edition of the *Diagnostic and Statistical Manual of Mental Disorders*.[22] Sample items ask participants how often in the past 2 weeks they have been bothered by "feeling down, depressed, or hopeless," "feeling tired or having little energy," and

"trouble concentrating on things, such as reading the newspaper or watching television."

For each question, participants responded using a 4-point Likert scale, with responses including not at all (0), several days (1), more than half the days (2), and nearly every day (3). Items were summed, with higher scores indicating greater severity of depression. As a measure of severity, the PHQ-9 can range from 0 to 27 because each of the nine items can be scored from 0 to 3. For the analyses presented herein, we defined depression status as follows: less than moderate depression (0–9) and moderate to severe depression (≥ 10).

The PHQ-9 has demonstrated evidence of reliability, with Cronbach's alpha ranging from 0.86 to 0.89 and a 48-hour test-retest correlation coefficient of 0.84.[21] Additionally, this cut-point of ≥ 10 has demonstrated evidence of validity, with a sensitivity of 88% and a specificity of 88% for clinical depression.[21] In the present sample, internal consistency of this questionnaire, as measured by Cronbach's alpha, was 0.84.

Measurement of hearing and vision impairment

In the 2005–2006 NHANES sample, participants self-reported hearing and vision functioning. For hearing assessment, participants were asked whether their hearing was excellent, good, a little trouble, moderate trouble, a lot of trouble, or deaf. The hearing variable was dichotomized into excellent or good hearing and a little or more hearing trouble. For vision assessment, participants were asked whether their eyesight, with glasses or contact lenses if worn, was excellent, good, fair, poor, or very poor. The vision variable was characterized as excellent, good or fair, and poor or worse vision. Participants with a little or more hearing trouble and poor or worse vision were classified as having dual sensory impairment. A categorical impairment variable was created with four groups including 1) excellent or good hearing and excellent, good, or fair vision; 2) a little or more hearing trouble; 3) poor or worse vision; and 4) dual

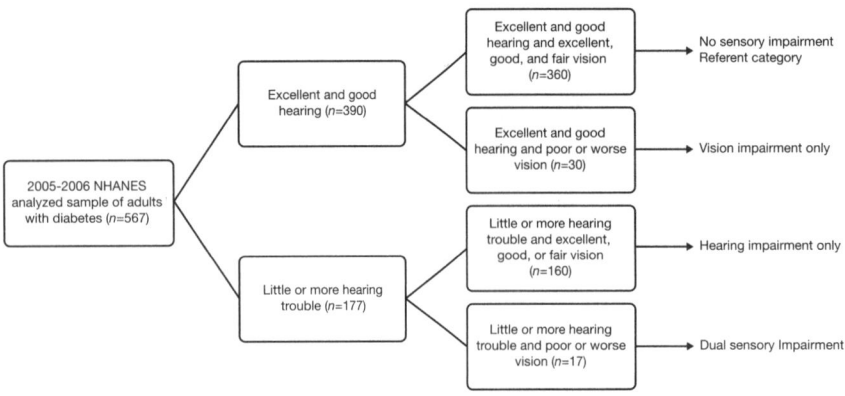

Figure 1. Classification of sensory impairment among adults with diabetes, NHANES 2005–2006.

sensory impairment. Note that the second and third categories were mutually exclusive in that participants classified as having a little or more hearing trouble did not have poor or worse vision, and those with poor or worse vision did not have a little or more hearing trouble (Figure 1).

Measurement of physical functioning

During a home interview and using the computer-assisted personal interviewing system, participants were asked several questions related to their physical functioning. To provide an assessment of physical functioning, participants were asked: "Because of a health problem, do you have difficulty walking without using any special equipment?" Response options were "yes" and "no." Participants were also asked how much difficulty they had walking for a quarter of a mile; walking up 10 steps without resting; stooping, crouching, or kneeling; lifting or carrying something as heavy as 10 lb; doing chores around the house; preparing meals; walking from one room to another on the same level; standing up from an armless straight chair; getting in or out of bed; eating, such as holding a fork, cutting food, or drinking from a glass; dressing, including tying shoes, working zippers, and fastening buttons; standing or being on their feet for ~ 2 hours; reaching up overhead; using their fingers to grasp or handle small objects; going out for activities such as shopping, movies, or sporting events; participating in social activities; and pushing or pulling large objects such

as a living room chair. Response options for these questions included "no difficulty," "some difficulty," "much difficulty," and "unable to do this activity."

With respect to physical functioning classification, participants were classified as "able to do activities" (i.e., they reported having no difficulty or some difficulty), "having much difficulty doing activities," and "unable to do activities." Participants were classified as "having much difficulty" if they said they had much difficulty for any of the above physical functioning questions. Participants were classified as "unable to do activities" if they answered "yes" to the question "Do you have difficulty walking without using any special equipment?" or if they reported being unable to do any of the above physical functioning questions.

Measurement of covariates

To control for potential confounding variables, covariates were examined in the analytical models. Participants completed questionnaires providing data on age, sex, race/ethnicity, and physical activity levels (whether they engaged in any moderate- or vigorous-intensity physical activity in the past 30 days for at least 10 minutes). Additionally, a comorbidity index variable was created, which included the following chronic diseases/events: arthritis, coronary heart disease, heart attack, congestive heart failure, stroke, cancer, emphysema, chronic bronchitis, and elevated blood pressure (systolic blood pressure ≥ 140 mmHg or diastolic blood pressure

≥ 90 mmHg). As a marker of active smoking status or as an index of environmental exposure to tobacco (i.e., passive smoking), serum cotinine was measured. Serum cotinine was measured by an isotope dilution high-performance liquid chromatography/atmospheric pressure chemical ionization tandem mass spectrometry. Other covariates included glycemic control as measured by A1C levels and BMI. During examination at the MECs, BMI was calculated from measured weight and height (weight in kilograms divided by the square of height in meters).

Data analysis

All analyses were performed using STATA (version 10.0, STATA Corp., College Station, Tex.). To provide demographic characteristics of the analyzed sample, means and standard errors were calculated for continuous variables, and proportions were calculated for categorical variables.

Mean depression scores across the impairment categorical variable and the physical functioning variable were calculated, and a one-way analysis of variance was used to test for a significant difference across groups. A χ^2 test was used to assess whether there was a difference in the proportion of individuals with depression across the impairment and physical functioning variables.

Two multivariate logistic regression models were computed. For both models, depression served as the outcome variable, with depression dichotomized into "less than moderate depression" (coded as 0) and "having moderate to severe depression symptoms" (coded as 1). The first multivariate logistic regression analysis was used to examine the association between the categorical impairment variable and depression while controlling for age, sex, race/ethnicity, comorbidity index, smoking, BMI, physical activity, and glycemic control. For the impairment categorical variable, "excellent or good hearing and excellent, good, or fair vision" served as the reference group. The second multivariate logistic regression was the same as the first model except the physical functioning variable was added to the model. Statistical significance was established as a nominal alpha level of 0.05.

In addition to examining the direct association between single and dual sensory impairment on depression symptoms, additive and multiplicative interaction for hearing and vision impairment was assessed. As described by Kalilani and Atashili,[23] multiplicative interaction exists when the joint effect of the risk factors differs from the product of the effects of the individual factors; additive interaction exists when the joint effect of the risk factors differs from the sum of the effects of the individual factors.

Additive interaction was tested by calculating the relative excess risk due to interaction (RERI), the attributable proportion due to interaction (AP), and the synergy index (S), using the methods described by Andersson et al.[24] RERI is the excess risk due to interaction relative to the risk without exposure;[23] AP is considered the attributable proportion of the outcome (in this case, depression) which is due to the interaction among individuals with both exposures (i.e., both hearing and vision impairment);[23] and S is the ratio of the combined effect and the sum of the individual effects.[25] To calculate these parameters, a logistic regression was computed with depression serving as the outcome variable. The regression coefficients from the single sensory hearing and vision variables, along with the dual sensory impairment variable, were entered into the Microsoft Excel spreadsheet developed by Andersson et al.[24] Then, the covariance matrix of the coefficients of the logistic model was computed with the appropriate covariances from the covariance matrix entered into the spreadsheet to provide an estimate of RERI, AP, and S. Statistical significance was evaluated with 95% confidence intervals with AP and RERI > 0 and S > 1.0 indicating additive interaction. Multiplicative interaction was tested by including a cross-product term for vision and hearing along with the main effect terms for each in the regression model.

The secondary purpose of this study was to examine the association between physical functioning and sensory impairment. To address this potential association, a multinomial logistic regression was employed, with sensory impairment serving as the outcome variable. Covariates included age, sex, race/ethnicity, comorbidity index, smoking, BMI, physical activity, glycemic control, and depression.

To ensure that NHANES results are representative of the U.S. population, the National Center for Health Statistics provides sample weights to correct for differential selection probabilities and to adjust for non-coverage and non-response. Sample sizes for some of our analyses were insufficient (i.e., $n < 35$) to provide reliable population estimates. Thus, our analyses are unweighted and reflect associations in NHANES participants and are not intended to represent the entire U.S. population.

Study Results
Characteristics of the study participants with diabetes are displayed in Table 1. Mean depression scores and percentages or participants with depression symptoms across the four categories of impairment and physical functioning are shown in Table 2. For sensory impairment, participants with excellent or good hearing and excellent, good, or fair vision had the lowest mean depression score (2.8, 95% CI 2.4–3.2), with participants having dual sensory impairment exhibiting the highest depression score (7.4, 95% CI 3.5–11.3, $P < 0.0001$). Participants with excellent or good hearing and

Table 1. Means and Proportions for Characteristics of People With Diabetes in NHANES 2005–2006 (n = 567)

Variable	Mean/Proportion (Standard Error)
Demographic and biological variables	
Age (years) (range 18–85 years)	60.6 (0.6)
Sex (% male)	50.7 (2.1)
BMI (kg/m²)	32.2 (0.3)
Race/ethnicity	
Mexican American (%)	24.3 (1.8)
Other Hispanic (%)	2.8 (0.6)
Non-Hispanic white (%)	38.9 (2.0)
Non-Hispanic black (%)	31.3 (1.9)
Other race (%)	2.4 (0.6)
Comorbidity Index	
0 comorbidities (%)	26.4 (1.8)
1 comorbidity (%)	34.5 (2.0)
2 comorbidities (%)	18.8 (1.6)
3 comorbidities (%)	10.7 (1.3)
4+ comorbidities (%)	9.4 (1.2)
Cotinine (ng/ml)	51.6 (5.4)
Those engaging in any moderate to vigorous physical activity within the past 30 days (%)	47.4 (2.0)
A1C (%)	7.3 (0.07)

Table 1. Means and Proportions for Characteristics of People With Diabetes in NHANES 2005–2006 (*n* = 567), *continued from p. 9*

Variable	Mean/Proportion (Standard Error)
Study variables	
Depression	3.4 (0.1)
Moderate to severe depression (%; *n* = 55)	9.7 (1.2)
Hearing	
Excellent (%; *n* = 184)	32.4 (1.9)
Good (%; *n* = 206)	36.3 (2.0)
A little trouble (%; *n* = 107)	18.8 (1.6)
Moderate trouble (%; *n* = 39)	6.8 (1.0)
A lot of trouble (%; *n* = 28)	4.9 (0.9)
Deaf (%; *n* = 3)	0.5 (0.3)
Vision	
Excellent (%; *n* = 123)	21.6 (1.7)
Good (%; *n* = 270)	47.6 (2.0)
Fair (%; *n* = 127)	22.3 (1.7)
Poor (%; *n* = 39)	6.8 (1.0)
Very poor (%; *n* = 8)	1.4 (0.4)
Impairment classification	
Excellent or good hearing and excellent, good, or fair vision (%; *n* = 360)	63.4 (2.0)
A little or more hearing trouble (%; *n* = 160)	28.2 (1.8)
Poor or worse vision (%; *n* = 30)	5.2 (0.9)
Dual sensory impairment (%; *n* = 17)	3.0 (0.7)
Physical functioning	
Able to do activities (%; *n* = 191)	45.4 (2.4)
Having much difficulty (%; *n* = 55)	13.0 (1.6)
Unable to do activities (%; *n* = 174)	41.4 (2.4)

excellent, good, or fair vision had the lowest prevalence of depression symptoms (6.9%, 95% CI 4.3–9.5%); participants with dual-sensory impairment had the highest prevalence (41.1%, 95% CI 17.0–65.3%, *P* < 0.001). For physical functioning, participants who were able to do activities had the lowest depression score (2.2, 95% CI 1.7–2.7), with participants who were unable to do activities having the highest depres-

sion score (5.7, 95% CI 4.8–6.5, *P* < 0.0001). Participants who were unable to do activities had a higher prevalence of depression (20.6%, 95% CI 14.6–26.7%) compared to participants who were able to do activities (5.7%, 95% CI 2.4–9.0%) and those having much difficulty (5.4%, 95% CI 0.0–11.5%).

The adjusted logistic regression analyses examining the association among depression, sensory impair-

ment, and physical functioning are shown in Table 3. In the first model, and after controlling for age, sex, race/ethnicity, comorbidity index, smoking, BMI, physical activity, and glycemic control, those with dual sensory impairment (odds ratio [OR] 11.21, 95% CI 3.30–37.99) were 11.2 times more likely to have depression symptoms compared to those with excellent or good hearing and excellent, good, or fair vision. For model 2, in which physical functioning was added to the model, the association between dual sensory impairment and depression was attenuated but still significant (OR 7.48, 95% CI 2.09–26.71). Independent of sensory impairment, participants unable to do activities (OR 3.21, 95% CI 1.28–8.08) were 3.21 times more likely to have depression symptoms than participants who were able to perform various activities. Although dual sensory impairment and physical functioning were both independent predictors of depression, the strength of the association was greater for dual sensory impairment.

To determine whether there was additive or multiplicative interaction between hearing and vision impairments on depression, further analyses were performed. The RERI (6.79, 95% CI –6.0 to 19.5) and S (3.07, 95% CI 0.57–16.53) were not significant. However, the AP was significant at 0.61 (95% CI 0.07–1.15), suggesting that a significant proportion of depression can be attributed to the additive interaction between hearing and vision. The cross-product term for hearing and vision to evaluate multiplicative interaction was not significant when added to the final model along with the main effect terms (*P* = 0.33).

The secondary purpose of this study was to examine the association between physical functioning and sensory impairment (Table 4). Participants who were unable to perform activities had a 1.73 (95% CI 0.94–3.19, *P* = 0.07), 2.78 (0.78–9.87, *P* = 0.11), and 2.21 (0.50–9.68, *P* = 0.29) nonsignificant greater odds, respectively, of having hearing, vision, and dual sensory impairment

Table 2. Mean Depression Scores and Percentages of Participants With Moderate to Severe Depression Symptoms Across the Impairment and Physical Functioning Variables Among People With Diabetes in NHANES 2005–2006

Variable	Mean Depression (95% CI)	P	Depressed (% [95% CI])	P
Impairment variable		< 0.0001		< 0.001
Excellent or good hearing and excellent, good, or fair vision (n = 360)	2.8 (2.4–3.2)		6.9 (4.3–9.5)	
A little or more hearing trouble (n = 160)	3.9 (3.1–4.7)		10.0 (5.3–14.6)	
Poor or worse vision (n = 30)	4.5 (2.9–6.1)		23.3 (7.9–38.7)	
Dual sensory impairment (n = 17)	7.4 (3.5–11.3)		41.1 (17.0–65.3)	
Physical functioning variable		< 0.0001		< 0.001
Able to do activities (n = 191)	2.2 (1.7–2.7)		5.7 (2.4–9.0)	
Having much difficulty (n = 55)	2.9 (2.0–3.8)		5.4 (0.0–11.5)	
Unable to do activities (n = 174)	5.7 (4.8–6.5)		20.6 (14.6–26.7)	

than participants who were able to perform activities.

Discussion

The purposes of this study were threefold: *1*) to examine the association between sensory impairment and depression among adults of all ages with diabetes, *2*) to examine whether dual sensory impairment and physical functioning are independently associated with depression, and *3*) to examine the association between physical functioning and sensory impairment. The major finding of this study was that both dual sensory impairment and physical functioning were independently associated with depression. Furthermore, we showed that there is additive interaction between hearing and vision on the association with depression.

Most previous research has examined the influence of diabetes on sensory impairment,[26–28] the association between single sensory impairment (i.e., hearing or vision alone) and health outcomes (e.g., depression) in the general population[29,30] among those with diabetes,[31] or the association between dual sensory impairment and depression in nondiabetic populations.[32] The examination of the correlates of dual sensory impairment is a relatively new line of inquiry among those with diabetes.

Our findings contribute to the literature by demonstrating that adults with diabetes who have both vision and hearing impairments (i.e., dual sensory impairment) have an increased odds of depression and that these dual sensory impairments have an additive effect on the odds of depression. Additionally, this study showed that physical functioning was marginally associated with dual sensory impairment among adults with diabetes. Similarly, our findings also indicated that glycemic control was independently associated with sensory impairment, which supports other research demonstrating that poor glycemic control among adults with diabetes is independently associated with functional limitations.[33] The independent association among glycemic control, sensory impairment, and functional limitations underscores the importance of glycemic control and of counseling patients about its importance.

Along these lines, it is reasonable to suggest that glycemic control may also be independently linked to depression symptoms, particularly because glycemic control is linked to factors (e.g., inflammation,[8,34] functional impairment,[33] and self-efficacy[35]) that are associated with depression. For example, those with poorer glycemic control may have greater systemic inflammation[36] and

functional impairment[33] and in turn may be at a greater risk for depression.[8,34,37] Moreover, Sacco and Bykowski[35] showed that glycemic control was indirectly associated with depression through diabetes adherence mastery (self-efficacy). Importantly, these findings only held true for adults with type 1 diabetes and not for those with type 2 diabetes.

In our study, glycemic control was not independently associated with depression symptoms. It was not possible to determine whether participants in the study had type 1 or type 2 diabetes. Given that type 2 diabetes is more common, however, it is plausible to suggest that a greater proportion of adults in this sample had type 2 diabetes, and if so, the null findings for this sample would support those reported by Sacco and Bykowski.[35] Our findings are also similar to those reported by McDonnall,[16] who showed that, among adults in the general population, physical status was associated with depression symptoms for individuals who had or who developed dual sensory loss.

To decrease the likelihood of developing depression, these findings underscore the importance of preventing sensory impairments and improving physical functioning among adults with diabetes.

Table 3. Association Among Depression (Dependent Variable), Impairment Classification Status, and Physical Functioning in People With Diabetes in NHANES 2005–2006

Variables	Those Having Depression (OR [95% CI])	
	Model 1 ($n = 514$)	Model 2* ($n = 375$)
Sensory impairment		
Excellent or good hearing and excellent, good, or fair vision	Referent	Referent
A little or more hearing trouble	1.14 (0.52–2.50)	0.73 (0.30–1.77)
Poor or worse vision	**4.13 (1.37–12.43)**	2.03 (0.55–7.47)
Dual sensory impairment	**11.21 (3.30–37.99)**	**7.48 (2.09–26.71)**
Covariates		
Age (years)	**0.96 (0.94–0.99)**	**0.93 (0.90–0.97)**
Sex		
Male	Referent	Referent
Female	1.25 (0.64–2.42)	1.08 (0.49–2.34)
Race/ethnicity		
Mexican American	Referent	
Non-Hispanic white	1.54 (0.62–3.83)	1.20 (0.41–3.51)
Non-Hispanic black	1.34 (0.51–3.48)	1.24 (0.42–3.61)
Other	0.54 (0.06–4.88)	0.48 (0.03–6.03)
Comorbidities		
0 comorbidities	Referent	Referent
1 comorbidity	2.56 (0.97–6.75)	2.39 (0.69–8.23)
2 comorbidities	1.61 (0.46–5.63)	1.23 (0.26–5.75)
3 comorbidities	2.49 (0.66–9.29)	1.66 (0.35–7.75)
4+ comorbidities	2.77 (0.69–11.03)	2.22 (0.44–11.08)
Smoking (ng/ml)	1.00 (0.99–1.00)	1.00 (0.99–1.00)
BMI (kg/m^2)	1.01 (0.96–1.05)	0.99 (0.94–1.04)
Physical activity		
Engaging in MVPA in past 30 days	Referent	Referent
Not engaging in MVPA in past 30 days	1.72 (0.85–3.49)	1.02 (0.44–2.37)
A1C (%)	0.94 (0.78–1.13)	0.92 (0.73–1.16)
Physical functioning		
Able to perform activities	NA	Referent
Having much difficulty	NA	0.94 (0.23–3.84)
Unable to perform activities	NA	**3.21 (1.28–8.08)**

Physical functioning now added to the model.
MVPA, moderate to vigorous physical activity; NA, not applicable. Bold indicates statistical significance ($P < 0.05$)

Table 4. Association Between Physical Functioning and Sensory Impairment in People With Diabetes in NHANES 2005–2006

Variables	Sensory Impairment Classification (OR [95% CI])*		
	A little or more hearing trouble	Poor or worse vision	Dual sensory impairment
Physical functioning			
Able to perform activities	Referent	Referent	Referent
Having much difficulty	1.76 (0.87–3.53)	1.25 (0.22–7.19)	0.80 (0.08–8.18)
Unable to perform activities	1.73 (0.94–3.19)	2.78 (0.78–9.87)	2.21 (0.50–9.68)
Covariates			
Age (years)	1.01 (0.99–1.04)	0.95 (0.90–1.00)	1.05 (0.98–1.12)
Sex			
Male	Referent	Referent	Referent
Female	0.74 (0.44–1.23)	1.02 (0.34–3.06)	0.62 (0.18–2.12)
Race/ethnicity			
Mexican American	Referent	Referent	Referent
Non-Hispanic white	1.14 (0.59–2.20)	0.23 (0.04–1.11)	1.72 (0.28–10.33)
Non-Hispanic black	0.86 (0.42–1.74)	0.87 (0.25–2.92)	1.36 (0.22–8.27)
Comorbidities			
0 comorbidities	Referent	Referent	Referent
1 comorbidity	1.00 (0.49–2.04)	2.82 (0.42–18.61)	0.49 (0.08–2.79)
2 comorbidities	0.71 (0.31–1.64)	6.47 (0.82–50.56)	0.58 (0.07–4.46)
3 comorbidities	1.64 (0.66–4.05)	7.53 (0.81–69.70)	0.80 (0.08–7.90)
4+ comorbidities	1.69 (0.65–4.40)	4.45 (0.40–49.44)	0.60 (0.06–5.75)
Smoking (ng/ml)	1.00 (0.99–1.00)	0.99 (0.99–1.00)	1.00 (0.99–1.00)
BMI (kg/m²)	0.99 (0.96–1.03)	0.96 (0.90–1.04)	1.03 (0.95–1.12)
Physical activity			
Engaging in MVPA in past 30 days	Referent	Referent	Referent
Not engaging in MVPA in past 30 days	1.18 (0.71–1.97)	2.37 (0.72–7.72)	2.40 (0.56–10.16)
Depression	1.02 (0.96–1.08)	1.03 (0.92–1.15)	**1.13 (1.02–1.25)**
A1C (%)	1.03 (0.88–1.21)	1.18 (0.89–1.56)	**1.43 (1.04–1.97)**

*Excellent or good hearing and excellent, good, or fair vision served as referent group.
MVPA, moderate to vigorous physical activity. Bold indicates statistical significance (P < 0.05).

Additionally, given the observed associations, interventions targeted at those who already experience dual sensory impairment may be needed to prevent or treat depression symptoms.

Given that some individuals with diabetes may be at risk for sensory impairment, physical dysfunction, and depression, effective preventive and rehabilitation programs are needed. Developing such programs is not an easy task, especially for adults with diabetes who suffer from these conditions.

It is not within the scope of this article to provide a detailed overview of programs for individuals suffering from these conditions. For a detailed review of rehabilitation measures for sensory impairment, readers are referred to the thorough review by Saunders and Echt.[10] Briefly, rehabilitation for individuals with dual sensory impairment should attempt to enhance communication by ensuring that the patient-provider environment is optimized, providing redundancy, speaking clearly, providing clear written or Braille materials, and providing assistive devices.[10]

Common treatment for depression may include counseling, antidepressant medication (e.g., selective serotonin reuptake inhibitors,[38] which may also help to regulate blood glucose levels[39]), and regular participation in physical activity.[40] Physical therapy, regular participation in home or fitness center–based structured exercise programs, and lifestyle physical activity may also serve as effective strategies to improve physical functioning among adults with diabetes.[41–43]

Based on our findings, clinicians should screen for physical functioning and depression in patients with diabetes and especially in those with hearing or vision impairments. Clinicians could use some of the described strategies in their practice to help prevent and improve depression symptoms, sensory impairment, and physical functioning. Additionally, implementation of said strategies in rehabilitation programs specializing in care for adults with diabetes may improve health outcomes, including physical functioning and psychological well-being, in this population.

Limitations of this study include the cross-sectional design, which precludes any ability to establish temporal sequence and determine causation. Also, sensory impairment and physical functioning were assessed using nonobjective measures. And finally, relatively few participants ($n = 17$) in the sample had dual sensory impairment. Notwithstanding these limitations, major findings of this study indicate that, among adults with diabetes, dual sensory impairment and severe physical dysfunction (i.e., individuals unable to perform various activities of daily living) are independently associated with depression.

The authors encourage future studies using a prospective design to provide evidence of cause and effect. If feasible, objectively measuring hearing and vision impairment is encouraged because it may reduce any sensory impairment misclas-

sification that may occur with a self-report methodology. Also, larger studies are needed to ensure a sufficient sample size for those with dual sensory impairment. Finally, identification and evaluation of strategies for prevention and reduction of depression among adults with diabetes is warranted.

In summary, our results suggest that people with diabetes who have more than one sensory impairment are more likely to be depressed and may be more likely to have physical functioning limitations. This highlights the importance of preventing and improving sensory impairments, depression, and physical functioning among adults with diabetes. Additionally, and as indicated by the American Association of Diabetes Educators,[44] clinicians are encouraged to screen for signs and symptoms of depression among people with diabetes.

References

[1]Bainbridge KE, Hoffman HJ, Cowie CC: Diabetes and hearing impairment in the United States: audiometric evidence from the National Health and Nutrition Examination Survey, 1999 to 2004. *Ann Intern Med* 149:1–10, 2008

[2]Zhang X, Gregg EW, Cheng YJ, Thompson TJ, Geiss LS, Duenas MR, Saaddine JB: Diabetes mellitus and visual impairment: National Health and Nutrition Examination Survey, 1999–2004. *Arch Ophthalmol* 126:1421–1427, 2008

[3]Bainbridge KE, Cheng YJ, Cowie CC: Potential mediators of diabetes-related hearing impairment in the U.S. population: National Health and Nutrition Examination Survey 1999–2004. *Diabetes Care* 33:811–816, 2010

[4]Antonetti DA, Barber AJ, Bronson SK, Freeman WM, Gardner TW, Jefferson LS, Kester M, Kimball SR, Krady JK, LaNoue KF, Norbury CC, Quinn PG, Sandiraseqarane L, Simpson IA: Diabetic retinopathy: seeing beyond glucose-induced microvascular disease. *Diabetes* 55:2401–2411, 2006

[5]Lin EH, Rutter CM, Katon W, Heckbert SR, Ciechanowski P, Oliver MM, Ludman EJ, Young BA, Williams LH, McCulloch DK, Von Korff M: Depression and advanced complications of diabetes: a prospective cohort study. *Diabetes Care* 33:264–269, 2010

[6]du Feu M, Fergusson K: Sensory impairment and mental health. *Adv Psychiatr Treat* 9:95–103, 2003

[7]Wexler DJ, Porneala B, Chang Y, Huang ES, Huffman JC, Grant RW: Diabetes differen-

tially affects depression and self-rated health by age in the U.S. *Diabetes Care* 35:1575–1577, 2012

[8]Stuart MJ, Baune BT: Depression and type 2 diabetes: inflammatory mechanisms of a psychoneuroendocrine co-morbidity. *Neurosci Biobehav Rev* 36:658–676, 2012

[9]Goldney RD, Phillips PJ, Fisher LJ, Wilson DH: Diabetes, depression, and quality of life: a population study. *Diabetes Care* 27:1066–1070, 2004

[10]Saunders GH, Echt KV: An overview of dual sensory impairment in older adults: perspectives for rehabilitation. *Trends Amplif* 11:243–258, 2007

[11]Schneider JM, Gopinath B, McMahon CM, Leeder SR, Mitchell P, Wang JJ: Dual sensory impairment in older age. *J Aging Health* 23:1309–1324, 2011

[12]Vitale S, Cotch MF, Sperduto RD: Prevalence of visual impairment in the United States. *JAMA* 295:2158–2163, 2006

[13]Shargorodsky J, Curhan SG, Curhan GC, Eavey R: Change in prevalence of hearing loss in US adolescents. *JAMA* 304:772–778, 2010

[14]Sinclair AJ, Conroy SP, Bayer AJ: Impact of diabetes on physical function in older people. *Diabetes Care* 31:233–235, 2008

[15]Russo A, Cesari M, Onder G, Zamboni V, Barillaro C, Pahor M, Bernabei R, Landi F: Depression and physical function: results from the aging and longevity study in the Sirente geographic area (ilSIRENTE Study). *J Geriatr Psychiatry Neurol* 20:131–137, 2007

[16]McDonnall MC: Physical status as a moderator of depressive symptoms among older adults with dual sensory loss. *Rehabil Psychol* 56:67–76, 2011

[17]Raina P, Wong M, Massfeller H: The relationship between sensory impairment and functional independence among elderly. *BMC Geriatr* 4:e3, 2004

[18]Keller BK, Morton JL, Thomas VS, Potter JF: The effect of visual and hearing impairments on functional status. *J Am Geriatr Soc* 47:1319–1325, 1999

[19]Brennan M, Horowitz A, Su YP: Dual sensory loss and its impact on everyday competence. *Gerontologist* 45:337–346, 2005

[20]Centers for Disease Control and Prevention: National Health and Nutrition Examination Survey. Available at: http://www.cdc.gov/nchs/nhanes/about_nhanes.htm. Accessed 6 December 2012

[21]Kroenke K, Spitzer RL, Williams JB: The PHQ-9: validity of a brief depression severity measure. *J Gen Intern Med* 16:606–613, 2001

[22]American Psychiatric Association: *Diagnostic and Statistical Manual of Mental Disorders: DSM-IV*. 4th ed. Washington, DC, American Psychiatric Association, 2000

[23]Kalilani L, Atashili J: Measuring additive interaction using odds ratios. *Epidemiol Perspect Innov* 3:5, 2006

[24]Andersson T, Alfredsson L, Kallberg H, Zdravkovic S, Ahlbom A: Calculating measures of biological interaction. *Eur J Epidemiol* 20:575–579, 2005

[25]Knol MJ, van der Tweel I, Grobbee DE, Numans ME, Geerlings MI: Estimating interaction on an additive scale between continuous determinants in a logistic regression model. *Int J Epidemiol* 36:1111–1118, 2007

[26]Zheng Y, He M, Congdon N: The worldwide epidemic of diabetic retinopathy. *Indian J Ophthalmol* 60:428–431, 2012

[27]Malucelli DA, Malucelli FJ, Fonseca VR, Zeigeboim B, Ribas A, Trotta Fd, Silva TP: Hearing loss prevalence in patients with diabetes mellitus type 1. *Brazilian J Otorhinolaryngol* 78:105–115, 2012

[28]Lerman-Garber I, Cuevas-Ramos D, Valdes S, Enriquez L, Lobato M, Osornio M, Escobedo AR, Pascual-Ramos V, Mehta R, Ramirez-Anguiano J, Gomez-Perez FJ: Sensorineural hearing loss: a common finding in early-onset type 2 diabetes mellitus. *Endocr Pract* 18:549–557, 2012

[29]Boi R, Racca L, Cavallero A, Carpaneto V, Racca M, Dall'Acqua F, Ricchetti M, Santelli A, Odetti P: Hearing loss and depressive symptoms in elderly patients. *Geriatr Gerontol Int* 12:440–445, 2012

[30]Kempen GI, Ballemans J, Ranchor AV, van Rens GH, Zijlstra GA: The impact of low vision on activities of daily living, symptoms of depression, feelings of anxiety and social support in community-living older adults seeking vision rehabilitation services. *Qual Life Res* 21:1405–1411, 2011

[31]Dowd KR: Could hearing loss be the link between diabetes and depression? *N C Med J* 72:402–404, 2011

[32]Bernabei V, Morini V, Moretti F, Marchiori A, Ferrari B, Dalmonte E, De Ronchi D, Rita Atti A: Vision and hearing impairments are associated with depressive-anxiety syndrome in Italian elderly. *Aging Ment Health* 15:467–474, 2011

[33]De Rekeneire N, Resnick HE, Schwartz AV, Shorr RI, Kuller LH, Simonsick EM, Vellas B, Harris TB: Diabetes is associated with subclinical functional limitation in nondisabled older individuals: the Health, Aging, and Body Composition study. *Diabetes Care* 26:3257–3263, 2003

[34]Krishnadas R, Cavanagh J: Depression: an inflammatory illness? *J Neurol Neurosurg Psychiatry* 83:495–502, 2012

[35]Sacco WP, Bykowski CA: Depression and hemoglobin A1c in type 1 and type 2 diabetes: the role of self-efficacy. *Diabetes Res Clin Pract* 90:141–146, 2010

[36]Gustavsson CG, Agardh CD: Inflammatory activity increases with haemoglobin A_{1c} in patients with acute coronary syndrome. *Scand Cardiovasc J* 43:380–385, 2009

[37]Hirsch JK, Sirois FM, Lyness JM: Functional impairment and depressive symptoms in older adults: mitigating effects of hope. *Brit J Health Psychol* 16:744–760, 2011

[38]Barbui C, Ostuzzi G, Cipriani A: SSRI plus supportive care more effective than supportive care alone for mild to moderate depression. *Evid Based Ment Health* 12:109, 2009

[39]Lustman PJ, Anderson RJ, Freedland KE, de Groot M, Carney RM, Clouse RE: Depression and poor glycemic control: a meta-analytic review of the literature. *Diabetes Care* 23:934–942, 2000

[40]Dunn AL, Trivedi MH, O'Neal HA: Physical activity dose-response effects on outcomes of depression and anxiety. *Med Sci Sports Exerc* 33(Suppl. 6):S587–S597; discussion 609–610, 2001

[41]Foy CG, Lewis CE, Hairston KG, Miller GD, Lang W, Jakicic JM, Rejeski WJ, Ribisl PM, Walkup MP, Wagenknecht LE: Intensive lifestyle intervention improves physical function among obese adults with knee pain: findings from the Look AHEAD trial. *Obesity (Silver Spring)* 19:83–93, 2011

[42]Manns PJ, Dunstan DW, Owen N, Healy GN: Addressing the nonexercise part of the activity continuum: a more realistic and achievable approach to activity programming for adults with mobility disability? *Phys Ther* 92:614–625, 2012

[43]Waryasz GR, McDermott AY: Exercise prescription and the patient with type 2 diabetes: a clinical approach to optimizing patient outcomes. *J Am Acad Nurse Pract* 22:217–227, 2010

[44]American Association of Diabetes Educators: Competencies for diabetes educators: a companion document to the guidelines for the practice of diabetes education. Available from http://www.Diabeteseducator. Org/export/sites/aade/_resources/pdf/compe-tencies.Pdf. Accessed 14 November 2012

Paul Loprinzi, PhD, is an assistant professor in the Exercise Science Program, and Gina Pariser, PT, PhD, is an associate professor of the Doctor of Physical Therapy Program at the Lansing School of Nursing and Health Sciences at Bellarmine University in Louisville, Ky. Ellen Smit, PhD, is an associate professor of the Program in Epidemiology, School of Biological and Population Health Sciences, College of Public Health and Human Sciences, at Oregon State University in Corvallis.

Better Glycemic Control and Weight Loss With the Novel Long-Acting Basal Insulin LY2605541 Compared With Insulin Glargine in Type 1 Diabetes

A randomized, crossover study

Julio Rosenstock, md[1]
Richard M. Bergenstal, md[2]
Thomas C. Blevins, md[3]
Linda A. Morrow, md[4]
Melvin J. Prince, md[5]

Yongming Qu, phd[5]
Vikram P. Sinha, phd[5]
Daniel C. Howey, md[5]
Scott J. Jacober, do[5]

OBJECTIVE—To compare effects of LY2605541 versus insulin glargine on daily mean blood glucose as part of a basal-bolus regimen for type 1 diabetes.

RESEARCH DESIGN AND METHODS—In this randomized, Phase 2, open-label, 2×2 crossover study, 137 patients received once-daily basal insulin (LY2605541 or glargine) plus mealtime insulin for 8 weeks, followed by crossover treatment for 8 weeks. Daily mean blood glucose was obtained from 8-point self-monitored blood glucose profiles. The noninferiority margin was 10.8 mg/dL.

RESULTS—LY2605541 met noninferiority and superiority criteria compared with insulin glargine in daily mean blood glucose (144.2 vs. 151.7 mg/dL, least squares mean difference = −9.9 mg/dL [90% CI −14.6 to −5.2], $P < 0.001$). Fasting blood glucose variability and A1C were reduced with LY2605541 compared with insulin glargine (both $P < 0.001$). Mealtime insulin dose decreased with LY2605541 and increased with insulin glargine. Mean weight decreased 1.2 kg with LY2605541 and increased 0.7 kg with insulin glargine ($P < 0.001$). The total hypoglycemia rate was higher for LY2605541 ($P = 0.04$) and the nocturnal hypoglycemia rate was lower ($P = 0.01$), compared with insulin glargine. Adverse events (including severe hypoglycemia) were similar, although more gastrointestinal-related events occurred with LY2605541 (15% vs. 4%, $P < 0.001$). Mean changes (all within normal range) were higher for alanine aminotransferase, aspartate aminotransferase, triglycerides, and LDL-cholesterol and lower for HDL-cholesterol with LY2605541 compared with insulin glargine (all $P < 0.02$).

CONCLUSIONS—In type 1 diabetes, compared with insulin glargine, LY2605541, a novel, long-acting basal insulin, demonstrated greater improvements in glycemic control, increased total hypoglycemia, and reduced nocturnal hypoglycemia, as well as reduced weight and lowered mealtime insulin doses.

Diabetes Care 36:522–528, 2013

The quest to prolong the action of insulin, which led to modern basal insulins, began in the 1930s with development of protamine zinc insulin (1,2). Basal insulins, such as protamine zinc, lente, isophane (NPH insulin), and ultralente insulins, were originally developed as suspensions to prolong action by delaying absorption (3,4). More recently, insulins glargine (GL) and detemir were developed to prolong subcutaneous absorption by altering amino acid structure (GL) or adding fatty acylated side chains (detemir) (4,5). Insulin degludec, a basal insulin in development, has the goal to achieve an effect longer than 24 h by prolonging subcutaneous absorption (6). Longer-acting insulins may be expected to reduce the need for twice-daily injections, variability, and the risk of hypoglycemia, as well as to provide minimal peak activity. Despite these refinements, current basal insulins cannot restore physiologic distribution of the twofold portal to systemic insulinemia because of subcutaneous systemic absorption, which results in similar portal and systemic levels. Thus, reduced hepatic insulin action must be balanced with excess peripheral insulin action to maintain glucose homeostasis.

LY2605541 is a novel, long-acting basal insulin consisting of insulin lispro covalently modified with a 20-kDa polyethylene glycol moiety. It is a solution-based basal insulin with a time-action profile that is believed to be modulated indirectly through slowed depot absorption and reduced clearance due to increased molecular size. LY2605541 has a duration of action of more than 36 h with low variability, acting considerably longer than insulin glargine (7).

This exploratory Phase 2 clinical trial was designed to determine if LY2605541 was noninferior to insulin GL for reduction of daily mean blood glucose (BG) in patients with type 1 diabetes on a basal-bolus regimen and to compare safety and efficacy of LY2605541 and insulin GL.

RESEARCH DESIGN AND METHODS—This Phase 2, multinational (Israel and U.S.), outpatient, open-label, randomized, two-arm crossover study compared LY2605541 with

From the [1]Dallas Diabetes and Endocrine Center at Medical City Dallas, Dallas, Texas; the [2]International Diabetes Center at Park Nicollet, Minneapolis, Minnesota; [3]Texas Diabetes and Endocrinology, Austin, Texas; the [4]Profil Institute for Clinical Research, Inc., Chula Vista, California; and [5]Eli Lilly and Company, Indianapolis, Indiana.
Corresponding author: Scott J. Jacober, jacober_scott_j@lilly.com.
Received 10 January 2012 and accepted 27 August 2012.
DOI: 10.2337/dc12-0067. Clinical trial reg. no. NCT01049412, clinicaltrials.gov.
This article contains Supplementary Data online at http://care.diabetesjournals.org/lookup/suppl/doi:10.2337/dc12-0067/-/DC1
D.C.H. is currently retired from Eli Lilly and Company, Indianapolis, Indiana.

insulin GL in patients with type 1 diabetes who had used GL once daily along with mealtime insulin, before the study. The primary objective was to determine if LY2605541 was noninferior to GL for daily mean BG after 8 weeks. The study was conducted from 4 February 2010 to 20 January 2011 in accordance with the International Conference on Harmonization Guidelines for Good Clinical Practice and the Declaration of Helsinki. All patients provided written informed consent.

Study inclusion criteria included type 1 diabetes duration $\geq$1 year, receiving GL treatment (maximum daily dose, 1 unit/kg) for $\geq$6 months, age 18 to 65 years, BMI 19 to 45 kg/m^2, and hemoglobin A$_{1c}$ (A1C) $\leq$10.5%. Exclusion criteria included treatment with GL twice daily in the past 30 days, treatment with oral or injectable diabetes medication other than insulins within the past 3 months, use of an insulin pump, more than one episode of severe hypoglycemia within the past 3 months or diagnosis of hypoglycemia unawareness, New York Heart Association class III or IV cardiac functional status, fasting triglycerides >500 mg/dL, liver disease or alanine aminotransferase (ALT)/aspartate aminotransferase (AST) levels twofold the upper limit of normal (ULN) or more, renal transplantation or serum creatinine >2.0 mg/dL, participation in a weight loss program, or more than one emergency department visit or hospitalization due to poor glucose control in the past 6 months.

Patients administering GL at any time other than prebreakfast were converted to a prebreakfast basal injection 2 weeks before randomization. Prebreakfast dosing was chosen to elicit potential differences in fasting BG (FBG) due to differences in the half-lives of LY2605541 and GL. Patients continued to use their prestudy mealtime insulin throughout the study.

The study randomization scheme in this open-label trial was stratified within each country by A1C ($\leq$ 8.5%, >8.5%) and baseline basal insulin dose ($\leq$0.4, >0.4 unit/kg). Patients were randomized to receive basal insulin (LY2605541 or GL) once daily plus mealtime insulin for 8 weeks, followed by crossover treatment for 8 weeks and a 4-week follow-up period (Supplementary Fig. 1).

Clinic visits occurred every 2 weeks, with telephone visits interspersed. Patients recorded their self-monitored FBG daily. Eight-point self-monitored BG (SMBG) profiles (measured premeal, 2 h postmeal, bedtime, and 3 A.M.) were

collected three times in the week before each clinic visit.

Hypoglycemia was defined as BG concentration $\leq$70 mg/dL, or if BG was not determined, as experiencing signs or symptoms associated with hypoglycemia (8). Severe hypoglycemia was defined as experiencing signs or symptoms of hypoglycemia with severe neurologic impairment requiring assistance from another person, with recovery after carbohydrate intake, glucagon administration, or intravenous glucose.

Initially, starting doses of LY2605541 were derived from patients' prior basal insulin doses using a conversion factor of 6 nmol LY2605541/unit of GL. After a prespecified interim analysis to assess LY2605541 dose conversion and adjustment, this was changed to 7 nmol LY2605541/unit of GL. LY2605541 concentration was approximately 1,000 nmol/mL, therefore LY2605541 doses were rounded to the nearest 10 nmol (the nearest 10 μL or volumetric unit) to allow accurate administration using a regular 100-unit syringe.

GL was initially transitioned to LY2605541 over 5 days. The total LY2605541 dose was administered each morning along with a full GL dose on the first morning. GL dose was tapered by 25% of the original dose on subsequent days and discontinued on the fifth day. After the interim assessment, this regimen was altered to taper GL over 4 days (75%, 50%, 25%, and 0% GL dose on days 1, 2, 3, and 4, respectively). To transition from LY2605541 back to GL, LY2605541 treatment was stopped, and 2 days later, GL was resumed in 25% daily increments over 4 days.

LY2605541 dose was increased at weekly intervals using the following algorithm: If the mean FBG of three consecutive mornings was 131 to 180 mg/dL, the LY2605541 dose was increased by 10 nmol (10 μL, 1 volumetric "unit"), and if >180 mg/dL, the LY2605541 dose was increased by 20 nmol (20 μL, 2 volumetric "units"). After the interim analysis, these increments were changed to 2 and 4 volumetric "units," respectively. The GL dose was adjusted at weekly intervals using the same algorithm with 2- and 4-unit increments throughout the study. If more than one episode of hypoglycemia occurred in a week, the GL dose was decreased by 2 units or the LY2605541 dose was decreased to 80% of the pre-event dose on the first day and then 90% thereafter.

Prandial insulin adjustments were made as needed, according to the clinical

judgment of the treating investigator, with the goal of maintaining preprandial BG between 90 and 130 mg/dL.

Blood samples were tested for the presence of antibodies against LY2605541 and categorized as negative or positive at baseline and at weeks 8 and 16. Percent binding <1.16% was classified as negative.

Statistical methods

SAS Drug Development system (SAS Institute, Cary, NC) was used to perform all statistical analyses. All analyses were based on a slightly modified intent-to-treatment principle in which all patients who took at least one dose of the study medication were included. All tests were performed for two-sided tests at $\alpha = 0.1$ and the corresponding 90% CIs were calculated. No adjustments for multiplicity were performed. The baseline value for all variables was the last nonmissing value before or at randomization, except that for the analysis of the change in body weight, the value at the beginning of each period was used as the baseline. Assuming no true treatment difference and the SD of within-patient difference of 35.8 mg/dL, the 108 patients who completed the study provided at least 90% power to show noninferiority of LY2605541 to GL at a noninferiority margin of 10.8 mg/dL with the two-sided $\alpha = 0.1$. If the upper limit of the 90% CI for the least squares (LS) mean difference between treatments was <10.8 mg/dL, LY2605541 was to be declared noninferior to GL. If it was <0 mg/dL, then LY2605541 was to be declared superior.

Daily mean BG was calculated from the three SMBG profiles performed before each visit. Three measures were used to quantify glucose variability: interday FBG (SD of the daily FBG measurements between this visit and the previous visit), interday SMBG variability (average of the interday SDs of the glucose at 8 individual points), and intraday BG variability (SD of SMBG profiles). Rates of hypoglycemia events adjusted for 30 days were calculated by the number of hypoglycemia events divided by patients' duration in the study, multiplied by 30.

All continuous variables, including the primary analysis variable, were analyzed using Grizzle's model (9), specifically, mixed-model repeated measures with independent variables of treatment, sequence, period, week since the beginning of each period, dose conversion (preinterim analysis, postinterim analysis), baseline A1C group, baseline basal insulin dose group, interaction between treatment and week, and a random effect for patient. To account for possible carry-over effect, body weight and A1C were also analyzed and plotted by sequence and period. Binary variables were analyzed using method of Nagelkerke et al. (10). Sequence groups were compared using the Fisher exact test. Hypoglycemia rate per patient for 30 days was analyzed using a negative binomial model with treatment, treatment sequence, period, and dose conversion as independent variables, and the unstructured variance-covariance was used to model the within-patient correlation.

RESULTS—Of 138 patients randomized to treatment, 137 received at least one dose of study drug and 108 completed the study. Patient decision was the most common reason for discontinuation from both sequence groups (Supplementary Fig. 2). Patient demographics for the two treatment sequence groups were well balanced (Table 1).

After 8 weeks of therapy, LY2605541 resulted in better daily mean ($\pm$ SE) BG (144.2 $\pm$ 2.5 mg/dL) compared with GL (151.7 $\pm$ 3.1 mg/dL; Table 2, Fig. 1). The LS mean difference (LY2605541 minus GL) was −9.9 mg/dL (90% CI −14.6 to −5.2 mg/dL, $P < 0.001$; Table 2). Because the upper limit of the 90% CI was less than 0, LY2605541 was demonstrated to be both statistically noninferior and superior to GL in controlling daily

mean BG. At 8 weeks, interday FBG variability was significantly lower with LY2605541 than with GL ($P < 0.001$), as were interday ($P = 0.061$) and intraday SMBG variabilities ($P = 0.004$).

The 8-point glucose profiles after 8 weeks are depicted in the insert in Fig. 1. FBG from SMBG profiles was not significantly different between LY2605541 and GL. Laboratory fasting plasma glucose, which was measured ~90 min later than FBG from SMBG, was significantly lower with LY2605541 than with GL (Table 2). LY2605541 treatment also resulted in significantly lower A1C (Table 2). During the first treatment period, both sequence groups showed similar reduction in A1C. During the second period, A1C levels rose slightly with GL but continued to fall with LY2605541 (Fig. 2A).

After 8 weeks of treatment, the mealtime insulin dose was ~24% lower with LY2605541 than with GL treatment (Table 2). The basal insulin doses were adjusted to optimize the SMBG FBG measurements using the algorithm noted above. The basal insulin dose for LY2605541 (Table 2) is presented in units per kilogram based on the definition of 1 unit = 9 nmol (7).

Patients had a mean weight loss of 1.20 kg ($P < 0.0001$) during LY2605541 treatment and a mean weight gain of 0.69 kg ($P = 0.0007$) during GL treatment (Fig. 2B). The LS mean difference was −1.89 kg ($P < 0.0001$). Change in weight over time is shown in Fig 2B.

ALT and AST increased during LY2605541 treatment and decreased slightly during GL treatment, resulting in a statistically significant treatment difference after 8 weeks of treatment (Table 2). Mean values for ALT and AST remained in the normal range. At the last visit of the second treatment period, one patient (1.9%) treated with LY2605541 had elevated ALT above three times ULN. This patient entered the study with elevated ALT and AST values of less than two times ULN. The patient's hepatitis serology was negative; a computed tomography scan demonstrated fatty liver.

There were significant differences in lipids after 8 weeks of treatment with LY2605541 or GL. LY2605541 treatment was associated with lower HDL-cholesterol and higher LDL-cholesterol and triglycerides (Table 2). LDL-cholesterol results were not significantly associated with differences in statin use or discontinuation. No other significant differences were observed in laboratory analytes.

Total hypoglycemic event rates (events/30 days) were 12% higher during LY2605541 treatment than during GL treatment during the 8-week treatment period ($P = 0.037$, Table 2). The nocturnal hypoglycemia rate was 25% lower ($P = 0.012$) for LY2605541 compared with GL (Table 2). Incidence of severe hypoglycemia was similar for both basal insulins (5 patients with 6 events with LY2605541 and 3 patients with 6 events with GL).

During LY2605541 treatment, six patients reported eight serious adverse events: severe hypoglycemia ($n = 5$, 6 events), as well as fall and facial bone fracture, both unrelated to hypoglycemia. During GL treatment, four patients reported eight serious adverse events: severe hypoglycemia ($n = 3$, 6 events), urosepsis, and urinary tract infection.

Treatment-emergent adverse events (TEAEs) were similar between groups, with 68 patients (54.8%) reporting one or more TEAEs during LY2605541 treatment and 62 patients (47.7%) reporting one or more TEAEs during GL treatment ($P = 0.691$). TEAEs that occurred in ≥5% of patients included upper respiratory tract infection in 12 (8.8%; $P = 1.00$ for between-treatment comparison), headache in 9 (6.6%; $P = 1.00$), and nasopharyngitis in 7 (5.1%; $P = 1.00$).

Events related to skin and subcutaneous tissue were more common during LY2605541 treatment ($n = 9$ [7.3%])

Table 1—Patient demographics and disease characteristics

	LY2605541/GL $n = 69$	GL/LY2605541 $n = 68$	P
Ethnicity			1.00
American Indian or Alaskan Native	—	1 (1.5)	
Asian	—	1 (1.5)	
Black	3 (4.3)	2 (2.9)	
Multiple	1 (1.4)	—	
Caucasian	65 (94.2)	64 (94.1)	
Hispanic or Latino	9 (13)	6 (8.8)	0.586
Country of residence			0.532
Israel	7 (10.1)	4 (5.9)	
U.S.	62 (89.9)	64 (94.1)	
Age (years)	36.8 $\pm$ 11.3	39.5 $\pm$ 12.3	0.181
Men	41 (59.4)	45 (66.2)	0.481
Weight (kg)	83.0 $\pm$ 15.7	83.1 $\pm$ 17.0	0.965
BMI (kg/m^2)	27.5 $\pm$ 4.4	27.1 $\pm$ 4.6	0.582
A1C (%)	7.73 $\pm$ 1.07	7.76 $\pm$ 0.95	0.890
Duration of diabetes (years)	16.8 $\pm$ 11.7	19.1 $\pm$ 11.5	0.258

Values are shown as mean $\pm$ SD or n (%). GL/LY2605541, patients who received 8 weeks of treatment with insulin GL, followed by 8 weeks of treatment with LY2605541; LY2605541/GL, patients who received 8 weeks of treatment with LY2605541, followed by 8 weeks of treatment with insulin GL.

Table 2—*Clinical assessments: values at baseline, after 8 weeks of treatment, and for LS mean difference of change from baseline*

| | Baseline | After 8 weeks of treatment | | LS mean (90% CI)* | P |
		LY2605541	Insulin GL		
Daily SMBG (mg/dL), mean ± SE	161.3 ± 2.9	144.2 ± 2.5	151.7 ± 3.1	−9.9 (−14.6 to −5.2)	<0.001
FBG (SMBG) (mg/dL), mean ± SE	187.4 ± 5.6	153.7 ± 4.1	154.8 ± 5.0	−4.3 (−14.2 to 5.4)	0.464
FPG (laboratory) (mg/dL), mean ± SE	197.8 ± 7.6	149.9 ± 6.8	178.6 ± 7.7	−26.3 (−44.1 to −8.3)	0.017
FBG interday variability, mean ± SE	61.7 ± 2.0	48.6 ± 1.8	56.9 ± 2.2	−8.5 (−12.4 to −4.5)	<0.001
SMBG variability, mean ± SE					
Interday	21.2 ± 1.6	17.6 ± 1.1	21.8 ± 1.6	−3.4 (−6.5 to −0.4)	0.061
Intraday	62.5 ± 1.6	52.2 ± 1.8	58.0 ± 2.2	−6.1 (−9.5 to −2.7)	0.004
A1C (%), mean ± SE	7.70 ± 0.09	7.07 ± 0.07	7.22 ± 0.08	−0.18 (−0.25 to −0.10)	<0.001
Cholesterol (mg/dL), mean ± SE					
HDL	60.3 ± 1.5	54.1 ± 1.5	59.2 ± 1.5	−5.4 (−7.3 to −3.1)	<0.001
LDL	96.1 ± 2.7	102 ± 3.1	92.4 ± 2.7	8.5 (2.7–14.3)	0.016
Triglycerides (mg/dL), mean ± SE	91.2 ± 4.4	113 ± 7.1	85.0 ± 4.4	29.2 (19.5–39.0)	<0.001
ALT (IU/L), mean ± SD	20.9 ± 10.8	27.4 ± 22.3	19.5 ± 9.7	8.6 (5.1–12.1)	<0.001
AST (IU/L), mean ± SD	21.1 ± 8.8	23.4 ± 11.9	20.1 ± 6.6	3.7 (1.9–5.6)	0.001
Rate of hypoglycemic events†					
Total events	3.78 ± 3.92	8.74 ± 7.70	7.36 ± 6.80	1.12‡ (1.03–1.23)	0.037
Nocturnal events	0.46 ± 1.13	0.88 ± 1.22	1.13 ± 1.42	0.75‡ (0.62–0.90)	0.012
Insulin dose (units/kg/day), mean ± SD					
Basal	0.36 ± 0.14	0.42 ± 0.18	0.43 ± 0.19	—	—
Mealtime	0.23 ± 0.17	0.19 ± 0.14	0.24 ± 0.18	−0.06 (−0.08 to −0.03)	<0.001

FPG, fasting plasma glucose. *Mean difference of change from baseline, which is based on mixed-model repeated-measures analyses. †Rate of events across 8 weeks of treatment, per 30 days. ‡These values are the ratios of the LY2605541 negative binomial mean to the insulin GL negative binomial mean.

compared with GL treatment (*n* = 2 [1.5%]), but the difference was not significant (*P* = 0.222). The most common TEAEs in this category were pruritus and rash, which occurred in two patients (1.5%) each. Gastrointestinal (GI)-related events were reported by more patients during LY2605541 treatment (*n* = 19 [15.3%]) than during GL treatment (*n* = 5 [3.8%]; *P* < 0.001). No individual GI-related TEAEs occurred in ≥5% of patients. The most prevalent were dyspepsia, nausea, and abdominal distension, which occurred in four patients each during LY2605541 treatment. Mean weight loss was 0.84 kg for LY2605541-treated patients who experienced a GI-related TEAE and 1.33 kg for LY2605541-treated patients who did not.

Pulse rate and blood pressure (BP) responses and comparisons were variable throughout the study. Systolic BP and pulse rate did not differ between treatments after 8 weeks, but diastolic BP was slightly higher for LY2605541 than for GL (75.0 ± 0.9 vs. 73.6 ± 0.8, Δ = 1.32 mmHg; *P* = 0.10).

The percentages of patients who were LY2605541 antibody-negative at baseline and became antibody-positive after 8 weeks of treatment was similar for LY2605541 and GL (Supplementary Table 1). Interpretation of antibody response during treatment period 2 is confounded due to the study's crossover design. Change in the antibody status (negative to positive or positive to negative) had no apparent effect on glycemic response.

CONCLUSIONS—The primary objective of this crossover Phase 2 study

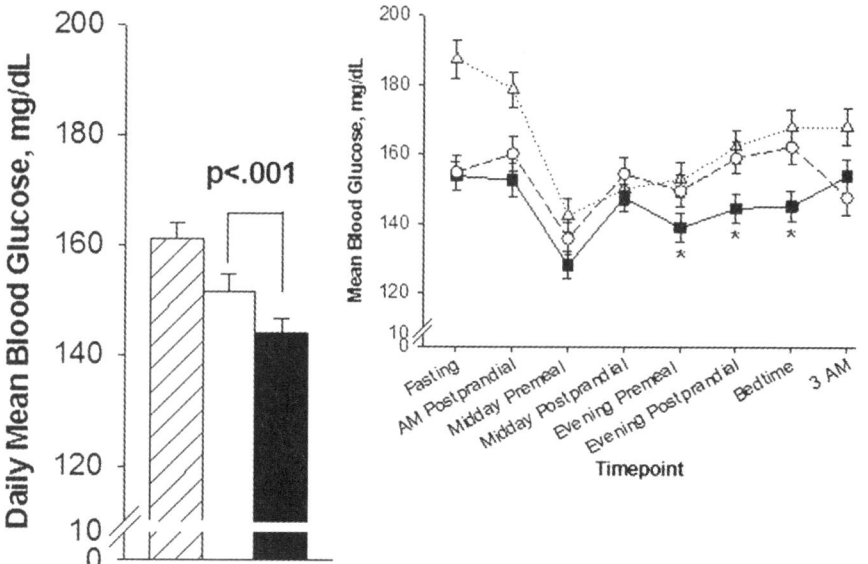

Figure 1—*Daily mean (± SE) BG at baseline and at 8 weeks for LY2605541 (LY) and insulin GL. Baseline for both treatments, ▧; insulin GL, ☐; LY2605541, ▪. Inset graph shows mean (± SE) 8-point SMBG profile at baseline and after 8 weeks of treatment for LY2605541 and GL. Baseline for both treatments, △; insulin GL, ○; LY2605541, ▪. *Times at which BG was significantly lower (P < 0.01) after 8 weeks of LY2605541 treatment compared with GL.*

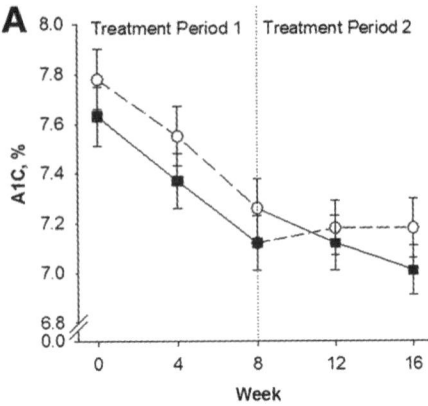

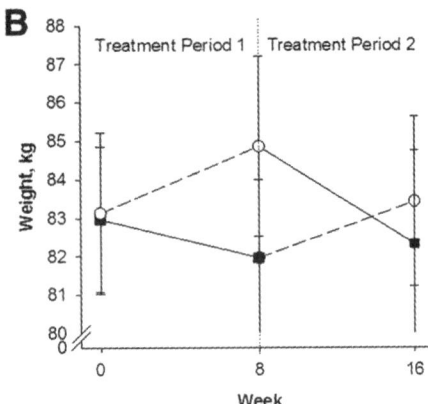

Figure 2—*Mean A1C and weight during treatment with LY2605541 and insulin GL. Patients received treatment with one basal insulin for the first 8-week treatment period and were switched to the other basal insulin for the second treatment period. Insulin GL, ○; LY2605541, ■. A: Mean (± SE) A1C throughout the two treatment periods. B: Mean (± SE) weight throughout the two treatment periods.*

was to compare the effect of two basal insulins, LY2605541 and GL, on mean BG of 8-point SMBG profiles after 8 weeks of treatment when used in basal-bolus insulin regimens in patients with type 1 diabetes. Mean BG was chosen rather than A1C because of the short duration of the study and the likelihood of a carryover effect in A1C. The study demonstrated LY2605541 was noninferior and superior to GL in achieving a lower mean BG after 8 weeks of treatment. LY2605541 also reduced A1C more than GL. Both sequence groups completed the study with mean values at or near guideline-recommended treatment goals for A1C, which attests to the robustness of study implementation.

In addition to improved glycemic control, LY2605541 achieved lower inter-day and intraday glycemic variability

compared with GL, possibly due to its longer duration and a lower peak-to-trough ratio compared with GL (7). These basal insulins were both administered before breakfast to compare the effect of their duration on fasting glucose. We anticipated that differences in fasting glycemia might be demonstrated because of difference in duration of action, but this was not observed in the fasting glucose from SMBG profiles.

The molar amount of LY2605541 equivalent to 1 unit of insulin was not known before this study. Because the final dose of LY2605541 in nanomoles per kilogram was empirically determined in this trial, and FBG from SMBG was similar between LY2605541 and GL after 8 weeks, the ratio of the basal insulin doses in nanomoles per kilogram at 8 weeks can be used as a reasonable dose conversion factor. This conversion indicates that 9 nmol LY2605541 has approximately the same effect on glycemic measures as 1 unit of insulin glargine. Similar results were seen in the type 2 diabetes trial (11). Thus, for Phase 3 trials, LY2605541 will be formulated at 900 nmol/mL to achieve a U-100 concentration.

The difference in laboratory fasting plasma glucose between treatments in this trial is likely to be artificial and not representative of the patient's glycemic pattern because these measurements were obtained later in the morning (~90 min after the recorded timing of the home-based SMBG FBG values). These laboratory measures were therefore typically obtained more than 24 h after the previous basal insulin dose and would not be representative of the patient's routine, but they do suggest a longer glucose-lowering action of LY2605541.

Patients required ~24% less meal-time insulin during LY2605541 treatment than during GL treatment. This was not a result of a relatively higher dose of LY2605541 compared with GL because fasting glycemia was not different between treatments but presumably is due to better daytime coverage from a longer-lasting basal insulin.

Despite morning administration, which should have minimized nocturnal hypoglycemia for the shorter-acting GL (12), LY2605541 was associated with a lower rate of nocturnal hypoglycemia than GL. However, overall rates of total hypoglycemia were higher during LY2605541 treatment. The higher rate of total hypoglycemia was not a result of a relatively higher dose of LY2605541

compared with GL, because fasting glycemia was not different between treatments and LY2605541 treatment resulted in lower nocturnal hypoglycemia events.

Different treat-to-target algorithms were used for dose titration and for reduction of the two basal insulins after hypoglycemia. The algorithm for LY2605541, while exploratory, was developed based on the pharmacokinetic and pharmacodynamic characteristics of that basal insulin (7). Further clinical experience will be needed to determine the optimal dose adjustment needed in instances of hypoglycemia with LY2605541 as well as the best use of meal-time insulin with this novel long-acting insulin.

Patients treated with LY2605541 lost weight while improving glycemic control. This observation was reaffirmed by sequential observations noted with the crossover design (Fig. 2B). Weight loss with improved glycemic control was also observed in a LY2605541 Phase 2 trial in patients with type 2 diabetes (11).

Patients in this study reported significantly more GI-related adverse events with LY2605541 compared with GL. The converse was noted in a study of LY2605541 in type 2 diabetes (11). Skin disorders were more common with LY2605541 in that study (11), but the difference between treatment groups in skin disorders was less pronounced in this study.

Patients treated with LY2605541 experienced increases in triglycerides and LDL-cholesterol and a reduction in HDL-cholesterol compared with baseline and GL treatment. Triglycerides returned to levels similar to baseline in the follow-up period, and cholesterol was not remeasured. A per-protocol analysis suggested that differences in statin use and discontinuation could not explain the LDL-cholesterol results. The combination of weight loss and lipid changes with improved glycemic control is in contrast to results typically observed with other therapeutically administered insulins. These findings of weight loss and triglycerides changes compared with GL were also observed in the LY2605541 type 2 diabetes study, although changes in LDL- and HDL-cholesterol were not (11).

Mean serum ALT and AST levels also increased from baseline and were higher than with GL, but were within the normal range. This increase in mean levels may reflect a hepatic adaptation reaction to the polyethylene glycolated insulin (13–15). Alternatively, this may reflect an increase in hepatic fat content, although serum enzyme elevations may not be a reliable indicator of this effect, and a similar magnitude of difference in ALT and AST was observed in the LY2605541 type 2 diabetes study (11). In future studies, additional hepatic monitoring will occur in larger populations with rigorous evaluation of elevations. Hepatic fat content will also be assessed in a subgroup of patients.

The effect of LY2605541 is intriguing in view of long-established precepts of insulin action. Our findings may indicate a significantly different physiological action of LY2605541 compared with other insulins. We speculate that the large molecular (and hydrodynamic) size (16) of this insulin contributes to this aspect of different action. This large size may reduce insulin transport (and thus action) into peripheral target tissues such as adipose tissue. The hepatic sinusoidal endothelium is fenestrated (17) and should permit less impeded transport into the liver. The net effect of these two differential aspects of insulin transport results in a hepatic preferential insulin, as was observed in a somatostatin and glucagon-infused, LY2605541-treated conscious dog model (17). LY2605541 may therefore have the potential to restore a more physiological insulin action and reduce the peripheral hyperinsulinemic action typical of exogenous insulin therapy. With potentially reduced peripheral action, patients converting to LY2605541 may experience decreased lipogenic insulin stimuli, increased lipolysis, and perhaps a transient increase in triglycerides with a concomitant but transient increase in LDL-cholesterol and decrease in HDL-cholesterol. Further, it could be hypothesized that increased lipid oxidation may lead to patients' weight loss. Lipid parameters and potential mechanisms of changes will be assessed in future studies of longer duration.

Results of this study are limited by the inherent nature of an open-label design, which is predominantly exploratory in nature, and of small population size. The short duration and crossover design, although permitting patients to be their own control, may confound observations for safety parameters. The study, however, was well implemented by the investigators, as is evident by end point A1C levels. Dosing variability may have occurred because both basal insulins were administered by vial and syringe, and patients had to reconstitute LY2605541.

In addition, different algorithms were used to adjust doses after hypoglycemia for the two basal insulins. Future Phase 3 studies will address these limitations.

In conclusion, LY2605541 basal insulin therapy for patients with type 1 diabetes has the potential to improve glycemic control, reduce weight, glucose variability, and nocturnal hypoglycemia, and lower prandial insulin requirements. LY2605541 was associated with an increase in total hypoglycemia. The reduction in prandial insulin dose from baseline to end point and the reduction in nocturnal hypoglycemia with LY2605541 suggest prandial insulin may be a major contributor to the increase in total hypoglycemia. Overall Phase 2 findings and preclinical results (18) suggest LY2605541 may have a novel mechanism of action. Phase 3 studies are underway to assess the observed benefits and further evaluate the clinical significance of changes in liver enzymes and lipids.

Acknowledgments—This study was funded by Eli Lilly and Company.

J.R. has served on scientific advisory panels for Roche Pharmaceuticals, sanofi-aventis, Novo Nordisk, Eli Lilly and Company, MannKind Corporation, GlaxoSmithKline, Takeda Pharmaceutical Company, Ltd., Daiichi-Sankyo, Johnson & Johnson, Novartis Pharmaceuticals Corporation, Boehringer Ingelheim Pharmaceuticals, Inc., Lexicon Pharmaceuticals, Inc.; has served as a consultant to Roche Pharmaceuticals, sanofi-aventis, Novo Nordisk, Eli Lilly and Company, MannKind Corporation, GlaxoSmithKline, Takeda Pharmaceutical Company, Ltd., Daiichi-Sankyo, Johnson & Johnson, Novartis Pharmaceuticals Corporation, Boehringer Ingelheim Pharmaceuticals, Inc., and Lexicon Pharmaceuticals, Inc.; and has received research support from Pfizer, Inc., sanofi-aventis, Novo Nordisk, Roche Pharmaceuticals, Bristol-Myers Squibb Company, Eli Lilly and Company, Forest Laboratories, Inc., GlaxoSmithKline, Takeda Pharmaceutical Company, Ltd., Novartis Pharmaceuticals Corporation, AstraZeneca LP, Amylin Pharmaceuticals, Inc., Johnson & Johnson, Daiichi-Sankyo, MannKind Corporation, Lexicon Pharmaceuticals, Inc., and Boehringer Ingelheim Pharmaceuticals, Inc.

R.M.B. has served on scientific advisory panels for Abbott Diabetes Care, Amylin Pharmaceuticals, Inc., Bayer Health Care, Eli Lilly and Company, Hygieia, Inc., Johnson & Johnson, Roche Pharmaceuticals, sanofi-aventis, and Valeritas; has served as a consultant to Abbott Diabetes Care, Amylin Pharmaceuticals, Inc., Bayer Health Care, Becton, Dickinson and Company, Boehringer Ingelheim Pharmaceuticals, Inc., Calibra Medical, Inc., Eli Lilly and Company, Halozyme Therapeutics, Helmsley Trust, Hygieia, Inc., Johnson & Johnson, Medtronic, ResMed, Roche Pharmaceuticals, sanofi-aventis, Takeda Pharmaceutical Company, Ltd., and Valeritas LLC; has received research support from Abbott Diabetes Care, Amylin Pharmaceuticals, Inc., Bayer Health Care, Becton, Dickinson and Company, Boehringer Ingelheim Pharmaceuticals, Inc., Calibra Medical, Inc., Dexcom, Inc., Eli Lilly and Company, Halozyme Therapeutics, Helmsley Trust, Hygieia, Inc., Intarcia Therapeutics, Inc., Johnson & Johnson, MannKind Corporation, Medtronic, National Institutes of Health, ResMed, Roche Pharmaceuticals, sanofi-aventis, and Takeda Pharmaceutical Company, Ltd.; and holds stock in Merck & Co.

T.C.B. has served on speaker bureaus for Eli Lilly and Company, Merck, Novo Nordisk, sanofi-aventis, Novartis, Bristol-Myers Squibb, Boehringer-Ingelheim, Amylin, and Medtronic; has received research support from Eli Lilly and Company, Novo Nordisk, sanofi-aventis, Novartis, Amylin, Halozyme, and Medtronic; and has served on a clinical advisory board for Eli Lilly and Company.

L.A.M. is an employee of and holds stock in Profil Institute for Clinical Research, which was contracted with Eli Lilly and Company to perform clinical research activities for this study. M.J.P., Y.Q., V.P.S., and S.J.J. are employees of and hold stock in Eli Lilly and Company. D.C.H. is a retired employee of Eli Lilly and Company and holds stock in Eli Lilly and Company. No other potential conflicts of interest relevant to this article were reported.

J.R., R.M.B., and L.A.M. participated in conducting the study, in the data analysis, in writing the manuscript, and approved the final manuscript. T.C.B. participated in the data analysis and in writing the manuscript and approved the final manuscript. M.J.P., V.P.S., and D.C.H. participated in the study design, in the data analysis, and in writing the manuscript and approved the final manuscript. Y.Q. participated in the study design, designed and conducted the statistical analyses, participated in the data analysis and in writing the manuscript, and approved the final manuscript. S.J.J. participated in the study design, in conducting the study, in the data analysis, and in writing the manuscript and approved the final manuscript. J.R. is the guarantor of this work and, as such, had full access to all data in the study and takes responsibility for the integrity of the data and the accuracy of the data analysis.

Parts of this study were presented at the 72nd Scientific Sessions of the American Diabetes Association, Philadelphia, Pennsylvania, 8–12 June 2012, and at the Annual Meeting of the European Association for the Study of Diabetes, Berlin, Germany, 1–5 October 2012.

The authors thank Dr. Jennie G. Jacobson, Eli Lilly and Company, for her expert assistance in the preparation of the manuscript.

References
1. Bliss M. *The Discovery of Insulin.* Chicago, IL, University of Chicago Press, 1982

2. Jersild M. Insulin zinc suspension; four years' experience. Lancet 1956;271:1009–1013

3. Binder C, Lauritzen T, Faber O, Pramming S. Insulin pharmacokinetics. Diabetes Care 1984;7:188–199

4. Bolli GB, Di Marchi RD, Park GD, Pramming S, Koivisto VA. Insulin analogues and their potential in the management of diabetes mellitus. Diabetologia 1999;42:1151–1167

5. Chapman TM, Perry CM. Insulin detemir: a review of its use in the management of type 1 and 2 diabetes mellitus. Drugs 2004; 64:2577–2595

6. Jonassen I, Havelund S, Ribel U, et al. Insulin degludec is a new generation ultra-long acting basal insulin with a unique mechanism of protraction based on multi-hexamer formation. Diabetes 2010;59(Suppl. 1):A11 [abstract]

7. Sinha VP, Howey DC, Soon DKW, et al. Single-dose pharmacokinetics (PK) and glucodynamics (GD) of the novel, long-acting basal insulin LY2605541 in healthy subjects. Diabetes 2012;61(Suppl. 1):A273 [abstract]

8. Workgroup on Hypoglycemia, American Diabetes Association. Defining and reporting hypoglycemia in diabetes: a report from the American Diabetes Association Workgroup on Hypoglycemia. Diabetes Care 2005;28:1245–1249

9. Grizzle JE. The two-period change-over design and its use in clinical trials. Biometrics 1965;21:467–480

10. Nagelkerke NJD, Hart AAM, Oosting J. The two-period binary response crossover trial. Biom J 1986;28:863–869

11. Bergenstal RM, Rosenstock J, Arakaki RF, et al. A randomized, controlled study of once-daily LY2605541, a novel long-acting basal insulin, versus insulin glargine in basal insulin-treated patients with type 2 diabetes. Diabetes Care 2012;35: 2140–2147

12. Hamann A, Matthaei S, Rosak C, Silvestre L; HOE901/4007 Study Group. A randomized clinical trial comparing breakfast, dinner, or bedtime administration of insulin glargine in patients with type 1 diabetes. Diabetes Care 2003;26:1738–1744

13. Au JS, Navarro VJ, Rossi S. Review article: drug-induced liver injury—its pathophysiology and evolving diagnostic tools. Aliment Pharmacol Ther 2011;34:11–20

14. Feldman M, Freidman LS, Brandt LJ. *Sleisenger and Fordtran's Gastrointestinal and Liver Disease*. 9th ed. Philadelphia, PA, Saunders Elsevier, 2010

15. Navarro VJ, Senior JR. Drug-related hepatotoxicity. N Engl J Med 2006;354:731–739

16. Hansen RJ, Cutler GB Jr, Vick A, et al. LY2605541: Leveraging hydrodynamic size to develop a novel basal insulin. Diabetes 2012;61(Suppl. 1):A228 [abstract]

17. Braet F, Wisse E. Structure and functional aspects of liver sinusoidal endothelial cell fenestrae: a review. Comp Hepatol 2002;1:1 Available at www.comparative-hepatology.com/content/1/1/1

18. Moore MC, Smith MS, Mace KF, et al. Novel pegylated basal insulin LY2605541 has a preferential hepatic effect on glucose metabolism. Diabetes 2012;61(Suppl. 1): A417 [abstract]

Assessment of Barriers to Improve Diabetes Management in Older Adults

A randomized controlled study

Medha N. Munshi, md[1,2,3]
Alissa R. Segal, pharmd, cde[1,4]
Emmy Suhl, rd, cde[1]
Courtney Ryan, bs[1]
Adrianne Sternthal, bs[1]
Judy Giusti, rd, cde[1]
Yishan Lee, ms[1]

Shane Fitzgerald, ms[1]
Elizabeth Staum, rd, cde[1]
Patricia Bonsignor, rn, cde[1]
Laura DesRochers, bs[1]
Richard McCartney, bs[1]
Katie Weinger, edd[1,3]

OBJECTIVE—To evaluate whether assessment of barriers to self-care and strategies to cope with these barriers in older adults with diabetes is superior to usual care with attention control. The American Diabetes Association guidelines recommend the assessment of age-specific barriers. However, the effect of such strategy on outcomes is unknown.

RESEARCH DESIGN AND METHODS—We randomized 100 subjects aged ≥69 years with poorly controlled diabetes (A1C >8%) in two groups. A geriatric diabetes team assessed barriers and developed strategies to help patients cope with barriers for an intervention group. The control group received equal amounts of attention time. The active intervention was performed for the first 6 months, followed by a "no-contact" period. Outcome measures included A1C, Tinetti test, 6-min walk test (6MWT), self-care frequency, and diabetes-related distress.

RESULTS—We assessed 100 patients (age 75 ± 5 years, duration 21 ± 13 years, 68% type 2 diabetes, 89% on insulin) over 12 months. After the active period, A1C decreased by −0.45% in the intervention group vs. −0.31% in the control group. At 12 months, A1C decreased further in the intervention group by −0.21% vs. 0% in control group (linear mixed-model, $P < 0.03$). The intervention group showed additional benefits in scores on measures of self-care (Self-Care Inventory-R), gait and balance (Tinetti), and endurance (6MWT) compared with the control group. Diabetes-related distress improved in both groups.

CONCLUSIONS—Only attention between clinic visits lowers diabetes-related distress in older adults. However, communication with an educator cognizant of patients' barriers improves glycemic control and self-care frequency, maintains functionality, and lowers distress in this population.

Diabetes Care 36:543–549, 2013

D iabetes is a major public health problem affecting an increasing number of older individuals (1). Treating older adults with diabetes is complicated by the presence of coexisting chronic conditions, including cognitive dysfunction, depression (2), physical disabilities (3), and polypharmacy (4). Although these conditions, collectively referred to as geriatric syndrome, are not specifically associated with diabetes, they may act as barriers by interfering with patients' abilities to perform self-care tasks such as glucose monitoring, understanding the role of diet and exercise on glucose excursions, and following complex insulin regimens (5,6). Some comorbidities have subtle presentations and may remain unidentified by medical providers (7). Unaddressed barriers in older adults may lead to nonadherence with diabetes self-care recommendations, treatment

complications such as hypoglycemia, and an overall decline in health and quality-of-life. The American Geriatrics Society (4) and the American Diabetes Association (8) recommend assessment for age-specific barriers in older adults to improve diabetes management. However, practical tools, methods of implementing this strategy, and the impacts of these recommendations on outcomes are unknown.

Older adults with diabetes frequently encounter fluctuations in their glucose levels when clinical (e.g., acute infections or exacerbation of heart disease or other chronic diseases), functional (e.g., falls or deconditioning), or social (e.g., illness or death in the family, caregiver stress of aging spouse) circumstances change. Strategies to adjust insulin regimens for fluctuations in blood glucose or dose-adjustment for sick-days commonly used in younger adults are difficult to follow for older patients with multiple medical co-morbidities, especially during times of stress. Consequently, when older adults are seen by their medical providers at an interval of 3 to 6 months, small changes made during clinic visits are frequently inadequate to improve overall glycemia.

Phone consultations and telemedicine are a frequently tested approach to improve outcomes in the management of chronic diseases, such as congestive heart failure, particularly when ongoing adjustments in doses of medications, such as diuretics, are required (9). In recent years, successful management of diabetes via telemedicine in older patients living in medically underserved areas has been shown to be successful (10). However, telephone follow-up between clinic visits is typically not used for glycemic management as part of chronic disease management in patients with diabetes. Community-living older adults with poorly controlled diabetes are a vulnerable population with a high risk of acute illnesses and hospitalizations. For these patients, phone calls by diabetes educators to adjust insulin doses or provide coping strategies to maintain self-care may be an effective and inexpensive method for decreasing wide glucose

• •

From the [1]Joslin Diabetes Center, Boston, Massachusetts; the [2]Beth Israel Deaconess Medical Center, Boston, Massachusetts; the [3]Harvard Medical School, Boston, Massachusetts; and the [4]Massachusetts College of Pharmacy for Health Sciences, Boston, Massachusetts.
Corresponding author: Medha N. Munshi, mmunshi@bidmc.harvard.edu.
Received 3 July 2012 and accepted 27 August 2012.
DOI: 10.2337/dc12-1303. Clinical trial reg. nos. NCT01480804 and NCT01486290, clinicaltrials.gov.

excursions from hyperglycemia and hypoglycemia.

In this study, we hypothesized that providing coping strategies for age-related barriers to self-care by phone contact between clinic visits would be superior to attention alone in improving glycemic control in older adults with poorly controlled diabetes.

RESEARCH DESIGN AND METHODS

—The institutional review boards of the Joslin Diabetes Center, the Beth Israel Deaconess Medical Center, and the Human Research Protection Office of the U.S. Department of Defense approved this study.

Participants

Participants were recruited from the Joslin Diabetes Center and the Beth Israel Deaconess Medical Center. Patients aged ≥69 years with type 1 or type 2 diabetes of at least 1-year duration, with poorly controlled diabetes (A1C >8%), were eligible. Exclusion criteria included terminal diseases, living >25 miles from Boston, living in an institutional setting (e.g., nursing home, group home), and inability to complete outcome assessments (e.g., poor vision, severe cognitive decline, unable to speak, read, or write English). Study participants continued to receive their medical care, including diabetes management, from their endocrinologists and/or primary care physicians throughout the study. All patients provided informed written consent.

Study design

Participants were followed up for 1 year. First, all patients were randomized to an intervention or attention control group. Then, the intervention group was further divided randomly to two groups, described below. Randomization was computer-generated and remained independent of participant enrollment. The adequacy of randomization was checked periodically, and patients were stratified once due to unequal number of patients with different durations of diabetes. During the first 6 months of the study, all patients received active intervention or attention as determined by their random assignment. From 6 to 12 months, all patients entered an "independence period" during which there was no contact between the study personnel and patients from either group. The independence period assessed the sustainability of the interventions' impact.

Group 1: Intervention group

The patients in this group underwent evaluation for barriers to self-care by a diabetes educator well versed with age-specific barriers. A geriatric diabetes team (GDT), consisting of a geriatric diabetologist, a diabetes educator, and a nutritionist, identified strategies to help patients cope with their barriers after consideration of patients' clinical and psychosocial environments and comorbid conditions. The strategies were designed to optimize patients' ability to perform self-care leading to better adherence with treatment recommendations given by their medical providers. Importantly, the study staff did not make changes to patients' diabetes treatment plans. This was important to protect the integrity of the study, particularly the ability to interpret the effect of management of barriers versus change in treatment regimen.

The strategies to cope with barriers were provided to the patients in intervention group via two methods by further randomizing patients into two groups. In one group, an office-based diabetes educator provided the strategy by phone calls, speaking with patients up to 11 times during the intervention period. The initial phone call included educating patients regarding their barriers and providing strategy options to cope with these barriers. Follow-up phone calls included continued assessment and encouragement to cope with barriers, as described in Table 1. In the second group, a non–health professional care manager, trained and briefed by the GDT, provided coping recommendations. The recommendations were conveyed to the patients in this group by the care manager. The care manager visited the patients' homes to assess safety issues or other needs not known to the study team and helped the patients and caregivers with all aspects of care coordination, including making medical appointments and arranging transportation. Patients in this group received phone contact from the care manager as often as needed during the intervention period.

Group 2: Attention control group

An educator (different from the one involved with the intervention), called participants in this group for total of 11 times within the first 6 months to provide similar attention time. The phone calls differed from the intervention calls in that the educator did not provide any diabetes-related advice or strategies and only discussed non–diabetes-related life events. Participants who asked specific questions related to diabetes management were advised to contact their medical providers.

Outcomes

All study participants underwent the outcome assessment at baseline and at 6 and 12 months, whereas the primary outcome (A1C) was measured at baseline and at 3, 6, and 12 months.

Clinical measures. The primary outcome of the study was glycemic control (A1C), before and after interventions. Other clinical outcomes included blood pressure, BMI, lipids, questionnaire for frequency of hypoglycemia and medication compliance, frequency of self-care activity (Self-Care Inventory-R [SCI-R]) (11), dietary assessment (Determine Your Nutritional Health checklist) (12), and cognition (clock-in-a-box test [7,13], Trail-Making Test A and B [14], and verbal fluency test [15]).

Functional measures. Functional measures included activities of daily living (16) and instrumental activities of daily living (17) number of falls and fear of falls, 6-min walk test (6MWT) (18), and the Tinetti test for gait and balance (19).

Psychosocial measures. Psychosocial measures included a Geriatric Depression Scale (GDS) (20) and/or a diagnosis of depression, diabetes-related distress (Problem Areas in Diabetes [PAID]) (21), and social resource assessment (Older Americans Resources and Services Multidimensional Functional Assessment Questionnaire) (22).

Economic measures. Economic measures included the number of emergency department (ED) visits, hospitalizations, and outpatient care utilization (clinic visits).

Statistical methods

We performed an intent-to-treat analysis with the last observation carried forward. We used paired t tests to assess changes within groups from baseline to 6 months and 12 months. We also compared between-group changes in outcomes at baseline, 6 months (end of intervention period), and 12 months (end of study) with mixed-models, using time and group as fixed factors, interaction between time and group, random intercepts, and an unstructured covariance matrix. A two-sided P value <0.05 indicated statistical significance. Results were confirmed using

Table 1—*Commonly found barriers and strategies recommended to overcome the barriers*

Barriers	Number of times the barrier was identified	Coping strategies
Inadequate mediations • Not adequate titrating • Unable to get provider appointment • Too complicated regimen to follow	87	• Facilitated earlier appointment with diabetes specialist/nurse practitioners or primary care providers
Lack of diabetes-related education/information • Inadequate previous education • Low health literacy	49	• Facilitated appointment with educator • Provided appropriate education material • Reinforcing information given by medical providers
Inadequate dietary information/understanding	52	• Facilitated appointment with nutritionist for dietary counseling
Inadequate physical activity	42	• Referral for exercise physiologist, physical therapy • Community exercise programs • Home exercise programs
Difficulty coping with comorbid conditions • Cognitive dysfunction • Depression • Visual impairment • Auditory impairment • Mobility/dexterity issues • Swallowing problems	61	• Assistance with blood glucose monitoring, meter use, schedule set up • Recommend and set up assistive devices including reminders for meals and monitoring, vision, gait • Recommend referral to audiology • Referral to memory clinic • Referral to mental health clinic • Recommend cognitive aids • Recommend referral to ophthalmology, podiatry
Hypoglycemia and fear of hypoglycemia	31	• Hypoglycemia education/reeducation

Social barriers
• Isolation
• Transportation difficulties
• Lack of motivation
• Caregiver stress
• Financial difficulties
• Major events self/family members interfering with self-care
• Difficulty with care coordination and facilitation
• Nonadherence
• Inadequate medical visits
• Inadequate monitoring
• Not integrating recommendations from providers
• Health beliefs interfering with therapy
	65	• Help to use community resources
		  –Health care services
		  –Patient/public assistance programs
		  –Social services
		  –Transportation
		• Medication-related assistance
		  –Help with discount meds
		  –Pharmacy delivery
		  –Education adherence aids
		  –Pharmacy assistance programs

multiple imputations (15) for missing data using PROC MI in SAS (the Markov chain Monte Carlo method).

RESULTS—Between August 2007 and May 2010, 103 patients were enrolled and 100 patients were randomized (3 patients dropped out after the screening but before the first study visit). Patients were randomized 2-to-1 in the intervention arm ($n = 70$ with care manager and $n = 35$ with office-based educator) versus control ($n = 30$). The Consolidated Standards of Reporting Trials study flow diagram is shown in Fig. 1.

The two intervention subgroups with different implementation strategies were compared for baseline characteristics and for all outcome measures. These subgroups did not differ in baseline characteristics or outcome variables at 6 or 12 months and were for this analysis.

Table 1 summarizes the types of barriers, the number of times these barriers were present, and the coping strategies recommended by the GDT. The most frequent barrier identified in intervention patients was "inadequate medications" due to lack of dose titration between the clinic visits. In addition, participants needed knowledge of insulin action, medication-adherence, and the effect of diet on blood glucose. Comorbidities interfering with diabetes management were another frequent barrier. Multiple social barriers were also identified.

Baseline characteristics
Table 2 reports the baseline characteristics of patients by group. The study population was an average age of 75 ± 5 years, duration of diabetes was 21 ± 13 years, 68% had type 2 diabetes, 54% were women, and 77% were Caucasian. Patients in the two groups did not differ on any baseline variable.

Intervention period
Changes in variables between the intervention and control groups from baseline to 6 months (during the intervention period) are as follows: Mean A1C was decreased by -0.45% (95% CI -0.7 to -0.2, $P < 0.007$) in the intervention group compared with -0.31% (-0.7 to

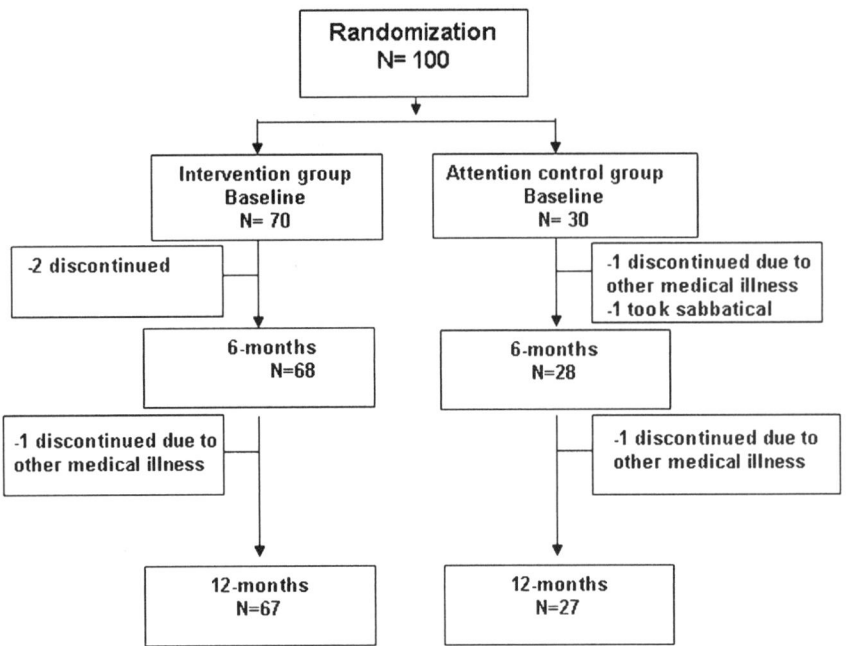

Figure 1—*Randomization and completion of the 6- and 12-month evaluations.*

−0.1, P = NS) in the control group. The mean SCI-R increased by 6.4 (4.2–8.5, P < 0.0001) in the intervention group but did not change the control group (1.2 [−1.7 to 4.1], P = NS). The Tinetti test and 6MWT scores worsened in the control group (−1.6 [−2.9 to −0.3], P = 0.02; and −42 [−86 to 2.6], P = 0.06, respectively) but remained unchanged in the intervention group (0.8 [−0.1 to 1.7], P = NS; and 4 [−10.7 to 19.2], P = NS, respectively). PAID scores decreased in the intervention (−7.9 [−11.4 to 4.4], P < 0.0001) and control groups (−5.2 [−9.5 to −0.9], P = 0.02).

Follow-up period
The change in variables between the intervention and control groups between 6 and 12 months are as follows (Fig. 2): The mean (95% CI) A1C decreased further in the intervention group by −0.21% (−0.4 to −0.04, P = 0.02) whereas no change (0%) occurred in the control group (−0.3 to 0.3, P = NS). In the control group, scores did not change on the SCI-R (−1.4 [−5.3 to 2.5], P = NS), PAID (1.3 [−2.9 to 5.6], P = NS), Tinetti (1.0 [−0.1 to 2.1], P = NS), or 6MWT (18 [−3 to 38], P = NS). The scores in the intervention group did not change on SCI-R (−0.2 [−1.7 to 1.4], P = NS) or PAID (1.5 [−1.4 to 4.4], P = NS). However, the scores on Tinetti and 6MWT declined in the intervention group

(−1.1 [−2 to 0.3], P = 0.007; and −27 [−46 to −8], P = 0.006, respectively) from the 6- to 12-month period. Figure 1 shows changes in variables during the intervention and the follow-up periods.

The linear mixed-models analysis examining each outcome over time found that the intervention group showed better outcomes for A1C (P < 0.03), SCI-R (P < 0.004), Tinetti (P < 0.009), and 6MWT (P < 0.01) than the control group. Scores on PAID did not differ between the groups (P = NS).

Utilization of medical resources
The GDT spent approximately 58 min/patient in the intervention group for the initial evaluation and assessment of barriers. The phone calls by an educator during the 6-month intervention lasted about 131 min/patient (11 phone calls of ~12 min). We evaluated utilization of outpatient medical services (e.g., ophthalmologists, podiatrists, primary care) and inpatient services (ED visits, hospitalizations) in both groups. The intervention and control groups did not differ in utilization of outpatient medical visits (3.8 vs. 3.9 visits/year). During the 12-month period, 5 of 70 participants from the intervention group reported eight diabetes-related ED visits (3 patients with multiple hypoglycemia and 2 with hyperglycemia), whereas none of the 30 participants

from the control group reported diabetes-related ED visits. One participant from intervention group was hospitalized with hypoglycemia. The difference between the numbers of hypoglycemic episodes between the two groups did not reach statistical significance.

Missing data
Overall, 3 of 70 patients dropped out from the intervention group and 4 of 30 from the control group.
Primary outcome. A1C data were available for 100% of the study population at the 6-month interval. For patients who dropped out, A1C data were collected from nonstudy visits in 6 subjects (3 from the intervention group and 3 from the control group). A1C data were missing in 3 of 70 in the intervention group and in 3 of 30 in the control group at 12 months.
Secondary outcomes. Eight subjects (4 from the intervention group and 4 from the control group) did not complete the 6-month or 12-month study visits for secondary outcomes. Some patients declined to complete assessments as follows: 6 participants from the intervention group and 7 from the control group refused PAID and SCI-R tests. The 6MWT and Tinetti test had a higher number of missing data because these tests require not only the questionnaire but also physical performance. Some subjects were unable to do these tests because of comorbidities such as arthritis and difficulty ambulating at various times. In the intervention group, data on the Tinetti test were missing in 7% at 6 months and in 13% at 12 months, whereas in the control group, data were missing in 10% at 6 months and in 13% at 12 months. Similarly, in the intervention group, the data were missing for 6MWT in 20% at 6 months and in 21% at 12 months. For the control group, data were missing in 10% at 6 months and in 13% at 12 months.

CONCLUSIONS—Assessment of age-specific barriers is recommended for management of diabetes in older adults (4). Our study is the first to evaluate the effect of assessing self-care barriers and recommending coping strategies in elderly in a randomized controlled fashion. We identified several self-care barriers in older adults with poorly controlled diabetes. The most common barrier was inadequate medications, primarily due to older patients' reluctance to make changes in insulin doses between clinic visits or during illnesses. The medical

Table 2—*Baseline characteristics of the subjects*

Characteristics	Attention control n = 30	Intervention group n = 70
Age (years)	75 ± 5	75 ± 5
Sex (%)		
Male	53	43
Female	47	57
Race (%)		
White	80	76
Nonwhite	20	24
BMI (kg/m^2)	32 ± 6	32 ± 7
Education (years)	14 ± 3	15 ± 3
Living alone (%)	30	21
Number of daily medications	9 ± 4	8 ± 4
A1C at baseline (%)	9 ± 0.8	9.3 ± 1.2
Diabetes duration (years)	23 ± 14	20 ± 12
Treatment (%)		
Oral agents	7	10
Insulin	57	44
Combination	37	46
Cognitive dysfunction (%)*	−0.07 ± 0.8	0.02 ± 0.8
Depression (%)	37	24
Independent in ADL	12 ± 0.3	12 ± 0.4
Independent in IADL	15.3 ± 1.2	15.3 ± 1.8
Score on		
Tinetti	24.5 ± 5.7	24.4 ± 4.6
6MWT (m)	317 ± 154	331 ± 107
SCI-R	69.5 ± 14	63.2 ± 15
PAID	24.7 ± 18	28 ± 17.6

Data are mean ± SD or as indicated. ADL, activities of daily living; IADL, instrumental activities of daily living.
*Calculated as combined z score for three tests of cognitive dysfunction: clock-in-a-box, Trail-Making Test A and B, and verbal fluency.

providers for most of the patients had prescribed insulin dose self-adjustment during a clinic visit, but the patients felt uncomfortable acting on the advice without talking to a health care provider. High glucose excursions were noted during many clinical and social life-events. In the intervention group, 24% of the patients had at least one unfavorable life-event (e.g., hospitalization, ED visits for non–diabetes-related conditions, surgeries, or death of close family members) that required additional medication adjustment during a 6-month period. We found that untoward clinical and psychosocial events occurred frequently, and even highly functional, independent older adults needed encouragement from a diabetes care provider to adjust medications. This strategy is more likely to benefit elderly patients who are taking insulin because they require dose adjustments with changes in overall health status. Further studies are also needed to see the efficacy of such an approach in older patients during vulnerable periods, such as after hospitalizations or rehabilitation,

where the need for insulin adjustment is unavoidable.

In our study, the intervention and control groups both showed improvement in glycemic control after contact with educators. However, the phone contact by an educator cognizant of patient's age-related barriers (intervention group) showed the additional benefit of maintaining functionality during the intervention period. The results of the 6MWT need caution in interpretation due to some older patients' inability or unwillingness to complete the test at each time period. Our results were unexpected because specific physical training programs were not included in coping strategies. Encouraging physical activity appropriate for the patient's overall health and social situation based on assessment of barriers may have helped improve compliance. We encouraged simple solutions, such as going to the senior center, joining a senior-friendly gym, or walking the hallways in apartment buildings, and using "exercise pedals" to maintain physical activities

during the inclement weather frequently seen in New England. Our results are very encouraging, because maintaining or improving functionality is a desired outcome for chronic disease management and leads to improvement in overall health and quality of life (23). During the independence period, functionality declined but remained above the baseline level. Our results underscore the need for periodical encouragement to improve functional capacity in elderly diabetic subjects, easily achievable by phone contact.

One of the strategies used for improving medication adjustment was encouraging earlier appointments with the health providers. We found that patients had difficulty navigating appointment systems and automated phone systems, and were hesitant or unable to send home monitoring numbers to providers for adjustment. Phone contact with the educators helped in facilitating communications. A large number of patients also lacked basic understanding of how medications work and/or dietary skills. Although most patients had previous education in these areas, they did not understand or remember the information. This was a discouraging finding in patients treated at a tertiary care diabetes clinic. Whether the need for reeducation is a function of aging should be studied further. This deficit in knowledge would likely be greater in communities where diabetes education is not readily available. In patients with adequate knowledge, we found that educator still needed to provide assurance regarding adjustment of insulin doses and encouragement to call providers when glucose levels were not well controlled. Thus, even though the control group educator did not perform an intervention, she encouraged contact with providers for any diabetes-related question. This may have led to therapeutic adjustments by patients' providers that would not have otherwise taken place. We believe this may be the reason why the primary outcome (A1C) improved in both arms in our study, albeit more clinically significant improvement occurred in the intervention arm.

As expected, diabetes-related distress improved in both groups. Talking to an educator helped lower the stress levels concerning diabetes in elderly patients. We also showed that during the independence period, distress scores worsened in both groups; however, they did not return to the patients' baseline levels. The frequency of self-care also improved in

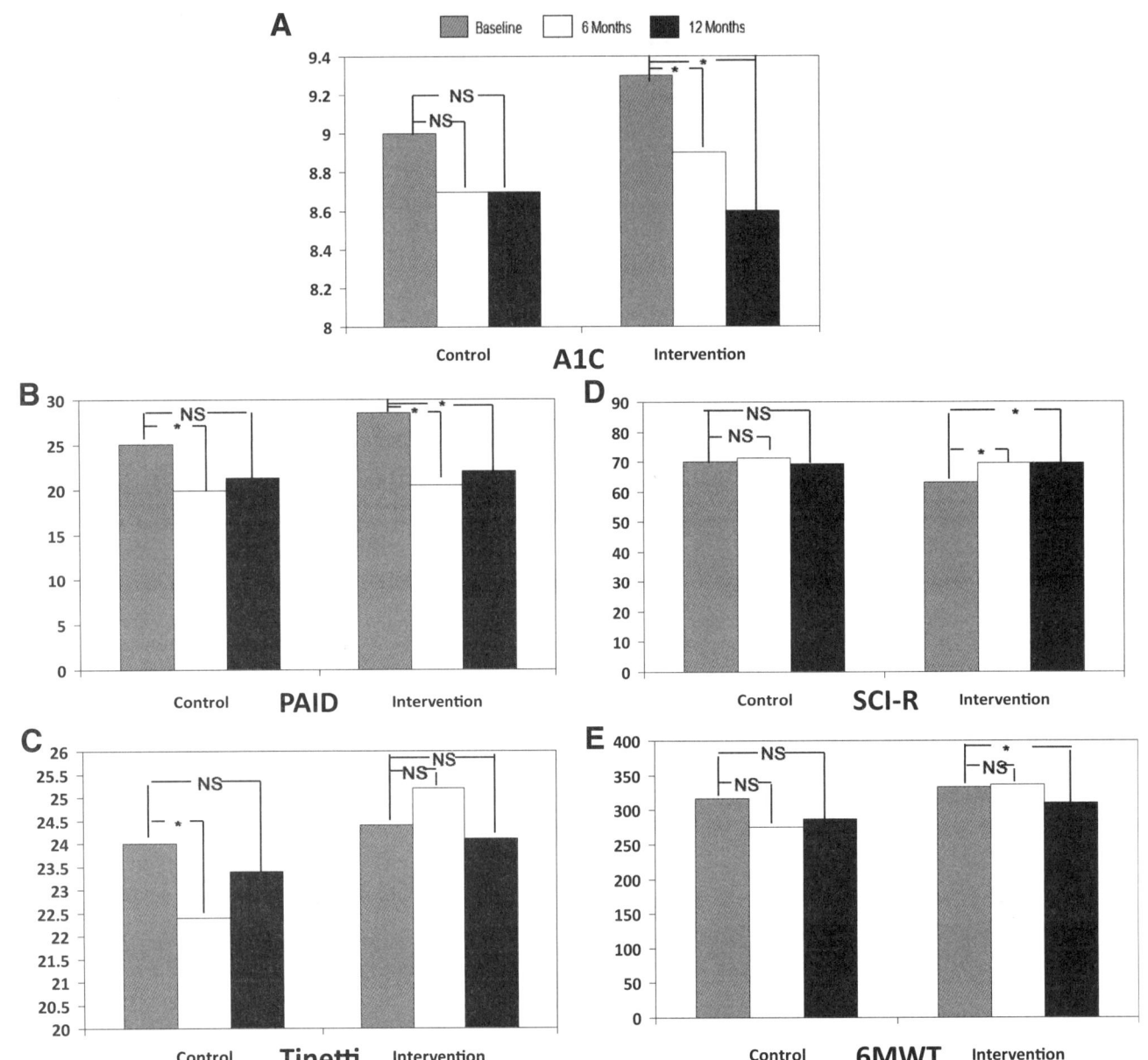

Figure 2—*Changes in variables from baseline to 6 and 12 months for A1C (A), PAID score (B), Tinetti scores (C), SCI-R (D), and 6MWT (E). *P ≤ 0.05.*

both groups during the intervention period, likely due to attention by the educators. The improvement was sustained only by the intervention group, probably due to the tailored strategies provided during the intervention period.

When we measured resource utilization, no difference in outpatient care was seen between the two groups. There were more diabetes-related ED visits and hospitalizations in the intervention group, although the numbers were too small to make definite conclusions. Our small sample size and relatively short study period limits the ability to generalize this information.

However, when comparing two high-risk groups, improvement in surrogate markers (improved functionality and self-care, reduced diabetes-related stress) indicate potential for cost-benefits in a large population over a longer period of time.

In this study, no changes were recommended to the diabetes treatment provided by patients' providers so that we could target the effect of overcoming barriers and not the change in treatment regimen. The interventions focused on optimizing patients' environment to enhance their ability to follow provider-led treatment recommendations. The study team felt that

many patients with multiple comorbidities were on complex regimens that were clearly beyond their coping abilities. Studies evaluating the effect of regimen change to accommodate individual barriers are needed to improve management in this population.

No difference was found between the two methods of providing strategies to the intervention group. We believe this was due to the nature of our study population, who were highly functional and well-educated individuals who used a tertiary care facility for diabetes management. This population was highly functional and did not require assistance once recommendations were provided by the study team. Thus, when strategies were suggested via phone calls by the educator, patients did as well as those who received additional assistance by care manager. These findings may differ for a frailer population that may require assistance to perform care-coordination and implement suggestions such as arranging transportation, finding exercise venues, and scheduling appointments with multiple providers. In this study, because the two methods for providing strategies were equally effective, simple phone calls by an educator cognizant of patients' barriers may prove to be a less costly approach. This area needs further investigation.

Our study highlights the complex challenge in studying older patients with multiple medical comorbidities. First, it was difficult to recruit and retain older patients with chronic medical conditions for a 12-month period. We also found that changes in A1C due to non–diabetes-related health issues and adverse medical and social events occurred in a large portion of our population beyond anyone's control. However, we believe this is a strength of the study, increasing its generalizability.

Our study indicates the importance of age-specific barrier assessment and provides a practical approach for intervention. The study also shows the important role of phone contact with an educator between clinic visits in elderly patients with diabetes. This inexpensive strategy, if proven beneficial in a larger population, would form the basis for long-term policy change.

Acknowledgments—The study was partly supported by a grant from a clinical research award from the American Diabetes Association, 1-07-CR-40 (M.N.M.), and partly from the U.S. Department of Defense Peer Reviewed Medical Research Program of the Office of the Congressionally Directed Medical Research Programs, W81XWH-07-1-0282 (M.N.M.).

M.N.M. received research funding from sanofi-aventis. No other potential conflicts of interest relevant to this article were reported.

M.N.M. researched data, contributed to discussion, and wrote the manuscript. A.R.S. researched data and edited the manuscript. E.Su., C.R., A.S., J.G., E.St., P.B., L.D.R., and R.M. researched data. Y.L. and S.F. analyzed data. K.W. researched data, contributed to discussion, and edited the manuscript. M.N.M. is the guarantor of this work and, as such, had full access to all the data in the study and takes responsibility for the integrity of the data and the accuracy of the data analysis.

Parts of this study were presented in poster form at the 71st Scientific Sessions of the American Diabetes Association, San Diego, California, 24–28 June 2011.

References

1. Centers for Disease Control and Prevention. U.S. Department of Health and Human Services. National Diabetes Fact Sheet: National Estimates and General Information on Diabetes and Prediabetes in the United States, 2011. Available from http://www.cdc.gov/diabetes/pubs/factsheet11.htm. Accessed 3 July 2012
2. Ciechanowski PS, Katon WJ, Russo JE. Depression and diabetes: impact of depressive symptoms on adherence, function, and costs. Arch Intern Med 2000; 160:3278–3285
3. Gregg EW, Beckles GL, Williamson DF, et al. Diabetes and physical disability among older U.S. adults. Diabetes Care 2000;23:1272–1277
4. Brown AF, Mangione CM, Saliba D, Sarkisian CA; California Healthcare Foundation/American Geriatrics Society Panel on Improving Care for Elders with Diabetes. Guidelines for improving the care of the older person with diabetes mellitus. J Am Geriatr Soc 2003;51(5 Suppl. Guidelines):S265–S280
5. Araki A, Ito H. Diabetes mellitus and geriatric syndromes. Geriatr Gerontol Int 2009;9:105–114
6. Huang ES, John P, Munshi MN. Multidisciplinary approach for the treatment of diabetes in the elderly. Aging Health 2009;5:207–216
7. Munshi M, Grande L, Hayes M, et al. Cognitive dysfunction is associated with poor diabetes control in older adults. Diabetes Care 2006;29:1794–1799
8. American Diabetes Association. Standards of medical care in diabetes—2012. Diabetes Care 2012;35(Suppl. 1):S11–S63
9. Anker SD, Koehler F, Abraham WT. Telemedicine and remote management of patients with heart failure. Lancet 2011; 378:731–739
10. Shea S, Weinstock RS, Teresi JA, et al.; IDEATel Consortium. A randomized trial comparing telemedicine case management with usual care in older, ethnically diverse, medically underserved patients with diabetes mellitus: 5 year results of the IDEATel study. J Am Med Inform Assoc 2009;16:446–456
11. Weinger K, Butler HA, Welch GW, La Greca AM. Measuring diabetes self-care: a psychometric analysis of the Self-Care Inventory-Revised with adults. Diabetes Care 2005;28:1346–1352
12. Posner BM, Jette AM, Smith KW, Miller DR. Nutrition and health risks in the elderly: the nutrition screening initiative. Am J Public Health 1993;83:972–978
13. Nishiwaki Y, Breeze E, Smeeth L, Bulpitt CJ, Peters R, Fletcher AE. Validity of the Clock-Drawing Test as a screening tool for cognitive impairment in the elderly. Am J Epidemiol 2004;160:797–807
14. Drane DL, Yuspeh RL, Huthwaite JS, Klingler LK. Demographic characteristics and normative observations for derived-trail making test indices. Neuropsychiatry Neuropsychol Behav Neurol 2002;15: 39–43
15. Abrahams S, Leigh PN, Harvey A, Vythelingum GN, Grisé D, Goldstein LH. Verbal fluency and executive dysfunction in amyotrophic lateral sclerosis (ALS). Neuropsychologia 2000;38:734–747
16. Katz S, Ford AB, Moskowitz RW, Jackson BA, Jaffe MW. Studies of illness in the aged. The Index of ADL: a standardized measure of biological and psychosocial function. JAMA 1963;185:914–919
17. Lawton MP, Brody EM. Assessment of older people: self-maintaining and instrumental activities of daily living. Gerontologist 1969;9:179–186
18. Bautmans I, Lambert M, Mets T. The six-minute walk test in community dwelling elderly: influence of health status. BMC Geriatr 2004;4:6
19. Tinetti ME. Performance-oriented assessment of mobility problems in elderly patients. J Am Geriatr Soc 1986;34:119–126
20. Montorio I, Izal M. The Geriatric Depression Scale: a review of its development and utility. Int Psychogeriatr 1996; 8:103–112
21. Polonsky WH, Anderson BJ, Lohrer PA, et al. Assessment of diabetes-related distress. Diabetes Care 1995;18:754–760
22. Fillenbaum GG, Smyer MA. The development, validity, and reliability of the OARS multidimensional functional assessment questionnaire. J Gerontol 1981; 36:428–434
23. Huang ES, Gorawara-Bhat R, Chin MH. Self-reported goals of older patients with type 2 diabetes mellitus. J Am Geriatr Soc 2005;53:306–311

Economic Costs of Diabetes in the U.S. in 2012

AMERICAN DIABETES ASSOCIATION

OBJECTIVE—This study updates previous estimates of the economic burden of diagnosed diabetes and quantifies the increased health resource use and lost productivity associated with diabetes in 2012.

RESEARCH DESIGN AND METHODS—The study uses a prevalence-based approach that combines the demographics of the U.S. population in 2012 with diabetes prevalence, epidemiological data, health care cost, and economic data into a Cost of Diabetes Model. Health resource use and associated medical costs are analyzed by age, sex, race/ethnicity, insurance coverage, medical condition, and health service category. Data sources include national surveys, Medicare standard analytical files, and one of the largest claims databases for the commercially insured population in the U.S.

RESULTS—The total estimated cost of diagnosed diabetes in 2012 is $245 billion, including $176 billion in direct medical costs and $69 billion in reduced productivity. The largest components of medical expenditures are hospital inpatient care (43% of the total medical cost), prescription medications to treat the complications of diabetes (18%), antidiabetic agents and diabetes supplies (12%), physician office visits (9%), and nursing/residential facility stays (8%). People with diagnosed diabetes incur average medical expenditures of about $13,700 per year, of which about $7,900 is attributed to diabetes. People with diagnosed diabetes, on average, have medical expenditures approximately 2.3 times higher than what expenditures would be in the absence of diabetes. For the cost categories analyzed, care for people with diagnosed diabetes accounts for more than 1 in 5 health care dollars in the U.S., and more than half of that expenditure is directly attributable to diabetes. Indirect costs include increased absenteeism ($5 billion) and reduced productivity while at work ($20.8 billion) for the employed population, reduced productivity for those not in the labor force ($2.7 billion), inability to work as a result of disease-related disability ($21.6 billion), and lost productive capacity due to early mortality ($18.5 billion).

CONCLUSIONS—The estimated total economic cost of diagnosed diabetes in 2012 is $245 billion, a 41% increase from our previous estimate of $174 billion (in 2007 dollars). This estimate highlights the substantial burden that diabetes imposes on society. Additional components of societal burden omitted from our study include intangibles from pain and suffering, resources from care provided by nonpaid caregivers, and the burden associated with undiagnosed diabetes.

Diabetes Care 36:1033–1046, 2013

D iabetes imposes a substantial burden on the economy of the U.S. in the form of increased medical costs and indirect costs from work-related absenteeism, reduced productivity at work and at home, reduced labor force participation from chronic disability, and premature mortality (1,2). In addition to the economic burden that has been quantified, diabetes imposes high intangible costs on society in terms of reduced quality of life and pain and suffering of people with diabetes, their families, and friends.

Improved understanding of the economic cost of diabetes and its major determinants helps to inform policymakers and to motivate decisions to reduce diabetes prevalence and burden. The previous cost of diabetes study by the American Diabetes Association (ADA) estimated that there were nearly 17.5 million people living in the U.S. with diagnosed type 1 or type 2 diabetes in 2007, at an estimated cost of $174 billion in higher medical costs and lost productivity (2).

The percentage of the population with diagnosed diabetes continues to rise, with one study projecting that as many as one in three U.S. adults could have diabetes by 2050 if current trends continue (3). In this updated cost of diabetes study, we estimate the total national economic burden of diagnosed diabetes in 2012 reflecting continued growth in prevalence of diabetes and its complications; changing health care practices, technology, and cost of treatment; and changing economic conditions.

RESEARCH DESIGN AND
METHODS—This study follows the methodology used in the 2002 and 2007 costs of diabetes studies by the ADA, with modifications to refine the analyses where appropriate (1,2). A prevalence-based approach is used to estimate the medical costs by demographic group, health service category, and medical condition. One difference from earlier studies is that for some analyses we now include race/ethnicity as a demographic dimension. We analyze the prevalence of diagnosed diabetes, utilization and costs attributable to diabetes by age-group (under 18, 18–34, 35–44, 45–54, 55–59, 60–64, 65–69, and over 70 years of age), sex, race/ethnicity (non-Hispanic white, non-Hispanic black, non-Hispanic other, and Hispanic), and insurance status (private; government including Medicare, Medicaid, Children's Health Insurance Program, and other government-sponsored coverage; and uninsured). State-specific estimates of prevalence and costs are provided in Supplementary Table 11.

• •

This report was prepared under the direction of the American Diabetes Association by Wenya Yang (The Lewin Group, Inc., Falls Church, Virginia); Timothy M. Dall (IHS Global Inc., Washington, DC); Pragna Halder (The Lewin Group, Inc.); Paul Gallo (IHS Global Inc.); Stacey L. Kowal (IHS Global Inc.); and Paul F. Hogan (The Lewin Group, Inc.).

Address correspondence to Matt Petersen, American Diabetes Association, 1701 N. Beauregard Street, Alexandria, VA 22311. E-mail: mpetersen@diabetes.org.

DOI: 10.2337/dc12-2625

This article contains Supplementary Data online at http://care.diabetesjournals.org/lookup/suppl/doi:10 .2337/dc12-2625/-/DC1.

See accompanying commentary, p. 775.

Major data sources analyzed include National Health Interview Survey (NHIS), American Community Survey (ACS), Behavioral Risk Factor Surveillance System (BRFSS), Medical Expenditure Panel Survey (MEPS), OptumInsight's de-identified Normative Health Information database (dNHI), the Medicare 5% sample Standard Analytical Files (SAFs), Nationwide Inpatient Sample (NIS), National Ambulatory Medical Care Survey (NAMCS), National Hospital Ambulatory Medical Care Survey (NHAMCS), National Nursing Home Survey (NNHS), National Home and Hospice Care Survey (NHHCS), and Current Population Survey (CPS). We use the most recent year's data available for each of these data sources, though for certain analyses we combine 3 years of data to achieve sufficient sample size. To estimate medical costs for less common health service categories such as hospital inpatient care, emergency care, home health, and podiatry, we combine 5 years of MEPS data to reduce variance in utilization and cost. The demographics of the U.S. population in 2012 with diabetes prevalence, epidemiological data, health care cost, and economic data are then combined into a Cost of Diabetes Model. Supplementary Table 1 describes how these data sources are used, along with their respective strengths and limitations, pertinent to this study. All cost and utilization estimates are extrapolated to the projected U.S. population in 2012 (4), with cost estimates calculated in 2012 dollars using the appropriate components of the medical consumer price index or total consumer price index (5).

Estimating the size of the population with diabetes

To estimate the number of people with diagnosed diabetes in 2012 we combined U.S. Census Bureau population numbers with estimated prevalence of diabetes by age-group, sex, race/ethnicity, insurance coverage, and whether residing in a nursing home.

Combining the 2009, 2010, and 2011 NHIS data produced a sample sufficient to estimate diabetes prevalence by demographic and insurance coverage ($n = 123,185$). Prevalence is based on respondents answering "yes" to the question, "Have you EVER been told by a doctor or health professional that you have diabetes or sugar diabetes?" We exclude gestational diabetes mellitus from the prevalence estimates. Previous research finds that self-report of a physician's diagnosis of diabetes is accurate in

estimating prevalence of diagnosed diabetes (6).

For the 2007 cost study, the estimated prevalence of diagnosed diabetes among the institutionalized population (24%) came from an analysis of the 2004 NNHS. There has been no update of the NNHS since 2004. Nearly one in three (32.8%) nursing home residents has diagnosed diabetes based on a nationally representative study that analyzed medical charts, minimum dataset records, and prescription claims files to identify people with diabetes (7). On the basis of this updated information on diabetes prevalence among nursing home residents, we estimate age-group–, sex-, and race/ethnicity–specific prevalence using the same distribution of the population demographic variables as shown in the 2004 NNHS survey data among the 1.6 million nursing home residents in 2012. Few data exist regarding the prevalence of diabetes among the noncivilian population or the institutionalized populations other than those in nursing homes (e.g., in prisons). We assume that the noncivilian population and the institutionalized populations other than those in nursing homes have diabetes prevalence similar to the noninstitutionalized population, controlling for demographics, based on the limited evidence available (8,9).

Combining the NHIS and NNHS data, we estimate the prevalence of diagnosed diabetes among population subgroups (by age-group, sex, race/ethnicity, and insurance coverage). Supplementary Table 3 shows that prevalence of diabetes increases with age, is somewhat higher for males than for females, and is highest among non-Hispanic blacks. Reflecting the high prevalence among the elderly population, 13.4% of the population with government-sponsored medical insurance (e.g., Medicare, Medicaid) has diagnosed diabetes as compared with 4.6% among the privately insured and 3.7% among the uninsured populations.

State-specific estimates of diabetes prevalence (Supplementary Table 11) come from combing the 2010 ACS, the 2009 and 2010 BRFSS, and the 2004 NNHS. We applied a statistical matching procedure that randomly matches each person in the 2010 ACS with a similar person either in the BRFSS (if not living in a nursing home) or in the NNHS (if living in a nursing home). Each noninstitutionalized person in the ACS is matched with a person in the BRFSS in the same state, sex, age-group (15 age-groups),

race/ethnicity, household income level (eight levels), and insured/uninsured status. Each person in the ACS in a nursing/residential facility is matched with a person in the NNHS in the same sex, age-group, and race/ethnicity. Our state prevalence estimates are slightly different from those reported by the U.S. Centers for Disease Control and Prevention (CDC) for 2010, which are based solely on the BRFSS (10).

Estimating the direct medical cost attributed to diabetes

We estimate health resource use among the population with diabetes in excess of resource use that would be expected in the absence of diabetes. Diabetes increases the risk of developing neurological, peripheral vascular, cardiovascular, renal, endocrine/metabolic, ophthalmic, and other complications (see Supplementary Table 2 for a more comprehensive list of comorbidities) (2). Diabetes also increases the cost of treating general conditions that are not directly related to diabetes (2,11–13). Therefore, a portion of health care expenditures for these medical conditions is attributed to diabetes.

As elaborated in the 2007 study, the approach used to quantify the increase in health resource use associated with diabetes was influenced by four data limitations: 1) absence of a single data source for all estimates, 2) small sample size in some data sources, 3) correlation of both diabetes and its comorbidities with other factors such as age and obesity, and 4) under-reporting of diabetes and its comorbidities in certain data sources. Because of these limitations we estimate diabetes-attributed costs using one of two approaches for each cost component.

For cost components estimated solely from the MEPS (ambulance services, home health, podiatry, diabetic supplies, and other equipment and supplies), we use a simple comparison of annual per capita health resource use for people with and without diabetes controlling for age, sex, and race/ethnicity. For nursing/residential facility use (which is not captured in the MEPS) and for cost components that rely on analysis of medical encounter data (hospital inpatient, emergency care, and ambulatory visits), we use an attributed risk methodology often used in disease-burden studies that relies on population etiological fractions (2,14). Etiological fractions estimate the excess use of health care services among the diabetic population relative to a similar population that does not have diabetes.

Both approaches are equivalent under a reasonable set of assumptions, but the first approach cannot be used with some national data sources analyzed (e.g., NIS) that are visit/hospital discharge level files, which might or might not identify the patient as having diabetes even if the patient does indeed have diabetes (2,14).

The attributable fraction approach combines etiological fractions (ε) with total projected U.S. health service use (U) in 2012 for each age-group (a), sex (s), medical condition (c), and care delivery setting (H)—hospital inpatient, emergency departments, and ambulatory visits (physician office visits combined with hospital outpatient/clinic visits):

$$\text{Attributed health resource use}_H$$
$$= \sum_{age} \sum_{sex} \sum_{\substack{medical \\ condition}} \varepsilon_{H,a,s,c} \times U_{H,a,s,c}$$

The etiological fraction is calculated using the diagnosed diabetes prevalence (P) and the relative rate ratio (R):

$$\varepsilon_{H,a,s,c} = \frac{P_{a,s} \times (R_{H,a,s,c} - 1)}{P_{a,s} \times (R_{H,a,s,c} - 1) + 1}$$

The rate ratio for hospital inpatient days, emergency visits, and ambulatory visits represents how annual per capita health service use for the population with diabetes compares to the population without diabetes:

$$R_{H,a,s,c}$$
$$= \frac{\text{annual per capita use for people with diabetes}_{a,s,c}}{\text{annual per capita use for people without diabetes}_{a,s,c}}$$

Diabetes and its comorbidities are correlated with other patient characteristics (e.g., demographics and body weight). To mitigate bias caused by correlation, we estimate age/sex/setting–specific etiological fractions for each medical condition. The primary data sources for calculating etiological fractions are OptumInsight's dNHI data (a consolidation of the Ingenix Research Data Mart and MCURE databases used in the 2007 study) and the 2010 5% sample Medicare SAFs. The dNHI data contains a complete set of medical claims for over 23 million commercially insured beneficiaries in 2011 and allows patient records to be linked during the year and across health delivery settings. This allows us to identify people with a diabetes ICD-9 diagnosis code (250.xx) in any of their medical claims during the year. The Medicare 5% sample SAFs

contain claims data filed on behalf of Medicare beneficiaries under both Part A and Part B, and like the dNHI we identify people with diabetes based on diabetes ICD-9 diagnosis codes. The large size of these two claims databases enables the generation of age/sex/setting–specific rate ratios for each medical condition, which are more stable than rates estimated using the MEPS.

Unlike the MEPS, the dNHI data and Medicare 5% claims data do not contain race/ethnicity and select patient characteristics that could affect both patients' health status and health seeking behaviors. For the 10 medical conditions—cataract, cellulitis, conduction disorders and cardiac dysrhythmias, general medical condition, heart failure, hypertension, myocardial infarction, other chronic ischemic heart disease, renal failure and its sequelae, and urinary tract infection—which are the largest contributors to the overall cost of diabetes, we estimated two multivariate Poisson regressions, using data from the MEPS, to determine the extent to which controlling only for age and sex might bias the rate ratios. First, we estimated a naïve model that produces diabetes-related rate ratios for hospital inpatient days, emergency visits, and ambulatory visits controlling for age and sex only. Then, we estimated a full model that includes diabetes status as the main explanatory variable and various known predictors of health service utilization including age, sex, education level, income, marital status, medical insurance status, and race/ethnicity as covariates. For the full model our focus is not on the relationship between health care use and the covariates (other than diabetes), but rather these covariates are included to control for patient characteristics not available in medical claims data that could be correlated with both medical conditions and health-seeking behavior. The full model omits indicators for the presence of co-existing conditions or complications of diabetes (e.g., hypertension), since including such variables could bias low the estimated relationship between diabetes and health care use for each of the 10 medical conditions. The rate ratio coefficients for the diabetes flag variable in the naïve and full models are then compared. The findings suggest statistically significant overestimates of the rate ratios for emergency visits when using the naïve model for five condition categories. For inpatient days, we found significant overestimates in the rate ratios for three

condition categories. For ambulatory visits, only hypertension was found to have a significantly higher rate ratio by comparing the MEPS-based naïve model and the full model.

To remedy the relative risk overestimation for these condition categories, we scaled the rate ratios estimated from dNHI and Medicare 5% sample using the regression results from the MEPS analysis by applying a scalar (with the scalar calculated as the full model rate ratio divided by the naïve model rate ratio) (2). For emergency department visits, claims-based rate ratios were scaled down for myocardial infarction (scale = 0.94), other chronic ischemic heart disease (0.93), hypertension (0.71), cellulitis (0.72), and renal failure (0.95). For inpatient days, claims-based rate ratios were scaled down for hypertension (0.62), cellulitis (0.93), and renal failure (0.90). Physician office visits were scaled down for hypertension (0.89). We did not find a significant overestimate of the rate ratios for general medical conditions for any of the three health service delivery settings comparing the MEPS-based naïve model and the full model. However, a comparison of the claims-based rate ratios with the rate ratios calculated from the MEPS-based naïve model found that the claims-based rate ratios for general conditions were significantly higher than the MEPS-based rate ratios for emergency department visits, hospital inpatient days, and ambulatory visits, respectively. Therefore, to be conservative in our cost estimates, we downward adjusted claims-based rate ratios for emergency department visits (0.70), hospital inpatient days (0.68), and ambulatory visits (0.66) for the general condition group by applying a scalar calculated as the MEPS-based naïve model rate ratio divided by the claims-based rate ratio.

Estimates of health resource use attributed to diabetes were combined with estimates of the average medical cost per event, in 2012 dollars, to compute total medical costs attributed to diabetes. For hospital inpatient days, office visits, emergency visits, and outpatient visits, we use average cost per visit/day specific to the medical conditions modeled. We combined the 2008–2010 MEPS files to estimate the average cost per event, except that for less common conditions or cost categories we combined the 2006–2010 MEPS files to obtain a larger sample and thereby produce more precise cost estimates. Although the MEPS contains both inpatient facility and professional expenditures and the NIS contains only facility charges (which are converted to costs using hospital-specific cost-to-charge ratios), the NIS has a much larger sample ($n = \sim 8$ million discharges in 2010) and also contains 5-digit diagnosis codes. Therefore, we use the 2010 NIS to estimate inpatient facility costs and the combined 2008–2010 MEPS to estimate the cost for professional services. The average costs per event or day by medical condition are shown in Supplementary Table 4.

Utilization of prescription medication (excluding insulin and other antidiabetic agents) for each medical condition is estimated from medications prescribed during physician's office, emergency department, and outpatient visits attributed to diabetes. The average number of medications prescribed during a visit for each age-sex-race stratum was estimated from 2008–2010 NAMCS and 2007–2009 NHAMCS data. We calculated the total number of people with diabetes that use insulin and other antidiabetic agents by combining diabetes prevalence and rate of use for these antidiabetic agents obtained from the 2009–2011 NHIS. The average cost per prescription filled, insulin, and oral and other antidiabetic agents were obtained from the combined MEPS 2008–2010. We combined the utilization of these medications with the average cost per prescription to estimate the cost by age, sex, race/ethnicity, and insurance status. The average per capita cost for diabetic supplies by age-sex-race stratum was calculated from the MEPS 2008–2010. Over-the-counter medications were not included owing to the lack of data on whether diabetes increases the use of such medications.

Consistent with the 2007 study, total nursing/residential facility days attributed to diabetes were estimated by combining the average length of stay and the nursing/residential facility population. Using 2004 NNHS, we calculated the number of residents with diabetes in each age-sex stratum, which was adjusted using the 32.8% diabetes prevalence estimate among nursing home residents, obtained from literature (7). Nursing/residential facility use attributed to diabetes was estimated using an attributable risk approach where the prevalence of diabetes among residents was compared with the prevalence of diabetes among the overall population in the same age-sex stratum. The analyses were conducted separately for short-stay, long-stay, and residential

facility residents to estimate total days of care. Similar to the 2007 study, cost per day was obtained from a geographically representative cost of care survey for 2012 (15).

Hospice days attributed to diabetes represents a combination of length of stay and diabetes prevalence among hospice residents. The 2007 NHHCS was used to calculate the number of hospice residents with diabetes and those that have a primary diagnosis of diabetes along with the average length of stay for each age-sex-race stratum. Cost per resident per day obtained from the Hospice Association of America was combined with hospice days attributed to diabetes to estimate the total cost of hospice care attributed to diabetes.

The 2006–2010 MEPS files were combined to increase the sample size to analyze the use of home health, podiatry, ambulance services, and other equipment and supplies. These cost components are estimated by comparing annual per capita cost for people with and without diabetes, controlling for age. Due to small sample size, sex and race/ethnicity were not included as a stratum when calculating costs per capita.

Estimating the indirect cost attributed to diabetes

The indirect costs associated with diabetes include workdays missed due to health conditions (absenteeism), reduced work productivity while working due to health conditions (presenteeism), reduced workforce participation due to disability, and productivity lost due to premature mortality (16–18). Productivity loss occurs among those in the labor force as well as among the nonemployed population. To estimate the value of lost productivity, we calculate the number of missed workdays resulting from absenteeism, reduced work productivity due to presenteeism, workforce participation reductions associated with chronic disability, and work years lost resulting from premature mortality associated with diabetes. This approach mirrors the one used in the 2007 study, with the exception of adding race/ethnicity as a dimension. More recent data sources were used with per capita productivity loss calculated by combining the estimates derived from the 2009–2011 NHIS and the average annual earnings from the 2011 CPS. Earnings were inflated to 2012 dollars using the overall consumer price index, and per capita estimates were applied to the number of people

with diabetes by age-group, sex, and race/ethnicity.

- **Absenteeism** is defined as the number of workdays missed due to poor health, and prior research finds that people with diabetes have higher rates of absenteeism than the population without diabetes (16–18). Estimates of excess absenteeism associated with diabetes range from 1.8 to 7% of total workdays (17,19–22). Ordinary least squares regression with the 2009–2011 NHIS shows that self-reported annual missed workdays are statistically higher for people with diabetes. Control variables include age-group, sex, race/ethnicity, diagnosed hypertension status (yes/no), and body weight status (normal, overweight, obese, unknown). Diabetes is entered as a dichotomous variable (diagnosed diabetes = 1; otherwise 0), as well as an interaction term with age-group. Controlling for hypertension and body weight produces more conservative estimates of the diabetes impact on absenteeism as comorbidities of diabetes are correlated with body weight status and a portion of hypertension is attributed to diabetes. Workers with diabetes average three more missed workdays than their peers without diabetes, with excess missed workdays varying by demographic group.

- **Presenteeism** is defined as reduced productivity while at work, and is generally measured through worker responses to surveys. These surveys rely on the self-reported inputs on the number of reduced productivity hours incurred over a given time frame. Multiple recent studies report that individuals with diabetes display higher rates of presenteeism than their peers without diabetes (19,21,22). The rate of presenteeism among the population with diabetes exceeds rates for their colleagues without diabetes—with the excess rates ranging from 1.8 to 38% of annual productivity (17,19–22). These estimates comparing presenteeism for employees with diabetes versus those without diabetes, however, fail to control for other factors that may be correlated with diabetes (e.g., age and weight status). Consequently, we model productivity loss associated with diabetes-attributed presenteeism using the estimate (6.6%) from the 2007 study that controls for the impact of factors correlated with diabetes (2).

- **Inability to work** associated with diabetes is estimated using a conservative approach that focuses on unemployment related to long-term disability. The CDC estimates that roughly 65,700 lower-limb amputations are performed each year on people with diabetes (23). These amputations and other comorbidities of diabetes can make it difficult for some people with diabetes to remain in the workforce or to find employment in their chosen profession (22,24). To quantify diabetes-related disability, we identify people in the 2009–2011 NHIS between ages 18 and 65 years who receive Supplemental Security Income (SSI) payments for disability. Using logistic regression, we estimate the relationship between diabetes and the receipt of SSI payments controlling for age-group, sex, race/ethnicity, hypertension, and weight. The results of this analysis suggest that people with diabetes have a 2.4 percentage point higher rate of being out of the workforce and receiving disability payments compared with their peers without diabetes. The diabetes effect increases with age and varies by demographic—ranging from 0.7 percentage points for non-Hispanic white males aged 65–69 years to 7.4 percentage points for non-Hispanic black females aged 55–59 years. Modeling disability-related unemployment is a conservative approach to modeling the employment effect of diabetes; regression analysis of the NHIS suggests that people with diabetes have actual labor force participation rates averaging approximately 10 percentage points lower than their peers without diabetes. The average daily earnings for those in the workforce are used as a proxy for the economic impact of reduced employment due to chronic disability. SSI payments are considered transfer payments and therefore are not included in the social cost of not working due to disability.

- **Reduced productivity for those not in the workforce** is included in our estimate of the national burden. This population includes all adults under 65 years of age who are not employed (including those voluntarily or involuntarily not in the workforce). The contribution of people not in the workforce to national productivity includes time spent providing child care, household activities, and other activities such as volunteering in the

community. Prior estimates of reduced productivity for those not in the workforce were based on estimates of "bed days" (which is defined as a day spent in bed because of poor health). The NHIS no longer collects data on bed days. Therefore, we use per capita absenteeism estimates for the working population as a proxy for reduced productivity days among the nonemployed population in a similar demographic. Whereas each workday lost due to absenteeism is based on estimated average daily earnings, there is no readily available measure of the value of a day lost for those not

in the workforce. Studies often use minimum wage as a proxy for the value of time lost, but this will underestimate the value of time. Using average earnings for their employed counterparts will overestimate the value of time. Similar to the 2007 study, we use 75% of the average earnings for people in the workforce as a productivity proxy for those under 65 years of age not in the labor force (which is close to the midpoint between minimum wage and the average hourly wage earned by a demographic similar to the unemployed under 65 years of age).

Table 1—*Health resource use in the U.S. by diabetes status and cost component, 2012 (in millions of units)*

| | Population with diabetes | | | | | |
| Health resource | Attributed to diabetes | | Incurred by people with diabetes | | Incurred by population without diabetes | U.S. total* |
	Units	% of U.S. total	Units	% of U.S. total		
Institutional care						
Hospital inpatient days	26.4	15.7%	43.1	25.7%	124.9	168.0
Nursing/residential facility days	101.3	16.4%	198.4	32.2%	418.0	616.4
Hospice days	0.2	0.3%	9.3	12.8%	63.1	—
Outpatient care						1,026.7
Physician office visits	85.7	8.3%	174.0	16.9%	852.8	128.7
Emergency department visits	7.3	5.7%	15.3	11.9%	113.5	100.7
Hospital outpatient visits	7.8	7.8%	15.0	14.9%	85.6	279.7
Home health visits	25.7	9.2%	64.9	23.2%	214.7	72.4
Medication prescriptions	361.4	11.8%	673.1	22.1%	2,377.9	3,051.1

Data sources: NIS (2010), NNHS (2004), NAMCS (2008–2010), NHAMCS (2007–2009), MEPS (2006–2010), and NHHCS (2007). *Numbers do not necessarily sum to totals because of rounding.

Table 2—*Health resource use attributed to diabetes in the U.S. by age-group and type of service, 2012 (in thousands of units)*

| | Age (years) | | | |
Health resource	<45 (n = 3.3 M)	45–64 (n = 10.2 M)	≥65 (n = 8.8 M)	Total* (N = 22.3 M)
Institutional care				
Hospital inpatient days	1,879 (<1%)	7,969 (37%)	16,535 (63%)	26,383
Nursing/residential facility days	1,456 (<1%)	18,587 (20%)	81,288 (80%)	101,331
Hospice days	0 (0%)	17 (9%)	168 (91%)	186
Outpatient care				
Physician office visits	8,077 (9%)	28,437 (33%)	49,212 (57%)	85,726
Emergency department visits	1,608 (22%)	2,589 (36%)	3,084 (42%)	7,280
Hospital outpatient visits	1,233 (16%)	3,241 (41%)	3,342 (43%)	7,817
Home health visits	3,249 (13%)	10,409 (40%)	12,076 (47%)	25,734
Medication prescriptions	27,839 (8%)	118,493 (33%)	215,105 (60%)	361,437

Data sources: NIS (2010), NNHS (2004), NAMCS (2008–2010), NHAMCS (2007–2009), MEPS (2006–2010), and NHHCS (2007). *Numbers do not necessarily sum to totals because of rounding.

- **Premature mortality** associated with diabetes reduces future productivity (and not just the current year productivity). Ideally, to model the value of lost productivity in 2012 associated with premature mortality one would calculate the number and characteristics of all people who would have been alive in 2012 but who died prior to 2012 because of diabetes. Data limitations prevent using this approach. Instead, we estimate the number of premature deaths associated with diabetes in 2012 and calculate the present value of their expected future earnings.

To estimate the total number of deaths attributable to diabetes we analyzed the CDC's 2009 Mortality Multiple Cause File to obtain mortality data by age, sex, and race/ethnicity for cardiovascular disease, cerebrovascular disease, renal failure, and diabetes. A literature review supports the 2007 ADA report estimate that ~16% of cardiovascular disease (excluding cerebrovascular disease) deaths can be attributed to diabetes (1,2,25). To estimate the fraction of cerebrovascular disease and renal failure deaths attributed to diabetes, we used etiological fractions for emergency department use as a proxy for mortality etiological fractions (2). Our estimates suggest that ~28% of deaths listing cerebrovascular disease as the primary cause and ~55% of deaths listing renal failure as the primary cause can be attributed to diabetes. The elderly represent the largest population group where deaths attributable to diabetes occur, with ~71% of deaths occurring among people aged ≥70 years and 8% of deaths occurring among people aged 65–69 years. To generate 2012 estimates, we grow the 2009 CDC mortality data using the annual diabetic population growth rate from 2009 to 2012 for each age, sex, and race/ethnicity group.

Productivity loss associated with early mortality is calculated by taking the net present value of future productivity (PVFP) for men and women by age and race/ethnicity using the same discount rate (3%), assumptions, and equation outlined in the 2007 ADA report (2). We combined the average annual earnings from the CPS, expected mortality rates from the CDC, and employment rates from the CPS by age, sex, and race/ethnicity to calculate the net present value of future earnings of a person who dies prematurely. Employment rates for 2007 (rather than

2012) are used to calculate PVFP as rates for 2007 are closer to the historical average (whereas rates for 2008–2012 are lower than average due to the recession). The results incorporate U.S. Bureau of Labor Statistics findings that many older workers are delaying retirement because of the economic downturn (with ~15% employed at age 65 years and diminishing to ~5% employed at age 70 years), with this pattern expected to exist even after the economy recovers (2).

RESULTS—In 2012, an estimated 22.3 million people in the U.S. were diagnosed with diabetes, representing about 7% of the population. This estimate is higher than but consistent with those published by the CDC for 2010 (23,26). The estimated national cost of diabetes in 2012 is $245 billion, of which $176 billion (72%) represents direct health care expenditures attributed to diabetes and $69 billion (28%) represents lost productivity from work-related absenteeism, reduced productivity at work and at home, unemployment from chronic disability, and premature mortality.

Health resource use attributed to diabetes

Table 1 shows estimates of health resource utilization attributed to diabetes and incurred by people with diabetes as a percentage of total national utilization. For example, of the projected 168 million hospital inpatient days in the U.S. in 2012, an estimated 43.1 million days (25.7%) are incurred by people with diabetes of which 26.4 million days are attributed to diabetes. About one-third of all nursing/residential facility days are incurred by people with diabetes, and over half of those are attributed to diabetes. About half of all physician office visits, emergency department visits, hospital outpatient visits, and medication prescriptions (excluding insulin and other antidiabetic agents) incurred by people with diabetes are attributed to their diabetes.

Table 2 shows that the population aged 65 years and older uses a substantially larger portion of services, especially hospital inpatient days, nursing/residential facility days, and hospice, compared with those under age 65 years. The significant increase in nursing/residential days attributed to diabetes from the 2007 study reflects both the increasing cost and the increased prevalence of diabetes

Table 3—Health resource use attributed to diabetes in the U.S. by medical condition and type of service, 2012 (in thousands of units)

Medical event	Diabetes	Neurological	Peripheral vascular	Chronic complications† Cardiovascular	Renal	Metabolic	Ophthalmic	Other‡	General medical^	Total*
Hospital inpatient days	839 (3%)	1,468 (6%)	971 (4%)	5,197 (20%)	1,701 (6%)	70 (0%)	11 (0%)	1,809 (7%)	14,318 (54%)	26,383 (100%)
Physician office visits	28,150 (33%)	2,077 (2%)	1,442 (2%)	12,823 (15%)	3,831 (4%)	1,211 (1%)	6,473 (8%)	1,511 (2%)	28,207 (33%)	85,726 (100%)
Emergency department visits	379 (5%)	209 (3%)	95 (1%)	747 (10%)	424 (6%)	46 (1%)	22 (0%)	414 (6%)	4,944 (68%)	7,280 (100%)
Hospital outpatient visits	3,038 (39%)	155 (2%)	341 (4%)	1,251 (16%)	241 (3%)	49 (1%)	283 (4%)	267 (3%)	2,192 (28%)	7,817 (100%)

Data sources: NIS (2010), NAMCS (2008–2010), NAMCS (2008–2010), and NHAMCS (2007–2009). †See Supplementary Table 2 for diagnosis codes for each category of complications. ‡Bacteremia, candidiasis of skin and nails, chronic osteomyelitis of the foot, other and unspecified noninfectious gastroenteritis and colitis, impotence of organic origin, infective otitis externa, degenerative skin disorders, candidiasis of vulva and vagina, cellulitis, diabetes with other specified manifestations, diabetes with unspecified complication, other bone involvement in disease classified elsewhere. ^Includes all other health care use that is not a known comorbidity of diabetes. *Numbers do not necessarily sum to totals because of rounding.

(32.8%) in general, and among the elderly in particular. Total utilization of prescription medications attributed to diabetes has more than doubled from the estimate in the 2007 study, reflecting a dramatic increase in the use of medications treating general conditions and diabetes comorbidities among people with diabetes. Supplementary Table 5 shows the per capita health resource use by demographic.

Analysis of health resource use attributed to diabetes by medical condition (Table 3), including diabetes, chronic complications of diabetes, and general medical conditions, shows that a large portion of health resource use attributed to diabetes—particularly hospital inpatient and emergency department visits—is for general medical conditions that are not chronic complications of diabetes. As discussed in the 2007 cost of diabetes study, diabetes contributes to longer hospital length of stay regardless of the reason for admission (and controlling for other factors that affect hospital length of stay) (2). In addition to general medical conditions, a substantial amount of attributed health resource use is for chronic complications of diabetes, particularly cardiovascular diseases and renal complications. Finally, more than one-third of physician office visits and nearly 40% of hospital outpatient visits have diabetes listed as the primary reason for the visit. Supplementary Table 8 shows the proportion of total health resource use attributed to diabetes for each medical condition.

Health care expenditures attributed to diabetes

Health care expenditures attributed to diabetes reflect the additional expenditures the nation incurs because of diabetes. This equates to the total health care expenditures for people with diabetes minus the projected level of expenditures that would have occurred for those people in the absence of diabetes. Table 4 summarizes the national expenditure for the cost components analyzed, accounting for over $1.3 trillion in projected expenditure for 2012. Approximately $306 billion of the total is incurred by people with diabetes, reflecting 23% of the total health care dollars. Costs attributed to diabetes total $176 billion, or 57% of the total medical costs incurred by people with diabetes. For the cost components analyzed, more than 1 in every 10 health care dollars is attributed to diabetes.

National health-related expenditures are projected to exceed $2.8 trillion in 2012, but slightly less than half of these expenditures are included in our analysis (27,28). These cost estimates omit national expenditures (and any portion of such expenditures that might be attributable to diabetes) for administering government health and private insurance programs, investment in research and infrastructure, over-the-counter medications, disease management and wellness programs, and office visits to nonphysician providers other than podiatrists (e.g., dentists and optometrists). Expenditures for health resources such as care in residential mental retardation facilities are likewise excluded from the analysis.

More than 40% of all health care expenditures attributed to diabetes come from higher rates of hospital admission and longer average lengths of stay per admission, constituting the single largest contributor to the attributed medical cost of diabetes. Of the projected $475 billion in national expenditures for hospital inpatient care (including both facility and professional services costs), approximately $124 billion (or 26%) is incurred by people who have diabetes, of which $76 billion is directly attributed to their diabetes. Medications as a whole (prescription medications, insulin, and other antidiabetic agents) represent over one-quarter (28%) of all health expenditures attributed to diabetes. Of the projected $286 billion in national cost for medications, $77 billion (27%) is incurred by people with diabetes, of which $50 billion is attributed to their diabetes.

Approximately 59% of all health care expenditures attributed to diabetes are for health resources used by the population aged 65 years and older, much of which is borne by the Medicare program (Table 5). The population 45–64 years of age incurs 33% of diabetes-attributed costs, with the remaining 8% incurred by the population under 45 years of age. The annual attributed health care cost per person with diabetes (Table 6) increases with age, primarily as a result of increased use of

Table 4—Health care expenditures in the U.S. by diabetes status and type of service, 2012 (in millions of dollars)

| Cost component | Population with diabetes | | | | Population without diabetes | Total* |
| | Attributed to diabetes | | Total incurred by people with diabetes | | | |
	Dollars	% of U.S. total	Dollars	% of U.S. total		
Institutional care						
Hospital inpatient	75,872	16%	123,726	26%	351,618	475,344
Nursing/residential facility	14,748	17%	28,622	32%	59,744	88,366
Hospice	32	0.3%	1,600	13%	10,889	12,489
Outpatient care						
Physician office	15,221	8%	31,443	17%	155,226	186,669
Emergency department	6,654	6%	14,119	12%	105,111	119,230
Ambulance services	218	11%	453	23%	1,534	1,987
Hospital outpatient	5,027	6%	11,354	13%	76,144	87,497
Home health	4,466	9%	11,269	23%	37,264	48,533
Podiatry	212	12%	458	25%	1,349	1,807
Outpatient medications and supplies						
Insulin	6,157	100%	6,157	100%	0	6,157
Diabetic supplies	2,296	100%	2,296	100%	0	2,296
Other antidiabetic agents†	12,137	100%	12,137	100%	0	12,137
Prescription medications	31,716	12%	59,067	22%	208,662	267,729
Other equipment and supplies‡	1,063	4%	3,593	15%	20,076	23,669
Total	175,819	13%	306,293	23%	1,027,617	1,333,910

Data sources: NIS (2010), NNHS (2004), NAMCS (2008–2010), NHAMCS (2007–2009), MEPS (2006–2010), NHHCS (2007), and NHIS (2009–2011). †Includes oral medications and noninsulin injectable antidiabetic agents such as exenatide and pramlintide. ‡Includes, but not limited to eyewear, orthopedic items, hearing devices, prosthesis, bathroom aids, medical equipment, and disposable supplies. *Numbers do not necessarily sum to totals because of rounding.

Table 5—Health care expenditures attributed to diabetes in the U.S. by age-group and type of service, 2012 (in millions of dollars)

Cost component	Age (years)			
	<45 (n = 3.3 M)	45–64 (n = 10.2 M)	≥65 (n = 8.8 M)	Total* (N = 22.3 M)
Institutional care				
Hospital inpatient	4,924 (6%)	22,934 (30%)	48,015 (63%)	75,872
Nursing/residential facility	211 (1%)	2,781 (19%)	11,757 (80%)	14,748
Hospice	0 (0%)	3 (9%)	29 (91%)	32
Outpatient care				
Physician office	1,334 (9%)	4,882 (32%)	9,005 (59%)	15,221
Emergency department	1,435 (22%)	2,363 (36%)	2,856 (43%)	6,654
Ambulance services	20 (9%)	169 (77%)	29 (13%)	218
Hospital outpatient	679 (13%)	1,943 (39%)	2,405 (48%)	5,027
Home health	564 (13%)	1,806 (40%)	2,096 (47%)	4,466
Podiatry	43 (20%)	61 (29%)	108 (51%)	212
Outpatient medications and supplies				
Insulin	1,102 (18%)	2,817 (46%)	2,239 (36%)	6,157
Diabetic supplies	238 (10%)	1,003 (44%)	1,056 (46%)	2,296
Other antidiabetic agents†	1,297 (11%)	5,767 (48%)	5,073 (42%)	12,137
Prescription medications	2,443 (8%)	10,398 (33%)	18,875 (60%)	31,716
Other equipment and supplies‡	117 (11%)	309 (29%)	637 (60%)	1,063
Total	14,406 (8%)	57,235 (33%)	104,178 (59%)	175,819

Data sources: NIS (2010), NNHS (2004), NAMCS (2008–2010), NHAMCS (2007–2009), MEPS (2006–2010), NHHCS (2007), and NHIS (2009–2011). †Includes oral medications and noninsulin injectable antidiabetic agents. ‡Includes but not limited to eyewear, orthopedic items, hearing devices, prosthesis, bathroom aids, medical equipment, and disposable supplies. *Numbers do not necessarily sum to totals because of rounding.

hospital inpatient and nursing facility resources, physician office visits, and prescription medications. Dividing the total attributed health care expenditures by the number of people with diabetes, we estimate the average annual excess expenditures for the population aged under 45 years, 45–64 years, and 65 years and above, respectively, at $4,394, $5,611, and $11,825. Total health care expenditures are attributed to diabetes by sex and race/ethnicity (Supplementary Table 6), insurance status (Supplementary Table 9 and 10), and state (Supplementary Table 11).

Table 7 summarizes diabetes-attributed health care expenditures for those cost components modeled by medical condition. Hospital inpatient is the largest component of attributed costs followed by physician office visit. Across different health care delivery settings, general medical conditions and cardiovascular disease categories are the two largest contributors of total health care expenditures attributed to diabetes in addition to diabetes itself. Together, the general medical conditions and cardiovascular disease categories are responsible for 78% of hospital inpatient costs attributed to diabetes,

47% of the cost for physician office visits, 82% of the cost for emergency department visits, and 52% of the cost for hospital outpatient.

Figure 1 summarizes the proportion of medical expenditures attributed to diabetes for each chronic complication over the total U.S. health care expenditure combining expenditures for hospital inpatient, hospital outpatient, emergency department visits, physician office visits, and prescription medications. Over a quarter of expenditures, in five out of the eight conditions shown in the chart, are attributed to diabetes. In addition, 7, 11, and 21% of national medical expenditures treating general conditions, endocrine/metabolic complications, and ophthalmic complications are attributable to diabetes.

The population with diabetes is older and sicker than the population without diabetes, and consequently annual medical expenditures are much higher (on average) than for people without diabetes (Table 8). After adjusting for age-sex differences in these two populations, people with diabetes have health care expenditures that are 2.3 times higher ($13,741 vs. $5,853) than expenditures would be

expected for this same population in the absence of diabetes. This suggests that diabetes is responsible for $7,888 in excess expenditures per year per person with diabetes. This 2.3 multiple is unchanged from the 2007 study.

Indirect costs attributed to diabetes

The total indirect cost of diabetes is estimated at $68.6 billion (Table 9). The majority of this burden comes from unemployment due to permanent disability ($21.6 billion), presenteeism ($20.8 billion), and premature mortality ($18.5 billion). Workdays absent ($5.0 billion) and reduced productivity for those not in the workforce ($2.7 billion) represent a relatively small portion of the total burden.

Our logistic regression analysis with NHIS data suggests that diabetes is associated with a 2.4 percentage point increase in the likelihood of leaving the workforce for disability. This equates to approximately 541,000 working-age adults leaving the workforce prematurely and 130 million lost workdays in 2012. For the population that leaves the workforce early because of diabetes-associated disability, we estimate that their average daily earnings would have been $166 per person (with the amount varying by demographic).

Presenteeism accounted for 30% of the indirect cost of diabetes. The estimate of a 6.6% annual decline in productivity attributed to diabetes (in excess of the estimated decline in the absence of diabetes) equates to 113 million lost workdays per year. The average daily earnings are $185 for the employed population with diabetes, which equates to $20.8 billion in annual cost attributed to diabetes (after factoring out absenteeism to prevent double counting).

The estimated number of deaths in 2012 attributable to diabetes is 246,000 (Table 10). For 73,000 deaths (30%), diabetes is listed as the primary cause. Of the 687,000 deaths where cardiovascular disease is listed as the primary cause, approximately 110,000 (16%) are attributable to diabetes. Approximately 38,000 cases where cerebrovascular disease is listed as the primary cause of death are attributable to diabetes, and 25,000 cases where renal disease is listed as the primary cause of death are attributable to diabetes. The average cost per premature death declines with age (reflecting fewer remaining expected working years), and across all premature deaths averaged approximately $75,100 per case.

Table 6—*Annual per capita health care expenditures attributed to diabetes in the U.S. by age-group and type of service, 2012 (in actual dollars)*

Cost component	Age (years)			
	<45 (n = 3.3 M)	45–64 (n = 10.2 M)	≥65 (n = 8.8 M)	All ages (N = 22.3 M)
Institutional care				
Hospital inpatient	1,502	2,248	5,450	3,404
Nursing/residential facility	64	273	1,334	662
Hospice	0.01	0.29	3	1
Outpatient care				
Physician office	407	479	1,022	683
Emergency department	438	232	324	299
Ambulance services	6	17	3	10
Hospital outpatient	207	191	273	226
Home health	172	177	238	200
Podiatry	13	6	12	10
Outpatient medications and supplies				
Insulin	336	276	254	276
Diabetic supplies	73	98	120	103
Other antidiabetic agents†	396	565	576	544
Prescription medications	745	1,019	2,142	1,423
Other equipment and supplies‡	36	30	72	48
Total*	4,394	5,611	11,825	7,888

Data sources: NIS (2010), NNHS (2004), NAMCS (2008–2010), NHAMCS (2007–2009), MEPS (2006–2010), NHHCS (2007), NHIS (2009–2011), and the U.S. Census Bureau (2012). †Includes oral medications and noninsulin injectable antidiabetic agents. ‡Includes but not limited to eyewear, orthopedic items, hearing devices, prosthesis, bathroom aids, medical equipment, and disposable supplies. *Numbers do not necessarily sum to totals because of rounding.

Figure 2 summarizes estimates of PVFP if a person dies at that age. PVFP is the value in 2012 of expected future lifetime earnings if the person had lived to the average age as the cohort born in the same year. The differences in PVFP by demographic reflect the differences in average earnings, the propensity to be in the workforce, and the number of years expected to remain in the workforce.

The cost of missed workdays due to absenteeism is estimated at $5.0 billion, representing 25 million days. If people not in the workforce have similar rates of days where they are unable to work due to poor health as their employed peers, this would equate to 20 million excess sick days with the estimated productivity loss valued at $2.7 billion. We do not count productivity loss for the population under age 18 years. While children constitute a small proportion of the population with diabetes, omitting productivity loss associated with diabetes among children will tend to bias low the cost estimates. For example, the economic cost associated with parents who take time off from work to take their children to the doctor for diabetes-related visits is omitted from these cost estimates.

The average annual productivity loss per person aged 18 years or older with diabetes is $3,100. Table 11 shows that per capita estimates range from a high of $6,844 for men aged 45–54 years to a low of $647 for women aged 70 years and older—reflecting differences by demographic in propensity to be in the workforce, average earnings, and mortality risk. Supplementary Table 7 shows the annual productivity loss per person with diabetes by cause and race/ethnicity.

CONCLUSIONS—This study found that there were more than 22.3 million people (about 7% of the U.S. population) with diagnosed diabetes in the U.S. in 2012. This is substantially higher than the 2007 estimate of 17.5 million people, reflecting changing demographics, increase in the prevalence of risk factors including obesity, decreasing mortality, and improvements in the detection of diabetes (29–32). Diabetes costs the nation a total of $245 billion, which includes $176 billion in direct medical cost and $69 billion in lost productivity. While the majority (59%) of direct medical cost is for the population aged 65 years and over, about 88% of indirect

cost is borne by the population under 65 years of age. We also found that after adjusting for age and sex, annual per capita health care expenditure is 2.3 times higher for people with diabetes than for those without diabetes. Diabetes is especially costly when it is associated with complications. While we were unable to calculate diabetes-attributed cost by complication groups for every cost component across the major health care delivery settings (hospital inpatient and outpatient, physician office, and emergency department), from 25% (emergency department) to 45% (hospital inpatient) of the diabetes-attributed medical expenditures were spent treating complications of diabetes. Other studies found that people with uncontrolled diabetes or with diabetes complications incur diabetes costs two to eight times more than people with controlled or nonadvanced diabetes (33,34).

For comparison, the $174 billion estimate of the total burden for 2007 published previously is equivalent to $202 billion when inflated to 2012 dollars using the average general inflation rate of 3%. The increase of $43 billion from the 2007 estimate in 2012 dollars to the new estimate of $245 billion reflects *1*) a 27% growth in diabetes prevalence, *2*) changing demographics of people with diabetes, *3*) growth in the utilization of certain types of health care services for treating diabetes and its comorbidities such as increased use of prescription medications and advanced treatment for cardiovascular disease, *4*) rising prices for medical goods and services above the general rate of inflation, and *5*) refinements to the data and methods used to calculate the cost of diabetes.

We found that the proportions of total national health services use attributed to diabetes and incurred by people with diabetes both increased from the estimates in the 2007 study, including utilization of nursing/residential facility days, physician office visits, emergency department visits, hospital outpatient visits, and prescription medications. The number of hospital inpatient days incurred by people with diabetes and those that are attributable to their diabetes have both increased from the 2007 level by about 6 and 9%, respectively, although the national utilization of hospital inpatient care has decreased by about 10% from 186 million days in 2007 to 168 million days in 2012 based on the analysis of NIS data.

Table 7—Health care expenditures attributed to diabetes in the U.S. by medical condition and type of service, 2012 (in millions of dollars)

Type of service	Diabetes	Chronic complications†							General medical^	Total*
		Neurological	Peripheral vascular	Cardiovascular	Renal	Metabolic	Ophthalmic	Other‡		
Hospital inpatient	1,979 (3%)	4,229 (6%)	2,813 (4%)	19,441 (26%)	3,807 (5%)	175 (0%)	28 (<1%)	4,002 (5%)	39,399 (52%)	75,872
Physician office	4,136 (27%)	413 (3%)	449 (3%)	2,196 (14%)	1,007 (7%)	176 (1%)	1,483 (10%)	295 (2%)	5,065 (33%)	15,221
Emergency department	301 (5%)	161 (2%)	86 (1%)	805 (5%)	324 (5%)	64 (1%)	16 (<1%)	262 (4%)	4,635 (70%)	6,654
Hospital outpatient	1,100 (22%)	115 (2%)	555 (11%)	635 (13%)	147 (3%)	18 (<1%)	314 (6%)	173 (3%)	1,971 (39%)	5,027

Data sources: NIS (2010), NAMCS (2008–2010), NHAMCS (2007–2009), and MEPS (2006–2010). †See Supplementary Table 2 for diagnosis codes for each category of complications. ‡Bacteremia, candidiasis of skin and nails, chronic osteomyelitis of the foot, other and unspecified noninfectious gastroenteritis and colitis, impotence of organic origin, infective otitis externa, degenerative skin disorders, candidiasis of vulva and vagina, cellulitis, diabetes with other specified manifestations, diabetes with unspecified complication, other bone involvement in disease classified elsewhere. ^Includes all other health care use that is not a known comorbidity of diabetes. *Numbers do not necessarily sum to totals because of rounding.

Additionally, even when using MEPS data that have been shown to underestimate costs when compared with claims data, especially for the privately insured (35), we found that the price of medical services per event (visit or day) has increased by 5–17% over the rate of general inflation from the 2007 level for hospital inpatient, hospital outpatient, emergency department, insulin, and other prescription medications. Due to the increase in diabetes prevalence, health resource utilization, and average per event cost of services, the $176 billion direct medical cost attributed to diabetes in 2012 is 30% higher than the general inflation-adjusted 2007 direct medical cost of $135 billion.

The indirect cost estimate of $69 billion for 2012 includes increased absenteeism ($5 billion) and reduced productivity while at work ($20.8 billion) for the employed population, reduced productivity for those not in the labor force ($2.7 billion), unemployment as a result of disease-related disability ($21.6 billion), and lost productive capacity due to early mortality ($18.5 billion). The $69 billion is only 3% higher than the inflation-adjusted 2007 estimate of $67 billion, despite the 27% growth in diabetes prevalence. Factors depressing the 2012 estimate include the decline in the number of people participating in the workforce in 2012 and the lower diabetes-attributed mortality estimates for 2012. Including race/ethnicity as a study

dimension also depressed the national indirect burden estimate relative to 2007, as Hispanics and non-Hispanic blacks have higher diabetes prevalence rates but lower labor force participation rates and lower average earnings. Since the 2007 study, the economic downturn has decreased overall rates of employment across all demographic groups regardless of diabetes status. A declining proportion of the adult population in the workforce depresses the estimates of absenteeism and presenteeism, while increasing the estimates of diabetes-related productivity losses for the population not in the workforce.

Our estimate of $245 billion only represents the economic cost of diagnosed diabetes. An earlier study found that 6.3 million U.S. adults have undiagnosed diabetes with an associated cost of $18 billion in 2007 (36). Furthermore, nearly 57 million adults in that study were estimated to have prediabetes, a precursor to diabetes, costing an additional $25 billion in higher medical spending (37,38). On the surface it appears that the financial burden of diabetes falls primarily on insurers who pay a substantial portion of medical costs, employers who experience productivity loss, and the people with diabetes and their families who incur higher out-of-pocket medical costs and reduced earnings potential or employment opportunities. Ultimately, though, the burden is passed along to all of society in the form of higher insurance premiums and taxes,

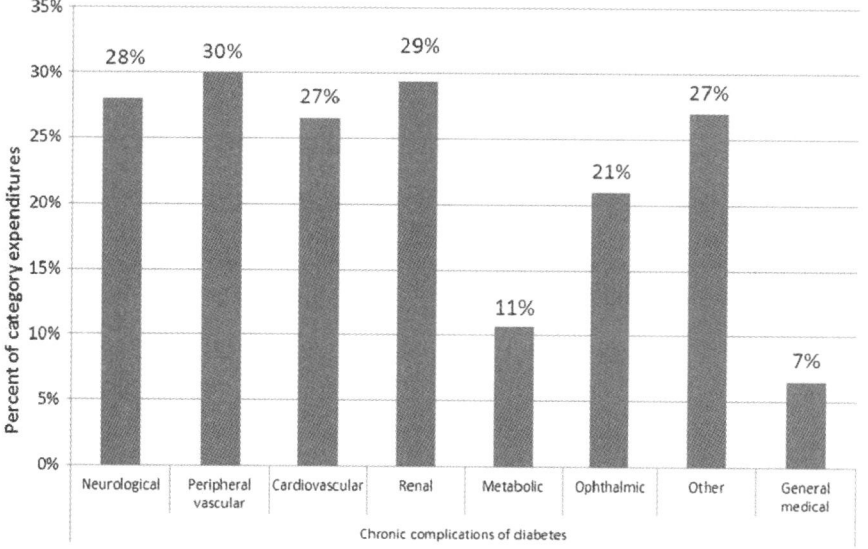

Figure 1—Percent of medical condition–specific expenditures associated with diabetes. Data sources: NIS (2010), NAMCS (2008–2010), NHAMCS (2007–2009), and MEPS (2006–2010 or 2008–2010). Note: See Supplementary Table 2 for diagnosis codes for each category of medical condition.

Table 8—*Annual per capita health care expenditures in the U.S. by diabetes status, 2012 (in actual dollars)*

		Unadjusted		Adjusted for age and sex		
Cost component	With diabetes ($)	Without diabetes ($)	Ratio with to without diabetes	Without diabetes ($)	Ratio with to without diabetes	Attributed to diabetes ($)
Institutional care						
Hospital inpatient	5,551	1,196	4.6	2,147	2.6	3,404
Nursing/residential facility	1,284	203	6.3	622	2.1	662
Hospice	N/A	N/A	N/A	N/A	N/A	N/A
Outpatient care						
Physician office	1,411	528	2.7	728	1.9	683
Emergency	633	357	1.8	335	1.9	299
Ambulance services	20	5	3.9	11	1.9	10
Hospital outpatient and freestanding ambulatory surgical center	509	259	2.0	284	1.8	226
Home health	506	127	4.0	305	1.7	200
Podiatry	21	5	4.5	11	1.9	10
Outpatient medications and supplies						
Insulin	276	NA	NA	NA	NA	276
Diabetic supplies	103	NA	NA	NA	NA	103
Other antidiabetic agents†	544	NA	NA	NA	NA	544
Prescription medications	2,650	710	3.7	1,227	2.2	1,423
Other equipment and supplies‡	161	68	2.4	113	1.4	48
Total	13,741	3,495	3.9	5,853	2.3	7,888

Data sources: NIS (2010), NNHS (2004), NAMCS (2008–2010), NHAMCS (2007–2009), MEPS (2006–2010), NHHCS (2007), NHIS (2009–2011), and the U.S. Census Bureau (2012). N/A, not available; NA, not applicable. †Includes antidiabetic agents such as exenatide and pramlintide. ‡Includes but not limited to eyewear, orthopedic items, hearing devices, prosthesis, bathroom aids, medical equipment, and disposable supplies.

reduced earnings, and reduced standard of living.

The cost estimates presented might be conservative for several reasons:

• Due to data limitations, we omitted from this analysis the potential increase in the use of over-the-counter medications and optometry and dental services. Diabetes increases the risk of periodontal disease, so one would expect dental costs to be higher for people with diabetes. We explored the MEPS data for the feasibility of capturing optometry and dental costs, but the small sample sizes prevented meaningful analyses. Also omitted from the cost estimates are expenditures for the prevention programs targeted to people with diabetes (e.g., disease management programs), research activities (e.g., to develop new drugs), and administration costs (e.g., to administer the Medicare and Medicaid programs, to process insurance claims). Administration costs for government health programs and private insurers are ~ $150 billion per year. Public and private expenditures for medical research and health infrastructure total over $130 billion per year (39). If a portion of these costs were attributed to diabetes,

the national cost of diabetes would be billions of dollars higher than our estimate suggests.

• Also omitted from the cost estimates are the intangible costs of diabetes such as pain, suffering, and reduced quality of life, as well as some of the nonmedical costs attributed to diabetes. Specifically, diabetic patients with advanced diabetic retinopathy, late-stage

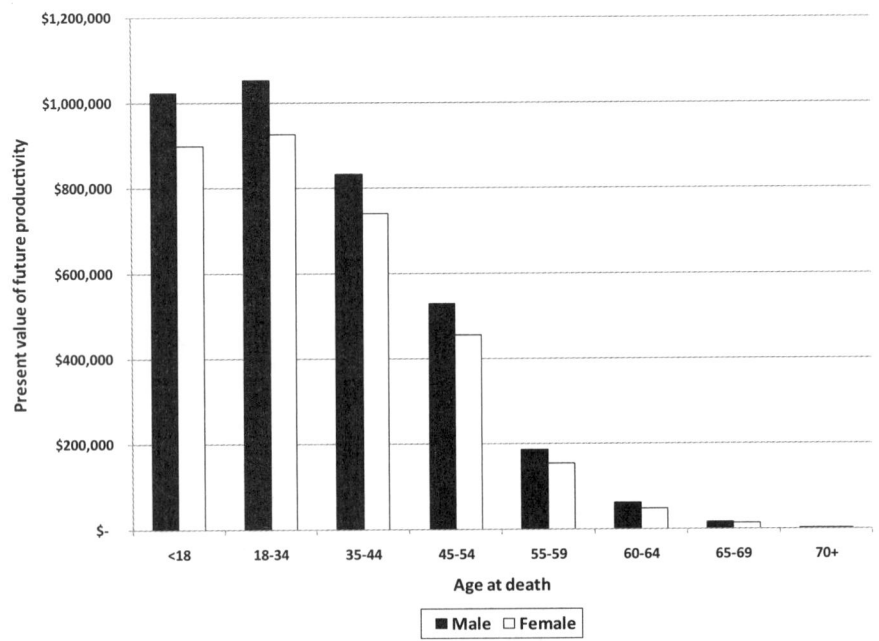

Figure 2—*Net present value of future lost earnings from premature death. Data sources: analysis of the NHIS (2009–2011), CPS (2011), and CDC mortality data.*

Table 9—Indirect burden of diabetes in the U.S., 2012 (in billions of dollars)

Cost component	Productivity loss	Total cost attributable to diabetes ($)	Proportion of indirect costs*
Workdays absent	25 million days	5.0	7%
Reduced performance at work	113 million days	20.8	30%
Reduced productivity days for those not in labor force	20 million days	2.7	4%
Reduced labor force participation due to disability	130 million days	21.6	31%
Mortality	246,000 deaths	18.5	27%
Total		68.6	100%

Data sources: analysis of the NHIS (2009–2011), CPS (2011), CDC mortality data, and the U.S. Census Bureau population estimates for 2010 and 2012. *Numbers do not necessarily sum to totals because of rounding.

renal complications, or lower-extremity amputations often require their homes and/or motor vehicles to be modified to accommodate their daily activity needs. Diabetes is the leading cause of new cases of blindness among adults aged 20–74 years (23), and the CDC estimates that roughly 65,700 lower-limb amputations are performed each year on people with diabetes (23). The nonmedical cost associated with these disabilities could further increase the total burden of diabetes.

- The lost productivity estimates are for those individuals with diagnosed diabetes and exclude lost productivity associated with the care for family members with diabetes. For example, the productivity loss associated with adults who take time off from work to care for a child or an elderly parent with diabetes is not included in the cost estimates. The value of informal caregiving is excluded from our cost estimate. Time and costs associated with traveling to doctor visits and other medical emergencies are omitted (except to the extent that such costs are partially

captured under ambulance costs and the absenteeism estimate for those in the workforce).

- Our estimate of lost productivity attributed to chronic disability from diabetes is also likely to be conservative due to three factors: 1) using SSI payments to identify cases of disability likely underestimates disability cases because the criteria for SSI eligibility include requirements for documentation of disability from a health professional and apply income limits; 2) these estimates omit the value of productivity loss that results in reduced earnings potential but does not prevent working; and 3) productivity loss associated with early retirement is not included, and a longitudinal study using the Health and Retirement Survey found that people with diabetes tend to retire ~1.2 years earlier than their peers without diabetes (40).

One challenge for this study was to control for the correlation between diabetes and the use of health resources for

reasons not directly attributed to diabetes. Health behavior that affects both the presence of diabetes and the presence of other comorbidities, unless controlled for, could result in an overestimation of the link between diabetes and the use of health resources. Controlling for age, sex, and race/ethnicity helps to control for this correlation. In addition, for the top 10 cost drivers, we conducted additional analysis controlling for other important explanatory variables using the MEPS data. Based on the results, we reduced the etiological fractions for several diabetes complications and for the general medical conditions group depending on the setting of care. This potential limitation also applies to the estimates of indirect costs attributed to diabetes, especially the estimated productivity loss due to presenteeism.

Other study limitations discussed previously include small sample size for some data sources used, the use of a data source (dNHI) that overrepresents the commercially insured population for the population younger than age 65 years, and the need to use different approaches to model different cost components because of data limitations. Another limitation common to claims-based analysis is the possibility of inaccurate diagnosis codes. Claims data tend to be less accurate than medical records in identifying patients with specific conditions due to reasons such as rule-out diagnosis, coding error, etc. The direction of such bias on our risk ratio calculations is unknown, although it is anticipated to be small as there is no reason to believe that the coding of comorbidities would be significantly different for people with and without diabetes.

Using a methodology that is largely consistent with our previous cost of diabetes study in 2007 with updated national survey and claims data from previous data sources, we estimated the total burden of diabetes in 2012. The estimates presented here show that diabetes places an enormous burden on society—both in the economic terms presented here and in reduced quality of life. The overall cost of diabetes estimates are consistent with earlier estimates after adjusting for the increasing prevalence of diabetes and price increases (though estimates for some cost components and medical conditions differ from the earlier study).

A recent study estimates that prevalence of diagnosed diabetes is likely to at least double between 2010 and 2050, and

Table 10—Mortality costs attributed to diabetes, 2012

		Deaths attributed to diabetes		
Primary cause of death	Total U.S. deaths (thousands)*	Deaths (thousands)	% of U.S. deaths in category	Value of lost productivity (millions of dollars)
Diabetes	73	73	100.0%	7,147
Renal disease	46	25	55.0%	2,004
Cerebrovascular disease	136	38	28.0%	1,484
Cardiovascular disease	687	110	16.0%	7,827
Total	N/A	246	N/A	18,462

*Data source: CDC National Vital Statistics Reports for total deaths in 2009 by primary cause of death, scaled to 2012 using the annual diabetic population growth rate from 2009 to 2012 for each age, sex, and race/ethnicity group (42).

Table 11—*Annual productivity loss per person with diabetes in the U.S. by age, sex, and cause, 2012 (in actual dollars)*

Sex	Age	Absenteeism	Presenteeism	Reduced productivity for those not in labor force	Unemployment from disability	Premature mortality	Total annual burden
Male	18–34	170	1,147	61	769	2,408	4,556
	35–44	403	2,187	117	1,341	2,442	6,490
	45–54	811	1,691	336	1,416	2,591	6,844
	55–59	419	1,816	221	1,577	1,116	5,149
	60–64	211	1,530	188	1,413	463	3,805
	65–69	89	878	—	417	209	1,593
	70+	—	305	—	503	68	876
Total		298	1,246	135	1,034	1,100	3,813
Female	18–34	114	769	66	798	1,100	2,847
	35–44	241	1,310	113	1,228	1,409	4,301
	45–54	436	908	297	1,241	1,340	4,222
	55–59	224	970	196	1,453	559	3,401
	60–64	93	679	142	1,224	256	2,394
	65–69	36	354	—	343	116	849
	70+	—	132	—	469	46	647
Total		149	614	111	901	548	2,322

Data sources: analysis of the NHIS (2009–2011), CPS (2011), and CDC mortality data. Note: Age <18 years is not included as no indirect costs are calculated for persons under the age of 18. For the age 70 years and older population, the rate of labor force participation is low so indirect costs are relatively low for this population despite high prevalence of diabetes. The NHIS sample size of employed people over age 70 years is small, and regression analysis with the NHIS found that diabetes is not associated with increased workdays absent for illness among the employed population aged 70 years and older. We conservatively assume that for the population aged 65 years and older and not in the workforce there is no loss in societal productivity (e.g., from volunteer work) associated with diabetes.

the prevalence of total diabetes (diagnosed and undiagnosed) may increase from the 2010 level of about one in nine adults to between one in five and one in three adults in 2050 (3,41).

This study highlights the large economic burden of diabetes and its complications on the individual and the health care system. Cost estimates from 2002, 2007, and now 2012 show that the burden is increasing—even after controlling for population growth and inflation. Cost comparisons by age-group show that the burden of diabetes increases with age. These trends underscore the importance of prevention and the efforts to mitigate the complications of diabetes.

Acknowledgments—No potential conflicts of interest relevant to this article were reported.

References

1. American Diabetes Association. Economic costs of diabetes in the U.S. in 2002. Diabetes Care 2003;26:917–932
2. American Diabetes Association. Economic costs of diabetes in the U.S. in 2007. Diabetes Care 2008;31:596–615
3. Boyle JP, Thompson TJ, Gregg EW, Barker LE, Williamson DF. Projection of the year 2050 burden of diabetes in the US adult population: dynamic modeling of incidence, mortality, and prediabetes prevalence. Popul Health Metr 2010;8:29
4. U.S. Census Bureau. Population Projections: 2008 National Population Projections [Internet], 2008. Available from http://www.census.gov/population/projections/data/national/2008.html. Accessed 16 January 2013
5. U.S. Bureau of Labor Statistics. Consumer Price Index: CPI Databases [Internet]. Available from http://www.bls.gov/cpi/data.htm. Accessed 16 January 2013
6. Okura Y, Urban LH, Mahoney DW, Jacobsen SJ, Rodeheffer RJ. Agreement between self-report questionnaires and medical record data was substantial for diabetes, hypertension, myocardial infarction and stroke but not for heart failure. J Clin Epidemiol 2004;57:1096–1103
7. Dybicz SB, Thompson S, Molotsky S, Stuart B. Prevalence of diabetes and the burden of comorbid conditions among elderly nursing home residents. Am J Geriatr Pharmacother 2011;9:212–223
8. American Diabetes Association. Diabetes management in correctional institutions (Position Statement). Diabetes Care 2011;34(Suppl. 1):S75–S81
9. Paris RM, Bedno SA, Krauss MR, Keep LW, Rubertone MV. Weighing in on type 2 diabetes in the military: characteristics of U.S. military personnel at entry who develop type 2 diabetes. Diabetes Care 2001;24:1894–1898
10. U.S. Centers for Disease Control and Prevention. CDC's State Surveillance Data. Available from http://www.cdc.gov/nceh/lead/data/state.htm. Accessed 16 January 2013
11. Osborn DP, Holt, R. Diabetes and mental health. In *Diabetes: Chronic Complications*. 3rd ed. Shaw KM, Cummings MH, Eds. Hoboken, NJ, John Wiley &Sons, Inc., 2012, p. 214–239
12. Vigneri P, Frasca F, Sciacca L, Pandini G, Vigneri R. Diabetes and cancer. Endocr Relat Cancer 2009;16:1103–1123
13. Egede LE, Zheng D, Simpson K. Comorbid depression is associated with increased health care use and expenditures in individuals with diabetes. Diabetes Care 2002;25:464–470
14. Benichou J. A review of adjusted estimators of attributable risk. Stat Methods Med Res 2001;10:195–216
15. Genworth Financial. Genworth 2012 Cost of Care Survey [Internet], 2012. Genworth Financial, Inc., Richmond, VA. Available from www1.genworth.com/content/etc/medialib/genworth_v2/pdf/ltc_cost_of_care.Par.40001.File.dat/2012%20Cost%20of%20Care%20Survey%20Full%20Report.pdf. Accessed 16 January 16 2013
16. Cawley J, Rizzo JA, Haas K. The association of diabetes with job absenteeism costs among obese and morbidly obese workers. J Occup Environ Med 2008;50:527–534
17. Fu AZ, Qiu Y, Radican L, Wells BJ. Health care and productivity costs associated with diabetic patients with macrovascular comorbid conditions. Diabetes Care 2009;32:2187–2192
18. Lee LJ, Yu AP, Cahill KE, et al. Direct and indirect costs among employees with diabetic retinopathy in the United States. Curr Med Res Opin 2008;24:1549–1559

19. DiBonaventura M, Link C, Pollack MF, Wagner J-S, Williams SA. The relationship between patient-reported tolerability issues with oral antidiabetic agents and work productivity among patients having type 2 diabetes. J Occup Environ Med 2011;53:204–210

20. Lamb CE, Ratner PH, Johnson CE, et al. Economic impact of workplace productivity losses due to allergic rhinitis compared with select medical conditions in the United States from an employer perspective. Curr Med Res Opin 2006;22:1203–1210

21. Loeppke R, Taitel M, Haufle V, Parry T, Kessler RC, Jinnett K. Health and productivity as a business strategy: a multiemployer study. J Occup Environ Med 2009;51:411–428

22. Rodbard HW, Fox KM, Grandy S; Shield Study Group. Impact of obesity on work productivity and role disability in individuals with and at risk for diabetes mellitus. Am J Health Promot 2009;23:353–360

23. U.S. Centers for Disease Control and Prevention. Diabetes Public Health Resource: 2011 National Diabetes Fact Sheet [Internet], 2011. Available from http://www.cdc.gov/diabetes/pubs/estimates11.htm. Accessed 16 January 2013

24. Wolf AM, Siadaty MS, Crowther JQ, et al. Impact of lifestyle intervention on lost productivity and disability: improving control with activity and nutrition. J Occup Environ Med 2009;51:139–145

25. Carnethon MR, Biggs ML, Barzilay J, et al. Diabetes and coronary heart disease as risk factors for mortality in older adults. Am J Med 2010;123:556.e1–e9

26. U.S. Centers for Disease Control and Prevention. Diabetes Data & Trends: Number (in Millions) of Civilian, Noninstitutionalized Persons with Diagnosed Diabetes, United States, 1980–2010 [Internet], 2011. Available from http://www.cdc.gov/diabetes/statistics/prev/national/figpersons.htm. Accessed 17 January 2013

27. Poisal JA, Truffer C, Smith S, et al. Health spending projections through 2016: modest changes obscure Part D's impact. Health Aff (Millwood) 2007;26:w242–w253

28. Smith C, Cowan C, Heffler S, Catlin A. National health spending in 2004: recent slowdown led by prescription drug spending. Health Aff (Millwood) 2006;25:186–196

29. U.S. Centers for Disease Control and Prevention. Overweight and Obesity: Adult Obesity Facts [Internet], 2012. Available from http://www.cdc.gov/obesity/data/adult.html. Accessed 16 January 2013

30. Hoyert DL. 75 Years of Mortality in the United States, 1935–2010. NCHS data brief, no. 88. Hyattsville, MD, National Center for Health Statistics, 2012

31. U.S. Preventive Services Task Force. Screening for Type 2 Diabetes Mellitus in Adults [Internet], 2008. Available from http://www.uspreventiveservicestaskforce.org/uspstf/uspsdiab.htm. Accessed 16 January 2013

32. Mokdad AH, Ford ES, Bowman BA, et al. Prevalence of obesity, diabetes, and obesity-related health risk factors, 2001. JAMA 2003;289:76–79

33. Kim S. Burden of hospitalizations primarily due to uncontrolled diabetes: implications of inadequate primary health care in the United States. Diabetes Care 2007;30:1281–1282

34. Brown JB, Pedula KL, Bakst AW. The progressive cost of complications in type 2 diabetes mellitus. Arch Intern Med 1999;159:1873–1880

35. Aizcorbe A, Liebman E, Pack S, Cutler DM, Chernew ME, Rosen AB. Measuring health care costs of individuals with employer-sponsored health insurance in the U.S.: a comparison of survey and claims data. Journal of the International Association for Official Statistics 2012;28:43–51

36. Zhang Y, Dall TM, Mann SE, et al. The economic costs of undiagnosed diabetes. Popul Health Manag 2009;12:95–101

37. Zhang Y, Dall TM, Chen Y, et al. Medical cost associated with prediabetes. Popul Health Manag 2009;12:157–163

38. Dall TM, Zhang Y, Chen YJ, Quick WW, Yang WG, Fogli J. The economic burden of diabetes. Health Aff (Millwood) 2010;29:297–303

39. Centers for Medicare & Medicaid Services. National Health Expenditure Projections 2010–2020: Forecast Summary. Available from https://www.cms.gov/Research-Statistics-Data-and-Systems/Statistics-Trends-and-Reports/NationalHealthExpendData/downloads/proj2010.pdf. Accessed 17 January 2013

40. Vijan S, Hayward RA, Langa KM. The impact of diabetes on workforce participation: results from a national household sample. Health Serv Res 2004;39(6 Pt 1):1653–1669

41. Narayan KM, Boyle JP, Geiss LS, Saaddine JB, Thompson TJ. Impact of recent increase in incidence on future diabetes burden: U.S., 2005–2050. Diabetes Care 2006;29:2114–2116

42. Hoyert DL, Xu JQ. Deaths: Preliminary Data for 2011. National Vital Statistics Reports, vol. 61, no. 6. Hyattsville, MD, National Center for Health Statistics, 2012

Update on the Antimicrobial Management of Foot Infections in Patients With Diabetes

Gregory T. Matsuura, PharmD, and Neil Barg, MD

Selecting appropriate antibiotics for the treatment of diabetic foot infections (DFIs) is crucial. Identifying the optimal antibiotic choice requires careful consideration of three major criteria: severity of infection, duration of wounds, and previous antibiotic exposure.

Chronic wounds can be colonized on the surface by a varied group of organisms, including aerobic gram-positive cocci (e.g., staphylococci, streptococci, and enterococci), enterobacteriaceae (e.g., *Escherichia coli, Klebsiella* spp., *Enterobacter* spp., and *Proteus* spp.), nonfermentive gram-negative rods (e.g., *Pseudomonas aeruginosa*), and anaerobic bacteria. Isolates from superficial swab cultures may not represent the underlying infecting pathogen.[1] Therefore, cultures obtained after the debridement of superficial debris, eschar, or calluses are best to guide targeted antibiotic therapy.[2] Once the probable pathogen(s) are isolated, de-escalation of empiric therapy can be guided by relevant culture results.

The severity of infection affects several treatment decisions. These include the route and choice of antibiotic, the need for hospital admission, consideration of surgical intervention, and overall length of therapy.

DFIs are characterized by the presence of at least two of the following clinical symptoms: localized edema, erythema, pain, and purulent discharge. Mild infections involve only the skin or subcutaneous tissue, and erythema, if present, is within 2 cm of an ulcer. Most mild infections and many moderate infections can be treated by narrow-spectrum antibiotics focused against staphylococcal and streptococcal bacteria.[3] Suggested treatment of mild DFIs consists of oral agents with activity against *Staphylococcus aureus* (Table 1).

Moderate infections refer to those with surrounding erythema > 2 cm or deeper infections that extend beyond the subcutaneous structures (e.g., deep abscesses, septic arthritis, or osteomyelitis). Severe infections are defined as cases with both local signs of infection and a systemic inflammatory response (e.g., leukocytosis, fever, hypotension, or tachycardia). Empiric treatment for moderate to severe DFIs includes an expansive assortment of options (Table 2).

The differing pharmacological properties of these agents must be thoughtfully considered when selecting antimicrobial therapy. For infections of greater severity, empiric therapy usually includes activity against both aerobic gram-positive and gram-negative organisms. Longstanding infections or infections with necrotic tissue often harbor anaerobic bacteria in addition to those listed above. Generally, these infections require the use of broad-spectrum antibiotics with additional activity against anaerobes such as *Bacteroides fragilis*.

Patient-specific factors also influence optimal antibiotic choice. Patients with diabetes are at a high risk of compromised skin integrity and impaired wound healing because of complications such as peripheral neuropathy, vascular insufficiency, and hyperglycemia.

DFIs without open skin wounds or with ulcers of limited duration are typically caused by gram-positive organisms, including *S. aureus* and β-hemolytic streptococci (Groups A, B, C, and G). In a study of 653 post-debridement samples from diabetic foot wounds,[4] aerobic gram-positive organisms accounted for 77% of all bacterial isolates, with staphylococci (43%) and streptococci (13%) representing the largest proportion

IN BRIEF

Foot infections are common problems in patients with diabetes and can lead to devastating complications and long-term morbidity. Although these infections invariably start in superficial soft tissues, they can involve deeper structures, including bone. Complications may include necrotizing fasciitis, soft tissue gangrene, septic arthritis, and osteomyelitis. This article reviews the factors involved in appropriate antibiotic selection and describes antimicrobial agents included in recently updated treatment guidelines from the Infectious Diseases Society of America.

Table 1. Spectrum of Activity of Suggested Oral Antibiotics for the Treatment of Mild DFIs

	Activity Against MSSA	Activity Against MRSA	Activity Against Enterobacteriaceae
Dicloxacillin	Yes	No	No
Clindamycin	Yes	Yes for community-acquired strains, inducible resistance reported (detected by D-test)	No
Cephalexin	Yes	No	Limited, but covers some strains of *E. coli*
Amoxacillin-clavulanate	Yes	No	Yes, but high rates of *E. coli* resistance
Minocycline	Yes	Yes	Limited
Trimethoprim-sulfamethoxazole	Yes	Yes	Limited
Levofloxacin	Only variable activity against MSSA	No	Yes, broad-spectrum activity

MRSA, methicillin-resistant S. aureus*; MSSA, methicillin-sensitive* S. aureus

of these organisms. Wounds of < 6 weeks' duration coincided with the greatest number of gram-positive infections. In contrast, gram-negative infections were more prevalent in patients with wounds present for ≥ 6 weeks.

The inclusion of anti-pseudomonal spectrum in the treatment of DFIs is common but controversial. Empiric antibiotic therapy with activity against *P. aeruginosa* (i.e., ceftazidime, cefepime, piperacillin-tazobactam, imipenem, or meropenem) is advised for patients with risk factors for this organism, those who have undergone recently failed nonpseudomonal therapy, and in cases of severe infection. Risk factors for *P. aeruginosa* infection include warm climate, open wounds that have been soaked in water, and a high local rate of pseudomonal infections.[3]

Surprisingly, clinical improvement in severe infections has been observed with regimens devoid of meaningful *P. aeruginosa* activity regardless of microbiological culture results.[5–7] For example, clinical response did not differ in a study that compared ertapenem, an agent lacking anti-pseudomonal activity, to piperacillin-tazobactam in 586 patients with moderate to severe DFIs.[5] Some caution is advised in interpreting this finding because only 28 cultures in this study isolated *P. aeruginosa*.

Patients with DFIs have numerous hospitalizations and are often exposed to multiple courses of antibiotics.[8] Previous antibiotic exposure can have a substantial influence on anticipated antimicrobial resistance. Kaye et al.[9] reported that patients with previous treatment with penicillin-based therapy had higher rates of *E. coli* resistance to the β-lactam/β-lactamase inhibitor combination ampicillin-sulbactam. Fluoroquinolone use has been associated with an increase in the acquisition of methicillin-resistant *S. aureus* (MRSA).[10,11] A common risk factor for the development of highly resistant bacteria is the previous use of broad-spectrum antimicrobials.[12,13] To minimize antibiotic exposure, chronic wounds without clinical signs of infection should not be cultured.[3] Unwarranted microbiological samples may encourage the use of antibiotic therapy and thereby increase the risk of harboring multi–drug-resistant organisms.

Expanded-Spectrum Penicillin–Based Therapy

Expanded-spectrum penicillin–based regimens include dicloxacillin and β-lactam/β-lactamase inhibitor combinations. Dicloxacillin, an oral penicillinase-resistant penicillin, is a recommended treatment for mild DFIs. This agent has excellent activity against methicillin-sensitive *S. aureus* (MSSA) and β-hemolytic streptococci but has no activity against gram-negative pathogens. Although inexpensive, dicloxacillin has variable oral absorption and requires dosing four times daily.

Other penicillin-based therapies consist of β-lactam/β-lactamase inhibitor combinations such as amoxicillin-clavulanate, ampicillin-

Table 2. Characteristics of Suggested Antibiotic Regimens for Moderate to Severe DFIs

	Available formulations	Once-Daily Dosing	Activity Against MRSA	Activity Against *P. aeruginosa*	Activity Against *B. fragilis*
Ampicillin-sulbactam	IV	No	No	No	Yes
Levofloxacin	IV and oral	Yes	No	Variable resistance rates	No
Ciprofloxacin plus clindamycin	IV and oral	No	Yes for clindamycin, but variable resistance rates	Yes for ciprofloxacin, but variable resistance rates	Yes for clindamycin, but variable resistance rates
Moxifloxacin	IV and oral	Yes	No	No	Yes, but rare resistance
Cefoxitin	IV	No	No	No	Yes, but some resistance
Ceftriaxone	IV	Yes	No	No	No
Ertapenem	IV	Yes	No	No	Yes
Piperacillin-tazobactam	IV	No	No	Yes	Yes
Imipenem	IV	No	No	Yes	Yes
Linezolid	IV and oral	No	Yes	No	No
Daptomycin	IV	Yes	Yes	No	No

IV, intravenous; MRSA, methicillin-resistant S. aureus

subactam, ticarcillin-clavulanate, and piperacillin-tazobactam. The addition of a β-lactamase inhibitor increases the spectrum of penicillin-based antibiotics to include MSSA, certain β-lactamase–producing gram-negatives, and anaerobes such as *B. fragilis*. Amoxacillin-clavulanate and ampicillin-sulbactam are almost identical with regard to spectrum, with activity against gram-positive organisms, enterobacteriaceae, and obligate anaerobes. Of note, isolates of *E. coli* can be resistant to these agents, particularly in patients with previous antibiotic exposure.[9] A recent study of *E. coli* bloodstream infections[14] observed an increase in ampicillin-sulbactam resistance over a 10-year period.

Piperacillin-tazobactam is a parenteral ureidopenicillin/β-lactamase inhibitor combination with broad-spectrum coverage of aerobic gram-positives, obligate anaerobes, and aerobic gram-negatives. In comparison to ampicillin-sulbactam, piperacillin-tazobactam has similar activity against gram-positive and anaerobic bacteria but has an increased spectrum against non-fermentive gram-negative rods including *P. aeruginosa*. This difference in gram-negative activity may not translate into a clinical advantage for all cases of DFIs. An open-label, randomized study[15] compared these two agents in 314 adult patients with moderate to severe infections of diabetic foot ulcers. The clinical efficacy rate for ampicillin-sulbactam was found to be statistically equivalent to piperacillin-tazobactam (83.1 vs. 81%,

respectively). Although ticarcillin-clavulanate has been studied in the treatment of DFIs, it has mainly been supplanted by piperacillin-tazobactam and is infrequently used.

Cephalosporins
Cephalosporins are semisynthetic β-lactams classified by generations. Generally, cephalosporins in higher generations have enhanced activity against gram-negative organisms but have varying degrees of activity against gram-positive cocci.

The spectrum of first-generation cephalosporins is focused against gram-positive bacteria. Cephalexin is an oral first-generation cephalosporin with activity against MSSA, streptococcus spp., and some strains of enteric gram-negative bacilli such as *E. coli*. This agent has been studied in the treatment of uncomplicated lower-extremity infections in diabetic patients.[16] Cephalexin usually requires dosing four times daily but offers a cost-effective option for mild DFIs.

Cefoxitin is a parenteral second-generation cephalosporin with activity against gram-positive, gram-negative, and anaerobic bacteria. This antimicrobial is usually given every 6 hours and, although active against obligate anaerobes, an increasing rate of *B. fragilis* resistance has been observed.[17]

Ceftriaxone is an injectable third-generation cephalosporin that provides broad-spectrum gram-positive and gram-negative activity. Ceftriaxone lacks clinically useful activity against bacteroides spp. and should be combined with an agent such as metronidazole if anaerobic pathogens are also suspected.[18] An open-label study[19] compared metronidazole plus ceftriaxone to ticarcillin/clavulanate as empiric treatment for diabetic lower-extremity infections in older men. Both regimens had similar treatment success rates (72 and 76%, respectively). Convenient once-daily dosing makes ceftriaxone an attractive parenteral option for outpatient therapy.

Carbapenems

Carbapenems are broad-spectrum parenteral antimicrobials that have activity against gram-positive, gram-negative, and anaerobic bacteria. Carbapenems should be reserved for treatment of infections likely to be caused by multi-antibiotic–resistant gram-negatives (e.g., when extended-spectrum β-lactamase [ESBL]–producing organisms are of particular concern). Both imipenem and meropenem have been studied for the treatment of diabetic foot infections in subsets of patients with complicated skin and skin structure infections.[20] The three available

carbepenems—imipenem, meropenem, and doripenem—have similar spectrums of activity that include ESBL-producing gram-negatives and *P. aeruginosa*.

Although also parenterally administered, ertapenem is the only carbapenem with once-daily dosing. With regard to therapeutic spectrum, ertapenem lacks clinical activity against enterococcus spp. and *P. aeruginosa*.[21] A difference in clinical outcomes was not observed in trials[5,22] comparing piperacillin-tazobactam to carbapenem-based therapy.

Carbapenem use has been associated with the emergence of multi-drug–resistant *P. aeruginosa* and *K. pneumonia*. Therefore, these antimicrobials must be used judiciously.[23-25] Involvement of an infectious diseases specialist should be considered for patients who require the use of these agents.

Fluoroquinolones

Ciprofloxacin, levofloxacin, and moxifloxacin are potential options for the empiric treatment of DFIs.[3] These fluoroquinolones are available in both oral and intravenous formulations, but differ with regard to antibacterial spectrum. Ciprofloxacin should be used in combination with clindamycin because of its relatively poor gram-positive activity. In contrast to ciprofloxacin, levofloxacin has improved gram-positive activity but is less potent against *P. aeruginosa*. Moxifloxacin possesses activity against obligate anaerobes, including *B. fragilis*, but lacks clinical utility for pseudomonal infections. Although levofloxacin and moxifloxacin can be used as empiric monotherapies, they may not provide reliable activity against *S. aureus*, particularly when MRSA is suspected.[26]

Most of the published fluoroquinolone DFI data have been derived from smaller subsets of patients

within larger studies of skin and skin structure infections. Graham et al.[27] compared levofloxacin in the treatment of complicated soft tissue infections to ticarcillin-clavulanate followed by oral amoxicillin-clavulanate. For the subset of 54 patients with DFIs, a clinical success rate of 69.2% for levofloxacin and 57.1% for ticarcillin-clavulanate/amoxicillin-clavulanate was observed. In two trials,[6,7] moxifloxacin monotherapy was shown to be clinically non-inferior to a regimen consisting of initial piperacillin-tazobactam therapy with a sequential switch to oral amoxicillin-clavulanate. Both studies included patients with DFIs, but these were smaller subsets within larger groups with skin and skin structure infections. For example, one study using moxifloxacin[6] included only 78 DFIs from among 617 patients enrolled in the original study. Because it has no demonstrated clinical superiority over other well-established treatment choices, empiric fluoroquinolone therapy should be reserved for β-lactam–allergic patients.

Agents Active Against MRSA

The prevalence of MRSA in DFIs has increased compared to historic rates and has been reported to be as high as 30%.[28] Risk factors for MRSA isolation from DFIs include chronic ulcers of > 6 weeks' duration, previous hospitalization, long-term antibiotic use, osteomyelitis, previous history of MRSA infection, and MRSA nasal colonization.[4,28-30] Empiric coverage of MRSA should be considered for patients with previous isolation of MRSA within the past year, high local MRSA rates (prevalence rates of 50% for mild infections and 30% for moderate infections), or severe infections while awaiting definitive culture results.[3]

For mild infections, oral agents with MRSA activity include

minocycline, trimethoprim-sul-famethoxazole (TMP-SMX), and clindamycin. Although TMP-SMX and minocycline have in vitro activity against many isolates of MRSA, their activity against streptococcal species is not uniform. For example, group B streptococci are intrinsically resistant to TMP-SMX, and tetracycline–resistant group A streptococci are widely prevalent. An additional agent such as amoxicillin should be added if β-hemolytic streptococci coverage is required.[30]

Clindamycin, a lincosamide, is available in both intravenous and oral formulations. This agent has activity against community acquired strains of MRSA, β-hemolytic streptococci, and anaerobic bacteria. However, MRSA isolates should be tested for inducible clindamycin resistance because treatment failures have been reported.[31]

Treatment options for moderate to severe DFIs with MRSA include vancomycin, daptomycin, and linezolid. Vancomycin, a glycopeptide antimicrobial, has been the traditional agent used to cover MRSA in more severe DFIs. Optimal dosing is important because patients with diabetes may have reduced penetration of vancomycin into soft tissue compared to patients without diabetes.[32] Additionally, some strains of *S. aureus*, compared to historic isolates, have shown a decreasing sensitivity to vancomycin.

The consensus recommendations published in 2009[33] offer guidance regarding the suggested dosing and monitoring for complicated MRSA infections. In the setting of vancomycin hypersensitivity or clinical failure, alternatives such as daptomycin or linezolid could be considered.

Linezolid, an oxazolidinone, has been studied in complicated skin and skin structure infections including DFIs. A pooled review[34] of 349

patients with diabetes receiving either linezolid or vancomycin for complicated skin and skin structure infections observed comparable rates of clinical success (74 and 71%, respectively). Linezolid is available in both intravenous and oral formulations and is active against aerobic gram-positive organisms, including MRSA and vancomycin-resistant enterococcus. This agent is well absorbed orally but considerably more expensive than the older oral antibiotics previously mentioned. Because of frequent myelosuppression, complete blood counts should be monitored for treatment courses > 14 days. One study[35] reported anemia (17.6%), thrombocytopenia (12.8%), and neutropenia (2.0%) associated with linezolid use. Furthermore, linezolid interacts with medications that increase concentrations of serotonin, resulting in rare but sometimes severe cases of serotonin syndrome.[36]

Daptomycin is a parenteral cyclic lipopeptide similar in spectrum to vancomycin with activity against gram-positive organisms. Once-daily dosing makes this an attractive outpatient option, but serial monitoring of creatine phosphokinase is recommended because of potential myopathy.[37] In a subset of 103 patients with DFIs, daptomycin had similar outcomes to either vancomycin or penicillinase-resistant semisynthetic penicillin (66 and 70%, respectively).[38]

Tigecycline is a parenteral broad-spectrum glycylcycline antibiotic. Although active against MRSA, this agent has been found to be inferior to other antimicrobials in the treatment DFIs.[39]

Mild DFIs involving MRSA can be treated with inexpensive oral options such as TMP-SMX, minocycline, or clindamycin. Vancomycin is still an appropriate choice for MRSA coverage in moderate to severe DFIs.

The superiority of alternative agents such as linezolid or daptomycin in the treatment of DFIs has not been demonstrated.

Conclusion

Identifying the appropriate antimicrobial treatment of DFIs is a complex process with many patient-specific considerations. Proper selection of antimicrobial therapy is imperative but often difficult because of polymicrobial colonization of chronic diabetic ulcers. Therapy must have activity against gram-positive organisms and, if risk factors are present, include coverage of MRSA. The role of *P. aeruginosa* therapy is less clear, and empiric antimicrobial coverage is not always necessary for this organism.

Regimens studied have not demonstrated meaningful superiority of any particular agent. The majority of published data pertain to the use of β-lactam–based regimens. Newer agents such as ertapenem and moxifloxacin are possible choices in the treatment of DFIs but should be considered only as alternative agents. Although linezolid and daptomycin are other potential treatment options for MRSA, no compelling evidence indicates the need to replace vancomycin for the treatment of DFIs. Linezolid and daptomycin generally should be reserved for cases of vancomycin failure or hypersensitivity.

The optimal antimicrobial treatment of DFIs has yet to be determined. Additional prospective, well-designed trials are needed to clarify which regimen(s) result in the best possible outcomes.

REFERENCES

[1]Senneville E, Melliez H, Beltrand E, Legout L, Valette M, Cazaubiel M, Cordonnier M, Caillaux M, Yazdanpanah Y, Mouton Y: Culture of percutaneous bone biopsy specimens for diagnosis of diabetic foot osteomyelitis: concordance with ulcer swab cultures. *Clin Infect Dis* 42:57–62, 2006

[2]Bowler PG, Duerden BI, Armstrong DG: Wound microbiology and associated approaches to wound management. *Clin Microbiol Rev* 14:244–269, 2001

[3]Lipsky BA, Berendt AR, Cornia PB, Pile JC, Peters EJ, Armstrong DG, Deery HG, Embil JM, Joseph WS, Karchmer AW, Pinzur MS, Senneville E: Executive summary: 2012 Infectious Diseases Society of America clinical practice guideline for the diagnosis and treatment of diabetic foot infections. *Clin Infect Dis* 54:1679–1684, 2012

[4]Yates C, May K, Hale T, Allard B, Rowlings N, Freeman A, Harrison J, McCann J, Wraight P: Wound chronicity, inpatient care, and chronic kidney disease predispose to MRSA infection in diabetic foot ulcers. *Diabetes Care* 32:1907–1909, 2009

[5]Lipsky BA, Armstrong DG, Citron DM, Tice AD, Morgenstern DE, Abramson MA: Ertapenem versus piperacillin/tazobactam for diabetic foot infections (SIDESTEP): prospective, randomised, controlled, double-blinded, multicentre trial. *Lancet* 366:1695–1703, 2005

[6]Lipsky BA, Giordano P, Choudhri S, Song J: Treating diabetic foot infections with sequential intravenous to oral moxifloxacin compared with piperacillin-tazobactam/amoxicillin-clavulanate. *J Antimicrob Chemother* 60:370–376, 2007

[7]Gyssens IC, Dryden M, Kujath P, Nathwani D, Schaper N, Hampel B, Reimnitz P, Alder J, Arvis P: A randomized trial of the efficacy and safety of sequential intravenous/oral moxifloxacin monotherapy versus intravenous piperacillin/tazobactam followed by oral amoxicillin/clavulanate for complicated skin and skin structure infections. *J Antimicrob Chemother* 66:2632–2642, 2011

[8]Fincke BG, Miller DR, Turpin R: A classification of diabetic foot infections using ICD-9-CM codes: application to a large computerized medical database. *BMC Health Serv Res* 10:192, 2010

[9]Kaye KS, Harris AD, Gold H, Carmeli Y: Risk factors for recovery of ampicillin-sulbactam-resistant Escherichia coli in hospitalized patients. *Antimicrob Agents Chemother* 44:1004–1009, 2000

[10]Cheng VC, Li IW, Wu AK, Tang BS, Ng KH, To KK, Tse H, Que TL, Ho PL, Yuen KY: Effect of antibiotics on the bacterial load of methicillin-resistant Staphylococcus aureus colonization in anterior nares. *J Hosp Infect* 70:27–34, 2008

[11]LeBlanc L, Pépin J, Toulouse K, Ouellette MF, Coulombe MA, Corriveau MP, Alary ME: Fluoroquinolones and risk for methicillin-resistant Staphylococcus aureus, Canada. *Emerg Infect Dis* 12:1398–1405, 2006

[12]Colodner R, Rock W, Chazan B, Keller N, Guy N, Sakran W, Raz R: Risk factors for the development of extended-spectrum β-lactamase-producing bacteria in non-hospitalized patients. *Eur J Clin Microbiol Infect Dis* 23:163–167, 2004

[13]Harris AD, McGregor JC, Johnson JA, Strauss SM, Moore AC, Standiford HC, Hebden JN, Morris JG Jr.: Risk factors for colonization with extended-spectrum β-lactamase-producing bacteria and intensive care unit admission. *Emerg Infect Dis* 13:1144–1149, 2007

[14]Al-Hasan MN, Lahr BD, Eckel-Passow JE, Baddour LM: Antimicrobial resistance trends of Escherichia coli bloodstream isolates: a population-based study, 1998–2007. *J Antimicrob Chemother* 64:169–174, 2009

[15]Harkless L, Boghossian J, Pollak R, Caputo W, Dana A, Gray S, Wu D: An open-label, randomized study comparing efficacy and safety of intravenous piperacillin/tazobactam and ampicillin/sulbactam for infected diabetic foot ulcers. *Surg Infect (Larchmt)* 6:27–40, 2005

[16]Lipsky BA, Pecoraro RE, Larson SA, Hanley ME, Ahroni JH: Outpatient management of uncomplicated lower-extremity infections in diabetic patients. *Arch Intern Med* 150:790–797, 1990

[17]Snydman DR, Jacobus NV, McDermott LA, Golan Y, Goldstein EJ, Harrell L, Jenkins S, Newton D, Pierson C, Rosenblatt J, Venezia R, Gorbach SL, Queenan AM, Hecht DW: Update on resistance of Bacteroides fragilis group and related species with special attention to carbapenems 2006–2009. *Anaerobe* 17:147–151, 2011

[18]Marshall WF, Blair JE. The cephalosporins. *Mayo Clin Proc* 74:187–195, 1999

[19]Clay PG, Graham MR, Lindsey CC, Lamp KC, Freeman C, Glaros A: Clinical efficacy, tolerability, and cost savings associated with the use of open-label metronidazole plus ceftriaxone once daily compared with ticarcillin/clavulanate every 6 hours as empiric treatment for diabetic lower-extremity infections in older males. *Am J Geriatr Pharmacother* 2:181–189, 2004

[20]Fabian TC, File TM, Embil JM, Krige JE, Klein S, Rose A, Melnick D, Soto NE: Meropenem versus imipenem-cilastatin for the treatment of hospitalized patients with complicated skin and skin structure infections: results of a multicenter, randomized, double-blind comparative study. *Surg Infect (Larchmt)* 6:269–282, 2005

[21]Zhanel GG, Wiebe R, Dilay L, Thomson K, Rubinstein E, Hoban DJ, Noreddin AM, Karlowsky JA: Comparative review of the carbapenems. *Drugs* 67:1027–1052, 2007

[22]Saltoglu N, Dalkiran A, Tetiker T, Bayram H, Tasova Y, Dalay C, Sert M: Piperacillin/tazobactam versus imipenem/cilastatin for severe diabetic foot infections: a prospective, randomized clinical trial in a university hospital. *Clin Microbiol Infect* 16:1252–1257, 2010

[23]Kwak YG, Choi SH, Choo EJ, Chung JW, Jeong JY, Kim NJ, Woo JH, Ryu J, Kim YS: Risk factors for the acquisition of carbapenem-resistant Klebsiella pneumoniae among hospitalized patients. *Microb Drug Resist* 11:165–169, 2005

[24]Hussein K, Sprecher H, Mashiach T, Oren I, Kassis I, Finkelstein R: Carbapenem resistance among Klebsiella pneumoniae isolates: risk factors, molecular characteristics, and susceptibility patterns. *Infect Control Hosp Epidemiol* 30:666–671, 2009

[25]Lautenbach E, Synnestvedt M, Weiner MG, Bilker WB, Vo L, Schein J, Kim M: Imipenem resistance in Pseudomonas aeruginosa: emergence, epidemiology, and impact on clinical and economic outcomes. *Infect Control Hosp Epidemiol* 31:47–53, 2010

[26]Tenover FC, Tickler IA, Goering RV, Kreiswirth BN, Mediavilla JR, Persing DH; MRSA Consortium: Characterization of nasal and blood culture isolates of methicillin-resistant Staphylococcus aureus from patients in United States Hospitals. *Antimicrob Agents Chemother* 56:1324–1330, 2012

[27]Graham DR, Talan DA, Nichols RL, Lucasti C, Corrado M, Morgan N, Fowler CL: Once-daily, high-dose levofloxacin versus ticarcillin-clavulanate alone or followed by amoxicillin-clavulanate for complicated skin and skin-structure infections: a randomized, open-label trial. *Clin Infect Dis* 35:381–389, 2002

[28]Eleftheriadou I, Tentolouris N, Argiana V, Jude E, Boulton AJ: Methicillin-resistant Staphylococcus aureus in diabetic foot infections. *Drugs* 70:1785–1797, 2010

[29]Stanaway S, Johnson D, Moulik P, Gill G: Methicillin-resistant Staphylococcus aureus (MRSA) isolation from diabetic foot ulcers correlates with nasal MRSA carriage. *Diabetes Res Clin Pract* 75:47–50, 2007

[30]Liu C, Bayer A, Cosgrove SE, Daum RS, Fridkin SK, Gorwitz RJ, Kaplan SL, Karchmer AW, Levine DP, Murray BE, J Rybak M, Talan DA, Chambers HF; Infectious Diseases Society of America: Clinical practice guidelines by the Infectious Diseases Society of America for the treatment of methicillin-resistant Staphylococcus aureus infections in adults and children. *Clin Infect Dis* 52:e18–e55, 2011

[31]Siberry GK, Tekle T, Carroll K, Dick J: Failure of clindamycin treatment of methicillin-resistant Staphylococcus aureus expressing inducible clindamycin resistance in vitro. *Clin Infect Dis* 37:1257–1260, 2003

[32]Skhirtladze K, Hutschala D, Fleck T, Thalhammer F, Ehrlich M, Vukovich T, Müller M, Tschernko EM: Impaired target site penetration of vancomycin in diabetic patients following cardiac surgery. *Antimicrob Agents Chemother* 50:1372–1375, 2006

[33]Rybak MJ, Lomaestro BM, Rotschafer JC, Moellering RC, Craig WA, Billeter M, Dalovisio JR, Levine DP: Vancomycin therapeutic guidelines: a summary of consensus recommendations from the Infectious Diseases Society of America, the American Society of Health-System Pharmacists, and the Society of Infectious Diseases Pharmacists. *Clin Infect Dis* 49:325–327, 2009

[34]Lipsky BA, Itani KM, Weigelt JA, Joseph W, Paap CM, Reisman A, Myers DE, Huang DB: The role of diabetes mellitus in the treatment of skin and skin structure infections caused by methicillin-resistant Staphylococcus aureus: results from three

randomized controlled trials. *Int J Infect Dis* 15:e140–e146, 2011

[35]Minson Q, Gentry CA: Analysis of linezolid-associated hematologic toxicities in a large veterans affairs medical center. *Pharmacotherapy* 30:895–903, 2010

[36]Lawrence KR, Adra M, Gillman PK: Serotonin toxicity associated with the use of linezolid: a review of postmarketing data. *Clin Infect Dis* 42:1578–1583, 2006

[37]Rivera AM, Boucher HW: Current concepts in antimicrobial therapy against select gram-positive organisms: methicillin-resistant Staphylococcus aureus, penicillin-resistant pneumococci, and vancomycin-resistant enterococci. *Mayo Clin Proc* 86:1230–1243, 2011

[38]Lipsky BA, Stoutenburgh U: Daptomycin for treating infected diabetic foot ulcers: evidence from a randomized, controlled trial comparing daptomycin with vancomycin or semi-synthetic penicillins for complicated skin and skin-structure infections. *J Antimicrob Chemother* 55:240–245, 2005

[39]Prasad P, Sun J, Danner RL, Natanson C: Excess deaths associated with tigecycline after approval based on noninferiority trials. *Clin Infect Dis* 54:1699–1709, 2012

Gregory T. Matsuura, PharmD, is a clinical assistant professor of pharmacotherapy at the Washington State University College of Pharmacy in Spokane and Yakima Valley Memorial Hospital in Yakima, Wash. Neil Barg, MD, is a clinical associate professor of medicine at the University of Washington School of Medicine in Seattle.

Hypoglycemia and Diabetes: A Report of a Workgroup of the American Diabetes Association and The Endocrine Society

Elizabeth R. Seaquist, MD[1]
John Anderson, MD[2]
Belinda Childs, ARNP, MN, BC-ADM, CDE[3]
Philip Cryer, MD[4]
Samuel Dagogo-Jack, MD, MBBS, MSC[5]

Lisa Fish, MD[6]
Simon R. Heller, MD[7]
Henry Rodriguez, MD[8]
James Rosenzweig, MD[9]
Robert Vigersky, MD[10]

OBJECTIVE—To review the evidence about the impact of hypoglycemia on patients with diabetes that has become available since the past reviews of this subject by the American Diabetes Association and The Endocrine Society and to provide guidance about how this new information should be incorporated into clinical practice.

PARTICIPANTS—Five members of the American Diabetes Association and five members of The Endocrine Society with expertise in different aspects of hypoglycemia were invited by the Chair, who is a member of both, to participate in a planning conference call and a 2-day meeting that was also attended by staff from both organizations. Subsequent communications took place via e-mail and phone calls. The writing group consisted of those invitees who participated in the writing of the manuscript. The workgroup meeting was supported by educational grants to the American Diabetes Association from Lilly USA, LLC and Novo Nordisk and sponsorship to the American Diabetes Association from Sanofi. The sponsors had no input into the development of or content of the report.

EVIDENCE—The writing group considered data from recent clinical trials and other studies to update the prior workgroup report. Unpublished data were not used. Expert opinion was used to develop some conclusions.

CONSENSUS PROCESS—Consensus was achieved by group discussion during conference calls and face-to-face meetings, as well as by iterative revisions of the written document. The document was reviewed and approved by the American Diabetes Association's Professional Practice Committee in October 2012 and approved by the Executive Committee of the Board of Directors in November 2012 and was reviewed and approved by The Endocrine Society's Clinical Affairs Core Committee in October 2012 and by Council in November 2012.

CONCLUSIONS—The workgroup reconfirmed the previous definitions of hypoglycemia in diabetes, reviewed the implications of hypoglycemia on both short- and long-term outcomes, considered the implications of hypoglycemia on treatment outcomes, presented strategies to prevent hypoglycemia, and identified knowledge gaps that should be addressed by future research. In addition, tools for patients to report hypoglycemia at each visit and for clinicians to document counseling are provided.

Diabetes Care 36:1384–1395, 2013

In 2005, the American Diabetes Association Workgroup on Hypoglycemia released a report entitled "Defining and Reporting Hypoglycemia in Diabetes" (1). In that report, recommendations were primarily made to advise the U.S. Food and Drug Administration (FDA) on how hypoglycemia should be used as an end point in studies of new treatments for diabetes. In 2009, The Endocrine Society released a clinical practice guideline entitled "Evaluation and Management of Adult Hypoglycemic Disorders," which summarized how clinicians should manage hypoglycemia in patients with diabetes (2). Since then, new evidence has become available that links hypoglycemia with adverse outcomes in older patients with type 2 diabetes (3–6) and in children with type 1 diabetes (7,8). To provide guidance about how this new information should be incorporated into clinical practice, the American Diabetes Association and The Endocrine Society assembled a new Workgroup on Hypoglycemia in April 2012 to address the following questions:

1. How should hypoglycemia in diabetes be defined and reported?
2. What are the implications of hypoglycemia on both short- and long-term outcomes in people with diabetes?
3. What are the implications of hypoglycemia on treatment targets for patients with diabetes?

From the [1]Department of Medicine, University of Minnesota, Minneapolis, Minnesota; [2]The Frist Clinic, Nashville, Tennessee; [3]Mid-America Diabetes Associates, Wichita, Kansas; the [4]Division of Endocrinology, Diabetes and Metabolism, Washington University School of Medicine, Saint Louis, Missouri; the [5]Division of Endocrinology, Diabetes and Metabolism, University of Tennessee Health Science Center, Memphis, Tennessee, [6]Diabetes, Metabolism and Endocrinology/Internal Medicine, Park Nicollet Clinic, Saint Louis Park, Minnesota; the [7]Academic Unit of Diabetes, Endocrinology and Metabolism, School of Medicine and Biomedical Sciences, University

of Sheffield, Sheffield, U.K.; the [8]Diabetes Center, University of South Florida College of Medicine, Tampa, Florida; [9]Diabetes Services, Boston Medical Center, Boston University School of Medicine, Boston, Massachusetts; and the [10]Diabetes Institute, Walter Reed National Military Medical Center, Bethesda, Maryland.

Corresponding author: Elizabeth R. Seaquist, seaqu001@umn.edu.

DOI: 10.2337/dc12-2480

This report was reviewed and approved by the American Diabetes Association's Professional Practice Committee in October 2012 and approved by the Executive Committee of the Board

of Directors in November 2012 and was reviewed and approved by The Endocrine Society's Clinical Affairs Core Committee in October 2012 and by Council in November 2012.

This article has been copublished in the *Journal of Clinical Endocrinology & Metabolism*.

A slide set summarizing this article is available online.

4. What strategies are known to prevent hypoglycemia, and what are the clinical recommendations for those at risk for hypoglycemia?
5. What are the current knowledge gaps in our understanding of hypoglycemia, and what research is necessary to fill these gaps?

How should hypoglycemia in diabetes be defined and reported?

—Hypoglycemia puts patients at risk for injury and death. Consequently the workgroup defines iatrogenic hypoglycemia in patients with diabetes as all episodes of an abnormally low plasma glucose concentration that expose the individual to potential harm. A single threshold value for plasma glucose concentration that defines hypoglycemia in diabetes cannot be assigned because glycemic thresholds for symptoms of hypoglycemia (among other responses) shift to lower plasma glucose concentrations after recent antecedent hypoglycemia (9–12) and to higher plasma glucose concentrations in patients with poorly controlled diabetes and infrequent hypoglycemia (13).

Nonetheless, an alert value can be defined that draws the attention of both patients and caregivers to the potential harm associated with hypoglycemia. The workgroup (1) suggests that patients at risk for hypoglycemia (i.e., those treated with a sulfonylurea, glinide, or insulin) should be alert to the possibility of developing hypoglycemia at a self-monitored plasma glucose—or continuous glucose monitoring subcutaneous glucose—concentration of ≤70 mg/dL (≤3.9 mmol/L). This alert value is data driven and pragmatic (14). Given the limited accuracy of the monitoring devices, it approximates the lower limit of the normal postabsorptive plasma glucose concentration (15), the glycemic thresholds for activation of glucose counterregulatory systems in nondiabetic individuals (15), and the upper limit of plasma glucose level reported to reduce counterregulatory responses to subsequent hypoglycemia (11). Because it is higher than the glycemic threshold for symptoms in both nondiabetic individuals and those with well-controlled diabetes (9,13,14), it generally allows time to prevent a clinical hypoglycemic episode and provides some margin for the limited accuracy of monitoring devices at low-glucose levels. People with diabetes need not always self-treat at an estimated glucose concentration of ≤70 mg/dL (≤3.9 mmol/L). Options other than

carbohydrate ingestion include repeating the test in the short term, changing behavior (e.g., avoiding driving or elective exercise until the glucose level is higher), and adjusting the treatment regimen. Although this alert value has been debated (9,13,14), a plasma concentration of ≤70 mg/dL (≤3.9 mmol/L) can be used as a cut-off value in the classification of hypoglycemia in diabetes.

Consistent with past recommendations (1), the workgroup suggests the following classification of hypoglycemia in diabetes:

1) **Severe hypoglycemia.** Severe hypoglycemia is an event requiring assistance of another person to actively administer carbohydrates, glucagon, or take other corrective actions. Plasma glucose concentrations may not be available during an event, but neurological recovery following the return of plasma glucose to normal is considered sufficient evidence that the event was induced by a low plasma glucose concentration.

2) **Documented symptomatic hypoglycemia.** Documented symptomatic hypoglycemia is an event during which typical symptoms of hypoglycemia are accompanied by a measured plasma glucose concentration ≤70 mg/dL (≤3.9 mmol/L).

3) **Asymptomatic hypoglycemia.** Asymptomatic hypoglycemia is an event not accompanied by typical symptoms of hypoglycemia but with a measured plasma glucose concentration ≤70 mg/dL (≤3.9 mmol/L).

4) **Probable symptomatic hypoglycemia.** Probable symptomatic hypoglycemia is an event during which symptoms typical of hypoglycemia are not accompanied by a plasma glucose determination but that was presumably caused by a plasma glucose concentration ≤70 mg/dL (≤3.9 mmol/L).

5) **Pseudo-hypoglycemia.** Pseudo-hypoglycemia is an event during which the person with diabetes reports any of the typical symptoms of hypoglycemia with a measured plasma glucose concentration >70 mg/dL (>3.9 mmol/L) but approaching that level.

The challenge of measuring glucose accurately

Currently, two technologies are available to measure glucose in outpatients: capillary measurement with point-of-care (POC) glucose meters (self-monitored blood glucose [SMBG]) and interstitial measurement with continuous glucose monitors (CGMs), both retrospective and real time. The International Organization for Standardization (ISO) and FDA standards

require that POC meters' analytical accuracy be within 20% of the actual value in 95% of samples with glucose levels ≥75 mg/dL and ±15 mg/dL for samples with glucose <75 mg/dL. Despite this relatively large permissible variation, Freckmann et al. (16) found that only 15 of 27 meters on the market in Europe several years ago met the current analytical standards of ±15 mg/dL in the hypoglycemia range, 2 of 27 met ±10 mg/dL, and none were capable of measuring ±5 mg/dL.

The need for accurate meters in the <75 mg/dL range is essential in insulin-treated patients, whether they are outpatients or inpatients, but it is less important in those outpatients who are on medications that rarely cause hypoglycemia. In critical care units, where the accuracy of POC meters is particularly crucial, their performance may be compromised by medications (vasopressors, acetaminophen), treatments (oxygen), and clinical states (hypotension, anemia) (17). Karon et al. (18) translated these measurement errors into potential insulin-dosing errors using simulation modeling and found that if there were a total measurement error of 20%, 1- and 2-step errors in insulin dose would occur 45% and 6% of the time, respectively, in a tight glycemic control protocol. Such imprecision may affect the safe implementation of insulin infusion protocols in critical care units and may account in part for the high hypoglycemia rates in most trials of inpatient intensive glycemic control.

Retrospective and real-time CGMs represent an evolving technology that has made considerable progress in overall (point + rate) accuracy. However, the accuracy of CGMs in the hypoglycemic range is poor as demonstrated by error grid analysis (19,20). With existing real-time CGMs, accuracy can be achieved in only 60–73% of samples in the range of 40–80 mg/dL (21,22). Because the accuracy of CGMs, like POC meters, is negatively affected by multiple factors in hospitalized patients and they are calibrated with POC meters affected by those same factors, CGMs are not recommended for glycemic management in hospitalized patients at this time (17).

What are the implications of hypoglycemia on both short- and long-term outcomes in people with diabetes?

—Iatrogenic hypoglycemia is more frequent in patients with profound endogenous insulin deficiency—type

1 diabetes and advanced type 2 diabetes—and its incidence increases with the duration of diabetes (23). It is caused by treatment with a sulfonylurea, glinide, or insulin and occurs about two to three times more frequently in type 1 diabetes than in type 2 diabetes (23,24). Event rates for severe hypoglycemia for patients with type 1 diabetes range from 115 (24) to 320 (23) per 100 patient-years. Severe hypoglycemia in patients with type 2 diabetes has been shown to occur at rates of 35 (24) to 70 (23) per 100 patient-years. However, because type 2 diabetes is much more prevalent than type 1 diabetes, most episodes of hypoglycemia, including severe hypoglycemia, occur in people with type 2 diabetes (25).

There is no doubt that hypoglycemia can be fatal (26). In addition to case reports of hypoglycemic deaths in patients with type 1 and type 2 diabetes, four recent reports of mortality rates in series of patients indicate that 4% (27), 6% (28), 7% (29), and 10% (30) of deaths of patients with type 1 diabetes were caused by hypoglycemia. A temporal relationship between extremely low subcutaneous glucose concentrations and death in a patient with type 1 diabetes who was wearing a CGM device and was found dead in bed has been reported (31). Although profound and prolonged hypoglycemia can cause brain death, most episodes of fatal hypoglycemia are probably the result of other mechanisms, such as ventricular arrhythmias (26). In this section, we will consider the effects of hypoglycemia on the development of hypoglycemia unawareness and how iatrogenic hypoglycemia may affect outcomes in specific patient groups.

Hypoglycemia unawareness and hypoglycemia-associated autonomic failure

Acute hypoglycemia in patients with diabetes can lead to confusion, loss of consciousness, seizures, and even death, but how a particular patient responds to a drop in glucose appears to depend on how frequently that patient experiences hypoglycemia. Recurrent hypoglycemia has been shown to reduce the glucose level that precipitates the counterregulatory response necessary to restore euglycemia during a subsequent episode of hypoglycemia (10–12). As a result, patients with frequent hypoglycemia do not experience the symptoms from the adrenergic response to a fall in glucose until the blood glucose reaches lower and lower levels. For

some individuals, the level that triggers the response is below the glucose level associated with neuroglycopenia. The first sign of hypoglycemia in these patients is confusion, and they often must rely on the assistance of others to recognize and treat low blood glucose. Such individuals are said to have developed hypoglycemia unawareness. Defective glucose counterregulation (the result of loss of a decrease in insulin production and an increase in glucagon release along with an attenuated increase in epinephrine) and hypoglycemia unawareness (the result of an attenuated increase in sympathoadrenal activity) are the components of hypoglycemia-associated autonomic failure (HAAF) in patients with diabetes. HAAF is a form of functional sympathoadrenal failure that is most often caused by recent antecedent iatrogenic hypoglycemia (25) and is at least partly reversible by scrupulous avoidance of hypoglycemia (32–34). Indeed, HAAF has been shown to be maintained by recurrent iatrogenic hypoglycemia (33,34). The development of HAAF is associated with a 25-fold (35) or greater (36) increased risk of severe hypoglycemia during intensive glycemic therapy. It is important to distinguish HAAF from classical autonomic neuropathy, which may occur as one form of diabetic neuropathy. Impaired sympathoadrenal activation is generally confined to the response to hypoglycemia, and autonomic activities in organs such as the heart, gastrointestinal tract, and bladder appear to be unaffected.

Clinically, HAAF can be viewed as both adaptive and maladaptive. On the one hand, patients with hypoglycemia unawareness and type 1 diabetes appear to perform better on tests of cognitive function during hypoglycemia than do patients who are able to detect hypoglycemia normally (37). In addition, the time necessary for full cognitive recovery after restoration of euglycemia appears to be faster in patients who have hypoglycemia unawareness than in patients with normal detection of hypoglycemia (37). The HAAF habituation of the sympathoadrenal response to recurrent hypoglycemic stress in humans (38) may be analogous to the phenomenon of habituation of the hypothalamic-pituitary-adrenocortical response to recurrent restraint stress in rats (39). Rats subjected to recurrent moderate hypoglycemia had less brain cell death (40) and less mortality (41) during or following marked hypoglycemia than those not subjected to recurrent hypoglycemia.

On the other hand, HAAF is clearly maladaptive since defective glucose counterregulation and hypoglycemia unawareness substantially increase the risk of severe hypoglycemia with its morbidity and potential mortality (26). A particularly low plasma glucose concentration might trigger a robust, potentially fatal sympathoadrenal discharge. Life-threatening episodes of hypoglycemia need not be frequent to be devastating.

Impact of hypoglycemia on children with diabetes

Hypoglycemia is a common problem in children with type 1 diabetes because of the challenges presented by insulin dosing, variable eating patterns, erratic activity, and the limited ability of small children to detect hypoglycemia. The infant, young child, and even the adolescent typically exhibit unpredictable feeding—not eating all the anticipated food at a meal and snacking unpredictably between meals—and have prolonged periods of fasting overnight that increase the risk of hypoglycemia. Selecting the correct prandial dose of insulin is therefore often difficult. Very low insulin requirements for basal and mealtime dosing in the infant and young child frequently require use of miniscule basal rates in pump therapy and one-half unit dosing increments with injections. Management rarely requires the use of diluted insulin, e.g., 10 units per mL. Infants and toddlers may not recognize the symptoms of hypoglycemia and lack the ability to effectively communicate their distress. Caregivers must be particularly aware that changes in behavior such as a loss of temper may be a sign of hypoglycemia.

Puberty is associated with insulin resistance, while at the same time the normal developmental stages of adolescence may lead to inattention to diabetes and increased risk for hypoglycemia. As children grow, they often have widely fluctuating levels of activity during the day, which puts them at risk for hypoglycemia. Minimizing the impact of hypoglycemia on children with diabetes requires the education and engagement of parents, patients, and other caregivers in the management of the disease (42,43).

The youngest patients are most vulnerable to the adverse consequences of hypoglycemia. Ongoing maturation of the central nervous system puts these children at greater risk for cognitive deficits as a consequence of hypoglycemia (44). Recent studies have examined the impact of hypoglycemia on cognitive function and cerebral structure in children and found that those who experience this complication before the age of 5 years seem to be more affected than those who do not have hypoglycemia until later (7). The long-term impact of hypoglycemia on cognition before the age of 5 years is unknown.

Impact of hypoglycemia on adults with type 1 diabetes

Landmark data on the impact of hypoglycemia on adults with type 1 diabetes come from the Diabetes Control and Complications Trial (DCCT) and its follow-up study, where cognition has been systematically measured over time. In this cohort, performance on a comprehensive battery of neurocognitive tests at 18 years of follow-up was the same in participants with and without a history of severe hypoglycemia (28). Despite such reassuring findings, recent investigation with advanced imaging techniques has demonstrated that adults with type 1 diabetes appear to call upon a greater volume of the brain to perform a working memory task during hypoglycemia (45). These findings suggest that adults with type 1 diabetes must recruit more regions to preserve cognitive function during hypoglycemia than adults without the disease. More work will be necessary to understand the significance of these observations on the long-term cognitive ability of adults with type 1 diabetes.

Impact of hypoglycemia on patients with type 2 diabetes

There is growing evidence that patients with type 2 diabetes might be particularly vulnerable to adverse events associated with hypoglycemia. Over the last decade, three large trials examined the effect of glucose lowering on cardiovascular events in patients with type 2 diabetes: ACCORD (Action to Control Cardiovascular Risk in Diabetes), ADVANCE (Action in Diabetes and Vascular Disease: Preterax and Diamicron MR Controlled Evaluation), and VADT (Veterans Affairs Diabetes Trial). Between them, a total of 24,000 patients with high cardiovascular risk were randomly assigned to either intensive glycemic control or standard therapy (3–5). In each, subjects who were randomly assigned to the intensive arm experienced more episodes of hypoglycemia than did those who were randomly assigned to the standard treatment arm. In the ACCORD trial, subjects who were

randomly assigned to the intensive arm also experienced a 20% increase in mortality, and the glycemic control study was stopped early due to this finding. A relationship between mortality and randomization to intensive glucose control was not observed in ADVANCE or VADT, although VADT was underpowered to explore this relationship. A number of explanations have been offered to explain the findings of ACCORD, including chance, greater weight gain, and specific medication effects, but perhaps the most convincing candidate was hypoglycemia, which was threefold higher in the intensive arm of ACCORD (4).

In the opinion of the blinded adjudication committee assigned to investigate mortality in ACCORD, hypoglycemia was judged to have a definite role in only one death, a probable role in three deaths, and a possible role in 38 deaths (46), which represents a role in less than 10% of the deaths recorded in the study population while the glycemic intervention was active. The investigators thus suggest that hypoglycemia at the time of death was probably not responsible for the increased mortality rate in the intensive arm of ACCORD. Since glycemia was not measured at the time of death in any of the ACCORD subjects, we may never know. However, the potential lethal mechanisms that might be provoked by hypoglycemia could cause mortality downstream of the hypoglycemic event, increasing the difficulty in establishing cause and effect.

All three trials clearly demonstrated that an episode of severe hypoglycemia was associated with an increased risk of subsequent mortality. In ACCORD, those who had one or more severe hypoglycemic episodes had higher rates of death than those without such episodes across both study arms (hazard ratio 1.41 [95% CI 1.03–1.93]) (46). One-third of all deaths were due to cardiovascular disease, and hypoglycemia was associated with higher cardiovascular mortality. In VADT, a recent severe hypoglycemic event was the strongest independent predictor of death at 90 days (3). In ADVANCE, where rates of hypoglycemia were low, a similar pattern was found (47). Of course, in post hoc analyses a causal relationship cannot be established with certainty. It is possible that the association between hypoglycemia and death may be merely an indicator for vulnerability for death from any cause.

The relationship between hypoglycemia and subsequent cognitive function in

patients with type 2 diabetes has also been investigated. In a large population study, hypoglycemic episodes that required hospitalization or a visit to the emergency department between 1980 and 2002 were associated with approximately double the risk of incident dementia after 2003 (6). However, since the study population did not undergo detailed tests of cognitive function prior to 2003, it is possible that those with incident dementia actually had mild cognitive dysfunction prior to experiencing the episode(s) of severe hypoglycemia. The possibility that mild cognitive dysfunction might increase the risk of experiencing severe hypoglycemia has been supported by analyses from the ACCORD study (48). In the ACCORD MIND (Memory IN Diabetes) study, in which cognitive function was assessed longitudinally, no difference was noted in the rate at which cognitive performance declined over time in subjects randomly assigned to the intensive versus the standard glucose arms despite the fact that they experienced three times as much hypoglycemia (49). Future investigation will need to address this question because the existing data are somewhat contradictory.

Impact of hypoglycemia on the elderly

Patients in the older age-groups are especially vulnerable to hypoglycemia. Epidemiological studies show that hypoglycemia is the most frequent metabolic complication experienced by older adults in the U.S. (50). Although severe hypoglycemia is common in older individuals with both type 1 and type 2 diabetes, patients with type 2 diabetes tend to have longer hospital stays and greater medical costs. The most significant predictors of this condition are advanced age, recent hospitalization, and polypharmacy, as shown in a study of Tennessee Medicare patients (51). Age-related declines in renal function and hepatic enzyme activity may interfere with the metabolism of sulfonylureas and insulin, thereby potentiating their hypoglycemic effects. The vulnerability of the elderly to severe hypoglycemia may be partially related to a progressive age-related decrease in β-adrenergic receptor function (52). Age-related impairment in counterregulatory hormone responses has been described in elderly patients with diabetes, especially with respect to glucagon and growth hormone (53). Symptoms of neuroglycopenia are more prevalent (54). With the prolonged duration of type 2 diabetes as is often seen in the elderly patient, the glucagon response to hypoglycemia is virtually absent (55). The intensification of glycemic control in the elderly patient is associated with an increased reduction in the plasma glucose thresholds for epinephrine release and for the appearance of hypoglycemia (56). As a result, changes in the level of glycemic control have a marked impact on the risk of developing hypoglycemia in the elderly.

Older adults with diabetes have a disproportionately high number of clinical complications and comorbidities, all of which can be exacerbated by and sometimes contribute to episodes of hypoglycemia. Older adults with diabetes are at much higher risk for the geriatric syndrome, which includes falls, incontinence, frailty, cognitive impairment, and depressive symptoms (57). The cognitive and executive dysfunction associated with the geriatric syndrome interferes with the patient's ability to perform self-care activities appropriately and follow the treatment regimen (58).

To minimize the risk of hypoglycemia in the elderly, careful education regarding the symptoms and treatment of hypoglycemia, with regular reinforcement, is extremely important because of the recognized gaps in the knowledge base of these individuals (59). In addition, it is important to assess the elderly for functional status as part of the overall clinical assessment in order to properly apply individualized glycemic control goals. Arbitrary short-acting insulin sliding scales, which are used much too often in long-term care facilities (60), should be avoided, and glyburide should be discontinued in favor of shorter-acting insulin secretagogues or medications that do not cause hypoglycemia. The recently published 2012 Beers list of prohibited medications in long-term care facilities specifically lists insulin sliding scales and glyburide as treatment modalities that should be avoided (61). Complex regimens requiring multiple decision points should be simplified, especially for patients with decreased functional status. In addition, caregivers and staff in long-term care facilities need to be educated on the causes and risks of hypoglycemia and the proper surveillance and treatment of this condition.

Impact of hypoglycemia on hospitalized patients

Persons with diabetes are three times more likely to be hospitalized than those without diabetes, and approximately 25% of hospitalized patients (including people without a history of diabetes) have hyperglycemia (62–65). Inpatient hyperglycemia has been associated with prolonged hospital length of stay and with numerous adverse outcomes including mortality (64,66–68). The understandable zeal to minimize the adverse consequences of inpatient hyperglycemia, together with the demonstration that intensive glycemic control improved outcomes in surgical intensive care unit (ICU) patients (69), led to widespread adoption of aggressive glucose management among ICU patients. However, subsequent studies showed that such aggressive lowering of glycemia in the ICU is not uniformly beneficial, markedly increases the risk of severe hypoglycemia, and may be associated with increased mortality (70–74).

The true incidence and prevalence of hypoglycemia among hospitalized patients with diabetes are not known precisely. In a retrospective study of 31,970 patients admitted to the general wards of an academic medical center in 2007, a total of 3,349 patients (10.5%) had at least one episode of hypoglycemia ($\leq$70 mg/dL) (75). In another review of 5,365 inpatients admitted to ICUs, 102 (1.9%) had at least one episode of severe hypoglycemia (<40 mg/dL) (76). The risk factors for inpatient hypoglycemia include older age, presence of comorbidities, diabetes, increasing number of antidiabetic agents, tight glycemic control, septic shock, renal insufficiency, mechanical ventilation, and severity of illness (75,76). With regard to impact, a retrospective analysis of 4,368 admissions involving 2,582 diabetic patients admitted to the general ward indicated that severe hypoglycemia ($\leq$50 mg/dL) was associated with increased length of stay and greater odds of inpatient death and death within 1 year of hospital discharge (77).

Impact of hypoglycemia during pregnancy

Maintaining blood glucose control in pregnancy as close to that of healthy pregnant women is important in minimizing the negative effects on the mother and the fetus (78). This is true for women with pregestational type 1 or type 2 diabetes, as well for those with gestational diabetes mellitus. Normal blood glucose levels during pregnancy are 20% lower than in nonpregnant women (79), making the definition and detection of hypoglycemia more challenging. For women with type 1 diabetes, severe hypoglycemia occurs 3–5 times more frequently in the first trimester and at a lower rate in the third trimester when compared with the incidence in the year preceding the pregnancy (80). Risk factors for severe hypoglycemia in pregnancy include a history of severe hypoglycemia in the preceding year, impaired hypoglycemia awareness, long duration of diabetes, low HbA$_{1c}$ in early pregnancy, fluctuating plasma glucose levels, and excessive use of supplementary insulin between meals. Surprisingly, nausea and vomiting during pregnancy did not appear to add significant risk. When pregnant and nonpregnant women are compared with CGM, mild hypoglycemia (defined by the authors as blood glucose <60 mg/dL) is more common in all pregnant women, but equally so regardless of whether or not they have diabetes, either pregestational or gestational (81). Hypoglycemia is generally without risk for the fetus as long as the mother avoids injury during the episode. For women with preexisting diabetes, insulin requirements rise throughout the pregnancy and then drop precipitously at the time of delivery of the placenta, requiring an abrupt reduction in insulin dosing to avoid postdelivery hypoglycemia. Breastfeeding may also be a risk factor for hypoglycemia in women with insulin-treated diabetes (82).

Impact of hypoglycemia on quality of life and activities of daily living

Hypoglycemia and the fear of hypoglycemia have a significant impact on quality-of-life measures in patients with both type 1 and type 2 diabetes (83). Nocturnal hypoglycemia in particular may impact one's sense of well-being on the following day because of its impact on sleep quantity and quality (84). Patients with recurrent hypoglycemia have been found to have chronic mood disorders including depression and anxiety (85,86), although it is hard to establish cause and effect between hypoglycemia and mood changes. Interpersonal relationships may suffer as a result of hypoglycemia in patients with diabetes. In-depth interviews of a small group of otherwise healthy young adults with type 1 diabetes revealed the presence of interpersonal conflict including fears of dependency and loss of control. These adults also reported difficulty talking about issues related to hypoglycemia with significant others (87). This difficulty may carry over to their work life, where hypoglycemia has been linked to reduced productivity (88). Hypoglycemia also impairs one's ability to drive a car (89–91), and many jurisdictions require documentation that severe hypoglycemia is not occurring before persons with diabetes are permitted to have a license to operate a motor vehicle (92). However, impaired awareness of hypoglycemia has not consistently been associated with an increased risk of car collisions (92–95).

What are the implications of hypoglycemia on treatment targets for patients with diabetes?

—The glycemic target established for any given patient should depend on the patient's age, life expectancy, comorbidities, preferences, and an assessment of how hypoglycemia might impact his or her life. This patient-centered approach requires that clinicians spend time developing an individualized treatment plan with each patient. For very young children, the risks of severe hypoglycemia on brain development may require a strategy that attempts to avoid hypoglycemia at all costs. For healthy adults with diabetes, a reasonable glycemic goal might be the lowest HbA_{1c} that does not cause severe hypoglycemia, preserves awareness of hypoglycemia, and results in an acceptable number of documented episodes of symptomatic hypoglycemia. With current therapies, a strategy that completely avoids hypoglycemia may not be possible in patients with type 1 diabetes who strive to minimize their risks of developing the microvascular complications of the disease. However, glycemic goals might reasonably be relaxed in patients with long-standing type 1 diabetes and advanced complications or in those who are free of complications but have a limited life expectancy because of another disease process. In such patients, the glycemic goal could be to achieve glucose levels sufficiently low to prevent symptoms of hyperglycemia.

For patients with type 2 diabetes, the risk of hypoglycemia depends on the medications used (96). Early in the course of the disease, most patients are treated with lifestyle changes and metformin, neither of which causes hypoglycemia. Therefore, an HbA_{1c} of <7% is appropriate for many patients with recent-onset type 2 diabetes. As the disease progresses, it is likely that medications that increase the risk of hypoglycemia will be added. This, plus the presence of complications or comorbidities that limit life expectancy, means that glycemic goals may

need to be less aggressive. While the benefits of achieving an HbA_{1c} of <7% may continue to be advocated for patients with type 2 diabetes at risk for microvascular complications and with sufficient life expectancy, less aggressive targets may be appropriate in those with known cardiovascular disease, extensive comorbidities, or limited life expectancy.

Older individuals with gait imbalance and frailty may experience a life-changing injury if they fall during a hypoglycemia episode, so avoiding hypoglycemia is paramount in such patients. Patients with cognitive dysfunction may have difficulty adhering to a complicated treatment strategy designed to achieve a low HbA_{1c} (48). Such patients will benefit from a simplification of the treatment strategy with a goal to prevent hypoglycemia as much as possible. Furthermore, the benefits of aggressive glycemic therapy in those affected are unclear.

What strategies are known to prevent hypoglycemia, and what are the clinical recommendations for those at risk for hypoglycemia?

—Recurrent hypoglycemia increases the risk of severe hypoglycemia and the development of hypoglycemia unawareness and HAAF. Effective approaches known to decrease the risk of iatrogenic hypoglycemia include patient education, dietary and exercise modifications, medication adjustment, careful glucose monitoring by the patient, and conscientious surveillance by the clinician.

Patient education
There is limited research related to the influence of self-management education on the incidence or prevention of hypoglycemia. However, there is clear evidence that diabetes education improves patient outcomes (97–99). As part of the educational plan, the individual with diabetes and his or her domestic companions need to recognize the symptoms of hypoglycemia and be able to treat a hypoglycemic episode properly with oral carbohydrates or glucagon. Hypoglycemia, including its risk factors and remediation, should be discussed routinely with patients receiving treatment with insulin or sulfonylurea/glinide drugs, especially those with a history of recurrent hypoglycemia or impaired awareness of hypoglycemia. In addition, patients must understand how their medications work so they can minimize the risk of

hypoglycemia. Care should be taken to educate patients on the typical pharmacokinetics of these medications. When evaluating a patient's report of hypoglycemia, it is important to adopt interviewing approaches that guide the patient to a correct identification of the precipitating factors of the episodes of hypoglycemia. Such a heuristic review of likely factors (skipped or inadequate meal, unusual exertion, alcohol ingestion, insulin dosage mishaps, etc.) in the period prior to the event can deepen the patient's appreciation of the behavioral factors that predispose to hypoglycemia.

There is convincing evidence that formal training programs that teach patients to replace insulin "physiologically" by giving background and mealtime/correction doses of insulin can reduce the risk of severe hypoglycemia. The Insulin Treatment and Training programs developed by Mühlhauser and Berger (100) have reported improved glycemic control comparable with DCCT while reducing the rates of severe hypoglycemia (101,102). These programs have been successfully delivered in other settings (103,104) with comparable reductions in hypoglycemic risk (105). Patients with frequent hypoglycemia may also benefit from enrollment in a blood glucose awareness training program. In such a program, patients and their relatives are trained to recognize subtle cues and early neuroglycopenic indicators of evolving hypoglycemia and respond to them before the occurrence of disabling hypoglycemia (106,107).

Dietary intervention
Patients with diabetes need to recognize which foods contain carbohydrates and understand how the carbohydrates in their diet affect blood glucose. To avoid hypoglycemia, patients on long-acting secretagogues and fixed insulin regimens must be encouraged to follow a predictable meal plan. Patients on more flexible insulin regimens must know that prandial insulin injections should be coupled to meal times. Dissociated meal and insulin injection patterns lead to wide fluctuations in plasma glucose levels. Patients on any hypoglycemia-inducing medication should also be instructed to carry carbohydrates with them at all times to treat hypoglycemia.

The best bedtime snack to prevent overnight hypoglycemia in patients with type 1 diabetes has been investigated without clear consensus (108–112). These conflicting reports suggest that the administration of bedtime snacks may need to be individualized and be part of a comprehensive strategy (balanced diet, patient education, optimized drug regimens, and physical activity counseling) for the prevention of nocturnal hypoglycemia.

Exercise management
Physical activity increases glucose utilization, which increases the risk of hypoglycemia. The risk factors for exertional hypoglycemia include prolonged exercise duration, unaccustomed exercise intensity, and inadequate energy supply in relation to ambient insulinemia (113,114). Postexertional hypoglycemia can be prevented or minimized by careful glucose monitoring before and after exercise and taking appropriate preemptive actions. Preexercise snacks should be ingested if blood glucose values indicate falling glucose levels. Patients with diabetes should carry readily absorbable carbohydrates when embarking on exercise, including sporadic house or yard work. Because of the kinetics of rapid-acting and intermediate-acting insulin, it may be prudent to empirically adjust insulin doses on the days of planned exercise, especially in patients with well-controlled diabetes with a history of exercise-related hypoglycemia.

Medication adjustment
Hypoglycemic episodes that are not readily explained by conventional factors (skipped or irregular meals, unaccustomed exercise, alcohol ingestion, etc.) may be due to excessive doses of drugs used to treat diabetes. A thorough review of blood glucose patterns may suggest vulnerable periods of the day that mandate adjustments to the current antidiabetes regimen. Such adjustments may include substitution of rapid-acting insulin (lispro, aspart, glulisine) for regular insulin, or basal insulin glargine or detemir for NPH, to decrease the risk of hypoglycemia. Continuous subcutaneous insulin infusion offers great flexibility for adjusting the doses and administration pattern of insulin to counteract iatrogenic hypoglycemia (115). For patients with type 2 diabetes, sulfonylureas are the oral agents that pose the greatest risk for iatrogenic hypoglycemia and substitution with other classes of oral agents or even glucagon-like peptide 1 analogs should be considered in the

event of troublesome hypoglycemia (96). Interestingly, successful transplantation of whole pancreata or isolated pancreatic islet cells in patients with type 1 diabetes (116–118) results in marked improvements in glycemic control and near abolition of iatrogenic hypoglycemia.

Patients who develop hypoglycemia unawareness do so because of frequent and recurrent hypoglycemia. To avoid such frequent hypoglycemia, adjustments in the treatment regimen that scrupulously avoid hypoglycemia are necessary (Table 1). In published studies, this has required frequent (almost daily) contact between clinician and patient, and adjustments to caloric intake and insulin regimen based on blood glucose values (10,119,120). With this approach, restoration of autonomic symptoms of hypoglycemia occurred within 2 weeks, and complete reversal of hypoglycemia unawareness was achieved by 3 months. In some but not all reports, the recovery of symptoms is accompanied by the improvement in epinephrine secretion (32,33,120,121). The return of hypoglycemic symptom awareness was associated with a modest increase (~0.5%)

in HbA$_{1c}$ values (33), but others have reported no loss of glycemic control (32,34).

Glucose monitoring
Glucose monitoring is essential in managing patients at risk for hypoglycemia. Patients treated with insulin, sulfonylureas, or glinides should check their blood glucose whenever they develop the symptoms of hypoglycemia in order to confirm that they must ingest carbohydrates to treat the symptoms and collect information that can be used by the clinician to adjust the therapeutic regimen to avoid future hypoglycemia. Patients on basal-bolus insulin therapy should check their blood glucose before each meal and figure this value into the calculation of the dose of rapid-acting insulin to take at that time. Such care in dosing will likely reduce the risk of hypoglycemia.

Recent technological developments have provided patients with new tools for glucose monitoring. Real-time CGM, by virtue of its ability to display the direction and rate of change, provides helpful information to the wearer leading to proactive measures to avoid hypoglycemia, e.g., when to think about having a

Table 1—*Approach to restore recognition of hypoglycemia in patients with HAAF*

Monitoring and goal setting
Encourage SMBG before meals, at bedtime, and during suggestive symptoms
Encourage SMBG between 2 A.M. and 5 A.M. at least three times weekly
Set targets for preprandial blood glucose levels at 100–150 mg/dL
Patient education
Educate patients on hypoglycemic symptoms and the role of recurrent hypoglycemia in the etiology of hypoglycemia unawareness
Reassure patients that hypoglycemia unawareness is reversible through avoidance of hypoglycemia
Train patients to recognize and respond promptly to early neuroglycopenic symptoms
Dietary intervention
Ensure adequate caloric intake
Recommend interprandial and bedtime snacks
Ensure access to readily absorbable carbohydrates at all times
Consider moderate amounts of xanthine beverages, if tolerated
Exercise counseling
Encourage SMBG before, during, and after exercise
Advise preexercise caloric intake if blood glucose is <140 mg/dL
Advise consumption of additional calories during and after exercise if blood glucose is <140 mg/dL
Medication adjustment
Adjust insulin regimen to achieve and maintain target glucose levels
Use rapid-acting insulin analogs (lispro, aspart, glulisine) to decrease the risk of interprandial hypoglycemia
Use basal insulin analogs (glargine, detemir) to decrease the risk of nocturnal hypoglycemia
Consider a continuous subcutaneous insulin infusion pump, as appropriate
Consider a CGM device

Adapted from reference 125.

snack or suspending insulin delivery on a pump. The CGM's audible and/or vibratory alarms may be particularly helpful in avoiding severe hypoglycemia at night and restoring hypoglycemic awareness. With the low-glucose alarms set at 108 mg/dL, 4 weeks of real-time CGM use restored the epinephrine response and improved adrenergic symptoms during a hyperinsulinemic hypoglycemic clamp in a small group of adolescents with type 1 diabetes and hypoglycemic unawareness (122).

The artificial pancreas, which couples a CGM to an insulin pump through sophisticated predictive algorithms, holds out the promise of completely eliminating hypoglycemia. Several internationally collaborative groups are working on various approaches to the artificial pancreas. The first step in this direction is the low-glucose suspend pump that is available in Europe and currently in clinical trials in the U.S. This device shuts off insulin delivery for up to 2 h once the interstitial glucose concentration reaches a preset threshold and reduces the duration of nocturnal hypoglycemia (123).

Clinical surveillance

Clinicians and educators must assess the risk of hypoglycemia at every visit with patients treated with insulin and insulin secretagogues. An efficient way to begin this assessment might be to have the patient complete the questionnaire shown in Table 2 while in the waiting room. Review of the completed questionnaire will help the clinician learn how often the patient is experiencing symptomatic and asymptomatic hypoglycemia, ensure the patient is aware of how to appropriately treat hypoglycemia, and remind both parties of the risks associated with driving while hypoglycemic. To ensure that hypoglycemia has been adequately addressed during a visit, providers may want to use the Hypoglycemia Provider Checklist (Table 3).

A careful review of the glucose log collected by the patient should also be done at each visit. The date, approximate time, and circumstances surrounding recent episodes of hypoglycemia should be noted, together with information regarding the awareness of the warning symptoms of hypoglycemia. A reliable history of impaired autonomic responses (tremulousness, sweating, palpitations, and hunger) during hypoglycemia may be the most practical

approach to making the diagnosis of hypoglycemia unawareness. If symptoms are absent or if frequent episodes of recurrent hypoglycemia occur within hours to days of each other, it is likely that the patient has HAAF. Other historical clues such as experiencing more than one episode of severe hypoglycemia that required the assistance of another over the preceding year or a family re-

port that they are recognizing more frequent episodes of hypoglycemia may also provide clues that the patient has developed hypoglycemia unawareness. A self-reported history of impaired or absent perception of autonomic symptoms during hypoglycemia correlates strongly with laboratory confirmation of hypoglycemia unawareness (33,121,124,125).

Table 2—Hypoglycemia Patient Questionnaire

Name _____

First　　　　　　　　Middle　　　　　　　　Last

Today's date _____

1. To what extent can you tell by your symptoms that your blood glucose is LOW?
____ Never ____ Rarely ____ Sometimes ____ Often ____ Always

2. In a typical week, how many times will your blood glucose go below 70 mg/dL?
_____ a week

3. When your blood glucose goes below 70 mg/dL, what is the usual reason for this?
_____

4. How many times have you had a severe hypoglycemic episode (where you needed someone's help and were unable to treat yourself)?
Since the last visit _____ times
In the last year _____ times

5. How many times have you had a moderate hypoglycemic episode (where you could not think clearly, properly control your body, had to stop what you were doing, but you were still able to treat yourself)?
Since the last visit _____ times
In the last year _____ times

6. How often do you carry a snack or glucose tablets (or gel) with you to treat low blood glucose? Check one of the following:
Never ___ Rarely ___ Sometimes___ Often___ Almost always___

7. How LOW does your blood glucose need to go before you think you should treat it?
Less than _____mg/dL

8. What and how much food or drink do you usually treat low blood glucose with?
_____

9. Do you check your blood glucose before driving? Check one of the following:
Yes, always___ Yes, sometimes ___ No___

10. How LOW does your blood glucose need to go before you think you should not drive?
_____mg/dL

11. How many times have you had your blood glucose below 70 mg/dL while driving?
Since the last visit _____ times
In the last year _____ times

12. If you take insulin, do you have a glucagon emergency kit?
Yes___/ No ___

13. Does a spouse, relative, or other person close to you know how to administer glucagon?
Yes___/ No ___

Table 3—*Hypoglycemia Provider Checklist*

Name _____

　　　First　　　　　　　　　Middle　　　　　　　　　Last

Today's date _____

1. __ Reviewed the Hypoglycemia Patient Questionnaire
2. __ Questioned the patient about circumstances surrounding severe or moderate hypoglycemia
3. __ Discussed strategies to avoid hypoglycemia with the patient
4. __ Made medication changes where clinically appropriate
5. __ Recommended carrying snack and/or glucose tablets where appropriate and provided instructions for how to use them (take 15 g glucose, wait 15 min, and remeasure blood glucose; repeat if hypoglycemia persists). A 1-page patient handout on treating hypoglycemia is available at http://clinical.diabetesjournals.org/content/30/1/38
6. __ Prescribed glucagon if appropriate

What are the current knowledge gaps in our understanding of hypoglycemia, and what research is necessary to fill these gaps?

—Since the publication of the previous report from the Workgroup on Hypoglycemia in 2005 (1), much has been learned about the impact of hypoglycemia on patient outcomes. However, hypoglycemia continues to cause considerable morbidity and even mortality in patients with diabetes. If patients are to benefit from the reduction in microvascular complications that follows from achieving near-normal levels of glycemia, additional research will be necessary to prevent them from experiencing hypoglycemia and HAAF. First, new surveillance methods that provide consistent ways of reporting hypoglycemia must be developed so that the impact of any intervention to prevent and treat hypoglycemia can be fully assessed. Greater attention must be focused on understanding which patients are most at risk for hypoglycemia and on developing new educational strategies that effectively reduce the number of episodes experienced by at-risk patients. New therapies that do not cause hypoglycemia, including an artificial pancreas, need to be developed for both type 1 and type 2 diabetes. The technologies used to monitor blood glucose must become more accurate, more reliable, easier to use, and less expensive. The mechanisms that render patients unable to increase glucagon secretion in response to hypoglycemia and that are responsible for the development of HAAF must be identified so strategies can be developed to ensure that patients always experience early warning signs of impending neuroglycopenia. The impact of hypoglycemia on short-term outcomes such as mortality and long-term outcomes such as cognitive dysfunction need to be better defined, and the mechanisms for these associations need to be understood. Focused research in these priority areas will address our knowledge gaps about hypoglycemia and ultimately reduce the impact of iatrogenic hypoglycemia on patients with diabetes.

Acknowledgments—The workgroup meeting was supported by educational grants to the American Diabetes Association from Lilly USA, LLC and Novo Nordisk and sponsorship to the American Diabetes Association from Sanofi. The sponsors had no input into the development of or content of the report. No other potential conflicts of interest relevant to this article were reported.

The workgroup members thank Stephanie Kutler and Meredith Dyer of The Endocrine Society and Sue Kirkman, MD, of the American Diabetes Association for staff support.

References

1. American Diabetes Association Workgroup on Hypoglycemia. Defining and reporting hypoglycemia in diabetes: a report from the American Diabetes Association Workgroup on Hypoglycemia. Diabetes Care 2005;28:1245–1249
2. Cryer PE, Axelrod L, Grossman AB, et al.; Endocrine Society. Evaluation and management of adult hypoglycemic disorders: an Endocrine Society Clinical Practice Guideline. J Clin Endocrinol Metab 2009; 94:709–728
3. Duckworth W, Abraira C, Moritz T, et al.; VADT Investigators. Glucose control and vascular complications in veterans with type 2 diabetes. N Engl J Med 2009;360:129–139
4. Gerstein HC, Miller ME, Byington RP, et al.; Action to Control Cardiovascular Risk in Diabetes Study Group. Effects of intensive glucose lowering in type 2 diabetes. N Engl J Med 2008;358:2545–2559
5. Patel A, MacMahon S, Chalmers J, et al.; ADVANCE Collaborative Group. Intensive blood glucose control and vascular outcomes in patients with type 2 diabetes. N Engl J Med 2008;358:2560–2572
6. Whitmer RA, Karter AJ, Yaffe K, Quesenberry CP, Jr, Selby JV. Hypoglycemic episodes and risk of dementia in older patients with type 2 diabetes mellitus. JAMA 2009; 301:1565–1572
7. Perantie DC, Lim A, Wu J, et al. Effects of prior hypoglycemia and hyperglycemia on cognition in children with type 1 diabetes mellitus. Pediatr Diabetes 2008;9: 87–95
8. Perantie DC, Koller JM, Weaver PM, et al. Prospectively determined impact of type 1 diabetes on brain volume during development. Diabetes 2011;60:3006–3014
9. Amiel SA, Sherwin RS, Simonson DC, Tamborlane WV. Effect of intensive insulin therapy on glycemic thresholds for counterregulatory hormone release. Diabetes 1988;37:901–907
10. Dagogo-Jack SE, Craft S, Cryer PE. Hypoglycemia-associated autonomic failure in insulin-dependent diabetes mellitus. Recent antecedent hypoglycemia reduces autonomic responses to, symptoms of, and defense against subsequent hypoglycemia. J Clin Invest 1993;91:819–828
11. Davis SN, Shavers C, Mosqueda-Garcia R, Costa F. Effects of differing antecedent hypoglycemia on subsequent counterregulation in normal humans. Diabetes 1997;46:1328–1335
12. Heller SR, Cryer PE. Reduced neuroendocrine and symptomatic responses to subsequent hypoglycemia after 1 episode of hypoglycemia in nondiabetic humans. Diabetes 1991;40:223–226
13. Boyle PJ, Schwartz NS, Shah SD, Clutter WE, Cryer PE. Plasma glucose concentrations at the onset of hypoglycemic symptoms in patients with poorly controlled diabetes and in nondiabetics. N Engl J Med 1988;318:1487–1492
14. Cryer PE. Preventing hypoglycaemia: what is the appropriate glucose alert value? Diabetologia 2009;52:35–37
15. Cryer P. The prevention and correction of hypoglycemia. In *Handbook of Physiology: Section 7, The Endocrine System, Volume II, The Endocrine Pancreas and Regulation of Metabolism*. Jefferson LS, Cherring AD, Eds. New York, Oxford University Press, 2001, p. 1057–1092
16. Freckmann G, Baumstark A, Jendrike N, et al. System accuracy evaluation of 27 blood glucose monitoring systems

according to DIN EN ISO 15197. Diabetes Technol Ther 2010;12:221–231

17. Klonoff DC, Buckingham B, Christiansen JS, et al.; Endocrine Society. Continuous glucose monitoring: an Endocrine Society Clinical Practice Guideline. J Clin Endocrinol Metab 2011;96:2968–2979

18. Karon BS, Boyd JC, Klee GG. Glucose meter performance criteria for tight glycemic control estimated by simulation modeling. Clin Chem 2010;56:1091–1097

19. Clarke WL, Cox D, Gonder-Frederick LA, Carter W, Pohl SL. Evaluating clinical accuracy of systems for self-monitoring of blood glucose. Diabetes Care 1987;10:622–628

20. Parkes JL, Slatin SL, Pardo S, Ginsberg BH. A new consensus error grid to evaluate the clinical significance of inaccuracies in the measurement of blood glucose. Diabetes Care 2000;23:1143–1148

21. DexCom Seven Plus Continuous Glucose Monitoring System User's Guide [article online], 2012. Available from http://dexcom.com/sites/dexcom.com/files/seven-plus/docs/SEVEN_Plus_Users_Guide.pdf and http://dexcom.com/sites/dexcom.com/files/LBL-011119_Rev_07_User's_Guide,_G4_US.pdf. Accessed 9 April 2012

22. Medtronic Guardian Real-Time Continuous Glucose Monitoring System User Guide [article online], 2012. Available from http://www.medtronicdiabetes.com/support/download-library/user-guides. Accessed 29 April 2012

23. Heller SR, Choudhary P, Davies C, et al.; UK Hypoglycaemia Study Group. Risk of hypoglycaemia in types 1 and 2 diabetes: effects of treatment modalities and their duration. Diabetologia 2007;50:1140–1147

24. Donnelly LA, Morris AD, Frier BM, et al.; DARTS/MEMO Collaboration. Frequency and predictors of hypoglycaemia in Type 1 and insulin-treated Type 2 diabetes: a population-based study. Diabet Med 2005;22:749–755

25. Cryer PE. The barrier of hypoglycemia in diabetes. Diabetes 2008;57:3169–3176

26. Cryer PE. Death during intensive glycemic therapy of diabetes: mechanisms and implications. Am J Med 2011;124:993–996

27. Patterson CC, Dahlquist G, Harjutsalo V, et al. Early mortality in EURODIAB population-based cohorts of type 1 diabetes diagnosed in childhood since 1989. Diabetologia 2007;50:2439–2442

28. Jacobson AM, Musen G, Ryan CM, et al.; Diabetes Control and Complications Trial/Epidemiology of Diabetes Interventions and Complications Study Research Group. Long-term effect of diabetes and its treatment on cognitive function. N Engl J Med 2007;356:1842–1852

29. Feltbower RG, Bodansky HJ, Patterson CC, et al. Acute complications and drug misuse are important causes of death for children and young adults with type 1 diabetes: results from the Yorkshire Register of Diabetes in Children and Young Adults. Diabetes Care 2008;31:922–926

30. Skrivarhaug T, Bangstad HJ, Stene LC, Sandvik L, Hanssen KF, Joner G. Long-term mortality in a nationwide cohort of childhood-onset type 1 diabetic patients in Norway. Diabetologia 2006;49:298–305

31. Tanenberg RJ, Newton CA, Drake AJ. Confirmation of hypoglycemia in the "dead-in-bed" syndrome, as captured by a retrospective continuous glucose monitoring system. Endocr Pract 2010;16:244–248

32. Cranston I, Lomas J, Maran A, Macdonald I, Amiel SA. Restoration of hypoglycaemia awareness in patients with long-duration insulin-dependent diabetes. Lancet 1994;344:283–287

33. Dagogo-Jack S, Rattarasarn C, Cryer PE. Reversal of hypoglycemia unawareness, but not defective glucose counterregulation, in IDDM. Diabetes 1994;43:1426–1434

34. Fanelli C, Pampanelli S, Epifano L, et al. Long-term recovery from unawareness, deficient counterregulation and lack of cognitive dysfunction during hypoglycaemia, following institution of rational, intensive insulin therapy in IDDM. Diabetologia 1994;37:1265–1276

35. White NH, Skor DA, Cryer PE, Levandoski LA, Bier DM, Santiago JV. Identification of type I diabetic patients at increased risk for hypoglycemia during intensive therapy. N Engl J Med 1983;308:485–491

36. Bolli GB, De Feo P, De Cosmo S, et al. A reliable and reproducible test for adequate glucose counterregulation in type I diabetes mellitus. Diabetes 1984;33:732–737

37. Zammitt NN, Warren RE, Deary IJ, Frier BM. Delayed recovery of cognitive function following hypoglycemia in adults with type 1 diabetes: effect of impaired awareness of hypoglycemia. Diabetes 2008;57:732–736

38. Arbelaez AM, Powers WJ, Videen TO, Price JL, Cryer PE. Attenuation of counterregulatory responses to recurrent hypoglycemia by active thalamic inhibition: a mechanism for hypoglycemia-associated autonomic failure. Diabetes 2008;57:470–475

39. Jaferi A, Nowak N, Bhatnagar S. Negative feedback functions in chronically stressed rats: role of the posterior paraventricular thalamus. Physiol Behav 2003;78:365–373

40. Puente EC, Silverstein J, Bree AJ, et al. Recurrent moderate hypoglycemia ameliorates brain damage and cognitive dysfunction induced by severe hypoglycemia. Diabetes 2010;59:1055–1062

41. Reno CM, Tanoli T, Puente EC, et al. Deaths due to severe hypoglycemia are exacerbated by diabetes and ameliorated by hypoglycemic pre-conditioning (Abstract). Diabetes 2011;60(Suppl. 1):A81

42. Clarke W, Jones T, Rewers A, Dunger D, Klingensmith GJ. Assessment and management of hypoglycemia in children and adolescents with diabetes. Pediatr Diabetes 2009;10(Suppl . 12):134–145

43. Silverstein J, Klingensmith G, Copeland K, et al.; American Diabetes Association. Care of children and adolescents with type 1 diabetes: a statement of the American Diabetes Association. Diabetes Care 2005;28:186–212

44. Hannonen R, Tupola S, Ahonen T, Riikonen R. Neurocognitive functioning in children with type-1 diabetes with and without episodes of severe hypoglycaemia. Dev Med Child Neurol 2003;45:262–268

45. Bolo NR, Musen G, Jacobson AM, et al. Brain activation during working memory is altered in patients with type 1 diabetes during hypoglycemia. Diabetes 2011;60:3256–3264

46. Bonds DE, Miller ME, Bergenstal RM, et al. The association between symptomatic, severe hypoglycaemia and mortality in type 2 diabetes: retrospective epidemiological analysis of the ACCORD study. BMJ 2010;340:b4909

47. Zoungas S, Patel A, Chalmers J, et al.; ADVANCE Collaborative Group. Severe hypoglycemia and risks of vascular events and death. N Engl J Med 2010;363:1410–1418

48. Punthakee Z, Miller ME, Launer LJ, et al.; ACCORD Group of Investigators; ACCORD-MIND Investigators. Poor cognitive function and risk of severe hypoglycemia in type 2 diabetes: post hoc epidemiologic analysis of the ACCORD trial. Diabetes Care 2012;35:787–793

49. Launer LJ, Miller ME, Williamson JD, et al.; ACCORD MIND Investigators. Effects of intensive glucose lowering on brain structure and function in people with type 2 diabetes (ACCORD MIND): a randomised open-label substudy. Lancet Neurol 2011;10:969–977

50. Bertoni AG, Krop JS, Anderson GF, Brancati FL. Diabetes-related morbidity and mortality in a national sample of U.S. elders. Diabetes Care 2002;25:471–475

51. Shorr RI, Ray WA, Daugherty JR, Griffin MR. Incidence and risk factors for serious hypoglycemia in older persons using insulin or sulfonylureas. Arch Intern Med 1997;157:1681–1686

52. Heinsimer JA, Lefkowitz RJ. The impact of aging on adrenergic receptor function:

clinical and biochemical aspects. J Am Geriatr Soc 1985;33:184–188

53. Meneilly GS, Cheung E, Tuokko H. Counterregulatory hormone responses to hypoglycemia in the elderly patient with diabetes. Diabetes 1994;43:403–410

54. Sinclair AJ, Paolisso G, Castro M, Bourdel-Marchasson I, Gadsby R, Rodriguez Mañas L; European Diabetes Working Party for Older People. European Diabetes Working Party for Older People 2011 clinical guidelines for type 2 diabetes mellitus. Executive summary. Diabetes Metab 2011;37(Suppl. 3):S27–S38

55. Segel SA, Paramore DS, Cryer PE. Hypoglycemia-associated autonomic failure in advanced type 2 diabetes. Diabetes 2002;51:724–733

56. Burge MR, Sobhy TA, Qualls CR, Schade DS. Effect of short-term glucose control on glycemic thresholds for epinephrine and hypoglycemic symptoms. J Clin Endocrinol Metab 2001;86:5471–5478

57. Bruce DG, Casey GP, Grange V, et al. Cognitive impairment, physical disability and depressive symptoms in older diabetic patients: the Fremantle Cognition in Diabetes Study. Diabetes Res Clin Pract 2003;61:59–67

58. Sinclair AJ, Conroy SP, Bayer AJ. Impact of diabetes on physical function in older people. Diabetes Care 2008;31:233–235

59. Strachan MWJ, Deary IJ, Ewing FME, Frier BM. Is type II diabetes associated with an increased risk of cognitive dysfunction? A critical review of published studies. Diabetes Care 1997;20:438–445

60. Pandya N, Thompson S, Sambamoorthi U. The prevalence and persistence of sliding scale insulin use among newly admitted elderly nursing home residents with diabetes mellitus. J Am Med Dir Assoc 2008;9:663–669

61. American Geriatrics Society 2012 Beers Criteria Update Expert Panel. American Geriatrics Society updated Beers Criteria for potentially inappropriate medication use in older adults. J Am Geriatr Soc 2012;60:616–631

62. American Diabetes Association. Economic costs of diabetes in the U.S. in 2007. Diabetes Care 2008;31:596–615

63. Aubert RE, Geiss L, Ballard DJ, Cocanougher B, Herman W. *Diabetes-Related Hospitalization and Hospital Utilization*. Bethesda, MD, National Institutes of Health, 1995

64. Clement S, Braithwaite SS, Magee MF, et al.; American Diabetes Association Diabetes in Hospitals Writing Committee. Management of diabetes and hyperglycemia in hospitals. Diabetes Care 2004;27:553–591

65. Umpierrez GE, Isaacs SD, Bazargan N, You X, Thaler LM, Kitabchi AE. Hyperglycemia: an independent marker of in-hospital mortality in patients with undiagnosed diabetes. J Clin Endocrinol Metab 2002;87:978–982

66. Bucerius J, Gummert JF, Walther T, et al. Impact of diabetes mellitus on cardiac surgery outcome. Thorac Cardiovasc Surg 2003;51:11–16

67. Capes SE, Hunt D, Malmberg K, Pathak P, Gerstein HC. Stress hyperglycemia and prognosis of stroke in nondiabetic and diabetic patients: a systematic overview. Stroke 2001;32:2426–2432

68. McCowen KC, Malhotra A, Bistrian BR. Stress-induced hyperglycemia. Crit Care Clin 2001;17:107–124

69. van den Berghe G, Wouters P, Weekers F, et al. Intensive insulin therapy in critically ill patients. N Engl J Med 2001;345:1359–1367

70. Brunkhorst FM, Engel C, Bloos F, et al.; German Competence Network Sepsis (SepNet). Intensive insulin therapy and pentastarch resuscitation in severe sepsis. N Engl J Med 2008;358:125–139

71. Finfer S, Chittock DR, Su SY, et al.; NICE-SUGAR Study Investigators. Intensive versus conventional glucose control in critically ill patients. N Engl J Med 2009;360:1283–1297

72. Griesdale DE, de Souza RJ, van Dam RM, et al. Intensive insulin therapy and mortality among critically ill patients: a meta-analysis including NICE-SUGAR study data. CMAJ 2009;180:821–827

73. Van den Berghe G, Wilmer A, Hermans G, et al. Intensive insulin therapy in the medical ICU. N Engl J Med 2006;354:449–461

74. Wiener RS, Wiener DC, Larson RJ. Benefits and risks of tight glucose control in critically ill adults: a meta-analysis. JAMA 2008;300:933–944

75. Boucai L, Southern WN, Zonszein J. Hypoglycemia-associated mortality is not drug-associated but linked to comorbidities. Am J Med 2011;124:1028–1035

76. Krinsley JS, Grover A. Severe hypoglycemia in critically ill patients: risk factors and outcomes. Crit Care Med 2007;35:2262–2267

77. Turchin A, Matheny ME, Shubina M, Scanlon JV, Greenwood B, Pendergrass ML. Hypoglycemia and clinical outcomes in patients with diabetes hospitalized in the general ward. Diabetes Care 2009;32:1153–1157

78. Metzger BE, Lowe LP, Dyer AR, et al.; HAPO Study Cooperative Research Group. Hyperglycemia and adverse pregnancy outcomes. N Engl J Med 2008;358:1991–2002

79. Yogev Y, Ben-Haroush A, Chen R, Rosenn B, Hod M, Langer O. Diurnal glycemic profile in obese and normal weight nondiabetic pregnant women. Am J Obstet Gynecol 2004;191:949–953

80. Ringholm L, Pedersen-Bjergaard U, Thorsteinsson B, Damm P, Mathiesen ER. Hypoglycaemia during pregnancy in women with Type 1 diabetes. Diabet Med 2012;29:558–566

81. Mazze R, Yogev Y, Langer O. Measuring glucose exposure and variability using continuous glucose monitoring in normal and abnormal glucose metabolism in pregnancy. J Matern Fetal Neonatal Med 2012;25:1171–1175

82. Riviello C, Mello G, Jovanovic LG. Breastfeeding and the basal insulin requirement in type 1 diabetic women. Endocr Pract 2009;15:187–193

83. Barendse S, Singh H, Frier BM, Speight J. The impact of hypoglycaemia on quality of life and related patient-reported outcomes in type 2 diabetes: a narrative review. Diabet Med 2012;29:293–302

84. King P, Kong MF, Parkin H, Macdonald IA, Tattersall RB. Well-being, cerebral function, and physical fatigue after nocturnal hypoglycemia in IDDM. Diabetes Care 1998;21:341–345

85. Gold AE, Deary IJ, Frier BM. Hypoglycaemia and non-cognitive aspects of psychological function in insulin-dependent (type 1) diabetes mellitus (IDDM). Diabet Med 1997;14:111–118

86. Strachan MW, Deary IJ, Ewing FM, Frier BM. Recovery of cognitive function and mood after severe hypoglycemia in adults with insulin-treated diabetes. Diabetes Care 2000;23:305–312

87. Ritholz MD, Jacobson AM. Living with hypoglycemia. J Gen Intern Med 1998;13:799–804

88. Davis RE, Morrissey M, Peters JR, Wittrup-Jensen K, Kennedy-Martin T, Currie CJ. Impact of hypoglycaemia on quality of life and productivity in type 1 and type 2 diabetes. Curr Med Res Opin 2005;21:1477–1483

89. Cox DJ, Gonder-Frederick L, Clarke W. Driving decrements in type I diabetes during moderate hypoglycemia. Diabetes 1993;42:239–243

90. Cox DJ, Gonder-Frederick LA, Kovatchev BP, Julian DM, Clarke WL. Progressive hypoglycemia's impact on driving simulation performance: occurrence, awareness and correction. Diabetes Care 2000;23:163–170

91. Quillian WC, Cox DJ, Gonder-Frederick LA, Driesen NR, Clarke WL. Reliability of driving performance during moderate hypoglycemia in adults with IDDM. Diabetes Care 1994;17:1367–1368

92. The DCCT Research Group. Epidemiology of severe hypoglycemia in the Diabetes Control and Complications Trial. Am J Med 1991;90:450–459

93. Cox DJ, Kovatchev B, Vandecar K, Gonder-Frederick L, Ritterband L, Clarke W. Hypoglycemia preceding fatal car collisions. Diabetes Care 2006;29:467–468

94. Eadington DW, Frier BM. Type 1 diabetes and driving experience: an eight-year

cohort study. Diabet Med 1989;6:137–141

95. Lave LB, Songer TJ, LaPorte RE. Should persons with diabetes be licensed to drive trucks?—Risk management. Risk Anal 1993;13:327–334

96. Inzucchi SE, Bergenstal RM, Buse JB, et al. Management of hyperglycemia in type 2 diabetes: a patient-centered approach. Position statement of the American Diabetes Association (ADA) and the European Association for the Study of Diabetes (EASD). Diabetes Care 2012;35:1364–1379

97. Deakin T, McShane CE, Cade JE, Williams RD. Group based training for self-management strategies in people with type 2 diabetes mellitus. Cochrane Database Syst Rev 2005;2:CD003417

98. Norris SL, Engelgau MM, Narayan KM. Effectiveness of self-management training in type 2 diabetes: a systematic review of randomized controlled trials. Diabetes Care 2001;24:561–587

99. Norris SL, Lau J, Smith SJ, Schmid CH, Engelgau MM. Self-management education for adults with type 2 diabetes: a meta-analysis of the effect on glycemic control. Diabetes Care 2002;25:1159–1171

100. Mühlhauser I, Berger M. Patient education—evaluation of a complex intervention. Diabetologia 2002;45:1723–1733

101. Bott S, Bott U, Berger M, Mühlhauser I. Intensified insulin therapy and the risk of severe hypoglycaemia. Diabetologia 1997;40:926–932

102. Sämann A, Mühlhauser I, Bender R, Kloos Ch, Müller UA. Glycaemic control and severe hypoglycaemia following training in flexible, intensive insulin therapy to enable dietary freedom in people with type 1 diabetes: a prospective implementation study. Diabetologia 2005;48:1965–1970

103. DAFNE Study Group. Training in flexible, intensive insulin management to enable dietary freedom in people with type 1 diabetes: dose adjustment for normal eating (DAFNE) randomised controlled trial. BMJ 2002;325:746

104. McIntyre HD, Knight BA, Harvey DM, Noud MN, Hagger VL, Gilshenan KS. Dose adjustment for normal eating (DAFNE)—an audit of outcomes in Australia. Med J Aust 2010;192:637–640

105. Hopkins D, Lawrence I, Mansell P, et al. Improved biomedical and psychological outcomes 1 year after structured education

in flexible insulin therapy for people with type 1 diabetes: the U.K. DAFNE experience. Diabetes Care 2012;35:1638–1642

106. Cox DJ, Gonder-Frederick L, Ritterband L, Clarke W, Kovatchev BP. Prediction of severe hypoglycemia. Diabetes Care 2007;30:1370–1373

107. Fritsche A, Stefan N, Häring H, Gerich J, Stumvoll M. Avoidance of hypoglycemia restores hypoglycemia awareness by increasing beta-adrenergic sensitivity in type 1 diabetes. Ann Intern Med 2001;134:729–736

108. Gray RO, Butler PC, Beers TR, Kryshak EJ, Rizza RA. Comparison of the ability of bread versus bread plus meat to treat and prevent subsequent hypoglycemia in patients with insulin-dependent diabetes mellitus. J Clin Endocrinol Metab 1996;81:1508–1511

109. Kalergis M, Schiffrin A, Gougeon R, Jones PJ, Yale JF. Impact of bedtime snack composition on prevention of nocturnal hypoglycemia in adults with type 1 diabetes undergoing intensive insulin management using lispro insulin before meals: a randomized, placebo-controlled, crossover trial. Diabetes Care 2003;26:9–15

110. Kaufman FR, Halvorson M, Kaufman ND. A randomized, blinded trial of uncooked cornstarch to diminish nocturnal hypoglycemia at diabetes camp. Diabetes Res Clin Pract 1995;30:205–209

111. Raju B, Arbelaez AM, Breckenridge SM, Cryer PE. Nocturnal hypoglycemia in type 1 diabetes: an assessment of preventive bedtime treatments. J Clin Endocrinol Metab 2006;91:2087–2092

112. Ververs MT, Rouwé C, Smit GP. Complex carbohydrates in the prevention of nocturnal hypoglycaemia in diabetic children. Eur J Clin Nutr 1993;47:268–273

113. Chipkin SR, Klugh SA, Chasan-Taber L. Exercise and diabetes. Cardiol Clin 2001;19:489–505

114. Zinman B, Ruderman N, Campaigne BN, Devlin JT, Schneider SH; American Diabetes Association. Physical activity/exercise and diabetes mellitus. Diabetes Care 2003;26(Suppl. 1):S73–S77

115. Linkeschova R, Raoul M, Bott U, Berger M, Spraul M. Less severe hypoglycaemia, better metabolic control, and improved quality of life in Type 1 diabetes mellitus with continuous subcutaneous insulin infusion (CSII) therapy; an observational study of 100 consecutive patients followed

for a mean of 2 years. Diabet Med 2002;19:746–751

116. Leitão CB, Tharavanij T, Cure P, et al. Restoration of hypoglycemia awareness after islet transplantation. Diabetes Care 2008;31:2113–2115

117. Meyer C, Hering BJ, Grossmann R, et al. Improved glucose counterregulation and autonomic symptoms after intraportal islet transplants alone in patients with long-standing type I diabetes mellitus. Transplantation 1998;66:233–240

118. Paty BW, Lanz K, Kendall DM, Sutherland DE, Robertson RP. Restored hypoglycemic counterregulation is stable in successful pancreas transplant recipients for up to 19 years after transplantation. Transplantation 2001;72:1103–1107

119. Amiel SA, Tamborlane WV, Simonson DC, Sherwin RS. Defective glucose counterregulation after strict glycemic control of insulin-dependent diabetes mellitus. N Engl J Med 1987;316:1376–1383

120. Fanelli CG, Epifano L, Rambotti AM, et al. Meticulous prevention of hypoglycemia normalizes the glycemic thresholds and magnitude of most of neuroendocrine responses to, symptoms of, and cognitive function during hypoglycemia in intensively treated patients with short-term IDDM. Diabetes 1993;42:1683–1689

121. Dagogo-Jack S, Fanelli CG, Cryer PE. Durable reversal of hypoglycemia unawareness in type 1 diabetes. Diabetes Care 1999;22:866–867

122. Ly TT, Hewitt J, Davey RJ, Lim EM, Davis EA, Jones TW. Improving epinephrine responses in hypoglycemia unawareness with real-time continuous glucose monitoring in adolescents with type 1 diabetes. Diabetes Care 2011;34:50–52

123. Choudhary P, Shin J, Wang Y, et al. Insulin pump therapy with automated insulin suspension in response to hypoglycemia: reduction in nocturnal hypoglycemia in those at greatest risk. Diabetes Care 2011;34:2023–2025

124. Smith CB, Choudhary P, Pernet A, Hopkins D, Amiel SA. Hypoglycemia unawareness is associated with reduced adherence to therapeutic decisions in patients with type 1 diabetes: evidence from a clinical audit. Diabetes Care 2009;32:1196–1198

125. Dagogo-Jack S. Hypoglycemia in type 1 diabetes mellitus: pathophysiology and prevention. Treat Endocrinol 2004;3:91–103

Treatment of Diabetes and Long-Term Survival After Insulin and Glucokinase Gene Therapy

David Callejas,[1,2,5] Christopher J. Mann,[1,2,5] Eduard Ayuso,[1,2,5] Ricardo Lage,[1,2,5] Iris Grifoll,[1,2,5] Carles Roca,[1,2,5] Anna Andaluz,[3] Rafael Ruiz-de Gopegui,[3] Joel Montané,[1,2] Sergio Muñoz,[1,2,5] Tura Ferre,[1,2,5] Virginia Haurigot,[1,2,5] Shangzhen Zhou,[6] Jesús Ruberte,[1,4,5] Federico Mingozzi,[6] Katherine A. High,[6,7] Felix Garcia,[3] and Fatima Bosch[1,2,5]

Diabetes is associated with severe secondary complications, largely caused by poor glycemic control. Treatment with exogenous insulin fails to prevent these complications completely, leading to significant morbidity and mortality. We previously demonstrated that it is possible to generate a "glucose sensor" in skeletal muscle through coexpression of glucokinase and insulin, increasing glucose uptake and correcting hyperglycemia in diabetic mice. Here, we demonstrate long-term efficacy of this approach in a large animal model of diabetes. A one-time intramuscular administration of adeno-associated viral vectors of serotype 1 encoding for glucokinase and insulin in diabetic dogs resulted in normalization of fasting glycemia, accelerated disposal of glucose after oral challenge, and no episodes of hypoglycemia during exercise for >4 years after gene transfer. This was associated with recovery of body weight, reduced glycosylated plasma proteins levels, and long-term survival without secondary complications. Conversely, exogenous insulin or gene transfer for insulin or glucokinase alone failed to achieve complete correction of diabetes, indicating that the synergistic action of insulin and glucokinase is needed for full therapeutic effect. This study provides the first proof-of-concept in a large animal model for a gene transfer approach to treat diabetes. **Diabetes 62:1718–1729, 2013**

D iabetes is a chronic disease for which there is currently no cure. Patients with type 1 diabetes need insulin replacement therapy to survive, but glycemia is not always properly regulated. Chronic hyperglycemia leads to development of diabetes-associated microvascular, macrovascular, and neurologic complications, which can be delayed by intensive insulin therapy (1). However, this treatment is not suitable for all diabetic patients because of its high risk of hypoglycemia secondary to excessive insulin dosage (1). Thus, precise regulation of glucose homeostasis is a major challenge in diabetes management. Therapeutic benefit has been obtained with islet transplantation (2), but access to human islets and the necessary immunosuppressive therapy are important limitations. Alternative cell- and gene-based therapies, centered around the engineering of nonpancreatic tissues to produce insulin, or the generation of stem cell-derived β cells, are undergoing investigation (3,4); however, long-term safety and efficacy data in large animal models are lacking.

Genetic engineering of skeletal muscle to counteract hyperglycemia is an attractive strategy to correct diabetes. Skeletal muscle is responsible for the disposal of ~70% of circulating glucose after a meal. In muscle, glucose utilization is controlled by insulin-stimulated glucose transport through the glucose transporter type 4 (GLUT4) (5) and phosphorylation by hexokinase II, which has a low K_m for glucose and is inhibited by glucose-6-phosphate, limiting glucose uptake (6). In diabetic muscle, because of the lack of insulin, GLUT4 translocation to the plasma membrane and hexokinase II activity both decrease. In contrast to hexokinase II, the liver enzyme glucokinase has a high K_m for glucose, is not inhibited by glucose-6-phosphate, and shows kinetic cooperation with glucose (7). When expressed in skeletal muscle of transgenic mice, glucokinase facilitates glucose uptake only when blood glucose is high (8). However, during diabetes, constant basal levels of insulin are required to ensure the presence of GLUT4 on the cell membrane (5). These observations led to the hypothesis that regulation of glycemia could be achieved by coexpression in skeletal muscle of glucokinase and low levels of insulin; in such a system, glucose influx is regulated by circulating glucose levels allowing glucose uptake only when hyperglycemia is present. Accordingly, intramuscular delivery of adeno-associated viral (AAV) vectors expressing insulin and glucokinase to diabetic mice resulted in disease correction (9).

AAV vectors are the vector of choice for in vivo gene therapy because of their excellent safety and efficacy profiles. Preclinical studies have shown that AAV-mediated gene transfer results in long-term gene expression in small and large animal models (10). Recently, these preclinical data have been successfully translated into humans (11,12). In the most clear-cut examples of success, clinical studies of hemophilia B (12) and Leber congenital amaurosis (11) were preceded by convincing studies of efficacy in large animal models (13,14). However, for most proof-of-concept studies in mice, no successful scale-up or long-term efficacy has been reported. This goal has yet to be demonstrated in large animal models of diabetes with gene and cell therapy approaches. Here, we used dogs treated with β-cell cytotoxic drugs as a model of experimental

From the [1]Center of Animal Biotechnology and Gene Therapy, Universitat Autònoma Barcelona, Bellaterra, Spain; the [2]Department of Biochemistry and Molecular Biology, School of Veterinary Medicine, Universitat Autònoma Barcelona, Bellaterra, Spain; the [3]Department of Animal Medicine and Surgery, School of Veterinary Medicine, Universitat Autònoma Barcelona, Bellaterra, Spain; the [4]Department of Animal Health and Anatomy, School of Veterinary Medicine, Universitat Autònoma Barcelona, Bellaterra, Spain; the [5]CIBER de Diabetes y Enfermedades Metabólicas Asociadas (CIBERDEM), Barcelona, Spain; the [6]Division of Hematology, Children's Hospital of Philadelphia, Philadelphia, Pennsylvania; and the [7]Howard Hughes Medical Institute, Philadelphia, Pennsylvania.

Corresponding author: Fatima Bosch, fatima.bosch@uab.es.

Received 17 August 2012 and accepted 28 January 2013.

DOI: 10.2337/db12-1113

This article contains Supplementary Data and videos online at http://diabetes .diabetesjournals.org/lookup/suppl/doi:10.2337/db12-1113/-/DC1.

D.C. and C.J.M. contributed equally to this study.

See accompanying commentary, p. 1396.

diabetes (15), because large animal models of autoimmune diabetes are not available. We demonstrate that after a single intramuscular injection of AAV1 vectors, insulin transgene (Ins) and glucokinase (Gck) transgene act synergistically to achieve tight control of glycemia. This represents the first proof-of-concept study of long-term correction of diabetes in a large animal model using gene transfer.

RESEARCH DESIGN AND METHODS

Animals. Male Beagle dogs were purchased from Isoquimen (Barcelona, Spain) and housed at Servei de Granges i Camps Experimentals of the Universitat Autònoma de Barcelona. Animals were fed individually once daily at 9:00 A.M. with 30 g/kg body weight of standard dry food (Nestle, Vevey, Switzerland) or twice daily at 9:00 A.M. and 9:00 P.M. with 15 g/kg body weight of diabetic food (Prescription Diets w/d; Hills, Topeka, KS) when indicated. Dogs were monitored regularly at the Universitat Autònoma de Barcelona Veterinary Clinical Hospital. C56Bl6 male mice (Harlan Teklad, Barcelona, Spain) were fed ad libitum with a standard diet (Harlan Teklad) and maintained in the specific pathogen free (SPF) mouse facility at the Center of Animal Biotechnology and Gene Therapy under a 12-h light–dark cycle (lights on at 8:00 A.M.). The Ethics Committee on Animal and Human Experimentation approved all procedures.

Diabetes induction. Experimental diabetes was induced in 6- to 12-month-old dogs by a single intravenous injection of a mixture of streptozotocin (35 mg/kg) and alloxan (40 mg/kg) (Sigma, St. Louis, MO) as described previously (15). When hyperglycemia developed, dogs were maintained without exogenous insulin treatment, unless indicated. Dogs receiving exogenous insulin were injected subcutaneously with Lantus (Sanofi-Aventis, Paris, France). When indicated, exogenous insulin treatment was optimized individually, increasing gradually the insulin dose up to the maximum tolerated dose that did not cause hypoglycemia. To induce diabetes in mice, animals aged 8 weeks were administered, for 5 consecutive days, an intraperitoneal injection of streptozotocin (45 mg/kg body weight) dissolved in 0.1 mol/L citrate buffer (pH 4.5) immediately before administration.

AAV production and administration. AAV vectors were produced by triple transfection of HEK293 cells and purified by a CsCl-based gradient method (16). Expression of an engineered human insulin gene containing an endoprotease furin cleavage signal and expression of rat glucokinase were driven by the cytomegalovirus (CMV) promoter in both vectors (9). For certain experiments as indicated, codon-optimized versions of human insulin (oIns; with furin cleavage sites) and human glucokinase cDNAs (oGck) were used. Vectors were delivered to a total of 12–25 sites on the lateral aspect of the thigh (with a five-prong needle syringe) and the craneolateral face of the leg (single point injections) of both hind limbs, with maximal vector dose per site of injection being $<6 \times 10^{11}$ vg (Supplementary Fig. 1). Dogs received a vector dose of 1×10^{12} vg/kg or 2×10^{12} vg/kg 2–4 weeks after diabetes induction (Supplementary Table 1). Mice were intramuscularly treated with 4×10^{12} vg/kg of AAV1-oGck 2 weeks after diabetes induction, distributed into tibialis cranealis, gastrocnemius, and quadriceps muscles of both hindlimbs.

Biodistribution. Total DNA was isolated from Dog3 with MasterPureDNA Purification Kit (Epicentre Biotechnologies, Madison, WI). Vector genome copy number was determined in 20 ng of genomic DNA by TaqMan quantitative PCR with primers and probe specific for the cytomegalovirus (CMV) promoter: forward primer, 5′-CACCAATGGGCGTGGATAGC-3′; reverse primer, 5′GCAGTTGTTACGACATTTTGGAAA-3′; and probe, 5′-ATTTCCAAGTCTC CACCC-3′.

RNA analysis. Liver and quadriceps total RNA was extracted (Qiagen, Valencia, CA) from dog and mouse samples and analyzed by Northern blot with radiolabeled (GE Healthcare UK, Buckinghamshire, UK) insulin or glucokinase cDNA probes or by quantitative RT-PCR for detection of glucokinase regulatory protein: forward primer, CAAGCACCAAGCGGTATCA; and reverse primer, GTCAGTGGGTTGGACTTCTCT.

Western blotting. Nuclear and cytoplasmatic protein fractions were obtained from skeletal muscle and liver extracted from starved mice, or 15 min after intraperitoneal glucose injection (3 g/kg body weight) as described (17). Fractioned or total protein lysates were subjected to SDS-PAGE, electrotransferred on polyvinylidene fluoride (Millipore) membranes, and probed with Akt (Cell Signaling, Danvers, MA), pAkt (Cell Signaling), Gck (Sigma), Histone 3 (Abcam, Cambridge, UK), and α-tubulin (Abcam) as previously described (18). All rabbit primary antibodies were immunodetected using horseradish peroxidase–conjugated polyclonal swine anti-rabbit immunoglobulins (Dako, Glostrup, Denmark). Loading was normalized by α-tubulin.

Morphological and immunohistochemical analysis. Dog samples were fixed in 10% formalin, embedded in paraffin, and sectioned. Double glucagon and insulin immunostaining was performed with mouse antiglucagon (Sigma) and guinea pig anti-insulin (Sigma) antibodies. Biotinylated horse anti-mouse (Vector Laboratories, Burlingame, CA) followed by streptavidin-conjugated Alexa488 (Molecular Probes, Leiden, the Netherlands) and Alexa568-conjugated goat anti-guinea pig (Molecular Probes) were used as secondary antibodies. The β-cell area was measured on four sections of pancreas biopsy samples, or multiple areas from the whole pancreas in necropsy samples, stained with anti-insulin and horseradish peroxidase–conjugated rabbit anti-guinea pig immunoglobulin (Dako, Glostrup, Denmark). Pancreatic β-cell area was calculated by dividing the area of insulin-positive cells by total pancreatic area of each section. To analyze muscle integrity, cross-sections were stained with hematoxylin and eosin or rabbit antilaminin (Dako, Glostrup, Denmark). Periodic acid-Schiff staining was used to evaluate muscle glycogen content (Sigma).

Hormone and metabolite determinations. Serum insulin was measured with human insulin radioimmunoassay (Millipore, Billerica, MA). Serum human C-peptide was determined with C-peptide radioimmunoassay (Millipore) that does not cross-react with insulin or with canine C-peptide. Serum glucagon was measured by radioimmunoassay (Millipore). Blood glucose levels were determined using a Glucometer Elite analyzer (Bayer, Leverkusen, Germany). Serum fructosamine concentration was measured by nitroblue tetrazolium reduction test. The concentration of glycogen in skeletal muscle was measured as previously described (9). Urine was analyzed by Multistix 10 SG Urinalysis Strips (Siemens, Munich, Germany).

Oral glucose tolerance test. Oral glucose tolerance tests (OGTTs) were performed in either 12- or 24-h fasted dogs. Briefly, animals were administered an oral gavage of glucose 1.75 g/kg body weight. Glycemia was determined at times 0, 15, and 30 min, and then every half hour up to 3 h after glucose administration.

Exercise test. Fasted dogs (24 h) were subjected to 37 min of exercise under increasing speed and slope on a variable speed belt treadmill (Starker Hund S.A.S., Padua, Italy). The protocol was as follows: 1) 5 min, 0 degrees, 4 km/h; 2) 5 min, 0 degrees, 8 km/h; 3) 5 min, 2.5 degrees, 8 km/h; 4) 5 min, 5 degrees, 8 km/h; 5) 5 min, 7.5 degrees, 8 km/h; 6) 5 min, 10 degrees, 8 km/h; 7) 5 min, 0 degrees, 10 km/h; and 8) 2 min, 0 degrees, 4 km/h. Dogs were allowed a recovery time equal to the exercise period (Video 1).

Glucokinase activity determination. To measure glucokinase activity in skeletal muscle, tissue biopsy samples were obtained from mice or from necropsy samples from Dog3. Frozen mouse gastrocnemius or dog quadriceps samples were homogenized in an ice-cold buffer (pH 7.4) containing 100 mmol/L Gly-Gly, 200 mmol/L ClK, 5 mmol/L DTT, and 65 mmol/L Tris. Samples were then centrifuged to pellet insoluble material. The glucose phosphorylation capacity was assayed in the supernatants at 30°C in a buffer containing 50 mmol/L Gly-Gly, 100 mmol/L KCl, 2.5 mmol/L DTT, glucose-6-phosphate dehydrogenase (1 units/mL), 0.5 mmol/L NADP, and 4.5 mmol/L ATP-Mg. Glucokinase activity was calculated as the difference between the glucose phosphorylation capacity at 100 and 0.5 mmol/L glucose. Protein content was measured by Bradford assay (Pointe Scientific) and glucokinase activity was expressed as mU/mg of protein.

Insulin sensitivity test in mice. Awake, fed AAV1-oGck– or AAV1-null–treated diabetic mice were intraperitoneally injected with 0.75 IU/kg body weight of insulin (Humulin regular; Eli Lilly). Glucose concentration was determined in blood samples obtained from tail vein before and at 0, 15, 30, 45, and 60 min after the insulin injection.

Statistical analysis. All values are expressed as means ± SEM. Differences between groups were compared by unpaired Student t test. $P < 0.05$ was considered statistically significant.

RESULTS

Glycemic control by insulin alone. After experimental diabetes induction, three dogs (DogDb1–3) were subjected to glycemic control with subcutaneous exogenous insulin according to hormone administration regimens and feeding protocols indicated for diabetic companion dogs. Despite therapy, fasting normoglycemia was not achieved in any of the animals (Fig. 1A–C); one of the animals, DogDb3, experienced severe fasting hyperglycemia. Exogenous insulin therapy prevented weight loss in all dogs (Fig. 1A–C). All these animals showed elevated fructosamine levels (Fig. 2A), a marker of glycosylated proteins in blood and an indicator of recent (3 weeks) glycemic control used in veterinary medicine (19–21). Finally, diabetic

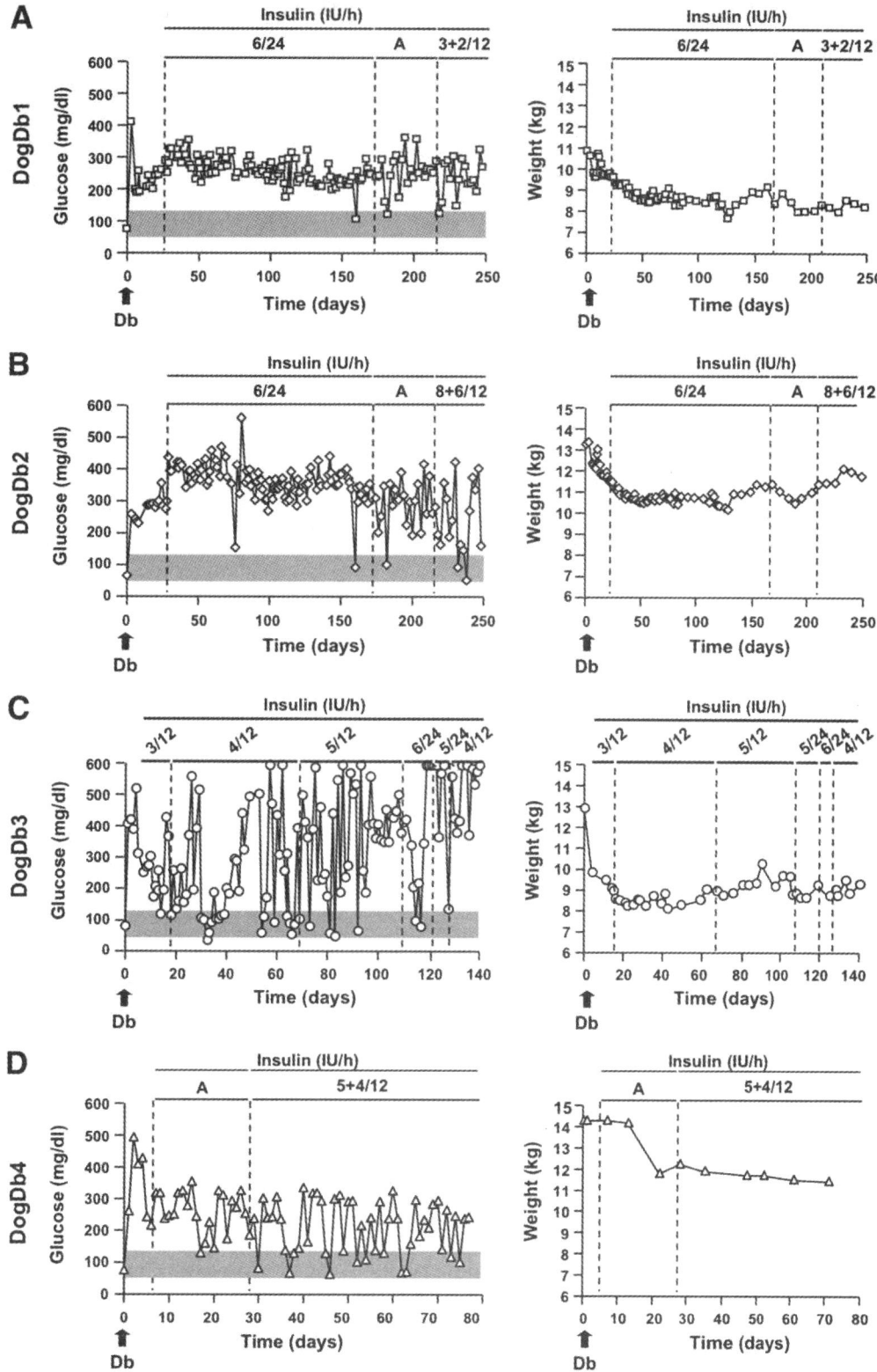

FIG. 1. Glycemic control by exogenous insulin. *A–D*: Follow-up of fasting glycemia and body weight of diabetic control dogs (DogDb1–4) treated daily with exogenous insulin (dosage [IU] and timing [24 h vs. 12 h] are shown). DogDb1, square; DogDb2, diamond; DogDb3, circle; DogDb4, triangle. Db, dog treatment with streptozotocin (STZ) plus alloxan. A indicates the period of adjustment of the insulin dosing regimen. Gray bar indicates fasting normoglycemia range in dogs (20).

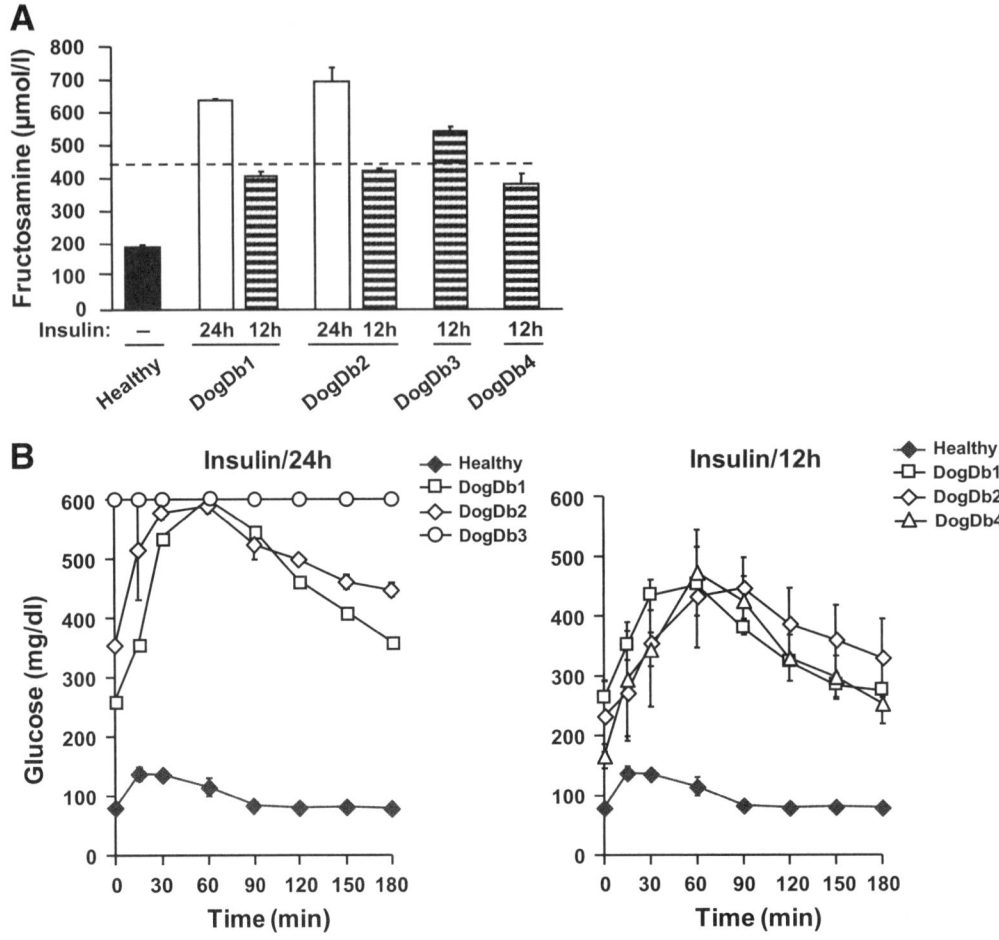

FIG. 2. Fructosamine levels and glucose disposal after a load in dogs treated with exogenous insulin. *A*: Monitoring of serum fructosamine in DogDb1–4 receiving exogenous insulin every 24 or 12 h. The fructosamine upper limit for good diabetes control in dogs is indicated with the dashed line. Fructosamine concentrations between 350 and 400 µmol/L indicate excellent glycemic control, concentrations between 400 and 450 µmol/L indicate good glycemic control, concentrations between 450 and 500 µmol/L indicate fair glycemic control, and concentrations >500 µmol/L indicate poor glycemic control (20). Results are shown as mean ± SEM of 2–4 determinations. *B*: OGTTs were performed at 1.75 g/kg glucose before (healthy) and after diabetes induction in DogDb1–3 treated with exogenous insulin every 24 h (*left*) or in DogDb1, DogDb2, and DogDb4 receiving insulin every 12 h (*right*). Mean ± SEM, *n* = 3. (A high-quality color representation of this figure is available in the online issue.)

dogs showed a marked and sustained increase in blood glucose compared with healthy animals when subjected to an OGTT at the American Diabetes Association–recommended standard dose of glucose (1.75 g/kg) (22) (Fig. 2*B*).

In an effort to further improve glycemic control, a new treatment regimen with exogenous insulin was established. In DogDb1 and DogDb2, and in an additional diabetic dog (DogDb4), insulin dosing was increased as much as possible without causing severe hypoglycemia; this was performed on an individual basis with twice-daily administrations. In addition, dogs were fed with diabetic food distributed in two servings. Despite treatment optimization, no major changes were observed in fasted glycemia (Fig. 1*A*, *B*, *D*), whereas the improvement in glycemic control resulted in lower fructosamine levels, which decreased to below the upper limit of good glycemic control (Fig. 2*A*) in veterinary medicine (450 µmol/L) (19–21) and improved OGTT (Fig. 2*B*).

When insulin alone was expressed in skeletal muscle of a diabetic dog by administration of 1×10^{12} vg/kg of AAV1-Ins vector (DogIns), partial correction of fasting glycemia

was achieved (Fig. 3*A*). This animal recovered the body weight initially lost after diabetes induction and had fructosamine levels that ranged between 250 and 300 µmol/L after gene transfer (Fig. 3*B*, *C*). Despite achieving normal levels of fasting insulinemia (Fig. 3*D*), the ability of DogIns to dispose of glucose after an OGTT was only moderately improved compared with diabetic dogs (Fig. 3*E*).

Ins and Gck gene transfer to skeletal muscle corrects diabetes in dogs. Five diabetic dogs (Dog1–4 and DogDb3+Ins/Gck) were intramuscularly administered with AAV1-Ins and AAV1-Gck vectors. Administration of 1×10^{12} vg/kg of each vector to Dog1 and Dog2 resulted in rapid return to fasting normoglycemia and normoinsulinemia, recovery of body weight (Fig. 4*A*, *B*, and Video 2), and long-term survival (>4 years, observation ongoing). The administration of a twice-high vector dose (2×10^{12} vg/kg) of each vector to Dog3 was also safe and resulted in correction of diabetes with no episodes of hypoglycemia (Fig. 4*C*, *D*). Thus, Ins and Gck gene transfer results in better control of diabetes than exogenous insulin therapy or gene transfer for Ins only. This result was further confirmed in DogDb3 (Fig. 1*C*), which was treated with AAV1-Ins and

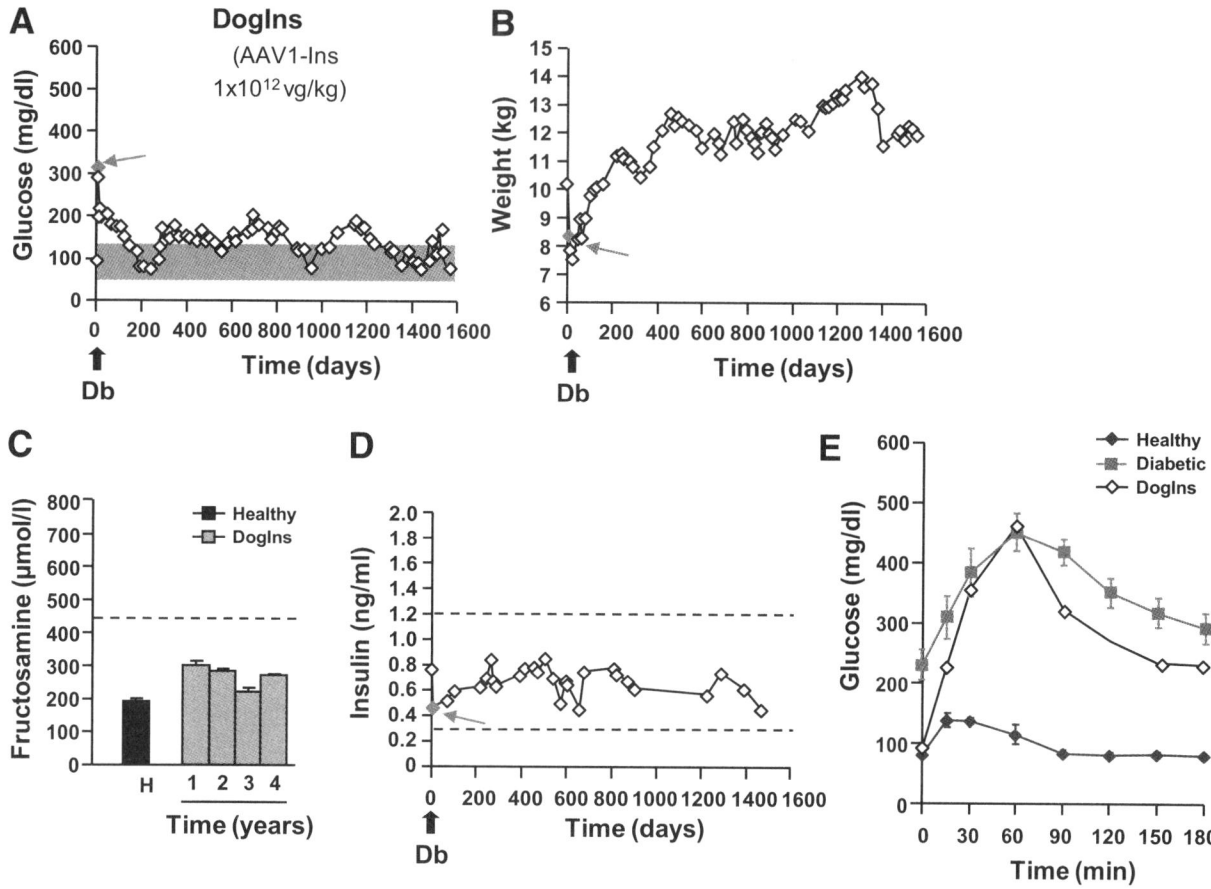

FIG. 3. Glycemic control by AAV1-Ins alone. Diabetic dog treated with AAV1-Ins (1×10^{12} vg/kg; DogIns) showed partial normalization of fasting blood glucose levels (*A*) and recovery of body weight loss (*B*). *C*: Fructosamine monitoring in DogIns. Results are shown as mean ± SEM of more than four measurements per year. *D*: Fasting insulinemia of DogIns. Dashed lines indicate average maximum and minimum fasting insulinemia values obtained by random measurements in six healthy dogs. *E*: No major improvement was observed in the ability of DogIns to dispose of glucose during an OGTT at 1.75 g/kg performed 4 years after gene transfer when compared with diabetic dogs under optimized exogenous insulin treatment. Db indicates dog treatment with streptozotocin (STZ) plus alloxan. Gray bar indicates fasting normoglycemia range in dogs (20). DogIns, diamond symbols in panels *A*, *B*, and *D*.

AAV1-Gck after 5 months of poorly controlled glycemia (now named DogDb3+Ins/Gck), resulting in normalization of glycemia without exogenous insulin administration. Codon-optimized versions of human transgenes also were tested to achieve better glycemic control at doses of 1×10^{12} vg/kg, because use of codon-optimized genes increases the production of proteins (23). Delivery of AAV1-oIns and AAV1-oGck to Dog4 led to rapid recovery of normoglycemia, normoinsulinemia, and body weight (Fig. 4*E*), with no signs of fasting hypoglycemia detected during the 5-month follow up.

In all Ins- and Gck-treated dogs, fructosamine levels remained within the range of 250–350 μmol/L (Fig. 5*A*). When an OGTT was performed at a dose of 1.75 g/kg, treated dogs showed only a small increase in glycemia after the load, followed by return to normoglycemia within 2 hours, a profile considered nondiabetic by American Diabetes Association guidelines (2-h plasma glucose <200 mg/dL) (22), with the exception of DogDb3+Ins/Gck, which was ~200 mg/dL at 120 min (Fig. 5*B*). Furthermore, Ins- and Gck-treated dogs showed improved glucose disposal even after high-dose (3 g/kg) glucose load; peak glycemia was lower than that of diabetic dogs and 2-h glycemia declined to <200 mg/dL (Supplementary Fig. 2). Importantly, Dogs1–4 and DogDb3+Ins/Gck showed good

glycemic control with exercise, with no development of hypoglycemia (Fig. 6). In agreement with normalization of glycemia, ketone bodies were never detected in the urine of these dogs (data not shown). Finally, Ins- and Gck-treated dogs did not show signs of secondary complications, whereas DogDb1–3 developed cataracts a few months after hyperglycemia development (Supplementary Table 2).

Both transgenes were expressed in skeletal muscle (Fig. 7*A*), and glucokinase was active in this tissue (Fig. 7*B*). Circulating insulin in AAV1-treated dogs derived from expression of Ins transgene in muscle, as documented by the lack of surviving β cells in pancreas biopsy samples (Fig. 7*A*, *C*, *D*) and with the detection of human C-peptide in serum (Fig. 7*E*). In contrast to healthy dogs, and in agreement with the lack of pancreatic insulin-producing cells, the first phase peak of insulin release after a meal was not observed in AAV1-treated dogs (Fig. 7*F*). Together, these findings suggest that circulating insulin detected in AAV1-treated dogs derives from the expression of the Ins transgene in skeletal muscle and not from residual expression from surviving β cells. All AAV1-Ins +Gck–treated diabetic dogs showed normal circulating glucagon levels (Fig. 7*G*), indicating preservation of α-cell function.

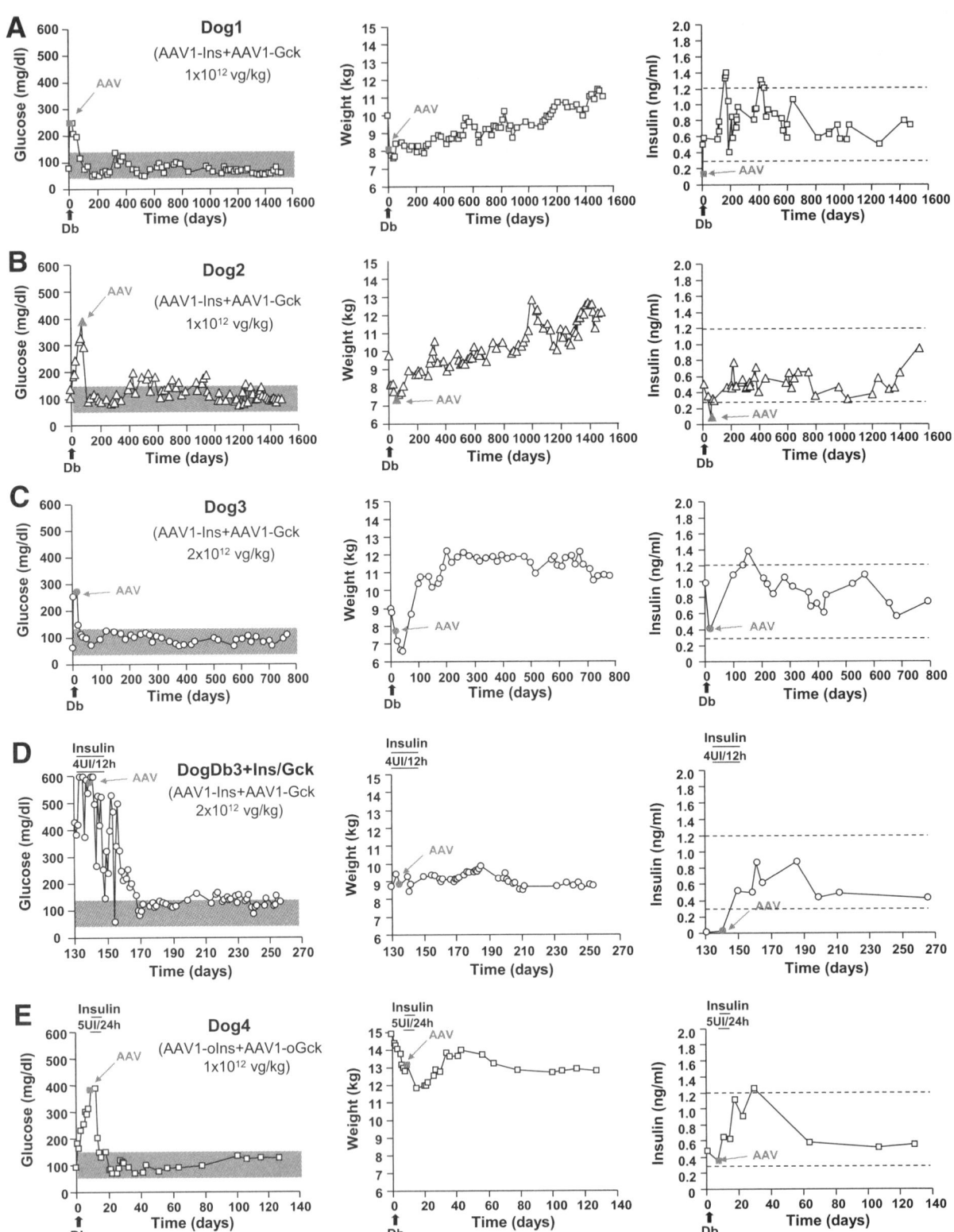

FIG. 4. Treatment with AAV1-Ins and AAV1-Gck corrects diabetes in dogs. *A–D*: Follow-up of glycemia, body weight, and insulinemia. Five diabetic dogs (Dog1–4 and DogDb3+Ins/Gck) were treated with AAV1-Ins and AAV1-Gck vectors at 1×10^{12} vg/kg each for Dog1 and Dog2 (*A* and *B*), at 2×10^{12} vg/kg each for Dog3 and DogDb3+Ins/Gck (*C* and *D*), or with AAV1-oIns and AAV1-oGck vectors at 1×10^{12} vg/kg each for Dog4 (*E*). Dogs had serum insulin levels that remained within the range of fasted healthy animals (dashed lines). Db indicates dog treatment with streptozotocin (STZ) plus alloxan. Gray bars indicate fasting normoglycemia range in dogs (20).

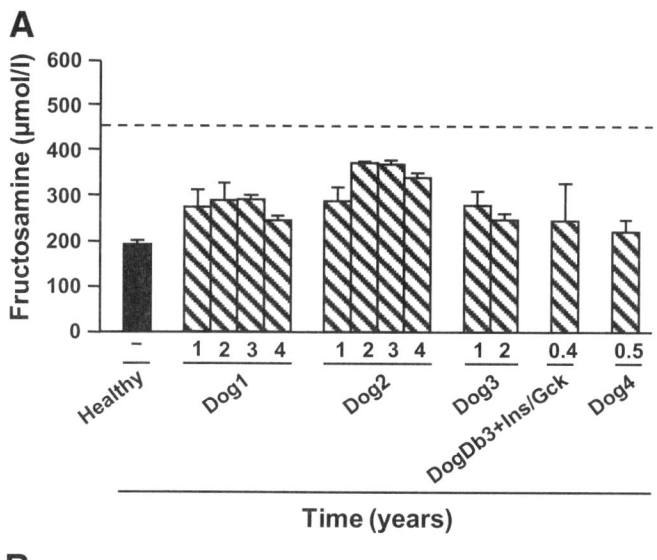

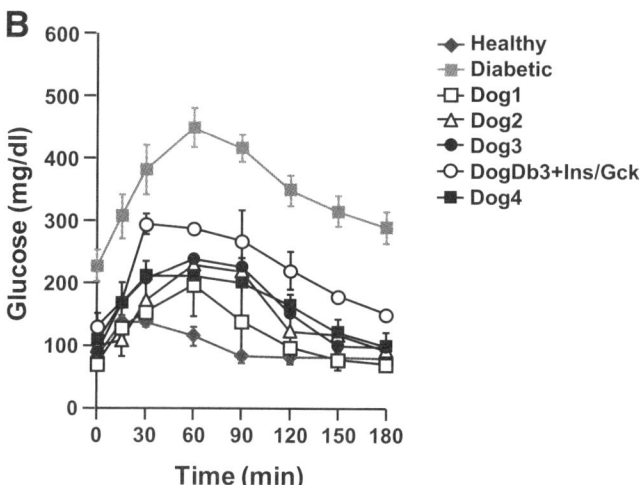

FIG. 5. AAV1-Ins and AAV1-Gck treatment normalizes serum fructosamine and recovers glucose disposal after a load. *A*: Dog1–4 and DogDb3+Ins/Gck had levels of serum fructosamine that ranged from 200 to 350 μmol/L. *B*: OGTT at a dose of glucose of 1.75 g/kg. Ins- and Gck-treated dogs showed a glucose profile similar to healthy animals and below the range for diabetes diagnosis according to American Diabetes Association guidelines (2-h plasma glucose <200 mg/dL). Data are represented as mean ± SEM of 2–3 OGTTs performed every year or during the study period in dogs with shorter follow-up. OGTTs for diabetic control dogs (red line) were performed during the period of intensive exogenous insulin treatment.

The production of insulin in skeletal muscle increased the phosphorylated AKT/total AKT ratio in muscle fibers, indicating that insulin activated its signaling in an autocrine/paracrine manner (Supplementary Fig. 3). Also, in agreement with the absence of glucokinase regulatory protein in skeletal muscle (data not shown) (24), glucokinase was detected only in the cytosol of AAV1-treated muscle fibers, even after a glucose challenge (Supplementary Fig. 4).

Dog3 was euthanized at 2.2 years after gene transfer, and vector genome biodistribution analysis confirmed that most of the detectable vector was present in injected muscles (Supplementary Table 3). Normal muscle morphology without glycogenosis was documented in AAV1-injected animals (Supplementary Fig. 5 and Supplementary Table 4).

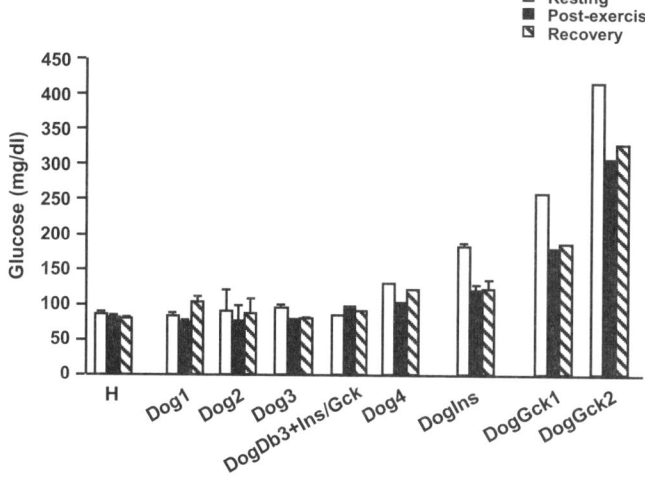

FIG. 6. Effect of exercise on glycemia. Blood glucose was measured in 24-h fasted dogs before, immediately after exercise, and during post-exercise recovery. None of the dogs was hypoglycemic over the periods analyzed. Dog1–4 and DogDb3+Ins/Gck showed good glycemic control under exercise, comparable with that of healthy dogs. A decline in blood glucose was observed after exercise in dogs treated with AAV1-Ins or with AAV1-oGck vectors only; these dogs had baseline glucose levels much higher than those of all other animals treated with AAV1-Ins and AAV1-Gck vectors.

Role of the glucokinase transgene in glycemic control. Two diabetic dogs were treated with AAV1-oGck vectors alone at 2×10^{12} vg/kg (DogGck1 and DogGck2). After vector delivery, both dogs remained hyperglycemic and required administration of exogenous insulin to reduce hyperglycemia and to stabilize weight loss (Fig. 8*A*, *B*), demonstrating that glucokinase expression alone is not sufficient to counteract hyperglycemia. Consistently, fructosamine was elevated in both dogs (Fig. 8*C*) and they developed cataracts a few months after hyperglycemia development (Supplementary Table 2). Dogs expressing glucokinase alone showed an impaired OGTT (1.75 g/kg), with glycemia curves similar to those of diabetic non-treated animals (Fig. 8*D*).

Similar to what it was performed with diabetic control dogs, exogenous insulin treatment was optimized on an individual basis in DogGck1 and DogGck2 with twice-daily administrations. Although no decline in fasted glycemia or fructosamine levels was observed (Fig. 8*A–C*), an improvement in OGTT was documented (Fig. 8*D*).

The higher sensitivity to exogenous insulin of DogsGck was, however, evidenced when an OGTT was performed with simultaneous subcutaneous injection of insulin. DogGck1 and DogGck2 had a faster glucose disposal than diabetic control dogs, with glycemia declining to <200 mg/dL in both animals (Fig. 8*E*). Increased sensitivity to exogenous insulin was also observed in diabetic mice treated with AAV1-oGck (Supplementary Fig. 6).

DISCUSSION

Since the 1922 breakthrough discovery of Banting and Best, who corrected hyperglycemia in dogs using pancreatic extracts, exogenous insulin administration has been the mainstay of diabetes therapy. Alternative therapies have been studied, but thus far only a few approaches, mainly involving allotransplantation or xenotransplantation of pancreatic islets, have reached clinical application (2).

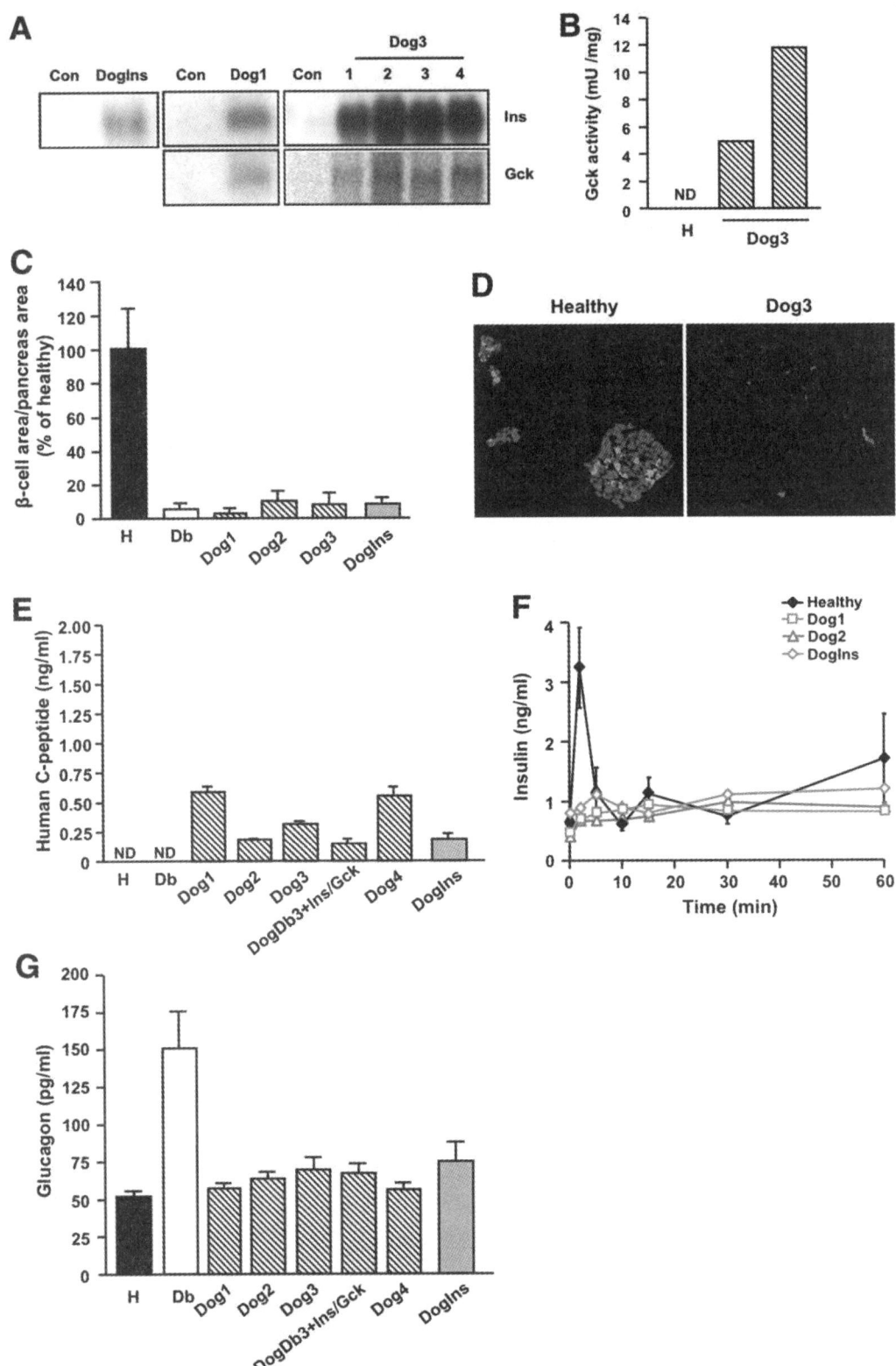

FIG. 7. Skeletal muscle is the source of insulin after AAV1-Ins and AAV1-Gck treatment. *A*: Transgene expression in skeletal muscle of AAV1-treated dogs. Northern blot analysis showing expression of insulin and glucokinase in skeletal muscle biopsy specimens from DogIns and Dog1, and necropsy samples from Dog3, obtained 9 months and 2.2 years after treatment, respectively. Uninjected muscle was used as a control. *B*: Measurement of glucokinase activity in skeletal muscle of healthy (H) dog and two different necropsy samples from Dog3. *C*: The β-cell area was quantified in necropsy samples (whole pancreas) from a healthy dog, a diabetic dog, and Dog3 (2.2 years after treatment), and in pancreas biopsy samples from Dog1, Dog2, and DogIns obtained 9 months after AAV1 administration. Diabetes induction led to >90% reduction in β-cell mass in all dogs. *D*: Representative images of pancreatic sections stained with insulin (red) and glucagon (green) illustrating the marked reduction of insulin-producing cells in Dog3 by 2.2 years after diabetes induction. Original magnification 200×. *E*: Human C-peptide was detectable in serum of all AAV1-Ins–treated dogs, but not in healthy (H) or untreated diabetic (Db) dogs, indicating that proinsulin was produced and processed in skeletal

In the clinical translation of bench results, the scale-up to a large animal model represents perhaps one of the most critical steps. This was demonstrated by the work performed in gene transfer for hemophilia B (12,25–27) and Leber congenital amaurosis (13,28), in which results for dogs were fully predictive of the outcome in humans.

Our novel approach to control hyperglycemia, through genetic engineering of a "glucose sensor" in skeletal muscle using AAV1 vectors, has permitted long-term, clinically meaningful regulation of glycemia in a large animal model of diabetes. Currently, the goal of normalization of glycemia is pursued through intensive insulin therapy, which can delay the onset and slow the progression of secondary complications of diabetes (1). However, this treatment is not suitable for all diabetic patients because of its high risk of hypoglycemia secondary to excessive insulin dosage (1). Additionally, cell therapies, including cadaveric and stem cell–derived islet transplantation, require life-long immunosuppression (2,29). Our approach circumvents a number of the challenges of diabetes therapy. In contrast to allotransplantation, in which supplies of human pancreatic islets are limiting, AAV vector manufacturing is robust and unlimited. Moreover, long-term (>10 years) transgene expression has been documented in humans after AAV vector administration to skeletal muscle (30).

The intramuscular delivery of AAV1 vectors to engineer the skeletal muscle results in expression of both transgenes in the target tissue, and not in the liver, the other tissue where vector genomes are detected, probably because of the silencing of the cytomegalovirus promoter (31). Our results support a model in which the production of insulin in skeletal muscle activates insulin signaling in an autocrine/paracrine manner, and the constant insulin production deriving from AAV1-Ins–transduced fibers is crucial for the system to work as a glucose sensor. Low basal levels of insulin are required to keep muscle capable of uptaking glucose by ensuring continuous GLUT4 translocation to the plasmatic membrane (9). Thus, glucose transport does not become a rate-limiting step to the system before a glucose challenge. However, because of the absence of glucokinase regulatory protein in muscle, the glucokinase produced in this tissue through gene transfer remains active in the cytosol (24). As a result, in a situation of hyperglycemia, glucokinase phosphorylates glucose efficiently, driving the uptake of large amounts of glucose through GLUT4 into the engineered muscle fibers. Then, AAV1-Ins alone is able to maintain good control of fasted glycemia, but AAV1-Gck is required to cope with a glucose overload, as shown by the OGTTs. The advantage of expressing both genes in the same muscle cell would be that by acting in an autocrine/paracrine manner, the levels of insulin required to achieve sufficient GLUT4 expression in the muscle fiber are low and therefore safe. Regarding the systemic action of insulin derived from the skeletal muscle, we have previously demonstrated that transgenic mice expressing insulin and glucokinase under the control of a muscle-specific promoter or diabetic mice treated with AAV1-Ins+Gck gene transfer have restored glucokinase and markedly reduced PEPCK expression in the liver (9). PEPCK is the most important enzyme in the

control of gluconeogenesis and is regulated mainly at transcriptional level, with its expression upregulated in starvation or diabetes (32). This evidence suggests that hepatic gluconeogenesis is reduced in Ins- and Gck-treated diabetic animals when compared with untreated diabetic controls, which would contribute to better glycemic control.

Insulin alone, either provided as exogenous therapy or expressed in muscle by an AAV1 vector, did induce glucose uptake; however, it did not guarantee tight control of glycemia, especially after a glucose challenge. Expression of glucokinase alone did not correct hyperglycemia either. Diabetic dogs treated with high doses of AAV1-Gck were hyperglycemic in fasting conditions. However, expression of glucokinase in muscle results in greater sensitivity to insulin, either when insulin is exogenously administered or when it is expressed at low, safe levels from an AAV1 vector. Furthermore, even if an intensive exogenous insulin treatment is adjusted on an individual basis for each diabetic control or AAV1-Gck–treated dog, the glycemic control achieved by Ins and Gck gene therapy is superior, as evidenced by the lower fasted glycemia and fructosamine levels, and improved glucose disposal in AAV1-Ins+Gck–treated animals. Thus, only the synergistic action of insulin and glucokinase allows for tight control of diabetic hyperglycemia.

Skeletal muscle has a number of key advantages as a target tissue for AAV-mediated gene transfer. Muscle is easily accessible by noninvasive procedures, and vector delivery leads to minimal systemic biodistribution (Supplementary Table 2). Moreover, gene delivery to muscle is not limited by the presence of preexisting neutralizing antibodies against AAV (33), a key aspect given the relatively high prevalence of anti-AAV antibodies in the general population (34). In addition, muscle has a metabolism highly based on glucose consumption and can efficiently secrete proteins into the bloodstream. Insulin can be produced, processed, and secreted as a mature protein from skeletal muscle, provided the gene has a genetic modification allowing the cleavage by the endoprotease furin (9). We have been unable to detect insulin within muscle fibers of transgenic or AAV1-treated mice, suggesting that the insulin produced in muscle fibers is not accumulated in vesicles and that its secretion is unlikely to be regulated by vesicle-mediated exocytosis (as in pancreatic β cells). In contrast, secretion from the skeletal muscle seems to be constitutive.

Long-term follow-up of treated dogs suggests that muscle expression of insulin and glucokinase is well-tolerated over a prolonged period. Studies confirmed the safety of the approach even under marked physical exertion, when high levels of glucose consumption increase the risk of hypoglycemic episodes. The use of a large animal model with a long life span allowed us to follow-up animals for early indicators of secondary complications. The absence of clinical findings, such as cataracts or urinary tract infection, and the reduction of biomarkers, such as glycosylated proteins (fructosamine), suggest that Ins and Gck gene transfer may prevent diabetes complications. Hence, normalization of glycemia with a one-time intervention

muscle. Results are shown as mean ± SEM (*n* = 23–56 measurements per dog). *F*: Time course of insulin secretion after a meal 4 years after AAV1 treatment of Dog1, Dog2, and DogIns. Basal levels correspond to a 24-h fasting period, after which animals were fed a 30-g/kg serving of standard diet. Only the healthy dogs showed the first peak of insulin release, which corresponds to pancreatic secretion of the insulin stored in secretory granules. *G*: Normal circulating glucagon levels were observed in AAV1-Ins– and AAV1-Gck–treated dogs indicating preservation of α-cell function. Results are shown as mean ± SEM (*n* = 5–6 measurements per dog). H, healthy; Db, diabetic; Con, control; ND, nondetected.

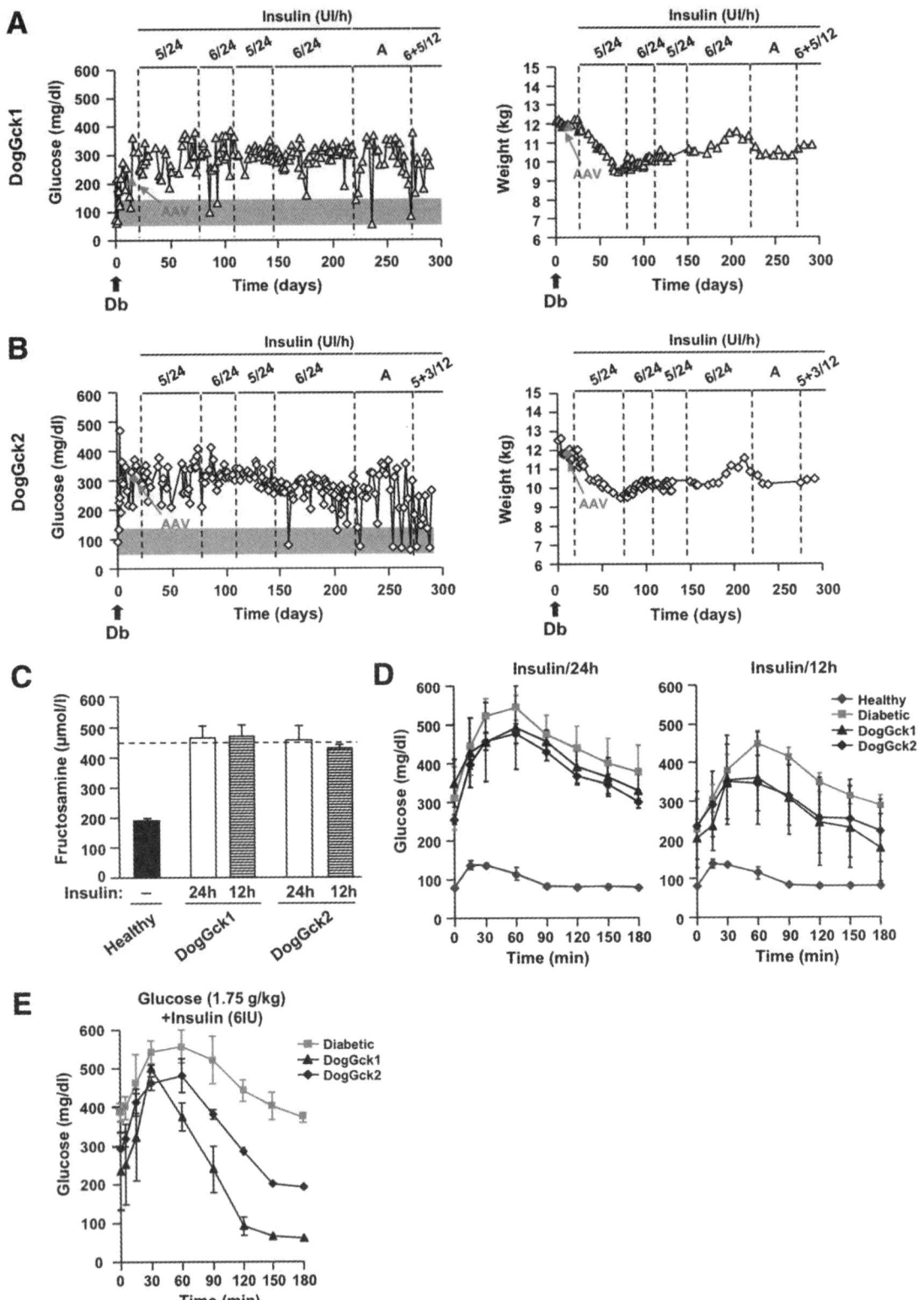

FIG. 8. Diabetic dogs treated with AAV1-oGck alone. Follow-up of glycemia and body weight of diabetic dogs treated with AAV1-oGck vectors (2×10^{12} vg/kg) in DogGck1 (*A*) and DogGck2 (*B*). DogGck remained hyperglycemic during fast and required daily administration of exogenous insulin (dosage [IU] and timing [24 h vs. 12 h] are shown). *C*: Fructosamine levels were altered in DogGck1 and DogGck2 receiving exogenous insulin every 24 or 12 h. Results are shown as mean ± SEM of 2–4 determinations. *D*: DogGck1 and DogGck2 showed similar OGTT profiles at 1.75 g/kg as diabetic untreated dogs when administered with exogenous insulin once daily. On implementation of the optimized treatment, OGTT improved. *E*: The synergistic effect of glucokinase and insulin. DogGck1 and DogGck2 and diabetic control dogs were administered a glucose load (1.75 g/kg) together with a subcutaneous injection of insulin (6 IU). Data are represented as mean ± SEM of 3 OGTTs. Db indicates dog treatment with streptozotocin (STZ) plus alloxan. Gray bars indicate fasting normoglycemia range in dogs (20).

could result in a substantial improvement in patient quality of life, particularly in populations with difficulties in diabetes management, such as brittle diabetes (35).

One possible limitation of the results presented here is that the dog model of diabetes used in this study does not fully mimic the immunological state of type 1 diabetic patients. However, although future studies in autoimmune models of diabetes are warranted, studies of mice (36), dogs (37), and humans (38) would suggest that targeting muscle with AAV vectors may at least partially escape immune recognition. This may be the result of lower levels of major histocompatibility complex class I presentation in this tissue, or the result of the induction of apoptosis of reactive T cells (36,38).

In summary, our data represent the first demonstration of long-term correction of diabetes in a large animal model using gene transfer. Future safety and efficacy studies will help to determine the range of Ins and Gck vector doses that are therapeutic, as well as the glucokinase/insulin expression ratio that is optimal for a tight control of glycemia. These studies will provide the basis for the initiation of a clinical veterinary study in companion animals with diabetes, a strategy also proposed for the clinical development of cancer therapeutics (39). The proposed clinical trial of diabetic dogs that are pets will greatly help define the safety and efficacy profiles of our approach in humans. One added advantage of this strategy is also related to the fact that large experimental animal models of autoimmune diabetes do not exist; thus, companion animals with naturally occurring diabetes constitute an extremely valuable and stringent model. In conclusion, this study lays the foundation for the clinical translation of this approach to veterinary medicine and possibly to humans.

ACKNOWLEDGMENTS

This work was supported by grants from Ministerio de Ciencia e Innovación, Plan Nacional I+D+I (SAF2008-00962 and SAF2011-24698), Generalitat de Catalunya (2009 SGR-224), Spain and European Commission (EUGENE2, LSHM-CT-2004-512013 and CLINIGENE, LSHB-CT-2006-018933), the National Institutes of Health grants 2P01-HL64190 and N01-HV78203, and the Howard Hughes Medical Institute.

D.C. and C.J.M. are recipients of predoctoral and postdoctoral fellowships from Ministerio de Ciencia e Innovación, Spain, respectively. F.B., D.C., and E.A. are inventors of a patent application regarding the use of insulin and glucokinase treatment of diabetes. F.M. and K.A.H. are inventors of a patent application of the AAV vector technology. No other potential conflicts of interest relevant to this article were reported.

D.C., C.J.M., and E.A. designed experiments, generated reagents, performed experiments, and wrote and edited the manuscript. R.L., I.G., C.R., A.A., R.R.-d.G., J.M., S.M., T.F., V.H., S.Z., J.R., F.M., and K.A.H. generated reagents and performed experiments. V.H., F.M., and K.A.H. wrote and edited the manuscript. F.G. designed experiments, generated reagents, and performed experiments. F.B. designed experiments and wrote and edited the manuscript. F.B. is the guarantor of this work and, as such, had full access to all the data in the study and takes responsibility for the integrity of the data and the accuracy of the data analysis.

The authors thank Malcolm Watford (Rutgers University), Sylvie Franckhauser (Universitat Autonoma de Barcelona, Spain), and Judith Storch (Rutgers University), for helpful discussions, and Juan Benitez (Universitat Autonoma de Barcelona, Spain), Marta Moya (Universitat Autonoma de Barcelona, Spain), and Luca Maggioni (Universitat Autonoma de Barcelona, Spain) for technical assistance.

REFERENCES

1. The Diabetes Control and Complications Trial Research Group. The effect of intensive treatment of diabetes on the development and progression of long-term complications in insulin-dependent diabetes mellitus. N Engl J Med 1993;329:977–986
2. Robertson RP. Islet transplantation a decade later and strategies for filling a half-full glass. Diabetes 2010;59:1285–1291
3. Kojima H, Fujimiya M, Matsumura K, et al. NeuroD-betacellulin gene therapy induces islet neogenesis in the liver and reverses diabetes in mice. Nat Med 2003;9:596–603
4. Kroon E, Martinson LA, Kadoya K, et al. Pancreatic endoderm derived from human embryonic stem cells generates glucose-responsive insulin-secreting cells in vivo. Nat Biotechnol 2008;26:443–452
5. Kahn BB. Lilly lecture 1995. Glucose transport: pivotal step in insulin action. Diabetes 1996;45:1644–1654
6. Printz RL, Koch S, Potter LR, et al. Hexokinase II mRNA and gene structure, regulation by insulin, and evolution. J Biol Chem 1993;268:5209–5219
7. Printz RL, Magnuson MA, Granner DK. Mammalian glucokinase. Annu Rev Nutr 1993;13:463–496
8. Otaegui PJ, Ferre T, Pujol A, Riu E, Jimenez R, Bosch F. Expression of glucokinase in skeletal muscle: a new approach to counteract diabetic hyperglycemia. Hum Gene Ther 2000;11:1543–1552
9. Mas A, Montané J, Anguela XM, et al. Reversal of type 1 diabetes by engineering a glucose sensor in skeletal muscle. Diabetes 2006;55:1546–1553
10. Mingozzi F, High KA. Therapeutic in vivo gene transfer for genetic disease using AAV: progress and challenges. Nat Rev Genet 2011;12:341–355
11. Maguire AM, High KA, Auricchio A, et al. Age-dependent effects of RPE65 gene therapy for Leber's congenital amaurosis: a phase 1 dose-escalation trial. Lancet 2009;374:1597–1605
12. Nathwani AC, Tuddenham EG, Rangarajan S, et al. Adenovirus-associated virus vector-mediated gene transfer in hemophilia B. N Engl J Med 2011;365:2357–2365
13. Acland GM, Aguirre GD, Ray J, et al. Gene therapy restores vision in a canine model of childhood blindness. Nat Genet 2001;28:92–95
14. Nathwani AC, Gray JT, Ng CY, et al. Self-complementary adeno-associated virus vectors containing a novel liver-specific human factor IX expression cassette enable highly efficient transduction of murine and nonhuman primate liver. Blood 2006;107:2653–2661
15. Anderson HR, Stitt AW, Gardiner TA, Lloyd SJ, Archer DB. Induction of alloxan/streptozotocin diabetes in dogs: a revised experimental technique. Lab Anim 1993;27:281–285
16. Ayuso E, Mingozzi F, Montane J, et al. High AAV vector purity results in serotype- and tissue-independent enhancement of transduction efficiency. Gene Ther 2010;17:503–510
17. Helenius M, Hänninen M, Lehtinen SK, Salminen A. Aging-induced up-regulation of nuclear binding activities of oxidative stress responsive NF-kB transcription factor in mouse cardiac muscle. J Mol Cell Cardiol 1996;28:487–498
18. Muñoz S, Franckhauser S, Elias I, et al. Chronically increased glucose uptake by adipose tissue leads to lactate production and improved insulin sensitivity rather than obesity in the mouse. Diabetologia 2010;53:2417–2430
19. Davison LJ, Herrtage ME, Catchpole B. Study of 253 dogs in the United Kingdom with diabetes mellitus. Vet Rec 2005;156:467–471
20. Nelson RW. Canine diabetes mellitus. In *Textbook of Veterinary Internal Medicine: Diseases of the Dog and the Cat.* 7th ed. Ettinger SJ, Feldman EC, Eds. St. Louis, MO, Saunders Elsevier, 2010, p. 1449–1474
21. Fracassi F, Boretti FS, Sieber-Ruckstuhl NS, Reusch CE. Use of insulin glargine in dogs with diabetes mellitus. Vet Rec 2012;170:52
22. American Diabetes Association. Standards of medical care in diabetes—2011. Diabetes Care 2011;34(Suppl. 1):S11–S61
23. Fath S, Bauer AP, Liss M, et al. Multiparameter RNA and codon optimization: a universal tool to assess and enhance autologous mammalian gene expression. PLoS ONE 2011;6:e17596

24. Shiota C, Coffey J, Grimsby J, Grippo JF, Magnuson MA. Nuclear import of hepatic glucokinase depends upon glucokinase regulatory protein, whereas export is due to a nuclear export signal sequence in glucokinase. J Biol Chem 1999;274:37125–37130

25. Manno CS, Pierce GF, Arruda VR, et al. Successful transduction of liver in hemophilia by AAV-Factor IX and limitations imposed by the host immune response. Nat Med 2006;12:342–347

26. Nathwani AC, Gray JT, McIntosh J, et al. Safe and efficient transduction of the liver after peripheral vein infusion of self-complementary AAV vector results in stable therapeutic expression of human FIX in nonhuman primates. Blood 2007;109:1414–1421

27. Mount JD, Herzog RW, Tillson DM, et al. Sustained phenotypic correction of hemophilia B dogs with a factor IX null mutation by liver-directed gene therapy. Blood 2002;99:2670–2676

28. Maguire AM, Simonelli F, Pierce EA, et al. Safety and efficacy of gene transfer for Leber's congenital amaurosis. N Engl J Med 2008;358:2240–2248

29. Van Belle T, von Herrath M. Immunosuppression in islet transplantation. J Clin Invest 2008;118:1625–1628

30. Buchlis G, Podsakoff GM, Radu A, et al. Factor IX expression in skeletal muscle of a severe hemophilia B patient 10 years after AAV-mediated gene transfer. Blood 2012;119:3038–3041

31. Al-Dosari M, Zhang G, Knapp JE, Liu D. Evaluation of viral and mammalian promoters for driving transgene expression in mouse liver. Biochem Biophys Res Commun 2006;339:673–678

32. Yang J, Reshef L, Cassuto H, Aleman G, Hanson RW. Aspects of the control of phosphoenolpyruvate carboxykinase gene transcription. J Biol Chem 2009;284:27031–27035

33. Manno CS, Chew AJ, Hutchison S, et al. AAV-mediated factor IX gene transfer to skeletal muscle in patients with severe hemophilia B. Blood 2003;101:2963–2972

34. Boutin S, Monteilhet V, Veron P, et al. Prevalence of serum IgG and neutralizing factors against adeno-associated virus (AAV) types 1, 2, 5, 6, 8, and 9 in the healthy population: implications for gene therapy using AAV vectors. Hum Gene Ther 2010;21:704–712

35. Bertuzzi F, Verzaro R, Provenzano V, Ricordi C. Brittle type 1 diabetes mellitus. Curr Med Chem 2007;14:1739–1744

36. Velazquez VM, Bowen DG, Walker CM. Silencing of T lymphocytes by antigen-driven programmed death in recombinant adeno-associated virus vector-mediated gene therapy. Blood 2009;113:538–545

37. Haurigot V, Mingozzi F, Buchlis G, et al. Safety of AAV factor IX peripheral transvenular gene delivery to muscle in hemophilia B dogs. Mol Ther 2010; 18:1318–1329

38. Mendell JR, Rodino-Klapac LR, Rosales-Quintero X, et al. Limb-girdle muscular dystrophy type 2D gene therapy restores alpha-sarcoglycan and associated proteins. Ann Neurol 2009;66:290–297

39. Gordon I, Paoloni M, Mazcko C, Khanna C; The Comparative Oncology Trials Consortium. The Comparative Oncology Trials Consortium: using spontaneously occurring cancers in dogs to inform the cancer drug development pathway. PLoS Med 2009;6:e1000161

In Brief

The usefulness of self-monitoring of blood glucose (SMBG) requires patients with diabetes to be competent and confident in their ability to carry out glucose testing and interpret its results to guide lifestyle choices and improve outcomes. SMBG instruction can be offered in a variety of settings by a wide array of health care professionals. However, patients too often receive no formal SMBG training. The two skills sets required to successfully perform SMBG include 1) operating a glucose meter and 2) appropriately interpreting SMBG data. Whenever diabetes education is provided, both skill sets, as well as potential barriers, should be assessed for all patients.

The Two Skill Sets of Self-Monitoring of Blood Glucose Education: The Operational and the Interpretive

Mary M. Austin, MA, RD, CDE, FAADE

Self-monitoring of blood glucose (SMBG) is an important aspect of treatment for all people with diabetes. It provides immediate feedback and data that enable people with diabetes to assess how their food choices, physical activity levels, and medications affect their blood glucose control. SMBG results can aid people with diabetes in evaluating their current diabetes management efforts by either reinforcing or calling into question their lifestyle choices.[1]

The last American Diabetes Association (ADA) consensus conference on SMBG was held in 1994.[2] Table 1 provides a list from that conference of potential applications for SMBG data.[2] Not surprisingly, many of these applications are directly related to insulin therapy.

More recently, other consensus panels have made recommendations related to SMBG use.[3,4] In 2009, the International Diabetes Federation (IDF) convened an international working group to consider SMBG recommendations for people with noninsulin-treated type 2 diabetes.[5] All six of its recommendations underscored the fact that, for SMBG to be useful for people with type 2 diabetes and effective in managing their diabetes (improving outcomes), it must be part of an educational program, individualized, and used in partnership with patients' health care providers (HCPs) (Table 2).

Although many health care professionals can teach the operational use of, and interpretive strategies for, SMBG, this article focuses on the role of diabetes educators in this process. Diabetes educators consider SMBG one outcome measurement component of "monitoring," which is included in the American Association of Diabetes Educators' AADE7

Table 1. Potential Applications for SMBG Data[1]

- Achieve and maintain target goals for blood glucose
- Prevent and detect hypoglycemia, including hypoglycemia unawareness
- Prevent and detect hyperglycemia and avoid diabetic ketoacidosis or hyperglycemic hyperosmolar syndrome
- Evaluate the glycemic response to types and amounts of food and physical activity
- Determine appropriate insulin-to-carbohydrate ratios, correction factors, and basal insulin rates for intensive management (multiple daily injections and insulin pumps)
- Adjust treatment in response to changes in lifestyle and the need to add, subtract, increase, or decrease dosages or types of pharmacological therapies
- Determine the need for adjustment in insulin dosages during illness
- Determine the need for insulin therapy in gestational diabetes

Table 2. SMBG Recommendations for People With Noninsulin-Treated Type 2 Diabetes[5]

- The purpose of performing SMBG and using SMBG data should be agreed on between the person with diabetes and the HCP and documented.
- Consider using SMBG at the time of diagnosis and as part of ongoing diabetes self-management education (DSME) to facilitate timely treatment and titration optimization.
- Consider SMBG as part of ongoing DSME to assist people with diabetes to better understand their disease and provide a means to actively and effectively participate in its control and treatment.
- SMBG should be used only when individuals with diabetes (and/or their caregivers) and/or their HCPs have the knowledge, skills, and willingness to incorporate SMBG monitoring and therapy adjustment into their diabetes care plan to attain treatment goals.
- SMBG protocols (intensity and frequency) should be individualized to address individuals' specific education/behavioral/clinical requirements.
- SMBG use requires an easy procedure for patients to regularly monitor the performance and accuracy of their glucose meter.

Self-Care Behaviors.[6] The other six diabetes self-care behaviors are being active, following a healthy eating plan, taking medications, practicing healthy coping strategies, reducing risks, and problem solving.

Components of SMBG Education
The goal of SMBG education is to ensure that people who use a blood glucose meter are competent and confident in their ability to perform blood glucose tests and interpret the resulting data to make lifestyle choices, which have an impact on clinical outcomes. Competence and confidence are necessary for people to use SMBG effectively as a tool in their diabetes self-management plan.

The two skill sets necessary for successful SMBG are 1) operational skills and 2) interpretive skills (Table 3). Because blood glucose meters can be obtained from a variety of sources,

Table 3. SMBG Education Checklist[1]

Operational Skills: Using the Meter
- Selecting a meter
- Ensuring meter accuracy
- Documenting SMBG data
- Addressing individual needs

Interpretation Skills: Using SMBG Data
- Knowing blood glucose targets
- Knowing the appropriate frequency and timing of glucose tests
- Using pattern management in decision-making

diabetes educators may not be directly involved initially in either teaching or assessing both of these skill sets. At the time of diabetes education, regardless of how long ago a person was prescribed a blood glucose meter, it is important for diabetes educators to assess both of these skill sets to uncover potential barriers to using the meter and SMBG data.

Operational skills
During education sessions in which the operational skills of monitoring are being taught, it is important that educators demonstrate the mechanics of performing a blood glucose test and then ask participants for a return demonstration. In addition to successfully performing blood glucose tests confidently and competently, individuals should learn how to use a lancet device, properly dispose of lancets and strips, use control solution, obtain an adequate blood sample, alternate testing sites, code the meter (if required), clean the meter, and document their SMBG results in a logbook or download blood glucose data from the meter. Educators should heed universal precautions when demonstrating how to operate a meter.[7] Other aspects of successfully operating a meter are discussed in detail in the following sections.

Selecting a meter. Many factors should be considered when choosing an appropriate meter for an individual with diabetes. These include patients' visual acuity, manual dexterity, and preferences, as well as meter size and readout options (e.g., back lighting, flagging, and messaging), calibration

(coding), and memory and downloading features. However, in many cases, meter selection is limited by patients' insurance coverage. If there is a choice of covered meters, the educator should present the available options, and the selection should be based on individuals' needs and preferences.

It is important for educators to evaluate whether the meter itself is a barrier to SMBG for each patient. This may be the result when patients' insurance plan switches approved meters without patients receiving additional training or education. Unless such patients are comfortable and confident using the replacement meter, continued SMBG may be jeopardized.

The nuances of insurance coverage for meters and test strips can also become a barrier to SMBG. Educators should encourage their patients to contact their insurance plan and ask if the blood glucose meter and strips are considered a pharmacy benefit or a durable medical equipment benefit. It is not unusual for patients to go to a pharmacy to obtain their meter and strips only to be told that these items are not a covered benefit. However, by asking the right questions of their insurers, patients sometimes find out that, although not covered under a pharmacy benefit, these items are covered if mail-ordered from a medical supply company.

Ensuring meter accuracy. The accuracy of the SMBG results depends on both meter capabilities and the human factor in performing a blood glucose test. The U.S. Food and Drug Administration requires all glucose meters to meet a minimum performance requirement set by the International Organization of Standardization (ISO). The international standard for glucose meters, known as ISO 15197, requires 95% of the meter results > 75 mg/dl to be within ± 20% of the true value as measured by a standardized laboratory blood glucose test system. For results < 75 mg/dl, 95% must be within ± 15 mg/dl of the true value.[8] It is expected that more stringent ISO standards for glucose meters will be released in the near future.

To ensure accurate data and limit human error when performing SMBG, educators should encourage individuals to:
- Store their meter and strips properly (Each meter has its own storage requirements; strips should

be stored with cap on bottle and not exposed to light, moisture, or temperature variations.)

- Use strips that are compatible, defect-free, and not expired (Expiration dates are not always provided when strips are supplied through a mail-order company.)
- Code their meter if the device requires coding
- Perform a control-solution check with every new container of strips and more often if necessary (if meter error is suspected because of unpredictable results). Control solution must be prescribed by a provider to be processed as a covered benefit.
- Use a meter that is clean and free of dried blood or debris
- Use an adequate-sized blood sample. Educators may need to teach patients techniques for obtaining an adequate blood droplet, including how to select a lancing device and appropriate puncture depth.
- Use clean, dry fingers (Using an alcohol swipe is not necessary.)

Documenting SMBG data. It is essential for SMBG results to be available in a format that allows people with diabetes to assess the relationship between their blood glucose results and their food intake, physical activity, and medication regimen. Meter memory features can be useful in verifying logbook accuracy, but used alone without a paper logbook may not provide patients with the opportunity to visualize multiple testing results over time.

For patients who have downloadable meters and the capability and capacity to download their results (usually displayed in various graphic formats), educators should review the downloading process to ensure that patients are interpreting the graphic displays correctly. If it is also possible to transmit blood glucose results by phone or electronically, patients and providers or educators should come to an agreement about how often and when transmission should occur.

Patients should be encouraged to bring their meter and blood glucose documentation to every medical visit. This provides the opportunity to review results, clean the meter, verify meter codes if necessary, and perform a control-solution test.

Addressing individual needs. Certain populations have specific needs related to meter selection and use. The elderly, children, and the visually impaired may have unique SMBG needs.

For the elderly, choice of meter and strips may be influenced by potential limitations in manual dexterity, slowed reaction time, or fluctuating vision.[9] How patients receive their monitoring supplies may affect their blood glucose testing. It may be more convenient and cost-effective for the elderly to receive their supplies via mail-order. Educators should address this option and remind patients that they must request shipments of their supplies because "auto-shipments" of meter supplies is no longer allowed.

Children may benefit from meters that require a small sample of blood

and lancing devices that hide the lancet and minimize discomfort. Parents often appreciate features such as back lighting for the display, which makes testing in the middle of the night easier, and a memory capacity to store multiple results. When children begin performing their own blood glucose checks, supervision should be provided to ensure that they are performing SMBG properly and recording results accurately.

People with visual impairments would benefit from a meter that is small, is portable, provides a clear speech output, has tactile markings on strips, and offers a method for consistent placement of the blood sample. A limited number of products offer these features. The National Federation for the Blind continuously evaluates products and services for people with diabetes who are blind and can be contacted through its Web site (http://nfb.org) for a list of currently available products.[10]

Interpretive skills

Interpreting SMBG results is considered a problem-solving self-care behavior. It is not uncommon for people who are testing their blood glucose, especially people with type 2 diabetes, to be proficient at and feel confident in their ability to perform tests, but to not use their SMBG data in lifestyle decision-making. Additionally, if patients' HCPs do not use the SMBG data in clinical decision-making, then SMBG is of no value and a waste of resources.

Table 4. ADA and AACE Target Blood Glucose Goals for Non-Pregnant Adults[10,11]

	ADA Guidelines	AACE Guidelines*
A1C (%)	• < 7.0; individualized based on duration of disease, age/life expectancy, comorbid conditions, known cardiovascular or advanced microvascular complications, hypoglycemia unawareness, and individual patient considerations • More (< 6.5) or less (8.0) stringent glycemic goals may be appropriate for individual patients	• ≤ 6.5 for most; individualized on the basis of age, comorbidities, and duration of disease • Closer to normal for healthy • Less stringent for "less healthy"
Fasting and preprandial blood glucose (mg/dl)	• 70–130	• < 110
Postprandial blood glucose (mg/dl)	• < 180 at "peak" levels, 1–2 hours after the start of a meal • Postprandial glucose may be targeted if A1C goal not met despite reaching preprandial glucose goals	• < 140, 2 hours after the start of a meal

As an analogy, one may know how a parachute works and how to wear it properly, but unless one uses a parachute when jumping out of a plane, the parachute is of no value. The same can be said for SMBG: it provides value when the data obtained are used. Using SMBG data depends on knowing blood glucose targets, understanding how often and when to test, and using glucose pattern management (GPM) in decision-making, not only for the people with diabetes, but also for their HCPs.

Knowing blood glucose targets. ADA[11] and the American Association of Clinical Endocrinologists (AACE)[12] have set guidelines for blood glucose targets. From a practical standpoint, it matters little which organization's blood glucose target guidelines are followed as long as patients who have been instructed to perform SMBG receive *some* blood glucose target recommendations.

HCPs have the responsibility to provide patients with blood glucose targets based on individual needs. ADA target blood glucose guidelines can be applicable to all people, given that tighter individual targets can be recommended that are within the ADA-recommended target range (Table 4).

The ADA postprandial peak value of < 180 mg/dl can be explained to individuals as aiming for a blood glucose that is no higher than 180 mg/dl, 1–2 hours after a meal. This range is helpful to individuals who find it difficult to check their blood glucose exactly 2 hours after the start of the meal.

HCPs should encourage individuals to write their targets in their blood glucose logbook or recording form; this helps to reinforce this information. Some meters with downloading capabilities can show results in a graphic format. The blood glucose targets that are individually set on the meter should be clearly stated to the person using the meter and written down somewhere for reference when tests are performed.

Knowing the appropriate frequency and timing of glucose tests. There are no universally accepted standards for frequency and timing of SMBG. Many factors must be considered when determining how often and when to test blood glucose. These factors include patients':
- Type of diabetes
- Willingness to perform SMBG
- Level of diabetes control
- Medication regimen
- Lifestyle and daily schedule with regard to activity, food, and work
- Physical ability to check blood glucose
- Ability to problem-solve and take action
- Financial limitations
- Comorbid conditions

Few doubt the value of SMBG for patients using a multiple daily injection (MDI) insulin regimen or insulin pump therapy because of its utility in detecting hypoglycemia and dosing insulin. For people with type 1 diabetes or those with type 2 diabetes using an MDI regimen, blood glucose testing should occur at least before meals and snacks, occasionally postprandially, at bedtime, before exercise, when hypoglycemia is suspected, after hypoglycemia treatment (until normoglycemia is attained), and before crucial tasks such as driving.[11]

However, what is more typically done in this population is testing while fasting and before meals to determine mealtime insulin doses. Occasionally, postprandial SMBG is performed to monitor the effect of a meal on the postmeal rise in blood glucose. To ensure safety, testing before bedtime and before driving are warranted for some individuals. Additional testing is useful during times of insulin dose adjustment, illness, pregnancy, strenuous physical activity, or prolonged exercise.

As with type 1 diabetes, there is no universal standard for testing frequency for type 2 diabetes. In this population, especially those who are not on insulin therapy, SMBG can be useful to reinforce lifestyle habits or changes and to monitor medication regimens. Schwedes et al.[13] showed that when individuals with type 2 diabetes who were not on insulin therapy checked meal-related glucose levels and participated in a structured counseling program, a majority significantly improved their glycemic control. Similarly, in a study by Barnett et al.[14] of patients with type 2 diabetes on oral medications showed that SMBG resulted in improved A1C levels.

The 2009 IDF SMBG guidelines for people with noninsulin-treated type 2 diabetes[5] have gone furthest in suggesting a testing regimen (timing and frequency) for type 2 diabetes (also called "structured testing"). These guidelines suggest numerous "focused" SMBG regimens based on the specific glucose data required (i.e., fasting vs. postprandial). Parkin et al.[15] examined studies involving structured testing as a component of comprehensive diabetes management and concluded that the results support the IDF's recommendations. In addition to these regimens, the *Type 2 BASICS* curriculum guide[16] of the International Diabetes Center in Minneapolis, Minn., suggests a 3-point profile to check fasting blood glucose and the effects of the largest meal.

Table 5 summarizes some of the possible testing regimens, all of which use a variation of paired testing. The 5- and 7-point regimens and the staggered-frequency regimen are considered meal-based testing schemes. The goal of these regimens is to discover the effect of food consumed on the rise in blood glucose after specific mealtimes. Educators can discuss these options with patients to decide which regimen they are willing to do. Patients who find performing SMBG seven times per day over several days unacceptable could instead perform fewer tests over several days at a specific mealtime and then rotate testing every several days until all mealtimes can be assessed. As patients test their blood glucose before and after meals, the resulting data should provide insight into when out-of-target blood glucose levels are occurring.

The 3-point testing regimen, which provides information about glucose control in the fasting state and around the largest meal of the day, can be particularly useful for newly diagnosed individuals with type 2 diabetes. Often patients with newly diagnosed type 2 diabetes are told to check their blood glucose only once per day, first thing in the morning. If their fasting blood glucose level is consistently within the target range, however, this offers little insight into their overall glycemic control. By testing both while fasting and before and after their largest meal, patients can begin to assess the impact of the food they eat on their glycemic control. This is particularly important for people who are working with a registered dietitian because meal-time monitoring is necessary to develop an individualized meal plan that will promote glycemic control.

Noninsulin-requiring people with type 2 diabetes typically only have

Table 5. Examples of SMBG Regimens[1]

	Pre-Breakfast	Post-Breakfast	Pre-Lunch	Post-Lunch	Pre-Supper	Post-Supper	Bedtime
Three-point SMBG profile to check fasting blood glucose and the effect of the largest meal							
Monday	×				×	×	
Tuesday	×				×	×	
Wednesday	×				×	×	
Thursday	×				×	×	
Friday	×				×	×	
Saturday	×				×	×	
Sunday	×				×	×	
Five-point SMBG profile							
Monday	×	×		×	×	×	
Tuesday	×	×		×	×	×	
Wednesday							
Thursday							
Friday							
Saturday							
Sunday	×	×		×	×	×	
Seven-point SMBG profile							
Monday							
Tuesday							
Wednesday							
Thursday	×	×	×	×	×	×	×
Friday	×	×	×	×	×	×	×
Saturday	×	×	×	×	×	×	×
Sunday							
Staggered SMBG profile							
Monday	×	×					
Tuesday			×	×			
Wednesday					×	×	
Thursday	×	×					
Friday			×	×			
Saturday					×	×	
Sunday	×	×					

Table 5. Examples of SMBG Regimens[1], *continued from p. 87*

Meal-based SMBG profile (less intensive)

Monday	×	×					
Tuesday							
Wednesday			×	×			
Thursday							
Friday							
Saturday					×	×	
Sunday							

SMBG profile to assess or detect fasting hyperglycemia

Monday							×
Tuesday	×						
Wednesday							×
Thursday	×						
Friday							×
Saturday	×						
Sunday							

insurance coverage for 30 test strips per month (unless their provider prescribes and justifies the need for more strips). It is important for educators to work with patients to determine how their monthly allotment of strips will be used to obtain actionable information. If their test strip allowance is limited, this may result in no SMBG testing on some days.

Using pattern management in decision-making. Some decisions such as treating hypoglycemia do not require multiple SMBG results to justify taking action. However, most clinical and lifestyle decisions, such as adjusting medication doses, changing food intake, or understanding the effects of exercise, will require three to four blood glucose results taken at the same time of day before taking action.

Pattern management involves both patients and providers performing a systematic review and analysis of the patients' recorded blood glucose levels. Some available meters and software programs provide automated pattern detection. Regardless of how patterns are detected, the goal is to proactively make changes in lifestyle or the therapeutic regimen to resolve consistent patterns of high or low blood glucose and attain blood glucose targets.[17]

A study by Wang et al.[18] suggested that teaching patients problem-solving skills to act on SMBG results is crucial to improving outcomes; testing blood glucose alone, without taking action based on the results, will not necessar-ily lead to improved clinical outcomes. Diabetes educators can play a key role in teaching problem-solving skills. Encouraging individuals to write their blood glucose values in a logbook that allows testing times and results to be recorded in a linear and vertical manner facilitates the process of reviewing results (Table 6). There are also meters available that can detect blood glucose patterns and provide users with feedback.

Additionally, the framework for interpreting SMBG records developed by Powers[19] provides the questions that need to be considered when assessing blood glucose results. (See related article in this issue, p. 91.) That framework groups questions in a three-step process: obtaining suf-

Table 6. Sample SMBG Log Recording Results in a Linear and Vertical Manner[1]

Target range 70–130 mg/dl fasting and before meals, < 180 mg/dl 2 hours after meals

	Pre-Breakfast	Post-Breakfast	Pre-Lunch	Post-Lunch	Pre-Dinner	Post-Dinner	Bedtime
Monday	128	256			188		
Tuesday	114	248					
Wednesday	118	212	122				
Thursday							
Friday						65	
Saturday							
Sunday							

ficient and accurate SMBG data; identifying all possible interpretations; and making individual plans and recommendations.

It is crucial for people with diabetes to understand all of the factors that can raise or lower their blood glucose. Unless this is clear, patients will not understand what action or lifestyle changes they need to undertake.

It is also important for patients and providers who are analyzing SMBG data to understand that the timing of a blood glucose test can provide valuable insight. For example, if fasting blood glucose results are not within the target range, this assesses the overnight effect of medication(s) taken the night before. If postmeal blood glucose levels are above target, this assesses the adequacy of premeal diabetes medications in light of the meal eaten; if no medications are taken before meals, this assesses the effect of the meal. Table 7 provides direction regarding what to assess when trying to problem-solve out-of-range blood glucose levels.

Paired testing, through which blood glucose is checked before and again 1–2 hours after a meal, has gained attention in recent years.[20] Postprandial testing provides insight on the effect of the meal, the efficacy of the medication(s), and the effect of physical activity on blood glucose levels. Research by Monnier et al.[21] concluded that, as A1C approaches a target of 7%, postprandial blood glucose contributes more to the A1C result than does fasting blood glucose. In such situations, diabetes educators should encourage individuals to focus their efforts on reaching their postprandial blood glucose targets.

It is important to remember that blood glucose testing alone is not sufficient to improve glycemic outcomes.[17] Patients should be educated not only about how to perform SMBG, but also about how to interpret the results, and providers may need SMBG education as well. A study by Rodbard et. al[22,23] showed that improvements in glycemic control occurred when structured SMBG was combined with comprehensive clinical education about SMBG data interpretation and use for medical providers.

Conclusion
Successful SMBG requires education; all patients who are prescribed a meter should also be provided with a referral

for diabetes self-management education. It is not enough to understand how to operate a blood glucose meter and successfully perform a test.

The educational components of SMBG include two types of skills: operational (how to operate the meter) and interpretive (how to interpret and act on SMBG results [i.e., GPM]). The value of monitoring is realized when people with diabetes are able to competently and confidently perform SMBG and then analyze the resulting data to make self-care choices

that positively affect their diabetes management.

It is crucial for SMBG results to be shared with patients' HCPs and considered when making clinical decisions. Between medical office visits, SMBG results may be the only feedback individuals have to critically assess their glycemic control and management. Educators and HCPs must not only teach patients how to correctly perform SMBG, but also be confident and competent in their own ability to interpret and use SMBG data

Table 7. Information Provided by SMBG at Different Times of Day[1]

SMBG Timing	Information Provided
Fasting	Assesses overnight effect of medications: • If fasting is higher than bedtime, possible nocturnal hypoglycemia or dawn effect
Premeal	Assesses basal insulin therapy needs
Postmeal	Assesses adequacy of premeal medications (rapid- or short-acting insulin or oral medications) in light of the meal eaten • If no premeal medications, it assesses effect of the meal
Bedtime	Assesses the effect of the evening meal and basal therapy needs
Random	Can help determine whether presenting symptoms are the result of blood glucose fluctuations (hypoglycemia)

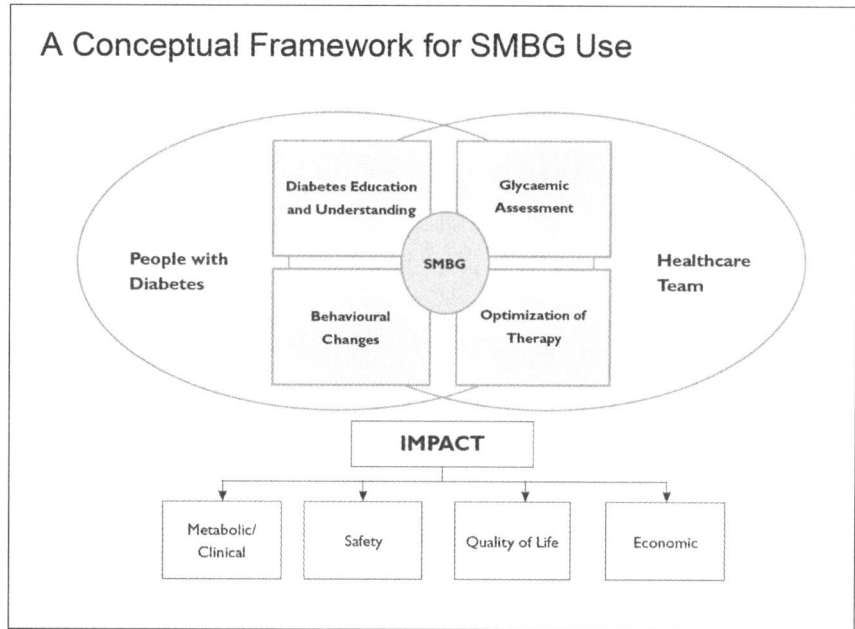

Figure 1. SMBG as a component of the education/treatment program. This figure illustrates and summarizes how SMBG can be used by individuals and HCPs and suggests the potential effect of SMBG on metabolic/clinical outcomes, safety, quality of life, and economic considerations. Reprinted with permission from ref. 5.

to teach problem-solving skills to their patients. Figure 1[5] illustrates and summarizes how SMBG can be used by individuals and HCPs and suggests the potential effect of SMBG on metabolic/clinical outcomes, safety, quality of life, and economic considerations.

References

[1]Austin MM, Powers MA: Monitoring. In *The Art and Science of Diabetes Self-Management Education Desk Reference*. 2nd ed. Mensing C, Ed. Chicago, American Association of Diabetes Educators, 2011, p. 167–194

[2]American Diabetes Association: Self-monitoring of blood glucose [consensus statement]. *Diabetes Care* 17:81–86, 1994

[3]Klonoff DC, Blonde L, Cembrowski G, Chacra AR, Charpentier G, Colagiuri, Dailey G, Gabbay RA, Heinemann L, Kerr D, Nicolucci A, Polonsky W, Schnell O, Vigersky R, Yale, JF: Census report: the current role of self-monitoring of blood glucose in non-insulin-treated type 2 diabetes. *J Diabetes Sci Technol* 5:1529–1548, 2011

[4]Hirsch IB, Bode BW, Childs BP, Close KL, Fisher WA, Gavin JR, Ginsberg BH, Raine CH, Verderese CA: Self-monitoring of blood glucose (SMBG) in insulin- and non-insulin-using adults in diabetes: accuracy, utilization, and research. *Diabetes Technol Ther* 10:419–439, 2008

[5]International Diabetes Federation: Guideline: self-monitoring of blood glucose in non-insulin-treated type 2 diabetes. Brussels, Belgium, International Diabetes Federation, 2009. Available from www.idf.org/webdata/docs/SMBG_EN2.pdf

[6]DeCoste K, Maurer L: The diabetes self-management education process. In *The Art and Science of Diabetes Self-Management Education Desk Reference*. 2nd ed. Mensing C, Ed. Chicago, American Association of Diabetes Educators, 2011, p. 21–69

[7]American Association of Diabetes Educators: Position statement: educating providers and persons with diabetes to prevent the transmission of blood borne infections and avoid injuries from sharps. *Diabetes Educ* 23:401–403, 1997

[8]International Organization for Standardization: In vitro diagnostic test systems: requirements for blood-glucose monitoring systems for self-testing in managing diabetes mellitus (ISO 15107). Geneva, International Organization for Standardization, 2003

[9]Peragallo-Dittko V: Clinical and educational usefulness of SMBG with the elderly. *Diabetes Spectrum* 8:17–19, 1995

[10]Bartos BJ, Cleary MJ, Kleinbeck C, Petzinger RA, Whittington A, Williams AS: Diabetes and disabilities: assistive tools, services and information. *Diabetes Educ* 34:600–605, 2008

[11]American Diabetes Association: Standards of medical care in diabetes—2013. *Diabetes Care* 36(Suppl. 1):S11–S66, 2013

[12]American Association of Clinical Endocrinologists: Medical guidelines for clinical practice for developing a diabetes mellitus comprehensive care plan. *Endocr Pract* 17 (Suppl. 2):1–53, 2011

[13]Schwedes U, Siebolds M, Mertes G: Meal-related structured self-monitoring of blood glucose: effect on diabetes control in non-insulin treated type 2 diabetic patients. *Diabetes Care* 25:1928–1932, 2002

[14]Barnett AH, Krentz AJ, Strojek K, Sieradzki J, Azizi F, Embong M, Imamoglu S, Perusicová J, Uliciansky V, Winkler G: The efficacy of self-monitoring of blood glucose in the management of patients with type 2 diabetes treated with a gliclazide modified release-based regimen: a multi-centre, randomized, parallel-group, 6-month evaluation (DINAMIC 1 study). *Diabetes Obes Metab* 10:1239–1247, 2008

[15]Parkin CG, Buskirk A, Hinnen DA, Axel-Schweitzer M: Results that matter: structured vs. unstructured self-monitoring of blood glucose in type 2 diabetes. *Diab Res Clin Pract* 97:6–15, 2012

[16]International Diabetes Center: *Type 2 Diabetes BASICS Curriculum Guide*. 3rd ed. Minneapolis, Minn., International Diabetes Center, 2009

[17]Hinnen D, Tomky D: Combating clinical inertia through pattern management and intensifying therapy. In *The Art and Science of Diabetes Self-Management Education Desk Reference*. 2nd ed. Mensing C, Ed. Chicago, American Association of Diabetes Educators, 2011, p. 531–575

[18]Wang J, Zgibor J, Matthews JT, Charron-Prochownik DM, Sereika S, Siminerio L: Self-monitoring of blood glucose is associated with problem-solving skills in hyperglycemia and hypoglycemia. *Diabetes Educ* 38:207–214, 2012

[19]Powers MA: *Handbook of Diabetes Medical Nutrition Therapy*. Aspen Publishers, 1996

[20]Polonsky WH, Fisher L, Schikman CH, Hinnen DA, Parkin CG, Jelsovsky Z, Petersen B, Schwitzer M, Wagner R: Structured self-monitoring of blood glucose significantly reduces A1C levels in poorly controlled, noninsulin-treated type 2 diabetes: results from the Structured Testing Program study. *Diabetes Care* 34:262–267, 2011

[21]Monnier L, Lapinski H, Colette C: Contributions of fasting and postprandial plasma glucose increments to the overall diurnal hyperglycemia of type 2 diabetic patients. *Diabetes Care* 26:881–885, 2003

[22]Rodbard HW, Schnell O, Unger J, Rees C, Amstutz L, Parkin CG, Jelsovsky Z, Wegmann N, Axel-Schweitzer M, Wagner R: Use of an automated decision support tool optimizes clinicians' ability to interpret and appropriately respond to structured self-monitoring of blood glucose data. *Diabetes Care* 35:693–698, 2012

[23]Rodbard HW, Schnell O, Unger J, Rees C, Amstutz L, Parkin CG, Jelsovsky Z, Wegmann N, Axel-Schweitzer M, Wagner R: Supplementary data: use of an automated decision support tool optimizes clinicians' ability to interpret and appropriately respond to structured self-monitoring of blood glucose data. Available from http://care.diabetes-journals.org/lookup/suppl/doi:10.2337/dc11-1351/-/DC1. Accessed 6 January 2013

Mary M. Austin, MA, RD, CDE, FAADE, is principal at The Austin Group, LLC, in Shelby Township, Mich.

Note of disclosure: Ms. Austin is a faculty member for the Johnson & Johnson Diabetes Institute, an educational entity funded by Johnson & Johnson, the parent company of glucose meter companies.

In Brief

Self-monitoring of blood glucose (SMBG) involves both the performance of glucose tests and glucose pattern management (GPM) and is a tool patients with diabetes can use to achieve their glucose goals. Seeing the effects that increased activity or modified carbohydrate intake can have on lowering glucose levels is a powerful motivator for patients and reinforces successful behaviors. This article describes how SMBG (including GPM) is integrated into a diabetes self-management education program to teach problem-solving skills and empower patients.

Glucose Pattern Management Teaches Glycemia-Related Problem-Solving Skills in a Diabetes Self-Management Education Program

Margaret A. Powers, PhD, RD, CDE, Janet Davidson, BSN, RN, CDE, and Richard M. Bergenstal, MD

People with diabetes make decisions every day that affect their glycemic control. Fortunately, a simple tool is available to help them with that decision-making: self-monitoring of blood glucose (SMBG). This article describes how the two components of SMBG (glucose testing and glucose pattern management [GPM]) help patients with type 2 diabetes achieve their glycemic goals. Too frequently, patients are taught how to perform glucose tests but not how to interpret and react to glucose patterns revealed in their results. This article demonstrates how GPM can be woven into a standard diabetes self-management education (DSME) curriculum for both newly diagnosed patients and those seeking ongoing education. Through GPM, patients learn how well their diabetes management is working and take steps to improve their glucose control.[1–5]

The GPM Process

GPM is the process of recognizing glucose patterns, analyzing what is causing out-of-target readings, and taking steps to bring readings back into the target range.[6] Sometimes referred to as "pattern control" or "glucose pattern control," this process provides patients with information to make decisions regarding their diabetes self-management. At the core of these decisions are glycemia-related problem-solving skills.

GPM is an integral component of patient-centered diabetes self-management because it:

- Educates patients about how well-controlled their glucose levels are
- Provides feedback on therapy and guides therapy changes
- Helps minimize the number of high and low glucose readings, thereby contributing to more stable glucose levels

GPM enables patients to understand how their day-to-day choices affect their glucose levels. Having this information empowers patients to make the decisions necessary to reach their goals.

Although quarterly or biannual A1C testing provides an overall average of glycemic control, it does not provide guidance on daily meal and activity decisions or medication adjustments. In addition, A1C levels may camouflage poor glycemic control because an optimum A1C level can be achieved even with wide glycemic fluctuations. In fact, such daily glycemic variability is a risk factor for hypoglycemia[7,8] and is being evaluated as a potential risk factor for other diabetes complications[9–12] and lower patient satisfaction/quality of life.[13]

Components of a DSME Program

The three essential components of DSME programs that integrate glucose testing and GPM are:

- A philosophical belief that glucose testing and GPM are necessary for understanding the impact of food, activity, and medications on daily glucose levels and, ultimately, on A1C levels
- Expert staff who can teach patients how to interpret their glucose data

and how to integrate these data into food, activity, and medication therapies
- Materials that guide data collection and interpretation

Patients who review glucose data and use GPM have the ability to choose the best therapy to help them to achieve their glycemic targets. Many providers focus on adding or increasing medication to the treatment plan, but patients may choose, appropriately, to pursue healthy eating and increased activity instead. By using GPM, the success of meal planning and increased activity can be readily verified in the glucose readings. It can safely and optimally assist patients in achieving their A1C goal.

A Curriculum Focus on GPM

The diabetes care team at the International Diabetes Center (IDC) in Minneapolis, Minn., developed the Type 2 Diabetes BASICS curriculum to facilitate teaching GPM to newly diagnosed patients with type 2 diabetes or individuals previously diagnosed but in need of a review or update.[6,14–17] The primary teaching strategy is to have patients record their glucose levels in a food and activity log so that they can see the direct cause-and-effect relationships. This exercise empowers patients to make their own decisions regarding lifestyle and medication. The curriculum encompasses the three essential DSME program components listed above, which support patient self-efficacy in using pattern management to achieve glucose goals.

The BASICS curriculum has four core sessions. The first two sessions can be described as survival-level education and are team-taught by a nurse and a dietitian. These sessions promote the basic knowledge and skills necessary to provide a safety net for living with diabetes. They also establish a focus on glucose management and problem-solving.

Research has shown that the curriculum results in reduced A1C levels and is as effective in group settings as in individual settings.[18] In a 6-month study, attendees in both settings significantly decreased their A1C levels—individuals by 1.7% ($P < 0.01$) and those in groups by 2.5% ($P < 0.01$). Body weight also significantly decreased—individuals by 10.4 lb ($P < 0.01$) and those in groups

by 5.8 lb ($P < 0.01$). Improvements in health-related quality-of-life measures were similarly positive. A recently presented study using the curriculum in a U.S. Department of Veterans Affairs group setting showed decreases in A1C levels and weight compared to a control group receiving only medical follow-up.[19]

A guide for teaching glucose testing and GPM in a DSME program, based on the IDC experience, is provided below.

Initial SMBG Education

Teaching SMBG (including both glucose testing and GPM) is based on the core philosophy that the majority of patients will ultimately succeed at GPM and that the practice will result in improved glucose control. At the end of the initial education session, patients should know their target glucose goals and recommended testing times and have an initial food plan.

As with all learning situations, it is best if unique patient needs are addressed before the delivery of content. Instructors might use these discussions to guide the flow of information. In one-on-one sessions, instructors may let patients lead the learning process so that the content makes the most sense to them. In group settings, the facilitator (a certified diabetes educator) addresses individual needs while keeping in mind the group dynamic. For the most part, individuals' questions correspond with the content delivered during the initial session. Common questions include, "Why do I have diabetes?," "Will I always have diabetes?," and "How is diabetes treated?"

With the above caveats recognizing the need to individualize DSME to alleviate such concerns, the following describes how glucose testing and GPM are addressed in an initial DSME session. Because this session builds a foundation for successful GPM, the educator(s) should agree on the importance of GPM, understand how they can support it, and be comfortable problem-solving a variety of pattern management questions.

The initial goals are to ensure that patients understand what diabetes is and what treatments are available and to define individual treatment goals. Patients learn what glucose testing entails, including blood glucose and A1C targets, and how carbohydrate and physical activity affect glucose

levels. To support discussion of these topics, it is helpful for patients to bring a 5- to 7-day food and activity record to the session.

Some DSME programs offer separate visits for teaching glucose testing and developing a food and activity plan. A prerequisite for teaching GPM is that patients must have a personalized food plan, so each program must decide how best to accomplish this. The IDC experience supports having a nurse/dietitian team co-teach an initial 2-hour session and blend glucose testing and GPM training throughout.

All educators need to have the same glycemic outcome goals and either use the same materials or be familiar with each others' materials. Education materials support the use of glucose data by highlighting the need for glucose control, listing target glucose goals, and providing logs for patients to record food, activity, and glucose data.

The IDC patient book begins with a definition of diabetes and how diabetes is diagnosed. It emphasizes the importance of glucose control, and, in so doing, sets the stage for introducing tools to manage glucose levels. Visual aids indicate that food and activity are always part of the treatment plan and that a variety of medications are available. The book states, "The best treatment plan is the one that keeps your glucose level in control."[17]

Develop an initial food plan

The initial food plan is typically based on carbohydrate counting, with carbohydrate choices or grams distributed among each day's meals and snacks. As eating behaviors change, so, too, will the food plan. Because patients have much to learn about carbohydrate counting, food preparation, and portion sizes before applying this knowledge to everyday situations, some programs prefer to have patients go through the learning phase before implementing glucose testing and GPM. Regardless, patients need a food plan to interpret glucose data. In addition, glucose data are needed to evaluate the food plan as it is being adjusted to best fit each patient's eating patterns, health needs, and glycemic goals.

Discuss glucose goals

Many patients ask what their glucose level should be. Glucose target goals for fasting, premeal, and, in

Table 1. Summary of Glucose Goals[10]

Test Time	Diabetes Target (mg/dl)	My Target	No Diabetes or Prediabetes (mg/dl)
Before a meal	70–120		< 100
Two hours after the start of a meal	< 160		< 140

Table 2. Diabetes Goal-Setting Worksheet Used in Primary Care

My Diabetes at a Glance	Aspirin Use (Y/N)	A1C (%)*	Blood Pressure (mmHg)	LDL Cholesterol (mg/dl)**	Tobacco Use (Y/N)	Eye Exam	Foot Exam	Urine Albumin: Creatinine Ratio (mg/g)
Most recent results								
Prior results								
My goal †	81 mg/day if you have heart disease or as recomended	< 7 or < 8	< 140/80	< 100 or 70	Tobacco free	Normal exam	Normal exam	< 30
How often to check	Take daily	3 months	Every clinic visit	Yearly	Never use	Yearly exam	Yearly exam	Yearly exam (more often if results are abnormal)

*A1C goal is < 7% unless factors exist that would contraindicate intensive control, including severe complications, frail elderly, history of severe hypoglycemia or hypoglycemia unawareness, limited support or agreement to participate in one's care, and limited life expectancy. Glucose targets for A1C goal of < 7% are 70–120 mg/dl premeal and < 160 mg/dl postmeal. Glucose targets for A1C goal of < 8% are 90–160 mg/dl premeal and < 200 mg/dl postmeal.

**LDL target is < 100 mg/dl unless there is known cardiovascular disease, in which case the target is < 70 mg/dl.

†Each patient should have goals reviewed and individualized.

©2013 Park Nicollet Health System, Minneapolis, Minn. Adapted with permission.

some cases, postmeal periods are discussed, and the patients' goals are written in their book. If a provider has not communicated A1C or prandial/postprandial glucose goals to patients, the educator discusses those and then communicates the goals to the provider. Primary care providers and their support team at Park Nicollet Clinic (the integrated health care system that includes IDC) use a patient handout, which is in the process of being integrated into the electronic health record as part of the post-visit summary. Called "My Diabetes Care Plan," the handout reviews glucose and other diabetes-related goals. It is important for discussion with patients to have a shared care plan (Table 1). The educator emphasizes that patients' food, activity, and medication plans are aimed at keeping glucose levels in target and that the only way to receive

immediate feedback on how well they are doing is through SMBG.

It is helpful for patients to understand that the glucose test is not a test in the sense that they will be graded. Rather, it is a test that alerts patients about what is helping them meet their target glucose goals and what is not. Glucose test results are labeled neither good nor bad but are provided as data for problem-solving and decision-making.

Patients learn that glucose levels will be out of target on occasion and that a reasonable goal is to have at least half of their glucose test results in their target range. Realizing that they are not expected to have every test result within range softens the nature of glucose testing as a "test" and eases patients' sense of perfectionism. Glycemic feedback is key to reaching long-term A1C goals (Table 2).

Recommend testing times

A typical testing routine after initial education is to have patients check their blood glucose three times a day: fasting and before and 2 hours after the start of their largest carbohydrate meal. The dietitian may recommend additional testing times based on patients' eating habits and activity patterns, and patients themselves may be interested in additional testing.

A consideration when recommending testing frequency is the number of glucose test strips a patient's insurance will reimburse. During the 2 weeks after the initial session and before the second session, patients will use 15–30 test strips, depending on the number of errors they have and any extra testing they perform.

Provide an integrated food/activity/glucose record

A food record form that includes a place to record glucose data, such as

Table 3. Framework for Interpreting SMBG Records*

Steps	Sample Questions to Consider
1. Obtain sufficient data.	*Food plan* • Is food plan followed or have adjustments been made? • Is carbohydrate counted correctly? • If food data are not available, determine why. *Physical activity* • Is activity plan followed or have adjustments been made? • If activity data are not available, determine why. *Medications* • Is medication taken as prescribed? • If medication dose is not available, determine why. *Other* • Are possible reasons for glucose excursions noted? • How are low blood glucose levels treated? Are the levels really low? How frequently do really low glucose levels occur and when? • Are more frequent blood glucose tests needed? • Can the patient answer questions or offer insights into schedule or lifestyle variations? Is there a trend in the results, or are fluctuations isolated?
2. Identify all possible interpretations.	*Food plan* • Does the patient understand and follow the food plan? • Could meals be spaced more appropriately? • Are meals consistent in composition and size? • Are snacks eaten and regular? *Physical activity* • Is the patient able to follow the activity plan? • Is physical activity irregular? *Medications* • If medication is taken, is the person taking the correct dose at the correct time? • Is any medication out of date? • Do diabetes medications provide inadequate or too much coverage for meals?
3. Collaborate with patient to integrate data and make individualized recommendations.	*Food plan* • Could changes be made to food/carbohydrate amounts or timing of intake to make it easier to follow? *Physical activity* • Could physical activity be more regular, increased, or decreased? *Medications* • Could the medication regimen be adjusted? A different amount or type, or at a different time? *Other* • What changes would the patient choose to make? • Should the glucose goals be changed?

These are initial questions to consider when reviewing and interpreting diabetes records. Additional questions should consider additional factors such as stress, financial needs that affect purchasing food and medications, and available support for implementing a diabetes care plan.
Adapted from Powers MA: Handbook of Diabetes Medical Nutrition Therapy. *Rockville, Md., Aspen Publishers, 1996, and from ref. 3.*

the one used in the BASICS program, facilitates the integration of glucose data and GPM. This is a key aspect of learning GPM (Tables 3 and 4). For most clinicians, this makes sense because it allows them to easily review food intake (amount of carbohydrate and type of food) as well as activity levels and corresponding glucose values. Patients can see that their carbohydrate intake, activity level, and medication, if taken, all contribute to

their glucose levels and, ultimately, their A1C.

Summarize the initial session(s)
As with all education sessions, it is important to end with a recap of the main points and personal goals. As part of the recap, it is helpful to review how to apply the information presented, what barriers might occur, how to deal with these barriers, and what support may be necessary to help patients reach their goals. Sample ques-

tions that focus on behavioral change include: What habits might be easy or difficult for me to change? What new behaviors would I like to start? What might get in my way of making these changes? What will facilitate change? Who will support me?

Activities between DSME sessions help patients focus on key aspects of diabetes management to reinforce what they can do to achieve glucose control. A checklist of activities might include:

Table 4. Checklist for Integrating Glucose Testing and GPM into a DSME Program

Concern	Activity
Care team expectations/ competencies	• Discuss and agree on philosophy about glucose testing and GPM • Train staff on interpretation and use of GPM • Have education materials that guide collection and interpretation of glucose data
Patient preparation for education	• Provider makes referral for medical nutrition therapy (MNT) and DSME* • Provider supports use of glucose testing and GPM • Patient completes one to two MNT visits before DSME or MNT is included in DSME; a food plan is needed for GPM
Initial glucose testing and GPM education	Patient will: • Know target glucose goals • Know recommended glucose testing times • Be able to follow initial food plan • Have forms to record food, activity, medication, and glucose data
Advancing GPM education	Patient will: • Identify glucose patterns • Discuss patterns in relation to food, activity, and medication • Adjust glucose testing times based on patterns • Have a plan for continuing MNT and DSME • Complete 3–7 days of food, activity, medication, and glucose records before each diabetes visit and as needed between visits

Referral guidelines and assistance in locating a registered dietitian and DSME program are available from http://professional.diabetes.org/erp_zip_search.aspx, http://www.diabeteseducator.org/DiabetesEducation/ Programs.html, and http://www.eatright.org/programs/rdfinder.

• Test your glucose level every day at the recommended testing times.
• Record your glucose readings.
• Complete your food and activity record for at least 3 days.
• Stay active or become more active.
• Think about the new behaviors you have started and your goals for the future.
• Make notes about the challenges of taking care of your diabetes.
• List what has been helpful.

Advancing Application of GPM

In the IDC's experience, two to four subsequent education sessions have been necessary to assess patients' knowledge, application of information, and resulting glucose levels to determine the appropriateness of therapy (nutrition, activity, and medication) and make changes, if needed. If patients are to successfully implement GPM, they should, by the end of the follow-up sessions, be able to assess their glucose data in relationship to their food, activity, and medication; know how to improve their glucose levels; and feel confident about making therapy changes or talking to their health care provider about changes to improve outcomes.

The first follow-up session is usually 2 weeks after patients begin to perform glucose testing and advances the interpretation of glucose values as patients begin to apply GPM. The goals of the session include reinforcing the content of the initial session(s) and discussing related questions, using glucose data to assess glycemic control, and evaluating patients' food plan, activity, and medication. Information may be provided on meter maintenance, obtaining accurate readings, high and low glucose levels, illness and stress, eating at a variety of places, alcohol, and physical activity.

After starting to implement their food plan and perform glucose testing, many patients begin to understand how glucose testing can give them useful feedback about their eating habits, activity level, and diabetes medications. Through GPM, they feel a sense of empowerment and confidence, which enables them to better engage and assist in the design of their diabetes care plan.

Find glucose patterns

A three-step framework for interpreting glucose records is detailed in Table 3 and provides guidance to health care providers who are new to reviewing diabetes records. The three steps are

1) obtain sufficient, accurate data; 2) identify all possible interpretations; and 3) make individualized recommendations and plans.

The first follow-up session engages patients in a discussion about glucose levels both in and out of target. The importance of knowing this information is emphasized. As noted in the IDC patient education book, "Your glucose test numbers show how well your diabetes treatment plan is working."[17]

Glucose records are reviewed for readings that are in target and above or below target. Patients are reminded that the goal is to have ~ 50% of their readings in the target range, and they or the educator performs this calculation. Specific glucose patterns are then examined. Patients are asked if they see any pattern that reflects when their glucose levels are in, above, or below target.

Patients can circle glucose numbers that are either low, high, or in target with different colored pens to more easily see their patterns. By reviewing numbers horizontally and vertically in their record books, they can identify glucose patterns of success and areas that need to be addressed.

Patients are reminded that glucose readings are not "good" or "bad," but rather are data on which to make clinical decisions. Finding patterns is a discovery process for both patients and the educator and promotes an ongoing collaborative relationship. Patients see the everyday impact of food and activity because they have access to their glucose values. They know their target glucose values, and they know how to review their food, activity, and glucose records.

Assess the food plan

In the IDC Food and Activity Record, patients list the foods they eat, the amounts they eat, and either the number of carbohydrate choices or the grams of carbohydrate at each meal and snack. They also record their glucose data. This information is used to assess patient understanding and application of the food plan, and, together, patients and the educator discuss glucose patterns. Some patients may have increased their glucose testing times to determine the effect of additional meals. This demonstrates the power of glucose feedback and engaged patients.

Because there are many aspects to a food plan, one or two visits with a registered dietitian for medical nutrition therapy (MNT) are recommended for initial teaching and another one or two visits are needed to evaluate and adjust therapy. As mentioned above, the IDC program typically combines the nutrition visit with the DSME visit (and bills as DSME), whereas other centers provide these services separately. All educators need to support and reinforce the principles of GPM.

Recommend testing times

After the initial education session, most patients check their glucose levels when fasting and before and 2 hours after the start of their largest carbohydrate meal. The general guidelines for testing after subsequent sessions are:

- If ≥ 50% of their glucose tests are within the target range, glucose testing can decrease to three times a day on 2–3 days/week.
- If their glucose results are within target goals < 50% of the time, patients are advised to perform glucose testing three times a day, every day until therapy modifications result in ≥ 50% of their glucose tests within the target range.
- If a specific time of day yields an elevated glucose pattern, but the patient still achieves ≥ 50% of his

or her glucose results within the target range, we address nutrition, activity, or medication modification for that time period, followed by additional testing to assess changes.

These recommendations may vary for patients who want to test more frequently; whose meal plan, activity level, or medication is changing; or who do not have enough test strips to perform SMBG as frequently as desired.

Some patients are surprised to discover that they have symptoms of hypoglycemia when their glucose is within target and not < 70 mg/dl. SMBG lets patients know whether their symptoms are the result of a low glucose level or the result of their body adjusting to better glycemic control. In this way, they avoid excess food intake based only on symptoms and know they are making an informed decision rather than a guess.

Patients must test often enough to attain the feedback they need to understand and refine their food and activity plan. SMBG should focus on times of day during which a recent pattern of high or low glucose levels has emerged.

Provide ongoing education

Ongoing education continues to focus on GPM, problem-solving, and behaviors that positively influence glucose levels and address challenges. Typical content includes:

- How diabetes changes over time
- Staying healthy
- Diabetes complications
- Smoking cessation
- Food choices and heart health (fats and sodium) when glucose numbers are puzzling
- Strategies for creating life balance
- How to know if your treatment plan needs changing
- Stress and depression
- Staying motivated
- Staying active

Key to ongoing education is a continued focus on GPM and increasing patient confidence in diabetes self-care. Patients are encouraged to keep complete diabetes records (food, activity, and glucose results) for 3–7 days before each diabetes clinic visit. If patients do not bring a food record with them, they are asked to complete a 1-day food recall as a basis for dis-

cussion. It is important to determine what is working and where changes might be needed—both important components of GPM.

Downloading meters provides more data, sometimes enabling patients to make more informed decisions related to their diabetes management. Meter downloads, particularly the "modal day" or "standard day" graphs, provide a collapsed summary of glucose data that shows immediately which glucose values are in or out of the target range. Of course, reviewing food, activity, and medication therapies along with the glucose data is a key to GPM.

Summary

GPM can increase patient confidence in diabetes self-management. Confidence comes from understanding how their glucose data compare to their target goals and knowing if and when they should make changes in their food choices or physical activity. Some patients use the data for discussions about possible adjustments to their medication.

This article has provided a roadmap for incorporating SMBG (glucose testing and GPM) into a DSME program based on the core principle that most patients benefit from knowing how to assess their care. The information patients' gain through GPM motivates them to take further steps to improve their self-care.

Acknowledgments

The authors thank the staff of the International Diabetes Center and the Park Nicollet primary care teams for their contributions to the development and implementation of the BASICS curriculum, diabetes support materials, and care processes.

References

[1]Virdi N, Daskiran M, Nigam S, Kozma C, Raja P: The association of self-monitoring of blood glucose use with medication adherence and glycemic control in patients with type 2 diabetes initiating non-insulin treatment. *Diabetes Technol Ther* 14:790–798, 2012

[2]Pearson J, Bergenstal R: Pattern management: an essential component of effective insulin management. *Diabetes Spectrum* 14:75–78, 2001

[3]Austin MM, Powers MA: Monitoring. In *The Art and Science of Diabetes Self-Management Education Desk Reference*. 2nd ed. Mensing C, Ed. Chicago, American

Association of Diabetes Educators, 2011, p. 167–193

[4]Polonsky WH, Fisher L, Schikman CH, Hinnen DA, Parken CG, Jelsovsky Z, Petersen B, Schweitzer M, Wagner R: Structured self-monitoring of blood glucose significantly reduces A1C levels in poorly controlled, noninsulin-treated type 2 diabetes. *Diabetes Care* 34:262–267, 2011

[5]Seibolds M, Gaedeke O, Schwedes U; SMBG Study Group: Self-monitoring of blood glucose: psychological aspects relevant to the changes in HbA1c in type 2 diabetic patients treated with diet or diet plus oral antidiabetic medication. *Patient Educ Couns* 62:104–110, 2006

[6]International Diabetes Center: *Blood Glucose Pattern Control.* Minneapolis, Minn., International Diabetes Center, 2008

[7]Monnier L, Wojtusciszyn A, Colette C, Owens D: The contribution of glucose variability to asymptomatic hypoglycemia in persons with type 2 diabetes. *Diabetes Technol Ther* 13:813–818, 2011

[8]Qu Y, Jacober S, Zhang Q, Wolka L, DeVries JH: Rate of hypoglycemia in insulin-treated patients with type 2 diabetes can be predicted from glycemic variability data. *Diabetes Technol Ther* 14:1008–1012, 2012

[9]Esposito K, Ciotola M, Carleo D, Schisano B, Sardelli L, Di Tommaso D, Misso L, Saccomanno F, Ceriello A, Giugliano D: Post-meal glucose peaks at home associate with carotid intima-media thickness in type 2 diabetes. *J Clin Endocrinol Metab* 2008;93:1345–1350

[10]Monnier L, Colette C, Leiter L, Ceriello A, Hanefeld M, Owens D, Tajima N, Tuomiletho J, Davidson J: The effect of glucose variability on the risk of microvascular complications in type 1 diabetes. *Diabetes Care* 30:185–186, 2007

[11]Siegelaar SE, Holleman F, Hoekstra JB, DeVries JH: Glucose variability; does it matter? *Endocr Rev* 31:171–182, 2012

[12]Rodbard D, Bailey T, Jovanovic L, Zisser H, Kaplan R, Garg SK: Improved quality of glycemic control and reduced glycemic variability with use of continuous glucose monitoring. *Diabetes Technol Ther* 11:717–723, 2009

[13]Testa MA, Blonde L, Gill J, Turner RR, Simonson DC: Patient satisfaction, quality of life and glycemic variability in type 1 and 2 diabetes: a cross-over trial of insulin glargine plus glulisine vs premix analog insulin. *J Clin Endocrinol Metab* 97:3504–3514, 2012

[14]International Diabetes Center: *Gestational Diabetes BASICS Curriculum Guide.* 2nd ed. Minneapolis, Minn., International Diabetes Center, 2011

[15]International Diabetes Center: *Insulin BASICS Patient Book.* 3rd ed. Minneapolis, Minn., International Diabetes Center, 2013

[16]Powers MA, Carstensen K, Colon K, Richeim P, Bergenstal RM: Diabetes BASICS: education, innovation, revolution. *Diabetes Spectrum* 19:90–98, 2006

[17]International Diabetes Center: *Type 2 BASICS Patient Book.* 3rd ed. Minneapolis, Minn., International Diabetes Center, 2010

[18]Rickheim PL, Weaver TW, Flader JL, Kendall DM: Assessment of group versus individual diabetes education. *Diabetes Care* 25:269–274, 2002

[19]North S, Palmer G: Outcome analysis of glycosylated hemoglobin, weight, and blood pressure in a Veterans' diabetes education program [Abstract]. Presented at the Academy of Nutrition and Dietetics' 2012 Food and Nutrition Conference and Expo, Philadelphia, Pa., 2012

Margaret A. Powers, PhD, RD, CDE, is a research scientist; Janet Davidson, BSN, RN, CDE, is director of patient services; and Richard M. Bergenstal, MD, is executive director of the International Diabetes Center in Minneapolis, Minn.

Note of disclosure: Dr. Bergenstal serves on an advisory board, is a consultant to, or performs clinical research for Abbott Diabetes Care, Bayer, DexCom, Johnson & Johnson, Medtronic, Roche, and Sanofi, all companies that manufacture glucose monitoring devices.

Personalized Management of Hyperglycemia in Type 2 Diabetes

Reflections from a *Diabetes Care* Editors' Expert Forum

Itamar Raz, md[1]
Matthew C. Riddle, md[2]
Julio Rosenstock, md[3]
John B. Buse, md, phd[4]
Silvio E. Inzucchi, md[5]
Philip D. Home, dm, dphil[6]
Stefano Del Prato, md[7]

Ele Ferrannini, md[8]
Juliana C.N. Chan, md[9]
Lawrence A. Leiter, md[10]
Derek LeRoith, md, phd[11]
Ralph DeFronzo, md[12]
William T. Cefalu, md[13]

In June 2012, 13 thought leaders convened in a *Diabetes Care* Editors' Expert Forum to discuss the concept of personalized medicine in the wake of a recently published American Diabetes Association/European Association for the Study of Diabetes position statement calling for a patient-centered approach to hyperglycemia management in type 2 diabetes. This article, an outgrowth of that forum, offers a clinical translation of the underlying issues that need to be considered for effectively personalizing diabetes care. The medical management of type 2 diabetes has become increasingly complex, and its complications remain a great burden to individual patients and the larger society. The burgeoning armamentarium of pharmacological agents for hyperglycemia management should aid clinicians in providing early treatment to delay or prevent these complications. However, trial evidence is limited for the optimal use of these agents, especially in dual or triple combinations. In the distant future, genotyping and testing for metabolomic markers may help us to better phenotype patients and predict their responses to antihyperglycemic drugs. For now, a personalized ("n of 1") approach in which drugs are tested in a trial-and-error manner in each patient may be the most practical strategy for achieving therapeutic targets. Patient-centered care and standardized algorithmic management are conflicting approaches, but they can be made more compatible by recognizing instances in which personalized A1C targets are warranted and clinical circumstances that may call for comanagement by primary care and specialty clinicians.

Diabetes Care 36:1779–1788, 2013

In April 2012, the American Diabetes Association (ADA) and the European Association for the Study of Diabetes (EASD) published a joint position statement titled "Management of Hyperglycemia in Type 2 Diabetes: A Patient-Centered Approach" (1). It was an important update to earlier guidelines (2–8), providing a thorough examination of the ever-more-complex therapeutic options for glycemic management, the benefits and risks of tight glycemic control, the efficacy and safety evidence for new drug classes, and the data supporting withdrawals of or restrictions on other agents. Furthermore, it placed great emphasis on patient-centered and personalized care.

These recommendations captured the attention of the *Diabetes Care* editorial team. On the one hand, the recommendations call for a more personalized approach, which, in theory, should be liberating for all health care providers (HCPs) involved in diabetes care. On the other hand, their "less prescriptive" nature has been viewed as providing insufficient guidance to some HCPs who may feel overwhelmed when trying to match the nuances of differences among the increasing number of antihyperglycemic medications to the nuances of each patient's preferences and medical characteristics.

To explore these issues, we convened a *Diabetes Care* Editors' Expert Forum in June 2012. Thirteen thought leaders from around the world convened and discussed approaches to personalized medicine, the rationale behind personalization in diabetes care, the tools necessary to implement such a strategy, and the current perceptions of personalized medicine. This narrative provides our view and clinical translation of the underlying issues that need to be considered for personalizing care and offers suggestions to stimulate future research in this area. Table 1 summarizes the main points discussed below.

PRACTICAL APPROACHES TO PERSONALIZED MEDICINE

From intervention trials to personalized targets

There can be little more than semantic differences among the terms "personalized medicine," "patient-centered care," and "clinical judgment." Factors such as patients' preferences, life expectancy, disease duration, comorbid conditions, socioeconomic status, and cognitive abilities have long played a role in the selection of optimal therapeutic options and,

From the [1]Diabetes Unit, Department of Internal Medicine, Hadassah Hebrew University Hospital, Jerusalem, Israel; the [2]Oregon Health and Science University, Portland, Oregon; the [3]Dallas Diabetes and Endocrine Center at Medical City and University of Texas Southwestern Medical Center, Dallas, Texas; the [4]University of North Carolina School of Medicine, Chapel Hill, North Carolina; the [5]Yale University School of Medicine and Yale-New Haven Hospital, New Haven, Connecticut; [6]Newcastle University, Newcastle upon Tyne, U.K.; the [7]Department of Clinical and Experimental Medicine, University of Pisa School of Medicine, Pisa, Italy; the [8]Department of Internal Medicine, University of Pisa School of Medicine, Pisa, Italy; the [9]Department of Medicine and Therapeutics, Hong Kong Institute of Diabetes and Obesity and Li Ka Shing Institute of Health Sciences, Chinese University of Hong Kong, Prince of Wales Hospital, China; [10]Keenan Research Centre in the Li Ka Shing Knowledge Institute of St. Michael's Hospital, and Departments of Medicine and Nutritional Sciences, University of Toronto, Toronto, Canada; the [11]Mount Sinai Medical School, New York, New York, and Rambam Technion Hospital, Haifa, Israel; the [12]University of Texas Health Science Center, San Antonio, Texas; and the [13]Pennington Biomedical Research Center, Louisiana State University System, Baton Rouge, Louisiana.
Corresponding author: William T. Cefalu, william.cefalu@pbrc.edu.
DOI: 10.2337/dc13-0512
A slide set summarizing this article is available online.

more recently, in the selection of therapeutic targets.

In 1998, the UK Prospective Diabetes Study (UKPDS) showed that treating patients with recently diagnosed type 2 diabetes reduced the risk of microvascular, but not macrovascular, complications (9). Of the three subsequent randomized controlled trials (RCTs) on glucose lowering and cardiovascular outcomes, two—ADVANCE (Action in Diabetes and Vascular Disease: Preterax and Diamicron MR Controlled Evaluation) and VADT (Veterans Affairs Diabetes Trial)—showed no statistically significant reduction in cardiovascular outcomes, while the glycemic intervention of the third—ACCORD (Action to Control Cardiovascular Risk in Diabetes)—was

Table 1—Summary of the main points from the Diabetes Care Editors' Expert Forum

- The complexity of management of type 2 diabetes is underappreciated.
- Its complications, once established, remain a largely intractable burden.
- The number of available antihyperglycemic agents has increased markedly during the past 2 decades, but trial evidence for their optimal use—especially in dual or triple combinations—is limited and unlikely to ever be complete.
- The availability of multiple pharmacological options should be instrumental to early, appropriate treatment to target, which is the only recognized strategy for the prevention of complications.
- In the more distant future, genotyping and testing for metabolomic markers may help to phenotype patients and predict their responses to antihyperglycemic drugs.
- At present, a personalized ("n of 1") approach may aid in achieving therapeutic targets.
- Patient-centered care and standardized, algorithmic management are conflicting approaches, but they can be made more compatible by recognizing instances in which personalized A1C targets are warranted and clinical circumstances that may call for primary care and specialty comanagement.
- Failure to achieve glycemic targets, failure to respond to therapy, recurrent hypoglycemia, drug intolerances/contraindications, the development of complications, hyperglycemia during hospitalization, pregnancy, and suspicion of unusual variants such as MODY, LADA, heavy proteinuria with short disease duration in the absence of other microvascular complications, or secondary diabetes all may serve as triggers for comanagement.

ended early because of increased mortality in participants randomized to intensive glycemic control (10–12). However, meta-analyses of the four intervention trials (UKPDS, ACCORD, ADVANCE, and VADT) have shown modest but statistically significant benefit of intensive glucose control on the risk for myocardial infarction, but not mortality (13).

Post hoc analyses seeking explanations for these results set the stage for today's new emphasis on personalized care. Suggestions that adverse effects of individual therapeutic agents or severe hypoglycemia were directly implicated in causing cardiovascular events were not supported by these analyses but cannot be ruled out because efforts to capture hypoglycemic events were probably inadequate, especially in individuals with hypoglycemia unawareness (13). However, individuals assigned to intensive therapy who failed to improve control to A1C levels <7.0% (<53 mmol/mol) in ACCORD fared poorly and had more severe hypoglycemia, and severe hypoglycemia was noted to be a risk marker for a wide range of medical conditions in ADVANCE (14,15). It was also suggested that individuals with long-standing type 2 diabetes, existing cardiovascular disease (CVD), and other comorbidities were unable to achieve cardiovascular benefit from better glucose lowering within the timeframe of these studies (16).

Accordingly, these trials and their subsequent analyses raised important questions about rigid, algorithm-based, "glucocentric" approaches to therapy. One message, then, is that "one size does not fit all" for glucose targets, choice of therapy, or number of therapies used in combination. However, some questions pertinent to personalization remain unanswered. What were the characteristics of the small group of individuals in ACCORD who failed to respond to further glucose-lowering therapy but who contributed much of the excess case fatality (12)? Similarly, what can these studies teach us about patients who benefitted most from the interventions? Gaining insight into the pathophysiological, genetic, lifestyle, adherence, comorbidity, or other factors responsible for these disparate responses could improve our ability to effectively personalize therapy.

The 2012 ADA/EASD position statement still recommends an A1C goal of <7.0% (<53 mmol/mol) for most individuals with type 2 diabetes if it can

be achieved safely in low-risk individuals with early diabetes or a relatively long life expectancy; it suggests an acceptance of higher A1C targets for individuals with a history of severe hypoglycemia, limited life expectancy, long-standing diabetes, or advanced micro- and macrovascular complications (1). Prior guidelines from multiple organizations (3–8) included recommendations about setting personalized glycemic targets based on phenotype and empirically matching "the right drugs to the right patients," but without hard evidence to substantiate such an approach. Personalized treatment was articulated more vigorously in the new position statement (1).

The challenges of personalized care

Patient-centered personalized therapy, although appealing, may be difficult to implement without a good understanding of the ever-changing glucose-lowering armamentarium. β-Cell dysfunction is progressive in type 2 diabetes (9), and thus monotherapy, or even combinations of oral agents, is not likely to control hyperglycemia indefinitely (17), although the ORIGIN (Outcome Reduction With Initial Glargine Intervention) trial demonstrated sustained normoglycemia with basal insulin glargine plus metformin and near-normoglycemia even with standard therapy using metformin plus a sulfonylurea over a 6–7 year period in early type 2 diabetes (18). At this time, the processes of assessing β-cell function and providing reliable clinical decisions based on this factor are less than optimal. Furthermore, so-called evidence-based guidelines may be limited in their ability to be more prescriptive given the lack of clinical trial evidence from properly conducted long-term RCTs comparing the effects of various agents on clinically important outcomes. Clinical inertia is also a problem, and most clinicians do not alter their patients' glucose-lowering regimens until A1C is significantly elevated (19). Developing and implementing personalized care plans may be especially daunting for those HCPs whose practice extends beyond diabetes alone and who must address these issues in the context of limited time and resources.

The need for translational tools

The task now at hand is clear: We should develop and make available tools that will enable effective translation of existing guidelines on targets and therapeutic options into practical clinical applications.

It is one thing to assess the efficacy of an intervention within the context of a structured clinical trial setting, but entirely different to evaluate that intervention in ordinary clinical practices with resource variations, variable patient adherence, and sociodemographic and cultural differences. Thus, the translation of results from RCTs to real-world situations is not an exact science. Until more hard evidence becomes available, clinicians need well-structured and user-friendly evidence summaries that outline safe and effective processes for therapeutic intensification, while still allowing for the personalization of care.

Although such an undertaking is beyond the scope of this discussion, we are providing a starting point that may guide the development of such tools to aid HCPs in personalizing both targets and therapeutic regimens. For target-setting, suggestions have been made in the past (20,21). Another possible starting place might be the decision-making scale developed by Ismail-Beigi et al. (22) and adapted for inclusion in the ADA/EASD position statement (1). That scale includes seven parameters to consider when determining glycemic targets. Expanding it or providing some means of rating each parameter for individual patients could help clinicians to better weigh factors such as life expectancy, duration of diabetes, risk from hypoglycemia, comorbidities, and availability of support systems. Such a tool could assist clinicians in choosing targets and help to involve patients in the decision-making process in an easily understood manner.

Tools are also needed to help HCPs in selecting appropriate agents and intensifying therapy. The ADA/EASD position statement leaves treatment-goal decisions to clinicians and patients (1). However, some believe that because of the vast and expanding array of available drugs, there should be a systematic way to prioritize the selection of drugs in relation to their efficacy, safety, and cost. It is most important to emphasize that the percentage of patients who show sufficient clinical response to any of these drugs varies widely. Nonadherence to treatment regimens may be as high as 50% in patients with chronic diseases such as diabetes (23), often because of the patients' lack of symptoms, negative emotions, and poor knowledge of their disease (24). Side effects are another cause of stopping or limiting treatment. Thus, patients must

be adequately monitored, especially after changes to their treatment regimen, to evaluate whether they have reached targets and to ensure that there are no major side effects or adherence issues. This information is crucial to make informed decisions regarding whether to continue, change, or add to the therapy regimen.

STATE OF THE ART FOR PERSONALIZING MEDICINE—

Personalized medicine can be defined in many ways. A shared decision-making approach that takes patient preferences and values into account in developing a management plan is widely endorsed. Another definition involves identifying a particular set of phenotypic and genotypic markers that would define ideal and nonideal therapies for individuals based, to whatever extent possible, on evidence rather than on clinical impressions. Perhaps the most relevant question is whether current science is at a stage where specific patient characteristics—genetic, pathophysiological, or phenotypic—might effectively guide us in more general diabetes practice.

Contributions from genetics: a distant hope

The field of genetics is not yet ready to contribute in these broader areas. Despite recent identification of monogenic forms of diabetes for which specific treatments seem to give benefit (25), for more typical type 2 diabetes, genetic information does not contribute greatly in guiding treatment choices. Recently, pharmacogenetic analysis has begun providing insights, finding possible links, for example, to poor responses to metformin (26,27) and glucagon-like peptide-1 (GLP-1) receptor agonists (28–30). Such research holds promise for eventually helping to identify individuals who are likely to be classified as "responders" or "nonresponders" to specific agents.

Human genome sequencing also offers some hope, but again, in the distant future (31). Because the development of diabetes, patients' responses to available therapies, and the risks for complications are all multifactorial and probably involve numerous genes, the chances are small that specific mutations will turn out to be powerful markers of diabetes risk or of variable treatment responses. Even assuming a significant increase in pharmacogenetics research and decreases in the costs associated with genome sequencing, for the

foreseeable future these efforts will not significantly improve our ability to predict, prevent, or diagnose diabetes or illuminate definitive pathways for selecting drug therapies for specific individuals.

What can we learn from pathophysiology?

Insulin resistance in the liver and muscle and islet β-cell failure represent the core pathophysiological defects in type 2 diabetes (32,33). Insulin resistance can often be demonstrated long before the onset of β-cell failure, but as long as the β-cells secrete sufficient amounts of insulin to offset the insulin resistance, glucose tolerance remains normal (32–36). With time, however, there is progressive β-cell failure, which leads to the development of impaired glucose tolerance and/or impaired fasting glucose and eventually type 2 diabetes (32–36). As the plasma insulin response declines, insulin resistance in the liver becomes manifest as an overproduction of glucose by the liver and the development of fasting hyperglycemia, while insulin resistance in muscle results in diminished glucose uptake and postprandial hyperglycemia (32,33).

Although the relative contributions of β-cell failure (possibly more severe in Asian populations) and insulin resistance (more severe in Westernized societies with a high prevalence of obesity) may vary among different ethnic groups (37), virtually all adults with type 2 diabetes have some combination of the two. Thus, antihyperglycemic agents that improve β-cell function and enhance hepatic and muscle insulin sensitivity may have a more durable effect in reducing A1C (38–45).

The importance of other pathophysiological disturbances in the development of type 2 diabetes is well recognized (32,33). These disturbances include

- Adipocyte insulin resistance, which leads to increased lipolysis, increased plasma free fatty acids, and eventual β-cell failure and muscle and hepatic insulin resistance (46)
- Excess glucagon secretion by α-cells and enhanced hepatic sensitivity to glucagon, leading to increased basal hepatic glucose production and impaired suppression of hepatic glucose production after meals (47,48)
- Dysfunction related to incretin hormones (GLP-1 and glucose-dependent insulinotropic peptide) (49), which are

responsible for ~50% of the insulin secreted in response to meals
- Possible renal adaptive mechanisms to hyperglycemia, which result in enhanced glucose reuptake leading to decreased urinary glucose clearance and the maintenance of established hyperglycemia (50)
- Central nervous system insensitivity to the anorectic effect of insulin and multiple neurotransmitter synaptic abnormalities resulting in excessive energy intake and obesity (33)

No single antihyperglycemic agent can correct all of these pathophysiological abnormalities. Thus, many patients may require multiple agents with different mechanisms of action to achieve their individualized A1C goal (33). Patients with type 2 diabetes who have a high initial A1C, in particular, may require two or more antihyperglycemic agents to achieve their A1C goal (1,4,7,8,33,51,52).

The precise choice of pharmacological agents to use remains a topic for debate, in part because of safety concerns involving several drug classes (53–55). But the basic point remains: To achieve durability of glycemic control, optimal regimens will likely need to address both insulin resistance and β-cell failure.

Does phenotype allow for personalized treatment?

The main characteristics that might influence approaches to treatment can be divided into two categories: patient features and disease features. Among the patient features are race/ethnicity, sex, age of onset or diagnosis, duration of diabetes, body weight, frailty/comorbidities, complications, propensity for side effects/drug tolerance, personality and aspirations, and psychosocial-economic context. Among the disease features are the balance between insulin deficiency and insulin insensitivity, fasting versus postprandial hyperglycemia, short versus long disease duration, and special circumstances such as maturity-onset diabetes of the young (MODY) or latent autoimmune diabetes in adulthood (LADA).

However, we are faced with a paucity of data on how patients with certain characteristics respond to specific therapies (56). We know that most glucose-lowering drugs for type 2 diabetes work in most patients. But we also know that there are nonresponders to any drug. Numerous post hoc studies have revealed some predictors of better responses, but

the data are inconclusive (57–60). Furthermore, those response differences tend to be small, and the strongest predictor remains baseline A1C, with the patients with higher A1C levels responding with greater reductions although not necessarily attaining target levels (58,61).

Indeed, the most fruitful phenotypic considerations for personalizing care today may be patients' propensity for side effects and tolerance of various medicines. There may be practical value to using a trial-and-error, or "n of 1," approach (62) based on the anticipation of a drug's efficacy (for example, "Pioglitazone will be highly effective in this very insulin-resistant patient"), a patient's need for certain added benefits ("A GLP-1 receptor agonist will help control hyperglycemia and may encourage weight loss in this obese patient"), and concerns about adverse events ("I will not prescribe a sulfonylurea for this elderly patient who lives alone and had a severe hypoglycemic episode a few years ago"). This is becoming standard clinical procedure for diabetes, just as it is for hypertension and numerous other chronic diseases.

The challenge is how to proceed in more complex situations. How, for example, would one select an appropriate pharmacological regimen for a 68-year-old man with diabetes of 14 years' duration who has coronary disease, obstructive sleep apnea, prostate cancer, and a history of possible pancreatitis; who is obese and has edema but no heart failure; who smokes and has a family history of bladder cancer; who has high fasting blood glucose and A1C levels; and who has some renal dysfunction and poorly controlled lipids? With so many competing comorbidities, what are this individual's targets and treatment options?

Table 2—Classes of antihyperglycemic agents

1. Insulins
2. Sulfonylureas
3. Metformin
4. α-Glucosidase inhibitors
5. Glinides
6. Pioglitazone
7. Pramlintide
8. GLP-1 receptor agonists
9. Dipeptidyl peptidase-4 inhibitors
10. Colesevelam
11. Bromocriptine
12. SGLT-2 inhibitors

Ultimately, clinicians must develop highly personalized care regimens, and, in the absence of other conclusive evidence, "n of 1" trials may prove to be the best approach, providing strong evidence of therapy effectiveness and safety at the individual level and incorporating shared decision making with patients.

ARE ADEQUATE THERAPEUTIC TOOLS AVAILABLE NOW FOR PERSONALIZED DIABETES CARE?

Multiple glucose-lowering medication classes: freedom or confusion?

We now have numerous classes of antihyperglycemic therapies (Table 2) and more are expected to be licensed. Does this extensive arsenal provide us with more flexibility in designing personalized diabetes regimens, or does it make the task more difficult by multiplying the options? For specialists, the answer is no doubt the former. But for many primary care providers who must simultaneously stay abreast of developments in numerous fields of medicine, the expanding array of choices may, at times, seem intimidating.

Recent meta-analyses have shown that there is not much difference among available therapies in glycemic control (e.g., A1C reduction and likelihood of achieving targets when adding an agent to metformin). However, when one considers other benefits, such as the risk of hypoglycemia and effects on body weight (63,64), there appears to be separation among the agents. In addition to these agents' relative glycemic efficacy and effects on body weight and hypoglycemia, HCPs immersed in diabetes care must balance the potential benefits of each agent against concerns that have been raised regarding possible associations between various agents and the risk of developing other diseases (65–67).

Difficulties in making benefit-risk judgments are further amplified by the fact that marketing may seek to create demand for drugs that is out of proportion to their efficacy. In addition, there remains a general lack of adequate comparative and exploratory controlled trials between the medications available, not to mention a lack of research into phenotype- and pathophysiology-based regimens.

Developing a straightforward algorithm that narrows the field of viable options will clearly require more evidence than is currently available. Without such evidence, we can offer only opinion, albeit opinion based on an understanding of pathophysiology, epidemiology, pharmacodynamics, toxicology, and costs. Unfortunately, the studies needed to make evidence-based treatment decisions—those that involve comparisons among multiple agents and are adequately powered for important, long-term clinical outcomes—have, for the most part, not been performed.

The upcoming GRADE (Glycemia Reduction Approaches in Diabetes: A Comparative Effectiveness Study) trial will address some of these points (68). In addition, studies on how best to combine the various agents, as well as the optimal timing (early combination therapy vs. the traditional step-wise approach), are urgently needed.

Furthermore, even the most carefully considered set of guidelines is based on averages—average A1C-lowering effect, average efficacy, average risk of adverse effects—without adequate consideration of the confidence intervals around those averages. Averages fail to identify subpopulations that respond better and have better tolerance to specific agents, and without these data, evidence-based personalized advice cannot be provided. For now, all HCPs, whether in specialty or primary care settings, should test the efficacy and weigh the safety risks of any given drug in each patient, ideally trying options over a period of months to see how well they work at the individual level.

How will new and emerging therapies enhance our ability to personalize care?

To complicate future decision making, there are many new therapies in the research and development pipeline, including newer and longer-acting injectable incretin-based drugs, newer basal insulins, oral sodium-glucose cotransporter-2 (SGLT-2) inhibitors, agents targeting the various peroxisome proliferator–activated receptors, and free fatty acid receptor agonists.

It is hoped that pharmaceutical companies developing new glucose-lowering agents will focus on providing some added value beyond what is already available by addressing unmet clinical needs such as the effects leading to a reduction in CVD risk factors and meaningful cardiovascular and other outcomes. Arguably, we lack what we seek most in a diabetes treatment: definitive demonstration

that an agent can safely lower A1C in a sustained and durable manner by definitively modifying disease progression, does so with minimal side effects (e.g., hypoglycemia), favorably improves CVD risk factors (e.g., weight, lipids, and blood pressure), and reduces cardiovascular and other morbidity and mortality.

As new drugs continue to be developed and submitted to regulatory agencies for approval, we should also consider the limitations of RCTs for informing a personalized approach to diabetes care (69,70). RCTs, at least as currently carried out, focus on selected populations and have restricted inclusion and exclusion criteria. They are generally of short duration, making it impossible to assess durability. They do not test individual responder rates and are not designed to identify responders who have a low safety risk. These trials are conducted in artificial environments, which pose problems for realistically measuring adherence. Finally, RCTs are not powered to assess subpopulations prospectively. Thus, efforts to personalize therapy are hindered by our reliance on trials that may be neither generalizable to the larger population nor individualized to specific patients.

Moving forward, there may be other informative data from these trials, not from the average results, but rather from outliers—the results from subjects who respond very well or not at all.

REGIONAL PERSPECTIVES ON PERSONALIZED MEDICINE—The

questions, concerns, and practical considerations discussed here pose difficult challenges for diabetes HCPs throughout the world. Because diabetes is a burgeoning pandemic, it behooves us to understand the issues from an international perspective.

The viewpoint that personalized diabetes care may be too complex to be implemented in many care settings is common in Europe, as it is in the United States and elsewhere. In Italy, for example, the Renal Insufficiency And Cardiovascular Events (RIACE) multicenter study, which included 15,773 patients with type 2 diabetes attending hospital-based diabetes clinics, showed that 40% of patients were taking metformin, 15% were managed through diet only, 24% were on insulin, 18% were taking sulfonylureas, and 3% were taking thiazolidinediones (71). Strikingly, this pattern did not change with age or with renal function,

duration of disease, or other stratifying criteria.

The story is much the same in other parts of the world, although patient characteristics differ. In China, key issues include rapid nutritional and lifestyle transitions, large patient populations, young age of onset, and heterogeneous phenotypes characterized by β-cell dysfunction, insulin resistance, and visceral obesity (72,73). High rates of kidney disease and diabetes-related cancer complicate diabetes care (72,74,75). All of these problems are compounded by a relative scarcity of research, low levels of awareness, an insufficient number of trained HCPs, and less-organized health care and financing systems.

Given the large population and finite resources, one may argue for using risk algorithms and biomarkers, including genetic variants, to identify high-risk subjects for early or intensified intervention, although the cost-effectiveness of such an approach will need to be formally tested. As elsewhere, patients with insulin-resistant features such as fatty liver, high triglycerides, and low HDL cholesterol may benefit from initial treatment with metformin, pioglitazone, and GLP-1 receptor agonists, whereas patients who are lean and face a long disease duration may benefit from dipeptidyl peptidase-4 (DPP-4) inhibitors or sulfonylureas with the early use of insulin. Other drugs such as α-glucosidase inhibitors and SGLT-2 inhibitors may help to lower A1C with a low risk of hypoglycemia and weight gain.

Although these phenotype-based therapies have a theoretical basis, clinical practice studies are needed to confirm their cost-effectiveness. There is also a need to empower medical and nonmedical personnel (diabetes educators) in clinics to collect patient data on demographics, risk factors, complications, social habits, emotional needs, self-care behaviors, compliance, expectations, and values to enable HCPs to personalize treatment goals, self-management strategies, and therapy regimens (76). These personnel should monitor patients' adherence to treatment, as well as their achievement of treatment goals.

In the United States, attempts to implement a concept as expansive as personalized care quickly run up against two opposing traditions that permeate not only the field of medicine, but indeed the entire U.S. culture. The first, rooted in American industrialism, is standardization, exemplified by the processes of production line efficiency and continuous quality improvement. One recognizes this tradition in the vision of industrialist Henry J. Kaiser, who founded the prototype non-profit health system Kaiser Permanente (77). The second tradition, embodied by the image of artist Norman Rockwell's humble country doctor, is personalization. This is apparent in the teachings of Dr. Francis W. Peabody, whose seminal dissertation on patient care concluded, "The secret of care of the patient is caring for the patient," (78) and in the work of Dr. Elliott P. Joslin, who wrote that " . . . unless the physician takes care, he will fall into schematic ways and forget that it is the patient who comes for treatment and not the diabetes. Each is a case unto itself" (79).

Recent guidelines for diabetes care in the United States have fallen somewhere along a continuum between these traditions. The ADA Standards of Care (80) have sought to straddle the line, whereas the algorithm-based 2009 ADA/EASD consensus statement (2) leaned more toward standardization, and the 2012 ADA/EASD position statement (1) evolved more toward personalized care.

ENHANCING PERSONALIZED CARE THROUGH COMANAGEMENT—Research has yielded strong evidence in favor of fairly standardized treatment goals and an algorithmic initial therapy pathway involving lifestyle modification, metformin, and the eventual addition of other oral agents

(sulfonylureas and basal insulin, in most cases). This approach allows many newly diagnosed patients to attain a reasonable blood glucose range and to maintain it for some period of time.

However, there will always be patients for whom the standard A1C target is not appropriate (Fig. 1). Likewise, patients' clinical circumstances often become more complicated over time, at which point the core treatment algorithm must give way to a more personalized approach. In such situations, the ideal course of action would be a patient-centered comanagement approach involving primary and specialty care providers as well as diabetes educators, dietitians, psychologists, and other HCPs as warranted by individual patient needs. Figure 2 depicts such an approach, which could be invoked by specific triggers such as failure to respond to treatment (14,81), failure to attain A1C targets, drug intolerances or contraindications, severe hypoglycemia, hyperglycemia during hospitalization, pregnancy, suspicion of unusual variants such as LADA, MODY, or secondary diabetes, heavy proteinuria with short disease duration in the absence of other microvascular complications, or other complicating circumstances.

Regardless of the final form such a process takes, it seems clear that personalizing diabetes care will require improved cooperation and comanagement of patients among HCPs in various disciplines. In such a paradigm, algorithmic care would

be both a useful starting place for most patients with type 2 diabetes and a framework on which to build more personalized therapy as needed.

CONCLUSIONS—Publication of the latest ADA/EASD position statement on type 2 diabetes management has generated strong interest in the concept of a personalized medical approach for individuals with diabetes (1). However, there are a multitude of pharmacological antihyperglycemic therapies now available, often with incomplete evidence concerning their long-term efficacy, effectiveness, tolerability, and safety. Accordingly, questions remain regarding the best ways to implement the recommendations of the position statement in the care of patients.

Emerging research in genetics, pathophysiology, metabolomics, and human behavior, as well as longer-term, randomized comparative trials could eventually yield new information to inform the personalization of care. In the meantime, we must develop tools to translate existing guidelines into practical clinical applications, and, more importantly, to develop processes that encourage the organized comanagement of patients by primary care providers, specialists, educators, dietitians, and other diabetes HCPs as patients' unique needs and risks require. Another consideration is how well the tools we develop can be implemented around the globe given the differences in pathophysiology among ethnic

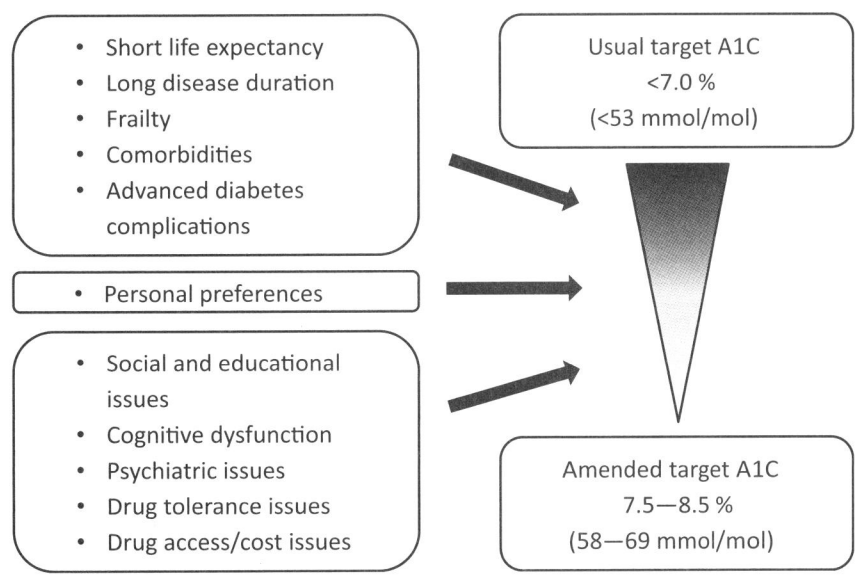

Figure 1—*Personalizing A1C targets for individuals with type 2 diabetes.*

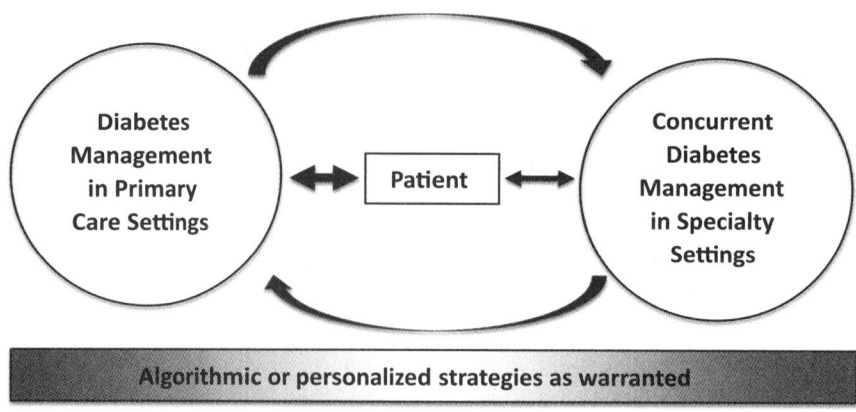

Figure 2—*A comanagement approach to personalized therapy for type 2 diabetes. The majority of patient care occurs in primary care settings with concurrent comanagement in specialty settings as warranted for individual patients. In such a model, the patient remains at the center of care, comanaging HCPs all provide algorithmic or personalized care as warranted, and communication occurs among all parties.*

groups, country-specific resources and medical care infrastructure, training level of providers, and knowledge of patients.

We hope these reflections have provided a broad overview of the evidence deficits and procedural challenges that will need to be overcome to ensure success in our efforts to implement effective, personalized therapy regimens for patients with type 2 diabetes.

Acknowledgments—I.R. has served on the advisory boards of AstraZeneca, Bristol-Myers Squibb, Eli Lilly, Merck (MSD), and Novo Nordisk; as a consultant for Andromeda, AstraZeneca/BMS, Eli Lilly, HealOr, Insuline, Johnson & Johnson, Teva, and TransPharma; and as a member of the speaker's bureau for AstraZeneca, Eli Lilly, Johnson & Johnson, Novo Nordisk, and Roche.

M.C.R. has received honoraria for consulting and/or research grant support through his institution from Amylin, Elcelyx, Eli Lilly, Sanofi, and Valeritas; these potential conflicts of interest have been reviewed and managed by Oregon Health and Science University.

J.R. has received grants or research support from Amylin, AstraZeneca, Boehringer Ingelheim, Bristol-Myers Squibb, Daiichi-Sankyo, Eli Lilly, GlaxoSmithKline, Johnson & Johnson, Lexicon, MannKind, Merck, Novartis, Novo Nordisk, Pfizer, Roche, Sanofi, and Takeda and has served on advisory boards for and received honoraria or consulting fees from Boehringer Ingelheim, Daiichi-Sankyo, Eli Lilly, GlaxoSmithKline, Johnson & Johnson, Lexicon, MannKind, Novo Nordisk, Sanofi, and Takeda.

J.B.B. is an investigator and/or consultant without direct financial benefit under contracts between his employer and the following companies: Abbott, Amylin, Andromeda, AstraZeneca, Bayhill Therapeutics, BD Research Laboratories, Boehringer Ingelheim, Bristol-Myers Squibb, Catabasis, Cebix, Diartis, Elcelyx, Eli Lilly, Exsulin, Genentech, GI Dynamics, GlaxoSmithKline, Halozyme, Hoffman-La Roche, Johnson & Johnson, LipoScience, Medtronic, Merck, Metabolic Solutions Development Company, Metabolon, Novan, Novella, Novartis, Novo Nordisk, Orexigen, Osiris, Pfizer, Rhythm, Sanofi, Spherix, Takeda, Tolerex, TransPharma, Veritas, and Verva.

S.E.I. has served as a consultant for Boehringer Ingelheim, Janssen, Merck, Novo Nordisk, and Takeda.

P.D.H. has received (or institutions with which he is associated have received) funding for his educational, advisory, and research activities from AstraZeneca/BMS Collaboration, Boehringer Ingelheim, Eli Lilly, GlaxoSmithKline, Janssen/Johnson & Johnson, Merck (MSD), Merck Serono, Novo Nordisk, Roche Diagnostics, Roche Pharmaceuticals, Sanofi, and Takeda.

S.D.P. has served as a consultant for AstraZeneca/BMS Collaboration, Boehringer Ingelheim, Eli Lilly, GlaxoSmithKline, Intarcia Therapeutics, Janssen/Johnson & Johnson, Merck (MSD), Merck Serono, Novartis, Novo Nordisk, Roche Pharmaceuticals, Sanofi, and Takeda and has received research support from Bristol-Myers Squibb, Merck (MSD), Novartis, Novo Nordisk, and Takeda.

E.F. has received honoraria for consulting and/or research grant support from AstraZeneca/BMS Collaboration, Boehringer Ingelheim, Daiichi-Sankyo, Eli Lilly, GlaxoSmithKline, Halozyme Therapeutics, Janssen/Johnson & Johnson, Merck (MSD), and Sanofi.

J.C.N.C. is a board member of the Asia Diabetes Foundation. She is a consultant for AstraZeneca, Bristol-Myers Squibb, Daiichi-Sankyo, GlaxoSmithKline, Merck (MSD), Pfizer, Qualigenics, and Sanofi. She has received honoraria, travel expenses, and/or payments for development of educational presentations from AstraZeneca, Bayer, Bristol-Myers Squibb, Daiichi-Sankyo, Eli Lilly, Glaxo-SmithKline, Merck Serono, Merck (MSD), Nestle Nutrition Institute, Novo Nordisk, Pfizer, Roche, Sanofi, and Takeda. Her institution, the Chinese University of Hong Kong, has received research grants from pharmaceutical companies for conducting clinical trials of drugs for individuals with diabetes and associated conditions.

L.A.L. has received research funding from, has provided continuing medical education on behalf of, and/or has acted as a consultant to AstraZeneca, Bristol-Myers Squibb, Boehringer Ingelheim, Eli Lilly, GlaxoSmithKline, Janssen, Merck, Novartis, Novo Nordisk, Roche, Sanofi, Servier, and Takeda.

D.L. is a consultant for AstraZeneca, Bristol-Myers Squibb, Janssen, Merck, and Sanofi.

R.D. serves on advisory boards or is a consultant for Amylin, Boehringer Ingelheim, Bristol-Myers Squibb, Lexicon, Novo Nordisk, and Takeda; receives grants from Amylin, Boehringer Ingelheim (pending), Bristol-Myers Squibb, and Takeda; and is a member of the speaker's bureau for Novo Nordisk.

W.T.C. has served as a consultant for AstraZeneca, Bristol-Myers Squibb, Halozyme Therapeutics, Intarcia Therapeutics, Johnson & Johnson, Lexicon, and Sanofi and has served as a principal investigator on research studies awarded to his institution from Astra-Zeneca, Bristol-Myers Squibb, Eli Lilly, Glaxo-SmithKline, Johnson & Johnson, Lexicon, and MannKind.

Writing and editing support services for this article were provided by Debbie Kendall of Kendall Editorial in Richmond, Virginia.

This article contains no data or data analysis and therefore there is no guarantor of these. All authors contributed to the thinking behind and the writing of the manuscript.

References

1. Inzucchi SE, Bergenstal RM, Buse JB, et al. Management of hyperglycemia in type 2 diabetes: a patient-centered approach. Position statement of the American Diabetes Association (ADA) and the European Association for the Study of Diabetes (EASD). Diabetes Care 2012;35: 1364–1379

2. Nathan DM, Buse JB, Davidson MB, et al.; American Diabetes Association; European Association for the Study of Diabetes. Medical management of hyperglycaemia in type 2 diabetes mellitus: a consensus algorithm for the initiation and adjustment of therapy: a consensus statement from the American Diabetes Association and the European Association for the Study of Diabetes. Diabetologia 2009;52:17–30

3. Bergenstal RM, Bailey CJ, Kendall DM. Type 2 diabetes: assessing the relative risks and benefits of glucose-lowering medications. Am J Med 2010;123:374. e9–374.e18

4. International Diabetes Foundation Clinical Guidelines Task Force. Global Guideline for Type 2 Diabetes. Brussels, International Diabetes Federation, 2012. Available from http://www.idf.org/global-guideline-type-2-diabetes-2012. Accessed 14 December 2012

5. Rodbard HW, Jellinger PS, Davidson JA, et al. Statement by an American Association of Clinical Endocrinologists/American College of Endocrinology consensus panel on type 2 diabetes mellitus: an algorithm for glycemic control. Endocr Pract 2009; 15:540–559

6. Canadian Diabetes Association Clinical Practice Guidelines Expert Committee. Canadian Diabetes Association 2008 clinical practice guidelines for the prevention and management of diabetes in Canada. Canadian Journal of Diabetes 2008;32 (Suppl. 1):S1–S201

7. National Institute for Health and Clinical Excellence. *Type 2 Diabetes: The Management of Type 2 Diabetes: NICE Clinical Guideline 87.* London, National Institute for Health and Clinical Excellence, 2009

8. Home P, Mant J, Diaz J, Turner C; Guideline Development Group. Management of type 2 diabetes: summary of updated NICE guidance. BMJ 2008;336:1306–1308

9. UK Prospective Diabetes Study (UKPDS) Group. Intensive blood-glucose control with sulphonylureas or insulin compared with conventional treatment and risk of complications in patients with type 2 diabetes (UKPDS 33). Lancet 1998;352: 837–853

10. Patel A, MacMahon S, Chalmers J, et al.; ADVANCE Collaborative Group. Intensive blood glucose control and vascular outcomes in patients with type 2 diabetes. N Engl J Med 2008;358:2560–2572

11. Duckworth W, Abraira C, Moritz T, et al.; VADT Investigators. Glucose control and vascular complications in veterans with type 2 diabetes. N Engl J Med 2009;360: 129–139

12. Gerstein HC, Miller ME, Byington RP, et al.; Action to Control Cardiovascular Risk in Diabetes Study Group. Effects of intensive glucose lowering in type 2 diabetes. N Engl J Med 2008;358:2545–2559

13. Control Group, Turnbull FM, Abraira C, Anderson RJ, et al. Intensive glucose control and macrovascular outcomes in type 2 diabetes. Diabetologia 2009;52:2288–2298

14. Riddle MC, Ambrosius WT, Brillon DJ, et al.; Action to Control Cardiovascular Risk in Diabetes Investigators. Epidemiologic relationships between A1C and all-cause mortality during a median 3.4-year follow-up of glycemic treatment in the ACCORD trial. Diabetes Care 2010;33: 983–990

15. Zoungas S, Patel A, Chalmers J, et al.; ADVANCE Collaborative Group. Severe hypoglycemia and risks of vascular events and death. N Engl J Med 2010;363:1410–1418

16. Skyler JS, Bergenstal R, Bonow RO, et al.; American Diabetes Association; American College of Cardiology Foundation; American Heart Association. Intensive glycemic control and the prevention of cardiovascular events: implications of the ACCORD, ADVANCE, and VA diabetes trials: a position statement of the American Diabetes Association and a scientific statement of the American College of Cardiology Foundation and the American Heart Association. Diabetes Care 2009; 32:187–192

17. Cook MN, Girman CJ, Stein PP, Alexander CM. Initial monotherapy with either metformin or sulphonylureas often fails to achieve or maintain current glycaemic goals in patients with type 2 diabetes in UK primary care. Diabet Med 2007;24: 350–358

18. Gerstein HC, Bosch J, Dagenais GR, et al.; ORIGIN Trial Investigators. Basal insulin and cardiovascular and other outcomes in dysglycemia. N Engl J Med 2012;367: 319–328

19. Karter AJ, Moffet HH, Liu J, et al. Glycemic response to newly initiated diabetes therapies. Am J Manag Care 2007;13: 598–606

20. Pozzilli P, Leslie RD, Chan J, et al. The A1C and ABCD of glycaemia management in type 2 diabetes: a physician's personalized approach. Diabetes Metab Res Rev 2010;26:239–244

21. Del Prato S, LaSalle J, Matthaei S, Bailey CJ; Global Partnership for Effective Diabetes Management. Tailoring treatment to the individual in type 2 diabetes practical guidance from the Global Partnership for Effective Diabetes Management. Int J Clin Pract 2010;64:295–304

22. Ismail-Beigi F, Moghissi E, Tiktin M, Hirsch IB, Inzucchi SE, Genuth S. Individualizing glycemic targets in type 2 diabetes mellitus: implications of recent clinical trials. Ann Intern Med 2011; 154:554–559

23. Wu JY, Leung WY, Chang S, et al. Effectiveness of telephone counselling by a pharmacist in reducing mortality in patients receiving polypharmacy: randomised controlled trial. BMJ 2006;333: 522

24. Fisher EB, Chan JCN, Nan H, Sartorius N, Oldenburg B. Co-occurrence of diabetes and depression: conceptual considerations for an emerging global health challenge. J Affect Disord 2012;142(Suppl):. S56–S66

25. Greeley SA, John PM, Winn AN, et al. The cost-effectiveness of personalized genetic medicine: the case of genetic testing in neonatal diabetes. Diabetes Care 2011; 34:622–627

26. Shu Y, Sheardown SA, Brown C, et al. Effect of genetic variation in the organic cation transporter 1 (OCT1) on metformin action. J Clin Invest 2007;117:1422–1431

27. Shu Y, Leabman MK, Feng B, et al.; Pharmacogenetics Of Membrane Transporters Investigators. Evolutionary conservation predicts function of variants of the human organic cation transporter, OCT1. Proc Natl Acad Sci USA 2003;100:5902–5907

28. Schäfer SA, Müssig K, Staiger H, et al. A common genetic variant in WFS1 determines impaired glucagon-like peptide-1-induced insulin secretion. Diabetologia 2009;52:1075–1082

29. Müssig K, Staiger H, Machicao F, et al. Association of type 2 diabetes candidate polymorphisms in KCNQ1 with incretin and insulin secretion. Diabetes 2009;58: 1715–1720

30. Smushkin G, Sathananthan M, Sathananthan A, et al. Diabetes-associated common genetic variation and its association with GLP-1 concentrations and response to exogenous GLP-1. Diabetes 2012;61: 1082–1089

31. Chen R, Mias GI, Li-Pook-Than J, et al. Personal omics profiling reveals dynamic molecular and medical phenotypes. Cell 2012;148:1293–1307

32. DeFronzo RA. Lilly lecture 1987. The triumvirate: beta-cell, muscle, liver. A collusion responsible for NIDDM. Diabetes 1988;37:667–687

33. DeFronzo RA. Banting Lecture. From the triumvirate to the ominous octet: a new paradigm for the treatment of type 2 diabetes mellitus. Diabetes 2009;58:773–795

34. Ferrannini E, Gastaldelli A, Miyazaki Y, Matsuda M, Mari A, DeFronzo RA. beta-Cell function in subjects spanning the range from normal glucose tolerance to overt diabetes: a new analysis. J Clin Endocrinol Metab 2005;90:493–500

35. Saad MF, Knowler WC, Pettitt DJ, Nelson RG, Mott DM, Bennett PH. The natural history of impaired glucose tolerance in the Pima Indians. N Engl J Med 1988; 319:1500–1506

36. Abdul-Ghani MA, Jenkinson CP, Richardson DK, Tripathy D, DeFronzo RA. Insulin secretion and action in subjects with impaired fasting glucose and impaired glucose tolerance: results from the Veterans Administration Genetic Epidemiology Study. Diabetes 2006;55:1430–1435

37. Abdul-Ghani MA, Matsuda M, Sabbah M, et al. The relative contributions of insulin resistance and beta cell failure to the transition from normal to impaired glucose tolerance varies in different ethnic groups. Diabetes Metab Syndr 2007;1:105–112

38. Bunck MC, Cornér A, Eliasson B, et al. Effects of exenatide on measures of β-cell function after 3 years in metformin-treated patients with type 2 diabetes. Diabetes Care 2011;34:2041–2047

39. Gastaldelli A, Ferrannini E, Miyazaki Y, Matsuda M, Mari A, DeFronzo RA. Thiazolidinediones improve beta-cell function in type 2 diabetic patients. Am J Physiol Endocrinol Metab 2007;292: E871–E883

40. Cusi K, Consoli A, DeFronzo RA. Metabolic effects of metformin on glucose and lactate metabolism in noninsulin-dependent diabetes mellitus. J Clin Endocrinol Metab 1996;81:4059–4067

41. Gastaldelli A, Miyazaki Y, Mahankali A, et al. The effect of pioglitazone on the liver: role of adiponectin. Diabetes Care 2006;29:2275–2281

42. Bajaj M, Baig R, Suraamornkul S, et al. Effects of pioglitazone on intramyocellular fat metabolism in patients with type 2 diabetes mellitus. J Clin Endocrinol Metab 2010;95:1916–1923

43. Klonoff DC, Buse JB, Nielsen LL, et al. Exenatide effects on diabetes, obesity, cardiovascular risk factors and hepatic biomarkers in patients with type 2 diabetes treated for at least 3 years. Curr Med Res Opin 2008;24:275–286

44. DeFronzo RA, Tripathy D, Schwenke DC, et al.; ACT NOW Study. Pioglitazone for diabetes prevention in impaired glucose tolerance. N Engl J Med 2011;364: 1104–1115

45. Kahn SE, Haffner SM, Heise MA, et al.; ADOPT Study Group. Glycemic durability of rosiglitazone, metformin, or glyburide monotherapy. N Engl J Med 2006; 355:2427–2443

46. Bays H, Mandarino L, DeFronzo RA. Role of the adipocyte, free fatty acids, and ectopic fat in pathogenesis of type 2 diabetes mellitus: peroxisomal proliferator-activated receptor agonists provide a rational therapeutic approach. J Clin Endocrinol Metab 2004;89:463–478

47. Unger RH, Aguilar-Parada E, Müller WA, Eisentraut AM. Studies of pancreatic alpha cell function in normal and diabetic subjects. J Clin Invest 1970; 49:837–848

48. Matsuda M, DeFronzo RA, Glass L, et al. Glucagon dose-response curve for hepatic glucose production and glucose disposal in type 2 diabetic patients and normal individuals. Metabolism 2002;51:1111–1119

49. Nauck MA, Vardarli I, Deacon CF, Holst JJ, Meier JJ. Secretion of glucagon-like peptide-1 (GLP-1) in type 2 diabetes: what is up, what is down? Diabetologia 2011;54:10–18

50. Abdul-Ghani MA, Norton L, DeFronzo RA. Role of sodium-glucose cotransporter 2 (SGLT 2) inhibitors in the treatment of type 2 diabetes. Endocr Rev 2011;32: 515–531

51. Rodbard HW, Jellinger PS, Davidson JA, et al. Statement by an American Association of Clinical Endocrinologists/American College of Endocrinology consensus panel on type 2 diabetes mellitus: an algorithm for glycemic control. Endocr Pract 2009; 15:540–559

52. Harrison LB, Adams-Huet B, Raskin P, Lingvay I. β-Cell function preservation after 3.5 years of intensive diabetes therapy. Diabetes Care 2012;35:1406–1412

53. Dormandy JA, Charbonnel B, Eckland DJ, et al.; PROactive investigators. Secondary prevention of macrovascular events in patients with type 2 diabetes in the PROactive Study (PROspective pioglitAzone Clinical Trial In macroVascular Events): a randomised controlled trial. Lancet 2005;366:1279–1289

54. Nissen SE, Wolski K. Rosiglitazone revisited: an updated meta-analysis of risk for myocardial infarction and cardiovascular mortality. Arch Intern Med 2010;170: 1191–1201

55. Lewis JD, Ferrara A, Peng T, et al. Risk of bladder cancer among diabetic patients treated with pioglitazone: interim report of a longitudinal cohort study. Diabetes Care 2011;34:916–922

56. Smith RJ, Nathan DM, Arslanian SA, Groop L, Rizza RA, Rotter JI. Individualizing therapies in type 2 diabetes mellitus based on patient characteristics: what we know and what we need to know. J Clin Endocrinol Metab 2010;95:1566–1574

57. Charpentier G, Vaur L, Halimi S, et al.; DIAMETRE. Predictors of response to glimepiride in patients with type 2 diabetes mellitus. Diabetes Metab 2001;27:563–571

58. Bloomgarden ZT, Dodis R, Viscoli CM, Holmboe ES, Inzucchi SE. Lower baseline glycemia reduces apparent oral agent glucose-lowering efficacy: a meta-regression analysis. Diabetes Care 2006;29:2137–2139

59. Nichols GA, Alexander CM, Girman CJ, Kamal-Bahl SJ, Brown JB. Treatment escalation and rise in HbA1c following successful initial metformin therapy. Diabetes Care 2006;29:504–509

60. Tomioka S, Ogata H, Tamura Y, et al. Clinical characteristics influencing the effectiveness of metformin on Japanese type 2 diabetes receiving sulfonylureas. Endocr J 2007;54:247–253

61. Topp BG, Waters SB, Alexander CM. Differences in reported efficacy between oral anti-hyperglycemic agents largely reflect differences in baseline A1C. Poster presented at the 68th Scientific Sessions of the American Diabetes Association, 6–10 June 2008, at the Moscone Convention Center, San Francisco, California

62. Tsapas A, Matthews DR. N of 1 trials in diabetes: making individual therapeutic decisions. Diabetologia 2008;51:921–925

63. Phung OJ, Scholle JM, Talwar M, Coleman CI. Effect of noninsulin antidiabetic drugs added to metformin therapy on glycemic control, weight gain, and hypoglycemia in type 2 diabetes. JAMA 2010;303:1410–1418

64. Liu SC, Tu YK, Chien MN, Chien KL. Effect of antidiabetic agents added to metformin on glycaemic control, hypoglycaemia and weight change in patients with type 2 diabetes: a network meta-analysis. Diabetes Obes Metab 2012;14: 810–820

65. Giovannucci E, Harlan DM, Archer MC, et al. Diabetes and cancer: a consensus report. Diabetes Care 2010;33:1674–1685

66. Noel RA, Braun DK, Patterson RE, Bloomgren GL. Increased risk of acute pancreatitis and biliary disease observed in patients with type 2 diabetes: a retrospective

cohort study. Diabetes Care 2009;32: 834–838

67. Elashoff M, Matveyenko AV, Gier B, Elashoff R, Butler PC. Pancreatitis, pancreatic, and thyroid cancer with glucagon-like peptide-1-based therapies. Gastroenterology 2011;141:150–156

68. George Washington University Biostatistics Center. The GRADE Study. Available from http://www2.bsc.gwu.edu/bsc/webpage.php?no=27. Accessed 14 December 2012

69. Woodcock J. The prospects for "personalized medicine" in drug development and drug therapy. Clin Pharmacol Ther 2007; 81:164–169

70. Brown PM. Personalized medicine and comparative effectiveness research in an era of fixed budgets. EPMA J 2010;1: 633–640

71. Solini A, Penno G, Bonora E, et al.; Renal Insufficiency And Cardiovascular Events (RIACE) Study Group. Diverging association of reduced glomerular filtration rate

and albuminuria with coronary and non-coronary events in patients with type 2 diabetes: the renal insufficiency and cardiovascular events (RIACE) Italian multicenter study. Diabetes Care 2012;35:143–149

72. Chan JC, Malik V, Jia W, et al. Diabetes in Asia: epidemiology, risk factors, and pathophysiology. JAMA 2009;301:2129–2140

73. Yoon KH, Lee JH, Kim JW, et al. Epidemic obesity and type 2 diabetes in Asia. Lancet 2006;368:1681–1688

74. Yang XL, Ma RC, Chan JC. Meta-analysis of trial data may support a causal role of hyperglycaemia in cancer. Diabetologia 2011;54:709–710; author reply 711–712

75. Sakuraba H, Mizukami H, Yagihashi N, Wada R, Hanyu C, Yagihashi S. Reduced beta-cell mass and expression of oxidative stress-related DNA damage in the islet of Japanese type II diabetic patients. Diabetologia 2002;45:85–96

76. So WY, Raboca J, Sobrepena L, et al.; JADE Program Research Team. Comprehensive

risk assessments of diabetic patients from seven Asian countries: The Joint Asia Diabetes Evaluation (JADE) program. J Diabetes 2011;3:109–118

77. Kaiser Permanente. Kaiser Permanente—more than 60 years of quality [article online]. Available from http://xnet.kp.org/newscenter/aboutkp/historyofkp.html. Accessed 8 October 2012

78. Peabody FW. Landmark article March 19, 1927: The care of the patient. By Francis W. Peabody. JAMA 1984;252:813–818

79. Joslin EP. *The Treatment of Diabetes Mellitus*. Philadelphia, Lea & Febiger, 1928, p. 557

80. American Diabetes Association. Standards of medical care in diabetes—2012. Diabetes Care 2012;35(Suppl. 1):S11–S63

81. Riddle MC, Karl DM. Individualizing targets and tactics for high-risk patients with type 2 diabetes: practical lessons from ACCORD and other cardiovascular trials. Diabetes Care 2012;35:2100–2107

A Critical Analysis of the Clinical Use of Incretin-Based Therapies

Are the GLP-1 therapies safe?

There is no question that incretin-based glucose-lowering medications have proven to be effective glucose-lowering agents. Glucagon-like peptide 1 (GLP-1) receptor agonists demonstrate an efficacy comparable to insulin treatment and appear to do so with significant effects to promote weight loss with minimal hypoglycemia. In addition, there are significant data with dipeptidyl peptidase 4 (DPP-4) inhibitors showing efficacy comparable to sulfonylureas but with weight neutral effects and reduced risk for hypoglycemia. However, over the recent past there have been concerns reported regarding the long-term consequences of using such therapies, and the issues raised are in regard to the potential of both classes to promote acute pancreatitis, to initiate histological changes suggesting chronic pancreatitis including associated preneoplastic lesions, and potentially, in the long run, pancreatic cancer. Other issues relate to a potential risk for the increase in thyroid cancer. There are clearly conflicting data that have been presented in preclinical studies and in epidemiologic studies. To provide an understanding of both sides of the argument, we provide a discussion of this topic as part of this two-part point-counterpoint narrative. In the point narrative below, Dr. Butler and colleagues provide their opinion and review of the data to date and that we need to reconsider the use of incretin-based therapies because of the growing concern of potential risk and based on a clearer understanding of the mechanism of action. In the counterpoint narrative following the contribution by Dr. Butler and colleagues, Dr. Nauck provides a defense of incretin-based therapies and that the benefits clearly outweigh any concern of risk.

—William T. Cefalu, md
Editor in Chief, *Diabetes Care*

The clinical value of new therapies for diabetes tends to be overestimated at launch, whereas the disadvantages emerge more slowly. Possible reasons include inflated expectations, marketing pressures, and the limited number of people exposed to the drug prior to launch. Full recognition of unwanted effects has also been delayed by inadequate postmarketing surveillance, especially when the unwanted effect is difficult to pinpoint or slow to emerge.

Off-target or unwanted effects pose a particular problem when a new class has wide-ranging effects. This was exemplified by the thiazolidinediones, nuclear receptor agonists with useful glucose-lowering properties but pleiotropic and unpredictable pathophysiological actions. Some undesirable outcomes such as osteopenia, redistribution of body fat, and fluid retention emerged as class effects, whereas others such as acute liver failure, increased cardiovascular morbidity, and bladder cancer appear specific to individual agents. Although the potential for unwanted effects was recognized at an early stage of development, it took years for them to be identified, analyzed, and acted upon. This meant that millions of people were exposed to agents whose potential long-term consequences were incompletely understood.

The glucagon-like peptide 1 (GLP-1)–based therapies have comparably pleiotropic actions. GLP-1 is a peptide hormone that enhances insulin secretion, inhibits glucagon release, delays gastric emptying, and suppresses appetite. Other potentially useful properties include enhanced growth and proliferation of pancreatic β-cells in immature (but not adult) rodents. GLP-1 receptors are however present in many other tissues, including thyroid, exocrine pancreas, meninges, renal tubules, and bone, and their activation results in changes entirely unrelated to glucose homeostasis. High levels of vigilance are therefore justified.

GLP-1 has a very short half-life and is therefore "seen" by its receptors in a transient and tightly regulated fashion in healthy individuals. The incretin effect is deficient in type 2 diabetes, and GLP-1–based therapy addresses this deficit. Its full glucose-lowering effect is however achieved at supraphysiological (DPP-4 inhibition) or pharmacological (GLP-1 mimetic) dosing levels. GLP-1 analogs thus achieve pharmacologic override of normal physiologic function and have the

potential to produce unexpected off-target effects, whereas DPP-4 inhibition enhances the release of gastric inhibitory polypeptide (GIP) as well as GLP-1, and the long-term impact of DPP-4 inhibition upon other regulatory systems is unknown.

Regulatory authorities have expressed concerns about the potential risk of acute pancreatitis, thyroid cancer, and renal failure with some or all of the GLP-1–based therapies, warnings that are (as appropriate) conveyed in every pack that is handed to a patient. These concerns are however largely discounted by the manufacturers and those representing their views to physicians, who typically maintain that the risk of pancreatic inflammation is illusory.

Pancreatitis: Now you see it, now you don't—Exenatide, the first GLP-1–based therapy, was launched in the U.S. on April 29, 2005. A single case report of acute pancreatitis appeared in 2006 and was spotted by investment advisors who conducted their own search of the U.S. Food and Drug Administration (FDA) database and reported a potential risk of acute pancreatitis on October 2, 2006. The company made a change to its label on October 8, but the FDA did not issue its first alert until October 2007 (1). This was followed by a series of publications, mostly sponsored by the manufacturers, which reported that pancreatitis is more common in established diabetes than previously appreciated, together with pharmacoepidemiological studies using administrative databases that indicated that pancreatitis is no more common with exenatide than with other therapies for diabetes (2–4).

It is not easy to estimate the prevalence of acute pancreatitis, let alone assign a probable cause, and there are genuine difficulties in ascertaining the prevalence of acute pancreatitis in a population with diabetes. Reverse causation is an important confounder since both acute and chronic pancreatitis may give rise to diabetes. Chronic pancreatitis may present with acute episodes of pancreatic pain. The formal criteria for diagnosis—typical pain, enzyme rises, and changes on computed tomography (CT) examination—may not be satisfied or adequately recorded in administrative databases, and unequivocal CT abnormalities may not be present. The source documentation is often inadequate and pharmacoepidemiologic analyses may reach differing rate estimates because of differing criteria. Last but not least, a plausible mechanism to explain the occurrence of pancreatitis was initially lacking. This is no longer the case.

Emergence of a mechanism

—GLP-1 receptors are abundantly expressed in the pancreatic ducts as well as in the pancreatic islets, and the intense interest in GLP-1–based therapies as a potential stimulus to β-cell regeneration has overshadowed the possibility that exocrine pancreatic cells might be similarly affected. Acinar and duct cells proliferate in response to GLP-1 therapy (5) and cause an increase in pancreatic weight (6,7) (Fig. 1). Such observations attracted little attention prior to 2009 when one of eight HIP rats, a model of type 2 diabetes, developed hemorrhagic pancreatitis following exposure to sitagliptin, and some of the remaining animals showed marked acinar to ductal metaplasia, a potentially premalignant change characteristic of chronic pancreatitis (7). Gier et al. (8) noted that the pancreatic duct gland (PDG) compartment of the pancreas is particularly responsive to the proproliferative actions of GLP-1 and confirmed that GLP-1 simulates proliferative signaling in human pancreatic ductal epithelium. Two short-term studies were subsequently performed at the request of the FDA. These studies were carried out with exenatide and liraglutide in the ZDF rat model of diabetes and were reassuring with respect to possible adverse effects of GLP-1 mimetic therapy on the exocrine pancreas. Notwithstanding, pancreatic enzymes rose in both studies: one of twelve animals treated with exenatide died of massive pancreatic necrosis, and pathological findings in treated animals included acinar to ductal metaplasia and foci of ductal hyperplasia (9,10).

Some of the relevant preclinical studies are summarized in Table 1 (5–13). In aggregate, they offer a plausible mechanism for the occurrence of acute pancreatitis in patients exposed to GLP-1–based therapies since duct proliferation might

lead to duct occlusion (particularly in the setting of existing dysplastic lesions), occlusion would generate back pressure, and back pressure would stress acinar cells thereby activating and releasing the digestive enzymes that they contain—a well-established causal mechanism for pancreatitis.

Human pancreatitis revisited

—Animal studies do not necessarily reflect the experience in humans, but the identification of a plausible mechanism is an important step toward establishing a potential hazard and indicates a need for more detailed analysis in humans. Observational and pharmacoepidemiologic studies have suggested that acute pancreatitis is more common than expected in the diabetic population and is not increased by exenatide relative to other therapies (2–4). Although space does not permit detailed consideration here, there are some anomalies. For example, Dore et al. (2) examined the frequency of pancreatitis in a claims database comprising 25,700 patients on exenatide (past or present users) as compared with 234,500 patients on other antihyperglycemic therapies. Overall, there were more cases of confirmed pancreatitis in past or present exenatide users as compared with other therapies (40/25,719 vs. 254/234,536 = 1.56/1,000 vs. 1.08/1,000 users). The study found a reduced frequency of pancreatitis in present users of exenatide, but a propensity-adjusted RR (relative risk) of 2.8 (CI 1.6–4.7) for past use. The latter observation was discounted because those being studied were no longer taking exenatide at the time of the episode, but the exclusion would not be valid if exenatide had been stopped because of premonitory symptoms of abdominal pain or if the proposed mechanism persisted in those no longer taking the drug. Garg et al. (14) found no evidence of an increased risk of pancreatitis with exenatide, but concede that "the limitations of this observational claims-based analysis cannot exclude the possibility of an increased risk." A recent case-control study addressed many of the limitations of previous reports, including inadequate power, and found that current and recent (1 month–2 years) users of GLP-1–based therapies had a twofold risk of acute pancreatitis (adjusted odds ratio 2.24 [95% CI 1.36–3.68] for current use and 2.01 [1.27–3.18] for recent use) (15).

Studies conducted by the manufacturer under the eyes of the regulators may

provide reliable information. A recent review identified 11 such reports in studies conducted by Novo Nordisk, the manufacturer of liraglutide. Seven occurred in the LEAD (Liraglutide Effect and Action in Diabetes) studies (16), two in other studies, and two in postmarketing reports. Adverse events from the FDA Serious Adverse Event (SAE) reports were not considered. The findings were considered to "implicate liraglutide as the cause in at least some of these cases" (17).

Further cause for concern comes from FDA MedWatch data. An excess of acute pancreatitis was already evident for exenatide within 1 year of launch (1), and an updated analysis in 2011 found that, as compared with other non-GLP-1–based diabetes therapies, the reporting rate for acute pancreatitis with exenatide was dramatically increased ($P < 2 \times 10^{-4}$) (18). This easily checked analysis has not been seriously challenged.

The FDA alert system was designed to identify potential safety problems, not to confirm them. Notwithstanding its limitations, to our knowledge there is no single instance in which a strong sustained signal has turned out to be entirely spurious. When Elashoff et al. (18) was published, there were 971 reported pancreatitis events for exenatide and 131 for sitagliptin. The corresponding numbers are now 2,327 and 718 (Table 2). Recognition of an adverse event undoubtedly increases the reporting frequency, but there was a signal for exenatide long before the first FDA alert was issued, and there was no reason to anticipate a similar problem with sitagliptin. Furthermore, there are now 888 reported pancreatitis events for liraglutide, 125 for saxagliptin, and 43 for linagliptin (Table 2). Every GLP-1–based therapy with sufficient market exposure has generated a signal for pancreatitis, and no other diabetes medication has done so.

We conclude that the balance of evidence does suggest an association between widely used GLP-1–based therapies and acute pancreatitis, suggesting a class effect, and that this is underpinned by a plausible mechanism.

What are the implications?

—The major concern is not pancreatitis, unpleasant though this is. The concern is that acute events may be no more than the tip of an iceberg, and that these agents might cause subclinical duct proliferation, acinar to ductal metaplasia, and subclinical pancreatitis in a much higher proportion of individuals. Pancreatitis,

Table 1—*Animal studies of GLP-1–based therapy on the exocrine pancreas*

Reference	Species/age	Treatment/day duration#	Pancreas weight	Pancreas enzymes	Histology	Replication/ method
Perfetti et al., 2000 (5)	Wistar rat 22 months	GLP-1 1.5 pmol/kg · min, 5 days	↑	→	NR	↑ Ducts and acinar cells PCNA
Koehler et al., 2009 (6)	Mice 9–12 weeks	Exenatide 48 nmol/kg, 4 wks	↑	→	NR	NR
	Mice 9–12 weeks	Liraglutide 75 μg/kg, 1 wk	↑	→	NR	NR
Matveyenko et al., 2009 (7)	HIP rats 2 months	Sitagliptin 200 mg/kg, 12 weeks	↑	NR	Pancreatitis (1/8) and acinar to ductal metaplasia (3/16)	↑ Ducts, Ki67
Nachnani et al., 2010 (12)	Rats 8 weeks	Exenatide 10 μg/kg, 11 weeks	NR	↑ Amylase	Exocrine inflammation	NR
Tatarkiewicz et al., 2010 (11)	Mice 10 weeks	Exenatide 7.2 nmol/kg, 4 weeks	→	→	No pancreatitis	→ Ducts Ki67
Vrang et al., 2012 (9)	ZDF rats 7 weeks	Exenatide 0.25 mg/kg, 13 weeks	→	↑ Amylase	1/12 death pancreatic necrosis; focal acinar hyperplasia;	→ Ducts Ki67*
		Liraglutide 1.0 mg/kg, 13 weeks	→	→	3/12 death by overdose, unexplained; increased ductal proliferation and acinar to ductal metaplasia	→ Ducts Ki67*
Nyborg et al., 2012 (13)	Cynomolgus monkeys age NR	Liraglutide 5 mg/kg, 87 weeks	NR	NR	Normal	NR
	Rats age NR	Liraglutide 1 mg/kg 26 weeks	NR	NR	Normal	NR
	Mice age NR	Liraglutide 3 mg/kg, 104 weeks	NR	NR	Normal	NR
Gier et al., 2012 (8)	Rats 10 weeks	Exenatide 10 μg/kg, 12 weeks	↑	→	PDG hyperplasia;	↑ PDG and ducts Ki67
	Pdx-1 Kras mice 6 weeks	Exenatide 5 nmol/kg, 12 weeks	↑	↑ Lipase	chronic pancreatitis and advanced PanINs	↑ Ducts Ki67
Tatarkiewicz et al., 2012 (10)	ZDF rats 8 wks	Exenatide 250 μg/kg, 12 weeks	→	↑ Amylase	Normal	→ Ducts Ki67*

Preclinical animal studies reporting the effects of GLP-1–based therapies on the exocrine pancreas. *Indicates pancreas fixed in formaldehyde for 24 h or more, typically denaturing proteins to the extent that measurement of cellular replication by Ki67 is unreliable. #Maximal dose and duration of GLP-1–based therapy included in each study is shown in the summary. NR, not recorded.

whether clinical or subclinical, is well known to predispose to pancreatic cancer, and there is a signal for cancer of the pancreas for exenatide in both the FDA and German regulatory databases and for sitagliptin in the FDA database (18,19). The signal has grown stronger with 258 pancreatic cancers reported for exenatide, 63 for liraglutide, 81 for sitagliptin, 18 for saxagliptin, and 1 for linagliptin (Table 2).

Low-grade asymptomatic chronic pancreatitis with associated proliferative changes is not uncommon in the middle-aged target population for this drug class (20), making it likely that the proproliferative actions of GLP-1 therapy will at times be superimposed upon low-grade pancreatitis and its associated dysplastic changes. Some insight into this possibility was gained in the chronic pancreatitis–prone Kras[G12D] mouse model in which exenatide therapy accelerated formation and growth of dysplastic intraepithelial neoplasia (PanIN) lesions as well as pancreatitis (8). To date, this is the only study of the actions of incretin treatment in a model of chronic pancreatitis (Fig. 1). In contrast, two studies of short-term GLP-1 exposure superimposed on acute toxin–induced pancreatitis were reported to show a protective effect, but such studies do not address the mechanism of relevance (6,11).

The incidence of pancreatic cancer, as of pancreatitis, is increased in type 2 diabetes (21). Work over the past decade has established that premalignant changes known as pancreatic intraepithelial (PanIN) lesions precede and predict the onset of pancreatic cancer. PanINs are present in up to 50% of the middle-aged population, although relatively few actually progress to cancer (20). Both PanINs and pancreatic cancer express the GLP-1 receptor in humans (8). Since progression of PanINs to pancreatic cancer is via the accumulation of additional somatic mutations, any driver of increased cellular replication in PanINs is likely to increase that probability. This theoretical risk was illustrated by the progression of PanINs in the exenatide-treated

Table 2—*FDA adverse event reports for GLP-1–based drugs*

Exenatide and sitagliptin vs. controls (04Q1 to 12Q2)

Drug	Pancreatitis events	Control events	OR	95% CI	P value
Exenatide	2,327	1,660	19.17	(16.41–22.50)	<2.2e-16
Sitagliptin	718	411	23.89	(19.76–28.93)	<2.2e-16
Controls	207	2,832			
Drug	Pancreatic cancer events	Control events	OR	95% CI	P value
Exenatide	258	1,660	2.99	(2.41–3.73)	<2.2e-16
Sitagliptin	81	411	3.80	(2.80–5.11)	<2.2e-16
Controls	147	2,832			
Drug	Thyroid cancer events	Control events	OR	95% CI	P value
Exenatide	74	1,660	3.94	(2.56–6.20)	1.67e-11
Sitagliptin	5	411	1.08	(0.33–2.81)	0.80
Controls	32	2,832			

Liraglutide vs. controls (10Q2 to 12Q2)

Drug	Pancreatitis events	Control events	OR	95% CI	P value
Liraglutide	888	259	56.81	(43.52–74.71)	<2.2e-16
Controls	84	1,393			
Drug	Pancreatic cancer events	Control events	OR	95% CI	P value
Liraglutide	63	259	5.64	(3.80–8.38)	<2.2e-16
Controls	60	1,393			
Drug	Thyroid cancer events	Control events	OR	95% CI	P value
Liraglutide	57	259	17.99	(10.12–33.56)	<2.2e-16
Controls	17	1,393			

Saxagliptin vs. controls (09Q4 to 12Q2)

Drug	Pancreatitis events	Control events	OR	95% CI	P value
Saxagliptin	125	65	30.96	(21.33–45.35)	<2.2e-16
Controls	100	1,618			
Drug	Pancreatic cancer events	Control events	OR	95% CI	P value
Saxagliptin	18	65	6.04	(3.21–10.95)	6.85e-8
Controls	74	1,618			
Drug	Thyroid cancer events	Control events	OR	95% CI	P value
Saxagliptin	0	65	0	(0.00–5.48)	>0.99
Controls	19	1,618			

Linagliptin vs. controls (11Q3 to 12Q2)

Drug	Pancreatitis events	Control events	OR	95% CI	P value
Linagliptin	43	14	42.36	(20.86–90.82)	<2.2e-16
Controls	43	601			
Drug	Pancreatic cancer events	Control events	OR	95% CI	P value
Linagliptin	1	14	1.79	(0.04–12.72)	0.45
Controls	24	601			
Drug	Thyroid cancer events	Control events	OR	95% CI	P value
Linagliptin	0	14	0	(0–27.80)	>0.99
Controls	8	601			

The updated adverse event reports from Elashoff et al. (18) to include most recent available quarters and GLP-1 drugs launched since the original Elashoff report. Since rosiglitazone (Avandia) is now rarely used in the U.S., the control drugs have been increased to include insulin preparations available in the U.S. The pattern of findings is comparable with or without these added controls. Control drugs include "AVANDIA," "ROSIGLITAZONE," "STARLIX," "NATEGLINIDE," "PRANDIN," "REPAGLINIDE," "NOVONORM," "GLIPIZIDE," "GLUCOTROL," "INSULIN DETEMIR," "LEVEMIR," "INSULIN ASPART," "NOVOLOG," "HUMULIN N," "HUMULIN R," "INSULIN LISPRO," "HUMALOG," "INSULIN GLARGINE," "LANTUS," "HUMULIN 70/30," and "NOVOLOG MIX 70/30." Pancreatitis events include "PANCREATITIS." Pancreatic cancer events include "PANCREATIC MASS," "PANCREATIC NEOPLASM," "ADENOCARCINOMA PANCREAS," and "PANCREATIC CARCINOMA." Thyroid cancer events include "THYROID CANCER," "THYROID GLAND CANCER," "THYROID NEOPLASM," and "THYROID MASS." Control events include "BACK PAIN," "CHEST PAIN," "COUGH," "SYNCOPE," and "URINARY TRACT INFECTION."

$Kras^{G12D}$ mouse model (8). It is worth noting here that such a potential link between GLP-1 therapy and risk for pancreatic cancer is analogous to estrogen therapy and breast cancer. Estrogen does not initiate breast cancer, but in individuals with pre-malignant dysplastic ductal changes that bear estrogen receptors, estrogen accelerates growth and malignant conversion in some individuals (22). Likewise, the very high concentration of insulin delivered to the bronchial tree with inhaled insulin was as-

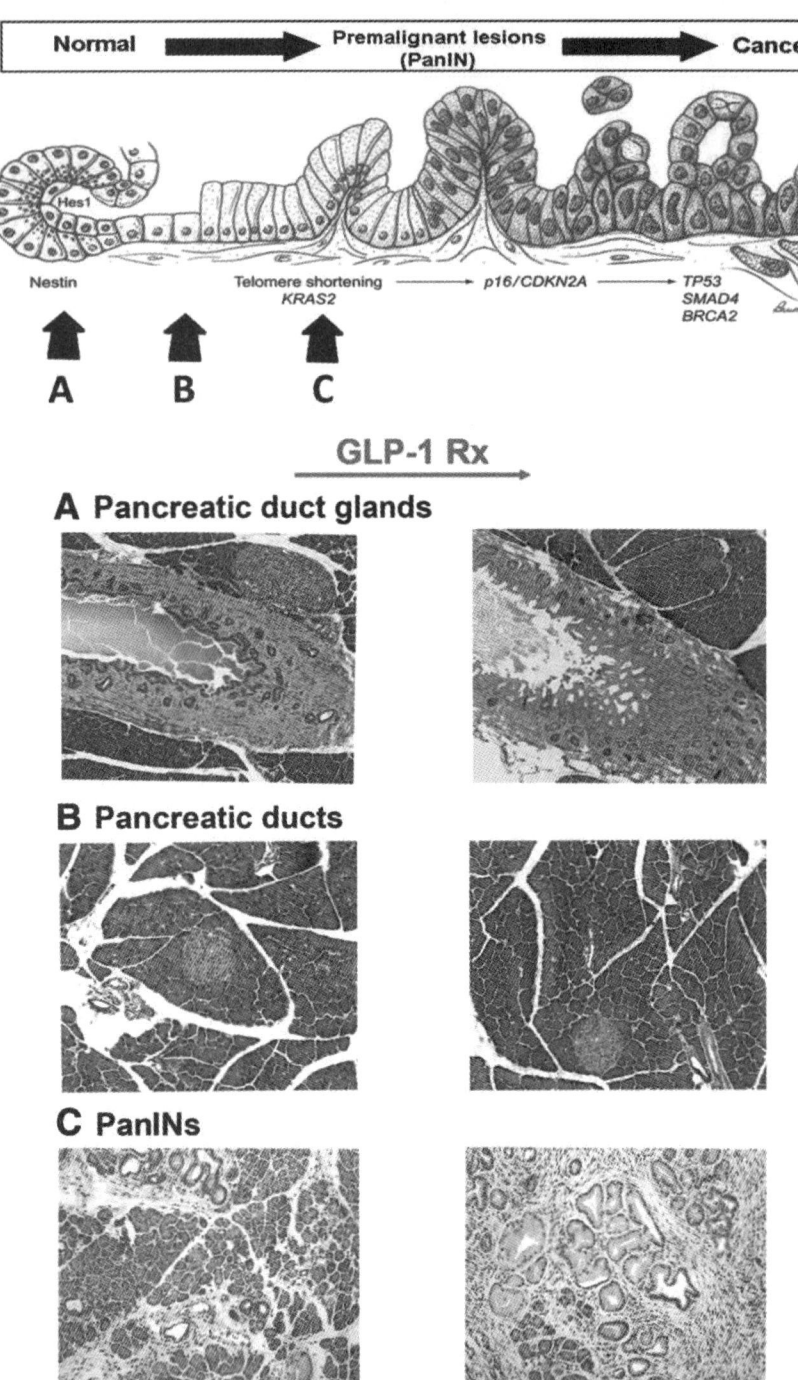

Figure 1—*GLP-1 actions on exocrine pancreas in animal studies depend on compartment studied and pancreas health. The histological characteristics of the transition from normal pancreas to premalignant changes (PanINs) typically present in the progression from asymptomatic chronic pancreatitis to cancer and, as established by human pathological and mouse genetic studies (top panel, modified from Maitra and Hruban [31]). In nondiabetic animal studies, exposure of pancreas to GLP-1 therapies has minimal discernible impact except in the pancreatic duct gland compartment where marked proliferation generates intraductal papillary projections (A: Pancreatic duct glands are markedly expanded in nondiabetic rats treated with exenatide 10 μg/kg daily for 12 weeks). However the pancreatic ducts show no obvious abnormalities in the same animals. B: In contrast, GLP-1 therapy accelerates pancreatitis and neoplasia in mice prone to chronic pancreatitis. C: Formation of PanINs and pancreatitis are markedly accelerated in the Pdx1-Cre; LSL-Kras^{G12D} mouse model treated with exenatide 5 nmol/kg for 12 weeks. A, B, and C used with permission from Gier et al. (8).*

sociated with an increased incidence of lung cancer (23). Are estrogen, insulin, or GLP-1 carcinogens? No, but all three can serve as growth factors, and when pharmacological stimulation of growth is imposed on dysplastic lesions, accelerated declaration of cancer is not unexpected.

Where do we go from here?—
The regulatory reflex, when presented with a safety concern, is to request further descriptive data from the manufacturers. Our view is that the request for further epidemiologic analysis misses the real point of concern and wastes valuable time. The answer lies in the human pancreas, and (until this answer is known) there are more relevant questions to ask.

One question is this: If subclinical pancreatitis is common (consistent with the episodes of abdominal pain or discomfort described by many users), we might anticipate subclinical increases in pancreatic enzymes. Anecdotally, many clinicians already know this to be the case, but there is only one published case series (24). We accept that pancreatic enzyme levels fluctuate in people with diabetes and that confirmation of increased levels in people exposed to GLP-1–based therapies does not in itself constitute evidence of subclinical pancreatitis, but if a signal is there, we need to know.

The debate has been conducted in the absence of a single report from the pancreas of a human exposed to GLP-1 therapies. This is where the answer lies (25). Most recently, the first data have become available from human pancreas following a year or more of incretin therapy; 7 individuals treated by sitagliptin and 1 by exenatide compared to 12 individuals with type 2 diabetes treated with other agents and nondiabetes (26). The pancreas was 40% enlarged with increased exocrine pancreas proliferation in incretin-treated individuals. Moreover, there was an increase in the number of PanIN (premalignant) lesions after prior incretin treatment, consistent with the findings in the Kras^{G12D} mouse model (8). A striking finding in the human pancreas after incretin treatment was marked α-cell hyperplasia with glucagon-expressing microadenomas in 3 of the 8 individuals, and a glucagon-expressing neuroendocrine tumor in 1 of the 8. Given the heavily promoted action of incretin therapy to suppress glucagon secretion, and the prior reports of α-cell hyperplasia and risk for progression to pancreatic neuroendocrine tumors (26), this finding,

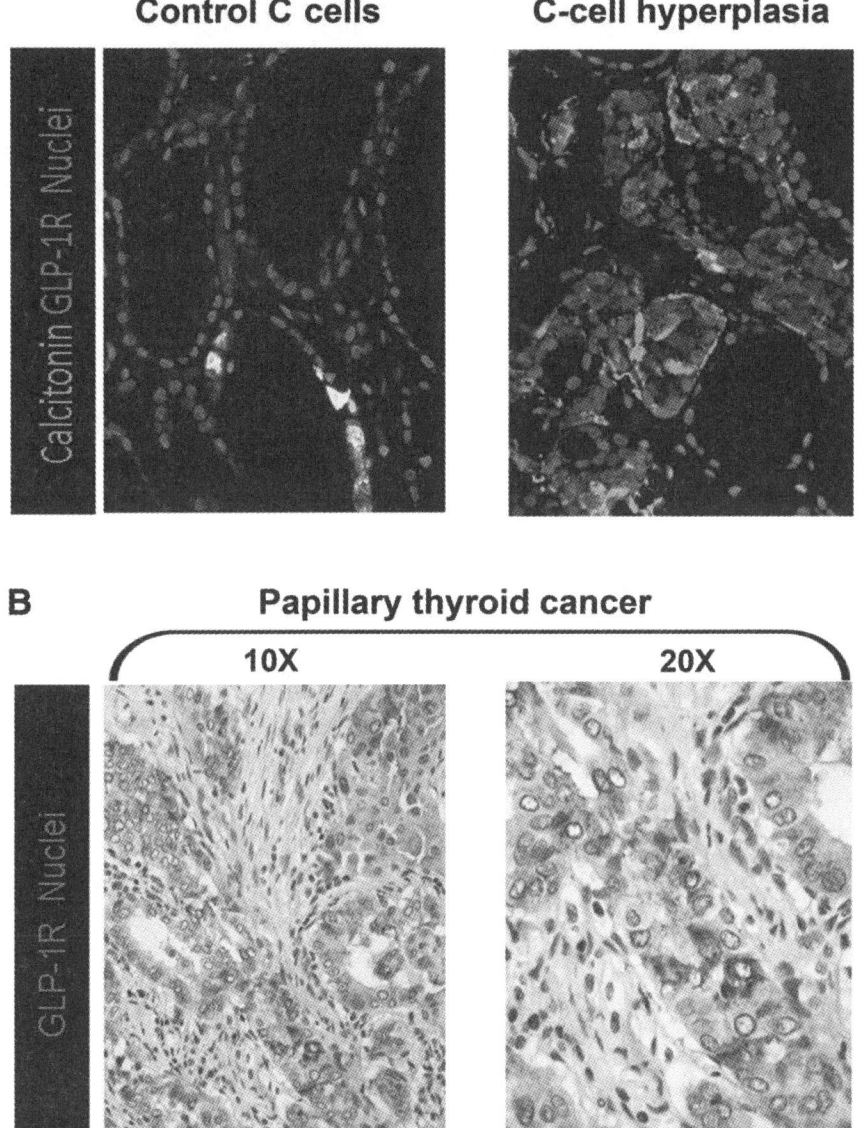

A

Control C cells   C-cell hyperplasia

Calcitonin GLP-1R Nuclei

B

Papillary thyroid cancer

10X   20X

GLP-1R Nuclei

Figure 2—*GLP-1 receptors (GLP-1R) are expressed in premalignant lesions in human thyroid. A: Human thyroid immunostained by immunofluorescence for calcitonin (green), GLP-1 receptor (red), and nuclei (blue) in a normal thyroid (left) and in C-cell hyperplasia (right). Yellow color indicates GLP-1 receptor expression in C cells, which is present occasionally in normal thyroid and frequently in C-cell hyperplasia. B: Human thyroid from papillary thyroid cancer (left and right panels) stained by immunohistochemistry for GLP-1 receptor (GLP-1R) (brown). GLP-1 receptor expression is present in ~20% of papillary thyroid cancers and most medullary thyroid cancers. Used with permission from Gier et al. (28).*

cancer—in individuals with type 2 diabetes. The model proposes acceleration of pancreatic dysplasia in the setting of low-grade chronic pancreatitis leading to sufficient ductal obstruction in a minority of individuals to provoke an episode of acute pancreatitis. Subclinical changes would be expected in a larger proportion of those exposed. The absence of pancreatitis or pancreatic dysplasia in nondiabetic models or short-term treatment of models of diabetes does not exclude the proposed mechanism. GLP-1 treatment, like estrogen in breast cancer, might promote development of pancreatic cancer in some individuals. Alternatively, periductal α-cell hyperplasia may cause duct obstruction and potentially progress to neuroendocrine neoplasia.

GLP-1 and thyroid cancer: Now you see it, now you don't

—Preclinical registration studies of liraglutide found an increased number of C-cell tumors of the thyroid in rodents. Studies sponsored by the manufacturers have suggested that C cells in humans do not express the GLP-1 receptor; that humans exposed to liraglutide have, in aggregate, little or no rise in calcitonin levels; and that nonhuman primates exposed to liraglutide do not develop thyroid tumors (27). In contrast, analysis of a much larger sample of human thyroid glands and C cells established that a subpopulation of C cells in humans does indeed express the GLP-1 receptor (28) (Fig. 2). It was further established that GLP-1 receptor expression was more abundant in C-cell hyperplasia, a potential precursor of medullary thyroid cancer. Moreover, GLP-1 receptor expression is also present in 20% of those with papillary thyroid cancer, a much more common tumor for which calcitonin levels would be irrelevant. While medullary thyroid cancer is rare (29), a relatively high proportion of the population has apparently quiescent micro foci of papillary thyroid cancer (30).

Once again we must ask whether relatively short-term negative studies of GLP-1 mimetic therapy and thyroid cancer in normal monkeys provide adequate reassurance against the risk of malignancy in humans. As in the pancreas, the concern is that proproliferative actions of GLP-1 superimposed on premalignant lesions (C-cell hyperplasia or micropapillary thyroid cancer) may accelerate the progression of these lesions toward cancer. And, once again, adverse event reporting shows a clear excess of reported thyroid cancer on both exenatide (74

while of concern, is perhaps not unexpected. No changes were reported in the exocrine pancreata of 10 monkeys that were treated with liraglutide for 87 weeks (13). Treatment was discontinued 2 weeks before the pancreata were obtained. The weight of the pancreata was not however reported (this would have been expected to increase). Long-term treatment of nondiabetic human primates with exenatide

has not been published. The concerns raised in this article go well beyond the scope of routine histologic analysis conducted for regulatory purposes, and a full review by independent experts in pancreatic pathology would now seem justified (25).

In summary, a plausible mechanism links GLP-1–based therapy with acute pancreatitis—and a potential risk of pancreatic thyroid cancer events) and liraglutide (57 thyroid cancer events), although there is currently no similar signal for the DPP-4 inhibitors (Table 2).

Conclusions: Déjà vu all over again?—The story is familiar. A new class of antidiabetic agents is rushed to market and widely promoted in the absence of any evidence of long-term beneficial outcomes. Evidence of harm accumulates, but is vigorously discounted. The regulators allow years to pass before they act. The manufacturers are expected—quite unrealistically—to monitor the safety of their own product. We should be thankful that those responsible for aircraft safety do not operate on the assumption that the absence of evidence is evidence of absence.

The safety of the GLP-1 therapies can no longer be assumed, and there will be rapid developments in this area. Drug safety can never be assumed, and the legal principle of "innocent until proved guilty" does not apply. The case presented here does not prove that these agents are unsafe, but it does suggest that the burden of proof now rests with those who wish to convince us of their safety.

PETER C. BUTLER, MD[1,2]
MICHAEL ELASHOFF, PHD[3]
ROBERT ELASHOFF, PHD[2,3]
EDWIN A.M. GALE, MD[4]

From the [1]Larry L. Hillblom Islet Research Center, University of California Los Angeles, David Geffen School of Medicine, Los Angeles, California; the [2]Jonsson Comprehensive Cancer Center, University of California Los Angeles, David Geffen School of Medicine, Los Angeles, California; the [3]Department of Biomathematics, University of California Los Angeles, David Geffen School of Medicine, Los Angeles, California; and the [4]University of Bristol, Bristol, U.K.
Corresponding author: Edwin A.M. Gale, edwin.gale@bristol.ac.uk.
DOI: 10.2337/dc12-2713

Acknowledgments—P.C.B. is funded by the National Institute of Diabetes and Digestive and Kidney Diseases (DK059579, DK061539, DK077967), The Larry L. Hillblom Foundation, and the Peter and Valerie Kompaniez Foundation. The reanalysis of the FDA database was supported by the National Institutes of Health (NIH)/National Center for Research Resources/National Center for Advancing Translational Sciences UCLA Clinical and Translational Science Institute Grant UL1TR000124. Its contents are solely the responsibility of the authors and do not necessarily represent the official views of the NIH.

E.A.M.G. has provided expert testimony in litigation concerning exenatide. No other potential conflicts of interest relevant to this article were reported.

The authors gratefully acknowledge the technical support of Chi-Hong Tseng (Department of Biomathematics, UCLA) and the editorial assistance of Bonnie Lui (Larry L. Hillblom Islet Research Center, UCLA).

• •

References

1. Gale EAM. Collateral damage: the conundrum of drug safety. Diabetologia 2009; 52:1975–1982
2. Dore DD, Bloomgren GL, Wenten M, et al. A cohort study of acute pancreatitis in relation to exenatide use. Diabetes Obes Metab 2011;13:559–566
3. Dore DD, Seeger JD, Arnold Chan K. Use of a claims-based active drug safety surveillance system to assess the risk of acute pancreatitis with exenatide or sitagliptin compared to metformin or glyburide. Curr Med Res Opin 2009;25:1019–1027
4. Girman CJ, Kou TD, Cai B, et al. Patients with type 2 diabetes mellitus have higher risk for acute pancreatitis compared with those without diabetes. Diabetes Obes Metab 2010;12:766–771
5. Perfetti R, Zhou J, Doyle ME, Egan JM. Glucagon-like peptide-1 induces cell proliferation and pancreatic-duodenum homeobox-1 expression and increases endocrine cell mass in the pancreas of old, glucose-intolerant rats. Endocrinology 2000;141:4600–4605
6. Koehler JA, Baggio LL, Lamont BJ, Ali S, Drucker DJ. Glucagon-like peptide-1 receptor activation modulates pancreatitis-associated gene expression but does not modify the susceptibility to experimental pancreatitis in mice. Diabetes 2009;58:2148–2161
7. Matveyenko AV, Dry S, Cox HI, et al. Beneficial endocrine but adverse exocrine effects of sitagliptin in the human islet amyloid polypeptide transgenic rat model of type 2 diabetes: interactions with metformin. Diabetes 2009;58:1604–1615
8. Gier B, Matveyenko AV, Kirakossian D, Dawson D, Dry SM, Butler PC. Chronic GLP-1 receptor activation by exendin-4 induces expansion of pancreatic duct glands in rats and accelerates formation of dysplastic lesions and chronic pancreatitis in the Kras[G12D] mouse model. Diabetes 2012;61:1250–1262
9. Vrang N, Jelsing J, Simonsen L, et al. The effects of 13 wk of liraglutide treatment on endocrine and exocrine pancreas in male and female ZDF rats: a quantitative and qualitative analysis revealing no evidence of drug-induced pancreatitis. Am J Physiol Endocrinol Metab 2012;303:E253–E264
10. Tatarkiewicz K, Belanger P, Gu G, Parkes D, Roy D. No evidence of drug-induced pancreatitis in rats treated with exenatide for 13 weeks. Diabetes Obes Metab 2013; 15:417–426
11. Tatarkiewicz K, Smith PA, Sablan EJ, et al. Exenatide does not evoke pancreatitis and attenuates chemically induced pancreatitis in normal and diabetic rodents. Am J Physiol Endocrinol Metab 2010;299:E1076–E1086
12. Nachnani JS, Bulchandani DG, Nookala A, et al. Biochemical and histological effects of exendin-4 (exenatide) on the rat pancreas. Diabetologia 2010;53:153–159
13. Nyborg NC, Mølck AM, Madsen LW, Knudsen LB. The human GLP-1 analog liraglutide and the pancreas: evidence for the absence of structural pancreatic changes in three species. Diabetes 2012;61:1243–1249
14. Garg R, Chen W, Pendergrass M. Acute pancreatitis in type 2 diabetes treated with exenatide or sitagliptin: a retrospective observational pharmacy claims analysis. Diabetes Care 2010;33:2349–2354
15. Singh S, Chang HY, Richards TM, et al. Glucagonlike peptide 1-based therapies and risk of hospitalization for acute pancreatitis in type 2 diabetes mellitus: a population-based matched case-control study. JAMA Intern Med 2013;173:534–539
16. Pratley RE, Nauck M, Bailey T, et al.; 1860-LIRA-DPP-4 Study Group. Liraglutide versus sitagliptin for patients with type 2 diabetes who did not have adequate glycaemic control with metformin: a 26-week, randomised, parallel-group, open-label trial. Lancet 2010;375:1447–1456
17. Franks AS, Lee PH, George CM. Pancreatitis: a potential complication of liraglutide? Ann Pharmacother 2012;46:1547–1553
18. Elashoff M, Matveyenko AV, Gier B, Elashoff R, Butler PC. Pancreatitis, pancreatic, and thyroid cancer with glucagon-like peptide-1-based therapies. Gastroenterology 2011;141:150–156
19. Spranger J, Gundert-Remy U, Stammschulte T. GLP-1-based therapies: the dilemma of uncertainty. Gastroenterology 2011;141:20–23
20. Sipos B, Frank S, Gress T, Hahn S, Klöppel G. Pancreatic intraepithelial neoplasia revisited and updated. Pancreatology 2009; 9:45–54
21. Wideroff L, Gridley G, Mellemkjaer L, et al. Cancer incidence in a population-based cohort of patients hospitalized with diabetes mellitus in Denmark. J Natl Cancer Inst 1997;89:1360–1365

22. Simpson PT, Reis-Filho JS, Gale T, Lakhani SR. Molecular evolution of breast cancer. J Pathol 2005;205:248–254

23. Kling J. Inhaled insulin's last gasp? Nat Biotechnol 2008;26:479–480

24. Lando HM, Alattar M, Dua AP. Elevated amylase and lipase levels in patients using glucagonlike peptide-1 receptor agonists or dipeptidyl-peptidase-4 inhibitors in the outpatient setting. Endocr Pract 2012;18:472–477

25. Gale EAM. GLP-1–based therapies and the exocrine pancreas: more light, or just more heat? Diabetes 2012;61:986–988

26. Butler AE, Campbell-Thompson M, Gurlo T, Dawson DW, Atkinson M, Butler PC. Marked expansion of exocrine and endocrine pancreas with incretin therapy in humans with increased exocrine pancreas dysplasia and the potential for glucagon-producing neuroendocrine tumors. Diabetes 2013;62:2595–2604

27. Bjerre Knudsen L, Madsen LW, Andersen S, et al. Glucagon-like peptide-1 receptor agonists activate rodent thyroid C-cells causing calcitonin release and C-cell proliferation. Endocrinology 2010;151: 1473–1486

28. Gier B, Butler PC, Lai CK, Kirakossian D, DeNicola MM, Yeh MW. Glucagon like peptide-1 receptor expression in the human thyroid gland. J Clin Endocrinol Metab 2012;97:121–131

29. Jemal A, Siegel R, Ward E, Hao Y, Xu J, Thun MJ. Cancer statistics, 2009. CA Cancer J Clin 2009;59:225–249

30. Bondeson L, Ljungberg O. Occult papillary thyroid carcinoma in the young and the aged. Cancer 1984;53:1790–1792

31. Maitra A, Hruban RH. Pancreatic cancer. Annu Rev Pathol 2008;3:157–88

A Critical Analysis of the Clinical Use of Incretin-Based Therapies

The benefits by far outweigh the potential risks

There is no question that incretin-based glucose-lowering medications have proven to be effective glucose-lowering agents. Glucagon-like peptide 1 (GLP-1) receptor agonists demonstrate an efficacy comparable to insulin treatment and appear to do so with significant effects to promote weight loss with minimal hypoglycemia. In addition, there are significant data with dipeptidyl peptidase 4 (DPP-4) inhibitors showing efficacy comparable to sulfonylureas but with weight neutral effects and reduced risk for hypoglycemia. However, over the recent past there have been concerns regarding the long-term consequences of using such therapies, and the issues raised are in regard to the potential of both classes to promote acute pancreatitis, to initiate histological changes suggesting chronic pancreatitis including associated preneoplastic lesions, and potentially, in the long run, pancreatic cancer. Other issues relate to an increase in thyroid cancer. There are clearly conflicting data that have been presented in preclinical studies and in epidemiologic studies. To provide an understanding of both sides of the argument, we provide a discussion of this topic as part of this two-part point-counterpoint narrative. In the point narrative preceding the counterpoint narrative below, Dr. Butler and colleagues provide their opinion and review of the data to date and that we need to reconsider use of incretin-based therapies because of the growing concern of potential risk and based on a clearer understanding of the mechanism of action. In the counterpoint narrative provided below, Dr. Nauck provides a defense of incretin-based therapies and that benefits clearly outweigh any concern of risk.

—William T. Cefalu, md
Editor in Chief, Diabetes Care

Glucagon-like peptide 1 (GLP-1)–based medications are GLP-1 receptor agonists (incretin mimetics) and inhibitors of the incretin-degrading and incretin-inactivating protease dipeptidyl peptidase-4 (DPP-4), which exclusively (GLP-1 receptor agonists) or predominantly (DPP-4 inhibitors) act by enhancing the stimulation of GLP-1 receptors (1). Their mechanisms of action (1–3) and clinical effects (1,2,4) have been reviewed extensively. With a lot of scientific data relevant to the judgment of these novel medications having accumulated over the past 6 years and the clinical experience of using them in patients with type 2 diabetes, this is a good moment in time to attempt a more general evaluation of the merits and risks associated with incretin-based medications. Such a judgment will have to take into account the core clinical effectiveness (control of glycemia, prevention of diabetes complications), additional effects that are or could be beneficial in type 2 diabetic patients (improvements in cardiovascular risk factors, e.g., weight loss and reductions in blood pressure), aspects of tolerability and safety, and costs. Among the critical

issues that have been raised against the use of GLP-1–based medications are their potential role as inducers of acute pancreatitis (5)—perhaps of chronic pancreatitis (6,7)—and in the long run promoting the development of preneoplastic lesions and thus raising the risk for pancreatic cancer (8). Rodent studies with longer-acting GLP-1 receptor agonists have raised the issue of a potential proliferative response of thyroid C-cells (9), giving rise to hyperplasia, adenomas, and, eventually, medullary thyroid carcinomas. Another point of concern is a small rise in pulse rate observed with some GLP-1 receptor agonists (but not with DPP-4 inhibitors) (10,11). In the point article of this point–counterpoint narrative that precedes this article, Butler et al. (12) cite their significant concerns with these adverse events and make a statement that continued human use may be problematic. With those stated concerns, this counterpoint narrative will discuss the current status of the incretin-based therapies and provide an opinion that the clinical benefits are clearly greater than the potential risks based on the evidence to date.

Special issues (rare findings of uncertain clinical importance)

In addition to the influence of GLP-1–based medications on those outcomes that typically determine the morbidity and mortality of patients with type 2 diabetes, i.e., that affect large proportions of such patients, there may be additional safety concerns of special interest. Some signals have suggested an untoward influence of such treatment on the risk for certain rare conditions. For GLP-1 receptor agonists and for DPP-4 inhibitors, these events of special interest are pancreatitis, pancreatic cancer, and thyroid carcinoma (Table 1). In addition, possible consequences of a rise in pulse rate with GLP-1 receptor agonists need to be discussed.

Pancreatitis

Cases of pancreatitis have been observed in animals (6,7,13) and patients (14) treated with incretin mimetics and DPP-4 inhibitors (5). The questions are whether pancreatitis occurs more often in association with treatment using GLP-1–based medications, and whether it is causally related to such treatment.

Pancreatitis in animal studies

Animal studies describe histological changes compatible with damage to the exocrine pancreas with exenatide (6,7) and sitagliptin (5). A similar study examining liraglutide did not confirm such damages induced by an incretin mimetic (13). Other studies find an amelioration of the course of experimentally induced acute pancreatitis in mice with exenatide (15) or an anti-inflammatory pattern of cytokines induced by liraglutide treatment (16). Another open question is whether these findings are representative of human acute or chronic pancreatitis.

Clinical acute pancreatitis with incretin-based glucose-lowering medications

Attempts to quantify the number of pancreatitis events while patients are

Table 1—*Contrasting clinical benefits and improved outcomes with adverse outcomes/risks associated with the use of incretin-based glucose-lowering medications (a, GLP-1 receptor agonists; b, inhibitors of DPP-4)*

Clinical benefits/improved outcomes from using incretin-based glucose-lowering medications	Adverse outcomes/risks from using incretin-based glucose-lowering medications
1. Effective lowering of fasting and postprandial glucose	1. a) Nausea, vomiting, diarrhea, and other "gastrointestinal" adverse events
a) Similar in magnitude to insulin treatment	• Leading to withdrawal of treatment in 3–8%
b) Similar in magnitude to sulfonylurea treatment	• Often improves with prolonged exposure
2. No stimulation of insulin secretion at low glucose = avoidance of hypoglycemia	2. b) DPP-4 = CD26, a marker of activated T cells; enzyme inhibition does not appear to affect immune function
3. No risk of body weight gain	3. Pancreatitis associated with the use of GLP-1 receptor agonists and DPP-4 inhibitors
a) Robust weight loss (2–4 kg) in most patients	• Animal studies controversial (both pro- and anti-inflammatory effects described)
b) No change in body weight or minor weight loss	• Epidemiology controversial (both increased and unchanged numbers reported)
4. Reduction systolic blood pressure	4. Pancreatic cancer hypothesized to be a long-term consequence of using incretin-based glucose-lowering drugs
a) By 2–5 mmHg	• No case reports reported
b) Only in patients with prior arterial hypertension	• Animal studies on potential to induce preneoplastic lesions highly controversial
	• Epidemiological data likely to be influenced by reporting bias
5. Durability better than with sulfonylureas (however, intrinsic improvement in durability due to lasting improvements in β-cell mass or function not proven)	5. C-cell proliferation (hyperplasia, adenomas, medullary thyroid cancer) induced by GLP-1 receptor agonists in rodents
	• No case reports of medullary thyroid carcinoma reported
	• In human subjects, no rise in calcitonin with exposure to GLP-1 receptor agonists
	• Epidemiological data likely to be influenced by reporting bias
	• Presence of GLP-1 receptors on non–C-cells (e.g., follicular cells) and in other thyroid tumors (e.g., papillary carcinoma) controversial
6. Prevention of microvascular diabetes complications based on glucose-lowering effects (supported by preclinical models and preliminary data from clinical trials)	6. Heart rate increased by 2–5 bpm with long-acting GLP-1 receptor agonists (mechanism unclear)
7. Potential to prevent cardiovascular events and mortality; see Fig. 1	

For appropriate literature citations, see text.

treated with GLP-1 receptor agonists or DPP-4 inhibitors have found odds ratios (ORs) around 1, however with relatively wide CIs (Fig. 1A and C) (17–21). Such data have been taken from claims databases and correlating the prescription of drugs used to treat diabetes with a diagnosis of acute pancreatitis. These analyses have made it clear that obese, type 2 diabetic subjects are more prone to developing acute pancreatitis than the nondiabetic population. On the other hand, one single study reports a more than tenfold excess of pancreatitis in patients using exenatide or sitagliptin (22). This notable exception is a study based on an analysis of the U.S. Food and Drug Administration (FDA) Adverse Event Reporting System (FAERS [formerly known as AERS]). This study, thus, is in obvious contradiction to other epidemiological data. It

summarizes reports to the FAERS from a period when publications and changes to drug labels had alerted the medical community to the fact that cases of acute pancreatitis had occurred in patients treated with exenatide and sitagliptin. This probably has prompted some reporting bias. The quality of the individual reports to the FAERS may also be questioned. The standards for the diagnosis of acute pancreatitis (at least two out of three criteria: *1*) typical severe abdominal pain, *2*) elevations in pancreas-specific enzymes such as amylase and lipase, and *3*) typical findings using appropriate imaging procedures [23]) may not always have been applied.

A recent case-control study reported a higher OR for the risk of hospitalization for a diagnosis of pancreatitis in patients taking "incretin-based medications,"

since a separate analysis for the use of exenatide (GLP-1 receptor agonist) or sitagliptin (DPP-4 inhibitor) did not yield significant findings (Fig. 1B and D). It cannot be excluded at present that a potential combination of stomach cramps, representing gastrointestinal adverse events of GLP-1 receptor agonists, and spontaneously elevated serum lipase activities were responsible for the hospitalizations and do not represent true pancreatitis episodes. Nevertheless, this small study analyzing only a few patients with pancreatitis is only the second study describing an elevated risk (24), however, only by combining exenatide and sitagliptin treatments as "incretin-based medications" and after adjusting for potential confounders. Figure 1B and D presents ORs and P values (all nonsignificant) calculated without adjustment for potential risk-modifying factors.

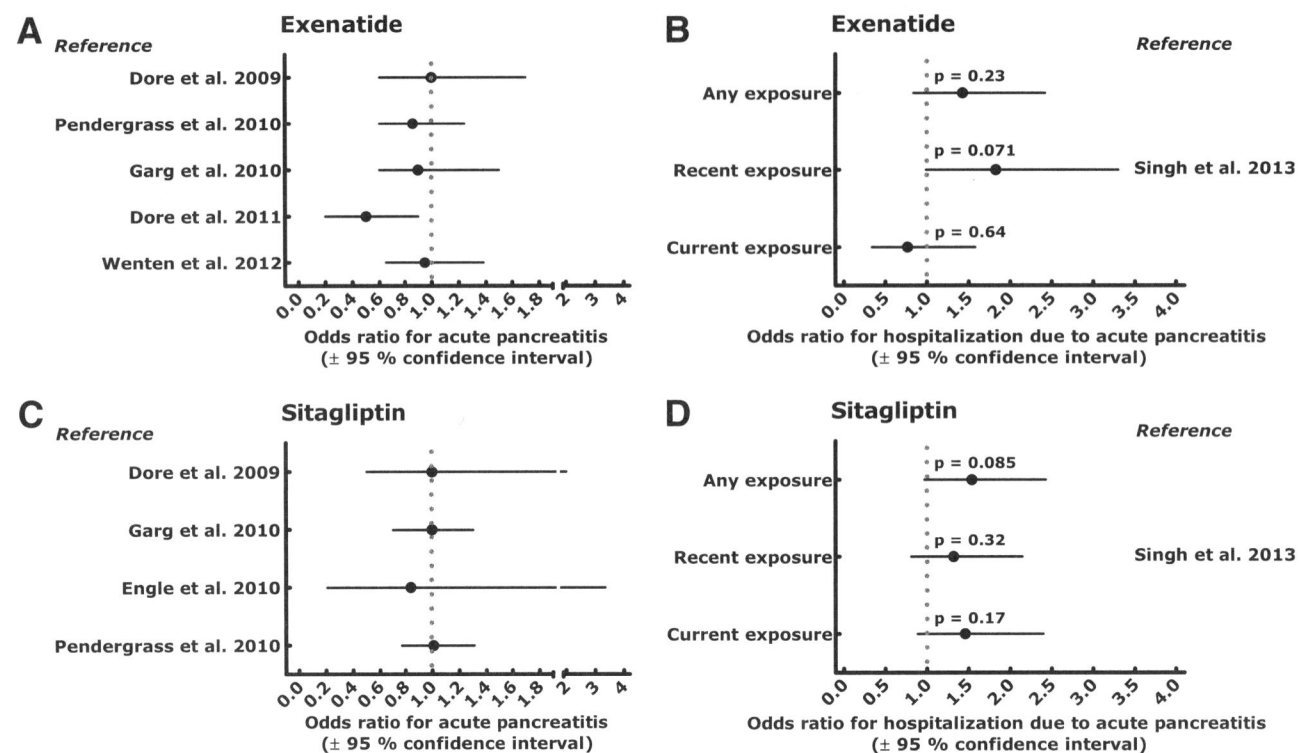

Figure 1—*ORs for the diagnosis of (A and C) or hospitalization for (B and D) acute pancreatitis in association with a medication of exenatide (GLP-1 receptor agonist, upper panels) or sitagliptin (DPP-4 inhibitor, lower panels). ORs and their 95% CIs and related P values were obtained directly or calculated (GraphPAD PRISM 5.02) from published analysis of claims databases. Data have been taken from the references quoted in the figure (17–21, 24, 50). Recent exposures: medication prescribed for use between 2 years and 30 days before hospitalization; current exposures: medication prescribed for use <30 days before hospitalization.*

Furthermore, treatment with the GLP-1 receptor agonist liraglutide can lead to elevations in lipase without associated symptoms of pancreatitis (25). Using such enzyme measurements to "screen" for pancreatitis may have resulted in false diagnoses of pancreatitis because elevations in pancreatic enzymes do not have the degree of specificity that would be necessary to make it a helpful screening instrument. Indeed, elevated lipase and amylase activity is found quite frequently in patients with type 2 diabetes with an absence of abdominal pain (26). Under these circumstances, most elevated amylase or lipase levels would be chance findings without any relationship to inflammatory changes within the exocrine pancreas. However, the nature of the elevation in serum lipase induced by liraglutide treatment needs to be explored so that we can understand its mechanism. At least this phenomenon indicates an interaction of GLP-1 receptor agonists with the exocrine pancreas, perhaps indicating the presence of GLP-1 receptors in this compartment. Effects of GLP-1 receptor stimulation on pancreatic enzyme synthesis, potential leakage into the circulation

rather than directional secretion into pancreatic digestive juice, and a potential induction of a chronic inflammatory response need to be studied. To date, it certainly cannot be taken as a fact that chronic stimulation of the GLP-1 receptor (as occurs during the treatment with incretin mimetics and DPP-4 inhibitors) induces acute or chronic inflammatory responses in the pancreas, nor that, based on a well-delineated mechanism and supported by convincing epidemiological data, the clinical use of incretin-based glucose-lowering medications would cause pancreatitis. Clinically, the development of typical chronic pancreatitis diagnosed because of typical morphological findings and exocrine insufficiency leading to maldigestion, nutritional deficiencies, and weight loss over and above what is expected from continued stimulation of brain GLP-1 receptors (1,27) in patients treated with GLP-1–based medications has never been described.

Incretin-based medications and chronic pancreatitis/pancreatic cancer
Regarding the related question of chronic changes in the exocrine pancreas leading

to pancreatic duct proliferation and the formation of preneoplastic lesions (like pancreatic intraepithelial neoplasms or pancreatic duct glands [28]), data from animal studies are similarly controversial with studies showing alterations of the exocrine pancreatic histology indicative of chronic pancreatitis with exenatide treatment (5–7), while another recent study using liraglutide did describe occasional pancreatitis as a rare finding—but not at all related to the dose of liraglutide—with similar numbers in placebo-treated rats, mice, and monkeys (13). It appears highly unlikely that there should be a difference intrinsic to the two GLP-1 receptor agonists used (exenatide vs. liraglutide). A recent finding reported that pancreas specimens from organ donors with type 2 diabetes, who had received treatment with the DPP-4 inhibitor sitagliptin ($n = 7$) or exenatide ($n = 1$), relative to patients with type 2 diabetes treated with other agents, had marked β-cell hyperplasia, β-cells coexpressing insulin and glucagon, hyperplasia of α-cells expressing glucagon, increased expression of proliferation markers, and an increased prevalence of preneoplastic lesions (29). This finding needs to be confirmed in a larger, representative sample of pancreas specimens obtained without preceding long-term critical illness, which alone may be responsible for some proliferative responses (30).

To put the state of this present discussion into perspective, it should be made clear that at most early proliferative or preneoplastic changes have been observed, which as such are not proof that eventually the process described will give rise to pancreatic cancer. Thus we have to discuss a *potential* risk (and certainly want to learn more about the long-term consequences of stimulating GLP-1 receptors for the exocrine pancreas), but not an actual threat to patients treated with incretin-based medications, based on a well-characterized mechanism with a risk clearly elevated based on sound epidemiological analyses. It is reassuring that no case of clinically evident chronic pancreatitis has been described after initiating treatment with incretin-based medications. Certainly, there is also no case report of pancreatic cancer diagnosed after exposing a patient to GLP-1 receptor agonists or DPP-4 inhibitors in a patient in whom there had previously been a morphologically tumor-free pancreas. Since pancreatic carcinomas develop slowly (31), one would probably not expect to see such a case after at most a few years of treatment, considering the recent introduction of the incretin-based medications, even if there were such a long-term risk.

Incretin-based medications and thyroid carcinoma

GLP-1 receptor agonists have the potential to induce proliferative changes in rodent thyroid C cells. Liraglutide increased the number of cases with C-cell hyperplasia, adenomas, and medullary thyroid carcinomas in mice and rats (9). In these species such abnormalities are also found spontaneously, i.e., in the absence of GLP-1 receptor stimulation, especially in male rats, in which medullary thyroid carcinoma developed in some animals treated with placebo (9). Accordingly, rodent C-cell lines in cell culture responded to GLP-1, exenatide, and liraglutide with acutely producing cyclic AMP and secreting calcitonin (9). Similar cell lines of human origin do not show such acute responses when GLP-1 receptors are stimulated (9). Whereas rodent C-cell lines are equipped with GLP-1 receptors at a high level of expression, this is not the case in their human counterparts (9). Along the same lines, long-term treatment in

obese human subjects with high liraglutide doses up to 3-mg per day does not lead to elevations in plasma calcitonin (32). Based on these results, the ability of GLP-1 receptor stimulation to induce proliferative responses in human C cells has been judged as probably absent. Medullary thyroid carcinomas are an extremely rare form of thyroid carcinomas in humans (33). No case report has been published describing a medullary thyroid carcinoma in a patient receiving a treatment with a GLP-1 receptor agonist who prior to such treatment had a morphologically normal thyroid gland and low calcitonin concentrations. Given the rare incidence of medullary thyroid carcinoma, *1*) the consequences of a potential elevation in the risk induced by incretin mimetics would still remain small, and 2) to prove or exclude such a relationship, efficient surveillance of extremely large numbers of patients would be needed.

The elevated risk for thyroid carcinoma in more general terms described in the study exploring the FAERS database (22) is difficult to reconcile. Similar reservations apply regarding reporting bias as mentioned for the pancreatitis/pancreatic carcinoma issue raised earlier (vide supra). Certainly, this would not be compatible with an explanation through a higher number of medullary carcinomas alone, which would need to increase by more than 30-fold in order to explain such numbers. However, whether follicular cells express GLP-1 receptors (9) or whether malignant cells from thyroid tumors of different histological varieties (e.g., papillary thyroid carcinomas) express the GLP-1 receptors (34) is controversial and may be related to the specificity of the antibody or the radioligand used for immunohistochemistry (35). The fact alone that some papillary thyroid carcinomas may show evidence of GLP-1 receptor expression (34) does not prove that such receptors and their stimulation by drugs may contribute to the genesis or proliferation of such tumors. Again, even a convincing case report is missing. Regarding the thyroid issues, certainly more investigations are required, but one hardly can conclude that, based on current knowledge, there is a definitely increased risk for medullary (or other types of) thyroid carcinoma with the use of GLP-1 receptor agonists. Nevertheless, patients with an individually elevate genetic risk should not be treated with such agents. An elevated risk when using DPP-4 inhibitors does not have to considered at all since no such findings have been reported (22).

Cardiovascular outcomes

In the absence of large-scale cardiovascular outcome trials, summaries of cardiovascular events reported as adverse events in clinical trials with incretin-based glucose-lowering medications and meta-analyses based thereon (36) are the best available source of information for an overall judgment at present. Phase 3 studies have accrued a number of cardiovascular events sufficient for a preliminary judgment based on trends. These trends observed for the incretin mimetics exenatide (37) and liraglutide (38) as well the DPP-4 inhibitors sitagliptin (39), vildagliptin (40), saxagliptin (41), linagliptin (42), and alogliptin (43) are surprisingly similar. As shown in Fig. 2, in all these analyses the relative risk for a combined end point composed of acute myocardial infarction, stroke, and cardiovascular death is reduced with any of the GLP-1–based medications relative to placebo or comparator treatment to a value below 1 (Fig. 2). However, the 95% CIs ranged to above 1.0 with most compounds, indicating that the number of events available for this analysis was too small to allow the definite conclusion of a significant improvement in cardiovascular prognosis with incretin-based glucose-lowering treatment.

A potential reduction in cardiovascular event rates with linagliptin treatment is further supported by a recent study comparing linagliptin with the sulfonylurea glimepiride (44).

There is some plausibility based on the influences of GLP-1–based drugs on cardiovascular risk factors (45). GLP-1 receptor agonists reduce body weight by reducing appetite and food intake. They also reduce systolic blood pressure by 2–5 mmHg, mechanistically explained by improved endothelial function and vasodilation, enhanced natriuresis, and fluid excretion. There is a potential for a reduction in postprandial triglyceride-rich lipoproteins, especially with those agents that have and preserve over time a prominent effect on gastric emptying. Effects on "nonclassical" cardiovascular risk factors point in the same direction. Furthermore, GLP-1 receptor stimulation has reduced the extent of myocardial necroses in animal experiments inducing acute myocardial infarction by coronary artery ligation. The results have been surprisingly uniform using different agents (GLP-1, exenatide, liraglutide, sitagliptin) in various species (45). In addition, in animal models of left ventricular failure,

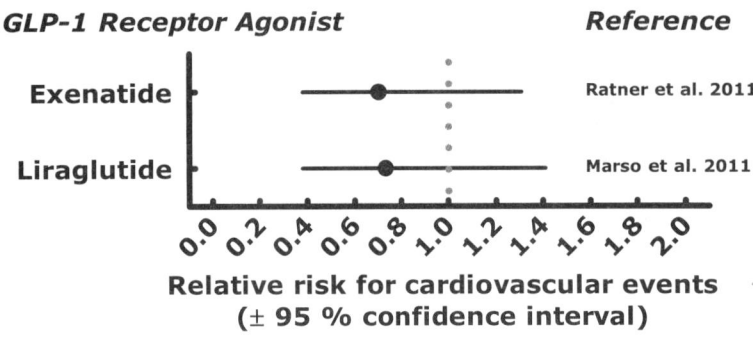

GLP-1 Receptor Agonist — **Reference**

Exenatide — Ratner et al. 2011

Liraglutide — Marso et al. 2011

Relative risk for cardiovascular events
(± 95 % confidence interval)

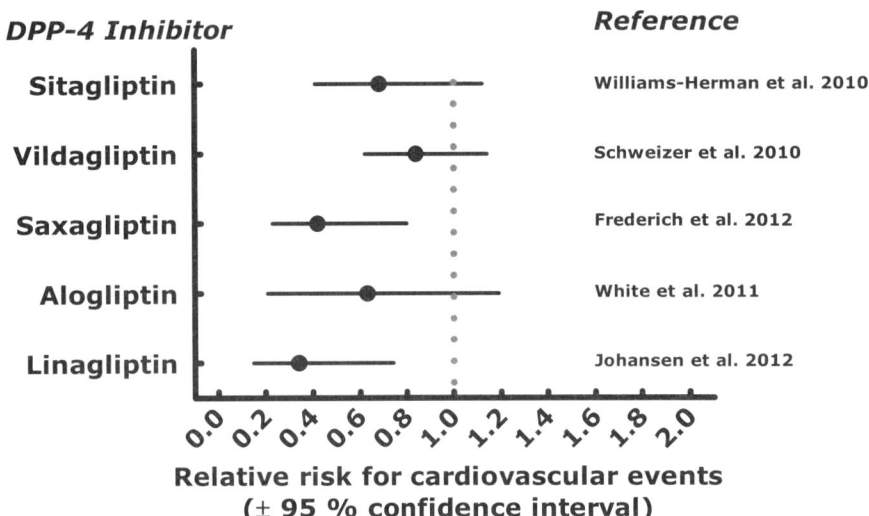

DPP-4 Inhibitor — **Reference**

Sitagliptin — Williams-Herman et al. 2010

Vildagliptin — Schweizer et al. 2010

Saxagliptin — Frederich et al. 2012

Alogliptin — White et al. 2011

Linagliptin — Johansen et al. 2012

Relative risk for cardiovascular events
(± 95 % confidence interval)

Figure 2—*Relative risk for major cardiovascular events reported as adverse events during phase 3 studies with the GLP-1 receptor agonists exenatide and liraglutide (upper panel) and with the DPP-4 inhibitors sitagliptin, vildagliptin, saxagliptin, alogliptin, and linagliptin (lower panel) compared with pooled comparators (placebo or active control medications). The relative risk is displayed together with the 95% CIs (bars). Data have been taken from the references quoted in the figure (37–43).*

GLP-1 and incretin mimetics may increase cardiac output by stimulating glucose and oxygen uptake into the myocardium. Clinical pilot trials support the notion that GLP-1 receptor stimulation may be beneficial in patients with acute coronary syndrome and chronic congestive heart failure (45). Therefore, one may be optimistic that cardiovascular outcome trials being performed to date, which will report

after the year 2015 (Table 2), will at least confirm cardiovascular safety with a potential to substantiate the beneficial effects in this important respect.

The greater picture—weighing benefits against potential risks and harms regarding the clinical use of incretin-based glucose-lowering medications

—Table 1 summarizes the beneficial effects of incretin-based glucose-lowering agents and their advantages over other antidiabetic pharmaceutical agents, but also the open issues discussed earlier in this article in order to define the balance of benefits on the one hand and the risks and harms on the other. Regarding the properties of incretin-based medications as antidiabetic drugs, they are effective in lowering glucose and avoid the problems of some other classes of glucose-lowering medications that are related to the induction of hypoglycemia and weight gain. Surrogate parameters indicate an improvement in the cardiovascular risk profile, and preliminary analyses of cardiovascular outcomes suggest the potential for benefit in this respect. Critical issues exist, but in many respects they are discussed in a controversial manner with only some data in support of an elevated risk (Table 1). Nausea and vomiting may be intolerable and lead to the discontinuation of treatment with GLP-1 receptor agonists. Putative interference of DPP-4 inhibitors with immune function does not lead to increased rates of common infections (39,46). Regarding the issues related to the potential short-term induction of acute and the putative long-term risk for chronic pancreatitis and eventually pancreatic cancer, data at hand today do not convincingly prove such risks. Thyroid issues related to GLP-1 receptors on C cells appear to mainly apply to rodents with a paucity of convincing human data that show a definite risk. This applies even more so to other forms of thyroid cancer. The fact that heart rate may increase with GLP-1 receptor agonists needs to be understood mechanistically. Potential explanations could be a reflex compensating for vasodilation (47) and lower blood pressure (10,11,48), a direct effect on the sinus node, or an increased relationship of sympathetic versus parasympathetic autonomous nervous system tone. Epidemiological findings relating higher heart rates to premature cardiovascular morbidity and mortality probably use pulse rate as a surrogate parameter for physical fitness (49). There is no reason to assume that incretin-based medications would lead to a reduced cardiorespiratory

Table 2—*Cardiovascular outcomes studies conducted with incretin-based glucose-lowering drugs*

Incretin-based medication	Name of clinical trial	Number of planned patients	Recruitment started	Trial completion expected	Identification number (ClinicalTrials.gov)
GLP-1R agonists					
Liraglutide	LEADER	8,754	8/2010	1/2016	NCT 01179048
Exenatide*	EXCEL	9,500	6/2010	3/2017	NCT 01144338
DPP-4 inhibitors					
Sitagliptin	TECOS	14,000	12/2008	12/2014	NCT 00790205
Saxagliptin	SAVOR-TIMI 53	16,500	5/2010	5/2015	NCT 01107886
Alogliptin	EXAMINE	5,400	9/2009	12/2014	NCT 00968708
Linagliptin	CAROLINA	6,000	10/2010	9/2018	NCT 01243424

*Once-weekly preparation; all data have been taken from ClinicalTrials.gov. GLP-1R, GLP-1 receptor.

fitness. A lower body weight speaks against this hypothesis.

Thus, while the benefits—expected or proven—from using incretin-based medications seem to be substantial and address risks central to patients with type 2 diabetes, the potential harms and risks typically refer to rare events and are discussed in a controversial manner, e.g., without certainty regarding a potential role of incretin-based medications to cause substantial harm. Obviously more needs to be learned regarding the open questions, but based on today's available knowledge, incretin-based medications can be considered effective and safe. Safety concerns related to the exocrine pancreas and the thyroid are not substantiated enough. Such considerations should not currently influence our treatment decisions regarding the potential prescription of GLP-1 receptor agonists or DPP-4 inhibitors within a treatment regimen for type 2 diabetes.

MICHAEL A. NAUCK, MD, PHD

From the Diabetes Center, Bad Lauterberg, Bad Lauterberg im Harz, Germany.
Corresponding author: Michael A. Nauck, nauck@diabeteszentrum.de.

DOI: 10.2337/dc12-2504

Acknowledgments—M.A.N. has received research grants (to his institution, the Diabeteszentrum Bad Lauterberg) from Berlin-Chemie AG/Menarini, Berlin, Germany; Eli Lilly & Co., Indianapolis, Indiana; Merck Sharp & Dohme, München, Germany; and Novartis Pharma AG, Basel, Switzerland (mono- or oligocentric studies); and from AstraZeneca, Södertälje, Sweden; Boehringer Ingelheim, Ingelheim, Germany; GlaxoSmithKline, King of Prussia, Pennsylvania; Lilly Deutschland GmbH, Bad Homburg, Germany; MetaCure Inc., Orangeburg, New York; Roche Pharma AG, Grenzach-Wyhlen, Germany; Novo Nordisk Pharma GmbH, Mainz, Germany; and Tolerx Inc., a Delaware Corporation, Cambridge, Massachusetts, for participation in multicentric clinical trials.

He has received consulting fees or/and honoraria for membership in advisory boards or/and honoraria for speaking from Amylin Pharmaceuticals, Inc., San Diego, California; AstraZeneca, Mjölndal, Sweden; Berlin-Chemie AG/Menarini, Berlin, Germany; Boehringer Ingelheim, Ingelheim, Germany; Bristol-Myers Squibb EMEA, Rueil-Malmaison, France; Diartis Pharmaceuticals, Inc., Redwood City, California; Eli Lilly & Co., Indianapolis, Indiana; F. Hoffmann-LaRoche Ltd., Basel, Switzerland; GlaxoSmithKline LLC, King of Prussia, Pennsylvania; Intarcia Therapeutics, Inc., Hayward, California; Lilly Deutschland GmbH, Bad Homburg, Germany; MannKind Corp., Danbury, Connecticut; Merck Sharp & Dohme GmbH, München, Germany; Merck Sharp & Dohme Corp., New Jersey; Novartis Pharma AG, Basel, Switzerland; Novo Nordisk A/S, Bagsværd, Denmark; Novo Nordisk Pharma GmbH, Mainz, Germany; Sanofi Pharma, Bad Soden/Taunus, Germany; Takeda, Deerfield, Illinois; Versartis, Sunnyvale, California; and Wyeth Research, Collegeville, Pennsylvania; including reimbursement for travel expenses in connection with the above-mentioned activities. He owns no stock and is employed by Diabeteszentrum Bad Lauterberg, Bad Lauterberg im Harz, Germany. No other potential conflicts of interest relevant to this article were reported.

The author thanks Ute Buss for help with retrieving literature and Marion Männel and Marion Masekowitz (all from Diabeteszentrum Bad Lauterberg) for secretarial assistance. The author also thanks Juris Meier (Division of Diabetology and Gastrointestinal Endocrinology, Medizinische Klinik I, St. Josef-Hospital, Klinikum der Ruhr-Universität Bochum, Bochum, Germany) for helpful discussions.

• •

References
1. Drucker DJ, Nauck MA. The incretin system: glucagon-like peptide-1 receptor agonists and dipeptidyl peptidase-4 inhibitors in type 2 diabetes. Lancet 2006;368:1696–1705
2. Nauck MA. Incretin-based therapies for type 2 diabetes mellitus: properties, functions, and clinical implications. Am J Med 2011;124(Suppl.):S3–S18
3. Deacon CF. Incretin-based treatment of type 2 diabetes: glucagon-like peptide-1 receptor agonists and dipeptidyl peptidase-4 inhibitors. Diabetes Obes Metab 2007;9(Suppl. 1):23–31
4. Deacon CF. Dipeptidyl peptidase-4 inhibitors in the treatment of type 2 diabetes: a comparative review. Diabetes Obes Metab 2011;13:7–18
5. Matveyenko AV, Dry S, Cox HI, et al. Beneficial endocrine but adverse exocrine effects of sitagliptin in the human islet amyloid polypeptide transgenic rat model of type 2 diabetes: interactions with metformin. Diabetes 2009;58:1604–1615
6. Nachnani JS, Bulchandani DG, Nookala A, et al. Biochemical and histological effects of exendin-4 (exenatide) on the rat pancreas. Diabetologia 2010;53:153–159
7. Gier B, Matveyenko AV, Kirakossian D, Dawson D, Dry SM, Butler PC. Chronic GLP-1 receptor activation by exendin-4 induces expansion of pancreatic duct glands in rats and accelerates formation of dysplastic lesions and chronic pancreatitis in the Kras(G12D) mouse model. Diabetes 2012;61:1250–1262
8. Butler PC, Matveyenko AV, Dry S, Bhushan A, Elashoff R. Glucagon-like peptide-1 therapy and the exocrine pancreas: innocent bystander or friendly fire? Diabetologia 2010;53:1–6
9. Bjerre Knudsen L, Madsen LW, Andersen S, et al. Glucagon-like peptide-1 receptor agonists activate rodent thyroid C-cells causing calcitonin release and C-cell proliferation. Endocrinology 2010;151:1473–1486
10. Pratley RE, Nauck M, Bailey T, et al.; 1860-LIRA-DPP-4 Study Group. Liraglutide versus sitagliptin for patients with type 2 diabetes who did not have adequate glycaemic control with metformin: a 26-week, randomised, parallel-group, open-label trial. Lancet 2010;375:1447–1456
11. Bergenstal RM, Wysham C, Macconell L, et al.; DURATION-2 Study Group. Efficacy and safety of exenatide once weekly versus sitagliptin or pioglitazone as an adjunct to metformin for treatment of type 2 diabetes (DURATION-2): a randomised trial. Lancet 2010;376:431–439
12. Butler PC, Elashoff M, Elashoff R, Gale EAM. A critical analysis of the clinical use of incretin-based therapies: are the GLP-1 therapies safe? Diabetes Care 2013;36:2118–2125
13. Nyborg NC, Mølck AM, Madsen LW, Knudsen LB. The human GLP-1 analog liraglutide and the pancreas: evidence for the absence of structural pancreatic changes in three species. Diabetes 2012;61:1243–1249
14. Ahmad SR, Swann J. Exenatide and rare adverse events. N Engl J Med 2008;358:1970-1971; discussion 1971-1972
15. Tatarkiewicz K, Smith PA, Sablan EJ, et al. Exenatide does not evoke pancreatitis and attenuates chemically induced pancreatitis in normal and diabetic rodents. Am J Physiol Endocrinol Metab 2010;299:E1076–E1086
16. Koehler JA, Baggio LL, Lamont BJ, Ali S, Drucker DJ. Glucagon-like peptide-1 receptor activation modulates pancreatitis-associated gene expression but does not modify the susceptibility to experimental pancreatitis in mice. Diabetes 2009;58:2148–2161
17. Garg R, Chen W, Pendergrass M. Acute pancreatitis in type 2 diabetes treated with exenatide or sitagliptin: a retrospective observational pharmacy claims analysis. Diabetes Care 2010;33:2349–2354
18. Dore DD, Seeger JD, Arnold Chan K. Use of a claims-based active drug safety surveillance system to assess the risk of acute pancreatitis with exenatide or sitaglip-

tin compared to metformin or glyburide. Curr Med Res Opin 2009;25:1019–1027

19. Dore DD, Bloomgren GL, Wenten M, et al. A cohort study of acute pancreatitis in relation to exenatide use. Diabetes Obes Metab 2011;13:559–566

20. Wenten M, Gaebler JA, Hussein M, et al. Relative risk of acute pancreatitis in initiators of exenatide twice daily compared with other anti-diabetic medication: a follow-up study. Diabetic Med 2012;29:1412–1418

21. Pendergrass M, Chen W. Association between diabetes, exenatide, sitagliptin and acute pancreatitis (Abstract). Diabetes 2010;59(Suppl. 1):A160

22. Elashoff M, Matveyenko AV, Gier B, Elashoff R, Butler PC. Pancreatitis, pancreatic, and thyroid cancer with glucagon-like peptide-1-based therapies. Gastroenterology 2011;141:150–156

23. Kiriyama S, Gabata T, Takada T, et al. New diagnostic criteria of acute pancreatitis. J Hepatobiliary Pancreat Sci 2010;17:24–36

24. Singh S, Chang H-Y, Richards TM, Weiner JP, Clark JM, Segal JB. *Glucagonlike peptide 1-based therapies and risk of hospitalization for acute pancreatitis in type 2 diabetes mellitus: a population-based matched case-control study.* JAMA Intern Med 2013;173:534–539

25. Steinberg W, De Vries H, Wadden TA, Bjørn Jensen C, Svendsen CB, Rosenstock J. Longitudinal monitoring of lipase and amylase in adults with type 2 diabetes and obesity: evidence from two phase 3 randomized clinical trials with the once-daily GLP-1 analog liraglutide (Abstract). Gastroenterol 2012;142(Suppl. 1):S850–S851

26. Steinberg W, Rosenstock J, De Vries H, Bloch Thomsen A, Svendsen CB, Wadden TA. Elevated serum lipase activity in adults with type 2 diabetes and no gastrointestinal symptoms (Abstract). Gastroenterol 2012;142(Suppl. 1):S93–S94

27. Flint A, Raben A, Astrup A, Holst JJ. Glucagon-like peptide 1 promotes satiety and suppresses energy intake in humans. J Clin Invest 1998;101:515–520

28. Vincent A, Herman J, Schulick R, Hruban RH, Goggins M. Pancreatic cancer. Lancet 2011;378:607–620

29. Butler AE, Campbell-Thompson M, Gurlo T, Dawson DW, Atkinson M, Butler PC. Marked expansion of exocrine and endocrine pancreas with incretin therapy in humans with increased exocrine pancreas dysplasia and the potential for glucagon-

producing neuroendocrine tumors. Diabetes 2013;62:2595–2604

30. In't Veld P, De Munck N, Van Belle K, et al. Beta-cell replication is increased in donor organs from young patients after prolonged life support. Diabetes 2010;59:1702–1708

31. Yachida S, Jones S, Bozic I, et al. Distant metastasis occurs late during the genetic evolution of pancreatic cancer. Nature 2010;467:1114–1117

32. Hegedüs L, Moses AC, Zdravkovic M, Le Thi T, Daniels GH. GLP-1 and calcitonin concentration in humans: lack of evidence of calcitonin release from sequential screening in over 5000 subjects with type 2 diabetes or nondiabetic obese subjects treated with the human GLP-1 analog, liraglutide. J Clin Endocrinol Metab 2011;96:853–860

33. Aschebrook-Kilfoy B, Ward MH, Sabra MM, Devesa SS. Thyroid cancer incidence patterns in the United States by histologic type, 1992-2006. Thyroid 2011;21:125–134

34. Gier B, Butler PC, Lai CK, Kirakossian D, DeNicola MM, Yeh MW. Glucagon like peptide-1 receptor expression in the human thyroid gland. J Clin Endocrinol Metab 2012;97:121–131

35. Waser B, Beetschen K, Pellegata NS, Reubi JC. Incretin receptors in non-neoplastic and neoplastic thyroid C cells in rodents and humans: relevance for incretin-based diabetes therapy. Neuroendocrinology 2011;94:291–301

36. Monami M, Ahrén B, Dicembrini I, Mannucci E. Dipeptidyl peptidase-4 inhibitors and cardiovascular risk: a meta-analysis of randomized clinical trials. Diabetes Obes Metab 2013;15:112–120

37. Ratner R, Han J, Nicewarner D, Yushmanova I, Hoogwerf BJ, Shen L. Cardiovascular safety of exenatide BID: an integrated analysis from controlled clinical trials in participants with type 2 diabetes. Cardiovasc Diabetol 2011;10:22

38. Marso SP, Lindsey JB, Stolker JM, et al. Cardiovascular safety of liraglutide assessed in a patient-level pooled analysis of phase 2: 3 liraglutide clinical development studies. Diab Vasc Dis Res 2011;8:237–240

39. Williams-Herman D, Engel SS, Round E, et al. Safety and tolerability of sitagliptin in clinical studies: a pooled analysis of data from 10,246 patients with type 2 diabetes. BMC Endocr Disord 2010;10:7

40. Schweizer A, Dejager S, Foley JE, Couturier A, Ligueros-Saylan M, Kothny W. Assessing the cardio-cerebrovascular safety of vildagliptin: meta-analysis of adjudicated

events from a large phase III type 2 diabetes population. Diabetes Obes Metab 2010;12:485–494

41. Frederich R, McNeill R, Berglind N, Fleming D, Chen R. The efficacy and safety of the dipeptidyl peptidase-4 inhibitor saxagliptin in treatment-naïve patients with type 2 diabetes mellitus: a randomized controlled trial. Diabetol Metab Syndr 2012;4:36

42. Johansen OE, Neubacher D, von Eynatten M, Patel S, Woerle HJ. Cardiovascular safety with linagliptin in patients with type 2 diabetes mellitus: a pre-specified, prospective, and adjudicated meta-analysis of a phase 3 programme. Cardiovasc Diabetol 2012;11:3

43. White JR. Alogliptin for the treatment of type 2 diabetes. Drugs Today (Barc) 2011;47:99–107

44. Gallwitz B, Rosenstock J, Rauch T, et al. 2-year efficacy and safety of linagliptin compared with glimepiride in patients with type 2 diabetes inadequately controlled on metformin: a randomised, double-blind, non-inferiority trial. Lancet 2012;380:475–483

45. Ussher JR, Drucker DJ. Cardiovascular biology of the incretin system. Endocr Rev 2012;33:187–215

46. Ligueros-Saylan M, Foley JE, Schweizer A, Couturier A, Kothny W. An assessment of adverse effects of vildagliptin versus comparators on the liver, the pancreas, the immune system, the skin and in patients with impaired renal function from a large pooled database of phase II and III clinical trials. Diabetes Obes Metab 2010;12:495–509

47. Nyström T, Gutniak MK, Zhang Q, et al. Effects of glucagon-like peptide-1 on endothelial function in type 2 diabetes patients with stable coronary artery disease. Am J Physiol Endocrinol Metab 2004;287:E1209–1215

48. Drucker DJ, Buse JB, Taylor K, et al.; DURATION-1 Study Group. Exenatide once weekly versus twice daily for the treatment of type 2 diabetes: a randomised, open-label, non-inferiority study. Lancet 2008;372:1240–1250

49. Stettler C, Bearth A, Allemann S, et al. QTc interval and resting heart rate as long-term predictors of mortality in type 1 and type 2 diabetes mellitus: a 23-year follow-up. Diabetologia 2007;50:186–194

50. Engel SS, Williams-Herman DE, Golm GT, et al. Sitagliptin: review of preclinical and clinical data regarding incidence of pancreatitis. Int J Clin Pract 2010;64:984–990

Feasibility of Outpatient Fully Integrated Closed-Loop Control

First studies of wearable artificial pancreas

Boris P. Kovatchev, phd[1]
Eric Renard, md, phd[2]
Claudio Cobelli, phd[3]
Howard C. Zisser, md[4]
Patrick Keith-Hynes, phd[1]
Stacey M. Anderson, md[1]
Sue A. Brown, md[1]
Daniel R. Chernavvsky, md[1]
Marc D. Breton, phd[1]
Anne Farret, md, phd[2]

Marie-Josée Pelletier, md[2]
Jérôme Place, msc[2]
Daniela Bruttomesso, md, phd[3]
Simone Del Favero, phd[3]
Roberto Visentin, msc[3]
Alessio Filippi, md[3]
Rachele Scotton, md[3]
Angelo Avogaro, md, phd[3]
Francis J. Doyle III, phd[5]

OBJECTIVE—To evaluate the feasibility of a wearable artificial pancreas system, the Diabetes Assistant (DiAs), which uses a smart phone as a closed-loop control platform.

RESEARCH DESIGN AND METHODS—Twenty patients with type 1 diabetes were enrolled at the Universities of Padova, Montpellier, and Virginia and at Sansum Diabetes Research Institute. Each trial continued for 42 h. The United States studies were conducted entirely in outpatient setting (e.g., hotel or guest house); studies in Italy and France were hybrid hospital–hotel admissions. A continuous glucose monitoring/pump system (Dexcom Seven Plus/Omnipod) was placed on the subject and was connected to DiAs. The patient operated the system via the DiAs user interface in open-loop mode (first 14 h of study), switching to closed-loop for the remaining 28 h. Study personnel monitored remotely via 3G or WiFi connection to DiAs and were available on site for assistance.

RESULTS—The total duration of proper system communication functioning was 807.5 h (274 h in open-loop and 533.5 h in closed-loop), which represented 97.7% of the total possible time from admission to discharge. This exceeded the predetermined primary end point of 80% system functionality.

CONCLUSIONS—This study demonstrated that a contemporary smart phone is capable of running outpatient closed-loop control and introduced a prototype system (DiAs) for further investigation. Following this proof of concept, future steps should include equipping insulin pumps and sensors with wireless capabilities, as well as studies focusing on control efficacy and patient-oriented clinical outcomes.

Diabetes Care 36:1851–1858, 2013

Automated closed-loop control of blood glucose, known as the "artificial pancreas," can have a tremendous impact on the health and lives of people with type 1 diabetes. Thus, the community of patients, families, diabetologists, and researchers have advocated strongly for the rapid commercialization of artificial pancreas technology for home use. To help facilitate this goal, the Food and Drug Administration has recently issued a guidance document to help industry and academic institutions achieve approval for outpatient evaluations of artificial pancreas technology as efficiently as possible. These studies necessarily begin in highly supervised hospital settings and progress through early feasibility, transitional, and, finally, pivotal trials, each with step-wise reduction in monitoring requirements as system performance and functionality are established under normal and stress conditions.

The components of the contemporary closed-loop control have been developed over the past 40 years, including subcutaneous insulin pump technology (1,2), continuous glucose monitoring (CGM) (3,4), and subcutaneous closed-loop control involving CGM coupled with insulin pump via a control algorithm (5–12). A comprehensive review of past and present research is presented in a recent Perspectives in Diabetes (13). However, the artificial pancreas control algorithms used by virtually all studies so far were based on laptop computers wired to a CGM and an insulin pump, a system limiting free movement and too cumbersome to be used beyond hospital confines (5–12). Nevertheless, feasibility of subcutaneous closed-loop control was demonstrated, the architecture of closed-loop control algorithms was improved, and the means for their in silico preclinical testing were introduced (14–16).

Further progress toward bringing closed-loop control to the outpatient setting depends on an artificial pancreas platform that is based on a readily available, inexpensive, wearable hardware, computationally capable of running closed-loop control algorithms, wirelessly connectable to CGM devices and insulin pumps, and capable of broadband communication for remote monitoring and safety supervision of the participants in outpatient clinical trials. A logical host for such a portable artificial pancreas platform is a contemporary smart phone, a consumer electronics device that meets virtually all of these

From the [1]Center for Diabetes Technology, Department of Psychiatry and Neurobehavioral Sciences, and Department of Medicine, Division of Endocrinology, University of Virginia, Charlottesville, Virginia; the [2]Montpellier University Hospital, Department of Endocrinology, Diabetes, and Nutrition, INSERM Clinical Investigation Centre 1001, Institute of Functional Genomics, CNRS UMR 5203, INSERM U661, University of Montpellier 1, Montpellier, France; the [3]Department of Information Engineering and Department of Internal Medicine, Unit of Metabolic Disease, University of Padova, Padova, Italy; the [4]Sansum Diabetes Research Institute, Santa Barbara, California; and the [5]University of California Santa Barbara, Santa Barbara, California.
Corresponding author: Boris P. Kovatchev, boris@virginia.edu.
Received 25 September 2012 and accepted 23 February 2013.
DOI: 10.2337/dc12-1965. Clinical trial reg. nos. NCT01578980, NCT01447992, and NCT01447979, clinicaltrials.gov.
This article contains Supplementary Data online at http://care.diabetesjournals.org/lookup/suppl/doi:10.2337/dc12-1965/-/DC1.
A slide set summarizing this article is available online.
B.P.K., E.R., C.C., and H.C.Z. contributed equally to this report.

aforementioned requirements. A recent report presented overnight inpatient closed-loop control in adolescents and young adults using a controller running on a Blackberry Storm smart phone (17).

In this study, we test the concept that a portable platform, the Diabetes Assistant (DiAs), running on a commercially available smart phone and fitted with a control and safety algorithms, can run closed-loop control in outpatient setting. The first pilot trials with this system were performed simultaneously in Padova and Montpellier on 26 October 2011 (18). We now present 2-day outpatient trials performed at four clinical centers. It should be emphasized that the primary goal of these trials was not a clinical outcome, but a demonstration that a contemporary smart phone is capable of running closed-loop control in outpatient setting.

RESEARCH DESIGN AND
METHODS—This study combines four coordinated protocols sharing the same DiAs artificial pancreas technology conducted at the Universities of Padova (Italy) and Montpellier (France), the University of Virginia (UVA), and the Sansum Diabetes Research Institute, Santa Barbara, California. To test whether a smart phone is capable of running outpatient closed-loop control, we have configured a system comprising available components, which were linked as follows: CGM → iDex ↔ DiAs (running all closed-loop computations, user interface, and communications to peripheral devices) ↔ iDex ↔ pump. The iDex is an experimental device manufactured by Insulet (Bedford, MA), which combines a DexCom Seven Plus receiver and OmniPod insulin pump. In addition, DiAs transferred data in real time to a central location allowing remote monitoring of patient state and system functions. The primary engineering end point was the percent time with all system communications working properly; the protocol criterion for success in this early feasibility study was this time reaching >80% of the total time of investigation. Secondary end points included the estimation of the failure rates of system components, frequency analysis of lost or inaccurate CGM records, and control algorithm performance. The clinical goal was to assess patients' and clinicians' subjective impressions of the system, i.e., the feasibility of its ambulatory use, including patient usability and wearability.

Subjects
A total of 20 adults (age 21–65 years) with type 1 diabetes were studied (5 subjects at each site). Before the tests, a pilot subject was performed in Italy, France, and in the United States. All participants were experienced insulin pump users and were required to have the following: prestudy HbA$_{1c}$ of 6–9%; predefined insulin pump parameters for basal rates, carbohydrate ratios, and insulin sensitivity factors; and proper mental status/cognition. The exclusion criteria were directed toward safety and included recent history of diabetic ketoacidosis or severe hypoglycemia, pregnancy, breastfeeding, or intention of becoming pregnant (females), uncontrolled arterial hypertension, and conditions that may increase the risk of hypoglycemia or infections.

Procedure
All protocols were approved by the review boards of the participating institutions. In addition, the United States–based studies received Food and Drug Administration approval (IDE #G120032) and the European studies received appropriate national-level certifications. All studies were registered with ClinicalTrials .gov (NCT01578980 for UVA/Sansum, NCT01447992 for Padova, and NCT01447979 for Montpellier). After consent and screening, subjects were trained to use the Omnipod insulin pump (Insulet) and participated in a 3- to 7-day pump initiation if needed. Two DexCom Seven Plus sensors (DexCom, San Diego, CA) were inserted 24–72 h before admission; throughout the trials, the sensors were calibrated per manufacturer's instructions using commercial glucometers. A calibration was performed before dinner at ~7:00 P.M., thereby allowing for further system-required calibrations to be performed during the timeframes before dinner and before breakfast. Per Food and Drug Administration recommendation, an additional (one-time) calibration was entered by the study staff if there was a discrepancy in the two sensor readings of ≥20% or if the CGM was reading <70 mg/dL and the Hemo-Cue value was >85 mg/dL.

Participants in Italy, France, and Virginia stayed at hotels, and participants in California resided at a guest house–like outpatient research unit of the Sansum consisting of a living room, kitchen, four bedrooms, and bathrooms. The participants in the European studies were admitted individually, one subject at a time; UVA had both single and double admissions; at Sansum, all five subjects were admitted concurrently. Subjects checked in by 5:00 P.M. and met with the study team, which confirmed that the subjects had brought their insulin, pump supplies, and regular medications. The subject's pump was removed and the study pump containing the subject's insulin was started. Connections were established between DiAs and one sensor designated as primary (via the iDex), the insulin pump (via the iDex), and the remote monitoring site. The subject was then introduced to DiAs operation; the orientation took ~15–20 min to complete. The DiAs user manual (Supplementary Data) and advice from the study team were available to the subjects at all times. After this introduction, the subjects were in charge of their interactions with DiAs, controlling the system via its graphical user interface.

The protocol continued for 42 h. During the first evening/night of study, DiAs was used in open-loop mode with the subject's home insulin parameters. At 7:00 A.M. on day 2, the system was switched into closed-loop mode and remained in closed-loop control for 29 h until the subject was discharged at 12:00 P.M. on day 3. Meals were delivered to the patient's room from local restaurants or consumed at local dining facilities (e.g., dining out at a restaurant in Padova or a hotel buffet breakfast at UVA). The carbohydrate content of the meals was estimated by the subject and proper entry of the desired carbohydrate amount into DiAs was confirmed by the study physician, but there were no dietary restrictions. When the subjects were outside of their room, they were accompanied by a member of the study team and DiAs were remotely monitored continually. Figure 1 describes the timeline of the studies in Europe and in the United States.

The two protocol differences between the European (Fig. 1A) and United States studies (Fig. 1B) were as follows: in Padova and Montpellier, the patient was moved to the hospital at 7:00 A.M. on day 2 of the study for initiation of closed-loop control and remained in the hospital for 10 h before returning to the hotel for the rest of the study; in the United States studies the control algorithm was switched into "safety-only" mode for the night (11:00 P.M. to 7:00 A.M.), as requested by the Food and Drug Administration.

Diabetes Care • July 2013 • 36:1851–1858

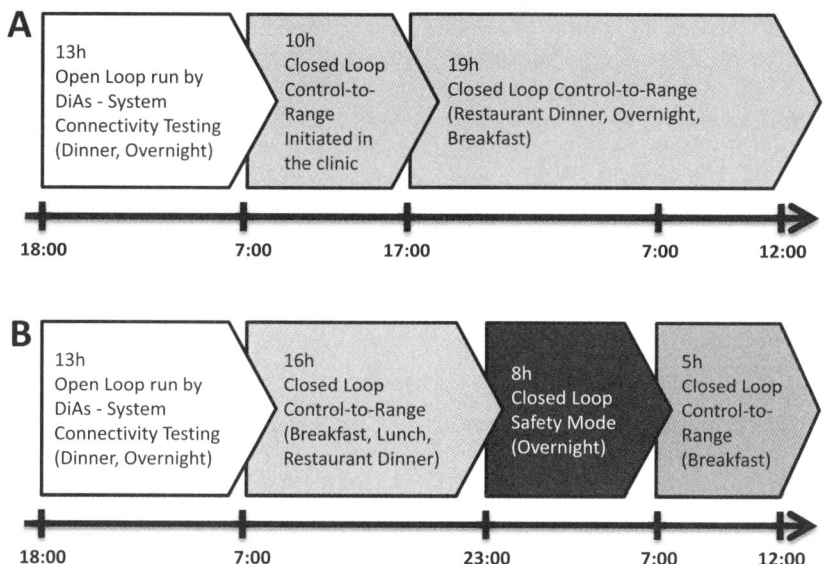

Figure 1—*Protocol design in European* (A) *and United States* (B) *investigation centers.*

Safety

A study physician, a nurse, and a technician were located in nearby rooms to provide assistance if needed. Patient data were monitored remotely via a password-protected Web site. Reference blood glucose readings were measured simultaneously by finger stick with a HemoCue (HemoCue AB, Ängelholm, Sweden) and a commercial glucometer beginning at 7:00 P.M. on the evening of admission and continuing every 2 h during the day. Overnight, there were no scheduled finger sticks; reference blood glucose measurements were taken only if DiAs or the secondary sensor alarm indicated hypoglycemia or hyperglycemia, or if the two sensors had readings diverging by >20%. Nursing staff checked DiAs and secondary CGM readings hourly overnight and system alarms were monitored remotely for the DiAs and with a baby monitor to capture alarms from the secondary CGM. Any DiAs hypoglycemia red-light warning triggered treatment with ~15 g fast-acting carbohydrate (e.g., juice), whereas hyperglycemia red-light warnings prompted checking the insulin pump for occlusion or malfunction. Any HemoCue reading >13.9 mmol/L (250 mg/dL) was followed by a β-hydroxybutyrate test (finger stick Precision Xtra β-Ketone measurement); confirmed β-hydroxybutyrate level >0.6 mmol/L was a criterion for discontinuation of the trial. In such a case, the subject could be rescheduled. Any HemoCue reading <80 mg/dL was followed-up with additional finger sticks at least every 15 min and any HemoCue blood glucose <70 mg/dL was treated with fast-acting glucose.

Technology

The hub of the DiAs system was an off-the-shelf smart phone running the Android operating system. To ensure the operation of the smart phone as a medical device, its operating system was modified to disable processes not related to closed-loop control operation and to include self-checks of system integrity. The communications between DiAs, the iDex, and the pump and the sensor were wireless, giving the patient the freedom to be fully detached from the DiAs controller. The system components worn by the patient included an Insulet OmniPod insulin pod and a DexCom Seven Plus sensor/transmitter. The patient additionally wore a pouch containing a communication box (either Viliv S5 Tablet or Galaxy Nexus phone) attached to the iDex. The iDex and the communication box were only needed for automated data transfer and pump control at this early feasibility stage. These devices did not have any computing or patient interaction functions and were abandoned in subsequent studies.

User interface

The subject controlled DiAs using graphical user interface, which allowed the following: initializing the system with the average daily insulin dose, basal rate, carbohydrate ratio, and correction factor; displaying CGM traces and insulin delivery graphs; and real-time interaction, such as entries of sensor calibrations,

meal carbohydrate content, premeal capillary glucose level, and other information the subject wished to provide (e.g., exercise or hypoglycemia treatment). Two traffic-light signals presented the degree of risks for hypoglycemia or hyperglycemia as follows: green light, no risks detected; yellow light, the system is working actively to mitigate the risks by either attenuating insulin delivery if hypoglycemia is anticipated or administering correction insulin if hyperglycemia is predicted; and red light, which signifies that risks cannot be eliminated by adjustment of insulin alone and intervention is required to either consume carbohydrate or ensure that insulin is delivered properly.

Control strategy

DiAs operated in two modes, open-loop (first 13 h of each study) controlling the pump per each patient's preset basal/bolus delivery instructions and displaying CGM and insulin delivery information or closed-loop (hours 14–42 of each study) running a closed-loop control algorithm. Both modes of operation included fully automated transfer of data from the sensor to DiAs and commands from DiAs to the insulin pump. User input was required only before meals and whenever the system signaled imminent risk for hypoglycemia or hyperglycemia. The closed-loop control algorithm included two modules: *1*) safety supervision responsible for prediction of hypoglycemia, attenuation, or discontinuation of insulin delivery if hypoglycemia is anticipated and warnings if hypoglycemia is imminent and cannot be prevented by insulin discontinuation alone (19) and *2*) range-correction module responsible for injecting correction boluses. The clinical use of this algorithm is described in detail in a recent publication as standard control to range (12); details on its engineering architecture also have been published (20). Occasional CGM data loss (up to 20 min) did not stop the operation of the controller; during loss of pump communication, insulin was not delivered.

Remote monitoring

In addition, DiAs transmitted data in real time through either 3G (telephone network) or WiFi to two servers (UVA and Montpellier), which allowed team members to log-in for remote observation from their locations. The server connections were one-directional: DiAs transmitted data out but could not be controlled from a remote location for safety reasons. The transmitted data contained glucose traces, insulin infusion by the pump, and technical information about the functioning of the control algorithm but did not contain any subject identifiers; the monitoring Web sites were password-protected.

Statistical analysis
Achieving statistical significance was not an objective of this early-feasibility investigation. The data analysis corresponded to the goals of the study and included estimation of the failure rates of system components, frequency analysis of lost or inaccurate CGM records, and percent time of active system operation. Post hoc analyses included t test and nonparametric comparisons of open versus closed-loop parameters of glucose control observed during the study; however, the study was not powered for this outcome. Before inclusion in the analyses, CGM data were sent through retrospective recalibration using reference blood glucose readings as discussed in a recent editorial (21).

RESULTS—The focus of this investigation was on the concept of using DiAs as a smart phone–based control algorithm and user interface host. All peripheral communication devices were secondary. We assessed Dias in terms of human factors and usability, system and component performance, performance of the control algorithm, utility of remote monitoring, and clinical events.

Human factors and usability
Before this study, a formative evaluation of the DiAs user interface was conducted to evaluate the feasibility of the design for patient use. Heuristic evaluation (expert review) was followed by three focus groups with type 1 diabetic patients with varying exposure to diabetes technology (n = 13). Feedback was gathered on various system components addressing user interaction, system features, and capabilities. Change recommendations were prioritized, and users were asked to rate the system on several criteria. Users indicated the importance of maintaining all existing insulin pump and CGM device functionalities (22).

The DiAs graphical user interface (Supplementary Data) proved to be reliable and well-understood by the subjects. All were able to easily navigate through the graphical user interface commands on their own in both open-loop and closed-loop modes of operation, view CGM and insulin information, and administer meal or correction boluses as needed. The subjects were free to move around the facility and in its vicinity. One subject used a hotel treadmill, one subject in Italy rode a bike, one subject in France walked to nearby museums, and five subjects took a shower with the pouch hanging just outside of the shower. Subjects also were free to entertain family and friends in their individual quarters.

System wearability was evaluated in relative terms, comparing DiAs to previous laptop-based systems. With the transition to a smart phone as a system hub and to wireless data transmission, the weight of a closed-loop control system was reduced several-fold. Figure 2A presents photos of DiAs displaying CGM and insulin delivery traces and the entire system worn by a study subject. DiAs communicated wirelessly with the iDex/communication box; these devices are placed in a pouch on the patient's belt. The iDex communicated wirelessly to an OmniPod insulin pump and to a DexCom sensor visible as attached on the subject. The communication range of the iDex with the insulin pod and DexCom sensor was ~5 inches, which necessitated the use of a belt pouch. With this set-up, the subjects were able to maintain activities of daily living, a necessary first step toward routine outpatient use.

System and component performance
Table 1 presents metrics of the technical performance of the artificial pancreas system overall and during the open-loop and closed-loop portions of the study. Two subjects described developed hyperglycemia with ketones because of pump site or pod failures in the initial open-loop portion of the study and were rescheduled. Only the completed second study data for the rescheduled subjects are included in this analysis. Additionally, the three pilot subjects for each country were not included in the analysis; the data of the first two from Italy and France were recently published (18). Overall, the artificial pancreas system was functional 98% of the time, which exceeded the initially set primary end point goal of 80%.

One element of system connectivity should be noted. In the European studies and in the first United States–based studies we used a Viliv S5 tablet to communicate with the iDex, which was then replaced by a more reliable Samsung Galaxy Nexus smart phone. As evident from Table 1, this replacement had a substantial effect on system reliability, reducing almost five-fold the number of unplanned system restarts because of loss of signal transmission. Because the communication box was dedicated solely to data transmission, its replacement did not affect the conceptual or the computing outcomes of the study.

Further, Table 1 presents data on the performance of the principal system components: the CGM, DiAs, and the insulin pump. Of particular importance for fully integrated closed-loop control is the stability of interdevice connections (sensor → iDex ↔ smart phone ↔ iDex ↔ insulin pump). Table 1 presents the availability of CGM and insulin pump communications with DiAs during the study.

Performance of the control algorithm
Although the study was not designed to test algorithm performance or to compare open-loop versus closed-loop, Table 2 presents a set of glycemic control metrics and certain post hoc comparisons of open-loop versus closed-loop nights using retrospectively recalibrated CGM data (21). The outpatient performance of the controller was similar to its inpatient performance of this same control algorithm observed in a previous study (standard control to range, 12); thus, first indications are that a different platform (e.g., a smart phone) under different outpatient conditions may achieve similar performance as a laptop-based system in the hospital. On open-loop versus closed-loop control, we observed 80 vs.72% time within target range (P = 0.22) and 0.53 vs. 0.27 hypoglycemic episodes ≤3.9 mmol/L (70 mg/dL) per 24 h (P = 0.16); in other words, there were no significant differences between open-loop and closed-loop control overnight, which is an expected result for standard control to range (12).

Utility of remote monitoring
Figure 2B presents a screenshot of the remote monitoring system operation during the study at Sansum. Each of the five subjects participating simultaneously in this study is represented by an icon on the computer screen. The icon summarizes real-time information, including patient identification number, current CGM reading and direction of change, the state of the hypoglycemia and hyperglycemia alerts, and a message informing the technician of possible risks or system malfunction. Safety supervision module was active for three patients (identification numbers 211, 212, and 214) as indicated

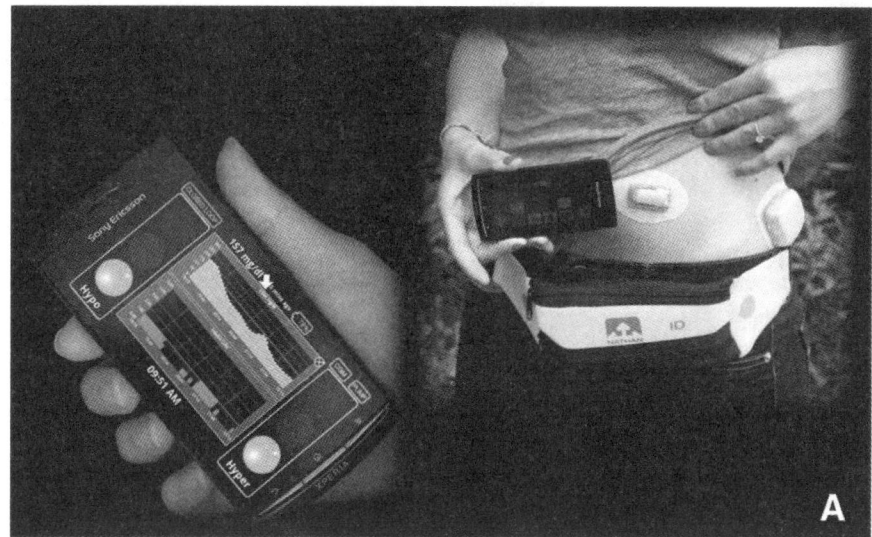

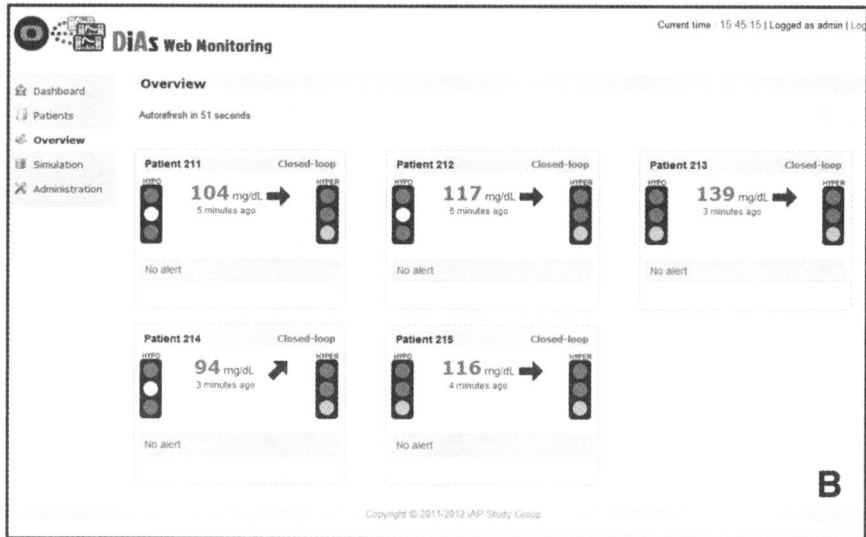

Figure 2—A: *Photos of the DiAs smart phone displaying CGM and insulin delivery traces (left) and the entire system worn by a study subject (right). B: Screenshot of the remote monitoring system operation during the trials at Sansum. Each of the five subjects participating simultaneously in these trials is represented by an icon on the computer screen. HYPER, hyperglycemia; HYPO, hypoglycemia.*

β-hydroxybutyrate level of 0.7 mmol/L 2 h after the insulin pump was initiated (consistent with pod compared with insertion site failure). Subject 2 dropped the communication tablet and attempts to restart it were unsuccessful. After the connection was reestablished with a new tablet, the insulin pod alarmed, prompting a pod change. The new pod occluded (blood noted in pod tubing), resulting in β-hydroxybutyrate of 1.3 mmol/L. Subject 3 experienced hyperglycemia to 295 mg/dL with β-hydroxybutyrate of 0.7 mmol/L at hour 36 of the study. At that time, DiAs was running in safety mode (Fig. 1) with the range controller switched off, delivering only basal rate (4.1 units in the previous 6 h). The subject's CGM glucose was noted to increase from 180 mg/dL to 295 mg/dL over the final 2 h, suggesting that a pod occlusion (unconfirmed) may have contributed to this event. These three patients were treated with subcutaneous insulin, resulting in prompt resolution of the mild ketosis.

CONCLUSIONS—Technology advancements in the past year made possible the development of DiAs, wearable ambulatory artificial pancreas platforms using an off-the-shelf smart phone as a computational hub. Besides more user-friendly touch-screen interface and wireless connectivity, one easily quantifiable result of the transition from a laptop-based to a phone-based closed-loop control is a significant reduction in the system weight, which brings the system one important step closer to ambulatory use. Ultimately, this would lead to "closing the loop" with a portable minimally invasive system suitable for home use. Industry is currently transitioning CGMs and pumps to include wireless connectivity; thus, DiAs is only the first of many portable devices that will be capable of wireless data exchange and fully integrated closed-loop control.

At the time of this outpatient trial, the DexCom Seven Plus and the OmniPod Insulet pump had short-range wireless capability to communicate with an iDex research platform. Also, for the iDex to establish wireless communication with DiAs, an intermediary tablet (or a cell phone) needed to be connected to the iDex. Hence, there was short-range wireless communication from the patient (wearing a pod and sensor/transmitter) to a pouch containing the iDex and tablet (or cell phone), and long-range wireless

by yellow hypoglycemia lights. There were no error messages. Each icon can be clicked during a monitoring session, which will display more detailed information for this subject, including detailed records of insulin delivery, glucose data, and the algorithm functions. Throughout the study, observation of the participants was performed mainly through the remote monitoring system, which proved to be a useful tool.

Clinical events
On six occasions during the study (two during open-loop and four during

closed-loop control), carbohydrate treatment was administered for blood glucose levels <3.3 mmol/L (60 mg/dL), for a total of 0.17 events per 24 h of system operation.

There were no instances of patient-initiated system shutdown, but the trials were discontinued by study staff on three occasions. The first two events occurred early, before initiation of closed-loop control, and the subjects were rescheduled for subsequent admissions, which concluded successfully. The third subject was discontinued at study hour 36 and was not rescheduled. Subject 1 experienced hyperglycemia of 260 mg/dL with

Table 1—*Performance metrics for the functioning of the artificial pancreas system used in these studies and of its primary components*

		Open-loop control	Closed-loop control	Combined
Overall system performance		274/277 h	533.5/549.5 h	807.5/826.5 h
Primary end point: Total duration of accurate DiAs communication functioning/total possible system time from patient admission to discharge and time of proper communication function		98.9%	97.1%	97.7%
Frequency of unplanned system resets or restarts, events/total time and events/24 h of DiAs operation	Viliv S5 tablet	25/167 h	35/331.5 h	60/498.5 h
		3.59	2.53	2.89
	Galaxy Nexus phone	1/110 h	7/218 h	8/328 h
		0.22	0.77	0.58
CGM and CGM–DiAs communication				
Reliability of CGM, number of nominal CGM cycles during study period for which the primary CGM was reporting data and percent of total		2,692/3,082	6,107/6,598	8,799/9,680
		87.3%	92.6%	90.9%
Frequency of CGM malfunction necessitating sensor replacement, events/total time and events/24 h of operation		0/277 h	1/549.5 h	1/826.5 h
		0.00	0.04	0.03
Frequency of sensor calibrations that were requested by the CGM, events/total time and events/24 h of operation		20/277 h	7/549.5 h	27/826.5 h
		1.73	0.31	0.78
Frequency of sensor calibrations that were forced by the user, events/total time and events/24 h of operation		29/277 h	57/549.5 h	86/826.5 h
		2.51	2.49	2.50
Reliability of CGM–DiAs communication, number and percent of total CGM cycles with values reported by the CGM and received by DiAs			6,010/6,107	
			98.4%	
DiAs platform				
Reliability of control algorithm, percent closed-loop control cycles in which control algorithm produced dosing recommendations, provided that CGM values were available in the past 20 min			100%	
Frequency of DiAs malfunction necessitating replacement of the smart phone platform, events/total time and events/24 h of operation		2/277 h	1/549.5 h	3/826.5 h
		0.17	0.04	0.09
Insulin pump				
Reliability of insulin pump components (pump occlusions or iDex malfunction leading to pod replacement), events/total time and events/24 h		2/277 h	2/549.5 h	4/826.5 h
		0.17	0.09	0.12
Reliability of DiAs insulin pump communication, number of microboluses delivered/expected per algorithm recommendation during open-loop and closed-loop	Viliv S5 tablet	1,679/2,121	3,268/3,576	4,947/5,697
		79.2%	91.4%	86.8%
	Galaxy Nexus phone	1,226/1,279	2,684/2,771	3,910/4,050
		95.9%	96.9%	96.5%

Data presented separately for the two communication boxes used throughout the study.

communication between the pouch and the DiAs artificial pancreas platform. These intermediate devices are now being phased out; communication boxes are no longer necessary. Such a technology improvement was anticipated in our study; thus, we focused on the smart phone computing and user-interface capabilities of the DiAs, assuming that this would be the device that is here to stay.

Special emphasis should be placed on the fact that the subjects were operating the system by themselves most of the time. To the best of our knowledge, this is the first trial in which the subjects were responsible for the oversight of their closed-loop systems, a step that is critical for outpatient deployment of closed-loop control. Based on this feedback, we conclude that the form factor of DiAs as an artificial pancreas platform is appropriate for outpatient use. However, before long-term efficacy studies comparing outpatient artificial pancreas with

Table 2—*Performance of the control algorithm*

	Open-loop control	Closed-loop control	Combined
Time within the target range of 3.9–10 mmol/L (70–180 mg/dL) during the day (7:00 A.M. to 11:00 P.M.)		68%	
Time below the target of 3.9 mmol/L (70 mg/dL) during the day (7:00 A.M. to 11:00 P.M.)		1.74%	
Time within the target range of 3.9–10 mmol/L (70–180 mg/dL) overnight (11:00 P.M. to 7:00 A.M.)	80%	72%	75%
Number of hypoglycemic episodes below the target of 3.9 mmol/L (70 mg/dL) overnight (11:00 P.M. to 7:00 A.M.), events/24 h	0.53	0.27	0.36
Time below the target of 3.9 mmol/L (70 mg/dL) overnight (11:00 P.M. to 7:00 a.m.)	1.6%	0.69%	0.99%

sensor-augmented pump therapy can proceed, system wearability during daily living and the reliability of device communications must be ensured. Testing of the system at four different sites in three countries and in a variety of hotel and restaurant settings using one, two, or five systems concurrently provided an opportunity to challenge DiAs with multiple scenarios that are likely to be encountered in nonhospital and, ultimately, home settings.

In general, the technical performance of the DiAs system with overall operational time of 98% exceeded the set goal of 80%. In retrospect, this goal may have been conservative, but before this study it was generally unclear whether a smart phone can run closed-loop control, and there was no experience to guide the choice of this goal. The principal system components—sensor, DiAs, and insulin pump—were reasonably reliable, with 0.03, 0.09, and 0.12 malfunction events necessitating device replacement per 24 h, respectively. Occasional CGM data points were lost (8.1%), but this did not result in skipping control cycles or discontinuation of the study; by design, control to range would function during transient absence of CGM data because the controller intervenes only if risks for hypoglycemia or hyperglycemia are detected (20).

Finally, we must emphasize the utility of remote monitoring, which was available on site and at remote locations (i.e., studies in Europe or in California were observed from Virginia and vice versa in real time). This was a critical aspect for patient safety that allowed close supervision so that intervention could occur quickly if needed. Our system allowed monitoring concurrently multiple patients, a feature

that was tested at Sansum with five patients simultaneously. This feature alone will allow acceleration of the number of subjects who could be studied at the same time, reducing staffing costs and making artificial pancreas research more efficient.

In summary, a wearable inexpensive closed-loop control platform (DiAs) was created and tested in early feasibility studies. Combined with real-time remote monitoring, this system opens the possibility for large pivotal trials that will establish the artificial pancreas as a viable mainstream treatment strategy in type 1 diabetes.

Acknowledgments—This study was supported by the JDRF Artificial Project, Award 22-2011-649, and by National Institutes of Health/National Institute of Diabetes and Digestive and Kidney Diseases grant RO1 DK 085623.

B.P.K., P.K.-H., and M.D.B. hold patents or patent applications related to the study technology. B.P.K. is a consultant/advisor for Animas and DexCom and received research grant and material support from Animas, Abbott, DexCom, Insulet, LifeScan, Tandem, and Sanofi. E.R. is a consultant/advisor for A. Menarini Diagnostics, Abbott, Cellnovo, Dexcom, Eli Lilly, Johnson & Johnson (Animas, LifeScan), Medtronic, Novo Nordisk, Roche Diagnostics, and Sanofi and received research grant/material support from Abbott, Dexcom, Insulet, and Roche Diagnostics. H.C.Z. is a consultant/advisor for Animas, Cellnovo, Insulet, MannKind, and Roche and received research grant/product support from Animas, Abbott, DexCom, Eli Lilly, GluMetrics, Insulet, LifeScan, Medtronic, Novo Nordisk, Roche, and Sanofi. S.M.A. received grant/material support from Animas and Beckton, Dickinson and Company. No other potential conflicts of interest relevant to this article were reported.

B.P.K. designed the study protocol, contributed to the technology design and to the clinical execution of the study, co-wrote the manuscript, and was the principal investigator of the project. E.R. was the principal investigator at the Montpellier site, co-designed the study protocol, contributed to the study approval and the clinical execution, and co-wrote the manuscript. C.C. co-designed the study protocol, contributed to the technology design and to the clinical execution of the study, co-wrote the manuscript, and was the principal investigator for the Italian studies. H.C.Z. co-developed the study protocol, directed the clinical trials in California, and co-wrote the manuscript. P.K.-H. was the chief engineer of the system used in the study responsible for all technical aspects of the outpatient artificial pancreas functioning. S.M.A. co-wrote the study protocol, was the study physician overseeing the execution of the clinical studies in Virginia, interpreted data, and co-wrote the manuscript. S.A.B. was the study physician responsible for the execution of the clinical studies in Virginia, interpreted data, and co-wrote the manuscript. D.R.C. coordinated all clinical aspects of the project design and execution, including on-site project management at University of Virginia and Sansum. M.D.B. co-designed the control algorithm and analyzed the data from this project. A.Fa. contributed to the clinical execution of the study and reviewed the manuscript. M.-J.P. contributed to the clinical execution of the study. J.P. was the primary designer of the remote monitoring system and was responsible for the technical execution of the study in France. D.B. was the study physician responsible for the execution of the clinical studies in Padova, interpreted data, and edited the manuscript. S.D.F. was responsible for technical aspects of the system functioning during the clinical studies in Padova, was involved in the testing phase of the system, and interpreted and processed data. R.V. (Padova) was co-responsible for technology oversight during the clinical trials in Padova and processed the data from Italy. A.Fi. was co-responsible for the execution of the clinical studies in Padova. R.S. was co-responsible for the execution of the clinical studies in Padova. A.A. directed the medical team in Padova and edited and revised the manuscript. F.J.D. was the principal investigator of the project in California and edited and revised the manuscript. B.P.K. is the guarantor of this work and, as such, had full access to all the data in the study and takes responsibility for the integrity of the data and the accuracy of the data analysis.

The authors thank Insulet (Bedford, MA) and Dexcom (San Diego, CA) for providing access to their technology. The authors acknowledge the University of Virginia engineering team that created the unique technology used by this study, including Lloyd Benton Mise and Najib Ben Brahim, who developed all system communications, and

Colleen Hughes Karvetski, PhD, and Stephen Patek, PhD, who co-designed the control algorithm. The authors acknowledge the clinical teams of this multisite project, including the following: Susan Demartini, MD (University of Virginia), who was the study physician responsible for the execution of the first clinical trial in Virginia; Christian Wakeman (University of Virginia), who orchestrated all data and maintained the primary database for this project; Mary Oliveri (University of Virginia), who was the primary contact for the United States regulatory submission; Hugues Chevassus, PharmD (Montpellier University Hospital), who contributed to the execution of the clinical studies in France; Wendy Bevier, PhD (University of California Santa Barbara), who coordinated clinical studies in Santa Barbara; and Eyal Dassau, PhD (University of California Santa Barbara), who was involved in the testing phase of the control system used in this study and in the study supervision in California.

References

1. Pickup JC, Keen H, Parsons JA, Alberti KG. Continuous subcutaneous insulin infusion: an approach to achieving normoglycaemia. BMJ 1978;1:204–207
2. Tamborlane WV, Sherwin RS, Genel M, Felig P. Reduction to normal of plasma glucose in juvenile diabetes by subcutaneous administration of insulin with a portable infusion pump. N Engl J Med 1979;300:573–578
3. Mastrototaro JJ. The MiniMed continuous glucose monitoring system. Diabetes Technol Ther 2000;2(Suppl. 1):S13–S18
4. Bode BW. Clinical utility of the continuous glucose monitoring system. Diabetes Technol Ther 2000;2(Suppl. 1):S35–S41
5. Bellazzi R, Nucci G, Cobelli C. The subcutaneous route to insulin-dependent diabetes therapy: closed-loop and partially closed-loop control strategies for insulin delivery and measuring glucose concentration. IEEE Eng Med Biol 2001;20:54–64
6. Hovorka R, Chassin LJ, Wilinska ME, et al. Closing the loop: the adicol experience. Diabetes Technol Ther 2004;6:307–318
7. Steil GM, Rebrin K, Darwin C, Hariri F, Saad MF. Feasibility of automating insulin delivery for the treatment of type 1 diabetes. Diabetes 2006;55:3344–3350
8. Weinzimer SA, Steil GM, Swan KL, Dziura J, Kurtz N, Tamborlane WV. Fully automated closed-loop insulin delivery versus semiautomated hybrid control in pediatric patients with type 1 diabetes using an artificial pancreas. Diabetes Care 2008;31:934–939
9. Hovorka R, Allen JM, Elleri D, et al. Manual closed-loop insulin delivery in children and adolescents with type 1 diabetes: a phase 2 randomised crossover trial. Lancet 2010;375:743–751
10. El-Khatib FH, Russell SJ, Nathan DM, Sutherlin RG, Damiano ER. A bihormonal closed-loop artificial pancreas for type 1 diabetes. Sci Transl Med 2010;2:27ra27
11. Kovatchev BP, Cobelli C, Renard E, et al. Multi-national study of subcutaneous model-predictive closed-loop control in type 1 diabetes: summary of the results. J Diabetes Sci Tech 2010;4:1374–1381
12. Breton MD, Farret A, Bruttomesso D, et al.; International Artificial Pancreas Study Group. Fully integrated artificial pancreas in type 1 diabetes: modular closed-loop glucose control maintains near normoglycemia. Diabetes 2012;61:2230–2237
13. Cobelli C, Renard E, Kovatchev BP. Artificial pancreas: past, present, future. Diabetes 2011;60:2672–2682
14. Kovatchev BP, Patek SD, Dassau E, et al.; Juvenile Diabetes Research Foundation Artificial Pancreas Consortium. Control to range for diabetes: functionality and modular architecture. J Diabetes Sci Tech 2009;3:1058–1065
15. Kovatchev BP, Breton MD, Man CD, Cobelli C. In silico preclinical trials: a proof of concept in closed-loop control of type 1 diabetes. J Diabetes Sci Tech 2009;3:44–55
16. Cobelli C, Man CD, Sparacino G, Magni L, De Nicolao G, Kovatchev BP. Diabetes: Models, Signals, and Control. IEEE Rev Biomed Eng 2009;2:54–96
17. O'Grady MJ, Retterath AJ, Keenan DB, et al. The use of an automated, portable glucose control system for overnight glucose control in adolescents and young adults with type 1 diabetes. Diabetes Care 2012;35:2182–2187
18. Cobelli C, Renard E, Kovatchev BP, et al. Pilot studies of wearable outpatient artificial pancreas in type 1 diabetes. Diabetes Care 2012;35:e65–e67
19. Hughes CS, Patek SD, Breton MD, Kovatchev BP. Hypoglycemia prevention via pump attenuation and red-yellow-green "traffic" lights using continuous glucose monitoring and insulin pump data. J Diabetes Sci Tech 2010;4:1146–1155
20. Patek SD, Magni L, Dassau E, Karvetski CH, Toffanin C, DeNicolao G. DelFaverok S, Breton M, Dalla Man C, Renard E, Zisser H, Doyle FJ III, Cobelli C, Kovatchev BP. Modular closed-loop control of diabetes. Trans Biomed Engineer 2012;29:2986–3000
21. Beck RW, Calhoun P, Kollman C. Challenges for outpatient closed loop studies: how to assess efficacy. Diabetes Technol Ther 2013;15:1–3
22. Hughes-Karvetski C, Guerlain S, Keith-Hynes P, McElwee M, Kovatchev B. Formative evaluation of the artificial pancreas user interface. 12th Annual Diabetes Technology Meeting. 8–10 November 2012. A-63

Social Media Made Easy: Guiding Patients to Credible Online Health Information and Engagement Resources

Susan E. Collins, MS, RD, CHES, and Dana M. Lewis, BA

Within the changing dynamic of health care, health care professionals (HCPs) are no longer the sole sources of health information. Recent estimates suggest that 83% of Internet users with chronic conditions such as diabetes go online to look for health information.[1] People with diabetes seek online information about the condition, treatment options, practical strategies and tools for managing diabetes in their daily lives, scientific breakthroughs, and advocacy efforts.[2] Yet, a Google search for "diabetes" returns 290 million results. A search for "diabetes online support" yields close to 36 million results. This can be overwhelming for anyone.

Some HCPs assist with this information overload by filtering and narrowing down online resources and search results for their patients. SurroundHealth, an online learning community for nonphysician HCPs, recently surveyed its members about the use of educational technology in health care. Many respondents reported that they used time during patient interactions to refer patients to online resources. Eighty-two percent of HCPs in private practice reported having referred patients to specific online resources, compared to 60% of HCPs in outpatient clinics and 52% of HCPs in hospital settings.

The HCPs who made referrals intended to help patients overcome common online obstacles such as difficulty distinguishing between high-quality information and material that is out of date, inaccurate, or overly promotional.[3] Connecting patients to credible online health information during office visits can facilitate more appropriate use of health care resources, shorter clinical encounters, more patient-centered decision-making, and, in some cases, reduced barriers to treatment adherence.[4,5]

This article explains how online health information and engagement resources are integrated into patients' overall health care experiences. In addition, it addresses common HCP concerns about patients accessing online resources and will outline steps that busy professionals can take to help connect patients to appropriate online resources.

Online Health Information Resources Versus Online Health Engagement Resources

Online health information resources push information out to the patient, whereas online health engagement resources promote the sharing of information, as well as support and interaction among patients.

Within an online health information resource, the information flows in one direction—from the content author to people with diabetes. The content reflects the perspectives and priorities of the author or author's organization. The author determines what information to share and when and how to share it. Typically conveyed in an objective manner, the information is usually vetted for factual accuracy before publication.

Examples of online health information resources for people with diabetes include Web sites of the American Diabetes Association (ADA; www.diabetes.org), the National Diabetes Education Program (www.ndep.nih.gov), and the Centers for Disease Control and Prevention's Diabetes Public Health Resource (www.cdc.gov/diabetes). In addition, people with diabetes can find credible health information resources via online learning centers affiliated with medical centers such as the Joslin Diabetes Center (www.joslin.org).

In contrast, online health engagement resources are social-networking tools and platforms (e.g., blogs, Twitter, Facebook, YouTube, and other online community sites) that allow active, two-way sharing of information (Table 1). Created by participants or community members, content often focuses on the real-life challenges of living with a particular disease or condition and offers emotional support, encouragement, coping, and problem-solving. People with diabetes often determine for themselves which specific health engagement resources are most useful and credible based on their life situation and learning needs. The information in health engagement resources is not guaranteed to be vetted for factual accuracy and may

Table 1. Comparison of Social Networking Tools and Platforms

Types of Platforms	Examples of Usage for Health Engagement	Key Benefits to Platform
Social networks (e.g., Facebook)	1. Patients share information with family and friends. 2. Patients join groups related to conditions and diseases. 3. Patients can "like" pages from organizations and causes and can access education and other resources shared by the organization.	Patients can determine the privacy of each piece of content that they post to their network and go back and change the privacy level if they change their mind about a post.
Microblogging (e.g., Twitter)	1. Patients share information with family and friends and potentially a larger audience of followers. 2. Patients can easily search using "hashtags," or key terms, to find resources or ongoing conversations about health topics. 3. Patients can find, join, or create mini-communities. 4. Patients can join scheduled chats about different health care topics. 5. Patients can get feedback and information by asking questions to their followers, which could include health care professionals or fellow patients.	Patients can find new communities and other patients regardless of their geographical location. Feedback and engagement is not reliant on preexisting networks; networks are easily expanded.
Blogs	1. Patients share information with family and friends and/or a potentially larger audience of followers or people who find their blogs via an Internet search. 2. Patients can embed content from other platforms (e.g., video) and use a variety of tools to tell their story.	Patients are not limited by space restraints (such as on Twitter) in sharing their thoughts or experiences.
Video platforms (e.g., YouTube)	1. Patients can chronicle their experience and share information via video. 2. As the #2 search engine after Google, YouTube offers thousands of health-related videos that patients can interact with and learn from, whether personal videos or organizations' educational videos.	Visual storytelling is compelling and engaging and can be used to demonstrate medical devices or other tools.
Health-specific social networks	1. Patients can join existing health-specific communities for support and resources. 2. Many communities have their own curated list of resources and recommendations for members and often provide formal or informal guidance from community members.	Content shared in health-specific networks is usually not shared with friends, family members, or coworkers unless it is cross-shared to another platform; this often gives patients a protected place to discuss and engage on health topics rather than with their other existing social networks.

reflect an individual's opinion or experiences.

Examples of online health engagement resources for people with diabetes include TuDiabetes. org (www.tudiabetes.org), Diabetes Social Media Advocacy (DSMA) (www.diabetessocmed.com), Children With Diabetes (www. childrenwithdiabetes.com), and You Can Do This Project (www.youcan-dothisproject.com). In general, the

Table 2. Comparison of Health Information and Health Engagement Resources

Characteristic	Health Information Resources	Health Engagement Resources
Flow of information	One way: pushed out from content author to people with diabetes	Two way: created by participants (people with diabetes, family, friends, and HCPs) using social media tools and platforms such as Twitter and YouTube
Tone	Objective, factual	Experiential, collaborative, and motivational
Accuracy	Content typically fact-checked before published	Informal self-policing of shared content among participants; most useful and credible resources gain validation and trust
Examples	www.diabetes.org www.ndep.nih.gov www.cdc.gov/diabetes www.joslin.org	www.tudiabetes.org www.diabetessocmed.com www.childrenwithdiabetes.com www.youcandothisproject.com

goal of health engagement resources is not to undermine the professional-patient therapeutic alliance or replace medical recommendations, but rather to serve as a source of inspiration, offer motivation and encouragement, and provide a sense of community.

Limited formal evidence exists of the effect of patients' involvement in social media on their overall health. However, research is underway to determine whether participation in a controlled social network of HCPs, patients, friends, and family members has a positive effect on knowledge, attitudes, and diabetes self-care management.[6] Although providers seek evidence to support the use of social media in improving diabetes care, people with diabetes view social media as tools to facilitate connecting with others, not as an intervention or a treatment approach.

Well-known blogger Kerri Sparling, who has type 1 diabetes, commented in a recent column titled "Proof Is in the People,"[7] on HCPs' interest in evidence: "Through connecting online, and in person, people living with diabetes have concrete proof that they are not alone, and that there is health worth fighting for, even after a diabetes diagnosis.

Social media . . . shows people that there isn't such a thing as a 'perfect diabetic,' but there can be an educated and determined one. It lets people know they aren't alone in the ebb and flow of their diabetes management. It doesn't encourage people to wallow in their troubles, but serves to inspire them to do the best they can, and to seek out the best healthcare they can find, both at home and in their doctor's offices."

Although the characteristics of health information resources differ from those of health engagement resources (Table 2), many people with diabetes consider both to be part of their overall online experience (Figure 1). In combination, online health information and health engagement resources represent informal learning and support that can complement the more formal information and education that

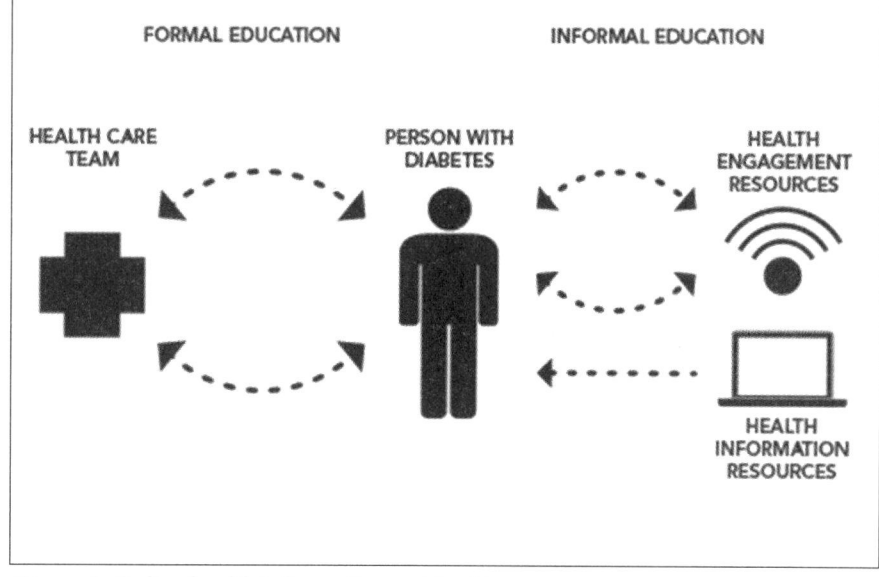

Figure 1. Online health information and health engagement resources represent informal education and support that can complement the more formal education people with diabetes receive from their health care team during office visits.

people with diabetes receive from their HCPs.

These resources are also there for HCPs' use. By going online and becoming acquainted with the different resources, HCPs may gain a better perspective on how their patients experience and learn from such sites. However, even with a deeper understanding of the value of online resources for patients, HCPs may struggle with concerns about protection of patient privacy, their professional responsibility, and the time constraints involved in staying up to date on available resources.

Overcoming Concerns About Privacy and Time

HCPs may hesitate to learn about or participate in social media because of concerns related to the Health Insurance Portability and Accountability Act (HIPAA) and uncertainty about how much to engage with people (possibly patients) online. HIPAA protects patients' privacy by limiting the ways in which their information is shared with others. Patients can choose to share or engage online and provide personal health information, whether about their care and treatment, health care decisions, or details of their patient-professional interactions. HCPs' reading of content that patients chose to share online does not violate HIPAA. However, commenting in a public setting to an individual patient without the patient's signed consent may be considered a HIPAA violation or cause concern that the patient's privacy is not being protected or respected.[8] Even if an HCP has a signed patient consent form, when commenting within a public viewable health engagement resource, the professional should provide only general health information and avoid specific, individualized medical advice. Privacy-protected e-mail is the best tool for direct online communication

about medical care with individual patients.

Lack of time is another deterrent to embracing social media for busy HCPs. In addition to more traditional avenues of continuing education (e.g., medical meetings, symposia, and peer-reviewed journals), HCPs may benefit from supplementing their education with social learning and curation. Curation is the process of evaluating a range of available resources and identifying specific ones that are most appropriate for patients' needs. Like a museum curator selecting pieces of art to include in a display, HPCs can identify and select online resources to share with their patients. Ultimately, the curated resources that professionals share with their patients can be an effective strategy to both enhance direct-to-patient education and save time during in-office education. In addition, posted patient experiences within the resources can help HCPs themselves learn about patients' challenges and insights related to new treatments and technologies.

Patients' Perceptions of HCPs' Involvement in Social Media

Because of the availability of social media tools, people with diabetes can now congregate and interact with each other online without restrictions of geographical location. Thus, online networking and engagement by people with diabetes is collectively referred to as "the diabetes online community." This online community also includes friends, family, and HCPs who work with people with diabetes.

DSMA holds weekly Twitter chats, known as #DSMA, for people with diabetes. During the 20 June 2012 chat, participants were asked to comment about whether having HCPs using social media was valuable. Responses included, "Yes, it will help them learn more about the

24/7 aspects to living with diabetes," "Yes, but I worry about 'big brother medical care'," and "Yes, to connect on a more human level, but no lecturing/knowing what's best." Overall, the #DSMA community consensus appeared to be that participation by HCPs in social media would be valuable and could help HCPs further their understanding of the complex issues that people with diabetes must deal with daily.[9]

Building the Bridge From Office Visit to Online Interaction: Time-Saving Approaches

Helping patients access online health engagement resources does not have to be a time-consuming endeavor, and professionals do not have to actively use all social media platforms and tools. Professionals can use the steps to curate credible resource suggestions for their patients.

1. Solicit and review recommendations. Ask staff members and patients to share their favorite online health information and engagement resources for diabetes. A listing of many health engagement resources can also be found at the Diabetes Advocates Web site (www.diabetes advocates.org; click on the tab for Members and Resources). Diabetes Advocates identifies a number of health engagement resources specifically for people with type 1 or type 2 diabetes, for parents of children with diabetes, and for Spanish-speaking people with diabetes.

Seeking input from patients regarding health engagement resources is crucial because HCPs may not have the necessary objectivity to identify the most useful engagement resources. People with diabetes of varying ages and life situations are sharing their experiences through health engagement resources. Relying on patients to help identify the most useful health engagement resources ensures a synergy between patients' needs and the recommended resources. Remember that self-policing among individuals within online diabetes communities also helps to ensure that the most credible and useful resources gain validation and trust.

HCPs should ask their staff members and patients the reasons the resources they recommend are highly preferred and use that rationale to inform their own recommendations. Seeking input positions HCPs as curators and navigators on behalf of patients and decreases the appearance of bias or of "endorsement" by professionals.

2. Create a list of credible online resources to proactively share with patients during office visits.

Before sharing the list, HCPs should first access and review the recommended online resources to become familiar with what they offer patients. HCPs or health care organizations that have their own Web sites can also share resource links via their sites.

HCPs should use the opportunity to emphasize to patients that a diabetes care plan is based on individual needs. If patients want to make changes to their plan based on online information or conversations, they should first discuss the proposed changes with their HCP.

HCPs should emphasize characteristics that indicate that a resource may not be credible. These include sites that:

Sell a specific product or service
- Display numerous advertisements, which may indicate potential for editorial bias
- Tout a quick fix or cure

- Use sensationalized stories and testimonials to persuade patients to take a specific action

Likewise, HCPs should teach patients how to recognize credible resources. These include sites that:
- Clearly identify the backgrounds and experience of the content author and the reason for sharing the information
- Offer a balanced perspective or information that is vetted and backed by a trusted organization such as the ADA
- Provide current and frequently updated content
- Seek input from credentialed medical advisors for any clinical content about diagnosis and treatment

3. Assess patients' use of online resources and level of health literacy.

Identify the health information and engagement resources patients are using, and gauge their level of understanding of such health information. Ask patients how the resources are helping them, and offer to address specific questions related to the information. Ask patients what tips and advice they would give other patients who want to reach out to online communities. Integrate this advice into ongoing discussions with other patients.

The number of patients who look online for diabetes-related information and resources is expanding. HCPs who proactively encourage patients to investigate reputable online health information and engagement resources may help improve their patients' problem-solving skills in managing diabetes day to day while also potentially strengthening the HCP-patient relationship.

REFERENCES

[1] Pew Internet & American Life Project: Profiles of health information seekers, 2011 [report online]. Available from http://www.pewinternet.org/Reports/2011/HealthTopics/Part-2.aspx?view=all. Accessed 26 November 2012

[2] Powers MA, March SB, Evert A: Use of Internet technology to support nutrition and diabetes self-management care. *Diabetes Spectrum* 21:91–99, 2008

[3] HealthEd Academy: Educational technology in the healthcare setting, 2012 [report online]. Available from http://www.healthedacademy.com/Home.aspx. Accessed 12 September 2012

[4] Wald HS, Dube CE, Anthony DC: Untangling the Web: the impact of Internet use on health care and the physician-patient relationship. *Patient Educ Couns* 63:218–224, 2007

[5] Ayers SL, Kronenfeld JJ: Chronic illness and health-seeking information on the Internet. *Health* 11:327–347, 2007

[6] University of California San Diego Health System: Social networking evaluated to improve diabetes self management [online press release]. Available from http://health.ucsd.edu/news/releases/Pages/2012-07-11-social-networking-and-diabetes.aspx. Accessed 24 January 2013

[7] DiaTribe: Proof is in the people [online blog post]. Available from http://diatribe.us/issues/50/sum-musings. Accessed 24 January 2013

[8] American Medical Association: AMA policy: Professionalism in the use of social media, 2012. Available from http://www.ama-assn.org/ama/pub/meeting/professionalism-social-media.shtml. Accessed 26 October 2012

[9] Diabetes Social Media Advocacy: #DSMA 20 June 2012 [Twitter chat]. Transcript available from http://bit.ly/RuNvdq. Accessed on 12 September 2012

Susan E. Collins, MS, RD, CHES, is senior vice president, health education, research and development, at HealthEd and a community leader for SurroundHealth (www.surroundhealth.net). Dana M. Lewis, BA, leads the international #hcsm (health care communications & social media) community on Twitter, manages digital strategy and internal communications at Swedish Medical Center in Seattle, Wash., and has type 1 diabetes.

Enhancing the Role of Medical Office Staff in Diabetes Care and Education

Melinda D. Maryniuk, RD, MEd, CDE, Carolé Mensing, RN, MA, CDE, FAADE, Sarah Imershein, MPH, Anne Gregory, MSM, and Richard Jackson, MD

Providing education for the 18.8 million people who have been diagnosed with diabetes in the United States is a challenge. Although there are now more than 17,000 certified diabetes educators (CDEs), only about one-third to one-half of the population with diabetes reports having ever received any type of formal diabetes education.[1,2] In addition, it is well recognized that, to maximize access to diabetes education, it needs to be available in convenient, community-based settings such as within primary care offices. Enhancing the role of medical office staff (MOS) in primary care to provide additional support for diabetes-related care and education activities can have beneficial results for patient outcomes and physician satisfaction.

Consider these facts:

- More than 90% of adults with diabetes are cared for by their primary care providers (PCPs).[3] Regardless of the settings in which PCPs work, they rarely have adequate time to provide necessary education to patients with diabetes.
- In a national survey of diabetes educators,[4] only 13% responded they worked in a "physician office" as their primary practice setting providing diabetes education.

The purposes of this article are to:
- Describe gaps in education in the primary care setting, as evidenced by both quantitative and qualitative research

- Describe an office-based program for training MOS to increase their basic understanding of, confidence in, and skills regarding diabetes, as well as to implement interventions to improve office systems
- Suggest specific ways in which PCPs can make small practice changes, particularly related to enhancing the role of MOS to improve care and outcomes

Alternatives for Provider Assistance

In 2010, the Joslin Diabetes Center collected and analyzed data to better understand the challenges and opportunities for improving diabetes care and education in primary care settings from the perspective of both patients and providers. Quantitative (surveys) and qualitative (focus groups) data were obtained. Analysis of survey data from 266 PCPs and 1,321 patients yielded the following insights:

- Sixty-two percent of the PCPs surveyed felt that they do not have enough time with patients during diabetes visits.
- Only 5.8% of patients and 6.0% of PCPs identified "diabetes educator" as a role of PCPs.
- Thirty-seven percent of PCPs reported that there is a lack of adequate support staff to teach about diabetes.
- More than half of the PCPs (58%) agreed that training office staff to help more in certain aspects of diabetes care and education would be helpful.

- PCPs reported that they do much of the education themselves; 61.7% reported that they are the primary person to give general diabetes education for newly diagnosed patients, and 65.0% responded that they provide ongoing diabetes education.

Ideally, and according to standards of medical care,[5] patients with newly diagnosed diabetes should be referred for both diabetes self-management education (DSME) and medical nutrition therapy (MNT). Instead of expecting patients to seek education services outside of their medical home, a variety of approaches have been described that effectively bring needed diabetes information and education services to primary care settings. For example, researchers at the University of Pittsburgh Diabetes Institute successfully implemented a program that involved placing part-time diabetes educators into primary care practices for specific "diabetes days" when office staff could schedule DSME appointments.[6]

Numerous programs employing community health workers (CHWs) have been introduced to facilitate diabetes self-management within primary care.[7,8] The use of CHWs has been particularly effective in underserved areas and those with ethnically diverse populations.[9] CHWs play an important role in helping to provide ongoing support, a crucial element of diabetes education as outlined by the national standards of DSME.[10]

CHWs can also be used effectively to draw attention to patients' key diabetes biomarkers (e.g., A1C, blood pressure, and LDL cholesterol) and thus facilitate dialogues between patients and providers that result in action.[11,12] In one community-based education project,[11] only 15% of 221 participants with diabetes demonstrated understanding or "awareness" of the A1C test (could recall a reasonable A1C value and give broad interpretation of the significance if it was above or below target). This awareness improved significantly compared to control subjects after delivery of targeted diabetes messages by CHWs.

Thus, as roles of nontraditional health care providers have been effectively increasing, and while the need for diabetes education in primary care settings remains high, it is logical to explore additional methods and office personnel who can work in concert with PCPs to ensure the delivery of accurate diabetes information and ongoing support.

Increasing MOS Roles in Diabetes Care

MOS (typically including medical assistants, licensed practical nurses, receptionists, laboratory personnel, and sometime nurses and other mid-level professionals) represent an often underutilized, yet readily available resource to assist the diabetes care team in providing basic education and self-management support in primary care settings.[13] Training in diabetes for MOS is often limited, which potentially affects both their confidence and skills. For example, one of the most important functions of diabetes care is measuring blood pressure. However, office-based blood pressure measurement is often inaccurate. Office-based blood pressure readings more often end in zero, resulting in the misclassi-

fication of patients and corresponding over- or under-treatment.[14] Part of this inaccuracy may be based in a lack of knowledge of the importance blood pressure plays in diabetes management.

Additionally, there are many other tasks associated with diabetes care and adherence to clinical guidelines that are not required to be performed by PCPs. Offices using flow sheets or templates have demonstrated improved adherence to clinical guidelines.[15] Checklists of quality measures, including whether routine laboratory tests or examinations have been performed and whether recommended counseling services have been provided, can be maintained by MOS either in the form of diabetes flow sheets in paper charts or corresponding templates in electronic health records (EHRs). With minimal training, MOS can effectively reduce the burden of such tasks on PCPs, help to ensure that high-quality diabetes care is delivered, and increase patient awareness of the importance of this care. Such training can empower MOS to be active members of the health care team.

A 2006 article[16] reported on the effectiveness of an intervention with MOS that involved CDEs delivering a 2-hour training program with follow-up ongoing support provided to 1,370 MOS in basic diabetes care and education. This initiative demonstrated a variety of improvements in both patients' confidence in self-care and A1C levels. In addition, participation in the program significantly and consistently increased MOS confidence in their ability to help patients manage their diabetes. The success of this project led to another pilot study, which is reported here.

Journey in Caring Pilot Study

The Journey in Caring (JIC) initiative involved training MOS to assist with

diabetes-related care tasks. At least one MOS was designated as a "diabetes champion" at each site to assist in the implementation and maintenance of the program. Materials and a 2-hour training curriculum were designed to improve MOS knowledge of diabetes, emphasize practical office procedures such as accurate measurement of blood pressure, and encourage the use of diabetes flow sheets based on American Diabetes Association clinical practice guidelines.[5] A set of basic diabetes education tear-sheets and a "Diabetes Care Plan" handout that could be individualized for each patient were also provided. Based on our work demonstrating the importance of helping increase patient awareness of diabetes biomarkers, emphasis was placed on helping MOS understand the rationale for these laboratory tests and how to talk about them to patients in the office setting. CDEs trained in program delivery implemented the programs and provided the training and follow-up to each office.

During the pilot phase, data were collected from 57 offices and 244 MOS. MOS completing the training not only showed significant improvements in knowledge and confidence, but also were more likely to talk with patients about the importance of dilated eye exams (26.6 vs. 43.0%, $P < 0.001$), foot care (39.8 vs. 59.4%, $P < 0.001$), and microalbumin tests (53.1 vs. 61.7%, $P < 0.001$). In addition, as shown in Figure 1, the pilot intervention showed that patients whose medical records incorporated flow sheets were more likely to experience an A1C reduction than patients whose medical records did not use diabetes flow sheets ($n = 56$, odds ratio 3.67, $P = 0.025$).[17]

Program Expansion

After a successful pilot test, JIC was extended nationally from 2009 to

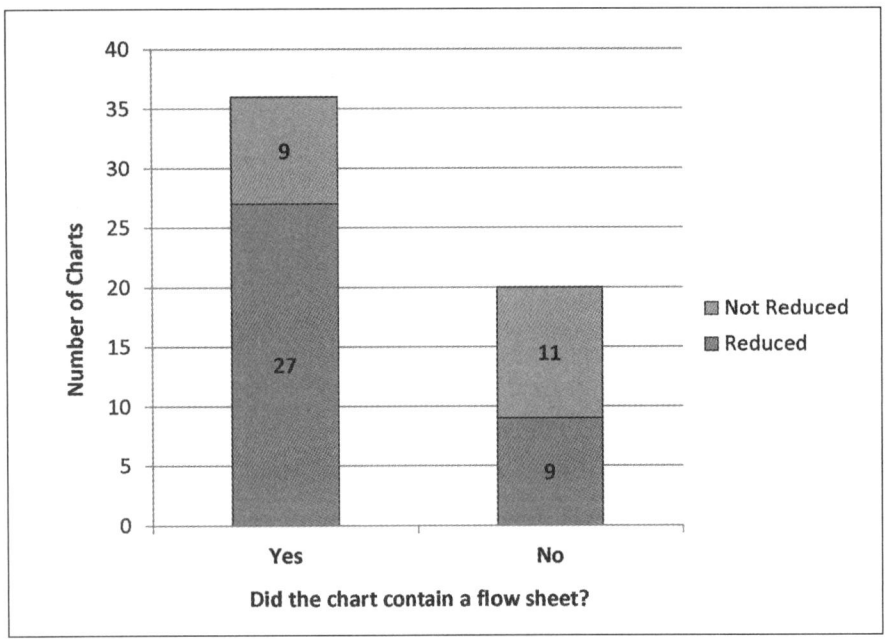

Figure 1. Patients whose charts incorporated flow sheets were more likely to experience A1C reduction than those whose charts did not include a flow sheet.

2011. The initiative was implemented in 189 medical offices reaching 1,623 MOS, of which the largest percentage were medical assistants (44%) and the remainder included a wide range of office employees including clinical (licensed practical nurses) and non-clinical (receptionists) staff. MOS team members who completed training received attendance certificates, and one individual earned the title of "diabetes champion" for his or her office.

Physician satisfaction with the program was high, and 96% of the 82 physicians who completed an evaluation survey reported improvement in MOS knowledge and skills related to diabetes care. MOS knowledge and confidence increased (particularly in the areas of meal planning and physical activity counseling), and there was a significant increase in the frequency with which MOS talked with patients about basic medical aspects of diabetes, self-monitoring of blood glucose (SMBG), meal planning, and exercise (Table 1).

Significant improvements were also shown in a number of diabetes office systems activities. Offices were assessed by CDEs and MOS for whether they performed specific activities "not at all," "somewhat," or "well" at the beginning of the program and again 6–8 weeks after the program. The number of offices that used a diabetes flow sheet "well" increased from 37% before the program to 63% after the program. Offices that were successful at making diabetes educational resources (including the handouts provided

as part of the program) available to patients improved from 48 to 85% (Figure 2).

Training MOS improves their confidence in the quality of their interactions with patients, which may ultimately translate into clinical benefits for patients. Training also results in improvements in office systems by improving documentation, communication, and consistency of messages to patients. A wait list–controlled study (in which randomized intervention offices receive the program immediately, whereas control offices wait for 6 months before receiving the program) is underway with a payer provider network to compare biometric outcomes, health care utilization, and costs between patients at offices that receive the JIC initiative and those at offices that do not have the program.

Takeaway Messages for PCPs

1. Complete an office gap analysis and create an action plan.
The diabetes office assessment provided in Table 2 can help PCPs identify gaps in care and areas in which to initiate quality improvement initiatives. Develop a plan for what your office might do to enhance diabetes care and education and to specifically enhance the role of MOS.

Table 1. MOS Survey Results for JIC Pilot and National Program Expansion			
	Pilot		**National**
MOS reporting that they were "satisfied" or "very satisfied" with how much they know about . . .	**Pre-program**	**Post-program**	**Post-program***
Basic medical aspects of diabetes (%)	52.4	95.3	90.8
SMBG (%)	68.8	96.9	91.7
Diabetes and nutrition/meal planning (%)	30.2	85.2	85.4
Diabetes and physical activity/exercise (%)	41.7	92.1	89.6
After successful outcomes were demonstrated in the pilot test, only post-program data were collected during the national rollout for scalability.			

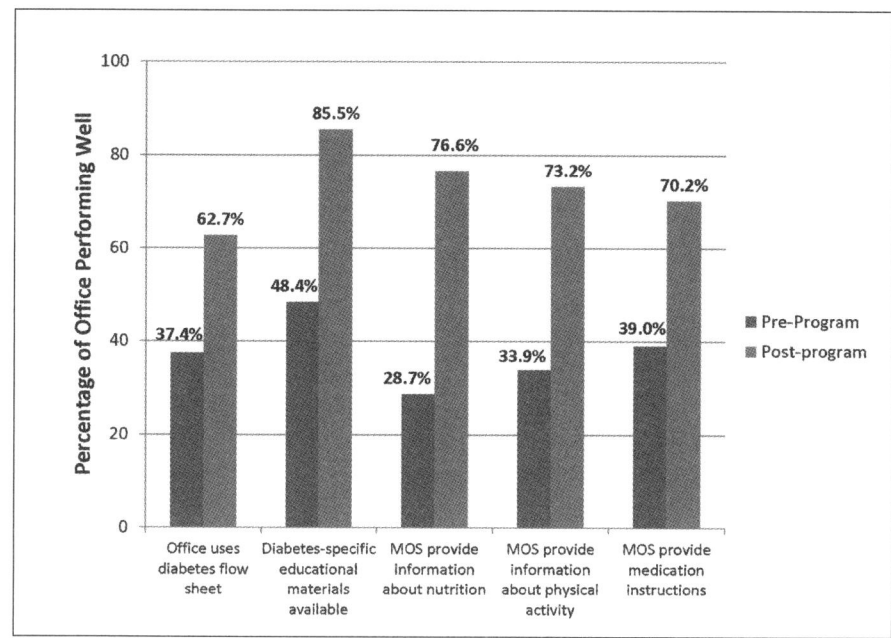

Figure 2. Offices that performed specific diabetes systems activities "well" before and after the JIC intervention.

Excellent free resources are available through the National Diabetes Information Clearinghouse (www.ndep.nih.gov). Other organizations such as the Joslin Diabetes Center also offer a wide variety of downloadable free resources for both office improvement and patient education. (See the Joslin Professional Education Consortium developed for PCPs at www.jpec.joslin.org.)

Consider applying for recognition for meeting minimum quality standards through the National Center for Quality Assurance diabetes recognition program (www.ncqa.org).

2. Plan routine diabetes staff training programs.
All members of the office practice team can benefit from periodic trainings and discussions about diabetes care. Dispel their misunderstandings. Many of them believe the same myths about diabetes that patients do, especially regarding the use of insulin. Although there are some online programs available for this purpose,[18] such education is best when

followed by team discussion to ensure that interpretation of the material is aligned with office practices. Discuss ways MOS can be more involved in sharing diabetes resources, providing ongoing support, or assisting in preparing patients for visits, including:
- Asking patients to think ahead about the diabetes questions they want to ask
- Reminding patients to complete laboratory work and eye and dental exams before their office visit
- Asking patients to encourage the eye and dental offices to send reports directly to their PCP
- Reminding patients that they will be asked to remove their shoes and socks for foot examinations
- Ensuring that pertinent test and examination results are recorded in patients' medical records, either on a diabetes flow sheet or the appropriate EHR templates

3. Focus on knowing the numbers.
When MOS know the targets for A1C, blood pressure, LDL cholesterol, microalbumin, and estimated glomer-

ular filtration rate, they can reinforce these for patients and have basic discussions when prepping patients for their medical visits. Ideally, obtaining point-of-care results, especially for A1C, can facilitate timely and relevant discussions.

When working with MOS, emphasize the importance of recording accurate height, weight, and blood pressure results (not rounding to the nearest 5 or 0) and sharing those results with patients. MOS are not expected to discuss the interpretation of the results with patients, but rather should encourage patients' awareness of the importance of such tests and prepare patients to discuss their results with their PCP during office visits.

4. Designate a diabetes champion.
Although the entire medical office team needs to be prepared to handle patients with diabetes, it is often helpful when one person is given recognition and responsibility related to diabetes activities. For example, the diabetes champion can be in charge of organizing diabetes education materials, stocking an insulin initiation teaching kit, and identifying local resources for diabetes education and support that can be used by other MOS members.

5. Identify community and other support resources.
Encourage the diabetes champion, with input from the entire team, to develop and maintain a list of resources, including diabetes education programs, diabetes educators, registered dietitians with expertise in diabetes care, diabetes support groups, insulin pump trainers, mall walking programs, weight control programs, YMCA prevention programs, online programs, and helpful smartphone applications. Online resources are available that organize local diabetes information into one

Table 2. PCP Office Assessment Tool for Diabetes Support Activities

Assess each diabetes activity and place a check mark (✓) in first column if present. Check at least two goals that are areas for improvement. Re-assess each diabetes activity in 3–6 months and place checks in the last column if improved.

Equipment and Procedures	Assess	✓ If goal	Re-check
Identify and mentor diabetes champion		☐	
Point-of-care A1C devices		☐	
Point-of-care lipid devices		☐	
Tape measures for waist circumference measurement		☐	
Monofilaments for foot checks		☐	
Culturally and linguistically appropriate educational materials		☐	
Diabetes flow sheet or EHR templates for completion of diabetes clinical guidelines		☐	
Computer and printer for meter, continuous glucose monitor, and insulin pump data downloads		☐	
Standing laboratory orders for routine diabetes tests (A1C, lipids, serum creatinine for estimated glomerular filtration rate, urine microalbumin-creatinine ratio)		☐	
Routine A1C or other glucose screening of people at risk for diabetes		☐	
Assess and Improve Skills for MOS	**Assess**	**✓ If goal**	**Re-check**
Blood pressure measurement skills		☐	
Accurate height and weight measurement		☐	
Fingerstick skills and operation of point-of-care devices		☐	
Diabetes basic ABCs (A1C, blood pressure, and cholesterol targets and testing frequencies)		☐	
Patient Education and Referral Follow-Up	**Assess**	**✓ If goal**	**Re-check**
Provide diabetes-specific education material		☐	
Refer to diabetes educators, DSME programs		☐	
Refer to registered dietitians for MNT		☐	
Obtain eye exam reports from ophthalmologist specializing in diabetes eye care		☐	
Remind all patients to obtain routine dental care		☐	
Maintain up-to-date list of local diabetes resources, support groups, and media (phone apps)		☐	
Provide smoking cessation information and referral		☐	
Has system to follow up if a referral was made and kept and if results are included in chart		☐	
Patient Information Given by MOS	**Assess**	**✓ If goal**	**Re-check**
Healthy eating information		☐	

Table 2. PCP Office Assessment Tool for Diabetes Support Activities , *continued from p. 120*			
Physical activity/exercise information		☐	
SMBG/meter teaching/ketone monitoring, as appropriate		☐	
Insulin/other injectable techniques		☐	
Oral medication use		☐	
Quality Improvement Activities	**Assess**	**✓ If goal**	**Re-check**
Conduct chart reviews of key performance measures; implement continuous quality improvement plan based on results		☐	
Use brief team meetings to discuss patient cases		☐	
Assess MOS knowledge and confidence in performing diabetes support activities		☐	
Complete application for National Center for Quality Assurance diabetes recognition program		☐	

searchable resource guide that can be modified for any practice and population (see www.diabeteslocal.org).

Summary

Although DSME is an essential component of high-quality diabetes care, most patients are never referred, never have access, or never attend formal diabetes education because of systems-level or behavioral barriers. MOS are an underutilized resource and, with minimal structured training in basic diabetes principles, can significantly affect the quality of care and health of patients with diabetes. Most medical encounters for people with diabetes occur in a primary care setting, and the MOS frequently interacts with diabetes patients. Thus, once they receive appropriate resources and training in basic diabetes principles, MOS can be an excellent addition to the care team.

ACKNOWLEDGMENTS

Journey in Caring is an educational program developed by the Joslin Diabetes Center and funded and distributed by Lilly USA, LLC. The Joslin Diabetes Center does not endorse products or services, including those of Lilly USA, LLC.

REFERENCES

[1]Peyrot M, Rubin RR, Funnell MM, Siminerio LM: Access to diabetes self-management education: results of national surveys of patients, educators, and physicians. *Diabetes Educ* 35:246–248, 252–246, 258–263, 2009

[2]U.S. Department of Health and Human Services: *Healthy People 2020.* Available from http://www.healthypeople.gov/2020/topicsobjectives2020/objectiveslist.aspx?topicId=8. Accessed 19 October 2012

[3]Beaser RS and the Staff of Joslin Diabetes Center: *Joslin's Diabetes Deskbook.* 2nd ed. Boston, Mass., Joslin Diabetes Center, 2010

[4]Martin AL: Changes and consistencies in diabetes education over 5 years: results of the 2010 National Diabetes Education Practice Survey. *Diabetes Educ* 38:35–46, 2012

[5]American Diabetes Association: Standards of medical care in diabetes—2013. *Diabetes Care* 36 (Suppl. 1):S11–S66, 2013

[6]Siminerio LM, Piatt GA, Emerson S, Ruppert K, Saul M, Solano F, Stewart A, Zgibor JC: Deploying the chronic care model to implement and sustain diabetes self-management training programs. *Diabetes Educ* 32:253–260, 2006

[7]Otero-Sabogal R, Arretz D, Siebold S, Hallen E, Lee R, Ketchel A, Li J, Newman J: Physician-community health worker partnering to support diabetes self-management in primary care. *Qual Prim Care* 18:363–372, 2010

[8]American Association of Diabetes Educators: Position Paper: Community health workers in diabetes management and prevention. *Diabetes Educ* 29:818, 821–814, 2003. Updated online in 2011. Available from http://www.diabeteseducator.org/DiabetesEducation/position/position_statements.html Accessed 19 October 2012

[9]Philis-Tsimikas A, Walker C, Rivard L, Talavera G, Reimann JO, Salmon M, Araujo R; Project Dulce: Improvement in diabetes care of underinsured patients enrolled in project dulce: a community-based, culturally appropriate, nurse case management and peer education diabetes care model. *Diabetes Care* 27:110–115, 2004

[10]Haas L, Maryniuk M, Beck J, Cox CE, Duker P, Edwards L, Fisher E, Hanson L, Kent D, Kolb L, McLaughlin S, Orzeck E, Piette JD, Rhinehart AS, Rothman R, Sklaroff S, Tomky D, Youssef G: National standards for diabetes self-management education and support. *Diabetes Care* 35:2393–2401, 2012

[11]Polonsky WH, Zee J, Yee MA, Crosson MA, Jackson RA: A community-based program to encourage patients' attention to their own diabetes care: pilot development and evaluation. *Diabetes Educ* 31:691–699, 2005

[12]Jackson R, Imershein S, Butkus S, Broughton S, Polonsky W: A1C and blood pressure awareness [abstract]. *Diabetes* 59 (Suppl. 1):A600, 2010

[13]Ruggiero L, Moadsiri A, Butler P, Oros SM, Berbaum ML, Whitman S, Cintron D: Supporting diabetes self-care in underserved populations: a randomized pilot study using medical assistant coaches. *Diabetes Educ* 36:127–131, 2010

[14]Broad J, Wells S, Marshall R, Jackson R: Zero end-digit preference in recorded blood pressure and its impact on classification of patients for pharmacologic management in primary care: PREDICT-CVD-6. *Br J Gen Pract* 57:897–903, 2007

[15]Hahn KA, Ferrante JM, Crosson JC, Hudson SV, Crabtree BF: Diabetes flow sheet

use associated with guideline adherence. *Ann Fam Med* 6:235–238, 2008

[16]Celeste-Harris S, Maryniuk M: Educating medical office staff: enhancing diabetes care in primary care offices. *Diabetes Spectrum* 19:84–89, 2006

[17]Mensing C, Maryniuk M, Reynolds L, Imershein S, Jackson R: Leveraging primary care office staff to enhance diabetes care [abstract]. *Diabetes* 58 (Suppl. 1):A318, 2009

[18]American Association of Diabetes Educators: Online course: Fundamentals of *Diabetes Care*. Available from www. diabeteseducator.org/ProfessionalResources/products/index.html#products. Accessed 19 October 2012

Melinda D. Maryniuk, RD, MEd, CDE, is the director of clinical education programs; Carolé Mensing, RN, MA, CDE, FAADE, is the manager of education and clinical services; Sarah Imershein, MPH, is an assistant director of program outcomes; and Anne Gregory, MSM, is an assistant director of education services at the Joslin Diabetes Center in Boston, Mass. Richard Jackson, MD, is director of medical affairs, healthcare services, and a senior physician at the Joslin Diabetes Center and is an assistant professor of medicine at Harvard Medical School in Boston, Mass.

Metabolic Effects of Bariatric Surgery in Patients With Moderate Obesity and Type 2 Diabetes

Analysis of a randomized control trial comparing surgery with intensive medical treatment

Sangeeta R. Kashyap, MD[1]
Deepak L. Bhatt, MD, MPH[2]
Kathy Wolski, MPH[3]
Richard M. Watanabe, PhD[4]
Muhammad Abdul-Ghani, MD, PhD[5]
Beth Abood, RN[1]

Claire E. Pothier, MPH[3]
Stacy Brethauer, MD[6]
Steven Nissen, MD[3]
Manjula Gupta, PhD[1]
John P. Kirwan, PhD[7]
Philip R. Schauer, MD[6]

OBJECTIVE—To evaluate the effects of two bariatric procedures versus intensive medical therapy (IMT) on β-cell function and body composition.

RESEARCH DESIGN AND METHODS—This was a prospective, randomized, controlled trial of 60 subjects with uncontrolled type 2 diabetes (HbA$_{1c}$ 9.7 ± 1%) and moderate obesity (BMI 36 ± 2 kg/m^2) randomized to IMT alone, IMT plus Roux-en-Y gastric bypass, or IMT plus sleeve gastrectomy. Assessment of β-cell function (mixed-meal tolerance testing) and body composition was performed at baseline and 12 and 24 months.

RESULTS—Glycemic control improved in all three groups at 24 months ($N = 54$), with a mean HbA$_{1c}$ of 6.7 ± 1.2% for gastric bypass, 7.1 ± 0.8% for sleeve gastrectomy, and 8.4 ± 2.3% for IMT ($P < 0.05$ for each surgical group versus IMT). Reduction in body fat was similar for both surgery groups, with greater absolute reduction in truncal fat in gastric bypass versus sleeve gastrectomy (−16 vs. −10%; $P = 0.04$). Insulin sensitivity increased significantly from baseline in gastric bypass (2.7-fold; $P = 0.004$) and did not change in sleeve gastrectomy or IMT. β-Cell function (oral disposition index) increased 5.8-fold in gastric bypass from baseline, was markedly greater than IMT ($P = 0.001$), and was not different between sleeve gastrectomy versus IMT ($P = 0.30$). At 24 months, β-cell function inversely correlated with truncal fat and prandial free fatty acid levels.

CONCLUSIONS—Bariatric surgery provides durable glycemic control compared with intensive medical therapy at 2 years. Despite similar weight loss as sleeve gastrectomy, gastric bypass uniquely restores pancreatic β-cell function and reduces truncal fat, thus reversing the core defects in diabetes.

Diabetes Care 36:2175–2182, 2013

Type 2 diabetes mellitus and obesity are closely interrelated chronic conditions growing in incidence worldwide, with diabetes-related deaths projected to double between 2005 and 2030 (1). The development of both insulin resistance and insulin secretory defects is the hallmark of type 2 diabetes, resulting in progressive hyperglycemia, subsequent microvascular complications, and macrovascular complications. Although lifestyle modifications and oral hypoglycemic agents improve glycemic control, the majority of patients do not achieve the optimal glycohemoglobin (HbA$_{1c}$) levels recommended by current guidelines (≤7.0%). The disease inexorably progresses in the majority of patients, ultimately requiring insulin replacement therapy. Most patients with type 2 diabetes are overweight or obese (BMI ≥30 kg/m^2), and abdominal adiposity, particularly, is tightly linked to induction of insulin resistance, metabolic syndrome, and increased cardiovascular risk. Many hypoglycemic agents, especially insulin, exacerbate weight gain and thwart lifestyle efforts, potentially contributing to the underlying pathophysiologic disorder.

Because of the limitations to medical therapy, surgical approaches for the treatment of obesity have increased 10-fold in the past decade. Roux-en-Y gastric bypass surgery is the most commonly performed in the United States, followed closely by the sleeve gastrectomy (2). Recently, two randomized controlled trials (3,4) demonstrated improved glycemic control in patients undergoing bariatric surgery compared with intensive medical therapy, resulting in the ability to withdraw or reduce glucose-lowering medications. The rapid rate of glucose lowering, disproportionate to degree of weight loss, suggests that bariatric surgery reverses the fundamental pathophysiological defects of type 2 diabetes. Animal studies suggest that bariatric surgery increases insulin secretion or improves enteroinsulinar responses, specifically the main incretin hormones glucagon like peptide-1 (GLP-1) and gastric inhibitory peptide (GIP) (5–7). Previous small-scale studies from matched case-control and observational studies in severely obese diabetic individuals have reported that weight loss improves insulin sensitivity, reduces hyperinsulinemia, and improves pancreatic β-cell function by

From the [1]Endocrinology and Metabolism Institute, Cleveland Clinic, Cleveland, Ohio; the [2]VA Boston Healthcare System, Brigham and Women's Hospital, and Harvard Medical School, Boston, Massachusetts; the [3]Miller Family Heart and Vascular Institute, Cleveland Clinic, Cleveland, Ohio; the [4]Department of Physiology and Biophysics, University of Southern California, Los Angeles, California; the [5]Diabetes Division, University of Texas Health Science Center, San Antonio, Texas; the [6]Bariatric and Metabolic Institute, Cleveland Clinic, Cleveland, Ohio; and the [7]Lerner Research Institute, Cleveland Clinic, Cleveland, Ohio.
Corresponding author: Sangeeta R. Kashyap, kashyas@ccf.org.
Received 7 August 2012 and accepted 13 January 2013.
DOI: 10.2337/dc12-1596. Clinical trial reg. no. NCT00432809, clinicaltrials.gov.
This article contains Supplementary Data online at http://care.diabetesjournals.org/lookup/suppl/doi:10.2337/dc12-1596/-/DC1.
A slide set summarizing this article is available online.

weight-independent mechanisms related to an incretin effect (8–10). However, there are no data from a randomized controlled trial examining the prolonged metabolic adaptations in conjunction with clinical efficacy outcomes after bariatric surgery relative to the effects of intensive medical therapy in moderately obese subjects with poorly controlled type 2 diabetes.

The STAMPEDE trial evaluated the efficacy and safety of intensive medical therapy (IMT) alone or intensive medical therapy combined with Roux-en-Y gastric bypass or sleeve gastrectomy to achieve a primary end point of HbA$_{1c}$ level of ≤6% (with or without medications) after 1 year of follow-up (11). The current report is a 2-year extension of a metabolic substudy of the STAMPEDE trial designed to thoroughly evaluate the effects of the three treatments on glucose regulation, pancreatic β-cell function (insulin secretion/sensitivity), and body composition in a subset of 60 subjects.

RESEARCH DESIGN AND METHODS

Study design
The STAMPEDE study rationale and design have been previously reported (3,11). The first consecutive 60 subjects randomized in the main trial, with ~20 randomized to each treatment group, were included in the substudy. STAMPEDE was a single-center study that randomized patients in a 1:1:1 ratio to intensive medical therapy alone or intensive medical therapy combined with either Roux-en-Y gastric bypass or sleeve gastrectomy with stratification by use of insulin at screening. Intensive medical therapy included the use of the latest lifestyle guidelines by the American Diabetes Association, frequent home monitoring and titration strategies, and use of the latest U.S. Food and Drug Administration–approved drug therapy including incretin analogs or mimetics and insulin sensitizers for treatment of hyperglycemia. Patients were examined in the outpatient clinic every 3 months by a diabetes specialist at the Cleveland Clinic (S.R.K.). The bariatric procedures were performed by a single primary surgeon (P.R.S.).

During the screening period, all patients received nutritional counseling by a certified diabetes educator. Subjects were encouraged to participate in Weight Watchers for additional nutritional counseling. Patients underwent a psychological evaluation before randomization

to assess qualification for bariatric surgery. Subjects randomized to bariatric surgery had periodic evaluation by nutrition, psychology, bariatricians, and the surgery team as clinically indicated. The Data and Safety Monitoring Board convened yearly to review progress and safety of the trial. The protocol was developed with the assistance of the Cleveland Clinic Coordinating Center for Clinical Research and was approved by the Cleveland Clinic Institutional Review Board. All participants provided written informed consent.

After randomization at the baseline visit and at 12 and 24 months after randomization, subjects underwent metabolic assessment with a liquid mixed-meal tolerance test and body composition measurements with dual-energy X-ray absorptiometry (iDXA; Lunar Prodigy, Madison, WI) scan.

Metabolic studies
The mixed-meal tolerance test was performed to assess glucose tolerance and metabolic measures of insulin sensitivity and secretion in response to a physiological stimulus. The liquid mixed meal consisted of a commercial product (Boost; 8 ounces, 350 kcal, 55% carbohydrate, 25% protein, 20% fat) and was consumed over 5 min after a 12- to 14-h overnight fast in a similar manner per protocol at baseline and 12 and 24 months. Fasting blood samples were obtained for glucose, C-peptide, insulin, lipids, HbA$_{1c}$, adipokines, and a complete metabolic panel. Blood was drawn every 30 min for 120 min during the mixed meal tolerance testing for determination of glucose, insulin, C-peptide, and free fatty acid responses. Additional blood was drawn at fasting and at 60 min after ingestion for determination of GLP-1 and GIP responses. Glucagon levels were determined at fasting and at 120 min. Diabetes medications were withheld for 24 h before study, including insulin administration.

Analytic determinations
Blood glucose was measured using the glucose oxidase method (YSI 2300 STAT Plus; YSI, Yellow Springs, OH). Plasma insulin was assayed by a double-antibody radioimmunoassay (RIA; Linco Research, St. Charles, MO). The intra-assay and interassay coefficients of variations were 2.6% and 3.0%, respectively. C-peptide was assayed using a chemiluminescence immunoassay (Linco Research). The intra-assay and interassay coefficients of variations were 3.5% and 7.2%, respectively. Blood

collected for GLP-1 (active) and GIP (total) analyses was treated immediately with a DPP4 and protease cocktail inhibitor (Sigma) and assayed using ELISA kits (ALPCO Diagnostics, Salem, NH). The intra-assay and interassay coefficients of variations were 3.6% and 9.3%, respectively. To correct for interassay variability, all premeasurements and postmeasurements for each individual were run on the same plate. Free fatty acid levels were determined by standard colorimetric methods (Wako Chemicals, Richmond, VA). The intra-assay and interassay coefficients of variation were 3.0% and 4.6%, respectively. Leptin was assayed using ELISA kits (R&D Systems, Minneapolis, MN). The intra-assay and interassay coefficients of variations were 3.6% and 5.3%, respectively.

Calculations
Insulin secretion rate (ISR) in vivo was reconstructed by deconvolution of plasma concentrations of C-peptide, a peptide with linear kinetics that is cosecreted with insulin but is not extracted by the liver as previously described (8,12). ISRs over each sampling period were derived by using a well-accepted twocompartment model described by Van Cauter et al. (12) of C-peptide distribution and degradation and standard parameters for C-peptide clearance estimated for each subject, taking into account body surface area, sex, and age. ISR was related to the glucose stimulus by dividing the incremental area under curve (AUC) for ISR by the incremental AUC for plasma glucose. Pancreatic β-cell function measured by the insulin secretion/insulin resistance (disposition) index was determined by dividing the ΔISR/Δglucose by the severity of insulin resistance (ΔISR [AUC] / ΔG [AUC] ÷ IR), as measured by the inverse of the Matsuda index (13). The Matsuda index incorporates both hepatic and muscle components of insulin resistance, correlates well with euglycemic insulin clamp, and was calculated as follows:

Matsuda index
$$= \frac{10,000}{\sqrt{(FPG \times FPI) \times (mean\ PG \times mean\ PI)}}$$

Of note, the Matsuda index was performed in those subjects not using exogenous insulin. The incremental AUC for ISR (ΔISR [AUC]) and the incremental AUC for plasma glucose (ΔG

[AUC]) were calculated according to the trapezoid rule. The incretin response during meal testing subtracted the fasting value from the meal value at 60 min.

Statistical analysis

This is a preplanned substudy with pre-specified analysis. However, because of the lack of published data in the literature regarding specified metabolic outcome measures at the time of trial design (2004–2005), and because of the exploratory nature of the substudy, no power calculations were performed for the substudy measures. Continuous variables with a normal distribution are reported as means and SDs. Variables with a non-normal distribution are reported as medians and interquartile ranges. Categorical variables were summarized using frequencies and were tested with the χ^2 statistic or Fisher exact test (two-tailed), as appropriate. One-way ANOVA was used to analyze continuous laboratory parameters, and comparisons between treatment groups were performed with either the Student t test or the Wilcoxon test. Glucose and insulin measures collected during the mixed-meal tolerance test were plotted graphically.

RESULTS

Patients

Sixty subjects enrolled in the substudy after randomization. At 24 months, 10% were lost to follow-up, with 17 subjects remaining in intensive medical therapy and 18 and 19 subjects remaining in the gastric bypass and sleeve gastrectomy groups, respectively. Baseline characteristics for the three study groups that were followed up for 24 months are shown in Table 1. The subjects were middle-aged, with a predominance of females, particularly in the sleeve gastrectomy group. The average BMI was 36 kg/m^2 with prolonged diabetes duration with mean baseline HbA$_{1c}$ levels of ~9%, indicating poor glycemic control despite using multiple glucose-lowering agents. Nearly half were insulin users, and a majority had hypertension and hyperlipidemia.

Glycemic and cardiovascular risk control

Table 2 shows glycemic and lipid outcomes at 12 and 24 months. Although glycemic control improved in all three arms at 24 months as compared with baseline, the gastric bypass group had significantly greater reduction in fasting glucose and HbA$_{1c}$ levels compared with IMT ($P < 0.05$) (Table 2). At 24 months, the proportion of patients with HbA$_{1c}$ ≤6% attenuated in the sleeve gastrectomy group from 26% to 11% but persisted in the gastric bypass group. The percent of patients using insulin at 24 months was markedly lower in gastric bypass and sleeve gastrectomy groups as compared with IMT. Large increases in HDL cholesterol and reductions in levels of triglycerides and high-sensitivity C-reactive protein were noted in both surgery groups as compared with the IMT group. Other laboratory parameters and medication usage are available in Supplementary Table 1.

Three subjects randomized to bariatric surgery required reoperation, including laparoscopy to assess nausea and vomiting, for cholecystectomy and for jejunostomy for feeding access to treat a gastric leak after sleeve gastrectomy. There were no deaths or episodes of serious hypoglycemia requiring intervention, malnutrition, or excessive weight loss among the three groups.

Body weight, body composition, and adipokines

Greater total body weight loss occurred after bariatric procedures compared with IMT at 12 months and was maintained at 24-month follow-up. A similar reduction in body weight, BMI, and absolute change in total body fat percent was observed between the sleeve gastrectomy and gastric bypass group at 24 months. However, despite similar weight loss, the absolute reduction in percent truncal fat was greater in the gastric bypass versus sleeve gastrectomy group (-16% vs. -10%; $P = 0.04$). Leptin levels reduced markedly after surgical weight loss, especially gastric bypass, compared with IMT. Suppression of free fatty acid concentration during mixed-meal testing was evident after both surgical procedures versus IMT (Supplementary Table 1).

Mixed-meal tolerance

Figure 1 demonstrates the median glucose and C-peptide levels during the mixed-meal tolerance test at baseline and 24 months. At 24 months, the shape of the glucose tolerance curve for gastric bypass normalized with a marked reduction in fasting and postprandial glucose levels. Intermediate effects on postprandial glucose lowering were noted in sleeve gastrectomy, and IMT showed the least change. Large reductions in fasting C-peptide levels were observed in sleeve gastrectomy and gastric bypass at

24 months but did not change in the IMT group. Postprandial C-peptide levels and insulin secretion rate at 30 and 60 min increased by more than two-fold in gastric bypass and sleeve gastrectomy, with greater increases noted with gastric bypass. The average AUC for insulin secretion rate at 24 months was significantly greater with both gastric bypass (4.4 ± 4 pmol/min) and sleeve gastrectomy (3.3 ± 2.5 pmol/min) than IMT (1.7 ± 2.4 pmol/min; both $P < 0.01$).

Insulin sensitivity

Median values for the insulin sensitivity (Matsuda index) in noninsulin-using subjects increased at 24 months after gastric bypass ($N = 9$) by 2.7-fold (3.8 vs. 1.4; $P < 0.001$) and 1.2-fold after sleeve gastrectomy ($N = 10$; 5.8 vs. 5.3) and did not change with IMT (2.6 vs. 2.4; $P =$ not significant). The absolute change in median insulin sensitivity (Matsuda index) at 24 months tended to be higher in gastric bypass compared with sleeve gastrectomy (2.3 [quartile 1: 0.9; quartile 3: 3.1] vs. 0.9 [quartile 1: -1.5; quartile 3: 4.6]), despite equivalent weight loss.

Pancreatic hormonal function

The absolute change in median values for pancreatic β-cell function (oral disposition index) at 24 months was markedly greater in gastric bypass than IMT (0.196 [quartile 1: 0.14; quartile 3: 0.29] vs. 0.027 [quartile 1: -0.011; quartile 3: 0.074]; $P = 0.001$) but not different between sleeve gastrectomy and medical therapy (0.058 [quartile 1: -0.009; quartile 3: 0.416] vs. 0.027 [quartile 1: -0.011; quartile 3: 0.074]; $P = 0.30$). A median 5.8-fold (quartile 1: -7.00; quartile Q3: 11.29) increase in β-cell function from baseline was noted in gastric bypass, with negligible increases in sleeve gastrectomy and IMT.

The change in β-cell function over 24 months for the substudy cohort correlated with the change in percentage of truncal fat ($r = 0.43$; $P = 0.0013$) and change in body weight ($r = 0.49$; $P < 0.001$). At 24 months, both percentage of truncal fat ($r = -0.32$; $P = 0.02$) and prandial free fatty acid levels ($r = -0.48$; $P = 0.0003$) were inversely correlated with β-cell function. In a multivariable analysis including both factors, prandial free fatty acid levels remained significant ($P = 0.004$), whereas percentage of truncal fat was no longer significant ($P = 0.41$).

Fasting glucagon concentrations were similar among the three groups at baseline. At 12 months, median glucagon

Table 1—*Baseline characteristics*

Parameter	All patients	IMT (N = 17)	Gastric bypass (N = 18)	Sleeve gastrectomy (N = 19)	P*
Age (years)	48.4 ± 9.3	50 ± 8.4	47.9 ± 9.7	47.5 ± 10.0	0.71
Female, n (%)	32 (59.3)	8 (47.1)	8 (44.4)	16 (84.2)	0.02
Caucasian, n (%)	39 (72.2)	14 (82.4)	11 (61.1)	14 (73.7)	0.37
Body weight (kg)	104.3 ± 15.1	107.9 ± 14.5	105.3 ± 13.6	100.0 ± 16.5	0.28
BMI (kg/m^2)	36.1 ± 2.9	35.8 ± 3.0	36.1 ± 2.6	36.4 ± 3.2	0.83
Duration of diabetes (years)	8.4 ± 5.0	10.5 ± 5.0	7.4 ± 5.0	7.6 ± 4.5	0.12
N of diabetes medications					0.68
1	2 (3.7)	1 (5.9)	0 (0.0)	1 (5.3)	
2	11 (20.4)	5 (29.4)	3 (16.7)	3 (15.8)	
≥3	41 (75.9)	11 (64.7)	15 (83.3)	15 (78.9)	
Insulin users, n (%)	25 (46.3)	8 (47.1)	8 (44.4)	9 (47.4)	0.98
History of dyslipidemia, n (%)	44 (81.5)	14 (82.4)	15 (83.3)	15 (78.9)	1.0
History of hypertension, n (%)	34 (63.0)	10 (58.8)	13 (72.2)	11 (57.9)	0.61

*P is for the overall comparison across treatment groups. The mean ± SD are reported for continuous variables. The BMI is calculated as weight in kilograms divided by the square of the height in meters. Race was self-reported.

levels tended to be lower in gastric bypass versus IMT (46 vs. 77 pg/mL; P = 0.07) and were reduced in sleeve gastrectomy versus IMT (38 vs. 77 pg/mL; P < 0.02). However, at 24 months fasting glucagon levels were not different among the three groups (~60 pg/mL).

Postprandial glucagon levels reduced in all three groups at 24 months from baseline values, but postprandial glucagon levels in gastric bypass were higher (77 pg/mL) than IMT (64 pg/mL; P < 0.05) and not different between sleeve gastrectomy (65 pg/mL) and IMT.

Incretin responses

Median levels of GLP-1 60 minutes after mixed-meal ingestion (taking into account fasting levels) increased dramatically 24 months after gastric bypass (12.5 vs. 2 pmol/L; P < 0.001) and sleeve gastrectomy (7.3 vs. 2.4 pmol/L; P < 0.01) and did not change with IMT (1.5 vs. 1.4 pmol/L; P = not significant). In contrast, median levels of GIP in response to mixed meal were reduced 24 months after gastric bypass (13.5 vs. 30.7 pmol/L; P < 0.01) and were significantly different (P < 0.01) from sleeve gastrectomy (36.9 pmol/L) and IMT (29.7 pmol/L). Both surgical groups had an overall increase in the incremental change in median GLP-1 response to mixed meal as compared with IMT at 24 months (gastric bypass 10.0 pmol/L [quartile 1: 5.2; quartile 3: 15.2] vs. sleeve gastrectomy 4.5 pmol/L [quartile 1: 2.9; quartile 3: 8.2]; P = 0.07; vs. IMT −0.4 pmol/L [quartile 1: −1.8; quartile 3: 1.1]; P < 0.001 for

both). However, a reduction in GIP response was noted in gastric bypass only at 24 months (gastric bypass, −20 pmol/L [quartile 1: −44.2; quartile 3: −10.2] vs. IMT 5.4 pmol/L [quartile 1: −6.3; quartile 3: 30.4]; P < 0.001 vs. sleeve gastrectomy 0.6 pmol/L [quartile 1: −18.6; quartile 3: 33.2]; P = NS).

Metabolic determinants of HbA$_{1c}$ ≤6% at 24 months

A multivariate logistic model of metabolic parameters that were associated with HbA$_{1c}$ ≤6% at 24 months in the substudy cohort demonstrated that the fold increase in the oral disposition index (β-cell function) was associated with an increased odds ratio of 1.67 (CI 1.012–1.124; P = 0.016), and the increase in truncal fat was associated with a lower odds ratio of 0.878 (CI 0.777–0.991; P = 0.036) to achieve glycemic control at 24 months.

CONCLUSIONS—Two recent bariatric surgery studies have shown markedly improved glycemic control in surgically treated patients with obesity and type 2 diabetes compared with medical therapy (3,4). In one of those studies, the STAMPEDE trial, 1 year after randomization, patients assigned to bariatric surgery were significantly more likely to achieve an HbA$_{1c}$ level of 6% compared with patients treated using IMT alone (3). In the current metabolic substudy, we extended follow-up of the STAMPEDE trial patients to 2 years and sought to determine the durability of the initial results and to examine the metabolic adaptations responsible

for the improved glycemic control observed with bariatric surgery. We measured a wide range of metabolic parameters at three time points, at baseline, after the original 1-year follow-up, and repeated measurements 2 years after initial randomization.

After 2 years, gastric bypass provided more durable glycemic control with little or no need for glucose-lowering agents in patients randomized to this strategy. Despite comparable weight loss compared with sleeve gastrectomy, more durable glycemic control was achieved in patients randomized to gastric bypass, with a substantially greater percentage of patients attaining the target HbA$_{1c}$ levels of ≤6%. Attenuation of improvement in diabetes control was noted in the sleeve gastrectomy treatment group despite persistent weight loss. Other long-term observational studies have documented greater relapse rates for glycemic control after gastric restrictive procedures such as sleeve gastrectomy, suggesting that surgical weight loss from enforced caloric restriction itself is insufficient to halt the disease (14,15). Our results extend the findings from our initial 12-month report and suggest factors beyond weight loss that are specific to intestinal bypass patients help regulate glucose levels and restore pancreatic β-cell function.

Striking metabolic changes were observed in patients randomized to bariatric surgery compared with intensive medical therapy, particularly in the gastric bypass treatment group. At baseline, all randomized patients exhibited poor pancreatic secretory function. After both 1 and 2

Table 2—*Clinical changes at 12 and 24 months: glycemic and lipid control*

	IMT (N = 17)	Gastric bypass (N = 18)	Sleeve gastrectomy (N = 19)	P*	P†	P‡
HbA$_{1c}$ ≤6 (12 months)	1/16 (6.25)	8/18 (44.44)	5/19 (26.32)	0.02	0.19	0.25
HbA$_{1c}$ ≤ 6 (24 months)	1/17 (5.9)	6/18 (33.3)	2/19 (10.5)	0.09	1.00	0.12
HbA$_{1c}$ (%)						
Baseline	9.5 ± 1.73	9.8 ± 1.35	9.7 ± 1.95	0.54	0.74	0.84
12 months	8.1 ± 2.34	6.3 ± 0.78	6.9 ± 1.11	0.004	0.05	0.08
24 months	8.4 ± 2.33	6.7 ± 1.23	7.1 ± 0.84	0.01	0.04	0.18
Change from baseline	−1.1 ± 1.99	−3.1 ± 1.38	−2.5 ± 2.39	0.001	0.06	0.37
Fasting plasma glucose, median, IQR (mg/dL)§						
Baseline	180 (159–241)	211 (181–252)	164 (112–224)	0.19	0.30	0.04
12 months	129 (103–212)	93 (78–133.0)	97 (81–137)	0.05	0.09	0.81
24 months	134 (90–160)	87 (75–105)	104 (80–113)	0.03	0.04	0.34
Change from baseline	−33.0 (−96 to −4)	−124 (−157 to −100)	−70 (−116 to −8.0)	0.001	0.31	0.03
N of subjects using insulin at 24 months	10 (59)	1 (5.6)	2/18 (11.1)	0.001	0.003	1.0
HDL cholesterol (mg/dL)						
Baseline	45.4 ± 11.9	40.5 ± 9.6	40.7 ± 8.2	0.19	0.17	0.95
24 months	50.2 ± 9.2	54.3 ± 13.5	57.5 ± 16.4	0.30	0.12	0.53
Change from baseline	4.8 ± 7.2	13.8 ± 8.8	16.8 ± 13.0	0.002	0.002	0.43
Triglycerides (mg/dL), median (IQR)§						
Baseline	155 (118–221)	161 (97–257)	154 (104–176)	0.99	0.69	0.61
24 months	127 (94–145)	126 (63–153)	119 (82–158)	0.49	0.89	0.45
Change from baseline	−56.0 (−81 to −8)	−56.0 (−131 to −11)	−2.0 (−61 to 9)	0.41	0.36	0.06
High-sensitivity C-reactive protein (mg/L), median (IQR)§						
Baseline	3.6 (2.4–5.1)	3.8 (2.0–5.8)	6.0 (2.9–9.9)	0.99	0.05	0.10
24 months	3.1 (2.1–5.5)	0.5 (0.3–2.0)	1.5 (0.6–3.6)	0.001	0.02	0.04
Change from baseline	−0.1 (−0.8 to 2.1)	−2.6 (−4.4 to −0.6)	−2.4 (−8.4 to −1.4)	0.001	0.002	0.75
Body weight (kg)						
Baseline	107.9 ± 14.5	105.3 ± 13.6	100.0 ± 16.5	0.58	0.14	0.30
12 months	106.3 ± 14.7	77.6 ± 10.0	75.8 ± 12.5	<0.001	<0.001	0.63
24 months	107.4 ± 14.9	79.9 ± 11.7	77.5 ± 14.3	<0.001	<0.001	0.58
Change from baseline	−0.5 ± 4.09	−25.4 ± 10.32	−22.5 ± 8.79	<0.001	<0.001	0.37
BMI (kg/m^2)						
Baseline	35.8 ± 2.9	36.1 ± 2.6	36.4 ± 3.2	0.74	0.57	0.77
12 months	35.3 ± 3.3	26.7 ± 2.5	27.6 ± 2.5	<0.001	<0.001	0.27
24 months	35.6 ± 3.1	27.4 ± 2.9	28.2 ± 3.1	<0.001	<0.001	0.46
Change from baseline	−0.2 ± 1.41	−8.7 ± 3.13	−8.2 ± 3.01	<0.001	<0.001	0.66
Total body fat (%)						
Baseline	42.2 ± 4.5	41.1 ± 4.7	46.1 ± 4.9	0.48	0.02	0.003
12 months	42.0 ± 6.7	27.0 ± 8.5	36.0 ± 6.3	<0.001	0.01	0.001
24 months	43.3 ± 5.2	30.5 ± 8.5	38.4 ± 6.1	<0.001	0.01	0.003
Change from baseline	1.1 ± 1.7	−10.6 ± 6.6	−7.7 ± 3.5	<0.001	<0.001	0.11
Truncal fat (%)						
Baseline	49.1 ± 4.23	50.0 ± 5.45	51.8 ± 4.62	0.59	0.07	0.27
12 months	47.9 ± 6.65	29.7 ± 10.02	39.1 ± 6.49	<0.001	<0.001	0.002
24 months	50.0 ± 5.04	34.1 ± 9.66	41.7 ± 5.93	<0.001	<0.001	0.006
Change from baseline	0.9 ± 2.3	−15.9 ± 10.7	−10.1 ± 5.0	<0.001	<0.001	0.04
Leptin (ng/mL)§						
Baseline	24.9 (15.6–30.8)	24.0 (15.1–31.0)	29.6 (21.4–49.5)	0.93	0.18	0.10
12 months	24.9 (16.2–33.4)	4.9 (3.1–12.8)	10.4 (7.6–21.5)	<0.001	0.003	0.02
24 months	29.3 (21.2–37.8)	7.2 (3.1–15.3)	19.1 (11.2–26.8)	<0.001	0.006	0.01
Change from baseline	4.7 (1.9–10.0)	−11.2 (−22.3 to −8.8)	−16.2 (−21.1 to −4.6)	<0.001	<0.001	0.99

Unless otherwise specified, data are expressed as mean ± SD. IQR, interquartile range. *P for IMT vs. gastric bypass. †P for IMT vs. sleeve gastrectomy. ‡P for gastric bypass vs. sleeve gastrectomy. §P values were generated using the Wilcoxon test; otherwise, the Student *t* test was used.

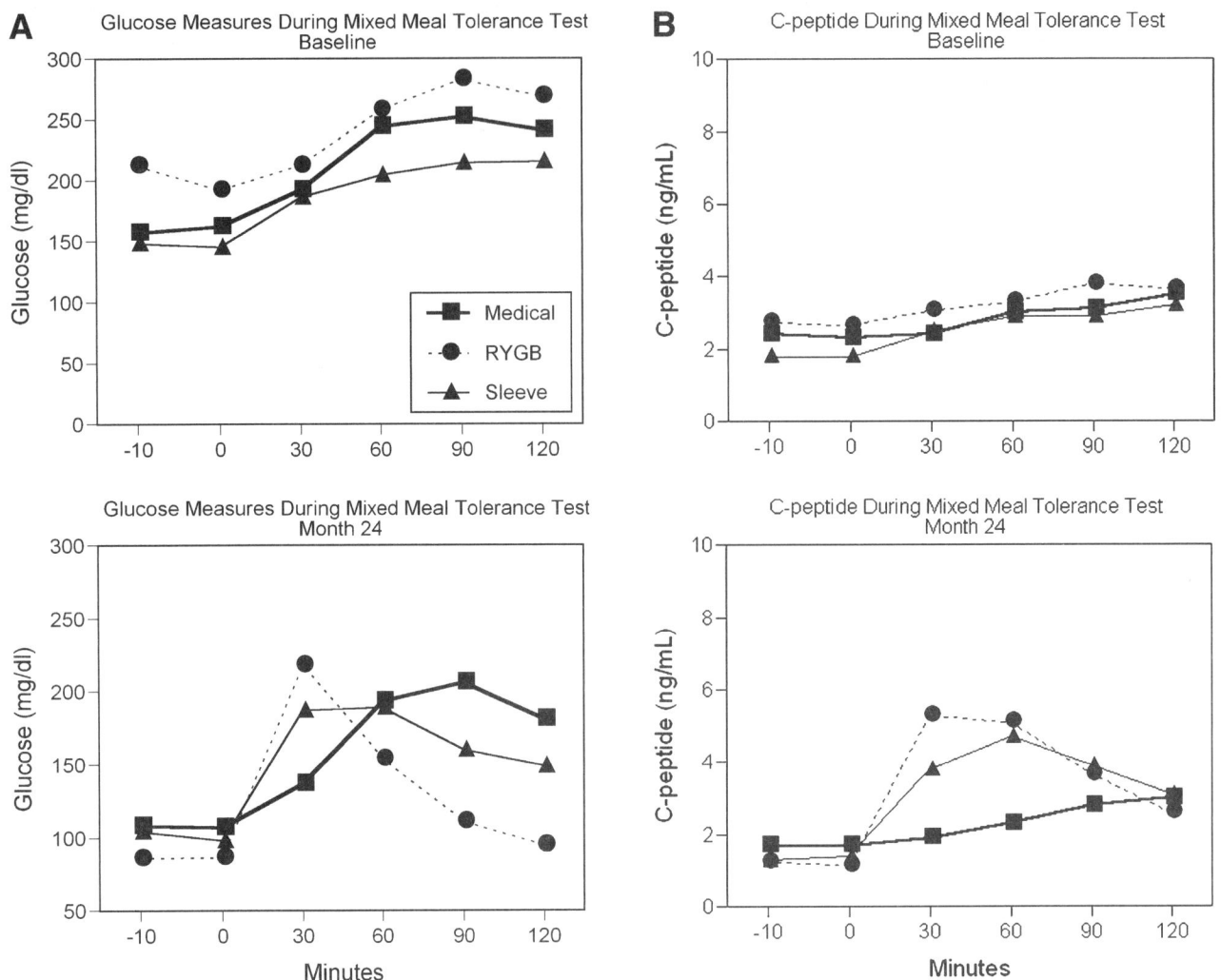

Figure 1—*Glucose* (A) *and C-peptide* (B) *during the mixed-meal tolerance test performed at time of randomization (baseline) and at 24 months after randomization for IMT, sleeve gastrectomy, and gastric bypass. Mixed meal consisted of Boost (8 ounces) with 30-min interval blood sampling for glucose and C-peptide values. Data are shown in median values. RYGB, Roux-en-Y gastric bypass.*

years of follow-up, gastric bypass patients achieved near-normal glucose tolerance after a physiological liquid mixed meal. These effects were associated with a remarkable 5.8-fold increase in overall pancreatic β-cell function. In gastric bypass patients, both insulin sensitivity and secretion components increased, but despite comparable weight loss in sleeve gastrectomy, insulin sensitivity was only partially restored and pancreatic β-cell function did not improve. Both bariatric surgery procedures stimulated incretins with markedly increased postprandial GLP-1 levels as noted in previous observational studies in obese patients with type 2 diabetes (8,9,16). However, divergence in postprandial GIP levels was noted, with a reduction seen only in gastric bypass that may be related to anatomical exclusion of the duodenum (which

produces GIP) or may be reflective of improved GIP action that is noted to be defective in type 2 diabetes (17).

The metabolic changes observed in these bariatric surgical patients are markedly different from previous studies performed in medically treated patients with type 2 diabetes and highlight the clinical value of improving β-cell function to achieve glycemic control. The UK Prospective Diabetes Study (UKPDS) demonstrated that pancreatic β-cell function continues to deteriorate over time despite diet, exercise, and administration of hypoglycemic agents (18). In UKPDS, the natural history of type 2 diabetes was characterized by an average increase in HbA$_{1c}$ level of 1% over 2 years despite the use of medications. In patients with well-controlled diabetes prescribed a single oral hypoglycemic agent, the mean

time of deterioration of glycemic control was 33–60 months (19). For patients using metformin and additionally prescribed a sulfonylurea, median HbA$_{1c}$ levels deteriorated as early as 6 months at a rate similar to that observed with metformin alone (20). These findings suggest that with continuing decline in β-cell function, single or even multiple agents are no longer sufficient to control blood glucose levels, which is why many patients ultimately require insulin therapy. For those who initiate insulin therapy, less than half achieve a desired HbA$_{1c}$ of ≤7% (21).

Although weight loss associated with hypocaloric diet has been shown to reduce insulin resistance, reduce hyperinsulinemia, and improve β-cell function (22–24), both bariatric surgery procedures displayed much larger postprandial insulinotropic effects compared with IMT. Greater insulin secretory effects of gastric bypass coupled with a nearly threefold improvement in insulin sensitivity likely account for complete normalization of postprandial glucose tolerance seen uniquely with gastric bypass patients. Lack of suppression of glucagon is known to contribute to postprandial hyperglycemia in diabetes (25), and, contrary to our expectation, bariatric surgery did not restore this defect. A slight increase in postprandial glucagon level was noted in gastric bypass, a finding consistent with a previous study (26).

Massive weight loss and reduction of adipose tissue mass clearly contribute to the major improvements in insulin sensitivity and cardiovascular risk profile observed after bariatric surgery. However, the marked improvements in insulin sensitivity and glycemic control observed in the gastric bypass group suggest factors specifically linked to the presence of abdominal (truncal) fat. Ectopic abdominal fat presence has long been recognized to induce insulin resistance, subclinical inflammation, and cardiovascular risk specific to type 2 diabetes (27,28). Previous studies also have demonstrated greater improvements in insulin sensitivity with intestinal bypass procedures (i.e., gastric bypass and biliopancreatic diversion) compared with BMI-matched nonsurgical patients, presumably because these procedures produce greater nutrient and fat malabsorption (29,30). In the current study, adipogenic inflammation was significantly reduced after both bariatric procedures, especially gastric bypass, mediated by factors such as free fatty acids, leptin, and C-reactive protein, which impair glucose uptake by insulin-dependent tissues (muscle and liver).

Although modest improvement in glycemic control, glucose metabolism, and clinical parameters was noted with IMT in our trial, more vigorous and behavioral/lifestyle modification strategies as used in the Look AHEAD trial (31) that aggressively target weight loss are clearly needed. Future randomized control trials are needed to compare such strategies results with bariatric surgery. However, maintaining weight loss in patients with diabetes who require insulin and other hypoglycemic agents is difficult in the "real world" clinical setting because conventional drug therapy generally results in weight gain. In addition, fear of hypoglycemia and patient burdens related to administration of multiple drugs

for diabetes and cardiovascular risk control presents significant barriers to implementing and adhering to IMT.

A limitation of this study is the validity of the incretin hormone responses that were obtained after the assigned interventions. Concentrations of GLP-1 and GIP were obtained at fasting and at 60 min after meal ingestion, and this likely underestimates the incretin surge that normally occurs rapidly (within 15 min) after meal ingestion. Nevertheless, large incremental changes in prandial GLP-1 levels and corresponding C-peptide levels were noted 2 years after both bariatric procedure types that were not observed with IMT. Further studies are warranted to thoroughly investigate the long-term effects of bariatric surgery on incretin responses and action to modulate insulin secretion. Additionally, insulin sensitivity determined by the Matsuda index was performed only in a subset of subjects not using exogenous insulin at baseline and followed trends similar to the whole cohort because insulin administration was withheld 24 h before meal testing.

In summary, bariatric surgery induces powerful metabolic effects in moderately obese patients with advanced type 2 diabetes inadequately controlled with currently available drug therapy. Bariatric surgery, particularly gastric bypass surgery, uniquely restores normal glucose tolerance and pancreatic β-cell function, presumably by targeting the truncal fat that represents the core metabolic defect involved in diabetes pathogenesis. Longer-term multicenter studies with safety outcomes are warranted to test the durability of these metabolic benefits.

Acknowledgments—Primary funding for the STAMPEDE trial is from Ethicon Endo-Surgery EES IIS 19900 (to P.R.S.). The American Diabetes Association clinical translational award (1-11-26 CT) to S.R.K. provided ancillary funding for STAMPEDE. A grant from the National Institutes of Health (R01-DK089547) to S.R.K., P.R.S., and J.P.K. was provided.

S.R.K. obtained research grants from Ethicon Endo-Surgery, National Institutes of Health, and American Diabetes Association. D.L.B. is a member of the Advisory Board for Medscape Cardiology, is on the Board of Directors for Boston VA Research Institute and Society of Chest Pain Centers, is the Chair of American Heart Association Get With The Guidelines Science Subcommittee, received honoraria from American College of Cardiology (Editor, Clinical Trials, Cardiosource), Duke Clinical Research Institute (clinical trial steering committees), Slack Publications

(Chief Medical Editor, Cardiology Today Intervention), and WebMD (CME steering committees), is the Senior Associate Editor of *Journal of Invasive Cardiology*, received research grants from Amarin, AstraZeneca, Bristol-Myers Squibb, Eisai, Ethicon, Medtronic, Sanofi, The Medicines Company, and FlowCo, and performed unfunded research for PLx Pharma and Takeda. D.L.B. receives honoraria from Ethicon Endo-Surgery as scientific advisory board member, consultant, and speaker, and has received honoraria from Covidien for speaking. J.P.K. receives grant funding from National Institutes of Health, Nestle Inc., and ScottCare. P.R.S. obtained research grants from Ethicon Endo-surgery, National Institutes of Health, and Bard-Davol; received educational grants from Stryker Endoscopy, Gore, Baxter, Covidien, and Allergan; and received honoraria from Ethicon Endo-surgery as a scientific advisory board member, consultant, and speaker. P.R.S. has been a consultant/advisory board member for RemedyMD, StrykerEndoscopy, Bard-Davol, Gore, Barosense, Surgiquest, and Carefusion. S.N. has consulted with Orexigen and Vivus. S.R.K., P.R.S., and the Cleveland Clinic Coordinating Center for Clinical Research had full and independent access to all of the data in the study. The sponsor participated in discussions regarding study design and protocol development and provided logistical support during the trial. The database, statistical analysis, and monitoring were all performed by the Cleveland Clinic Coordinating Center for Clinical Research. The manuscript was prepared by the corresponding author and modified after consultation with co-authors. The sponsor was permitted to review the manuscript and suggest changes, but the final decision on content and submission was exclusively retained by the academic authors. J. Michael Henderson, MD (Chair), James B. Young, MD, and Venu Menon, MD, Cleveland Clinic, Cleveland, Ohio, are members of the Data and Safety Monitoring Board. No other potential conflicts of interest relevant to this article were reported.

S.R.K. was responsible for the study concept and design, acquired data, provided administrative technical or material support, performed study supervision, analyzed and interpreted data, drafted the manuscript, and obtained funding. D.L.B. was responsible for the study concept and design and analysis, interpreted data, critically revised the manuscript for important intellectual content, provided administrative technical or material support, performed study supervision, and drafted the manuscript. K.W. analyzed and interpreted data, performed statistical analysis, and drafted the manuscript. R.M.W. analyzed and interpreted data. M.A-.G. analyzed and interpreted data. B.A. was responsible for subject recruitment and for carrying out the mixed-meal testing and DXA scan procedures. C.E.P. was responsible for the study concept and design, drafted the manuscript, and provided administrative technical or material support. S.B. was responsible for the study concept and design. S.N. was responsible for the study concept and design, analyzed and interpreted data, and critically revised manuscript for important intellectual content. M.G. acquired data. J.P.K. analyzed and interpreted data and critically revised the manuscript for important intellectual content. P.R.S. was responsible for study concept and design, acquired data, analyzed and interpreted data, critically revised the manuscript for important intellectual content, obtained funding, provided administrative technical or material support, and performed study supervision. S.R.K. is the guarantor of this work and, as such, had full access to all the data in the study and takes responsibility for the integrity of the data and the accuracy of the data analysis.

This work was presented as a late-breaking poster at the 72nd Scientific Sessions of the American Diabetes Association, Philadelphia, Pennsylvania, 8–12 June 2012.

The authors are grateful for the skilled nursing care provided by Sharon O'Keefe and to Chytaine Hall, both affiliated with the Endocrinology Institute at Cleveland Clinic, for performing the metabolic studies. The authors appreciate the skilled technical expertise of Sarah Neal (Lerner Institute, Cleveland Clinic) and the laboratory staff of Preventive Research Laboratory, a core reference laboratory under the guidance of Stanley Hazen, MD, PhD (Heart and Vascular Institute and Lerner Institute, Cleveland Clinic), for performing all gut and adipose cytokines. The authors thank Rose Lounsbury, BS, Clinical Endocrinology Laboratory (Endocrinology Institute, Cleveland Clinic), for performing the assays related to fatty acids and glucagon.

References

1. Danaei G, Finucane MM, Lu Y, et al.; Global Burden of Metabolic Risk Factors of Chronic Diseases Collaborating Group (Blood Glucose). National, regional, and global trends in fasting plasma glucose and diabetes prevalence since 1980: systematic analysis of health examination surveys and epidemiological studies with 370 country-years and 2·7 million participants. Lancet 2011; 378:31–40

2. Buchwald H, Oien DM. Metabolic/bariatric surgery Worldwide 2008. Obes Surg 2009;19:1605–1611

3. Schauer PR, Kashyap SR, Wolski K, et al. Bariatric surgery versus intensive medical therapy in obese patients with diabetes. N Engl J Med 2012;366:1567–1576

4. Mingrone G, Panunzi S, De Gaetano A, et al. Bariatric surgery versus conventional medical therapy for type 2 diabetes. N Engl J Med 2012;366:1577–1585

5. Gatmaitan P, Huang H, Talarico J, et al. Pancreatic islet isolation after gastric bypass in a rat model: technique and initial results for a promising research tool. Surg Obes Relat Dis 2010;6:532–537

6. Rubino F, Gagner M, Gentileschi P, et al. The early effect of the Roux-en-Y gastric bypass on hormones involved in body weight regulation and glucose metabolism. Ann Surg 2004;240:236–242

7. Rubino F, Forgione A, Cummings DE, et al. The mechanism of diabetes control after gastrointestinal bypass surgery reveals a role of the proximal small intestine in the pathophysiology of type 2 diabetes. Ann Surg 2006;244:741–749

8. Kashyap SR, Daud S, Kelly KR, et al. Acute effects of gastric bypass versus gastric restrictive surgery on beta-cell function and insulinotropic hormones in severely obese patients with type 2 diabetes. Int J Obes (Lond) 2010;34:462–471

9. Korner J, Bessler M, Inabnet W, Taveras C, Holst JJ. Exaggerated glucagon-like peptide-1 and blunted glucose-dependent insulinotropic peptide secretion are associated with Roux-en-Y gastric bypass but not adjustable gastric banding. Surg Obes Relat Dis 2007;3:597–601

10. Laferrère B, Teixeira J, McGinty J, et al. Effect of weight loss by gastric bypass surgery versus hypocaloric diet on glucose and incretin levels in patients with type 2 diabetes. J Clin Endocrinol Metab 2008; 93:2479–2485

11. Kashyap SR, Bhatt DL, Schauer PR; STAMPEDE Investigators. Bariatric surgery vs. advanced practice medical management in the treatment of type 2 diabetes mellitus: rationale and design of the Surgical Therapy And Medications Potentially Eradicate Diabetes Efficiently trial (STAMPEDE). Diabetes Obes Metab 2010;12:452–454

12. Van Cauter E, Mestrez F, Sturis J, Polonsky KS. Estimation of insulin secretion rates from C-peptide levels. Comparison of individual and standard kinetic parameters for C-peptide clearance. Diabetes 1992;41:368–377

13. Kanat M, Mari A, Norton L, et al. Distinct β-cell defects in impaired fasting glucose and impaired glucose tolerance. Diabetes 2012;61:447–453

14. Buchwald H, Estok R, Fahrbach K, et al. Weight and type 2 diabetes after bariatric surgery: systematic review and meta-analysis. Am J Med 2009;122:248–256, e5

15. Pournaras DJ, Aasheim ET, Søvik TT, et al. Effect of the definition of type II diabetes remission in the evaluation of bariatric surgery for metabolic disorders. Br J Surg 2012;99:100–103

16. Laferrère B, Heshka S, Wang K, et al. Incretin levels and effect are markedly enhanced 1 month after Roux-en-Y gastric bypass surgery in obese patients with type 2 diabetes. Diabetes Care 2007;30:1709–1716

17. Nauck MA, Heimesaat MM, Orskov C, Holst JJ, Ebert R, Creutzfeldt W. Preserved incretin activity of glucagon-like peptide 1 [7-36 amide] but not of synthetic human gastric inhibitory polypeptide in patients with type-2 diabetes mellitus. J Clin Invest 1993;91:301–307

18. U.K. Prospective Diabetes Study Group. U.K. prospective diabetes study 16. Overview of 6 years' therapy of type II diabetes: a progressive disease. Diabetes 1995;44:1249–1258

19. Kahn SE, Haffner SM, Heise MA, et al.; ADOPT Study Group. Glycemic durability of rosiglitazone, metformin, or glyburide monotherapy. N Engl J Med 2006;355: 2427–2443

20. Cook MN, Girman CJ, Stein PP, Alexander CM, Holman RR. Glycemic control continues to deteriorate after sulfonylureas are added to metformin among patients with type 2 diabetes. Diabetes Care 2005;28: 995–1000

21. Koro CE, Bowlin SJ, Bourgeois N, Fedder DO. Glycemic control from 1988 to 2000 among U.S. adults diagnosed with type 2 diabetes: a preliminary report. Diabetes Care 2004;27:17–20

22. Henry RR, Gumbiner B. Benefits and limitations of very-low-calorie diet therapy in obese NIDDM. Diabetes Care 1991;14: 802–823

23. Hofsø D, Jenssen T, Bollerslev J, et al. Beta cell function after weight loss: a clinical trial comparing gastric bypass surgery and intensive lifestyle intervention. Eur J Endocrinol 2011;164:231–238

24. Lim EL, Hollingsworth KG, Aribisala BS, Chen MJ, Mathers JC, Taylor R. Reversal of type 2 diabetes: normalisation of beta cell function in association with decreased pancreas and liver triacylglycerol. Diabetologia 2011;54:2506–2514

25. Shah P, Basu A, Basu R, Rizza R. Impact of lack of suppression of glucagon on glucose tolerance in humans. Am J Physiol 1999;277:E283–E290

26. Salehi M, Prigeon RL, D'Alessio DA. Gastric bypass surgery enhances glucagon-like peptide 1-stimulated postprandial insulin secretion in humans. Diabetes 2011;60:2308–2314

27. Azrad M, Gower BA, Hunter GR, Nagy TR. Intra-abdominal adipose tissue is independently associated with sex-hormone binding globulin in premenopausal women. Obesity (Silver Spring) 2012;20:1012–1015

28. Heshka S, Ruggiero A, Bray GA, et al.; Look AHEAD Research Group. Altered body composition in type 2 diabetes mellitus. Int J Obes (Lond) 2008;32:780–787

29. Bikman BT, Zheng D, Pories WJ, et al. Mechanism for improved insulin sensitivity after gastric bypass surgery. J Clin Endocrinol Metab 2008;93:4656–4663

30. Guidone C, Manco M, Valera-Mora E, et al. Mechanisms of recovery from type 2 diabetes after malabsorptive bariatric surgery. Diabetes 2006;55:2025–2031

31. Wadden TA, West DS, Delahanty L, et al.; Look AHEAD Research Group. The Look AHEAD study: a description of the lifestyle intervention and the evidence supporting it. Obesity (Silver Spring) 2006; 14:737–752

In Brief

The obesity paradox (survival advantage in overweight/obese patients with type 2 diabetes) has called into question the importance of weight loss in overweight people with diabetes. A systematic review of weight loss studies with a minimum of 1-year outcomes in people with diabetes reported inconsistent beneficial effects of weight loss on A1C, lipids, and blood pressure. To lower the risk of cardiovascular disease, a better nutrition therapy intervention may be reducing energy intake, which may or may not lead to weight loss, and selecting cardioprotective foods in appropriate portion sizes. However, any nutrition therapy intervention must be based on lifestyle changes the person with diabetes is willing and able to make.

The Obesity Paradox and Diabetes

Marion J. Franz, MS, RD, CDE

It is being called the "obesity paradox": research findings that people with obesity-related illnesses and who are overweight or obese have better outcomes, including less mortality, than their normal-weight peers.[1] These seemingly contradictory results have also been shown to apply to people with acute coronary syndrome, stroke, and diabetes.[2–9] The consequences of obesity are clear: increased risk for diabetes, high blood pressure, heart disease, stroke, and kidney disease.[10] So, the question of emerging interest becomes why, then, once the disease develops, does being overweight appear to be beneficial?

Flegal et al.,[1] in a systematic review and meta-analysis, reported that, in the general public, severe obesity was associated with an increased risk for death from all causes but that lesser amounts of excess weight either did not increase this risk or were protective. They concluded, ". . . excess mortality in obesity may predominantly be due to elevated mortality at higher body mass index (BMI) levels. Overweight was associated with significantly lower all-cause mortality." They further noted that these results are consistent with previous findings that have also shown lower mortality among overweight and moderately obese patients. Possible explanations include earlier medical care and aggressive risk factor treatment given to heavier patients, cardioprotective metabolic effects of increased body fat, and/or beneficial effects of higher metabolic reserves.[1]

A U-shaped association of weight with mortality is reported in people with diabetes. In a recent study,[4] the records of 106,640 people with type 2 diabetes in Scotland were reviewed and BMI recorded around the time of diagnosis and mortality throughout the next ~ 5 years was assessed. Mortality risk was higher in people with a BMI of 20 to < 25 kg/m^2 and in those with a BMI ≥ 35 kg/m^2. Vascular mortality was also higher for each 5-kg/m^2 increase in BMI > 30 kg/m^2 but was lower below this level. Another study[5] assessed the relationships between BMI and all-cause mortality in African-American and white men with type 2 diabetes and observed a significantly higher mortality risk (70%) in those with a BMI within the normal range (18.5–24.9 kg/m^2) than in heavier subjects, with a higher mortality rate in African Americans (95%) than in whites (53%). In a study of patients who developed diabetes,[6] total, cardiovascular, and noncardiovascular mortality rates were higher among normal-weight than among obese subjects. This finding was true regardless of diabetes type. Two other recent studies, Translating Research into Action for Diabetes[7] and the

PROactive trial,[8] also observed that participants who were of normal weight at the baseline examination or who lost weight during the trial (PROactive) experienced higher mortality than participants who were overweight or obese. This obesity paradox (survival advantage in obese patients with type 2 diabetes) was also shown to exist in patients with diabetes and cancer.[9] Similar findings had been reported in two earlier studies.[11,12] All of the above brings into question the role of weight management in people with chronic diseases, especially in people with diabetes.

Weight Loss/Management: Prevention Versus Treatment of Diabetes

The research results described above suggest that, perhaps, guidelines recommending weight loss should apply primarily to prevention and not necessarily to treatment of chronic diseases, including diabetes. Strong evidence exists for the benefits of moderate weight loss for the prevention of type 2 diabetes.[13] The question becomes, what are the benefits from weight loss as glycemic impairments progress from prediabetes to overt type 2 diabetes?

The goals of medical nutrition therapy (MNT) for individuals with diabetes include achieving and maintaining blood glucose levels in the normal range or as close to normal as is safely possible, a lipid and lipoprotein profile that reduces the risk for cardiovascular disease (CVD), and blood pressure levels in the normal range or as close to normal as is safely possible.[13] To achieve these goals, weight loss has been recommended for all overweight or obese individuals who have diabetes or are at risk for diabetes, with the level of evidence rated A (clear evidence from well-conducted, generalizable, randomized, controlled trials that are adequately powered).[14] But perhaps the benefits of weight loss in the treatment of type 2 diabetes need to be reexamined. An inconclusive picture emerges from review of the benefits of weight loss on A1C, lipids, and blood pressure in people with type 2 diabetes. This also brings into question the effects of weight loss on risk factors for the prevention and treatment of CVD in people with diabetes.

Weight Loss and Diabetes-Related Outcomes

A PubMed search was conducted to determine the outcomes from baseline to study completion of nutrition therapy weight loss interventions in overweight or obese adults with type 2 diabetes. Research was reviewed from 1 January 2000 to 1 February 2013. Eleven randomized, clinical trials with a completion rate of ≥ 70% and 12-month laboratory data reported were identified and are included in Table 1.[15–27] Because the duration of trials affects their outcomes, and to better compare outcomes among studies, 1-year outcomes are presented in the table for all trials. However, also included are data from two trials reporting 18-month data,[18,19] two with 2-year data,[23,24] and two with 4-year data.[21,25–27] One trial[21] did not report the statistical significance of intervention changes from baseline to study end, and one trial[25] reported statistical significance for the intervention arm only; however, both trials are included in the intervention summaries.

Eight of the studies compared varying weight loss interventions (10 different interventions),[17–24] and three studies compared the intervention to usual care or to a control group.[15,16,25,27] Weight loss interventions implemented in 19 study arms included meal replacements (2 studies),[15,17] individualized food plans (2 studies),[16,17] one study with two group behavioral weight management arms,[18] low fat (3 studies),[20,21,24] high monounsaturated fat (MUFA),[19] high carbohydrate (CHO) (3 studies),[19,22,23] low CHO (2 studies),[20,24] high protein (2 studies),[22,23] Mediterranean-style diet (MED),[21] and intensive lifestyle intervention (ILI).[25–27] Although physical activity was suggested or encouraged in several studies,[16,18,19,20,22] only two studies, those testing MED and ILI, included physical activity recommendations and measured and reported adherence.[21,25,27] Four studies[15,17,23,24] did not mention physical activity.

Weight changes

Weight losses from interventions ranged from 1.9 to 8.4 kg at 12 months; 16 of the interventions[15–24] reported weight losses ranging from 2.4 to 4.8 kg. The MED and ILI interventions reported the largest weight loss at 1 year, 6.2 and 8.4 kg, respectively,[21,25] and a low-CHO intervention reported the smallest, 1.9 kg.[24] In the trials reporting data collected for > 1 year, none of the average weight losses were back to baseline by the end of the studies.

A1C results

All of the studies reported the effect of weight loss on 1-year A1C values. Improvements in A1C were reported from eight of the weight loss interventions.[15,18,21,22,25] However, one of the trials extending to 18 months[18] reported significant improvements in A1C at 12 months that were not maintained to 18 months. The MED reported the largest improvement in A1C at 1 year, –1.2%,[21] and the ILI reported the second largest, –0.64%.[25] Significant improvements in A1C were also reported from the use of meal replacements[15] and one low-fat,[21] one high-protein,[22] and one high-CHO[22] study. At 4 years, the MED and ILI reported continued improvements in A1C, –0.9 and –0.36%, respectively.[21,27] Perhaps of equal importance is that nonsignificant changes in A1C were reported from 11 weight loss interventions at 1 year [16,17,19,20,23,24] and from one study at 18 months.[18]

Also of interest, five trials compared weight loss interventions with differing macronutrient percentages (high-MUFA vs. high-CHO,[19] low-CHO vs. low-fat,[20] high-protein vs. high-CHO,[22,23] and low-CHO vs. low-fat[24]). All five reported that weight changes did not differ statistically between arms, and weight losses ranged from 1.9 to 4.0 kg. Furthermore, eight of the intervention arms reported nonsignificant changes in A1C from baseline to study end,[19,20,23,24] and only two intervention arms (in one study) reported significant but modest changes in A1C.[22] These findings support a conclusion that a variety of eating patterns with differing macronutrient percentages are moderately effective for weight loss but may not improve A1C levels.

Weight loss interventions reporting improvements in A1C at 1 year had weight losses of 4.8, 4.2, 3.0, 2.7, 2.2, and 1.0 kg, with the MED (–6.2 kg, 7.2%) and ILI (8.4 kg, 8.6%) having larger weight losses. Weight loss interventions reporting no statistically significant improvement in A1C at 1 year had similar weight losses ranging from 1.9 to 4.4 kg. Although there is overlap in the weight loss effect on A1C, it does appear that larger amounts of weight lost are more likely to improve A1C; weight losses of ~ 7–8% are needed.

Lipid levels

Ten of the trials (11 weight loss intervention arms) measured lipid levels. The most consistently reported positive change was in HDL cholesterol. However, all but the ILI and MED reported nonsignificant changes in various lipids as a result of weight loss. HDL was reported for 17 of the interventions; 10 reported positive changes in HDL,[15,17,19,20–22,24,25] and 7 reported nonsignificant changes. Triglycerides were also reported for 17 interventions; 6 reported lowering of triglycerides,[17,21,22,25] and 11 reported nonsignificant changes. LDL cholesterol was reported from 15 interventions, with only the ILI reporting a positive change.[25] Total cholesterol was reported for 16 interventions, and only the MED resulted in a positive change.[21]

Blood pressure

Eight studies (14 weight loss interventions) reported the effect of weight loss on blood pressure. Five studies reported positive blood pressure changes,[15,19,21,24,25] and three studies reported no changes.[20,22,23]

Medication-related effects

Weight loss may also have an effect on dosage of anti-diabetes, lipid, and blood pressure medications. However, changes in these medications can also confound results of the nutrition therapy intervention. Limited data are available on medications taken at baseline and whether medication adjustments were made as a result of weight loss. Four trials did not report on medication changes;[15,18,19,23] two studies reported no change in medications in one study arm.[17,22] General decreases in medications were reported in seven studies from weight loss interventions.[16,17,20–22,24,25] Only one study reported an increase in medications and that was in the Look AHEAD trial control group for lipids and is noted in the next section.[27]

Look AHEAD (Action for Health in Diabetes) Trial

Because of its size and duration, it is important to summarize the Look AHEAD trial.[25–27] The trial, conducted in 16 centers in the United States and planned to last 11.5 years, was designed to test whether a lifestyle intervention resulting in weight loss would reduce rates of heart disease, stroke, and CVD deaths in overweight and obese people with type 2 diabetes, a group at increased risk for such events. Half of the 5,145 people enrolled in the study were randomly assigned to receive an ILI, and the other half were assigned to a control group that received a general program of diabetes support and education (DSE). Both groups received routine medical care from their own health care providers. Participants randomized to the ILI received meal replacements or structured food plans, were encouraged to achieve 175 minutes of physical activity per week, and attended three to four education/counseling sessions per month. At 4 years, participants in the ILI group averaged a weight loss of 4.7 kg compared to 1.1 kg in the control group.[27]

In September 2012, the National Institutes of Health stopped the ILI group early, acting on the recommendation of the study's data and safety monitoring board.[28] The independent advisory board found that the ILI did no harm but was not on a trajectory that would result in greater decreases in cardiovascular events compared to the control group. The board recommended continuing to follow all Look AHEAD participants to identify other potential longer-term effects of the intervention.

The benefits on A1C, HDL cholesterol, triglycerides, and blood pressure were significantly greater in the ILI group compared to the DSE group after 4 years (weight $P < 0.001$, A1C $P < 0.001$, HDL cholesterol $P < 0.001$, triglycerides $P < 0.001$, systolic blood pressure $P < 0.001$, and diastolic blood pressure $P = 0.01$), but reductions in LDL cholesterol were greater in the DSE group ($P = 0.009$) because of more aggressive use of medications to lower lipid levels in the this group.[27] It is encouraging and important to note that both groups had a lower number of cardiovascular events compared to previous studies of people with diabetes.[27]

MNT for Diabetes

So, if weight loss is not the complete nutrition therapy answer for improvements in cardiometabolic outcomes for diabetes, what other interventions have been reported to be beneficial? A systematic review was conducted to determine the effectiveness of MNT provided by a registered dietitian (or nutritionist) independently or as part of an overall diabetes self-management education (DSME) program. Although weight loss is sometimes reported, it is not the primary goal of the nutrition therapy interventions. Eleven studies published after 2000 reported improvements in A1C with independent MNT interventions, and seven studies showed improvement when MNT was part of DSME.[29] Randomized, clinical studies and observational outcome studies documented decreases in A1C of ~ 1–2% (range −0.5 to −2.6%), depending on the type and duration of diabetes and the baseline A1C value.

Of interest are the types of nutrition therapy interventions that are most effective. Interventions for people with type 2 diabetes include reduced energy/fat intake, individualized MNT, portion control and healthy food choices, and carbohydrate counting, and for people with type 1 diabetes, carbohydrate counting and matching insulin to carbohydrate intake. Although it is clear that there is not one nutrition therapy intervention that applies to all people with diabetes, a consistent theme for individuals with type 2 diabetes is that a reduced energy intake, which may or may not lead to substantial weight loss, consistently improves glycemic control.

An eating pattern designed to both lower glucose and improve lipids and blood pressure, along with regular physical activity, is the cornerstone of diabetes care.[30,31] A cardioprotective eating pattern provides 25–35% of calories from fat, with < 7% of calories from saturated and *trans* fatty acids. The majority of the fat intake is from unsaturated fatty acids. Cholesterol intake is ideally < 200 mg/day. Evidence indicates that this type of eating pattern can reduce total cholesterol by 7–21%, LDL cholesterol by 7–22%, and triglycerides by 11–31%.[32] In addition, controlling sodium intake to 2,400 mg/day has an approximate systolic blood pressure–lowering range of 2–8 mmHg.[31]

Although the ILI in the Look AHEAD trial resulted in weight loss and improved A1C, some lipids, and blood pressure, it did not improve these risk factors enough to result in better CVD protection than standard diabetes (education/medical) care. Equally important, it is not clear how

Table 1. Diabetes Weight Loss Trials: Outcomes of Interventions at 1 Year Compared to Baseline Values (Five Trials With > 1 Year Outcomes Also Reported)

Study	Subjects Enrolled (n [n of completers, percentage of completers])	Interventions	Weight Loss (kg)	A1C (%)	Lipids (mg/dl)	Blood Pressure (mmHg)
Metz et al.[15]	119 (92, 77%)	1. Prepared meal plan (meal replacements) 2. Usual care (reduced energy intake)	1. ↓3.0 ± 5.4 2. ↓1.0 ± 3.8	1. ↓0.24 ± 1.52 (P < 0.001) 2. ↓0.2 ± 1.30 (P < 0.001)	1. TC ↓6.2 ± 29.2, LDL ↑7.0 ± 26.7, HDL ↑1.9 ± 5.7, TG ↓14.2 ± 126 (all NS) 2. TC ↑1.0 ± 41.7, LDL ↓0.3 ± 24.6, HDL ↑0.3 ± 5.2, TG↑5.1 ± 274.0 (all NS)	1. SBP ↓8.8 ± 12.6 1. DBP↓5.1 ± 5.6 (both P < 0.001) 2. SBP ↓ .9 ± 13.2 2. DBP ↓3.8 ± 6.2 (both P < 0.001)
Wolf et al.[16]	144 (115, 80%)	1. Case management (individualized food plan) 2. Usual care	1. ↓2.4 (↓4.1 to ↓0.6) 2. ↑0.6 (↑1.0 to ↑2.2)	1. ↓0.1 (NS) 2. ↓0.09 (NS)	TC, LDL, HDL, TG (both groups NS changes)	Not reported
Li et al.[17]	104 (82, 79%)	1. Soy-based meal replacement 2. Individualized food plan	1. ↓4.4 ± 0.8 (P < 0.0001) 2. ↓2.4 ± 0.8 (P = 0.038)	1. ↓0.30 (NS) 2. ↓0.15 (NS)	1. TC ↓10.7, LDL ↓6.1, HDL ↑1.0 (all NS); TG ↓28 (P = 0.038) 2. TC ↓5.3, LDL ↑8.8, TG ↓28 (all NS); HDL ↑2.3 (P = 0.012)	Not reported
West et al.[18]	217 (195, 90% at 12 months)	1. Group behavioral weight management 2. Group behavioral weight management plus motivational interviewing	1. ↓2.7 ± 0.6 2. ↓4.8 ± 0.6	1. ↓0.6 ± 0.1 (P < 0.0001) 2. ↓0.4 ± 0.01 (P < 0.0001)	Not reported	Not reported
	217 (202, 90% at 18 months)		1. ↓1.7 ± 0.6 2. ↓3.5 ± 0.6	1. ↓0.2 ± 0.1 (NS) 2. ↓0.1 ± 0.1 (NS)		
Brehm et al.[19]	124 (95, 77% at 12 months)	1. High monounsaturated fat 2. High carbohydrate	1. ↓4.0 ± 0.8 (P < 0.01) 2. ↓3.8 ± 0.6 (P < 0.01)	1. ↑0.1 (NS) 2. No change (NS)	1. TC ↓5, LDL ↓3. TG ↓1 (all NS); HDL ↑5 (P < 0.01) 2. TC ↓2, LDL ↓3, HDL ↑5, TG ↓5 (all NS); HDL ↑5 (P < 0.01)	1. SBP ↓2 (NS) 1. DBP ↓5 (P < 0.01) 2. SBP ↓1 (NS) 2. DBP ↓4 (P < 0.01)
	57 (38, 67% at 18-month extension)		No significant change from 12 months	No significant change from 12 months	No significant changes from 12 months	No significant changes from 12 months
Davis et al.[20]	105 (85, 81%)	1. Low carbohydrate 2. Low fat	1. ↓3.1 ± 4.8 (P = 0.005) 2. ↓3.1 ± 5.8 (P = 0.005)	1. ↓0.02 ± 0.89 (NS) 2. ↑0.24 ± 1.4 (NS)	1. TC ↑3.9 ± 29.4, LDL ↓1.5, TG ↓13.3 (all NS); HDL ↑6.2 (P = 0.002) 2. TC ↓5.0 ± 27.1, LDL ↓7.0, TG ↓1.0, HDL ↑2.3 (all NS)	1. SBP ↑2.0 ± 15.6 1. DBP ↓2.9 ± 9.4 2. SBP ↓1.8 ± 22.6 2. DBP ↓2.3 ± 11.6 (all NS)

Study	n	Intervention			Lipids	Blood pressure
Esposito et al.[21]*	215 (195, 91% at 1 year)	1. Mediterranean-style diet (MED) 2. Low fat	1. ↓6.2 ± 3.2 2. ↓4.2 ± 1.9	1. ↓1.2 ± 1.0 2. ↓0.6 ± 0.6	1. TC ↓15.1 ± 14.7, HDL ↑3.9 ± 4.6, TG ↓39.0 ± 50.5 2. TC ↓5.8 ± 6.6, HDL ↑1.0 ± 0.8, TG ↓19.4 ± 40.0	1. SBP ↓5.1 ± 4.2 1. DBP ↓4.0 ± 3.0 2. SBP ↓2.0 ± 1.9 2. BP ↓1.0 ± 1.0
	215 (195, 91% at 4 years)		1. ↓3.8 ± 2.0 2. ↓3.2 ± 1.9	1. ↓0.9 ± 0.6 2. ↓0.5 ± 0.4	1. TC ↓9.7 ± 7.7, HDL ↑3.5 ± 3.1, TG ↓24.8 ± 24.6 2. TC ↓3.9 ± 7.9, HDL ↑1.0 ± 0.1, TG ↓6.2 ± 8.9	1. SBP ↓2.5 ± 2.6 1. DBP ↓2.9 ± 1.9 2. SBP ↓1.0 ± 1.0 2. DBP ↓1.5 ± 1.4
Larsen et al.[22]	108 (99, 92% at 1 year)	1. High protein 2. High carbohydrate	1. ↓2.2 (P < 0.001) 2. ↓2.2 (P < 0.001)	1. ↓0.23 (P < 0.001) 2. ↓0.28 (P < 0.001)	1. TC ↓5.8 (NS), LDL ↓1.9 (NS), HDL ↑3.1 (P = 0.008), TG ↓41.6 (P < 0.001) 2. TC ↓0.4 (NS), LDL ↓1.5 (NS), HDL ↑3.1 (P = 0.008), TG ↓26.6 (P < 0.001)	1. SBP ↓5.0 1. DBP ↓0.2 2. SBP ↓0.8 2. SBP ↓0.7 (all NS)
Krebs et al.[23]	419 (310, 74% at 12 months)	1. High protein 2. High carbohydrate	1. ↓3.2 (P < 0.001) 2. ↓2.4 (P < 0.001)	1. ↓0.18 (NS) 2. ↓0.20 (NS)	1. TC ↓3.9, LDL ↓2.3, HDL ↑0.8, TG ↓9.7 (all NS) 2. TC ↓2.7, LDL ↓3.1, HDL ↑0.8, TG ↑1.8 (all NS)	1. SBP ↓0.2 1. DBP ↓0.1 2. SBP ↓0.5 2. DBP ↓0.5 (all NS)
	419 (294, 70% at 24 months)		1. ↓3.9 (P < 0.001) 2. ↓3.0 (P < 0.001)	1. ↑0.1 (NS) 2. ↑0.1 (NS)	1. TC ↓9.2 (P = 0.02), LDL ↓6.6 (NS), HDL ↓0.4 (NS), TG ↓3.5 (NS) 2. TC ↓12.8 (P = 0.02), LDL ↓7.7 (NS), HDL ↑0.7 (NS), TG ↓0.9 (NS)	1.SBP ↑2.0 1. DBP ↓0.3 2. SBP ↑1.0 2. DBP ↓0.4 (all NS)
Guldbrand et al.[24]	61 (54, 89% at 12 months)	1. Low carbohydrate 2. Low fat	1. ↓1.9 (P < 0.001) 2. ↓3.9 (P < 0.001)	1. ↓0.2 (NS) 2. ↑0.1 (NS)	1. TC ↓7.7 (NS), LDL ↓7.7 (NS), HDL ↑4.3 (P = 0.024), TG ↓26.6 (NS) 2. TC 0.0 (NS), LDL ↓3.9 (NS), HDL ↑3.1 (P = 0.029), TG ↓8.9 (NS)	1. SBP ↓8 (P = 0.003) 1. DBP ↓6 (P = 0.002) 2. SBP ↓10 (P < 0.001) 2. DBP ↓8 (P < 0.001)
	61 (47, 77% at 24 months)		1. ↓2.0 (P = 0.020) 2. ↓2.9 (P = 0.002)	1. 0.0 (NS) 2. ↑0.2 (NS)	1. TC ↓3.9 (NS), LDL ↓11.6 (P = 0.020), HDL ↑8.9 (P < 0.001), TG ↓17.7 (NS) 2. TC ↓11.6 (NS), LDL ↓11.6 (P = 0.017), HDL ↑4.3 (P = 0.050), TG ↓8.9 (NS)	1. SBP ↓9 (P = 0.012) 1. DBP ↓5 (P = 0.004) 2. SBP ↓11 (P < 0.001) 2. DBP ↓6 (P = 0.001)
Look AHEAD Research Group[25-27]**	5,145 (4,959, 96% at 1 year)	1. Intensive lifestyle intervention (ILI) 2. Diabetes support/education (control)	1. ↓8.7 ± 6.9 (P < 0.0001) 2. ↓0.7 ± 4.8	1. ↓0.64 ± 1.02 (P < 0.0001) 2. ↓0.14	1. LDL ↓5.2 ± 28.63, HDL ↑3.4 ± 0.2, TG ↓30.3 ± 2.0 (all P < 0.0001) 2. LDL ↓5.7 ± 0.6, HDL ↑1.4 ± 0.1, TG ↓14.6 ± 1.8	1. SBP ↓6.8 ± 0.4 1. DBP ↓3.0 ± 0.2 (both P < 0.0001) 2. SBP ↓2.8 ± 0.3 2. DBP ↓1.8 ± 0.2
	5,145 (4,815, 94% at 4 years)		1. ↓4.7 ± 0.2 2. ↓1.1 ± 0.2	1. ↓0.36 (0.4–0.33) 2. ↓0.09 (0.13–0.06)	1. LDL ↓8.8 (12.1–10.4), HDL ↑3.7 (3.43–3.91), TG ↓25.6 (27.9–23.2) 2. LDL ↓9.2 (10.0–8.4), HDL ↑2.0 (1.73–2.22), TG ↓19.8 (22.11–23.21)	1. SBP ↓5.3 (5.8–4.96) 1. DBP ↓2.9 (3.2–2.7) 2. SPB ↓3.0 (3.4–2.5) 2. DBP ↓2.5 (2.8–2.2)

*Statistical significance from baseline not reported.
**Statistical significance from baseline only reported for 1-year ILI.
DBP, diastolic blood pressure; HDL, HDL cholesterol; LDL, LDL cholesterol; NS, not significant; PA, physical activity; SBP, systolic blood pressure; TC, total cholesterol; TG, triglycerides.

the intervention package might be delivered in a real-world medical setting. It involved weekly sessions for the first 6 months, sessions three times per month for the next 6 months, and, for years 2–4, at least monthly contact by telephone or e-mail, as well as a variety of ancillary group classes in between contacts.[27]

In contrast, the MED (plus physical activity) intervention, which also improved A1C, lipids, and blood pressure, involved monthly sessions for the first year and bimonthly sessions thereafter. An interesting side note is that, although the authors described the Mediterranean-style eating plan as low carbohydrate, the actual intent was to have the carbohydrate content be < 50% of the reduced daily energy, with added fat being 30–50 g of olive oil.[21] Reported intake at 1 year included an average carbohydrate intake of 43% of calories, protein 28%, polyunsaturated fats 29%, and saturated fats 10%. This could better be described as a moderate-carbohydrate eating pattern, which is typical of people with type 2 diabetes.[33]

In summary, the most common nutrition advice given to people with type 2 diabetes involves weight loss. But weight loss is atypically substantial (< 5%) over the long term and, even if successful, may not result in cardiometabolic outcomes as strong as clinicians and individuals with diabetes would like to see. More realistic and helpful nutrition advice for overweight individuals with diabetes may be to pay less attention to the scale and concentrate more on eating smaller portions while choosing healthy foods such as fruits, vegetables, whole grains, legumes, low-fat dairy products, lean meats, and unsaturated fats in appropriate portion sizes.

To prevent and treat CVD, nutrition therapy for diabetes, instead of focusing on weight loss, should focus on 1) nutrition interventions shown to improve metabolic outcomes (glycemia, lipids, and blood pressure), 2) prioritizing goals for individuals, 3) negotiating lifestyle changes individuals are willing and able to make, and 4) assisting patients in choosing appropriate portion sizes of foods shown to have health benefits.

References

[1]Flegal K, Kit B, Graubard B: Association for all-cause mortality with overweight and obesity using standard body mass index categories: systematic review and meta-analysis. *JAMA* 309:71–82, 2013

[2]Angerås O, Albertsson P, Karason K, Råmanddal T, Matejka G, James S, Lagervist B, Rosengren A, Omerovis E: Evidence for obesity paradox in patients with acute coronary syndrome: a report from the Swedish Coronary Angiography and Angioplastry Registry. *Eur Heart J* 34:345–353, 2013

[3]Doehner W, Schenkel J, Anke S, Springer J, Audebert H: Overweight and obesity are associated with improved survival, functional outcomes, and stroke recurrence after acute stroke or transient ischaemic attack: observations from the TEMPiS trial. *Eur Heart J* 34:268–277, 2013

[4]Logue J, Walker JJ, Leese G, Lindsay R, McKnight J, Morris A, Philip S, Wild S, Sattar N, on behalf of the Scottish Diabetes Research Network Epidemiology Group: Association between BMI measured within a year after diagnosis of type 2 diabetes and mortality. *Diabetes Care* 36:887–893, 2013

[5]Kokkinos P, Myers J, Faselies C, Doumas M, Kheifbek R, Nylen E: BMI-mortality paradox and fitness in African American and Caucasian men with type 2 diabetes. *Diabetes Care* 35:1021–1027, 2012

[6]Carnethon MR, De Chavez PJ, Biggs ML Lewis CE, Pankow JS, Bertoni AG, Golden SH, Liu K, Mukamal KJ, Campbell-Jenkins B, Dyer AR: Association of weight status with mortality in adults with incident diabetes. *JAMA* 308:581–590, 2012

[7]McEwen LN, Kim C, Karter AJ, Haan MN, Ghosh D, Llantz PM, Mangione CM, Thompson TJ, Herman WH: Risk factors for mortality among patients with diabetes. *Diabetes Care* 30:1736–1741, 2007

[8]Doehner W, Erdman E, Cairns R, Clark AL, Dormandy JA, Ferrannini E, Anker SD: Inverse relation of body weight and weight change with mortality and morbidity in patients with type 2 diabetes and cardiovascular co-morbidity: an analysis of the PROactive study population. *Int J Cardiol* 162:20–26, 2012

[9]Tseng CH: Obesity paradox: differential effects on cancer and noncancer mortality in patients with type 2 diabetes mellitus. *Atherosclerosis* 226:186–192, 2013

[10]Centers for Disease Control and Prevention: Overweight and obesity: causes and consequences. Available from http://www.cdc.gov/obesity/adult/causes/index.html. Accessed 10 February 2013

[11]Klein R, Klein BE, Moss SE: Is obesity related to microvascular and macrovascular complications in diabetes? The Wisconsin Epidemiologic Study of Diabetic Retinopathy. *Arch Intern Med* 157:650–656, 1997

[12]Ross C, Langer RD, Barrett-Connor E: Given diabetes, is fat better than thin? *Diabetes Care* 20:650–652, 1997

[13]American Diabetes Association: Nutrition recommendations and interventions for diabetes: a position statement of the American Diabetes Association. *Diabetes Care* 31 (Suppl. 1):S61–S78, 2008

[14]American Diabetes Association: Standards of medical care in diabetes—2013 (Position Statement). *Diabetes Care* 36 (Suppl. 1):S11–S66, 2013

[15]Metz JA, Stern JS, Kris-Etherton P, Reusser ME, Morris CD, Hatton DC, Haynes B, Resnick LM, Pi-Sunyer X, Clark S, Chester L, McMahon M, Snyder GW, McCarron DA: A randomized trial of improved weight loss with a prepared meal plan in overweight and obese patients. *Arch Intern Med* 160:2150–2158, 2000

[16]Wolf AM, Conaway MR, Crowther JQ, Hazen KY, Nadler JL, Oneida B, Bovbjerg VE: Translating lifestyle intervention to practice in obese patients with type 2 diabetes. *Diabetes Care* 27:1570–1576, 2004

[17]Li Z, Hong K, Saltsman P, DeShields S, Bellman M, Thames G, Liu Y, Wang H-J, Elashoff R, Heber D: Long-term efficacy of soy-based meal replacement vs an individualized diet plan in obese type II DM patients: relative effects on weight loss, metabolic parameters, and C-reactive protein. *Eur Jr Clin Nutr* 59:411–418, 2005

[18]West DS, DiLillo V, Bursac Z, Gore SA, Greene PG: Motivational interviewing improves weight loss in women with type 2 diabetes. *Diabetes Care* 30:1081–1087, 2007

[19]Brehm BJ, Lattin BL, Summer SS, Boback JA, Gilchrist GM, Jandacek RJ, D'Alessio DA: One-year comparison of a high-monounsaturated fat diet with a high-carbohydrate diet in type 2 diabetes. *Diabetes Care* 32:215–220, 2009

[20]Davis NJ, Tomuta N, Schechter C, Isasi CR, Segal-Isaacson CJ, Stein D, Zonszein JZ, Wylie-Rosett J: Comparative study of the effects of a 1-year dietary intervention of a low-carbohydrate diet versus a low-fat diet on weight and glycemic control in type 2 diabetes. *Diabetes Care* 32:1147–1152, 2009

[21]Esposito K, Maiorino MI, Ciotola M, Di Paol C, Scognamiglio P, Gicchino M, Petrizzo M, Saccomanno F, Beneduce F, Ceriello A, Giufliano D: Effects of a Mediterranean-style diet on the need for antihyperglycemic drug therapy in patients with newly diagnosed type 2 diabetes: a randomized trial. *Ann Intern Med* 151:306–314, 2009

[22]Larsen RN, Mann NJ, Maclean E, Shaw JE: The effect of a high-protein, low-carbohydrate diets in the treatment of type 2 diabetes: a 12 month randomized controlled trial. *Diabetologia* 54:731–740, 2011

[23]Krebs JD, Elley CR, Parry-Strong A, Lunt H, Drury PL, Bell DA, Robinson E, Moyes SA, Mann JI: The Diabetes Excess Weight Loss (DEWL) Trial: a randomized controlled trial of high-protein versus high-carbohydtate diets over 2 years in type 2 diabetes. *Diabetologia* 55:905–914, 2012

[24]Guldbrand H, Dizdar B, Bunjaku B, Lindström T, Bachrach-Lindström M, Fredrikson M, Fredrikson M, Östgren CJ, Nystrom FH: In type 2 diabetes, randomization to advice to follow a low-carbohydrate diet transiently improves glycaemic control compared with advice to follow a low-fat diet producing similar weight loss. *Diabetologia* 55:2118–2127, 2012

[25]Look AHEAD Research Group: Reduction in weight and cardiovascular disease risk factors in individuals with type 2 diabetes: one-year results of the Look AHEAD trial. *Diabetes Care* 30:1374–1383, 2007

[26]Wing RR, Lang W, Wadden TA, Safford M, Knowler WC, Bertoni AG, Hill JO, Brancati FL, Peters A, Wagenknecht L, The Look AHEAD Research Group: Benefits of modest weight loss in improving cardiovascular risk factors in overweight and obese individuals with type 2 diabetes. *Diabetes Care* 34:1481–1486, 2011

[27]Look AHEAD Research Group: Long-term effects of a lifestyle intervention on weight and cardiovascular risk factors in individuals with type 2 diabetes mellitus: four-year results of the Look AHEAD trial. *Arch Intern Med* 170:1566–1575, 2010

[28]National Institute of Diabetes and Digestive and Kidney Diseases: Weight loss does not lower heart disease risk from type 2 diabetes.

Available from http://www.nih.gov/news/health/oct2012/niddk-19.htm. Accessed 13 February 2013

[29]Pastors JG, Franz MJ: Effectiveness of medical nutrition therapy in diabetes. In *American Diabetes Association Guide to Nutrition Therapy for Diabetes*. 2nd ed. Franz MJ, Evert AB, Eds. Alexandria, Va., American Diabetes Association, 2012, p. 1–18

[30]Karmally E, Zimmerman JS: Nutrition therapy for diabetes and lipid disorders. In *American Diabetes Association Guide to Nutrition Therapy for Diabetes*. 2nd ed. Franz MJ, Evert AB, Eds. Alexandria Va., American Diabetes Association, 2012, p. 265–294

[31]Aebersold K, Ostrovsky N, Wylie-Rosett J: Nutrition therapy for diabetes and hypertension. In *American Diabetes Association Guide to Nutrition Therapy for Diabetes*. 2nd ed. Franz MJ, Evert AB, Eds. Alexandria

Va., American Diabetes Association, 2012, p. 295–306

[32]Academy of Nutrition and Dietetics: Disorders of lipid metabolism evidence-based nutrition practice guidelines update, 2010. Available from http://www.adaevidence library.com/topic.ctm?cat=4528. Accessed 20 February 2013

[33]Vitolins MZ, Anderson AM, Delahanty L, Raynor H, Miller GD, Mobley C, Reeves R, Yamamoto M, Champagne C, Wing RR, Mayer-Davis E, and the Look AHEAD Research Group: Action for Health in Diabetes (Look AHEAD) Trial: baseline evaluation of selected nutrients and food groups. *J Am Diet Assoc* 109:1367–1375, 2009

Marion J. Franz, MS, RD, CDE, is a nutrition/health consultant at Nutrition Concepts by Franz, Inc., in Minneapolis, Minn.

In Brief

Diabetes is considered a risk equivalent for coronary heart disease (CHD). The use of statins for primary and secondary prevention in patients with diabetes is well established and supported by robust data from randomized, controlled trials and national guidelines. The American Diabetes Association recommends that individuals with diabetes and a history of cardiovascular disease (CVD), as well as those > 40 years of age without CVD but with CVD risk factors, should be treated with a statin regardless of their baseline LDL cholesterol concentration. This review explains the rationale behind considering diabetes a CHD risk equivalent and summarizes the data for statin use in adults with diabetes without (primary prevention) and with (secondary prevention) established CVD. Although individuals with diabetes are at an increased risk for CVD and benefit from statin therapy, the risk of CVD in people with diabetes is heterogeneous. It therefore may be reasonable to match the intensity of statin therapy with patients' baseline CVD risk.

The Role of Statins in Diabetes Treatment

Bishnu H. Subedi, MD, Rajesh Tota-Maharaj, MD, Michael G. Silverman, MD, C. Michael Minder, MD, Seth S. Martin, MD, M. Dominique Ashen, NP, Roger S. Blumenthal, MD, and Michael J. Blaha, MD, MPH

Diabetes is a leading public health concern. More than 8% of the U.S. population has diabetes, with the incidence and prevalence expected to increase during the next several years.[1,2] Of particular concern is the increased risk of developing incident coronary heart disease (CHD) and the increased risk of cardiac death.[3] In fact, two out of three adults with diabetes who are > 65 years of age die as a result of CHD, and this risk increases steeply with the addition of other risk factors.[4,5]

Based on observations that patients with type 2 diabetes and no history of myocardial infarction (MI) have the same risk of MI and CHD mortality as patients without diabetes with a prior MI,[6] current guidelines consider diabetes a CHD risk equivalent, thereby elevating it to the highest risk group in terms of predicted 10-year event rates.[7,8] Although most long-term observation studies have consisted of patients with type 2 diabetes, a similar increased risk of cardiovascular disease (CVD) has been shown among patients with type 1 diabetes.[9]

Guidelines for Statin Therapy in Diabetes
The classification of diabetes as a CHD risk equivalent has had implications for CVD prevention strategies. Joint American Heart Association and American Diabetes Association (ADA) guidelines[10] recommend adding a statin to lifestyle changes regardless of baseline lipid levels in patients with diabetes who are > 40 years of age and have one or more traditional risk factors. For patients < 40 years of age who have multiple CVD risk factors, guidelines suggest consideration of a statin in addition to lifestyle therapy if LDL cholesterol remains > 100 mg/dl. If treated patients do not reach the above targets on maximal tolerated statin therapy, a reduction in LDL cholesterol of 30–40% from baseline is an alternative therapeutic target. For adults with diabetes who have overt CVD, there are uniform recommendations for targeting an LDL cholesterol of < 100 mg/dl with an optional goal of < 70 mg/dl using higher-potency statins.[10,11]

Heterogeneity of CVD Risk
Although people with diabetes have an increased CVD risk, not all individuals with diabetes carry an identical increased risk. The highest-risk group includes those with prior ischemic events, followed by those with stable atherosclerosis and those with diabetes and multiple risk factors without identifiable CVD. Tailoring therapy based on individual risk, rather than follow-

ing a uniform treatment approach for diabetes patients, may result in better treatment outcomes, fewer medication side effects, and a more cost-effective therapy regimen.[12] Therefore, risk stratification remains vital to finding those patients at highest risk who could benefit from a more aggressive strategy.

An individualized risk approach is also important to optimize treatment in people who are already on drug therapy. One recent study[13] found that 14% of Veteran Affairs patients were "over-treated" with statins without any indication of being at higher risk,

implying the need for adjusting the intensity of treatment to the level of risk with the use of appropriate clinical performance measures.

Evidence for the Use of Statins in Patients With Diabetes

Primary prevention trials in diabetes
Current clinical practice is based on relatively few randomized, control trials. Among these studies[14-22] are the Heart Protection Study (HPS),[14] the Collaborative Atorvastatin Diabetes Study (CARDS),[15] the Anglo-Scandinavian Cardiac Outcomes Lipid Lowering Arm (ASCOT-LLA),[16]

the Antihypertensive and Lipid Lowering Treatment to Prevent Heart Attack (ALLHAT) study,[17] and the Management of Elevated Cholesterol in the Primary Prevention Group of Adult Japanese (MEGA) trials.[18] All of these studies included a substantial portion of subjects with diabetes. A few key primary prevention trials are summarized in Table 1.

The HPS provided initial evidence for the routine use of statin therapy in diabetes patients at risk for major CVD events. Patients with nonfasting total cholesterol > 135 mg/dl were randomized to 40 mg simvas-

Table 1. Summary of Nine Primary Prevention Trials in Diabetes

Clinical Trials	Publication Year	Age at Enrollment (years)	Study Group	Diabetes Subjects (n)		Statin Type and Dose	Mean Follow-Up (years)	Sites
				Type 1	Type 2			
WOSCOPS[19]	1996	45–64	Primary prevention (men)	8	68	Pravastatin, 40 mg	4.9	Scotland
AFCAPS[20]	2000	Male: 45–73 Female: 55–73	Primary prevention	0	155	Lovastatin, 20–40 mg	5.2	United States
HPS[14]	2003	40–80	High-risk	615	5,348	Simvastatin, 40 mg	5.3	United Kingdom
PROSPER[21]	2002	70–82	Elderly	51	572	Pravastatin, 40 mg	3.2	Scotland, Ireland, and the Netherlands
ALLHAT[17]	2002	> 55	Hypertension	0	3,638	Pravastatin, 20–40 mg	4.8	United States and Canada
ASCOT-LLA[16]	2003	40–79	Hypertension	0	2,527	Atorvastatin, 10 mg	3.3	United Kingdom, Ireland, and Nordic countries
CARDS[15]	2004	40–75	Type 2 diabetes	3	2,835	Atorvastatin, 10 mg	4	United Kingdom and Ireland
MEGA[18]	2006	40–70	Hyperlipidemia	0	3,866	Pravastatin, 10–20 mg	5.3	Japan
ASPEN[22]	2006	40–75	Primary prevention	0	2,410	Atorvastatin, 10 mg	4	Europe, Australia, and North America

AFCAPS, Air Force/Texas Coronary Atherosclerosis Prevention Study; ALLHAT, Antihypertensive and Lipid Lowering Treatment to Prevent Heart Attack; ASCOT-LLA, Anglo-Scandinavian Cardiac Outcomes—Lipid Lowering Arm; ASPEN, Atorvastatin Study for Prevention of CHD Endpoints in Non-Insulin-Dependent Diabetes; CARDS, Collaborative Atorvastatin Diabetes Study; HPS, Heart Protection Study; MEGA, Management of Elevated Cholesterol in the Primary Prevention Group of Adult Japanese; PROSPER, Prospective Study of Pravastatin in the Elderly at Risk; WOSCOPS, West of Scotland Coronary Prevention Study.

tatin daily versus a matching placebo. Statin-treated diabetes patients had a 22% (95% CI 13–30%) relative risk reduction (event rate 20.2 vs. 25.1%). Similar reductions were seen in those without baseline occlusive arterial disease and those with baseline LDL cholesterol levels < 116 mg/dl.[14]

The ASCOT-LLA addressed lipid lowering in hypertensive patients in a 2 × 2 factorial analysis with atorvastatin, 10 mg, versus placebo. A baseline diagnosis of diabetes was present in 2,532 participants. Over a median follow-up of 3.3 years, there were 116 major CVD events (9.2%) in atorvastatin-allocated diabetes patients and 151 events (11.9%) in the placebo group (hazard ratio [HR] 0.77, 95% CI 0.61–0.98).[16]

The CARDS trial enrolled patients with type 2 diabetes with at least one additional risk factor, including hypertension, retinopathy, proteinuria, or smoking. This trial randomized 2,838 patients to atorvastatin, 10 mg daily, versus placebo. Relative risk reductions by individual outcomes were 36% for acute coronary events, 31% for coronary revascularizations, and 48% for stroke. Treatment would be expected to prevent 37 major vascular events (MVEs) per 1,000 patients treated for 4 years. Compared to placebo, the absolute risk reduction with atorvastatin was similar in patients with LDL cholesterol concentrations > 120 or < 120 mg/dl (reduction from 9.5 to 6.1% vs. reduction from 8.5 to 3.6%). Like HPS, CARDS supported treatment of patients with type 2 diabetes and other CVD risks with statin therapy regardless of their baseline LDL cholesterol level.[15]

The MEGA trial[18] assigned 8,214 men and postmenopausal women with a total cholesterol of 220–270 mg/dl to receive diet therapy or diet plus pravastatin, 10–20 mg/day, over a mean of 5.3 years. Interestingly, the diabetes group had a nonsignificant reduction in events. However, in further analysis,[23] when authors included the "impaired fasting glucose" group and made a large group called "abnormal fasting glucose," the reduction in events became significant (HR 0.68, 95% CI 0.48–0.96) with a number needed to treat (NNT) of 42. These results may suggest that the relative benefits of statin therapy in an Asian population are similar to those seen in American and European populations.

The Steno-2 Study[24] showed that a multifactorial intervention (lipid-lowering therapy, aspirin, renin-angiotensin inhibition, and tight glucose control) significantly reduced CVD mortality (HR 0.43, 95% CI 0.19–0.94) and events (0.41, 0.25–0.67) among 160 patients with type 2 diabetes and microalbuminuria over a mean of 7.8 years. This study demonstrated that early implementation of statin treatment as part of a multifaceted approach to risk reduction achieves large reductions in absolute risk and thus a lower NNT. This made primary prevention strategies incorporating statin therapy as part of a multifactorial approach in diabetes patients a key therapy in modern medicine.

The ASPEN trial[22] did not find a significant difference in composite CVD or CHD outcomes when atorvastatin, 10 mg, versus placebo was used in a population with type 2 diabetes over a mean of 4 years. The negative results may be related to the overall study design, the lower statin dose, the nature of the primary endpoint, and the protocol changes required because of changing treatment guidelines.

Secondary prevention trials in diabetes

Among secondary prevention trials, A to Z,[25] PROVE- IT TIMI 22 (Pravastatin or Atorvastatin Evaluation and Infection Therapy—Thrombolysis in Myocardial Infarction 22),[26] TNT (Treating to New Targets),[27] and IDEAL (Incremental Decrease in End Points through Aggressive Lipid Lowering)[28] comprise the preponderance of evidence in contemporary clinical practice. Other relevant secondary prevention trials are summarized in Table 2.[29–35]

In diabetes patients with an acute coronary syndrome, the early initiation of aggressive statin treatment results in a favorable trend toward reduction of major CVD events with an NNT of 77 over a median of 2 years.[25] Additionally, intensive therapy to maintain an LDL cholesterol level < 70 mg/dl provides greater protection against recurrent major events than moderate lipid lowering. In the PROVE-IT TIMI 22 trial,[26] patients were randomized to 40 mg pravastatin or 80 mg atorvastatin after an ST segment elevation MI, a non-ST segment

elevation MI, or high-risk unstable angina; 18% of the trial population had diabetes. The median LDL cholesterol level achieved during treatment was 95 mg/dl in the standard-dose pravastatin group and 62 mg/dl in the high-dose atorvastatin group (P < 0.001). Over a mean 24 months of follow-up, a 16% reduction in the HR in favor of atorvastatin in the entire cohort (P = 0.005) was observed with a nonsignificant 5.8% reduction in the diabetes subgroup.

In the TNT (Treating to New Targets) trial,[27] 1,501 patients with diabetes, stable CHD, and LDL cholesterol levels < 130 mg/dl were randomized to 10 or 80 mg atorvastatin and followed for a median of 4.9 years. A 25% reduction in rates of serious events was observed in the high-dose group (HR 0.75, 95% CI 0.58–0.97). This finding reinforced the benefit of intensive lipid lowering, even in patients with stable CHD.

In the IDEAL trial,[28] 8,888 patients with a history of acute MI were randomized to receive high-dose atorvastatin (80 mg) or usual-dose simvastatin (20 mg), and 12% of the patients in each arm had diabetes. A total of 10.4% of the simvastatin group had significant coronary events, as opposed to 9.3% in the atorvastatin group (HR 0.89, 95% CI 0.78–1.01). Nonfatal acute MI occurred in 7.2 and 6.0% in the two groups, respectively (HR 0.83, 95% CI 0.71–0.98). Although there was no statistical difference in outcomes between 20 mg simvastatin and 80 mg atorvastatin, this study cautiously concluded that patients who have had an MI may benefit from intensive lowering of LDL cholesterol without an increase in non-CVD mortality or other serious adverse reactions.

Meta-analyses of statin trials in diabetes

Several meta-analyses have clearly shown the benefits of statin therapy for either short-term (< 5 years) or long-term (> 10 years) cardiovascular outcomes in primary prevention.[36] These benefits not only apply to people at higher risk (> 10%) but also to the lower-risk population.[37] This argument is especially valid in people with diabetes.[38]

In 2008, the Cholesterol Treatment Trialists (CTT) group[39] analyzed 14 trials to ascertain the effects of statins on patients with diabe-

Table 2. Summary of Seven Secondary Prevention Trials

Clinical Trials	Publication Year	Age at Enrollment (years)	Study Group	Diabetes Subjects		Statin Type	Mean Follow-Up (years)	Sites
				Type 1	Type 2			
4S[29]	1994	35–70	CHD	24	178	Simvastatin, 20–40 mg	5.4	Scandinavia
CARE[30]	1998	21–75	Post-MI	193	393	Pravastatin, 40 mg	5	United States and Canada
Post-CABG[31]	1999	54–69	CABG	27	89	Lovastatin, 2.5–80 mg	4.3	United States
LIPID[32]	1998	31–75	CHD	106	676	Pravavastin, 40 mg	6.1	Australia and New Zealand
GISSI-P[33]	2004	60	Post-MI	120	462	Pravastatin, 20 mg	2	Italy
LIPS[34]	2005	60–70	Post-PCI	39	163	Fluvastatin, 80 mg	3.9	Europe, Canada, and Brazil
ALERT[35]	2003	40–60	Renal transplant	280	116	Fluvastatin, 40 mg	5.1	Europe and Canada

4S, Scandanavian Simvastatin Survival Study; ALERT, Assessment of Lescol in Renal Transplant; CABG, Coronary Artery Bypass Graft; CARE, Cholesterol and Recurrent Events; GISSI-P, Gruppo Italiano per lo Studio della Sopravvivenza nell'Infarto Miocardico-Prevenzione; LIPID, Long-Term Intervention with Pravastatin in Ischemic Disease; LIPS, Lescol Intervention Prevention Study

tes. Four primary prevention trials (HPS, ASCOT-LLA, CARDS, and ALLHAT-LLT; see Table 1) accounted for 14,996 (83%) of the 18,686 patients with diabetes. During a mean follow-up of 4.3 years, per 39 mg/dl lowering of LDL cholesterol, the proportional reduction in all-cause mortality was 9% (rate ratio 0.91, 99% CI 0.82–1.01). This outcome was primarily driven by a significant 21% reduction in vascular mortality (rate ratio 0.87, 99% CI 0.76–1.00) with no effect on nonvascular mortality (rate ratio 0.97, 99% CI 0.82–1.16). However, this study did not include major adverse events from microvascular complications (neuropathy or retinopathy) or metabolic disturbances (incidence of diabetic ketoacidosis or nonketotic hyperglycemia). The proportional effects of statins in people with diabetes with vascular disease (secondary prevention) or without vascular disease (primary prevention) were similar. After 5 years, 42 (95% CI 30–55) fewer people had MVEs per 1,000 among those considered to be at high risk (> 10%).

A 2009 study[40] reviewed 10 primary prevention trials for benefits of statins across age, sex, and lower-risk diabetes populations. Over a mean follow-up of 4.1 years, treatment with statins significantly reduced the risk of all-cause mortality (odds ratio [OR] 0.88, 95% CI 0.81–0.96), major coronary events (OR 0.70, 95% CI 0.61–0.81), and major cerebrovascular events (OR 0.81, 95% CI 0.71–0.93) similarly among all clinical subgroups.

A 2012 study[41] explored the net effects of statins in people at low risk of vascular events. In this analysis, 7% of subjects with diabetes had a risk of < 5%, and 10% of subjects with diabetes had risk of 5–10%. There were significant reductions in MVEs in both lower-risk groups (among the < 5% group, rate ratio 0.61, 99% CI 0.45–0.81); among the 5–10% group, rate ratio 0.66, 99% CI 0.57–0.77) over a median of 5 years.

A recent review[42] meticulously examined the patients with diabetes without known CVD in seven primary prevention trials. It showed that statin therapy was associated with a significant reduction of major CVD and cerebrovascular events (OR 0.79, 95% CI 0.66–0.95), but no statistical difference in all-cause mortality.

These three meta-analyses indicate that there likely are some benefits of treating even low-risk people with diabetes. Some experts have suggested that it may be important to revise guidelines to address the important population of patients at low to intermediate risk who could substantially benefit from statins.

In 2010, the CTT[43] also analyzed the effects of intensive versus standard statin regimens (five trials, 39,612 individuals, median follow-up 5.1 years) and of statin versus control (21 trials, 129,526 individuals, median follow-up 4.8 years). Fourteen percent of people in the more versus less intensive regimen and 19% of people in the statin versus control group had diabetes. Among diabetes patients, an intensive regimen was associated with significant reduction in CVD events compared to standard treatment in both type 1 (4.5 vs. 6.0%; rate ratio 0.77, 99% CI 0.58–1.01) and type 2 diabetes (4.2 vs. 5.1%, rate ratio 0.80, 99% CI 0.74–0.86). Regardless of whether patients with at least one risk factor have documented CHD, the use of a higher-potency generic statin in lowering of LDL cholesterol to < 70 mg/dl appears to be both safe and efficacious. These benefits accrue without increasing noncoronary mortality.[44]

It should be noted that a 2010 review[45] showed that there was no definite statistically significant difference in all-cause mortality across 11 primary prevention trials. In contrast to the 2008 analysis performed by the CTT, this review included the ASPEN trial, a negative clinical outcome trial in people with diabetes. Notably, this 2010 article did not examine nonfatal CVD or CHD outcomes. Because of methodological differences in the populations included and the statistical models, other recent meta-analyses[46,47] do show a statistically significant decrease in total mortality with statin therapy in the primary prevention setting.

Non-LDL Targets of Statin Therapy in Diabetes

Although a 20–30% relative CVD reduction is impressive, this means that 70–80% of residual CVD risk persists despite statin treatment.[48] The residual risk in treated patients with diabetes can be attributed to a number of factors, some of which may be potentially related to lipoproteins, including apolipoprotein B (Apo-B) or LDL particle concentration, but the vast majority of the residual risk is likely related to nonlipid factors. Apo-B is considered the key atherogenic moiety.[49] In an analysis studying markers of CVD risk, Apo-B (risk ratio 1.43, 95% CI 1.35–1.51) outperformed non-HDL (1.34, 1.24–1.44), which outperformed LDL (1.25, 1.18–1.33).[50]

Patients with diabetes often have normal LDL levels but increased triglycerides, non-HDL cholesterol, and Apo-B, which may contribute to their high vascular risk despite largely normal LDL levels.[51] This suggests that the risk in those patients with elevated levels of LDL particles may be underestimated by solely measuring cholesterol levels, although routinely calculated LDL for guiding treatment is less accurate compared to direct measurement, especially in hypertriglyceridemia.[52] Apo-B or LDL particle concentration may be

Table 3. ADA/ACC Consensus Targets: Lipoprotein Therapy[53]

Cardio-Metabolic Risk	Goals		
	LDL (mg/dl)	Non-HDL (mg/dl)	Apo-B (mg/dl)
Highest-risk patients, including those with 1. Known CVD or 2. Diabetes plus one or more additional major CVD risk factors	< 70	< 100	< 80
High-risk patients, including those with 1. No diabetes or known clinical CVD but two or more additional major CVD risk factors or 2. Diabetes but no other major CVD risk factors	< 100	< 130	< 90

Other major risk factors (beyond dyslipoproteinemia) include smoking, hypertension, and family history of premature CAD.

set as additional targets for many patients after lipoprotein cholesterol targets have been reached. An ADA and American College of Cardiology statement[53] recommends consideration of measuring Apo-B in addition to LDL and non-HDL cholesterol in patients on lipid-lowering therapy. It further recommends an Apo-B target of < 80 mg/dl (Table 3).

Approach to Statin Intensification, Statin Intolerance, and Patient Preference

When it is unclear whether a patient has CHD and might benefit from an LDL goal of < 70 mg/dl, one should assess whether there is potential benefit from statin intensification. Use of coronary artery calcium (CAC) may prove helpful in guiding the intensity of statin therapy in diabetes. CAC is related to ongoing disease burden[54] and is an independent predictor of CVD in diabetes.[55,56] The absence of CAC remains associated with an excellent 7-year prognosis, whereas CAC > 100 portends a worse prognosis.[57] Prediction of CHD events in diabetes is improved by CAC compared to traditional risk factors (HR 6.2 vs. 2.9, P < 0.05).[58] In patients reporting side effects in association with statin therapy or hesitating to initiate therapy, CAC might be used to better quantify CVD risk and guide more informed risk-benefit discussions between patients and providers.

For example, based on a recent meta-analysis,[59] people with a CAC of < 10 are 6.8 times less likely to a have a CVD event. These patients do not

meet conventional criteria for high risk or even intermediate risk, reinforcing the heterogeneity of risk in diabetes. At this time, a CAC score of 0 among individuals with diabetes may lead a provider to withhold aspirin therapy.[57] However, it should not lead to withholding of statin therapy based on the robust data at all levels of risk.[36] A less potent statin may be a reasonable choice for people with mild intolerance and those who would not prefer statin therapy because of low CAC scores.

Role of Statins in Diabetes With Renal Disease

Dyslipidemia is common in people with diabetes and chronic kidney disease (CKD). CVD events are a frequent cause of morbidity and mortality in this population. A 2009 review[60] showed that statins significantly reduce the risk of all-cause and CVD mortality in CKD patients who are not receiving renal replacement therapy. A 2011 trial[61] suggested that lowering LDL with statins reduces the risk of major atherosclerotic events in patients with moderate to severe kidney disease, including those with diabetes. Guidelines[62] recommend using statins to reduce the risk of major CVD events in patients with diabetes and CKD, including those who have received a kidney transplant. However, it is recommended that statins not be initiated in patients with diabetes who are already treated by dialysis, mainly because of a more than fivefold increased risk of hemorrhagic strokes in this population.[63]

Statins and Incident Diabetes Risk

Statin therapy is associated with an increase in the risk of hyperglycemia and diabetes. In one meta-analysis, statins were associated with a 9% increased risk (an absolute difference of about 0.4%) of developing diabetes. To cause a new case of diabetes, 255 patients would have to be treated for a mean of 4 years.[64] Compared to low-dose therapy, intensive therapy is associated with a 12% increase in risk of diabetes with a number needed to harm of 498 per year.[65] People > 65 years of age are more susceptible to this unwanted effect.[66] In a post hoc analysis of the Women's Health Initiative study,[67] statin treatment among postmenopausal women was associated with increased risk of diabetes (HR 1.48, 95% CI 1.38–1.59). A 2013 meta-analysis[68] showed that various types and doses of statins show different potential to increase the incidence of diabetes; more potent statin therapy increases the risk of statin-induced hyperglycemia.

The statin and diabetes link was investigated in the Justification for the Use of Statins in Prevention: an Intervention Trial Evaluating Rosuvastatin (JUPITER) study, which found a 27% increase in physician-reported, new-onset diabetes in patients receiving rosuvastatin.[69] A 2012 analysis[70] of the trial showed that individuals with at least one diabetes risk factor were at higher risk of developing diabetes during the study. Overall, the time to diagnosis of diabetes was accelerated by 5.4 weeks in the rosuvastatin group. However, this trial has potential for reporting bias among the placebo arm. For example, it is possible that patients on statin therapy could have experienced more contact with their care providers because of unreported side effects

from statins (e.g., myalgias), leading to earlier diagnosis of diabetes.[71]

Statin therapy may accelerate the eventual expected rise of glucose values in people with multiple components of the metabolic syndrome. In the JUPITER study, 77% of participants had impaired fasting glucose, and a significant number of participants had metabolic syndrome and prediabetes (A1C > 5.7%) at baseline in the rosuvastatin arm.[66] In a review of three atorvastatin trials,[72] four risk factors independently predicted new-onset diabetes: fasting glucose > 100 mg/dl, triglycerides > 150 mg/dl, BMI > 30 kg/m^2, and history of hypertension).

A recent study[73] examined the incidence of diabetes and CVD events according to these baseline risk factors. Compared to lower-dose therapy, atorvastatin, 80 mg/day, did not increase the incidence of diabetes in patients with none or one risk factor but did, by 24%, among patients with two to four risk factors. However, the number of CVD events was significantly reduced with atorvastatin, 80 mg/day, in both risk groups. Several analyses have shown that cardiovascular and mortality benefits of statin therapy exceed the diabetes risk, including in participants at high risk of developing diabetes.[66,70]

From a clinical standpoint, there is no evidence that elevation in blood glucose while taking statins is associated with an increased risk of CVD events or that it attenuates the beneficial effects of the statin therapy.[70,73] The evidence from individual clinical trials is mixed. Clinicians must interpret this information cautiously because many potentially confounding factors are involved. There is a lack of data for microvascular disease and glycemic control in patients with

existing diabetes. All statin trials have been less than rigorous in terms of diagnosing diabetes. (Almost all relied on physician report or nontraditional means of diagnosis.) None of these trials was designed to look for diabetes.[71]

Perhaps statin therapy uncovers diabetes only in people at risk for diabetes. Improved survival benefit with statins may allow more people at risk for diabetes to live long enough to actually develop and have it diagnosed, whereas those without statins may die before ever developing or being diagnosed with diabetes.[74]

There is still no clear mechanism for the increased risk for diabetes. Although statin-prescribing practices should not change because of the modest diabetes risk, it is clear that patients being prescribed statins should be informed of their potential future diabetes risk, and this may provide added incentive to undertake sustained lifestyle changes. Following such advice could help to alleviate their diabetes risk and further reduce their CVD risk.[75]

Conclusions

There are clear benefits of statins as a class effect in patients with diabetes. In primary prevention, guidelines maintain that diabetes is often a CHD risk equivalent, and this strategy guides a generally aggressive approach to statin therapy. The benefits of statin therapy among individuals with diabetes and elevated CVD risk are clearly established.

Importantly, not all patients with diabetes have an identically elevated risk. Thus, additional risk stratification is an option to ensure identification of the highest-risk individuals who would benefit most from an aggressive primary prevention strategy. Advanced risk stratification, for example, with

Table 4. Key Clinical Practice Points

- Statins provide risk reduction in a wide range of patients with diabetes who either have established CVD or are at high risk of developing atherothrombosis.
- All patients with diabetes and established CHD should be prescribed a statin unless contraindicated.
- All diabetes patients who are at a higher risk of CVD should receive a statin regardless of their baseline lipid levels. Men > 50 years and women > 60 years who have diabetes and one other CVD risk factor should probably get a statin.
- The main goal of statin therapy is to achieve an LDL level of < 100 mg/dl and, ideally, < 70 mg/dl using higher-dose statins or 30–40% LDL reduction when earlier targets cannot be met with maximum tolerated therapy.
- Diabetes patients at apparent low to low-intermediate risk could be considered for further risk stratification, for example, with coronary artery calcium scoring.
- At every patient encounter, lifestyle modification should be addressed emphatically to help reduce the incident diabetes risk from statins as well as overall CVD risks.

CAC testing, can integrate risk factor information and potentially identify patients for earlier intervention.

Such risk stratification also has a potential role in the clinical approach to statin intensification, statin intolerance, and patient reluctance to take statins. Most patients in randomized clinical trials have been 40–80 years of age and had similar reductions in CVD morbidity and mortality irrespective of sex, race, geographical location, or other CVD risk factors. The absolute benefit will vary based on patients' underlying risk.

Despite treatment with statins, a large burden of residual risk remains. Some degree of residual risk may be addressed by personalizing statin therapy through more accurate lipoprotein cholesterol assessment, using targets such as non-HDL, Apo-B, and LDL lipoprotein particle size. Nevertheless, residual risk may also be attributed to other risk factors. At this time, it is probably most cost-effective to strive for non-HDL targets with a potent generic statin.

Ultimately, careful risk-benefit analysis should guide the use of statin therapy. Regarding potential risks, there is evidence of mild hyperglycemia and a small risk of incident diabetes, particularly among patients with metabolic syndrome who are prescribed high-potency statins. However, pooled analyses from existing trials have demonstrated that the benefit accrued from statin therapy far outweighs the small potential risk of hyperglycemia or diabetes, particularly in those at the highest CVD risk. (Key clinical points are summarized in Table 4.)

References

[1]Centers for Disease Control and Prevention: National diabetes fact sheet, 2011. Available from http://www.cdc.gov/diabetes/pubs/pdf/ndfs_2011.pdf. Accessed 27 May 2013

[2]National Institute of Diabetes and Digestive and Kidney Diseases: National diabetes statistics, 2011. Available from http://diabetes.niddk.nih.gov/dm/pubs/statistics. Accessed 31 December 2012

[3]Sarwar N, Gao P, Seshasai SR, Gobin R, Kaptoge S, Di Angelantonio E, Ingelsson E, Lawlor DA, Selvin E, Stampfer M, Stehouwer CD, Lewington S, Pennells L, Thompson A, Sattar N, White IR, Ray KK, Danesh J: Diabetes mellitus, fasting blood glucose concentration, and risk of vascular disease: a collaborative meta-analysis of 102 prospective studies. Lancet 375:2215–2222, 2010

[4]Udell JA, Scirica BM, Braunwald E, Raz I, Steg PG, Davidson J, Hirshberg B, Bhatt DL: Statin and aspirin therapy for the prevention of cardiovascular events in patients with type 2 diabetes mellitus. Clin Cardiol 35:722–729, 2012

[5]Stamler J, Wentworth D, Vaccaro O, Neaton JD: Diabetes, other risk factors and 12-yr cardiovascular mortality for men screened in the Multiple Risk Factor Intervention Trial. Diabetes Care 16:434–444, 1993

[6]Haffner SM, Lehto S, Rönnemaa T, Pyörälä K, Laakso M: Mortality from coronary heart disease in subjects with type 2 diabetes and in nondiabetic subjects with and without prior myocardial infarction. N Engl J Med 339:229–234, 1998

[7]Expert Panel on Detection, Evaluation, and Treatment of High Blood Cholesterol in Adults: Third report of the Expert Panel on Detection, Evaluation, and Treatment of High Blood Cholesterol in Adults (Adult Treatment Panel III). Circulation 106:3143–3421, 2002

[8]Perk J, De Backer G, Gohlke H, Graham I, Reiner Z, Verschuren M, Albus C, Benlian P, Boysen G, Cifkova R, Deaton C, Ebrahim S, Fisher M, Germano G, Hobbs R, Hoes A, Karadeniz S, Mezzani A, Prescott E, Ryden L, Scherer M, Syvänne M, Scholte op Reimer WJ, Vrints C, Wood D, Zamorano JL, Zannad F: European guidelines on cardiovascular disease prevention in clinical practice (version 2012). The Fifth Joint Task Force of the European Society of Cardiology and Other Societies on Cardiovascular Disease Prevention in Clinical Practice. Eur Heart J 223:1635–1701, 2012

[9]Krolewski AS, Kosinski EJ, Warram JH, Leland OS, Busick EJ, Asmal AC, Rand LI, Christlieb AR, Bradley RF, Kahn CR: Magnitude and determinants of coronary artery disease in juvenile-onset, insulin-dependent diabetes mellitus. Am J Cardiol 59:750–755, 1987

[10]Buse JB, Ginsberg HN, Bakris GL, Clark NG, Costa F, Eckel R, Fonseca V, Gerstein HC, Grundy S, Nesto RW, Pignone MP, Plutzky J, Porte D, Redberg R, Stitzel KF, Stone NJ: Primary prevention of cardiovascular diseases in people with diabetes mellitus: a scientific statement from the American Heart Association and the American Diabetes Association. Circulation 115:114–126, 2007

[11]Reiner Z, Catapano AL, De Backer G, Graham I, Taskinen MR, Wiklund O, Agewall S, Alegria E, Chapman MJ, Durrington P, Erdine S, Halcox J, Hobbs R, Kjekshus J, Filardi PP, Riccardi G, Storey RF, Wood D: ESC/EAS guidelines for the management of dyslipidaemias: the Task Force for the Management of Dyslipidaemias of the European Society of Cardiology (ESC) and the European Atherosclerosis Society (EAS). Eur Heart J 32:1769–1818, 2011

[12]Madanieh R, Hasan RK, Anusionwu OF, Blumenthal RS, Blaha MJ: Cardiovascular disease prevention: matching evidence-based algorithms with individualized care. Clin Pharmacol Ther 93:2–4, 2013

[13]Beard AJ, Hofer TP, Downs JR, Lucatorto M, Klamerus ML, Holleman R, Kerr EA: Assessing appropriateness of lipid management among patients with diabetes mellitus: moving from target to treatment. Circ Cardiovasc Qual Outcomes 6:66–74, 2013

[14]Collins R, Armitage J, Parish S, Sleigh P: MRC/BHF Heart Protection Study of cholesterol-lowering with simvastatin in 5963 people with diabetes: a randomised placebo-controlled trial. Lancet 361:2005–2016, 2003

[15]Colhoun HM, Betteridge DJ, Durrington PN, Hitman GA, Neil HA, Livingstone SJ, Thomason MJ, Mackness MI, Charlton-Menys V, Fuller JH: Primary prevention of cardiovascular disease with atorvastatin in type 2 diabetes in the Collaborative Atorvastatin Diabetes Study (CARDS): multicentre randomised placebo-controlled trial. Lancet 364:685–696, 2004

[16]Sever PS, Dahlöf B, Poulter NR, Wedel H, Collins R, Beevers G, Caulfield M, Kjeldsen SE, Kristinsson A, McInnes GT, Mehlsen J, Nieminen M, O'Brien E, Ostergren J: Prevention of coronary and stroke events with atorvastatin in hypertensive patients who have average or lower-than-average cholesterol concentrations in the Anglo-Scandinavian Cardiac Outcomes Trial — Lipid Lowering Arm (ASCOT-LLA): a multicentre randomized trial. Lancet 361:1149–1158, 2003

[17]ALLHAT Collaborative Research Group: Major outcomes in moderately hypercholesterolemic, hypertensive patients. JAMA 288:2998–3007, 2002

[18]Nakamura H, Arakawa K, Itakura H: Primary prevention of cardiovascular disease with pravastatin in Japan (MEGA Study): a prospective randomised controlled trial. Lancet 368:1155–1163, 2006

[19]Davis DR: Prevention of coronary heart disease with pravastatin in men with hypercholesterolemia. N Engl J Med 334:1302–1306, 1996

[20]Gotto AM Jr, Whitney E, Stein EA, Shapiro DR, Clearfield M, Weis S, Jou JY, Langendörfer A, Beere PA, Watson DJ, Downs JR, de Cani JS: Relation between baseline and on-treatment lipid parameters and first acute major coronary events in the Air Force/Texas Coronary Atherosclerosis Prevention Study (AFCAPS/TexCAPS). Circulation 101:477–484, 2000

[21]Shepherd J, Blauw GJ, Murphy MB, Bollen EL, Buckley BM, Cobbe SM, Ford I, Gaw A, Hyland M, Jukema JW, Kamper AM, Macfarlane PW, Meinders AE, Norrie J, Packard CJ, Perry IJ, Stott DJ, Sweeney BJ, Twomey C, Westendorp RG: Pravastatin in Elderly Individuals at Risk of Vascular Disease (PROSPER): a randomised controlled trial. Lancet 3560:1623–1630, 2002

[22]Knopp RH, D'Emden M, Smilde JG, Pocock SJ: Efficacy and safety of atorvastatin in the prevention of cardiovascular end points in subjects with type 2 diabetes: the Atorvastatin Study for Prevention of Coronary Heart Disease Endpoints in Non-Insulin-Dependent Diabetes Mellitus (ASPEN). Diabetes Care 29:1478–1485, 2006

[23]Tajima N, Kurata H, Nakaya N, Mizuno K, Ohashi Y, Kushiro T, Teramoto T, Uchiyama S, Nakamura H: Pravastatin reduces the risk for cardiovascular disease in Japanese hyper-

cholesterolemic patients with impaired fasting glucose or diabetes: diabetes subanalysis of the Management of Elevated Cholesterol in the Primary Prevention Group of Adult Japanese. *Atherosclerosis* 199:455–462, 2008

[24]Gaede P, Lund-Andersen H, Parving H-H, Pedersen O: Effect of a multifactorial intervention on mortality in type 2 diabetes. *N Engl J Med* 358:580–591, 2008

[25]de Lemos JA, Blazing MA, Wiviott SD, Lewis EF, Fox KA, White HD, Rouleau JL, Pedersen TR, Gardner LH, Mukherjee R, Ramsey KE, Palmisano J, Bilheimer DW, Pfeffer MA, Califf RM, Braunwald E: Early intensive vs a delayed conservative simvastatin strategy in patients with acute coronary syndromes: phase Z of the A to Z trial. *JAMA* 292:1307–1316, 2004

[26]Cannon CP, Bruanwald E, McCabe C, Rader DJ, Rouleau JL, Belder R, Joyal SV, Hill KA, Pfeffer MA, Skene AM: Intensive versus moderate lipid lowering with statins after acute coronary syndromes. *N Engl J Med* 350:1495–1504, 2004

[27]Waters DD, Guyton JR, Herrington DM, McGowan MP, Wenger NK, Shear C: Treating to New Targets (TNT) study: does lowering low-density lipoprotein cholesterol levels below currently recommended guidelines yield incremental clinical benefit? *Am J Cardiol* 93:154–158, 2004

[28]Pedersen TR, Faergeman O, Kastelein JJP, Olsson AG, Tikkanen MJ, Holme I, Larsen ML, Bendiksen FS, Lindahl C, Szarek M, Tsai J: High-dose atorvastatin vs usual-dose simvastatin for secondary prevention after myocardial infarction: the IDEAL study: a randomized controlled trial. *JAMA* 294:2437–2445, 2005

[29]Scandinavian Simvastatin Survival Study Group: Randomised trial of cholesterol lowering in 4444 patients with coronary heart disease: the Scandinavian Simvastatin Survival Study (4S). *Lancet* 344:1383–1389, 1994

[30]Goldberg RB, Mellies MJ, Sacks FM, Moyé LA, Howard BV, Howard WJ, Davis BR, Cole TG, Pfeffer MA, Braunwald E: Cardiovascular events and their reduction with pravastatin in diabetic and glucose-intolerant myocardial infarction survivors with average cholesterol levels: subgroup analyses in the Cholesterol And Recurrent Events (CARE) trial. *Circulation* 98:2513–2519, 1998

[31]Hoogwerf BJ, Waness A, Cressman M, Canner J, Campeau L, Domanski M, Geller N, Herd A, Hickey A, Hunninghake DB, Knatterud GL, White C: Effects of aggressive cholesterol lowering and low-dose anticoagulation on clinical and angiographic outcomes in patients with diabetes: the Post Coronary Artery Bypass Graft Trial. *Diabetes* 48:1289–1294, 1999

[32]Keech A, Colquhoun D, Best J, Kirby A, Simes RJ, Hunt D, Hague W, Beller E, Arulchelvam M, Baker J, Tonkin A: Secondary prevention of cardiovascular events with long-term pravastatin in results from the LIPID trial. *Diabetes Care* 26:2713–2721, 2003

[33]Tavazzi L, Tognoni G, Franzosi MG, Latini R, Maggioni AP, Marchioli R, Nicolosi GL, Porcu M: Rationale and design of the GISSI heart failure trial: a large trial to assess the effects of n-3 polyunsaturated fatty acids and rosuvastatin in symptomatic congestive heart failure. *Eur J Heart Fail* 6:635–641, 2004

[34]Arampatzis CA, Goedhart D, Serruys PW, Saia F, Lemos PA, de Feyter P: Fluvastatin reduces the impact of diabetes on long-term outcome after coronary intervention: a Lescol Intervention Prevention Study (LIPS) substudy. *Am Heart J* 149:329–335, 2005

[35]Holdaas H, Fellström B, Cole E, Nyberg G, Olsson AG, Pedersen TR, Madsen S, Grönhagen-Riska C, Neumayer HH, Maes B, Ambühl P, Hartmann A, Staffler B, Jardine AG: Long-term cardiac outcomes in renal transplant recipients receiving fluvastatin: the ALERT extension study. *Am J Transplant* 5:2929–2936, 2005

[36]Minder CM, Blaha MJ, Horne A, Michos ED, Kaul S, Blumenthal RS: Evidence-based use of statins for primary prevention of cardiovascular disease. *Am J Med* 125:440–446, 2012

[37]Minder M, Blaha MJ, Tam LM, Muñoz D, Michos ED, Kaul S, Blumenthal RS: Making the case for selective use of statins in the primary prevention setting. *Arch Intern Med* 171:1593–1594, 2011

[38]Joshi PH, Chaudhari S, Blaha MJ, Jones SR, Martin SS, Post WS, Cannon CP, Fonarow GC, Wong ND, Amsterdam E, Hirshfeld JW, Blumenthal RS: A point-by-point response to recent arguments against the use of statins in primary prevention. *Clin Cardiol* 35:404–409, 2012

[39]Cholesterol Treatment Trialists Collaborators: Efficacy of cholesterol-lowering therapy in 18,686 people with diabetes in 14 randomised trials of statins: a meta-analysis. *Lancet* 371:117–125, 2008

[40]Brugts JJ, Yetgin T, Hoeks SE, Gotto AM, Shepherd J, Westendorp RG, de Craen AJ, Knopp RH, Nakamura H, Ridker P, van Domburg R, Deckers JW: The benefits of statins in people without established cardiovascular disease but with cardiovascular risk factors: meta-analysis of randomised controlled trials. *BMJ* 338:b2376, 2009

[41]Mihaylova B, Emberson J, Blackwell L, Keech A, Simes J, Barnes EH, Voysey M, Gray A, Collins R, Baigent C: The effects of lowering LDL cholesterol with statin therapy in people at low risk of vascular disease: meta-analysis of individual data from 27 randomised trials. *Lancet* 380:581–590, 2012

[42]Chen Y-H, Feng B, Chen Z-W: Statins for primary prevention of cardiovascular and cerebrovascular events in diabetic patients without established cardiovascular diseases: a meta-analysis. *Exp Clin Endocrinol Diabetes* 120:116–120, 2012

[43]Baigent C, Blackwell L, Emberson J, Holland LE, Reith C, Bhala N, Peto R, Barnes EH, Keech A, Simes J, Collins R: Efficacy and safety of more intensive lowering of LDL cholesterol: a meta-analysis of data from 170,000 participants in 26 randomised trials. *Lancet* 376:1670–1681, 2010

[44]Cheung BMY, Lauder IJ, Lau C-P, Kumana CR: Meta-analysis of large randomized controlled trials to evaluate the impact of statins on cardiovascular outcomes. *Br J Clin Pharmacol* 57:640–651, 2004

[45]Ray KK, Seshasai SRK, Erqou S, Sever P, Jukema JW, Ford I, Sattar N: Statins and all-cause mortality in high-risk primary prevention: a meta-analysis of 11 randomized controlled trials involving 65,229 participants. *Arch Intern Med* 170:1024–1031, 2010

[46]Taylor F, Huffman MD, Macedo AF, Moore TH, Burke M, Davey Smith G, Ward K, Ebrahim S: Statins for the primary prevention of cardiovascular disease. *Cochrane Database Syst Rev* CD004816, 2013

[47]Tonelli M, Lloyd A, Clement F, Conly J, Husereau D, Hemmelgarn B, Klarenbach S, McAlister FA, Wiebe N, Manns B: Efficacy of statins for primary prevention in people at low cardiovascular risk: a meta-analysis. *CMAJ* 183:E1189–E1202, 2011

[48]Matikainen N, Kahri J, Taskinen M-R: Reviewing statin therapy in diabetes: towards the best practice. *Prim Care Diabetes* 4:9–15, 2010

[49]Song SH, Gray TA: Early-onset type 2 diabetes: higher burden of atherogenic apolipoprotein particles during statin treatment. *QJM* 105:973–980, 2012

[50]Sniderman AD, Williams K, Contois JH, Monroe HM, McQueen MJ, de Graaf J, Furberg CD: A meta-analysis of low-density lipoprotein cholesterol, non-high-density lipoprotein cholesterol, and apolipoprotein B as markers of cardiovascular risk. *Circ Cardiovasc Qual Outcomes* 4:337–345, 2011

[51]Martin SS, Qasim AN, Mehta NN, Wolfe M, Terembula K, Schwartz S, Iqbal N, Schutta M, Bagheri R, Reilly MP: Apolipoprotein B but not LDL cholesterol is associated with coronary artery calcification in type 2 diabetic whites. *Diabetes* 58:1887–1892, 2009

[52]Martin SS, Blaha MJ, Elshazly MB, Brinton EA, Toth PP, McEvoy JW, Joshi PH, Kulkarni KR, Mize PD, Kwiterovich PO, Defilippis AP, Blumenthal RS, Jones SR: Friedewald estimated versus directly measured low-density lipoprotein cholesterol and treatment implications. *J Am Coll Cardiol.* Electronically published ahead of print on 20 March 2013 (doi:10.1016/j.jacc.2013.01.079)

[53]Brunzell JD, Davidson M, Furberg CD, Goldberg RB, Howard BV, Stein JH, Witztum JL.Lipoprotein management in patients with cardiometabolic risk: consensus conference report from the American Diabetes Association and the American College of Cardiology Foundation. *J Am Coll Cardiol* 51:1512–1524, 2008

[54]Blaha MJ, Budoff MJ, Blumenthal RS, Nasir K: Coronary artery calcium for guiding statin treatment: authors' reply. *Lancet* 379:312–313, 2012

[55]Becker A, Leber AW, Becker C, von Ziegler F, Tittus J, Schroeder I, Steinbeck G, Knez A: Predictive value of coronary calcifications for future cardiac events in asymptomatic patients with diabetes mellitus: a prospective study in 716 patients over 8 years. *BMC Cardiovasc Disord* 8:27, 2008. Available

pdf/1471-2261-8-27.pdf. Accessed 27 May 2013

[56]Elkeles RS, Godsland IF, Feher MD, Rubens MB, Roughton M, Nugara F, Humphries SE, Richmond W, Flather MD: Coronary calcium measurement improves prediction of cardio-vascular events in asymptomatic patients with type 2 diabetes: the PREDICT study. *Eur Heart J* 29:2244–2251, 2008

[57]Silverman MG, Blaha MJ, Budoff MJ, Rivera JJ, Raggi P, Shaw LJ, Berman D, Callister T, Rumberger JA, Rana JS, Blumenthal RS, Nasir K: Potential implications of coronary artery calcium testing for guiding aspirin use among asymptomatic individuals with diabetes. *Diabetes Care* 35:624–626, 2012

[58]Malik S, Budoff MJ, Katz R, Blumenthal RS, Bertoni AG, Nasir K, Szklo M, Barr RG, Wong ND: Impact of subclinical athero-sclerosis on cardiovascular disease events in individuals with metabolic syndrome and diabetes: the multi-ethnic study of atheroscle-rosis. *Diabetes Care* 34:2285–2290, 2011

[59]Kramer CK, Zinman B, Gross JL, Canani LH, Rodrigues TC, Azevedo MJ, Retnakaran R: Coronary artery calcium score prediction of all cause mortality and cardiovascu-lar events in people with type 2 diabetes: systematic review and meta-analysis. *BMJ* 346:f1654, 2013

[60]Navaneethan SD, Pansini F, Perkovic V, Manno C, Pellegrini F, Johnson DW, Craig JC, Strippoli GF: Statins for people with chronic kidney disease not requiring dialysis. *Cochrane Database Syst Rev* CD007784, 2009

[61]Baigent C, Landray MJ, Reith C, Emberson J, Wheeler DC, Tomson C, Wanner C, Krane V, Cass A, Craig J, Neal B, Jiang L, Hooi LS, Levin A, Agodoa L, Gaziano M, Kasiske B, Walker R, Massy ZA, Feldt-Rasmussen B, Krairittichai U, Ophascharoensuk V, Fellström B, Holdaas H, Tesar V, Wiecek A, Grobbee D, de Zeeuw D, Grönhagen-Riska C, Dasgupta T, Lewis D, Herrington W, Mafham M, Majoni W, Wallendszus K, Grimm R, Pedersen T, Tobert J, Armitage J, Baxter A, Bray C, Chen Y, Chen Z, Hill M, Knott C, Parish S, Simpson D, Sleight P, Young A, Collins R: The effects of lowering LDL cholesterol with simvastatin plus ezeti-mibe in patients with chronic kidney disease (Study of Heart and Renal Protection): a randomised placebo-controlled trial. *Lancet* 377:2181–2192, 2011

cal practice guideline for diabetes and CKD: 2012 update. *Am J Kidney Dis* 60:850–886, 2012

[63]Holdaas H, Holme I, Schmieder RE, Jardine AG, Zannad F, Norby GE, Fellström BC: Rosuvastatin in diabetic hemodialysis patients. *J Am Soc Nephrol* 22:1335–1341, 2011

[64]Sattar N, Preiss D, Murray HM, Welsh P, Buckley BM, de Craen AJ, Seshasai SR, McMurray JJ, Freeman DJ, Jukema JW, Macfarlane PW, Packard CJ, Stott DJ, Westendorp RG, Shepherd J, Davis BR, Pressel SL, Marchioli R, Marfisi RM, Maggioni AP, Tavazzi L, Tognoni G, Kjekshus J, Pedersen TR, Cook TJ, Gotto AM, Clearfield MB, Downs JR, Nakamura H, Ohashi Y, Mizuno K, Ray KK, Ford I: Statins and risk of incident diabetes: a col-laborative meta-analysis of randomised statin trials. *Lancet* 375:735–742, 2010

[65]Preiss D, Seshasai SRK, Welsh P, Murphy SA, Ho JE, Waters DD, DeMicco DA, Barter P, Cannon CP, Sabatine MS, Braunwald E, Kastelein JJ, de Lemos JA, Blazing MA, Pedersen TR, Tikkanen MJ, Sattar N, Ray KK: Risk of incident diabetes with intensive-dose compared with moderate-dose statin therapy: a meta-analysis. *JAMA* 305:2556–2564, 2011

[66]Minder CM, Santos RD, Blumenthal RS: Statins and diabetes: rethinking the data. Available from http://www.cardiosource.org/Science-And-Quality/Hot-Topics. Accessed 28 November 2012

[67]Culver AL, Ockene IS, Balasubramanian R, Olendzki BC, Sepavich DM, Wactawski-Wende J, Manson JE, Qiao Y, Liu S, Merriam PA, Rahilly-Tierny C, Thomas F, Berger JS, Ockene JK, Curb JD, Ma Y: Statin use and risk of diabetes mellitus in postmenopausal women in the Women's Health Initiative. *Arch Intern Med* 172:144–152, 2012

[68]Navarese EP, Buffon A, Andreotti F, Kozinski M, Welton N, Fabiszak T, Caputo S, Grzesk G, Kubica A, Swiatkiewicz I, Sukiennik A, Kelm M, De Servi S, Kubica J: Meta-analysis of impact of different types and doses of statins on new-onset diabetes mellitus. *Am J Cardiol* 111:1123–1130, 2013

[69]Food and Drug Administration: Drug safety communication: important safety label changes to cholesterol-lowering statin drugs. Available from http://www.fda.gov/Drugs/DrugSafety/ucm293101.htm. Accessed 19 January 2013

[70]Libby P, Glynn RJ: Cardiovascular benefits and diabetes risks of statin therapy in primary prevention: an analysis from the JUPITER trial. *Lancet* 380:565–571, 2012

[71]Axsom K, Berger JS, Schwartzbard AZ: Statins and diabetes: the good, the bad, and the unknown. *Curr Atheroscler Rep* 15:299, 2013

[72]Waters DD, Ho JE, DeMicco DA, Breazna A, Arsenault BJ, Wun CC, Kastelein JJ, Colhoun H, Barter P: Predictors of new-onset diabetes in patients treated with atorvastatin: results from 3 large randomized clinical tri-als. *J Am Coll Cardiol* 57:1535–1545, 2011

[73]Waters DD, Ho JE, Boekholdt SM, DeMicco DA, Kastelein JJ, Messig M, Breazna A, Pedersen TR: Cardiovascular event reduction versus new-onset diabetes during atorvastatin therapy: effect of baseline risk factors for diabetes. *J Am Coll Cardiol* 61:148–152, 2013

[74]Rocco MB: Statins and diabetes risk: fact, fiction, and clinical implications. *Cleve Clin J Med* 79:883–893, 2012

[75]Sattar N, Taskinen M-R: Statins are diabe-togenic: myth or reality? *Atheroscler Suppl* 13:1–10, 2012

Bishnu H. Subedi, MD, is a research affiliate at Johns Hopkins Hospital and an internal medicine resident at the Greater Baltimore Medical Center in Baltimore, Md. Rajesh Tota-Maharaj, MD, is a cardiol-ogy fellow at Danbury Hospital in Danbury, Conn. Michael G. Silverman, MD, is a research fel-low; C. Michael Minder, MD, and Seth S. Martin, MD, are cardiology fellows; and M. Dominique Ashen, NP, is a nurse practitioner in the Department of Preventive Cardiology at Johns Hopkins Hospital. Roger S. Blumenthal, MD, is a profes-sor of medicine in Johns Hopkins University School of Medicine and director of the Johns Hopkins Ciccarone Preventive Cardiology Center. Michael J. Blaha, MD, MPH, is a clinical/research fellow in the Division of Cardiology at Johns Hopkins Hospital.

Association of Self-Efficacy and Self-Care With Glycemic Control in Diabetes

Carla Moore Beckerle, DNP, APRN, ANP-BC, and Mary Ann Lavin, DSc, APRN, ANP-BC, FNI, FAAN

Abstract

Successful daily self-management of diabetes is essential to the achievement of positive health outcomes. Basic to successful self-management of any disease is a sense of self-efficacy, or the feeling of confidence in one's self-management abilities. This study examined the association of these variables on the achievement of glycemic control, specifically A1C levels.

This study used a retrospective cohort design to evaluate the predictive relationship of self-efficacy and self-care behaviors on A1C level. After Institutional Review Board approval was obtained, 60 medical records were accessed of people ≥ 18 years of age with type 1 or type 2 diabetes who were seen consecutively in a primary care practice located in an urban setting.

Data analysis revealed no statistically significant relationships between global measures of self-efficacy and self-care and A1C levels. However, there were two questions from the Stanford Diabetes Self-Efficacy for Diabetes Scale found to be significantly related to A1C ($P < 0.009$). Those whose diabetes was well controlled were confident in selecting appropriate foods when hungry and in their ability to exercise for 15–30 minutes, four to five times per week. These findings, if replicated in future studies, may provide clinicians an opportunity to develop and test targeted self-management interventions yielding the highest probability of improved glycemic control.

The incidence of diabetes has escalated in the United States, with the estimated number of those diagnosed with the disease doubling in the past several years to 8.3% of the population.[1] Successful daily management of diabetes and the use of self-management techniques require a positive expectation of outcomes and confidence in one's ability to manage the disease. Factors that influence diabetes control include the association between self-efficacy and self-care behaviors.[2] When diabetes control is achieved, micro- and macrovascular complications decline.[3]

According to the American Diabetes Association (ADA) Standards of Medical Care in Diabetes,[4] achieving adequate glycemic control requires behavioral changes to increase activity levels, change eating patterns, comply with medication regimens, perform self-monitoring of blood glucose, and monitor carbohydrate intake. An explanation of how such behavioral changes require self-efficacy and self-care management is appropriate.

Bandura[5] defined self-efficacy as "people's beliefs about their capabilities to produce designated levels of performance that exercise influence over events that affect their lives." Self-efficacy beliefs determine how people feel, think, motivate themselves, and behave over time. A judgment regarding self-efficacy may determine how much effort a person expends when confronted by challenges. This means that people with an adequate sense of self-efficacy feel

Address correspondence to Carla Moore Beckerle, DNP, APRN, ANP-BC, Vice President of Clinical Programs, Esse Health, 12655 Olive Blvd., St. Louis, MO 63141.

confident in their ability to perform, whether that means administering their medications correctly, adjusting their diet as indicated, preventing hypoglycemia, or exercising appropriately. A strong sense of self-efficacy is necessary to master challenges inherent in these activities. The perception of being capable influences the thought patterns necessary to perform such tasks.

Bandura advocates evaluating self-efficacy beliefs in terms of judgments of capability ("I am capable of . . ." or "I feel confident that I can . . .").[6] He further recommends that people's judgment about their capability be measured across realms or domains of activity, with different degrees of task difficulty and under different situational circumstances. For people with type 1 or type 2 diabetes, a sense of confidence in their ability to performing daily self-care activities seems basic to successful glycemic control.

According to Bandura, "self-care behavior is the end result of cognitive processes that people employ when acquiring knowledge."[7] Knowledge acquisition, in turn, is the result of a teaching and learning process. The aim of self-care is to appropriately fulfill the daily regimen of tasks that individuals need to carry out to manage diabetes. Self-care behavioral skills in people with diabetes can be challenging for individuals because self-care poses many demands regarding such areas as dietary choices, exercise, glucose monitoring, and medication adherence.[8]

Although self-efficacy and self-care influence the choices people make, some people may have a high degree of both but may still choose unhealthy behaviors. Two examples would be a physician with diabetes who does not adhere to dietary recommendations or a registered nurse with diabetes who does not take steps to decrease portion sizes. Yet, these individuals would answer that they have confidence in their ability to implement these behaviors. Still, enhancing self-efficacy and self-care is thought to be a strategy for accelerating the implementation of new behaviors.

This study evaluates self-efficacy and self-care and its predictive relationship to A1C levels. Its hypothesis is that, as self-care and self-efficacy increase, A1C levels decrease.

Background

A literature review was performed using the key words self-efficacy, diabetes, glycosylated hemoglobin levels, and self-care. Databases searched included PubMed, OVID, and CINAHL.

The stability of self-efficacy and self-care behaviors has been examined in people with diabetes. In one study of 221 participants,[9] self-efficacy and self-care behaviors were evaluated at three points in time over 9 months. Participants' beliefs about their abilities (i.e., self-efficacy) in general were unchanged, but their reported ability to perform diabetes self-care increased over time. Outcomes were limited to patient reports. No measures of glycemic control were obtained. However, the authors did make an important distinction between self-efficacy (a person's beliefs about or confidence in his or her abilities around specific disease management behaviors) and self-care (actual

---

Table 1. Self-Efficacy for Diabetes Scale

I would like to know how confident you are in doing certain activities. For each of the following questions, please choose the number that corresponds to your confidence that you can do the tasks regularly at the present time.

1. How confident do you feel that you can eat your meals every 4 to 5 hours every day, including breakfast every day?	Not at all 1 2 3 4 5 6 7 8 9 10 Confident
2. How confident do you feel that you can follow your diet when you have to prepare or share food with other people who do not have diabetes?	Not at all 1 2 3 4 5 6 7 8 9 10 Confident
3. How confident do you feel that you can choose the appropriate foods to eat when you are hungry (for example, snacks)?	Not at all 1 2 3 4 5 6 7 8 9 10 Confident
4. How confident do you feel that you can exercise 15 to 30 minutes, 4 to 5 times a week?	Not at all 1 2 3 4 5 6 7 8 9 10 Confident
5. How confident do you feel that you can do something to prevent your blood sugar level from dropping when you exercise?	Not at all 1 2 3 4 5 6 7 8 9 10 Confident
6. How confident do you feel that you know what to do when your blood sugar level goes higher or lower than it should be?	Not at all 1 2 3 4 5 6 7 8 9 10 Confident
7. How confident do you feel that you can judge when the changes in your illness mean you should visit the doctor?	Not at all 1 2 3 4 5 6 7 8 9 10 Confident
8. How confident do you feel that you can control your diabetes so that it does not interfere with the things you want to do?	Not at all 1 2 3 4 5 6 7 8 9 10 Confident

This scale is free to use without permission. Stanford Patient Education Research Center, 1000 Welch Road, Suite 204, Palo Alto, CA 94304. Funded by the National Institute of Nursing Research.

---

implementation of specific disease management behaviors).

Self-care education may benefit from standardization and prioritization. Preferred methods now in use may become standardized practices in the future. These include the use of lifestyle coaches located within community settings,[10,11] who cover a variety of topics (i.e., wellness behavior, relaxation techniques, person-provider communication, and self-reported health status methods)[12,13] and who employ written action plans to achieve greater glycemic control.[14,15] Although self-care education for chronic illness (including diabetes) and the resultant heightening of self-efficacy appear to be associated with positive health outcomes,[16–21] we do not know the amount of variance in specific outcomes (e.g., glycemic control) brought about by improvements in self-efficacy. This study examines how well self-care and self-efficacy measures predict A1C values.

Study Methods
The study site, Esse Health, comprises 31 private primary care offices in a large, Midwestern suburb. Esse Health serves patients with Medicare and commercial insurance, as well as those who self-pay for health care.

Esse Health encourages innovation to improve chronic disease care. A quality improvement committee oversees the design and implementation of numerous projects at these sites. At the time of this study, one of the innovations was the inclusion of the Stanford Self-Efficacy for Diabetes Scale (SES) (Table 1)[22] and the Self-Care Inventory (SCI) (Table 2)[23] in the assessment process. The Esse Health dietitians were responsible for documentation of the two surveys in the health care records of people with type 1 or type 2 diabetes.

This innovation prompted analyses of baseline self-efficacy and self-care management data and their relationship to glycemic control. The specific questions asked were:
1. What is the association between self-efficacy and self-care? Does the risk of poor self-care increase as self-efficacy decreases?

2. What is the association between self-efficacy and A1C? Does the risk of poor glycemic control increase as self-efficacy decreases?
3. What is the association between self-care and A1C? Does the risk of poor glycemic control increase as self-care decreases?
4. Given that the above associations are positive, what percentage of the variance in A1C values is accounted for by self-care or self-efficacy measures?

To answer these questions, archived data were retrieved for all cognitively unimpaired people, aged ≥ 18 years, with type 1 or type 2 diabetes seen between 10 February and 10 March 2012. The specific data reviewed included SES and SCI scores and all A1C results conducted within the 12-month period preceding the visit that occurred between 10 February and 10 March 2012. Charts missing the required data were excluded. For adequate power, it was determined that 60 records were needed for a sample size large enough to detect a 33% improve-

ment in the proportion of people with well-controlled glycemia a level of $\alpha = 0.05$. All data collected were de-identified and entered into SPSS Statistics for Windows, version 17 (SPSS Inc., Chicago, Ill.) for analysis.

The study focused on two independent variables and one dependent, or outcome, variable. The independent variables were the SES and SCI scores. The SES is an eight-item questionnaire. Each item requires a response on a 10-point Likert scale, with 1 being "not at all confident" and 10 being "totally confident." The SCI is a 14-item questionnaire with a 5-point Likert scale with 1 being "I do not do what is recommended" and 5 being "I always do what is recommended." The dependent, or outcome, variable was glycemic control, defined as the ADA-recommended A1C value of < 7.0%. Lack of glycemic control refers to a value ≥ 7.0%. If A1C is within the target range, the recommended frequency of testing is every 6 months; if it is not, the recommended testing frequency is every 3 months. Patients' mean A1C

Table 2. Self-Care Inventory

Please rate each of the items according to how well you followed your prescribed regimen for diabetes care in the past month.

Scale: 1 = Never do it; 2 = Sometimes follow recommendations, mostly not; 3 = Follow recommendations about 50% of the time; 4 = Usually do this as recommended, occasional lapses; 5 = Always do this as recommended without fail; and NA = Cannot rate this item/not applicable

1. Glucose testing 1 2 3 4 5 NA

2. Glucose recording 1 2 3 4 5 NA

3. Administering correct insulin dose 1 2 3 4 5 NA

4. Administering insulin at right time 1 2 3 4 5 NA

5. Adjusting insulin intake based on blood glucose values 1 2 3 4 5 NA

6. Eating the proper foods; sticking to meal plan 1 2 3 4 5 NA

7. Eating meals on time 1 2 3 4 5 NA

8. Eating regular snacks 1 2 3 4 5 NA

9. Carrying quick-acting sugar to treat reactions 1 2 3 4 5 NA

10. Coming in for appointments 1 2 3 4 5 NA

11. Wearing a medic alert ID 1 2 3 4 5 NA

12. Exercising regularly 1 2 3 4 5 NA

13. Exercising strenuously 1 2 3 4 5 NA

was, therefore, usually based on a minimum of two values per year. If only one value was available in the medical record, this single value was used in lieu of a mean.

Data analysis addressed each of the study questions. Pearson χ^2 and Fishers exact tests were used to determine the association between high and low self-care and self-efficacy scores and A1C levels $\geq 7.0\%$ and $< 7.0\%$ (uncontrolled and controlled glycemia, respectively). These results were also stratified to examine age and sex effects. The influence of ethnicity was not examined, because this information was not collected by Esse Health at the time of the project.

The distribution of the self-care and self-efficacy scores were plotted to examine how well self-care and self-efficacy scores predicted A1C values. If the distribution appeared normal, then the variables were to be evaluated as continuous variables. If the distributions did not appear normal, then the relationship was to be tested using nonparametric statistics (Spearman's correlation coefficient).

Study Results

Initially, 60 medical records were evaluated, but only 57 contained completed data. Therefore, 57 medical records were reviewed and included. Table 3 presents the age and sex distribution of people comprising the retrospective cohort. There was relatively even distribution between the sexes. Age was distributed by adults (18–62 years), older adults (63–74 years), and very old adults (75–99 years). This distribution was established to generally

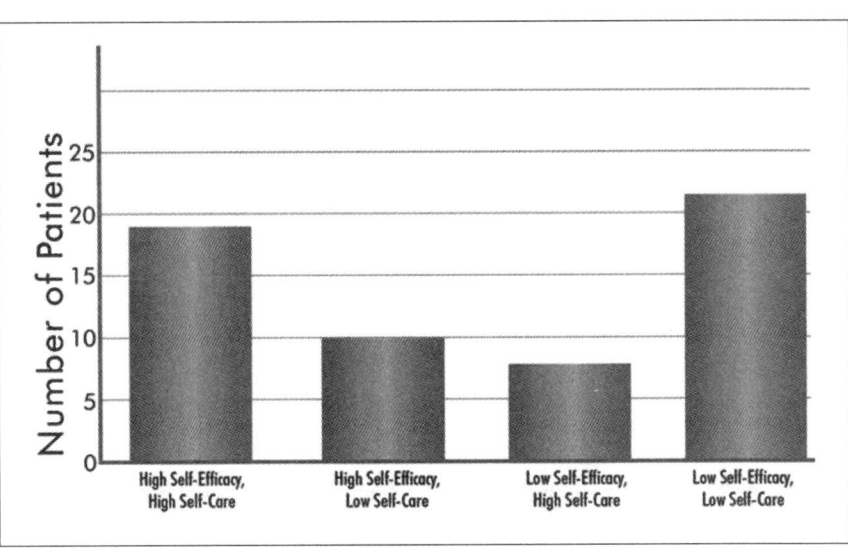

Figure 1. Distribution of SES and SCI scores by number of patients included in study. $\chi^2 = 7.86$, $df = 1$, P = < 0.001; $\rho = 0.537$, P < 0.000 (two-tailed).

reflect the working population (18–62 years) and the younger and older retired populations. It was thought that members of the older retired population may experience an escalating number of chronic illnesses and a decreased ability to self-manage their diabetes. If such differences existed, the investigators wanted to identify them. χ^2 analyses were used to determine the associations between controlled versus uncontrolled A1C and sex (male vs. female) and each of the three age categories. No statistically significant findings were detected.

Figure 1 addresses the first question: What is the association between self-efficacy and self-care? The distribution of SES and SCS responses were examined. Note that self-efficacy and self-care vary together ($\chi^2 = 7.86$, degrees of free-

dom [df] 1, $P < 0.009$; Spearman's correlation coefficient [ρ] = 0.537, $P < 0.000$). In other words, high SES is associated with high SCI and vice versa. This supports Bandura's work among people with diabetes.

The second question asked whether there was a difference in mean A1C values between patients with high and low self-efficacy and self-care scores. No significant differences were found. Self-efficacy and self-care scores varied together.[10]

These findings evoked a closer examination of the SES and SCI items and why they may or may not be related to glycemic control. The question asked was: Why would self-care items such as how well a person obtains or records glucose values in the past month be poorly correlated with A1C? The answer may be that, regardless of how well glucose values are recorded, they will yield glycemic control if the prescribed regimen was less than optimal.

This study did not examine provider compliance with ADA guidelines. For example, it did not look at records to see whether metformin dosages were increased in response to high A1C levels. Similarly, the frequency with which a person obtains and records glucose values will not yield better A1C values if the person was nonadherent to a prescribed regimen. Unfortunately, a medication possession ratio was

Table 3. Age and Sex Distribution of the Retrospective Study Cohort*

Age (Years)	Sex		Total
	Male (52%)	Female (48%)	
18–62	7	8	15
63–74	14	16	30
75–99	5	7	12
Total	26	31	57

*At the time of this study, Esse Health did not collect data on race and ethnicity. Therefore, these parameters were not included.

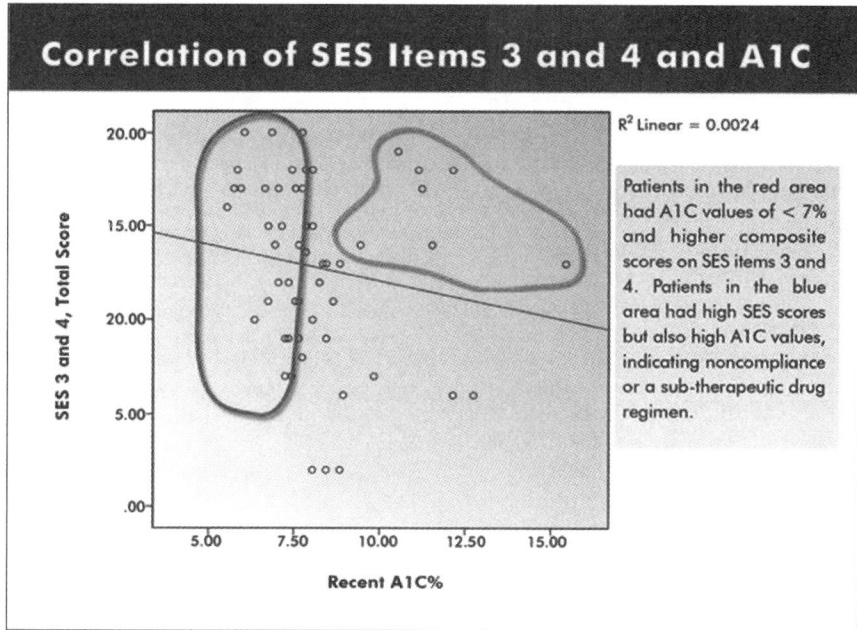

Correlation of SES Items 3 and 4 and A1C

R^2 Linear = 0.0024

Patients in the red area had A1C values of < 7% and higher composite scores on SES items 3 and 4. Patients in the blue area had high SES scores but also high A1C values, indicating noncompliance or a sub-therapeutic drug regimen.

Figure 2. Correlation of composite scores for items 3 and 4 in the SES and A1C.

not included in the records of study participants.[11,24]

Thus, if A1C outcomes are to be used, then only self-care measures that are directly related to A1C (e.g., "I take my medication as prescribed") must be used, with the response checked against a medication possession ratio for reliability.

A deeper analysis of the relationship between SES and A1C was also undertaken. Even if not all items were associated with greater glycemic control, perhaps specific items on the SES were directly related to glycemic control. Therefore, each item was evaluated independently.

The results indicated that two items may serve as proxy measures for self-efficacy in general among people with diabetes. The first (item 3) was: How confident are you that you can choose the appropriate foods to eat when you are hungry? Although the association with A1C

Table 4. Clinical Decision-Making Based on Self-Efficacy Assessment, Diagnosis, and A1C Outcomes and Related Interventions

Self-Efficacy Assessment (answers to SES items 3 and 4)	Self-Efficacy Diagnosis	A1C Outcomes and Related Interventions	
		Controlled	Uncontrolled
Both responses positive	High self-efficacy	Continue to reinforce patient's confidence in self-management.	Initiate interventions to check medication possession ratio. If the patient is compliant, check the adequacy of the provider's adherence to ADA recommendations for drug therapy and adjust as needed.
One response positive, the other negative	Moderate self-efficacy	Continue to reinforce patient's confidence to self-manage well with the one variable. Initiate interventions to build self-confidence in the other variable.	Continue to build confidence in the patient's ability to self-manage, while also checking patient's medication possession ratio. If the patient is compliant, check the adequacy of the provider's adherence to ADA recommendations for drug therapy and adjust as needed.
Both responses negative	Low self-efficacy	Congratulate patient on the degree of glycemic control, while initiating interventions to build self-confidence in these two self-management areas.	Continue to build confidence in the patient's ability to self-manage, while also checking the patient's medication possession ratio. If the patient is compliant, check the adequacy of the provider's adherence to ADA recommendations for drug therapy and adjust as needed.

was not statistically significant, the responses approached significance ($P < 0.06$). The second item (item 4) was: How confident do you feel that you can exercise 15–30 minutes, four to five times per week? The association here with A1C was statistically significant ($P < 0.016$).

When the two items were computed together as a composite score, they yielded a probability of < 0.009 (Figure 2). Those who scored high on the composite score of items 3 and 4 were more likely to have an A1C of $< 7\%$. The slope of the line indicated that, as scores decrease, so too does glycemic control, manifested by higher A1C values. Finally, the blue area in Figure 2 indicates that there were some patients who scored well on the composite items (above the slope) but still had poorly controlled glycemia (A1C values well above 7%). These were people who felt confident in their ability to exercise and properly portion their food but who may not do so or who may have a subtherapeutic drug regimen.

Figure 2 also raises questions applicable to future research. For example, assuming appropriate medication possession ratios and a therapeutic, guideline-based drug regimen, could time and money be saved and effectiveness boosted by using these two items to gauge patients' self-efficacy? Could interventions aimed at increasing patients' confidence in incorporating exercise into their routine and selecting appropriate foods enhance glycemic control more effectively than current standard care?

There were some limitations involved in the implementation of this study. Although each item was read to patients at the time of patients' interview with the dietitian, some patients may not have fully understood how to scale their responses. The ability to scale responses may require a conceptual clarity that some patients did not possess. In future studies, it is recommended that the intra-rater reliability of patient responses be evaluated and enrollment limited to the records of patients with acceptable reliability scores.

Another possible limitation involved the SCI. It is possible that people may have found it difficult to report to a dietitian who is part of the health care team that they did not do what the team recommended. This may have been especially true when patients saw that their responses were to be recorded in their health record.

Summary

This retrospective chart review suggests that increased confidence of patients with diabetes with regard to selecting appropriate foods when hungry (SES item 3) and working exercise into their daily routine (SES item 4) seems to be correlated with improved glycemic control. On the basis of these results, these two questions were inserted into the nutrition screening tool at Esse Health, and their relationship to glycemic control will continue to be evaluated. In addition, a clinical decision-making tool was developed (Table 4).

This tool is a simple assessment and diagnosis of self-efficacy and its relationship to glycemic control and related interventions. Future studies will report on the results obtained through the use of this tool. The evaluation of such an approach is an important area for future research.

Finally, when glycemic control is the outcome variable being evaluated for clinical or research purposes, it is highly recommended that medication possession ratios and the adequacy of patients' therapeutic regimen be considered variables that should be controlled, if results are to be interpreted correctly. Clinically, medication possession ratios and the adequacy of patients' therapeutic regimen should be evaluated at each clinic visit at which it is determined that glycemic control has not been achieved. This study suggests that a two-item self-efficacy assessment (Table 4) should also be performed at these same visits.

References

[1]Expert Committee on the Diagnosis and Classification of Diabetes Mellitus: Follow-up report on the diagnosis of diabetes mellitus. *Diabetes Care* 26:3160–3167, 2003

[2]Glasgow R, Toobert D, Riddle M, Donnelly J, Mitchell D, Calder D: Diabetes-specific social learning variable and self-care behaviors among persons with type II diabetes. *Health Psychol* 8:285–303, 1989

[3]World Health Organization: Definition and diagnosis of diabetes mellitus and intermediate hyperglycemia. Available from http://www.who.int/diabetes/publications/Definition%20and%20diagnosis%20of%20diabetes_new.pdf, 2006. Accessed 23 March 2012

[4]American Diabetes Association: Standards of medical care in diabetes—2013. *Diabetes Care* 36 (Suppl. 1):S11–S66, 2013

[5]Bandura A: *Self-Efficacy: The Exercise of Control.* New York, Prentice-Hall, 1994

[6]Bandura A: *Social Foundations of Thought and Action: A Social Cognitive Theory.* Englewood Cliffs, N.J., Prentice-Hall, 1986

[7]Bernal H, Woolley S, Schensul J, Dickinson J: Correlations of self-efficacy in diabetes self-care among Hispanic adults with diabetes. *Diabetes Educ* 26:673–680, 2000

[8]Bandura A: Health promotion by social cognitive means. *Health Educ Behav* 31:143–164, 2004

[9]Rapley P, Passmore A, Phillips M: Review of psychometric properties of the diabetes self-efficacy scale: Australian longitudinal study. *Nurs Health Sci* 5:289–297, 2003

[10]Sousa V, Zauszniewski J, Musil C, Price LP, Davis S: Relationships among self-care agency, self-efficacy, self-care, and glycemic control. *Res Theory Nurs Pract* 19:217–230, 2005

[11]Norris S, Nichols P, Caspersen C, Glasgow R, Engelgau M, Synder S, Carande-Kulis K, Isham G, Garfield S, Briss P, McCulloch D: Increasing diabetes self-management education in community settings: a systematic review. *Am J Prev Med* 22:39–66, 2002

[12]Lorig K, Ritter P, Villa F, Armas J: Community-based peer-led diabetes self-management: a randomized trial. *Diabetes Educ* 35:641–651, 2009

[13]Diabetes Prevention Program Research Group: The Diabetes Prevention Program (DPP): description of lifestyle intervention. *Diabetes Care* 25:2165–2171, 2002

[14]Handley M, MacGregor K, Schillnger D, Sharifi C, Wong S, Bodenheimer T: Using action plans to help primary care patients adopt healthy behaviors: a descriptive study. *J Am Board Fam Med* 19:224–231, 2006

[15]Connell C, Davis W, Gallant M, Sharpe P: Impact of social support, social cognitive variable, and perceived threat on depression among adults with diabetes. *Health Psychol* 13:263–273, 1994

[16]Judge T, Erez A, Bono J, Thoresen C: Are measures of self-esteem, neuroticism, locus of control, and generalized self-efficacy indicators of a common core construct? *J Pers Soc Psychol* 83:693–710, 2002

[17]Clark M, Hampson S, Avery L, Simpson R: Effects of a brief tailored intervention on the

process and predictors of lifestyle behavior change in patients with type 2 diabetes. *Psychol Health Med* 9:440–449, 2004

[18]Siebolds M, Gaedeke O, Schwedes U: Self-monitoring of blood glucose: psychological aspects relevant to changes in HbA1c in type 2 diabetic patients treated with diet or diet plus oral antidiabetic. *J Behav Med* 22:345–351, 2006

[19]Lo R: Adherence to health regime self-efficacy scale. *J Adv Nurs* 30:418–421, 1999

[20]Anderson M, Funnel M, Butler M, Fitzgerald T, Fesse C: Patients' empowerment: results of a randomized controlled trial. *Diabetes Care* 18:943–949, 1995

[21]Mulcahy K, Maryniuk M, Peeples M, Peyrot M, Tomky D, Weaver T, Yarborough P: Diabetes self-management education core outcomes measures. *Diabetes Educ* 29:768–770, 773–784, 2003

[22]Stanford Patient Education Research Center: Diabetes self-efficacy scale. Available from http://patienteducation.stanford.edu/research/sediabetes.html. Accessed 5 July 2013

[23]Weinger K, Butler HA, Welch GW, LaGreca AM: Measuring diabetes self-care: a psychometric analysis of the Self-Care Inventory-revised with adults. *Diabetes Care* 28:1346–1352, 2005

[24]Ward W, Armbrecht E, Lavin MA: Medication possession and glycemic control among uninsured type 2 diabetics. *J Nurse Pract* 8:528–533, 2012

Carla Moore Beckerle, DNP, APRN, ANP-BC, is vice president of clinical programs at Esse Health in St. Louis, Mo. Mary Ann Lavin, DSc, APRN, ANP-BC, FNI, FAAN, is an associate professor at the St. Louis University School of Nursing in Missouri.

Mechanisms and Management of Diabetic Painful Distal Symmetrical Polyneuropathy

Solomon Tesfaye, md[1]
Andrew J.M. Boulton, md[2]
Anthony H. Dickenson, phd[3]

Although a number of the diabetic neuropathies may result in painful symptomatology, this review focuses on the most common: chronic sensorimotor distal symmetrical polyneuropathy (DSPN). It is estimated that 15–20% of diabetic patients may have painful DSPN, but not all of these will require therapy. In practice, the diagnosis of DSPN is a clinical one, whereas for longitudinal studies and clinical trials, quantitative sensory testing and electrophysiological assessment are usually necessary. A number of simple numeric rating scales are available to assess the frequency and severity of neuropathic pain. Although the exact pathophysiological processes that result in diabetic neuropathic pain remain enigmatic, both peripheral and central mechanisms have been implicated, and extend from altered channel function in peripheral nerve through enhanced spinal processing and changes in many higher centers. A number of pharmacological agents have proven efficacy in painful DSPN, but all are prone to side effects, and none impact the underlying pathophysiological abnormalities because they are only symptomatic therapy. The two first-line therapies approved by regulatory authorities for painful neuropathy are duloxetine and pregabalin. α-Lipoic acid, an antioxidant and pathogenic therapy, has evidence of efficacy but is not licensed in the U.S. and several European countries. All patients with DSPN are at increased risk of foot ulceration and require foot care, education, and if possible, regular podiatry assessment.

Diabetes Care 36:2456–2465, 2013

The neuropathies are the most common long-term microvascular complications of diabetes and affect those with both type 1 and type 2 diabetes, with up to 50% of older type 2 diabetic patients having evidence of a distal neuropathy (1). These neuropathies are characterized by a progressive loss of nerve fibers affecting both the autonomic and somatic divisions of the nervous system. The clinical features of the diabetic neuropathies vary immensely, and only a minority are associated with pain. The major portion of this review will be dedicated to the most common painful neuropathy, chronic sensorimotor distal symmetrical polyneuropathy (DSPN). This neuropathy has major detrimental effects on its sufferers, confirming an increased risk of foot ulceration and Charcot neuroarthropathy as well as being associated with increased mortality (1).

In addition to DSPN, other rarer neuropathies may also be associated with painful symptoms including acute painful neuropathy that often follows periods of unstable glycemic control, mononeuropathies (e.g., cranial nerve palsies), radiculopathies, and entrapment neuropathies (e.g., carpal tunnel syndrome). By far the most common presentation of diabetic polyneuropathy (over 90%) is typical DSPN or chronic DSPN.

The Toronto Diabetic Neuropathy Expert Group recently defined DSPN as "a symmetrical, length-dependent sensorimotor polyneuropathy attributable to metabolic and microvessel alterations as a result of chronic hyperglycemia exposure and cardiovascular risk covariates" (2). An abnormality of nerve conduction (NC) tests, which is frequently subclinical, appears to be the first objective quantitative indication of the condition. The occurrence of diabetic retinopathy and nephropathy in a given patient strengthen the case that the polyneuropathy is attributable to diabetes. DSPN results in insensitivity of the feet that predisposes to foot ulceration (1) and/or neuropathic pain (painful DSPN), which can be disabling.

Clinical features of painful DSPN—The onset of DSPN is usually gradual or insidious and is heralded by sensory symptoms that start in the toes and then progress proximally to involve the feet and legs in a stocking distribution. When the disease is well established in the lower limbs in more severe cases, there is upper limb involvement, with a similar progression proximally starting in the fingers. As the disease advances further, motor manifestations, such as wasting of the small muscles of the hands and limb weakness, become apparent. In some cases, there may be sensory loss that the patient may not be aware of, and the first presentation may be a foot ulcer. Approximately 50% of patients with DSPN experience neuropathic symptoms in the lower limbs including uncomfortable tingling (dysesthesia), pain (burning; shooting or "electric-shock like"; lancinating or "knife-like"; "crawling", or aching etc., in character), evoked pain (allodynia, hyperesthesia), or unusual sensations (such as a feeling of swelling of the feet or severe coldness of the legs when clearly the lower limbs look and feel fine, odd sensations on walking likened to "walking on pebbles" or "walking on hot sand," etc.). There may be marked pain on walking that may limit exercise and lead to weight gain. Painful DSPN is characteristically more severe at night and often interferes with normal sleep (3). It also has a major impact on the ability to function normally (both mental and physical functioning, e.g., ability to maintain work, mood, and quality of life [QoL]) (3,4).

In one study from the U.S., the burden of painful DSPN was found to be considerable, resulting in a persistent discomfort despite polypharmacy and

From the ¹Diabetes Research Unit, Sheffield Teaching Hospitals, Royal Hallamshire Hospital, Sheffield, U.K.; the ²Institute for Endocrinology and Diabetes, University of Manchester, Manchester, U.K.; and ³Neuroscience, Physiology and Pharmacology, University College London, London, U.K.
Corresponding author: Andrew J.M. Boulton, aboulton@med.miami.edu.
DOI: 10.2337/dc12-1964

high resource use and led to limitations in daily activities and poor satisfaction with treatments (4). The unremitting nature of the pain can be distressing, resulting in mood disorders including depression and anxiety (4). The natural history of painful DSPN has not been well studied, and there is a need for large, population-based, prospective studies looking at the natural history and potentially modifiable risk factors, if any. However, it is generally believed that painful symptoms may persist over the years (5), occasionally becoming less prominent as the sensory loss worsens (6).

Epidemiology—There have been relatively few epidemiological studies that have specifically examined the prevalence of painful DSPN, which range from 10–26% (7–9). In a recent study of a large cohort of diabetic patients receiving community-based health care in northwest England (n = 15,692), painful DSPN assessed using neuropathy symptom and disability scores was found in 21% (7). In one population-based study from Liverpool, U.K., the prevalence of painful DSPN assessed by a structured questionnaire and examination was estimated at 16% (8). Notably, it was found that 12.5% of these patients had never reported their symptoms to their doctor and 39% had never received treatment for their pain (8), indicating that there may be considerable underdiagnosis and undertreatment of painful neuropathic symptoms compared with other aspects of diabetes management such as statin therapy and management of hypertension.

Risk factors for DSPN per se have been extensively studied, and it is clear that apart from poor glycemic control, cardiovascular risk factors play a prominent role (10): risk factors for painful DSPN are less well known. Preliminary epidemiological studies suggest clinical correlates for painful DSPN compared with painless DSPN to include weight (11), obesity (12), waist circumference (13), peripheral arterial disease (11,13), and triglycerides (12). However, one limitation of these studies was that assessment of both DSPN and painful DSPN was carried out using screening methods (Michigan Neuropathy Screening Instrument) questionnaire (11,13) or the Douleur Neuropatique en 4 questions (12) for neuropathic pain, and the neurological examination of Michigan Neuropathy Screening Instrument (11,13) or Neuropen (12) for assessment of DSPN.

Diagnosing and assessing the severity of DSPN and painful DSPN

—A broad spectrum of presentations may occur in patients with DSPN, ranging from one extreme of the patient with very severe painful symptoms but few signs, to the other when patients may present with a foot ulcer having lost all sensation without ever having any painful or uncomfortable symptoms; when pressed, such patients may admit to the feet feeling somewhat "numb" or "dead." Thus, it is well recognized that the severity of symptoms may not relate to the severity of the deficit on clinical examination (1).

Diagnosing and assessing severity of DSPN

The American Diabetes Association Consensus Statement (14) recommended that the diagnosis of painful DSPN in clinical practice be a clinical one, relying on the patient's description of pain and typical features of peripheral neuropathy manifesting in reduction of sensory modalities and absence/reduction of ankle/knee reflexes. Because DSPN is a diagnosis of exclusion, a careful clinical history and a peripheral neurological and vascular examination of the lower limbs are essential to exclude other causes of neuropathic pain and leg/foot pain such as peripheral vascular disease, arthritis, malignancy, alcohol abuse, spinal canal stenosis, etc. NC studies are rarely helpful in clinical practice but might help in excluding other causes of pain such as entrapment syndromes. Patients with asymmetrical symptoms and/or signs (such as loss of an ankle jerk in one leg only), rapid progression of symptoms, or predominance of motor symptoms and signs should be carefully assessed for other causes of the findings.

For longitudinal studies and clinical trials in which a more accurate quantification of neuropathy is required, the Toronto Diabetic Neuropathy Consensus Panel suggested a reliable objective and quantitative measure; that is, NC abnormality as the minimal criteria for the diagnosis of DSPN (2). When NC values have not been assessed, the Consensus Panel recommended that it is not possible to provide a "confirmed" diagnosis of DSPN—only a "possible" or "probable" diagnosis.

However, subjects with pure small-fiber neuropathy may be diagnosed by quantitative sensory testing (QST) to assess the psychophysical thresholds for cold and warm sensations, heat and cold pain, and pain to pin prick; or by cutaneous vasomotor function to measure skin blood flow as a marker of c-fiber neurovascular dysfunction (15). However, the gold standard for assessing small fiber function remains quantification of intraepidermal nerve fibers from punch skin biopsy immunostained by PGP9.5 (16). Indeed, QST has also been routinely used in some clinics to diagnose general neuropathy (e.g., the 10-g monofilament is widely used in diabetic clinics to screen for DSPN), and recently, the German Pain Network has developed QST to characterize the somatosensory phenotype of patients with neuropathic pain (17), though the Toronto Consensus Panel recognized its limitation of essentially being subjective and the potential for bias by perceptual/cognitive factors. Recent advances in small fiber neuropathy assessment include brain-evoked potentials with electrical and laser stimulation (laser-evoked potentials) (18), and contact heat–evoked potential—a measure of cerebral responses of A-delta fiber–mediated thermonociceptive stimuli (19).

There are several instruments that evaluate combinations of neuropathy symptoms, signs, and neurophysiological test abnormalities giving scores for severity of DSPN (20–24). However, clinical examination is not always reproducible, and recent studies emphasize the importance of the proficiency of the clinical neurological assessment (24). For controlled clinical trials of DSPN, the Toronto Consensus Panel advocated the use of an NC test as an early and reliable indicator of the occurrence of this neuropathy (2). The group also emphasized that to be reliable the test must be carried out rigorously, using appropriate reference values corrected for applicable variables (2).

Assessing neuropathic pain severity

The frequency and severity of painful symptoms can be assessed by a number of simple numeric rating scales (25). The use of simple scales such as the visual analog scale or the numerical rating scale, such as an 11-point Likert scale (0 = no pain to 10 = worst pain imaginable) is recommended. These scales can then be used to monitor response to treatment in clinical practice or research context. Other validated scales and questionnaires include 1) the modified Brief Pain Inventory Short Form (BPI-MSF) (26) recently used as the primary end point in pharmacological treatment trials of painful

DSPN; 2) the neuropathic pain symptom inventory (27), which evaluates the different symptoms and dimensions of neuropathic pain; 3) the neuropathic pain questionnaire (28), which consists of 12 items, including 10 related to sensations and or sensory responses and 2 related to affect; 4) the LANNS pain scale (29), which contains five symptom and two clinical examination items and is easy to score within clinical settings; 5) painDETECT, a screening tool that incorporates an easy to use, patient based (self-report) questionnaire with nine items that do not require a clinical exam (30); and 6) the McGill Pain Questionnaire, which measures the sensory and affective components of pain, often used in its shortened format (31).

QoL might be assessed by generic instruments that may allow cross comparison with other chronic medical conditions. However, it is also important to use validated, neuropathy-specific measures of QoL, such as the NeuroQol (32), that reliably capture the key dimensions of patients' experience of DSPN and is a valid tool for studying the impact of neuropathy and foot ulceration on QoL. Another neuropathy-specific measure of QoL is the Norfolk Quality of Life Scale (33), which is a validated patient-reported outcome measure, sensitive to the different features of diabetic neuropathy including small-fiber, large-fiber, and autonomic function. There are a number of scales that might assess pain behavior and sleep interference and the prediction of response to therapy (34). Finally, the impact of painful symptoms on mood can be assessed using the Hospital Anxiety and Depression Scale (35) and Beck's Depression Inventory (36).

Mechanism of neuropathic pain in diabetes

We will now consider the changes at central and peripheral levels induced by DSPN that relate to the sensory changes experienced by patients and the mechanisms that treatments are thought to modulate.

The exact pathophysiological mechanisms of neuropathic pain in diabetes remain elusive although several mechanisms have been postulated (Table 1) (37). Other potential mechanisms include the association of increased blood glucose instability in the genesis of neuropathic pain (38), an increase in peripheral nerve epineurial blood flow (39), altered foot skin microcirculation (40), reduced intraepidermal nerve fiber density in the context of early neuropathy

Table 1—Mechanisms of neuropathic pain

Peripheral mechanisms
  Changes in sodium channel distribution and expression
  Changes in calcium channel distribution and expression
  Altered neuro-peptide expression
  Sympathetic sprouting
  Loss of spinal inhibitory control
  Altered peripheral blood flow
  Axonal atrophy, degeneration, or regeneration
  Damage to small fibers
  Increased glycemic flux
Central mechanisms
  Central sensitization
  Changes in the balance of facilitation/ inhibition within descending pathways
  Increased thalamic vascularity

Adapted with permission from Tesfaye and Kempler (37).

(41), increased thalamic vascularity (42), and autonomic dysfunction (43).

The fact that diabetes induces neuropathy and that in a proportion of patients this is accompanied by pain despite the loss of input and numbness, suggests that marked changes occur in the processes of pain signaling in the peripheral and central nervous system. Neuropathic pain is characterized by ongoing pain together with exaggerated responses to painful and nonpainful stimuli, hyperalgesia, and allodynia. These combinations of loss and gain of function have been recently characterized by sensory testing by Maier et al. (44), and five subgroups of patients emerge with many of the signs and symptoms overlapping with those seen in patients with postherpetic neuralgia. This suggests common mechanisms but importantly, the subgroups may turn out to have different responses to pharmacological agents and so lead to a prediction of analgesic response. Nevertheless, the changes seen suggest altered peripheral signaling and central compensatory changes perhaps driven by the loss of input. Indeed, the descriptors used, such as electric shock, burning, and lancinating indicate that diabetes induces changes in the way peripheral signals are processed.

Capsaicin in chili peppers evokes burning pain due to activation of transient receptor potential channel (TRP) V1, a receptor situated on small peripheral fibers and part of the family of 27 TRP channels cloned in humans (45), some of

which are thought to transduce thermal signals (46) and include TRPM8 and TRPA1, important in cold hypersensitivity (47). Local application of capsaicin can be analgesic in localized painful neuropathies, and polymorphisms in TRPV1 can explain some of the variation in pain seen after neuropathy in patients (48).

There are many other less understood or characterized peripheral sensors, including the P2X receptors for ATP, released from all damaged cells suggesting further potential targets for therapies (49). Very clear evidence points to the key role of changes in ion channels as a consequence of nerve damage and their roles in the disordered activity and transduction in damaged and intact fibers (50).

Sodium channels depolarize neurons and generate an action potential. Following damage to peripheral nerves, the normal distribution of these channels along a nerve is disrupted by the neuroma and "ectopic" activity results from the accumulation of sodium channels at or around the site of injury. Other changes in the distribution and levels of these channels are seen and impact upon the pattern of neuronal excitability in the nerve. Inherited pain disorders arise from mutated sodium channels, notably gain and loss of functions of the sodium channel Nav 1.7 (51,52), and polymorphisms in this channel impact on the level of pain in patients, indicating that inherited differences in channel function might explain some of the variability in pain between patients with DSPN (53). Following peripheral nerve damage, levels of another sodium channel, Nav 1.3, in dorsal root ganglia increase and are thought to support ectopic neuronal firing. Blockers of these pain-related channels and also the very important Nav1.8 have been produced but have yet to reach the clinic. Thus, treatments revolve around nonselective sodium channel blockers including local anesthetics such as lidocaine and the anticonvulsant carbamazepine in trigeminal neuralgia (54).

A recent study (55) proposes a mechanism for the observed neuropathic changes that follow diabetes. The levels of the glycolytic metabolite methylglyoxal distinguished between diabetic patients with pain and those without pain. Methylglyoxal activated peripheral nerves and altered the function of Nav 1.8. and Nav 1.7. In animals, the metabolite was found to slow NC, increase release of calcitonin gene-related peptide from nerves, and cause thermal and mechanical hyperalgesia.

This hyperalgesia was reflected by functional changes in pain-related areas of the brain (55).

Where sodium channels act to generate action potentials, potassium channels serve as the molecular brakes of excitable cells, playing an important role in modulating neuronal hyperexcitability. The drug retigabine, a potassium channel opener acting on the channel (K_V7, M-current) opener, blunts behavioral hypersensitivity in neuropathic rats (56) and also inhibits C and Aδ-mediated responses in dorsal horn neurons in both naïve and neuropathic rats (57), but has yet to reach the clinic as an analgesic although it has recently been approved by the FDA as an add-on treatment of partial seizures (58).

There are likely many other changes in potassium channels after neuropathy, and their importance is underscored by the fact that opioids act to open these channels and suppress activity in pain pathways by actions at both spinal and brain sites.

The third channel set in neuronal events is made up of voltage-gated Ca channels, which serve to release transmitter.

In the case of afferent sensory fibers, these are glutamate and peptides such as substance P. Following nerve injury, $\alpha_2\delta$ subunits of these channels are slowly upregulated in the central terminals of peripheral nerves, so favoring increased release of these transmitters into the spinal cord (59). This will therefore compensate for the loss of afferent fibers produced by the neuropathy. Gabapentin and pregabalin target the $\alpha_2\delta$ subunit and by preventing its trafficking into the membrane reduce the abnormal transmitter release (59).

A further permissive factor in the actions of these drugs is activity in spinal 5-hydroxytryptamine 3 receptors, themselves driven by activity in descending pathways from the brain; this rapidly switching circuit may not only explain the actions of $\alpha_2\delta$ ligands after nerve injury but also their acute effects such as those seen after surgery (60).

Central excitatory mechanisms

Aδ and C fibers terminate primarily in the superficial laminae of the dorsal horn where the large majority of neurons are nociceptive specific (Fig. 1). Some of these neurons gain low threshold inputs after neuropathy and these cells project predominantly to limbic brain areas such as the periaqueductal gray, lateral parabrachial nucleus, thalamus, nucleus tractus solitarius, and the medullary reticular formation. Within deeper lamina V, neurons are wide-dynamic range, responding to both innocuous and noxious stimuli, and so candidates for abnormal coding of low-threshold inputs and hence allodynia, exhibiting wind-up and projecting to sensory areas of the brain such as the thalamus and thence the cortex, where the sensory component of pain is represented (Fig. 2). Thus, spinal cord neurons provide parallel outputs to the affective and sensory areas of the brain. Changes induced in these neurons by repeated noxious inputs underpin central sensitization where the resultant hyperexcitability of neurons leads to greater responses to all subsequent inputs—innocuous and noxious—expanded receptive fields and enhanced outputs to higher levels of the brain (Fig. 2). These changes may then alter descending controls (Fig. 2). The spinal mechanisms involve the actions of glutamate

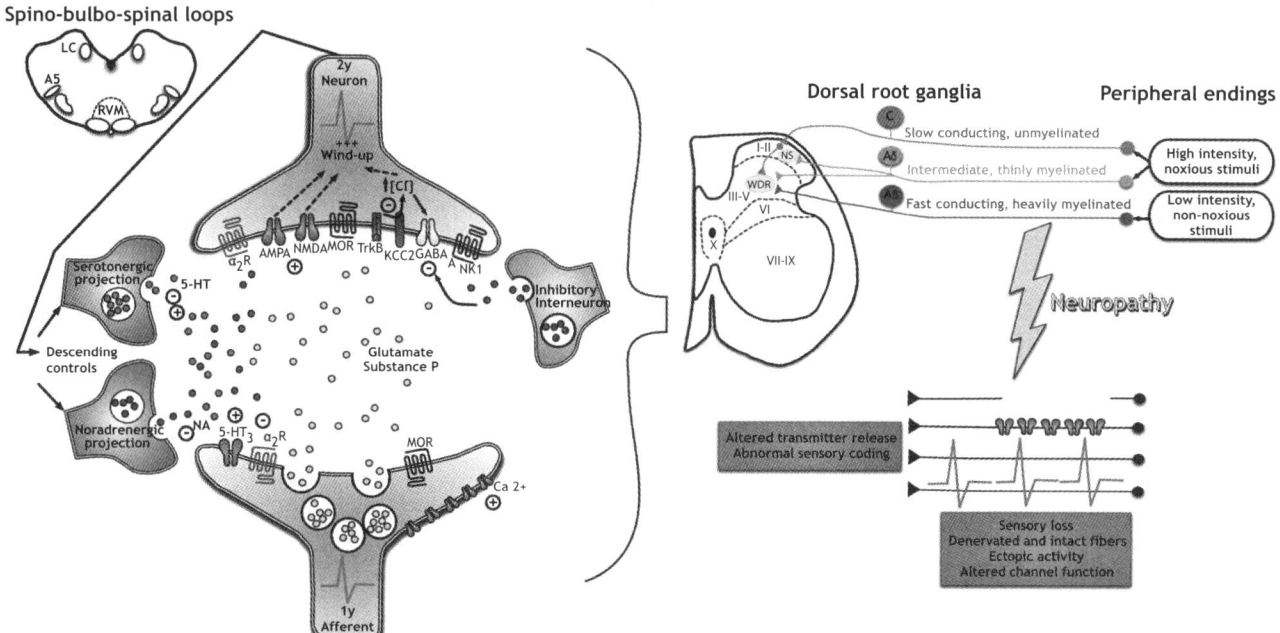

Figure 1—*A representation of the central spinal and peripheral changes that accompany neuropathy. The existence of a lesion or disease of a peripheral sensory nerve alters the conduction and transmission of sensory messages. The normal transfer of modalities (top right) onto spinal nociceptive specific (NS) and wide-dynamic range (WDR) neurons is changed by ectopic activity, sensory loss, and changes in ion channels. Spinal cord neurons are subject to many receptor-mediated events, but increases in Ca channel function lead to increased transmitter release so that glutamate causes an enhanced activation of AMPA and NMDA receptors. Substance P acts on neurokinin 1 (NK1) receptors to add to the excitation. Reduced spinal inhibition through γ-aminobutyric acid (GABA) and the transporter potassium-chloride transporter member 5 (KCC2) aids enhanced pain messages. Reduced noradrenaline (NA) descending inhibition via α-2 adrenoceptors and increased 5-hydroxytryptamine (5HT) descending excitation via 5HT3 receptors add to the dominance of excitatory transmission. μ-Opioid receptors (MOR) are found on this circuitry.*

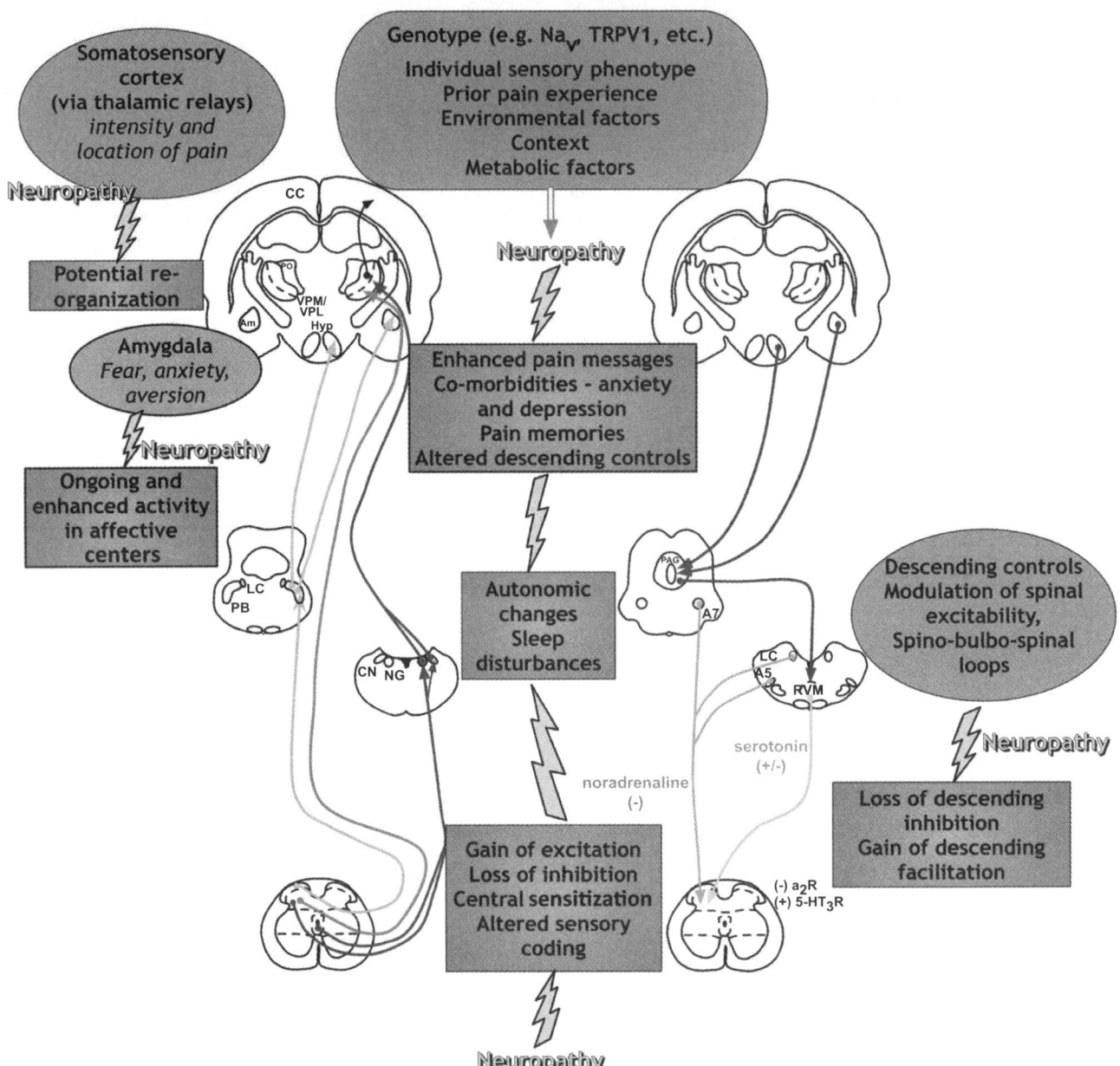

Figure 2—*An overview of the ascending* (left) *and descending* (right) *pain pathways. From the spinal cord there are spinoreticular projections and dorsal column pathways to the cuneate nucleus (CN) and nucleus gracilis (NG). Other limbic projections relay in the parabrachial nucleus (PB) and then project to the hypothalamus (Hyp) and amygdala (Am), where central autonomic function and fear/anxiety are processed. Spinothalamic pathways run to the ventrobasal medial (VPM) and lateral (VPL) areas and then run to the somatosensory part of the cerebral cortex (CC) where the location and the sensory components of pain are generated. Limbic brain areas (Am and Hyp) project down to the periqueductal gray (PAG) and to the locus coereleus (LC), A5 and A7 nuclei, and the rostroventral medial medulla (RVM). Thence, descending noradrenaline (NA) inhibition via α-2 adrenoceptors and increased 5-hydroxytryptamine (5HT) descending excitation via 5HT3 receptors modulates spinal cord activity. The changes induced by peripheral neuropathy on these brain functions are depicted together with comorbidities, and genotypic and phenotypic factors are shown.*

and its coreleased transmitter substance P permitting *N*-methyl-D-aspartate (NMDA) receptor activation, resulting in the wind-up of dorsal horn neurons. The analgesic effects of ketamine result from its ability to modulate this activity through blocks of the NMDA receptor (Fig. 1). However, similar mechanistic events underlie memory,

cognitive, and related functions and so the side effects of ketamine result from a lack of selectivity for spinal-pain related NMDA functions (61).

As a consequence of these changes in the sending of nociceptive information within the peripheral nerve and then the spinal cord, the information sent to the

brain becomes amplified so that pain ratings become higher. Alongside this, the persistent input into the limbic brain areas such as the amygdala are likely to be causal in the comorbidities that patients often report due to ongoing painful inputs disrupting normal function and generating fear, depression, and sleep problems

(Fig. 2). Of course, many patients report that their pains are worse at night, which may be due to nocturnal changes in these central pain processing areas. Finally, the neuropathic pain alters function and activity in the descending controls, which relay information from higher brain centers via the midbrain and brainstem to the spinal cord. In healthy volunteers and patients, a loss of inhibition or gain of facilitation promotes pain whereas evoking inhibition reduces pain (60). Preclinical studies suggest that the bases for this are descending noradrenergic, mostly inhibitory, and certain serotonergic controls that facilitate pain (Figs. 1 and 2). These monoamine descending controls regulate spinal neuronal activity bidirectionally and underlie the efficacy of antidepressants for the treatment of pain (60).

The increased analgesic effect of tapentadol, recently shown to be effective in animals and patients with diabetic neuropathy, likely resides in synergistic interactions between its weak opioid actions at spinal and supraspinal sites coupling to enhancing noradrenergic controls and so reducing opioid load (62). Interestingly, changes in the balance of control from the brain—the gain in descending facilitation coupled with a loss of inhibition—occur in the later stages after peripheral injury suggestive of a role in maintaining but not initiating the pain state. Furthermore, animal studies suggest that the recruitment of descending inhibitions may be protective and so can override the pain initiated by the neuropathic damage to the peripheral nerve (63).

So, overall, the mechanisms of pain in diabetic neuropathy extend from altered channel function in peripheral nerves through enhanced spinal processing and finally to changes in many higher centers (Fig. 2).

Management of painful

DSPN—The assessment and treatment of painful DSPN should ideally involve a multidisciplinary team that may include a diabetologist, a neurologist, the pain clinic team, specialist nurses, podiatrists, psychologists, physiotherapists, occupational therapists, and others. However, in most clinical settings this is not possible, and the management falls mainly to the diabetes physician, the primary care physician, or the neurologist. When treatment is started, a realistic objective would be to achieve around 50% reduction in

pain intensity. However, being "realistic" shouldn't be interpreted as less aggressive pursuit of maximum pain relief. Secondary objectives should include restoration or improvement in functional measures, QoL, sleep, and mood. Although it is hoped that improvement in pain will be followed by improvement in functionality, this may not be the case as many of these patients may have other comorbidities. Moreover, the multidisciplinary team should discuss potential interventions in addition to pharmacotherapy to help patients optimize function in the presence of residual pain.

Although strong evidence implicates poor glycemic control as a pathogenetic mechanism in the etiology of DSPN, there is no proof from randomized, controlled trials that this is the case for neuropathic pain in diabetes. However, as increased blood glucose flux has been reported to contribute to pain in DSPN (38), there is a general consensus that good blood glucose control should be the first step in the management of any form of diabetic neuropathy. Additionally, as cardiovascular disease is common in patients with DSPN (10) and vascular risk factors (hypertriglyceridemia, hypertension, visceral obesity etc.) appear to be implicated in the pathogenesis of DSPN (10,64), there is a good rationale for management of vascular risk factors beyond glycemic control.

Pharmacological treatment

Several pharmacological treatments have proven efficacy in the management of painful DSPN, although only duloxetine and pregabalin are approved for the treatment of neuropathic pain in diabetes by both the Food and Drugs Administration of the U.S. and the European Medicines Agency.

Pharmacological treatment of painful DSPN is not entirely satisfactory because currently available drugs are often ineffective and complicated by adverse events. Tricyclic compounds (TCAs) have been used as first-line agents for many years, but their use is limited by frequent side effects that may be central or anticholinergic, including dry mouth, constipation, sweating, blurred vision, sedation, and orthostatic hypotension (with the risk of falls particularly in elderly patients). For this reason, low-dose amitriptyline or imipramine 10 mg taken at night may be started. Depending upon efficacy and side effects, the dose can gradually be increased to

75 mg/day and on occasions even up to 150 mg/day (1). Higher doses have been associated with an increased risk of sudden cardiac death, and caution should be taken in any patient with a history of cardiovascular disease (65).

The selective serotonin noradrenalin reuptake inhibitors (SNRI) duloxetine and venlafaxine have been used for the management of painful DSPN (65). SNRIs relieve pain by increasing synaptic availability of 5-hydroxytryptamine and noradrenalin in the descending pathways that inhibit pain impulses. The efficacy of duloxetine in painful DSPN has been investigated in three identical trials, and pooled data from these shows that the 60 mg/day and 120 mg/day doses are effective in relieving painful symptoms, starting within 1 week and lasting the full treatment period of 12 weeks (66). The main side effects include nausea, somnolence, dizziness, constipation, dry mouth, and reduced appetite, although these tend to be mild to moderate and are transient. It is advisable to start at 30 mg/day taken with food for the first week and then increase to the standard dose of 60 mg/day. Venlafaxine (150–225 mg/day) is also effective in relieving painful DSPN, although cardiovascular adverse events limit its use in diabetes (67).

The anticonvulsant gabapentin, which binds to the $\alpha2\delta$ subunit of the calcium channel thereby reducing neurotransmitter release in the hyperexcited neuron, gradually titrated from 100 mg t.i.d. to 3,600 mg/day is also effective (68). More recently, there have been several clinical trials involving pregabalin in painful DSPN, and these showed clear efficacy in management of painful DSPN (69). Unlike gabapentin, pregabalin has linear pharmacokinetics, doesn't require a long titration period, and is started at 75 mg b.i.d. for about a week and increased to 150 mg b.i.d. maintenance dose with a maximum dose of 600 mg/day (55). The side effects include dizziness, somnolence, peripheral edema, headache, and weight gain.

Other effective but generally considered second line drugs (65) for painful DSPN include other anticonvulsants,in particular carbamazepine (65), although it has troublesome side effects including dizziness, somnolence and gait disturbance; tramadol, a weak opioid and weak inhibitor of noradrenaline and serotonin reuptake (65); the strong opioid oxycodone controlled release (65); and topical treatments including the substance-P depleter, topical capsaicin and the lidocaine patch (65). Refractory cases of patients with painful DSPN may be treated with intravenous lignocaine (5 mg/kg over 30 min) (65). Of the pathogenetically oriented treatments for painful DSPN only the antioxidant, α-lipoic acid administered intravenously over 3 weeks (600 mg i.v. per day) has been proven to be efficacious (2,70).

Recent guidelines for pharmacological treatment

The European Federation of Neurological Societies proposed that first-line treatments might comprise of TCAs, SNRIs, gabapentin, or pregabalin (71). The U.K. National Institute for Health and Care Excellence guidelines on the management of neuropathic pain in nonspecialist settings proposed that duloxetine should be the first-line treatment with amitriptyline as an alternative, and pregabalin as a second-line treatment for painful DSPN (72). However, this recommendation of duloxetine as the first-line therapy was not based on efficacy but rather cost-effectiveness. More recently, the American Academy of Neurology recommended that pregabalin is "established as effective and should be offered for relief of [painful DSPN] (Level A evidence)" (73), whereas venlafaxine, duloxetine, amitriptyline, gabapentin, valproate, opioids, and capsaicin were considered to be "probably effective and should be considered for treatment of painful DSPN (Level B evidence)" (63). However, this recommendation was primarily based on achievement of greater than 80% completion rate of clinical trials, which in turn may be influenced by the length of the trials. Finally, the International Consensus Panel on Diabetic Neuropathy recommended TCAs, duloxetine, pregabalin, and gabapentin as first-line agents having carefully reviewed all the available literature regarding the pharmacological treatment of painful DSPN (65), the final drug choice tailored to the particular patient based on demographic profile and comorbidities.

Tailoring treatment to individual requirements

The initial selection of a particular first-line treatment will be influenced by the assessment of contraindications, evaluation of comorbidities (including sleep disturbance, mood disorders, and other chronic medical/diabetes complications), and cost (65). For example, in diabetic patients with a history of heart disease,

elderly patients on other concomitant medications such diuretics and antihypertensives, and patients with comorbid orthostatic hypotension TCAs have relative contraindications. In patients with liver disease, duloxetine should not be prescribed, and in those with peripheral edema, pregabalin or gabapentin should be avoided. Moreover, although pharmaceutical companies may recommend a particular starting dose for their drugs based on their clinical trials, one has to appreciate that the clinical practice scenario is different from clinical trial scenario because many elderly patients with multiple comorbidities would have been excluded from trials. Therefore, treatment has to be individualized to take patient comorbidities including occupation, renal impairment, etc. into account, and caution is advised to start at lower than recommended doses and titrate gradually.

Comparator and combination trials

A major deficiency in the area of the treatment of neuropathic pain in diabetes is the relative lack of comparative or combination studies. Virtually all previous trials have been of active agents against placebo, whereas there is a need for more studies that compare a given drug with an active comparator and indeed lower-dose combination treatments (64). These issues have been highlighted by recent consensus guidelines from international institutions that have emphasized the need for large comparative and combination treatment trials in painful DSPN as a matter of priority (74,75).

Comparator trials. Bansal et al. (76) compared amitriptyline with pregabalin in painful DSPN in a small, randomized, double-blind, crossover trial. This study confirmed that whereas there was little difference in efficacy, pregabalin was the preferred drug because of a superior adverse event profile. However, a major drawback of this study was its small size, involving 51 patients only with many patients failing to complete the study.

Another recent small crossover study from the same group as the above study has compared duloxetine with amitriptyline (77). The study found that both drugs were equally efficacious although of the reported adverse events, dry mouth was more common with amitriptyline than duloxetine (55 vs. 24%; $P < 0.01$). Numerically, more patients preferred duloxetine although this was

not statistically significant (48 vs. 36%; $P = 0.18$).

The lack of direct comparator studies led to an indirect comparison of the efficacy and tolerability of duloxetine with that of pregabalin and gabapentin in participants with painful DSPN, using placebo as a common comparator (78). Efficacy criteria were reduction in 24-h pain severity for all three treatments, and treatment response rate ($\geq$50% pain reduction), and overall health improvement (as measured on the Patient Global Impression of Improvement/Change questionnaire) for duloxetine and pregabalin only. Indirect comparison between duloxetine and gabapentin found no statistically significant differences. Comparing duloxetine with pregabalin, the authors found significant differences in overall health improvement, favoring pregabalin, and in dizziness, favoring duloxetine. There was no significant difference in 24-h pain severity between duloxetine and pregabalin (78).

Combination trials. Gilron et al. (79) studied nortriptyline and gabapentin either in combination or alone in a randomized trial and confirmed that when given together, they were more efficacious than either drug given alone. In another crossover study by the same group, low-dose combination therapy with gabapentin and morphine was significantly more effective than higher doses of either (80).

COMBO-DN study. The COMBO-DN study that has just been completed (81) is the largest combination trial in painful DSPN and assessed whether combining standard doses of duloxetine and pregabalin is superior to increasing each drug to its maximum recommended dose in patients with incomplete pain relief. Patients with painful DSPN with a daily pain score of at least 4 (scale 0–10) were randomly assigned in a 1:1:1:1 ratio to one of four groups. For the 8-week initial treatment period, patients in groups 1 and 2 were treated with 60 mg duloxetine/day; patients in groups 3 and 4 received 300 mg pregabalin/day. Thereafter, only nonresponders (<30% improvement in pain relief) received double-blind treatment for further 8 weeks of the combination versus high-dose monotherapy treatment period with duloxetine 120 mg/day for group 1, duloxetine 60 mg/day + pregabalin 300 mg/day for groups 2 and 3, and pregabalin 600 mg/day for group 4. The primary outcome was change in the 24-h average pain (an item from BPI-MSF) after combination versus high-dose monotherapy period (groups 1, 4 pooled versus groups 2, 3 pooled).

Eight-hundred and four patients were evaluated in the initial period and 339 in the combination versus high-dose monotherapy treatment period, respectively. The difference between combination and monotherapy in the mean change of BPI-MSF average pain during combination versus high-dose monotherapy treatment period was not statistically significant (combination, −2.35; monotherapy, −2.16; $P = 0.37$) (81). Proportions of patients with treatment emergent adverse events were however similar: 36.7% (Combination) and 33.5% (Monotherapy). As a secondary end point the COMBO-DN study also compared the efficacy of standard doses of duloxetine and pregabalin as initial treatment for painful DSPN, and duloxetine was found to have superior efficacy compared with pregabalin, without any safety findings of concern. At the end of the combination versus high-dose monotherapy treatment period, although the groups are no longer randomized, 50% pain relief was found in 46.9% of subjects on 600 mg/day pregabalin compared with 28.4% on 120 mg/day of duloxetine.

Taken together, even though the primary end point was not met, the COMBO-DN study demonstrated that at standard doses duloxetine has better efficacy than pregabalin as an initial treatment for painful DSPN, without any safety findings of concern. However, pregabalin catches up with duloxetine in terms of efficacy as the doses are increased to maximum.

Conclusion—A simple algorithm was suggested by the Toronto International Neuropathy Consensus meeting (Fig. 3) to help practitioners in the management of patients with painful DSPN (2,65). After exclusion of other causes and optimization of glycemic control, first-line therapies would include either an antidepressant (a tricyclic or duloxetine) or an anticonvulsant (gabapentin or pregabalin). These therapies all have level A evidence for efficacy and a clear pathway of progression if initial therapies fail is provided. Those patients with the severest neuropathic pain unresponsiveness to antidepressant or anticonvulsant therapy might require short-term treatment with opioid or opioid-like drugs such as tramadol or controlled release oxycodone. Finally, it must always be emphasized that all patients with any form of diabetic neuropathy are at increased risk of foot ulceration and require education in self foot care and, if possible, regular podiatry assessment and treatment.

Acknowledgments—S.T. has received honoraria for invited lectures from Eli Lilly and Pfizer. A.J.M.B. has received honoraria from Eli Lilly and Pfizer and has served on an advisory board for Pamlab. A.H.D. is a speaker and is on the advisory board panels for Astellas, Grunenthal, and Pfizer and Lilly. A.H.D. is supported by the Wellcome Trust London Pain Consortium. No other potential conflicts of interest relevant to this article were reported.

The authors gratefully acknowledge the production of figures by Dr. Shafaq Sikandar.

References
1. Boulton AJM, Malik RA, Arezzo JC, Sosenko JM. Diabetic somatic neuropathies. Diabetes Care 2004;27:1458–1486
2. Tesfaye S, Boulton AJM, Dyck PJ, et al.; Toronto Diabetic Neuropathy Expert Group. Diabetic neuropathies: update on definitions, diagnostic criteria, estimation of severity, and treatments. Diabetes Care 2010;33:2285–2293
3. Zelman DC, Brandenburg NA, Gore M. Sleep impairment in patients with painful diabetic peripheral neuropathy. Clin J Pain 2006;22:681–685
4. Gore M, Brandenburg NA, Dukes E, Hoffman DL, Tai KS, Stacey B. Pain severity in diabetic peripheral neuropathy is associated with patient functioning, symptom levels of anxiety and depression, and sleep. J Pain Symptom Manage 2005;30:374–385
5. Boulton AJM, Armstrong WD, Scarpello JHB, Ward JD. The natural history of painful diabetic neuropathy—a 4-year study. Postgrad Med J 1983;59:556–559
6. Benbow SJ, Chan AW, Bowsher D, MacFarlane IA, Williams G. A prospective study of painful symptoms, small-fibre function and peripheral vascular disease in chronic painful diabetic neuropathy. Diabet Med 1994;11:17–21
7. Abbott CA, Malik RA, van Ross ER, Kulkarni J, Boulton AJ. Prevalence and characteristics of painful diabetic neuropathy in a large community-based diabetic population in the U.K. Diabetes Care 2011; 34:2220–2224
8. Daousi C, McFarlane IA, Woodward A, Nurmikko TJ, Bendred PE, Benbow SJ. Chronic painful peripheral neuropathy in an urban community: a control comparison of people with and without diabetes. Diabet Med 2004;21:976–982
9. Davies M, Brophy S, Williams R, Taylor A. The prevalence, severity, and impact of painful diabetic peripheral neuropathy in type 2 diabetes. Diabetes Care 2006;29:1518–1522
10. Tesfaye S, Chaturvedi N, Eaton SEM, et al.; EURODIAB Prospective Complications Study Group. Vascular risk factors

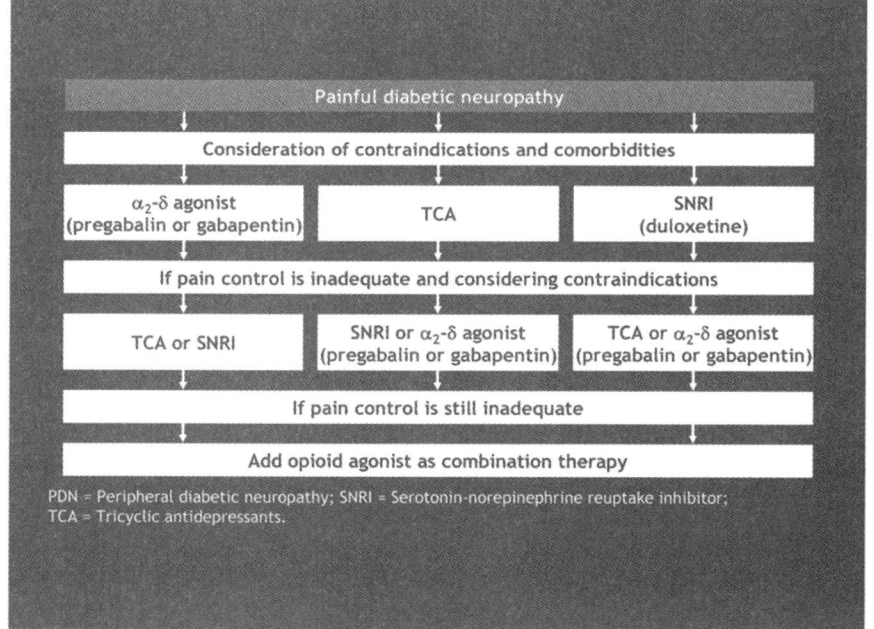

Figure 3—*Treatment algorithm for painful DSPN. Adapted with permission from Tesfaye et al. (65).*

and diabetic neuropathy. N Engl J Med 2005;352:341–350

11. Ziegler D, Rathmann W, Dickhaus T, Meisinger C, Mielck A; KORA Study Group. Neuropathic pain in diabetes, pre-diabetes and normal glucose tolerance: the MONICA/KORA Augsburg Surveys S2 and S3. Pain Med 2009;10:393–400

12. Van Acker K, Bouhassira D, De Bacquer D, et al. Prevalence and impact on quality of life of peripheral neuropathy with or without neuropathic pain in type 1 and type 2 diabetic patients attending hospital outpatients clinics. Diabetes Metab 2009; 35:206–213

13. Ziegler D, Rathmann W, Meisinger C, Dickhaus T, Mielck A; KORA Study Group. Prevalence and risk factors of neuropathic pain in survivors of myocardial infarction with pre-diabetes and diabetes. The KORA Myocardial Infarction Registry. Eur J Pain 2009;13:582–587

14. Boulton AJ, Vinik AI, Arezzo JC, et al.; American Diabetes Association. Diabetic neuropathies: a statement by the American Diabetes Association. Diabetes Care 2005; 28:956–962

15. Vinik AI, Erbas T, Park TS, Pierce KK, Stansberry KB. Methods for evaluation of peripheral neurovascular dysfunction. Diabetes Technol Ther 2001;3:29–50

16. Malik R, Veves A, Tesfaye S, et al.; on behalf of the Toronto Consensus Panel on Diabetic Neuropathy. Small fiber neuropathy: role in the diagnosis of diabetic sensorimotor polyneuropathy. Diabetes Metab Res Rev 2011;27:678–684

17. Rolke R, Baron R, Maier C, et al. Quantitative sensory testing in the German Research Network on Neuropathic Pain (DFNS): standardized protocol and reference values. Pain 2006;123:231–243

18. Ragé M, Van Acker N, Knaapen MW, et al. Asymptomatic small fiber neuropathy in diabetes mellitus: investigations with intraepidermal nerve fiber density, quantitative sensory testing and laser-evoked potentials. J Neurol 2011;258:1852–1864

19. Chao C-C, Tseng MT, Lin YJ, et al. Pathophysiology of neuropathic pain in type 2 diabetes: skin denervation and contact heat-evoked potentials. Diabetes Care 2010;33:2654–2659

20. Young MJ, Boulton AJM, MacLeod AF, Williams DR, Sonksen PH. A multicentre study of the prevalence of diabetic peripheral neuropathy in the United Kingdom hospital clinic population. Diabetologia 1993;36:150–154

21. Bril V, Perkins BA. Validation of the Toronto Clinical Scoring System for diabetic polyneuropathy. Diabetes Care 2002;25: 2048–2052

22. Feldman EL, Stevens MJ, Thomas PK, Brown MB, Canal N, Greene DA. A practical two-step quantitative clinical and electrophysiological assessment for the diagnosis

and staging of diabetic neuropathy. Diabetes Care 1994;17:1281–1289

23. Dyck PJ. Detection, characterization, and staging of polyneuropathy: assessed in diabetics. Muscle Nerve 1988;11:21–32

24. Dyck PJ, Overland CJ, Low PA, et al. Signs and symptoms versus nerve conduction studies to diagnose diabetic sensorimotor polyneuropathy: Cl vs. NPhys trial. Muscle Nerve 2010;42:157–164

25. Cruccu G, Sommer C, Anand P, et al. EFNS guidelines on neuropathic pain assessment: revised 2009. Eur J Neurol 2010;17:1010–1018

26. Zelman DC, Gore M, Dukes E, Tai KS, Brandenburg N. Validation of a modified version of the brief pain inventory for painful diabetic peripheral neuropathy. J Pain Symptom Manage 2005;29:401–410

27. Bouhassira D, Attal N, Fermanian J, et al. Development and validation of the Neuropathic Pain Symptom Inventory. Pain 2004;108:248–257

28. Backonja MM, Krause SJ. Neuropathic pain questionnaire—short form. Clin J Pain 2003;19:315–316

29. Bennett M. The LANSS Pain Scale: the Leeds assessment of neuropathic symptoms and signs. Pain 2001;92:147–157

30. Freynhagen R, Baron R, Gockel U, Tölle TR. painDETECT: a new screening questionnaire to identify neuropathic components in patients with back pain. Curr Med Res Opin 2006;22:1911–1920

31. Melzack R. The short-form McGill pain questionnaire. Pain 1987;30:191–197

32. Vileikyte L, Peyrot M, Bundy C, et al. The development and validation of a neuropathy- and foot ulcer-specific quality of life instrument. Diabetes Care 2003;26: 2549–2555

33. Vinik EJ, Hayes RP, Oglesby A, et al. The development and validation of the Norfolk QOL-DN, a new measure of patients' perception of the effects of diabetes and diabetic neuropathy. Diabetes Technol Ther 2005;7:497–508

34. Vinik A. The approach to the management of the patient with neuropathic pain. J Clin Endocrinol Metab 2010;95:4802–4811

35. Zigmond AS, Snaith RP. The hospital anxiety and depression scale. Acta Psychiatr Scand 1983;67:361–370

36. Beck AT, Steer RA, Brown GK. *Manual for the Beck Depression Inventory-II.* San Antonio, TX, Psychological Corporation, 1996, p. 38

37. Tesfaye S, Kempler P. Painful diabetic neuropathy. Diabetologia 2005;48:805–807

38. Oyibo SO, Prasad YDM, Jackson NJ, Jude EB, Boulton AJ. The relationship between blood glucose excursions and painful diabetic peripheral neuropathy: a pilot study. Diabet Med 2002;19:870–873

39. Eaton SE, Harris ND, Ibrahim S, et al. Increased sural nerve epineurial blood flow

in human subjects with painful diabetic neuropathy. Diabetologia 2003;46:934–939

40. Quattrini C, Harris ND, Malik RA, Tesfaye S. Impaired skin microvascular reactivity in painful diabetic neuropathy. Diabetes Care 2007;30:655–659

41. Sorensen L, Molyneaux L, Yue DK. The relationship among pain, sensory loss, and small nerve fibers in diabetes. Diabetes Care 2006;29:883–887

42. Selvarajah D, Wilkinson ID, Gandhi R, Griffiths PD, Tesfaye S. Microvascular perfusion abnormalities of the Thalamus in painful but not painless diabetic polyneuropathy: a clue to the pathogenesis of pain in type 1 diabetes. Diabetes Care 2011;34:718–720

43. Gandhi RA, Marques JLB, Selvarajah D, Emery CJ, Tesfaye S. Painful diabetic neuropathy is associated with greater autonomic dysfunction than painless diabetic neuropathy. Diabetes Care 2010; 33:1585–1590

44. Maier C, Baron R, Tölle TR, et al. Quantitative sensory testing in the German Research Network on Neuropathic Pain (DFNS): somatosensory abnormalities in 1236 patients with different neuropathic pain syndromes. Pain 2010;150:439–450

45. Venkatachalam K, Montell C. TRP channels. Annu Rev Biochem 2007;76:387–417

46. Caterina MJ, Schumacher MA, Tominaga M, Rosen TA, Levine JD, Julius D. The capsaicin receptor: a heat-activated ion channel in the pain pathway. Nature 1997; 389:816–824

47. Colburn RW, Lubin ML, Stone DJ Jr, et al. Attenuated cold sensitivity in TRPM8 null mice. Neuron 2007;54:379–386

48. Binder A, May D, Baron R, et al. Transient receptor potential channel polymorphisms are associated with the somatosensory function in neuropathic pain patients. PLoS One 2011; 6:e17387

49. Honore P, Kage K, Mikusa J, et al. Analgesic profile of intrathecal P2X(3) antisense oligonucleotide treatment in chronic inflammatory and neuropathic pain states in rats. Pain 2002;99:11–19

50. Dickenson AH, Matthews EA, Suzuki R. Neurobiology of neuropathic pain: mode of action of anticonvulsants. Eur J Pain 2002;6(Suppl. A):51–60

51. Yang Y, Wang Y, Li S, et al. Mutations in SCN9A, encoding a sodium channel alpha subunit, in patients with primary erythermalgia. J Med Genet 2004;41:171–174

52. Cox JJ, Reimann F, Nicholas AK, et al. An SCN9A channelopathy causes congenital inability to experience pain. Nature 2006; 444:894–898

53. Reimann F, Cox JJ, Belfer I, et al. Pain perception is altered by a nucleotide polymorphism in SCN9A. Proc Natl Acad Sci USA 2010;107:5148–5153

54. Harvey VL, Dickenson AH. Mechanisms of pain in nonmalignant disease. Curr Opin Support Palliat Care 2008;2:133–139

55. Bierhaus A, Fleming T, Stoyanov S, et al. Methylglyoxal modification of Nav1.8 facilitates nociceptive neuron firing and causes hyperalgesia in diabetic neuropathy. Nat Med 2012;18:926–933

56. Blackburn-Munro G, Jensen BS. The anticonvulsant retigabine attenuates nociceptive behaviours in rat models of persistent and neuropathic pain. Eur J Pharmacol 2003;460:109–116

57. Passmore GM, Selyanko AA, Mistry M, et al. KCNQ/M currents in sensory neurons: significance for pain therapy. J Neurosci 2003;23:7227–7236

58. Harris JA, Murphy JA. Retigabine (ezogabine) as add-on therapy for partial-onset seizures: an update for clinicians. Ther Adv Chronic Dis 2011;2:371–376

59. Bauer CS, Nieto-Rostro M, Rahman W, et al. The increased trafficking of the calcium channel subunit alpha2delta-1 to presynaptic terminals in neuropathic pain is inhibited by the alpha2delta ligand pregabalin. J Neurosci 2009;29:4076–4088

60. Bannister K, Bee LA, Dickenson AH. Preclinical and early clinical investigations related to monoaminergic pain modulation. Neurotherapeutics 2009;6:703–712

61. D'Mello R, Dickenson AH. Spinal cord mechanisms of pain. Br J Anaesth 2008; 101:8–16

62. Bee LA, Bannister K, Rahman W, Dickenson AH. Mu-opioid and noradrenergic $\alpha(2)$-adrenoceptor contributions to the effects of tapentadol on spinal electrophysiological measures of nociception in nerve-injured rats. Pain 2011;152:131–139

63. De Felice M, Sanoja R, Wang R, et al. Engagement of descending inhibition from the rostral ventromedial medulla protects against chronic neuropathic pain. Pain 2011;152:2701–2709

64. Ziegler D. Current concepts in the management of diabetic polyneuropathy. Curr Diabetes Rev 2011;7:208–220

65. Tesfaye S, Vileikyte L, Rayman G, et al.; Toronto Expert Panel on Diabetic Neuropathy. Painful diabetic peripheral neuropathy: consensus recommendations on diagnosis,

assessment and management. Diabetes Metab Res Rev 2011;27:629–638

66. Kajdasz DK, Iyengar S, Desaiah D, et al. Duloxetine for the management of diabetic peripheral neuropathic pain: evidence-based findings from post hoc analysis of three multicenter, randomized, double-blind, placebo-controlled, parallel-group studies. Clin Ther 2007;29(Suppl.):2536–2546

67. Rowbotham MC, Goli V, Kunz NR, Lei D. Venlafaxine extended release in the treatment of painful diabetic neuropathy: a double-blind, placebo-controlled study. Pain 2004;110:697–706

68. Backonja MM, Beydoun A, Edwards KR, et al. Gabapentin for the symptomatic treatment of painful neuropathy in patients with diabetes mellitus: a randomized controlled trial. JAMA 1998;280:1831–1836

69. Freeman R, Durso-Decruz E, Emir B. Efficacy, safety, and tolerability of pregabalin treatment for painful diabetic peripheral neuropathy: findings from seven randomized, controlled trials across a range of doses. Diabetes Care 2008;31:1448–1454

70. Ziegler D, Nowak H, Kempler P, Vargha P, Low PA. Treatment of symptomatic diabetic polyneuropathy with the antioxidant alpha-lipoic acid: a meta-analysis. Diabet Med 2004;21:114–121

71. Attal N, Cruccu G, Baron R, et al.; European Federation of Neurological Societies. EFNS guidelines on the pharmacological treatment of neuropathic pain: 2010 revision. Eur J Neurol 2010;17:1113–e88

72. NICE Clinical Guideline 96: Neuropathic Pain. The pharmacological management of neuropathic pain in adults in non-specialist settings. March 2010. Available from www.nice.org.uk

73. Bril V, England J, Franklin GM, et al.; American Academy of Neurology; American Association of Neuromuscular and Electrodiagnostic Medicine; American Academy of Physical Medicine and Rehabilitation. Evidence-based guideline:

Treatment of painful diabetic neuropathy: report of the American Academy of Neurology, the American Association of Neuromuscular and Electrodiagnostic Medicine, and the American Academy of Physical Medicine and Rehabilitation. Neurology 2011;76:1758–1765

74. Vorobeychik Y, Gordin V, Mao J, Chen L. Combination therapy for neuropathic pain: a review of current evidence. CNS Drugs 2011;25:1023–1034

75. O'Connor AB, Dworkin RH. Treatment of neuropathic pain: an overview of recent guidelines. Am J Med 2009;122(Suppl.):S22–S32

76. Bansal D, Bhansali A, Hota D, Chakrabarti A, Dutta P. Amitriptyline vs. pregabalin in painful diabetic neuropathy: a randomized double blind clinical trial. Diabet Med 2009;26:1019–1026

77. Kaur H, Hota D, Bhansali A, Dutta P, Bansal D, Chakrabarti A. A comparative evaluation of amitriptyline and duloxetine in painful diabetic neuropathy: a randomized, double-blind, cross-over clinical trial. Diabetes Care 2011;34:818–822

78. Quilici S, Chancellor J, Löthgren M, et al. Meta-analysis of duloxetine vs. pregabalin and gabapentin in the treatment of diabetic peripheral neuropathic pain. BMC Neurol 2009;9:6

79. Gilron I, Bailey JM, Tu D, Holden RR, Jackson AC, Houlden RL. Nortriptyline and gabapentin, alone and in combination for neuropathic pain: a double-blind, randomised controlled crossover trial. Lancet 2009;374:1252–1261

80. Gilron I, Bailey JM, Tu D, Holden RR, Weaver DF, Houlden RL. Morphine, gabapentin, or their combination for neuropathic pain. N Engl J Med 2005;352:1324–1334

81. Tesfaye S, Wilhelm S, Lledo A, et al. Duloxetine and pregabalin: high-dose monotherapy or their combination? The "COMBO-DN study" - a multinational, randomized, double-blind, parallel-group study in patients with diabetic peripheral neuropathic pain. Pain. 31 May 2013 [Epub ahead of print]

Very Low–Calorie Diet Mimics the Early Beneficial Effect of Roux-en-Y Gastric Bypass on Insulin Sensitivity and β-Cell Function in Type 2 Diabetic Patients

Clifton Jackness,[1] Wahida Karmally,[2] Gerardo Febres,[1] Irene M. Conwell,[1] Leaque Ahmed,[3] Marc Bessler,[3] Donald J. McMahon,[1] and Judith Korner[1]

Marked improvement in glycemic control occurs in patients with type 2 diabetes mellitus shortly after Roux-en-Y gastric bypass surgery (RYGB) and before there is major weight loss. The objective of this study was to determine whether the magnitude of this change is primarily due to caloric restriction or is unique to the surgical procedure. We studied eleven subjects who underwent RYGB and fourteen subjects mean-matched for BMI, HbA$_{1c}$, and diabetes duration who were admitted to our inpatient research unit and given a very low–calorie diet (VLCD) of 500 kcal/day with a macronutrient content similar to that consumed by patients after RYGB. Frequently sampled intravenous glucose tolerance tests were performed before and after interventions. Both groups lost an equivalent amount of weight over a mean study period of 21 days. Insulin sensitivity, acute insulin secretion after intravenous glucose administration, and β-cell function as determined by disposition index improved to a similar extent in both groups. Likewise, changes in fasting glucose and fructosamine levels were similar. Based on these data, VLCD improves insulin sensitivity and β-cell function just as well as RYGB in the short term. *Diabetes* **62:3027–3032, 2013**

The prevalence of obesity and the associated health consequences, including type 2 diabetes mellitus (T2DM), continues to rise (1). The typical progression of T2DM is one of deteriorating β-cell function that requires an increasing amount of oral medical therapy and finally insulin treatment to achieve adequate glycemic control (2). Ultimately, there is pancreatic β-cell failure (3). Calorie restriction and subsequent weight loss have been shown to be effective treatment modalities of T2DM (4). Caloric restriction can improve hyperglycemia through regulation of hepatic glucose production (5). In addition to cumulative weight loss, the rapidity with which the weight loss is achieved also exerts an effect on glycemic control (6). Unfortunately, most individuals are unable to maintain a reduced body weight through diet alone (7). In contrast, weight loss achieved by bariatric surgery has been shown to result in a lesser degree of recidivism than nonsurgical treatments and is associated with marked improvement of glycemic control (8).

While Roux-en-Y gastric bypass surgery (RYGB) produces profound weight loss, glycemic control improves within the first 2–3 weeks after the procedure and before much of the weight loss occurs, leading to the hypothesis that factors in addition to weight loss are involved (9,10). In an animal study of nonobese Goto-Kakizaki rats, bypass of the duodenum and jejunum has been shown to control hyperglycemia unrelated to weight reduction (11), leading to the hypothesis that routing nutrients away from the proximal small intestine produces an antidiabetes effect. Rapid delivery of nutrients to the distal small intestine also enhances postprandial secretion of the incretin glucagon-like peptide-1 (GLP-1). Substantial changes in GLP-1 levels have been observed after RYGB but not after gastric banding or equivalent weight loss achieved by diet (12–14), thus providing another mechanism for improvement in glucose homeostasis after RYGB.

We have previously demonstrated that there was less improvement in β-cell function of subjects with T2DM on an 800 kcal/day low-calorie diet compared with a matched cohort of RYGB subjects when assessed with an intravenous glucose challenge after equivalent weight reduction (15). A limitation of the study was that the low-calorie diet group took longer than the surgery group to achieve equivalent weight loss, indicating that the degree of caloric restriction was not equivalent to the RYGB group. The difference in caloric intake confounds interpretation of the results because the degree of caloric restriction in addition to the amount of weight loss affects glucostatic parameters. For example, Wing et al. (16) demonstrated that an 11% reduction in body weight with a 400 kcal/day diet resulted in significantly greater insulin sensitivity compared with the same weight reduction achieved over a longer period of time on a 1,100 kcal/day diet. Henry et al. (4) demonstrated that on 330 kcal/day, the majority of improvement in fasting plasma glucose occurred within the first 10 days of caloric restriction preceding most of the weight loss. Minimal further improvement followed after continued weight loss, thus demonstrating that most of the improvement in glucose occurs within the first few days of caloric restriction.

Based on our previous study, we were unable to rule out the possibility that the greater improvement in β-cell function after RYGB was due to the surgical procedure itself as opposed to greater caloric restriction. Therefore,

From the [1]Department of Medicine, Columbia University College of Physicians and Surgeons, New York, New York; the [2]Irving Institute for Clinical and Translational Research, Columbia University, New York, New York; and the [3]Department of Surgery, Columbia University College of Physicians and Surgeons, New York, New York.

Corresponding author: Judith Korner, jk181@columbia.edu.

Received 14 December 2012 and accepted 17 April 2013.

DOI: 10.2337/db12-1762. Clinical trial reg. no. NCT00627484, clinicaltrials.gov.

See accompanying commentary, p. 3017.

in this study, we sought to confirm our previous finding by changing the diet to a very low–calorie diet (VLCD) of 500 kcal/day, which is similar to the typical intake in the early post-RYGB period. This VLCD resulted in the same amount of weight loss over the same period of time as the RYGB group. β-Cell function was assessed by frequently sampled intravenous glucose tolerance tests (fsIVGTTs) before and at a mean of 21 days after the interventions.

RESEARCH DESIGN AND METHODS

Two groups of subjects with a self-reported history of T2DM were recruited, consisting of individuals who were scheduled to undergo RYGB ($n = 11$) or willing to participate in a nonsurgical inpatient VLCD program ($n = 14$). The decision to undergo surgery was made between patient and physician, independent of this research protocol. Subjects for the VLCD were recruited by word of mouth and flyers placed throughout the Medical Center. Main inclusion criteria were HbA$_{1c}$ 6.5–12% (48–108 mmol/mol), age 18–65 years, and BMI >35 kg/m^2. Major exclusion criteria were the use of thiazolidinedione or insulin at a dose of >60 units/day, use of dipeptidyl peptidase-4 inhibitor or GLP-1 receptor agonist for >12 months, fasting triglycerides >400 mg/dL, weight change >5% in the previous 3 months, or significant illness. Of study participants, 16% were Caucasian, 44% African American, and 40% Hispanic. The study was approved by the Columbia University Institutional Review Board, and written informed consent was obtained from all subjects.

After an overnight fast, volunteers in the VLCD group were admitted as inpatients for the duration of the study to the Clinical Research Resource in the Irving Institute of Clinical and Translational Research and were placed on a clear diet equivalent to the inpatient postoperative RYGB diet of 360 kcal for the day. On day 2 and the next 14–24 days (duration depended upon subjects' personal schedules), a diet similar in amount and macronutrient content that is recommended by the bariatric dietitians during this early postoperative period was provided. The diet consisted of 500 kcal/day (50% protein, 35% carbohydrate, and 15% fat) consumed as six mini-meals prepared with low-fat milk, pureed fruit and vegetables, Crystal Light, and Jell-O pudding mixes (Kraft Foods, Northfield, IL). Protein intake was met with the incorporation of UNJURY whey protein isolate (ProSynthesis Laboratories, Sterling, VA). Appropriate vitamin and mineral supplementation was provided as well as noncaloric noncarbonated caffeine-free beverages, sugar-free chewing gum, and sodium-free flavored bouillon. After the first 4 days, subjects were allowed day passes to leave the unit when needed to run personal errands, and if necessary, were provided a cooler containing a meal to ensure adherence to diet and schedule. RYGB was performed as previously described (13). Although patients were encouraged to lose weight prior to surgery, none of our participants were on a reduced-calorie diet at the time of the first fsIVGTT or experienced weight change between the time of testing and the day of surgery.

fsIVGTT procedure and calculations. fsIVGTT was performed prior to and postintervention. Subjects were instructed to avoid strenuous exercise for 2 days prior to the procedure. Oral diabetes medications were held 2–3 days prior to testing and injectable medications held 1 day prior. After a 10-h fast, blood samples were collected for hormone and metabolic analyses. Glucose (0.3g/kg body wt as dextrose 50 g/dL) was administered intravenously within 2 min at $t = 0$, and subsequent samples were obtained at 2, 3, 4, 5, 6, 8, 10, 12, 14, 16, 19, 22, 24, 25, 27, 30, 40, 50, 60, 70, 90, 100, 120, 140, 160, and 180 min. At 20 min, an intravenous injection of regular insulin (0.05 units/kg body wt) was administered to increase the accuracy of measuring insulin sensitivity in diabetic subjects (17). Insulin sensitivity was assessed using the Bergman minimal model analysis (MINMOD Millennium 6.02 software) of fsIVGTT (18,19). The equations of this model provide measures of glucose-dependent glucose elimination, the sensitivity of glucose elimination to insulin (S_i), and the acute insulin response to glucose (AIR). Disposition index (DI) is derived from the product of S_i and AIR and is a measure of insulin secretion in relation to insulin sensitivity. Acute C-peptide response (ACPR) is the relative mean increase (in percent) from fasting in C-peptide levels 3–5 min after glucose administration. Homeostasis model assessment of insulin resistance (HOMA-IR) was calculated as reported by Matthews et al. (20).

Analytic assays. Serum insulin, C-peptide, and high-sensitivity C-reactive protein (CRP) were measured with the Immulite Analyzer (Siemens, Los Angeles, CA). Leptin, total ghrelin, and glucose were measured as previously described (21). Total PYY was measured by ELISA (Millipore, St. Charles, MO) with a sensitivity of 10 pg/mL and 2.3% intra-assay and 7.2% interassay coefficients of variation. Total GLP-1 was measured by radioimmunoassay after alcohol extraction according to the manufacturer's protocol (Millipore). Sensitivity of the assay is 3 pmol/L, and recovery in each assay was tested by parallel extraction of standards. High–molecular weight adiponectin was quantified by ELISA (Millipore) with an assay sensitivity of 0.5 ng/mL and 2.4%

intra-assay and 5.5% interassay coefficients of variation. All samples analyzed by radioimmunoassay or ELISA were run in duplicate.

Statistical analysis. Based on our previous work, we estimated that ΔDI for VLCD versus RYGB would equal 160 with an estimated SD equal to 120. Nine subjects in each group would provide 80% probability of detecting this estimated difference with a P α < 0.05% (15). SAS version 9.2 software (Cary, NC) was used for statistical analysis. Group differences in the distribution of continuous variables at baseline were tested with a Student independent t test, as were group differences at end point. Within-group differences between pre- and posttreatment were tested with dependent t tests. The between-group differences in the change from pre- to posttreatment were tested with independent t tests. All tests were two tailed, with P values <0.05 considered statistically significant. No adjustment of the critical value of the test statistic was made for the separate tests of different peptides or for HOMA-IR. Model estimated means and SEs are presented.

RESULTS

Clinical characteristics. Baseline clinical characteristics of study subjects were similar between groups (Table 1). The study cohort had a mean BMI of 41.2 kg/m^2. The mean duration of diabetes was 5.7 ± 0.9 years (range 0.5–15), and the mean HbA$_{1c}$ was 8.4 ± 0.3% (6.2–11.1) (68 ± 3 mmol/mol [range 44–98]). All subjects except one person in the VLCD were taking antihyperglycemic medications, with two subjects in each group on additional insulin therapy. Table 2 shows that there was no difference in the time period (21 ± 1 days) needed to achieve a similar loss of body weight (7.6 ± 0.4%) between treatment groups.

Glucostatic parameters before and after interventions. Baseline glucostatic parameters, with the exception of fasting insulin concentrations, were similar in both groups and are presented in Table 2. Decreases in fasting glucose and C-peptide concentrations and increases in S_i, AIR, ACPR, and DI occurred in both groups to a similar extent (Table 2 and Figs. 1 and 2). While the insulin–to–C-peptide ratio was different between groups, the decrease in these values was not different ($P = 0.26$). Within-group change in fructosamine was significant in VLCD group but did not reach significance in RYGB group ($P = 0.057$). However, the change in fructosamine when adjusted for baseline values was not significant between groups ($P = 0.33$). After interventions, three RYGB and four VLCD subjects remained on antihyperglycemic medication.

Linear regression was used to determine whether baseline characteristics correlated with changes in DI. Duration of diabetes was not predictive of change in DI in RYGB (β = −1.66; $P = 0.29$) or VLCD (β = −1.56; $P = 0.33$), and the initial value of HbA$_{1c}$ was not predictive either (β = −4.8, $P = 0.29$, and β = 7.6, $P = 0.26$, in RYGB and VLCD, respectively). Baseline DI was not associated with change in DI (β = −1.9, $P = 0.19$, and β = −0.2, $P = 0.86$). Baseline S_i and AIR were not predictive of the change in DI in either group (data not shown). The amount of weight loss was not correlated with change in DI in either the RYGB ($P = 0.92$) or VLCD ($P = 0.99$) group.

TABLE 1
Subject characteristics at baseline

Parameter	RYGB	VLCD
N (female/male)	11 (7/4)	14 (8/6)
Age (years)	44.6 ± 3.0	51.9 ± 2.0
Body weight (kg)	121.4 ± 6.7	114.2 ± 6.6
BMI (kg/m^2)	43.2 ± 2.3	39.2 ± 1.0
T2DM duration (years)	5.9 ± 1.6	5.5 ± 1.1
HbA$_{1c}$ (%; mmol/mol)	8.2 ± 0.5; 66 ± 2	8.5 ± 0.3; 69 ± 1

Data are means ± SEM.

TABLE 2
Weight loss and glucostatic parameters before and after interventions

Parameter	RYGB		VLCD		P^a
	Pre-intervention	Postintervention	Pre-intervention	Postintervention	
Weight loss period (days)		22.9 ± 1.8		19.6 ± 1.0	0.10
Weight loss (%)		8.1 ± 0.7		7.2 ± 0.4	0.27
Glucose (mg/dL)	179 ± 21	$125 \pm 12^{**}$	184 ± 12	$110 \pm 6^{***}$	0.32
Fructosamine (μmol/L)	273 ± 1.8	241 ± 11	299 ± 12	$250 \pm 8^{***}$	0.33
C-peptide (ng/mL)	3.72 ± 0.41	$2.95 \pm 0.32^{*}$	3.59 ± 0.40	$2.55 \pm 0.36^{**}$	0.51
Insulin (μIU/mL)	$\mathbf{23.1 \pm 3.8}$	$\mathbf{12.7 \pm 2.4^{**}}$	$\mathbf{13.8 \pm 2.1}$	$\mathbf{6.8 \pm 1.5^{***}}$	0.23
Insulin–to–C-peptide ratio	$\mathbf{6.30 \pm 0.67}$	$\mathbf{4.08 \pm 0.54^{**}}$	$\mathbf{3.80 \pm 0.33}$	$\mathbf{2.45 \pm 0.25^{***}}$	0.26
HOMA-IR	9.5 ± 1.6	$\mathbf{3.5 \pm 0.6^{**}}$	6.2 ± 1.1	$\mathbf{1.8 \pm 0.4^{***}}$	0.35
S_g (min^{-1})	0.011 ± 0.001	0.014 ± 0.003	0.013 ± 0.002	0.011 ± 0.002	0.22
S_i (mL · μU^{-1} · min^{-1})	1.03 ± 0.25	$1.66 \pm 0.27^{*}$	1.26 ± 0.20	$2.11 \pm 0.29^{*}$	0.59
AIR (mL^{-1} · μU · min)	33.7 ± 13.0	$124.0 \pm 36^{**}$	32.4 ± 14.7	$97.3 \pm 28.3^{**}$	0.45
ACPR (%)	12.1 ± 2.8	$28.5 \pm 21.0^{*}$	12.1 ± 5.3	$24.0 \pm 17.7^{**}$	0.99
DI	30.1 ± 15.6	$201 \pm 62^{*}$	31.0 ± 15.7	$168 \pm 59^{*}$	0.71

Data are presented as mean $\pm$ SEM. S_g, glucose-dependent glucose elimination. Boldface data at pre- or postintervention are different between groups: $P < 0.05$. $^a P$ value for independent t test of group difference in change from pre- to posttreatment. $^*P < 0.05$, $^{**}P < 0.01$, $^{***}P < 0.001$, within-group differences between pre- and posttreatment.

Plasma hormone and lipid levels. There were significant increases in adiponectin and GLP-1 in the RYGB group, and the difference in change from baseline between groups approached significance (Table 3) ($P = 0.05$ and 0.10 for change in adiponectin and GLP-1, respectively). There were no significant changes in fasting plasma levels of ghrelin and PYY. As expected, with both methods of weight loss plasma leptin levels decreased. CRP levels did not change in either group.

Baseline and posttreatment measurements of lipids were similar between groups, although there was some variation in the pattern of changes (Table 3). Three subjects in the RYGB group and four in the VLCD were taking cholesterol-lowering medication. Free fatty acid levels increased after RYGB and VLCD ($P = 0.029$ and 0.062, respectively).

DISCUSSION

Contrary to our expectations, this study demonstrates that RYGB in subjects with T2DM does not result in greater improvement in β-cell function compared with equivalent weight loss achieved over the same time period by VLCD. As evaluated by fsIVGTT, both groups demonstrated significant and similar increases in acute insulin secretion and insulin sensitivity. We previously demonstrated a greater improvement in DI in subjects with T2DM after RYGB compared with individuals who achieved equivalent weight loss on an outpatient low-calorie diet (15). However, the degree to which calories were restricted was not equivalent to the RYGB, and therefore, the rate of weight loss for the RYGB was greater. Based on studies of caloric restriction, the degree of caloric restriction is a major factor that exerts a glucose-lowering effect independent from the amount of weight loss (4,16). This is the first study of individuals with T2DM that compares RYGB to a diet group matched for both the amount and rate of weight loss. Others have evaluated β-cell function after surgery, but there has not been a simulation of a gastric bypass diet without the surgery in patients with T2DM. Isbell et al. (22), for example, evaluated RYGB with matched obese subjects on a VLCD 2–7 days after intervention. There was in both groups a 25% improvement in insulin sensitivity as quantified by HOMA-IR, but a significant decrease in fasting glucose levels was demonstrated in

the diet group only. These results are somewhat difficult to interpret given that the groups were a mix of subjects with and without T2DM, and there may be a confounding effect of residual inflammation in this very early postoperative state.

Differences in the methods used to assess β-cell function, characteristics of the patient population, and differences in operative procedures among surgeons also make it difficult to compare studies with sometimes seemingly conflicting outcomes. For example, with use of the hyperglycemic clamp it was found that 4 weeks after RYGB there was an increase in insulin sensitivity, but DI remained unchanged (23). An explanation for this finding in comparison with our study is that metabolic testing was carried out when subjects were consuming an 800-calorie liquid diet prior to surgery. It is also unclear whether diabetes medications, including metformin and thiazolidinediones, were held prior to testing. Similar to our results, Lin et al. (24) showed that DI improved 23-fold (from 23 to 403) 1 month after RYGB. Nannipieri et al. (25) also showed that β-cell glucose sensitivity improved (but did not normalize) 45 days after RYGB in patients with T2DM. Interestingly, insulin sensitivity but not β-cell glucose sensitivity improved in proportion to weight loss. Certainly, duration of diabetes also influences β-cell function (26). Lim et al. (27) studied patients with T2DM and restricted caloric intake to 600 kcal/day for 8 weeks and demonstrated not just improvement but normalization of both β-cell function and hepatic insulin sensitivity. The duration of diabetes, however, was <4 years, which limits comparison with our study cohort with a longer duration of diabetes. In the absence of a gold standard for assessing β-cell function and the inclusion of a diverse population, comparison of different studies is indeed problematic (28).

Similar to dietary interventions (4,6), there is considerable variability in the glycemic response after RYGB. From a clinical perspective, it would be helpful to predict the glycemic response to surgery from known or easily measureable baseline characteristics. In retrospective studies, it appears that patients with a longer history of diabetes or on insulin therapy were less likely to achieve euglycemia off antihyperglycemic medications (29,30). Magnitude of weight loss has been associated with better glycemic outcome (29–31). From our data, it appears that

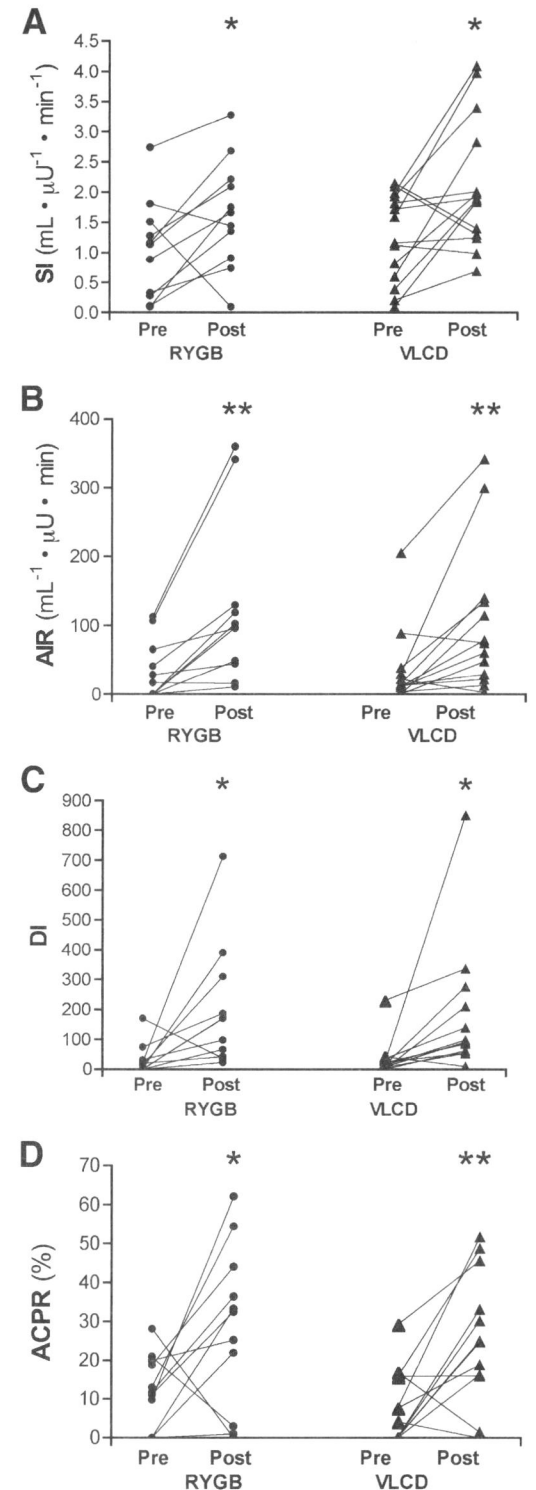

FIG. 1. Changes in S_i (*A*), AIR (*B*), DI (*C*), and ACPR (*D*) for all subjects shown individually. *$P < 0.05$, **$P < 0.01$, ***$P < 0.001$ vs. baseline.

changes, as weight tends to increase with time, and deterioration of glycemic control, even with maintenance of weight loss, has been observed (30,32–34).

It has been well documented that RYGB produces profound postprandial stimulation of GLP-1 secretion and a greater incretin effect than observed with diet-induced weight loss (14). RYGB also alters glucose absorption, causing a marked increase in the early rate of appearance of ingested glucose into the systemic circulation that would be expected to alter the pattern of insulin secretion (35). For these reasons, we evaluated β-cell function in the absence of enteral nutrient passage and without the confounding effect of altered glucose kinetics. Although gut hormones were not measured during the fsIVGTT, others have demonstrated that there is negligible change in GLP-1 concentrations upon intravenous glucose infusion (14,36). Thus, the findings in our study suggest that there are changes in β-cell function, independent of glucose absorption from the gut and the incretin effect, that occur to a similar extent after RYGB and VLCD. Because of the incretin effect, however, we did expect that overall glycemic control would improve to a greater extent after RYGB. Contrary to our expectations, decreases in fructosamine levels from baseline were of similar magnitude between RYGB and VLCD. It is likely that the greater incretin effect noted after larger meal challenges in RYGB patients may not have provided much advantage in the setting of very small meals and less demand for prandial insulin secretion. In this vein, it has been noted that β-cell function (15) and clinical outcome after RYGB (14) are better than equivalent weight loss achieved by LCD; however, the caloric intake and duration of the weight loss periods were greater in the diet groups of both studies.

Another component of insulin and glucose metabolism is insulin clearance, which has been demonstrated to increase after 11% weight loss on a 500–600 kcal/day diet (37). We did not directly measure insulin clearance, but given that fasting insulin was greater in the RYGB group at baseline while C-peptide levels were nearly identical it appears that insulin clearance may have been greater in the VLCD group. It is unclear why there was a difference, since groups were fairly well matched for some of the factors that are associated with clearance such as S_i, AIR, fasting glucose, and BMI (38,39). Unfortunately, we do not have measurements of waist circumference or visceral adipose tissue that could conceivably be different in this relatively small sample size and might affect insulin clearance. Nevertheless, the change in the insulin–to–C-peptide ratio was nearly identical between groups, suggesting that the interventions do not differentially affect clearance.

Limitations of this study are the nonrandomized intervention scheme, as well as the relatively small sample size. The study was designed to detect a 1.3-SD difference in change in DI between groups. Smaller differences may not have been detected, but the clinical significance of smaller differences is somewhat questionable. It is possible that with more subjects changes in some of the secondary end points would reach statistical significance, such as the increase in adiponectin in the VLCD group and decrease in fructosamine after RYGB. Although the groups were matched for duration of diabetes, this was a self-reported time of diagnosis that likely varies from the actual onset of the disease. Another factor to consider is that acute inflammation, even with a minimally invasive laparoscopic procedure, could have increased insulin resistance blunting the response of the RYGB patients. We

duration of T2DM, baseline β-cell function, or HbA$_{1c}$ and the amount of weight loss did not correlate with changes in DI. However, in this short-term study we are unable to assess the maximal improvement in glycemic parameters, as it has been shown that S_i continues to improve with further weight loss between 6 and 24 months after surgery (24). Likewise, we cannot predict the durability of these

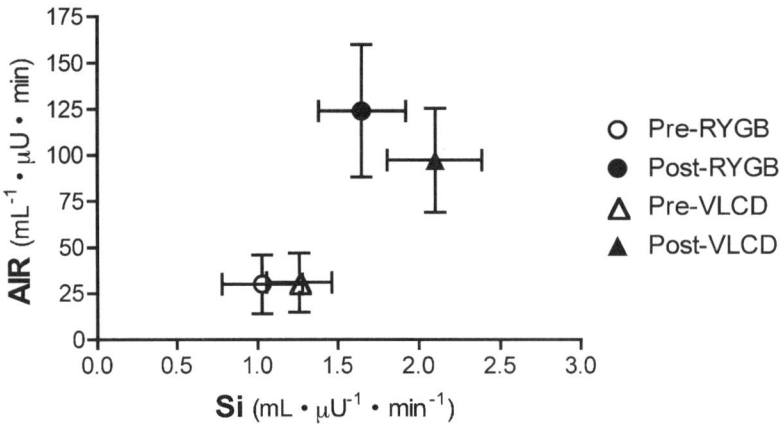

FIG. 2. Graphic representation of the relationship between insulin sensitivity and insulin secretion before and after interventions.

did not perform detailed assessment of residual inflammation; however, CRP levels were not statistically different between both groups. Physical activity levels were not monitored, although given the inpatient setting we were able to limit the activity in the VLCD group to that expected of postsurgical patients. The RYGB group was not studied under inpatient observation because the surgical procedure itself imposes limitation of caloric intake to ~500 kcal/day in the first 2–3 weeks after surgery.

These data indicate that the changes in glucose homeostasis that occur within 2–3 weeks after RYGB are primarily due to very low energy intake as opposed to specific surgically-induced hormonal effects. Clearly, this does not mean that RYGB is not more beneficial in the long term, since the degree of caloric restriction required to mimic surgical results cannot be maintained in most individuals. As in our prior study, even when the diet was 800 kcal/day instead of 500 kcal/day less improvement in β-cell function was noted. It would be expected that in the longer term, the average blood glucose would begin to increase in the VLCD group as caloric intake was liberalized even if the weight loss were maintained (4,5). The RYGB group may maintain or further their improvements by virtue of continued weight loss. Furthermore, even if it were possible to match caloric intake with RYGB for a much longer period, there may be

changes in nutrient absorption (i.e., amino acids, fatty acids) and bile acid secretion specific to the bypass procedure that could affect clinical outcome independent of weight loss and calorie restriction.

In summary, our data suggest that RYGB is not superior to VLCD with regard to early changes in β-cell function in obese subjects with T2DM when tested in the absence of an enteral nutrient stimulus. Observing glucostatic parameters in the longer term would be useful to investigate the durability of these changes. Certainly, incretins play a role in improving glucose homeostasis after RYGB, but there are likely nonenteral mechanisms associated with glycemic control in the short and longer term that result from calorie restriction. Further study is required in order to define preoperative characteristics that could better predict an individual's response to surgical interventions for the treatment of type 2 diabetes.

ACKNOWLEDGMENTS

This work was supported by National Institutes of Health (NIH) Grant DK072011 (to J.K.), National Center for Research Resources (NCRR) Grant UL1 RR024156, and a pilot grant from the Columbia Diabetes Research Center (NIH Grant DK63608). C.J. was supported by NIH T32 Training Grant DK07271.

TABLE 3
Plasma hormone levels and lipids before and after interventions

| | RYGB | | VLCD | | |
	Pre-intervention	Postintervention	Pre-intervention	Postintervention	P^a
Leptin (ng/mL)	27.4 ± 2.2	15.6 ± 1.8***	31.3 ± 5.3	24.7 ± 3.9**	0.66
CRP (mg/L)	11.6 ± 2.7	10.9 ± 3.1	11.4 ± 2.5	10.8 ± 4.5	0.96
Adiponectin (μg/mL)	2,893 ± 327	3,830 ± 364*	2,876 ± 534	2,909 ± 484	0.05
GLP-1 (pmol/L)	13.3 ± 2.8	21.1 ± 6.4*	21.1 ± 3.4	20.2 ± 3.4	0.10
Ghrelin (pg/mL)	305 ± 42	298 ± 37	341 ± 20	371 ± 23	0.25
PYY (pg/mL)	79.2 ± 20.4	**78.6 ± 15.3**	69.7 ± 13.7	**42.4 ± 8.8**	0.16
Lipids					
Total cholesterol (mg/dL)	164 ± 7	126 ± 11**	181 ± 11	154 ± 10***	0.31
HDL (mg/dL)	40.4 ± 2.4	**30.2 ± 1.0*****	41.5 ± 2.5	**35.1 ± 1.5*****	0.14
Total/HDL	4.26 ± 0.35	4.16 ± 0.32	4.50 ± 0.33	4.48 ± 0.37	0.86
LDL (mg/dL)	99.3 ± 6.0	77.4 ± 10.1*	108 ± 11	99.5 ± 10.0	0.17
Triglycerides (mg/dL)	119 ± 21	96.6 ± 8.0	143 ± 19	94.9 ± 9.1*	0.36
FFA (mmol/L)	0.69 ± 0.05	0.91 ± 0.05*	0.67 ± 0.05	0.83 ± 0.04	0.64

Data are means ± SEM. FFA, free fatty acids. Boldface data at pre- or postintervention are different between groups: $P < 0.05$. [a]P value for independent t test of group difference in change from pre- to posttreatment. ***$P < 0.001$, **$P < 0.01$, *$P < 0.05$, within-group differences between pre- and posttreatment.

J.K. has received research grant support from Covidien and payment for serving on the Scientific Advisory Board of Nutrisystem. No other potential conflicts of interest related to this article were reported.

C.J. was responsible for patient recruitment and care and data management and participated in manuscript preparation. W.K. designed food menus and supervised the bionutrition staff. G.F. was responsible for patient recruitment and performance of glucose tolerance tests. I.M.C. performed all hormone assays and assisted with sample preparation and data entry. L.A. and M.B. assisted with patient recruitment. D.J.M. performed data analysis. J.K. conceived and designed the study, supervised the experiments and collection of data, and prepared the manuscript. J.K. is the guarantor of this work and, as such, had full access to all the data in the study and takes responsibility for the integrity of the data and the accuracy of the data analysis.

Parts of this study were presented in abstract form at the 30th Annual Scientific Meeting of the Obesity Society, San Antonio, Texas, 20–24 September 2012.

The bionutrition staff of the NCRR were invaluable for the performance of this study. The authors also thank the participants in this study; Nancy Restuccia, MS, RD, CDN (Columbia University Medical Center, New York, New York), for guidance with bariatric nutrition guidelines; and Dr. Leona Plum (Profil Institut für Stoffwechselforschung, Neuss, Germany) for critical review of the manuscript.

REFERENCES

1. Finkelstein EA, Khavjou OA, Thompson H, et al. Obesity and severe obesity forecasts through 2030. Am J Prev Med 2012;42:563–570
2. DeFronzo RA, Bonadonna RC, Ferrannini E. Pathogenesis of NIDDM. A balanced overview. Diabetes Care 1992;15:318–368
3. Leahy JL, Hirsch IB, Peterson KA, Schneider D. Targeting beta-cell function early in the course of therapy for type 2 diabetes mellitus. J Clin Endocrinol Metab 2010;95:4206–4216
4. Henry RR, Scheaffer L, Olefsky JM. Glycemic effects of intensive caloric restriction and isocaloric refeeding in noninsulin-dependent diabetes mellitus. J Clin Endocrinol Metab 1985;61:917–925
5. Kelley DE, Wing R, Buonocore C, Sturis J, Polonsky K, Fitzsimmons M. Relative effects of calorie restriction and weight loss in noninsulin-dependent diabetes mellitus. J Clin Endocrinol Metab 1993;77:1287–1293
6. Watts NB, Spanheimer RG, DiGirolamo M, et al. Prediction of glucose response to weight loss in patients with non-insulin-dependent diabetes mellitus. Arch Intern Med 1990;150:803–806
7. Wadden TA. Treatment of obesity by moderate and severe caloric restriction. Results of clinical research trials. Ann Intern Med 1993;119:688–693
8. Schauer PR, Kashyap SR, Wolski K, et al. Bariatric surgery versus intensive medical therapy in obese patients with diabetes. N Engl J Med 2012;366:1567–1576
9. Moo TA, Rubino F. Gastrointestinal surgery as treatment for type 2 diabetes. Curr Opin Endocrinol Diabetes Obes 2008;15:153–158
10. Cummings DE. Endocrine mechanisms mediating remission of diabetes after gastric bypass surgery. Int J Obes (Lond) 2009;33(Suppl. 1):S33–S40
11. Rubino F, Marescaux J. Effect of duodenal-jejunal exclusion in a non-obese animal model of type 2 diabetes: a new perspective for an old disease. Ann Surg 2004;239:1–11
12. Korner J, Bessler M, Inabnet W, Taveras C, Holst JJ. Exaggerated glucagon-like peptide-1 and blunted glucose-dependent insulinotropic peptide secretion are associated with Roux-en-Y gastric bypass but not adjustable gastric banding. Surg Obes Relat Dis 2007;3:597–601
13. Korner J, Inabnet W, Febres G, et al. Prospective study of gut hormone and metabolic changes after adjustable gastric banding and Roux-en-Y gastric bypass. Int J Obes (Lond) 2009;33:786–795
14. Laferrère B, Teixeira J, McGinty J, et al. Effect of weight loss by gastric bypass surgery versus hypocaloric diet on glucose and incretin levels in patients with type 2 diabetes. J Clin Endocrinol Metab 2008;93:2479–2485
15. Plum L, Ahmed L, Febres G, et al. Comparison of glucostatic parameters after hypocaloric diet or bariatric surgery and equivalent weight loss. Obesity (Silver Spring) 2011;19:2149–2157
16. Wing RR, Blair EH, Bononi P, Marcus MD, Watanabe R, Bergman RN. Caloric restriction per se is a significant factor in improvements in glycemic control and insulin sensitivity during weight loss in obese NIDDM patients. Diabetes Care 1994;17:30–36
17. Welch S, Gebhart SS, Bergman RN, Phillips LS. Minimal model analysis of intravenous glucose tolerance test-derived insulin sensitivity in diabetic subjects. J Clin Endocrinol Metab 1990;71:1508–1518
18. Bergman RN, Ider YZ, Bowden CR, Cobelli C. Quantitative estimation of insulin sensitivity. Am J Physiol 1979;236:E667–E677
19. Saad MF, Anderson RL, Laws A, et al. A comparison between the minimal model and the glucose clamp in the assessment of insulin sensitivity across the spectrum of glucose tolerance. Insulin Resistance Atherosclerosis Study. Diabetes 1994;43:1114–1121
20. Matthews DR, Hosker JP, Rudenski AS, Naylor BA, Treacher DF, Turner RC. Homeostasis model assessment: insulin resistance and beta-cell function from fasting plasma glucose and insulin concentrations in man. Diabetologia 1985;28:412–419
21. Korner J, Bessler M, Cirilo LJ, et al. Effects of Roux-en-Y gastric bypass surgery on fasting and postprandial concentrations of plasma ghrelin, peptide YY, and insulin. J Clin Endocrinol Metab 2005;90:359–365
22. Isbell JM, Tamboli RA, Hansen EN, et al. The importance of caloric restriction in the early improvements in insulin sensitivity after Roux-en-Y gastric bypass surgery. Diabetes Care 2010;33:1438–1442
23. Kashyap SR, Daud S, Kelly KR, et al. Acute effects of gastric bypass versus gastric restrictive surgery on beta-cell function and insulinotropic hormones in severely obese patients with type 2 diabetes. Int J Obes (Lond) 2010;34:462–471
24. Lin E, Liang Z, Frediani J, et al. Improvement in ß-cell function in patients with normal and hyperglycemia following Roux-en-Y gastric bypass surgery. Am J Physiol Endocrinol Metab 2010;299:E706–E712
25. Nannipieri M, Mari A, Anselmino M, et al. The role of beta-cell function and insulin sensitivity in the remission of type 2 diabetes after gastric bypass surgery. J Clin Endocrinol Metab 2011;96:E1372–E1379
26. Clauson P, Linnarsson R, Gottsäter A, Sundkvist G, Grill V. Relationships between diabetes duration, metabolic control and beta-cell function in a representative population of type 2 diabetic patients in Sweden. Diabet Med 1994;11:794–801
27. Lim EL, Hollingsworth KG, Aribisala BS, Chen MJ, Mathers JC, Taylor R. Reversal of type 2 diabetes: normalisation of beta cell function in association with decreased pancreas and liver triacylglycerol. Diabetologia 2011;54:2506–2514
28. Ferrannini E, Mingrone G. Impact of different bariatric surgical procedures on insulin action and beta-cell function in type 2 diabetes. Diabetes Care 2009;32:514–520
29. Schauer PR, Burguera B, Ikramuddin S, et al. Effect of laparoscopic Roux-en Y gastric bypass on type 2 diabetes mellitus. Ann Surg 2003;238:467–484; discussion 84–85
30. Arterburn DE, Bogart A, Sherwood NE, et al. A multisite study of long-term remission and relapse of type 2 diabetes mellitus following gastric bypass. Obes Surg 2013;23:93–102
31. Sugerman HJ, Wolfe LG, Sica DA, Clore JN. Diabetes and hypertension in severe obesity and effects of gastric bypass-induced weight loss. Ann Surg 2003;237:751–756; discussion 757–758
32. Sjöström L, Lindroos AK, Peltonen M, et al.; Swedish Obese Subjects Study Scientific Group. Lifestyle, diabetes, and cardiovascular risk factors 10 years after bariatric surgery. N Engl J Med 2004;351:2683–2693
33. DiGiorgi M, Rosen DJ, Choi JJ, et al. Re-emergence of diabetes after gastric bypass in patients with mid- to long-term follow-up. Surg Obes Relat Dis 2010;6:249–253
34. Chikunguwo SM, Wolfe LG, Dodson P, et al. Analysis of factors associated with durable remission of diabetes after Roux-en-Y gastric bypass. Surg Obes Relat Dis 2010;6:254–259
35. Bradley D, Conte C, Mittendorfer B, et al. Gastric bypass and banding equally improve insulin sensitivity and β cell function. J Clin Invest 2012;122:4667–4674
36. Haltia LT, Savontaus E, Vahlberg T, Rinne JO, Kaasinen V. Acute hormonal changes following intravenous glucose challenge in lean and obese human subjects. Scand J Clin Lab Invest 2010;70:275–280
37. Svendsen PF, Jensen FK, Holst JJ, Haugaard SB, Nilas L, Madsbad S. The effect of a very low calorie diet on insulin sensitivity, beta cell function, insulin clearance, incretin hormone secretion, androgen levels and body composition in obese young women. Scand J Clin Lab Invest 2012;72:410–419
38. Lee CC, Haffner SM, Wagenknecht LE, et al. Insulin Clearance and the Incidence of Type 2 Diabetes in Hispanics and African Americans: the IRAS Family Study. Diabetes Care 2013;36:901–907
39. Goodarzi MO, Cui J, Chen YD, Hsueh WA, Guo X, Rotter JI. Fasting insulin reflects heterogeneous physiological processes: role of insulin clearance. Am J Physiol Endocrinol Metab 2011;301:E402–E408

Practical Use of Glucagon-Like Peptide-1 Receptor Agonist Therapy in Primary Care

Timothy S. Reid, MD

Glucagon-like peptide-1 (GLP-1) receptor agonists are one of the newer classes of medications for the treatment of adults with type 2 diabetes. The GLP-1 receptor agonist class became available in 2005 in the United States with the approval of short-acting exenatide by the U.S. Food and Drug Administration (FDA). There are now three GLP-1 receptor agonists available: exenatide for twice-daily administration (BID), exenatide for once-weekly administration (QW), and liraglutide for once-daily administration. Other GLP-1 receptor agonists are in development.

The 2012 American Diabetes Association (ADA)/European Association for the Study of Diabetes position statement on a patient-centered approach to treating patients with type 2 diabetes[1] recommends GLP-1 receptor agonists as one of several choices for two- and three-drug combinations after initial treatment with lifestyle modification, exercise, diet, and metformin. GLP-1 receptor agonists are also recommended if metformin is contraindicated or not tolerated.

GLP-1 receptor agonists are one of five classes of medications recommended for two- and three-drug combinations (i.e., with a sulfonylurea [or meglitinide], thiazolidinedione, insulin, or dipeptidyl peptidase-4 [DPP-4] inhibitor), so selecting among the five classes can be challenging.[1] In addition to these five classes, other options include the α-glucosidase inhibitors, bromocriptine, colesevelam, and pramlintide. This article reviews some of the benefits and limitations of the GLP-1 receptor agonist class, including differences within the class; describes how these agents allow for individualization of treatment; and offers some suggestions regarding practical considerations when using this class of medications.

Overview of Benefits and Limitations of GLP-1 Receptor Agonists

Pharmacological overview

The GLP-1 receptor agonist class has five important actions for patients with type 2 diabetes. The first is an increase in glucose-mediated insulin production by pancreatic β-cells.[2–6] "Glucose-mediated" is an important nuance because insulin production and release remains under the control of the glucose-sensing mechanisms of β-cells and only occurs during hyperglycemia. As a consequence, there is a low incidence of hypoglycemia. In rat and mouse models, there is a

---

IN BRIEF

The glucagon-like peptide-1 (GLP-1) receptor agonist class of medications has distinct benefits and limitations that provide an opportunity to individualize the treatment of patients with type 2 diabetes. Many strategies can be used to improve patient acceptance of and self-management with a GLP-1 receptor agonist.

---

slowing of β-cell death.[7–10] Conflicting data in humans involving a variety of measures of β-cell function make it unclear whether this is also a phenomenon in humans.[11–15] Other actions include a decrease or no change in fasting endogenous glucose release via a reduction in glycogenolysis but not gluconeogenesis and a reduction in glucagon secretion.[3,16,17] The gastric emptying rate is also slowed, thereby slowing the absorption of carbohydrate, leading to a lower rise in plasma glucose.[3,18] GLP-1 receptor agonists also act via the central nervous system, resulting in a sensation of satiety and reduced food intake.[19–21] This effect explains, in part, the added benefit that many patients lose weight when taking a GLP-1 receptor agonist.[11,15,22–26]

By comparison, DPP-4 inhibitors, which also act on the incretin system, do not slow the gastric emptying rate, promote satiety, reduce food intake, or promote weight loss.[27] These differences between DPP-4 inhibitors and GLP-1 receptor agonists are thought to result from differences in how the two classes exert their actions on the incretin system. DPP-4 inhibitors work indirectly by inhibiting the metabolism of native GLP-1 produced in the gut, thereby raising the level of endogenous GLP-1 to ~ 10 pmol/L.[28] By comparison, GLP-1 receptor agonists act directly on the GLP-1 receptor, providing a level of GLP-1 activity of ≈ 60 pmol/L of GLP-1.[29] From this, it is

Table 1. Head-to-Head Clinical Trials Comparing GLP-1 Receptor Agonists			
	Exenatide BID	**Exenatide QW**	**Liraglutide**
Magnitude of lowering:[14,31–34]			
A1C (%)	0.8–1.5	1.3–1.9	1.1–1.5
FPG (mg/dl)	11–25	32–41	19–38
PPG (mg/dl)	124	95	Not rated
Gastric emptying rate	Slow	Slow	Little effect
Dosing frequency	Twice daily	Once weekly	Once daily
Dosing in relation to eating	Within 60 minutes of two major meals, at least 6 hours apart	Any time during the day regardless of meals	Any time during the day regardless of meals
Ease of administration	Prefilled pen; 29-, 30-, or 31-gauge needle	Kit that requires assembly; 23-gauge needle	Prefilled pen; 30- or 32-gauge needle
Onset of action	Days	Several weeks	Days
FBG, fasting blood glucose; PPG, postprandial glucose.			

clear that DPP-4 inhibitors should not be considered an oral form of GLP-1 receptor agonist.

Benefits of GLP-1 receptor agonists
Beyond the low associated incidence of hypoglycemia and weight loss effects, GLP-1 receptor agonists offer several advantages that may be useful in individualizing therapy.

A1C reduction
A reduction in A1C of 0.5–1.5% has been reported with GLP-1 receptor agonists as monotherapy.[11,15,22–24,30] Head-to-head clinical trials show significantly greater lowering of A1C with exenatide QW compared to exenatide BID,[31,32] 1.8 mg liraglutide compared to exenatide BID,[14,33] and 1.8 mg liraglutide compared to exenatide QW[34] (Table 1).

Effects on fasting and postprandial glucose
Although A1C reduction results from a lowering of both fasting blood glucose (FBG) and postprandial glucose (PPG), there are differences among the three GLP-1 receptor agonists. A 30-week comparison showed a

significantly greater reduction in FBG with exenatide QW compared to exenatide BID (reduction of 41 vs. 25 mg/dl, respectively, $P < 0.0001$). Both treatments resulted in significant improvements in seven-point self-monitoring of blood glucose (SMBG) profiles.[32] Another investigation showed that exenatide BID resulted in a significantly greater reduction than liraglutide in PPG after breakfast and supper but not after lunch, whereas liraglutide resulted in a significantly greater reduction than exenatide BID in FBG.[14] A 26-week comparison of exenatide QW and 1.8 mg liraglutide once daily showed reductions in A1C of 1.28 and 1.48% (95% CI 0.08–0.33), respectively.[35]

Effects on cardiovascular biomarkers
Another benefit of GLP-1 receptor agonists is their impact on cardiovascular risk factors and biomarkers. GLP-1 receptor agonists cause a reduction of 1–7 mmHg in systolic blood pressure but have no significant effect on diastolic blood pressure.[11,14,15,23,33,36–42] Improvements in lipid profile are also observed,

notably a reduction in triglycerides of 12–40 mg/dl.[11,14,23,25,36,38–42] It is unclear whether these changes will have a beneficial outcome on cardiovascular event risk reduction. Long-term cardiovascular outcome trials are in progress with most GLP-1 receptor agonists.

Limitations of GLP-1 receptor agonists
As with all medications used to treat type 2 diabetes, GLP-1 receptor agonists have some limitations that should be discussed with patients when considering treatment options. Although hypoglycemia is common with many glucose-lowering agents, the occurrence of hypoglycemia with GLP-1 receptor agonists is generally low (Table 2). Focusing on the limitations that patients are more likely to experience (e.g., transient gastrointestinal [GI] adverse events) and how these limitations will be addressed is helpful in minimizing patients' concerns. Providing patient education materials and involving other members of the diabetes health care team can further reassure patients that the limitations of GLP-1 receptor

Table 2. Hypoglycemia Rates in Head-to-Head Clinical Trials Comparing GLP-1 Receptor Agonists

	Exenatide BID Versus Liraglutide[14] (*n* = 464)	Exenatide BID Versus Liraglutide[33] Extension (*n* = 389)	Exenatide BID Versus Exenatide QW[31] (*n* = 252)	Exenatide BID Versus Exenatide QW[32] (*n* = 295)	Exenatide QW Versus Liraglutide[34] (*n* = 911)
Hypoglycemia	Minor: 2.600 vs. 1.932 episodes/ patient-year Major: 2 vs. 0 episodes/ patient-year	Minor: 1.30 vs. 0.74 episodes/ patient-year	Minor: 3.3 vs. 3.9% Major: none	Minor: 5.4 vs. 6.1% Major: none	Minor: 15 vs. 12%* 4 vs. 3%** Major: none

*In those taking a concomitant sulfonylurea.
**In those not taking a concomitant sulfonylurea.

agonists will be addressed as needed to improve self-management.

Transient GI adverse events
Each of the GLP-1 receptor agonists, to varying degrees, can cause transient nausea and diarrhea. As monotherapy, nausea occurs in 8, 11, and 28% of patients treated with exenatide BID, exenatide QW, and liraglutide, respectively, whereas diarrhea is experienced by < 2, 11, and 17%, respectively.[43–45] Similar GI adverse effects can occur with metformin; nausea/vomiting occurs in 26%, whereas diarrhea has been reported to lead to discontinuation in 6%.[46]

GI adverse events are usually self-limiting. Nausea is usually mild and peaks within 8 weeks of starting exenatide BID and 4–8 weeks of starting liraglutide. Nausea resolves in all but ~ 10% within 28 weeks with exenatide BID and in 8 weeks with liraglutide.[23,47,48] For exenatide QW, nausea peaks soon after initiation and resolves within 10 weeks in nearly all patients.[15]

These possible GI adverse events are important to discuss with patients because patients who are not expecting such situations may stop the medication believing that it

is a permanent problem. In addition, protracted vomiting, should it occur, may lead to pre-renal azotemia.

The most common approach to minimizing the risk and severity of nausea includes using a dose escalation strategy for exenatide BID and liraglutide; dose escalation is not needed for exenatide QW. Exenatide BID should be initiated at a dose of 5 µg twice daily and increased to 10 µg twice daily after 1 month based on clinical response. Exenatide BID should be taken within 60 minutes before the morning and evening meals. Liraglutide should be initiated at a dose of 0.6 mg once daily for 1 week and then increased to 1.2 mg once daily. If the 1.2-mg dose does not result in acceptable glycemic control, the dose can be increased to 1.8 mg once daily. One modification of this dose escalation strategy that is not described in the approved package inserts but that the author has found useful is to lengthen the time period during which dose escalation occurs.

Other strategies to help minimize the risk of nausea not described in the approved package insert include self-administering exenatide BID < 60 minutes before mealtime, temporarily

reducing the dose, or stopping eating when patients feel full.[49–51] Patients should be educated to avoid administering a GLP-1 receptor agonist close to a large or high-fat meal because doing so is likely to cause nausea. An advantage of exenatide QW and liraglutide is that they can be administered without regard to meal times.

Injection site reactions
Another possible limitation is the local irritation and nodule formation around the injection site that occurs most frequently with exenatide QW. The nodules, which are generally not visible but can be felt, typically last only a few weeks. Local irritation or nodule formation is usually a minor issue that can be prevented or managed by rotating injection sites in the abdomen, thigh, and upper arms.

Infrequent adverse events
As with other medications, infrequent adverse events are possible with glucose-lowering medications, including the GLP-1 receptor agonists. Although these adverse events may not be routinely discussed with patients, if questions arise, they should be discussed at a depth and in a manner appropriate for the patients based on their questions and previous

discussions and as part of a risk-benefit discussion. Patients should also be referred to the medication guide for each product for additional information.

Pancreatitis

One possible but infrequent adverse event is pancreatitis, which has been reported in post-marketing surveillance for all marketed GLP-1 receptor agonists and DPP-4 inhibitors. In clinical trials of liraglutide, 13 cases of pancreatitis (9 acute and 4 chronic) were reported in patients treated with liraglutide and 1 case was reported in a patient treated with glimepiride (2.7 vs. 0.5 cases/1,000 patient-years).[45]

Analyses of two insurance claims databases show rates of pancreatitis that are similar among the glucose-lowering agents examined.[52,53] In one analysis ($n = 786,656$), the incidence rates (cases per 1,000 patient-years) were 5.7 for exenatide BID, 5.6 for sitagliptin, and 5.6 for metformin, sulfonylureas, or thiazolidinediones.[52] Similar rates of acute pancreatitis over 1 year were observed in a second analysis among patients treated with exenatide BID, sitagliptin, metformin, or glyburide.[53]

In contrast, an association between GLP-1 receptor agonist therapy and an increased risk of pancreatitis was found in two other analyses. In one, which examined the FDA database of reported adverse events from 2004 to 2009, the use of exenatide BID or sitagliptin increased the odds ratio for reported pancreatitis sixfold compared to other glucose-lowering agents.[54] In the other, Singh et al.[55] found an increased risk of acute pancreatitis with current or recent (within 2 years) use of a GLP-1 receptor agonist. These findings were based on the health records of 1,269 patients hospitalized with acute pancreatitis and matched controls.

The findings by Singh et al. were quickly challenged in a joint response from the ADA and the American Association of Clinical Endocrinologists (AACE),[56] which stated that this analysis "does not provide the basis for changing treatment in people with diabetes." The joint statement by ADA and AACE noted that further clarity on this issue should come from nine prospective, controlled trials of GLP-1 receptor agonist therapy involving > 65,000 subjects. In the meantime, patients should be encouraged to speak to their providers to assess which treatments are best for them and to not stop therapy without consulting their provider.

The association of GLP-1 receptor agonists with pancreatitis is difficult to assess because of the nearly threefold greater risk of pancreatitis in people with type 2 diabetes compared to those without type 2 diabetes.[57] Until this issue is resolved, it is important to explain to patients the difference between the symptoms of pancreatitis and the minor, transient nausea described above. In addition, in patients with a history of pancreatitis, glucose-lowering agents other than exenatide BID[43] and exenatide QW[44] should be used, and liraglutide should be used with caution, according to the package inserts for each of these agents.[45]

Potential risk of thyroid C-cell neoplasms

Although very rare in humans, another possible safety concern relates to the risk of thyroid C-cell neoplasms, which were found in preclinical studies with rats and mice but not with monkeys.[58,59] Thyroid C-cell tumors were also observed in rodents not exposed to a GLP-1 receptor agonist, and expression of GLP-1 receptors in the thyroid C-cell tissues of humans and monkeys is low.[59]

One of the conditions required by the FDA for making exenatide QW and liraglutide commercially available was to create a national registry of patients with thyroid tumors. The registry will allow monitoring to identify increases in the incidence of this problem in humans. If patients have a history of medullary C-cell tumors or multiple endocrine neoplasia-2 (thyroid, parathyroid, and pheochromocytoma tumors), they should not be treated with a GLP-1 receptor agonist.[44,45]

Role of GLP-1 Receptor Agonists in Therapy

There are several clinical situations in which patients with type 2 diabetes may benefit from treatment with a GLP-1 receptor agonist. This includes patients who are taking metformin, a sulfonylurea, or a thiazolidinedione (alone or in combination) but are not at their glycemic goal, as well as patients with an A1C of 7–9%. However, for patients with an A1C > 9%, the addition of basal insulin should be strongly considered until glycemic control has improved. At that time, a decision can be made as to whether to continue basal insulin. Of the three GLP-1 receptor agonists, liraglutide and exenatide BID are indicated for use in combination with basal insulin.[43,45]

Selection of a GLP-1 receptor agonist should be based on various clinical parameters. For example, if FBG is the primary target, exenatide QW or liraglutide are preferred over exenatide BID. Conversely, if PPG is the primary target, exenatide BID is preferred. Of course, other issues, including frequency of administration; side effects such as nausea, injection site reactions, and nodule formation; and patients' ability to use the administration devices are also important considerations.

It is important to realize that a small percentage of patients experience no or a minimal reduction in their blood glucose with a GLP-1 receptor agonist. Although the reason for this is unknown in most patients, in some it may be because they have been skipping doses or have reduced their dose. Because adverse events are a frequent reason for poor adherence, inquiring about medication difficulties such as adverse events at all follow-up visits can be helpful and provides an opportunity to find solutions that are acceptable to patients. It is most helpful to discuss with patients at the time of therapy initiation how to deal with common adverse events.

Other situations in which a GLP-1 receptor agonist might be a good choice include in older patients with type 2 diabetes, who are more likely to experience hypoglycemia unawareness.[60] In addition, limited data from clinical trials indicate that people ≥ 65 years of age experienced no difference in efficacy or safety compared to younger patients.[43–45] However, assessment of renal function before initiation of a GLP-1 receptor agonist is suggested because older patients may experience a reduction in renal function.

Patients with renal impairment or end-stage renal disease (creatinine clearance < 30 ml/min) should not use exenatide BID or exenatide QW. Liraglutide can be used without dosage reduction but should be used with caution because data are limited regarding its use in patients with various stages of renal impairment.

Another group for whom a GLP-1 receptor agonist might be a good choice includes patients who experience excessive hunger or weight gain. It is not uncommon for patients to describe a sensation of "always being hungry." GLP-1 receptor agonists have been noted clinically by some providers to blunt that sensation.

Finally, although the U.S. Federal Aviation Administration does not allow insulin use for commercial pilots,[61] and the U.S. Department of Transportation does not allow insulin use for commercial truck drivers,[62] GLP-1 receptor agonists are allowed for pilots and are not mentioned in the list of medications of concern for commercial truck drivers.

Patients generally should not be placed on concurrent treatment with a GLP-1 receptor agonist and a DPP-4 inhibitor (i.e., alogliptin, linagliptin, saxagliptin, or sitagliptin). Although there are differences between the two classes of medications, both act on the incretin system. There is, however, preliminary evidence that the addition of exenatide BID to the combination of sitagliptin plus metformin produces additional (0.3%) A1C reduction beyond the combination of exenatide BID and metformin over 20 weeks.[63] Nonetheless, patients who are taking a DPP-4 inhibitor should discontinue it at the start of GLP-1 therapy.

Some additional patients also should not be considered for GLP-1 receptor agonist treatment. Such a therapy would not be appropriate in patients who have severe GI disease (e.g., gastroparesis).[43,44] Patients who are pregnant or nursing should be excluded from using a GLP-1 receptor agonist, which are classified as pregnancy category C agents, unless the benefits outweigh the risks to the fetus.[43–45] Because exenatide is cleared primarily by the kidneys, blood concentrations of exenatide (BID or QW) are not expected to be altered in patients with hepatic impairment.[43,44] Liraglutide should be used cautiously, although no dose adjustment is recommended in patients with hepatic impairment.[45]

Managing Expectations and Maximizing Acceptance of GLP-1 Receptor Agonist Therapy

Managing patient expectations from the outset is key to maximizing benefits and minimizing limitations associated with GLP-1 receptor agonist. One problem noted by the author with some frequency is that patients expect immediate results with this type of therapy. With exenatide BID and liraglutide, it is not uncommon to see glucose-lowering within the first few days. However, exenatide QW requires a few weeks to begin showing effects; maximal benefit may not be seen for up to 10 weeks.

In addition to patients' glycemic control expectations, it is especially important to manage their expectations with regard to weight. It is not uncommon for patients to ask about "those new medications that cause weight loss." GLP-1 receptor agonists should not be presented to patients as weight loss drugs. It must be made clear that, although weight loss occurs in ~ 80% of patients,[64] it is not possible to identify which patients will lose weight before initiating the therapy.

In the author's experience, patients fit into one of three groups with respect to the weight effects of the GLP-1 receptor agonists. The first is the small percentage of patients who do not lose weight but have the expected 0.5–1.5% reduction in A1C. For these patients, the lack of a weight effect should not be viewed as a clinical failure. The second group is those who experience a 2- to 5-lb weight loss, and the third group includes those who have a greater weight loss, perhaps as much as 20–40 lb. Some patients in the third group subsequently regain some of their lost weight.

Although patients with a BMI > 30 or 35 kg/m² are generally those who experience the greatest weight loss,[65] this has not always been the case in the author's experience, in which some patients with a BMI < 30 kg/m² have been observed to lose 15–20 lb. The loss in weight usually plateaus in about 8 weeks with exenatide BID and 8–12 weeks with liraglutide.

Consideration of a GLP-1 receptor agonist should involve discussing with patients their comfort with delivering a medication subcutaneously. This can be a significant issue for patients and providers, with concerns similar to those that arise when considering starting insulin.[66] Patient concerns include having to use a needle and give a "shot," the social stigma associated with using an injected medication, the perceived complexity of the delivery system, and the belief that this in some way signifies that the disease process is getting worse. Providers also have concerns, including feeling that it takes more time to educate patients about using a subcutaneous medication, the availability and qualification of staff to teach patients how to use these medications, and concerns that patients will not accept their recommendation to use a GLP-1 receptor agonist. Such concerns on the part of patients and providers can create an environment of reluctance to advance diabetes care, thereby making it difficult for patients to attain glycemic control.[67]

Addressing patient barriers
Numerous strategies can be implemented to address potential patient barriers. First, it may be helpful to ask patients if they have any concerns or issues they would like to discuss. Many patients with type 2 diabetes have searched for information online, talked with neighbors, or have otherwise gained some secondhand knowledge about these medications.

Once patients' concerns are identified, it is much easier to address them. It may not be pos-

sible to address more than two or three issues during a clinic visit, but patients should be assured that remaining issues will be addressed in subsequent visits or, alternatively, by other members of the diabetes health care team.

It is also important to avoid suggesting that advancing to this (or any other) glucose-lowering medication signifies that the disease is getting worse. Rather it is important to make clear that diabetes is a progressive illness that requires medication adjustment to maintain management goals.

Clinicians may find it especially helpful to discuss with patients the benefits and limitations of GLP-1 receptor agonists, noting that they are much less likely than insulin therapy to cause hypoglycemia or weight gain. The potential of losing weight with a GLP-1 receptor agonist can be a strong motivator for patients who have struggled with weight gain while using other glucose-lowering agents. Similarly, learning that the risk of hypoglycemia is much lower than with insulin or a secretagogue may help relieve patients' anxiety. It can also be valuable to have patients check their FBG and PPG levels a few times for the week or two after starting GLP-1 receptor agonist therapy. Seeing these levels decrease can be another motivating factor that can blunt initial concerns regarding issues such as self-injection and GI adverse effects.

Two of the GLP-1 receptor agonists, liraglutide and exenatide QW, do not require dose timing with meals. Remembering to take a medication in advance of a meal, as is necessary for exenatide BID, can be challenging for some patients.

All three of the GLP-1 receptor agonists have administration devices/systems that make both the dosing and teaching of the medica-

tions relatively simple. Liraglutide and exenatide BID are delivered with pen devices with 31- or 32-gauge needles, whereas exenatide QW has a delivery kit that simplifies the mixing of diluent and powdered medication but requires a syringe with an 8-mm, 23-gauge needle. Despite the larger-gauge administration needle required with exenatide QW, some patients may decide that the once-weekly administration is a key benefit because they can select the day of the week that they want to administer their dose and stick with it. Other patients may decide they like the once-daily administration of liraglutide because they do not need to worry about timing their dose with a meal.

Because patients usually have concerns about giving themselves an injection, avoiding use of the word "shot" is suggested. Patients associate shots with painful antibiotic and vaccine injections they have had in the past. It is also helpful to acknowledge that not wanting to "stick holes" in themselves is a very rational decision. Differentiating subcutaneous administration from intramuscular injection is important. GLP-1 receptor agonists use much smaller, shorter needles and are delivered into the subcutaneous fat. They are not intramuscular injections.

It is often helpful to patients to make a connection between doing something that they perceived as unpleasant and attaining the goals that they want to attain. Although it is important to establish and follow achievement of the numeric goals of diabetes control, it is also important to emphasize the greater sense of well-being patients may feel when they achieve improved blood glucose control.

Addressing these issues and educating people with type 2 diabetes is a team process. The author typically discusses treatment options with patients, explaining the benefits and limitations of each choice. Once a decision is made, much of the detailed patient education is provided by clinic staff. For this reason, it is important to work with staff to develop a coordinated process that can be followed when patients begin therapy with a GLP-1 receptor agonist or other glucose-lowering therapy. It is important that the teaching is consistent from both providers and support staff

when providing patient education. In addition, it is important for those involved in providing patient education to be knowledgeable about the disease and the treatments, including how each delivery device works. For the three GLP-1 receptor agonists, understanding—and demonstrating—the differences among the devices is crucial before presenting to patients.

Local diabetes education programs and certified diabetes educators can be quite helpful

with this process. More information about how to find a local diabetes educator may be found at the American Association of Diabetes Educators website (http://www.diabeteseducator.org/DiabetesEducation/Find.html). In addition, a wide variety of patient education resources are available from the ADA (http://www.diabetes.org/living-with-diabetes/?loc=GlobalNavLWD) and AACE (http://resources.aace.com).

Table 3. Strategies to Improve Patient Acceptance and Self-Management With a GLP-1 Receptor Agonist

Manage patient expectations before initiating GLP-1 receptor agonist therapy.
- Avoid presenting GLP-1 receptor agonists as weight loss medications.

Investigate concerns (e.g., needle phobia, cost, and perceived complexity) before initiating therapy.

To allay concerns for patients with needle phobia:
- Familiarize patients (and yourself) with pen devices or delivery kit.
- Avoid use of the word "shot."
- Differentiate between subcutaneous and intramuscular injections.
- Have patients self-inject the first dose in the office; alternatively, just use the needle.

To enhance patient motivation for initiating GLP-1 receptor agonist therapy:
- Help patients make the connection between doing something that is perceived as unpleasant and the goals they want to attain, including a greater sense of well-being.
- Discuss benefits such as weight loss and the low incidence of hypoglycemia.
- Encourage patients to perform SMBG a few times daily for a week or two after initiating to see reductions in FBG and PPG levels.
- Involve a dietitian to help patients identify strategies to maximize the potential for weight loss.
- Explain that GLP-1 receptor agonists help patients lose weight by promoting satiety, leading to decreased caloric intake, and not by altering metabolism.
- Advise patients to eat meals without distractions such as television.
- Advise patients to eat a small portion and then wait 30 minutes before eating more, to allow satiety to occur.
- Counsel patients to stop eating when they feel full.

To address nausea:
- Before initiation, educate patients that transient nausea is possible.
- Use a dose escalation strategy for exenatide BID or liraglutide, but not for exenatide QW, as described in package inserts.
  - Consider lengthening the time over which the dose is escalated.
- Administer exenatide BID < 60 minutes before the meal.
- Temporarily reduce the dose.
- Counsel patients to stop eating when they feel full.
- Avoid administering the medication close to a large or high-fat meal.

Educate patients regarding the possibility of localized irritation or nodule formation at injection site. Advise rotating injection among sites in the abdomen, thigh, and upper arms.

Assess adherence if the glycemic response is less than expected (e.g., A1C reduction < 0.5%).

Summary

The GLP-1 receptor agonist class of medications offers health care providers an important novel treatment option with distinct benefits and limitations compared to other classes of glucose-lowering medications. Working in collaboration with patients, providers and their staff can individualize treatment and implement strategies to improve patient acceptance and self-management with a GLP-1 receptor agonist (Table 3). Doing so will undoubtedly help patients with type 2 diabetes attain their metabolic and treatment goals.

ACKNOWLEDGMENTS

Funding for the development of this article was provided by Novo Nordisk to the Primary Care Education Consortium, which provided editorial assistance to the author. The author received no financial compensation for this article. The author independently made the decision to submit his article and is solely responsible for all content.

REFERENCES

[1]Inzucchi SE, Bergenstal RM, Buse JB, Diamant M, Ferrannini E, Nauck M, Peters AL, Tsapas A, Wender R, Matthews DR: Management of hyperglycemia in type 2 diabetes: a patient-centered approach. Position statement of the American Diabetes Association (ADA) and the European Association for the Study of Diabetes (EASD). *Diabetes Care* 35:1364–1379, 2012

[2]Drucker DJ: The biology of incretin hormones. *Cell Metab* 3:153–165, 2006

[3]Naslund E, Bogefors J, Skogar S, Gryback P, Jacobsson H, Holst JJ, Hellstrom PM: GLP-1 slows solid gastric emptying and inhibits insulin, glucagon, and PYY release in humans. *Am J Physiol* 277:R910–R916, 1999

[4]Fehmann HC, Habener JF: Insulinotropic hormone glucagon-like peptide-I(7-37) stimulation of proinsulin gene expression and proinsulin biosynthesis in insulinoma beta TC-1 cells. *Endocrinology* 130:159–166, 1992

[5]Kreymann B, Williams G, Ghatei MA, Bloom SR: Glucagon-like peptide-1 7-36: a physiological incretin in man. *Lancet* 2:1300–1304, 1987

[6]Nauck MA, Heimesaat MM, Behle K, Holst JJ, Nauck MS, Ritzel R, Hufner M, Schmiegel WH: Effects of glucagon-like peptide 1 on counterregulatory hormone responses, cognitive functions, and insulin secretion during hyperinsulinemic, stepped hypoglycemic clamp experiments in healthy volunteers. *J Clin Endocrinol Metab* 87:1239–1246, 2002

[7]Bulotta A, Hui H, Anastasi E, Bertolotto C, Boros LG, Di MU, Perfetti R: Cultured pancreatic ductal cells undergo cell cycle redistribution and beta-cell-like differentiation in response to glucagon-like peptide-1. *J Mol Endocrinol* 29:347–360, 2002

[8]Farilla L, Bulotta A, Hirshberg B, Li CS, Khoury N, Noushmehr H, Bertolotto C, Di MU, Harlan DM, Perfetti R: Glucagon-like peptide 1 inhibits cell apoptosis and improves glucose responsiveness of freshly isolated human islets. *Endocrinology* 144:5149–5158, 2003

[9]Xu G, Stoffers DA, Habener JF, Bonner-Weir S: Exendin-4 stimulates both beta-cell replication and neogenesis, resulting in increased beta-cell mass and improved glucose tolerance in diabetic rats. *Diabetes* 48:2270–2276, 1999

[10]Zhou J, Wang X, Pineyro MA, Egan JM: Glucagon-like peptide 1 and exendin-4 convert pancreatic AR42J cells into glucagon- and insulin-producing cells. *Diabetes* 48:2358–2366, 1999

[11]Moretto TJ, Milton DR, Ridge TD, Macconell LA, Okerson T, Wolka AM, Brodows RG: Efficacy and tolerability of exenatide monotherapy over 24 weeks in antidiabetic drug-naive patients with type 2 diabetes: a randomized, double-blind, placebo-controlled, parallel-group study. *Clin Ther* 30:1448–1460, 2008

[12]Bunck MC, Diamant M, Corner A, Eliasson B, Malloy JL, Shaginian RM, Deng W, Kendall DM, Taskinen MR, Smith U, Yki-Jarvinen H, Heine RJ: One-year treatment with exenatide improves beta-cell function, compared with insulin glargine, in metformin-treated type 2 diabetic patients: a randomized, controlled trial. *Diabetes Care* 32:762–768, 2009

[13]Mari A, Degn K, Brock B, Rungby J, Ferrannini E, Schmitz O: Effects of the long-acting human glucagon-like peptide-1 analog liraglutide on beta-cell function in normal living conditions. *Diabetes Care* 30:2032–2033, 2007

[14]Buse JB, Rosenstock J, Sesti G, Schmidt WE, Montanya E, Brett JH, Zychma M, Blonde L: Liraglutide once a day versus exenatide twice a day for type 2 diabetes: a 26-week randomised, parallel-group, multinational, open-label trial (LEAD-6). *Lancet* 374:39–47, 2009

[15]Russell-Jones D, Cuddihy RM, Hanefeld M, Kumar A, Gonzalez JG, Chan M, Wolka AM, Boardman MK: Efficacy and safety of exenatide once weekly versus metformin, pioglitazone, and sitagliptin used as monotherapy in drug-naive patients with type 2 diabetes (DURATION-4): a 26-week double-blind study. *Diabetes Care* 35:252–258, 2012

[16]Degn KB, Juhl CB, Sturis J, Jakobsen G, Brock B, Chandramouli V, Rungby J, Landau BR, Schmitz O: One week's treatment with the long-acting glucagon-like peptide 1 derivative liraglutide (NN2211) markedly improves 24-h glycemia and alpha- and beta-cell function and reduces endogenous glucose release in patients with type 2 diabetes. *Diabetes* 53:1187–1194, 2004

[17]Seghieri M, Rebelos E, Gastaldelli A, Astiarraga BD, Casolaro A, Barsotti E, Pocai A, Nauck M, Muscelli E, Ferrannini E: Direct effect of GLP-1 infusion on endogenous glucose production in humans. *Diabetologia* 56:156–161, 2013

[18]Delgado-Aros S, Kim DY, Burton DD, Thomforde GM, Stephens D, Brinkmann BH, Vella A, Camilleri M: Effect of GLP-1 on gastric volume, emptying, maximum volume ingested, and postprandial symptoms in humans. *Am J Physiol Gastrointest Liver Physiol* 282:G424–G431, 2002

[19]Gutzwiller JP, Goke B, Drewe J, Hildebrand P, Ketterer S, Handschin D, Winterhalder R, Conen D, Beglinger C: Glucagon-like peptide-1: a potent regulator of food intake in humans. *Gut* 44:81–86, 1999

[20]Gutzwiller JP, Drewe J, Goke B, Schmidt H, Rohrer B, Lareida J, Beglinger C: Glucagon-like peptide-1 promotes satiety and reduces food intake in patients with diabetes mellitus type 2. *Am J Physiol* 276:R1541–R1544, 1999

[21]DeFronzo RA, Okerson T, Viswanathan P, Guan X, Holcombe JH, MacConell L: Effects of exenatide versus sitagliptin on postprandial glucose, insulin and glucagon secretion, gastric emptying, and caloric intake: a randomized, cross-over study. *Curr Med Res Opin* 24:2943–2952, 2008

[22]Nelson P, Poon T, Guan X, Schnabel C, Wintle M, Fineman M: The incretin mimetic exenatide as a monotherapy in patients with type 2 diabetes. *Diabetes Technol Ther* 9:317–326, 2007

[23]Garber A, Henry R, Ratner R, Garcia-Hernandez PA, Rodriguez-Pattzi H, Olvera-Alvarez I, Hale PM, Zdravkovic M, Bode B: Liraglutide versus glimepiride monotherapy for type 2 diabetes (LEAD-3 Mono): a randomised, 52-week, phase III, double-blind, parallel-treatment trial. *Lancet* 373:473–481, 2009

[24]Garber A, Henry RR, Ratner R, Hale P, Chang CT, Bode B: Liraglutide, a once-daily human glucagon-like peptide-1 analogue, provides sustained improvements in glycaemic control and weight loss for 2 years as monotherapy compared with glimepiride in patients with type 2 diabetes. *Diabetes Obes Metab* 13:348–356, 2011

[25]Taylor K, Gurney K, Han J, Pencek R, Walsh B, Trautmann M: Exenatide once weekly treatment maintained improvements in glycemic control and weight loss over 2 years. *BMC Endocr Disord* 11:9, 2011

[26]Nauck M, Frid A, Hermansen K, Thomsen AB, During M, Shah N, Tankova T, Mitha I, Matthews DR: Long-term efficacy and safety comparison of liraglutide, glimepiride and placebo, all in combination with metformin in type 2 diabetes: 2-year

results from the LEAD-2 study. *Diabetes Obes Metab* 15:204–212, 2013

[27]Morales J: The pharmacologic basis for clinical differences among GLP-1 receptor agonists and DPP-4 inhibitors. *Postgrad Med* 123:189–201, 2011

[28]Herman GA, Bergman A, Stevens C, Kotey P, Yi B, Zhao P, Dietrich B, Golor G, Schrodter A, Keymeulen B, Lasseter KC, Kipnes MS, Snyder K, Hilliard D, Tanen M, Cilissen C, De Smet M, de Lepeleire I, Van Dyck K, Wang AQ, Zeng W, Davies MJ, Tanaka W, Holst JJ, Deacon CF, Gottesdiener KM, Wagner JA: Effect of single oral doses of sitagliptin, a dipeptidyl peptidase-4 inhibitor, on incretin and plasma glucose levels after an oral glucose tolerance test in patients with type 2 diabetes. *J Clin Endocrinol Metab* 91:4612–4619, 2006

[29]Holst JJ, Deacon CF: Glucagon-like peptide-1 mediates the therapeutic actions of DPP-IV inhibitors. *Diabetologia* 48:612–615, 2005

[30]Vilsboll T, Zdravkovic M, Le Thi T, Krarup T, Schmitz O, Courreges JP, Verhoeven R, Buganova I, Madsbad S: Liraglutide, a long-acting human glucagon-like peptide-1 analog, given as monotherapy significantly improves glycemic control and lowers body weight without risk of hypoglycemia in patients with type 2 diabetes. *Diabetes Care* 30:1608–1610, 2007

[31]Blevins T, Pullman J, Malloy J, Yan P, Taylor K, Schulteis C, Trautmann M, Porter L: DURATION-5: exenatide once weekly resulted in greater improvements in glycemic control compared with exenatide twice daily in patients with type 2 diabetes. *J Clin Endocrinol Metab* 96:1301–1310, 2011

[32]Drucker DJ, Buse JB, Taylor K, Kendall DM, Trautmann M, Zhuang D, Porter L: Exenatide once weekly versus twice daily for the treatment of type 2 diabetes: a randomised, open-label, non-inferiority study. *Lancet* 372:1240–1250, 2008

[33]Buse JB, Sesti G, Schmidt WE, Montanya E, Chang CT, Xu Y, Blonde L, Rosenstock J: Switching to once-daily liraglutide from twice-daily exenatide further improves glycemic control in patients with type 2 diabetes using oral agents. *Diabetes Care* 33:1300–1303, 2010

[34]Buse JB, Nauck M, Forst T, Sheu WH, Shenouda SK, Heilmann CR, Hoogwerf BJ, Gao A, Boardman MK, Fineman M, Porter L, Schernthaner G: Exenatide once weekly versus liraglutide once daily in patients with type 2 diabetes (DURATION-6): a randomised, open-label study. *Lancet* 381:117–124, 2013

[35]Buse JB, Nauck M, Forst T, Sheu WH, Shenouda SK, Heilmann CR, Hoogwerf BJ, Gao A, Boardman MK, Fineman M, Porter L, Schernthaner G: Exenatide once weekly versus liraglutide once daily in patients with type 2 diabetes (DURATION-6): a randomised, open-label study. *Lancet* 381:117–124, 2013

[36]Pratley RE, Nauck M, Bailey T, Montanya E, Cuddihy R, Filetti S, Thomsen AB, Sondergaard RE, Davies M: Liraglutide versus sitagliptin for patients with type 2

diabetes who did not have adequate glycaemic control with metformin: a 26-week, randomised, parallel-group, open-label trial. *Lancet* 375:1447–1456, 2010

[37]Bergenstal RM, Wysham C, MacConell L, Malloy J, Walsh B, Yan P, Wilhelm K, Malone J, Porter LE: Efficacy and safety of exenatide once weekly versus sitagliptin or pioglitazone as an adjunct to metformin for treatment of type 2 diabetes (DURATION-2): a randomised trial. *Lancet* 376:431–439, 2010

[38]Blonde L, Klein EJ, Han J, Zhang B, Mac SM, Poon TH, Taylor KL, Trautmann ME, Kim DD, Kendall DM: Interim analysis of the effects of exenatide treatment on A1C, weight and cardiovascular risk factors over 82 weeks in 314 overweight patients with type 2 diabetes. *Diabetes Obes Metab* 8:436–447, 2006

[39]Zinman B, Hoogwerf BJ, Garcia SD, Milton DR, Giaconia JM, Kim DD, Trautmann ME, Brodows RG: The effect of adding exenatide to a thiazolidinedione in suboptimally controlled type 2 diabetes: a randomized trial. *Ann Intern Med* 146:477–485, 2007

[40]Russell-Jones D, Vaag A, Schmitz O, et al.: Liraglutide vs insulin glargine and placebo in combination with metformin and sulfonylurea therapy in type 2 diabetes mellitus (LEAD-5 met+SU): a randomised controlled trial. *Diabetologia* 52:2046–2055, 2009

[41]Zinman B, Gerich J, Buse JB, Lewin A, Schwartz S, Raskin P, Hale PM, Zdravkovic M, Blonde L: Efficacy and safety of the human glucagon-like peptide-1 analog liraglutide in combination with metformin and thiazolidinedione in patients with type 2 diabetes (LEAD-4 Met+TZD). *Diabetes Care* 32:1224–1230, 2009

[42]Nauck MA, Duran S, Kim D, Johns D, Northrup J, Festa A, Brodows R, Trautmann M: A comparison of twice-daily exenatide and biphasic insulin aspart in patients with type 2 diabetes who were suboptimally controlled with sulfonylurea and metformin: a non-inferiority study. *Diabetologia* 50:259–267, 2007

[43]Byetta package insert. San Diego, Calif., Amylin Pharmaceuticals, 2011

[44]Bydureon package insert. San Diego, Calif., Amylin Pharmaceuticals, 2012

[45]Victoza package insert. Princeton, N.J., Novo Nordisk, 2012

[46]Glucophage package insert. Princeton, N.J., Bristol-Myers Squibb, 2011

[47]DeFronzo RA, Ratner RE, Han J, Kim DD, Fineman MS, Baron AD: Effects of exenatide (exendin-4) on glycemic control and weight over 30 weeks in metformin-treated patients with type 2 diabetes. *Diabetes Care* 28:1092–1100, 2005

[48]Nauck M, Frid A, Hermansen K, Shah NS, Tankova T, Mitha IH, Zdravkovic M, During M, Matthews DR: Efficacy and safety comparison of liraglutide, glimepiride, and placebo, all in combination with metformin, in type 2 diabetes: the LEAD (liraglutide

effect and action in diabetes)-2 study. *Diabetes Care* 32:84–90, 2009

[49]Cobble ME: How to implement incretin therapy. *J Fam Pract* 57:S26–S31, 2008

[50]Freeman JS: Optimizing outcomes for GLP-1 agonists. *J Am Osteopath Assoc* 111:eS15–eS20, 2011

[51]Unger JR, Parkin CG: Glucagon-like peptide-1 (GLP-1) receptor agonists: differentiating the new medications. *Diabetes Ther* 2:29–39, 2011

[52]Garg R, Chen W, Pendergrass M: Acute pancreatitis in type 2 diabetes treated with exenatide or sitagliptin: a retrospective observational pharmacy claims analysis. *Diabetes Care* 33:2349–2354, 2010

[53]Dore DD, Seeger JD, Arnold CK: Use of a claims-based active drug safety surveillance system to assess the risk of acute pancreatitis with exenatide or sitagliptin compared to metformin or glyburide. *Curr Med Res Opin* 25:1019–1027, 2009

[54]Elashoff M, Matveyenko AV, Gier B, Elashoff R, Butler PC: Pancreatitis, pancreatic, and thyroid cancer with glucagon-like peptide-1-based therapies. *Gastroenterology* 141:150–156, 2011

[55]Singh S, Chang HY, Richards TM, Weiner JP, Clarke JM, Segal JB: Glucagonlike peptide 1-based therapies and risk of hospitalization for acute pancreatitis in type 2 diabetes mellitus: a population-based matched case-conttrol study. *JAMA Intern Med.* Electronically published in 2013 (doi:10.1001/jamainternmed.2013.2720)

[56]American Association of Clinical Endocrinologists, American Diabetes Association issue joint response to published *JAMA* article [article online]. Available from http://media.aace.com/press-release/correcting-and-replacing-american-association-clinical-endocrinologists-american-diabe. Accessed 16 August 2013

[57]Noel RA, Braun DK, Patterson RE, Bloomgren GL: Increased risk of acute pancreatitis and biliary disease observed in patients with type 2 diabetes: a retrospective cohort study. *Diabetes Care* 32:834–838, 2009

[58]Parks M, Rosebraugh C: Weighing risks and benefits of liraglutide: the FDA's review of a new antidiabetic therapy. *N Engl J Med* 362:774–777, 2010

[59]Knudsen LB, Madsen LW, Andersen S, Almholt K, de Boer AS, Drucker DJ, Gotfredsen C, Egerod FL, Hegelund AC, Jacobsen H, Jacobsen SD, Moses AC, Molck AM, Nielsen HS, Nowak J, Solberg H, Thi TD, Zdravkovic M: Glucagon-like peptide-1 receptor agonists activate rodent thyroid C-cells causing calcitonin release and C-cell proliferation. *Endocrinology* 151:1473–1486, 2010

[60]Bremer JP, Jauch-Chara K, Hallschmid M, Schmid S, Schultes B: Hypoglycemia unawareness in older compared with middle-aged patients with type 2 diabetes. *Diabetes Care* 32:1513–1517, 2009

[61]Guide for aviation medical examiners. Pharmaceuticals (Therapeutic medications) [article online]. Available from http://www.

faa.gov/about/office_org/headquarters_
offices/avs/offices/aam/ame/guide/pharm.
Accessed 16 August 2013

[62]Medical examination report for
commercial driver fitness determination
[article online]. Available from http://www.
fmcsa.dot.gov/documents/safetyprograms/
medical-report.pdf. Accessed 16 August 2013

[63]Violante R, Oliveira JH, Yoon KH,
Reed VA, Yu MB, Bachmann OP, Ludemann
J, Chan JY: A randomized non-inferiority
study comparing the addition of exenatide
twice daily to sitagliptin or switching from
sitagliptin to exenatide twice daily in
patients with type 2 diabetes experiencing
inadequate glycaemic control on metformin
and sitagliptin. *Diabet Med* 29:e417–e424, 2012

[64]Klonoff DC, Buse JB, Nielsen LL,
Guan X, Bowlus CL, Holcombe JH,
Wintle ME, Maggs DG: Exenatide effects
on diabetes, obesity, cardiovascular risk
factors and hepatic biomarkers in patients
with type 2 diabetes treated for at least
3 years. *Curr Med Res Opin* 24:275–286,
2008

[65]Niswender K, Pi-Sunyer X, Buse J,
Jensen KH, Toft AD, Russell-Jones D,
Zinman B: Weight change with liraglutide
and comparator therapies: an analysis of
seven phase 3 trials from the liraglutide
diabetes development programme. *Diabetes
Obes Metab* 15:42–54, 2013

[66]Polonsky WH, Fisher L, Guzman
S, Villa-Caballero L, Edelman SV:
Psychological insulin resistance in
patients with type 2 diabetes: the scope
of the problem. *Diabetes Care* 28:2543-2545

[67]Koerbel G, Korytkowski M:
Insulin-therapy resistance: another form of
insulin resistance in type 2 diabetes.
Practical Diabetology 22:36–40, 2003

---

*Timothy S. Reid, MD, is medical
director of Mercy Diabetes Center
in Janesville, Wis.*

*Note of disclosure: Dr. Reid has
served on speakers bureaus and as a
consultant for Amylin/Bristol-Myers
Squibb, Novo Nordisk, Sanofi, and
Boehringer Ingelheim/Eli Lilly, all of
which manufacture or are developing
GLP-1 receptor agonist products.*

Educating Patients About Hypoglycemia Prevention and Self-Management

Jeff Unger, MD

Case Presentation

Mrs. B was a 68-year-old, Asian-American woman with a 15-year history of type 2 diabetes. Her coexisting medical conditions included unilateral intraductal carcinoma of the breast, which was treated with a modified radical mastectomy 6 years ago and showed no evidence of recurrence. Although there was no history of alcohol use, her liver function studies had been elevated to two times the upper limit of normal for several years. A liver biopsy revealed the presence of nonalcoholic steatohepatitis (NASH). She was admitted to the hospital on one occasion within the past year for bleeding esophageal varices.

Mrs. B had no history of macrovascular disease, chronic kidney disease, retinopathy, or neuropathy. For the past 10 years, she had taken 10 mg glyburide daily. Her primary care provider (PCP) was concerned that her A1C had increased from 7.4 to 7.9% in the past 6 months.

Her family members stated that they rarely spoke about diabetes, self-monitoring of blood glucose (SMBG), or diabetes-related complications. In fact, the patient's 72-year-old husband also has type 2 diabetes and is undergoing dialysis. In the past year, Mr. B has had at least two episodes of severe hypoglycemia that required hospitalization. He blames his end-stage renal disease on medication he is taking to control his blood glucose levels.

Because of concerns about Mrs. B's increasing A1C, her PCP asked her to consult with a local endocrinol-ogist who added basal insulin to her diabetes treatment regimen. She was not provided with any specific instructions about how to inject the basal insulin or when to perform SMBG. Her son noted that she tended to get "confused," but he did not attribute this to her blood glucose level because he never saw her checking her glucose. Her handwritten glucose log showed several readings in the low 50 to 60 mg/dl range, but a pattern of hypoglycemia could not be determined.

One month after beginning the combination therapy of glyburide and basal insulin, Mrs. B was observed to be driving 90 mph in the wrong direction on a residential street. After swerving to miss several cars, she lost control of her vehicle, hit a tree, and was killed on impact.

Spontaneous hypoglycemia is uncommon in the nondiabetic population but constitutes the primary barrier to optimal glycemic control in people with diabetes.

The pathogenesis of type 1 diabetes can be viewed as a bihormonal defect. Patients experience an absolute deficiency of insulin production and secretion as a result of autoimmune destruction of pancreatic β-cells coupled with exaggerated excretion of glucagon production by pancreatic α-cells. Over time, the loss of glucose counterregulation results in a higher likelihood of developing hypoglycemia that cannot be reversed by endogenous hormonal interventions.

Patients with type 2 diabetes can experience hypoglycemia resulting from medications that trigger insulin release in a glucose-independent manner. Over time, counterregulatory communication between the glucagon-producing α-cells and the insulin-producing β-cells becomes physiologically dysfunctional, thereby increasing the risk of hypoglycemia.

Patients with coexisting disorders such as cirrhosis, eating disorders, chronic kidney disease, cardiovascular disease, and advanced age are at high risk for mortality because of acute, severe hypoglycemic events.

Physicians and ancillary practitioners have the responsibility to teach patients with diabetes how to predict, avert, and correctly manage hypoglycemia. Patients with hypoglycemia awareness adrenergic failure (HAAF) should be encouraged to use continuous glucose monitoring (CGM) devices, which can proactively alert them to impending hypoglycemic events.

Definition of Hypoglycemia

A hypoglycemia and diabetes work group of the American Diabetes Association and The Endrocrine Society has recommended that a plasma concentration ≤ 70 mg/dl should be the cut-off value for defining the upper boundary of hypoglycemia.[1] Although this value is higher than the threshold of hypoglycemia symptoms, patients can prepare to take corrective action

Table 1. Subclassification of Hypoglycemia[1]		
Classification of Hypoglycemia	**Plasma Concentration**	**Description**
Severe hypoglycemia	May not be known to patient, but neurological recovery after the glucose correction is considered evidence that the event was induced by hypoglycemia	Requires the assistance of another person to actively administer carbohydrate or glucagon or to take other corrective actions
Documented symptomatic hypoglycemia	≤ 70 mg/dl	Typical symptoms of hypoglycemia are accompanied by a documented plasma glucose level ≤ 70 mg/dl
Asymptomatic hypoglycemia	≤ 70 mg/dl	No symptoms noted, but blood glucose is noted to be ≤ 70 mg/dl
Probable symptomatic hypoglycemia	—	Symptoms typical of hypoglycemia are not accompanied by a plasma glucose determination but are presumed to be associated with a plasma level ≤ 70 mg/dl
Pseudo-hypoglycemia	≥ 70 mg/dl	Patient reports symptoms typical of hypoglycemia, yet the blood glucose levels are ≥ 70 mg/dl

when their blood glucose levels drop to < 70 mg/dl before developing defective hormonal counterregulation. The subclassifications of hypoglycemia are shown in Table 1.

Prevalence of Hypoglycemia

Patients with type 1 diabetes may experience plasma glucose concentrations < 50 mg/dl as often as 10% of the time. Defective glucose counterregulation may occur within 1 year of being diagnosed with type 1 diabetes. Typical patients with type 1 diabetes will experience two episodes of symptomatic hypoglycemia weekly and thousands of events during their lifetime.[2,3]

The frequency and severity of hypoglycemia in patients with type 2 diabetes is often underestimated by clinicians. Unfortunately, patients fear the adrenergic symptoms associated with treatment-emergent hypoglycemia. Once they become a "victim" of hypoglycemia, they may be reluctant, or even resistant, toward intensified regimens designed to achieve recommended glycemic goals.[4]

The risk of hypoglycemia in patients with insulin-requiring type 2 diabetes is equal to that in patients with type 1 diabetes. The Diabetes Audit and Research in Tayside, Scotland study[5] determined that the prevalence of hypoglycemia among people with type 1 diabetes was 7.1%, compared to 7.3% in its cohort of people with insulin-treated type 2 diabetes. Thus, patients with type 2 diabetes of long duration who require insulin are at higher risk of developing hypoglycemia than are treatment-naive individuals starting insulin for the first time.[4]

The incidence of hypoglycemia is particularly high among patients treated with insulin over extended periods of time, again reinforcing the idea that advanced disease progression and increased insulin use subsequently escalate the risk of hypoglycemia. The U.K. Hypoglycemia Study Group found that the incidence of severe hypoglycemia in patients with type 1 diabetes treated with insulin for > 15 years was three times higher than in those treated with insulin for < 5 years. The prevalence of

hypoglycemia in patients with type 2 diabetes exposed to insulin therapy for > 5 years is 25%, a threefold increased risk compared to individuals exposed to insulin for < 2 years.[2] Clinicians and educators should reinforce the importance of hypoglycemia prevention, detection, and reversal for all patients with type 1 diabetes and for those with type 2 diabetes who have used insulin for > 5 years.

Consequences of Hypoglycemia

Effect of hypoglycemia on morbidity and mortality rates

Hypoglycemia increases the risk of cardiovascular and all-cause mortality in patients with diabetes.[6] Severe hypoglycemia is associated with a macrovascular events hazards ratio (HR) of 2.88 and a microvascular events HR of 1.81. The mortality HR for a hypoglycemic event in patients with type 2 diabetes is 2.69.[6]

Hypoglycemia during hospital admissions is associated with increased lengths of stay and with increased 1-year mortality and inpatient mortality rates (2.96%

for patients who had at least one hypoglycemic episode during the hospitalization vs. 0.82% for patients who had none).[7]

Neurological impairment after a hypoglycemic event

Because the brain depends on glucose as an obligate energy source, a reduction in available glucose reserves can result in serious neurological consequences. Both mood and memory are impaired after a single episode of hypoglycemia.[8]

Plasma blood glucose levels of < 40 mg/dl will result in neuroglycopenia, which is associated with altered levels of consciousness, coma, and death. Severe neurological sequellae are relatively rare, even in patients who experience frequent hypoglycemia. Glucose levels < 50 mg/dl can interfere with patients' ability to perform everyday tasks, resulting in cognitive deterioration, irritability, belligerent behavior, fatigue, visual failure, dysarthria, disorientation, coma, and seizures.[9] Hypoglycemia-induced dementia has been observed in elderly patients, although the mechanism by which cognitive impairment occurs is not clear.[10]

Recurrent hypoglycemia lowers or even eliminates the blood glucose concentration threshold at which patients develop a sympathetic response likely to prompt them to take evasive action in time to reverse an impending event. Elderly patients may lose their balance without warning, falling to the ground. The subsequent confusion after such a fall is likely to be attributed to "the aging process" rather than to deficient glucose counterregulation.

Prolongation of a hypoglycemic event is likely to result in subsequent episodes within a 24-hour period. Aberrant behavior and structural damage to the brain may occur with repeated episodes of hypoglycemia.

Hypoglycemia awareness autonomic failure

Repeated hypoglycemic events can lead to HAAF, a neurological condition affecting one's ability to perceive the autonomic features of low blood glucose levels. Patients with HAAF become defenseless and unable to reverse an impending event. Adults with type 1 diabetes who have impaired awareness of hypoglycemia are much more likely to be exposed to asymptomatic hypoglycemia and are at higher risk of developing severe hypoglycemia than those who are able to detect a drop in plasma glucose.

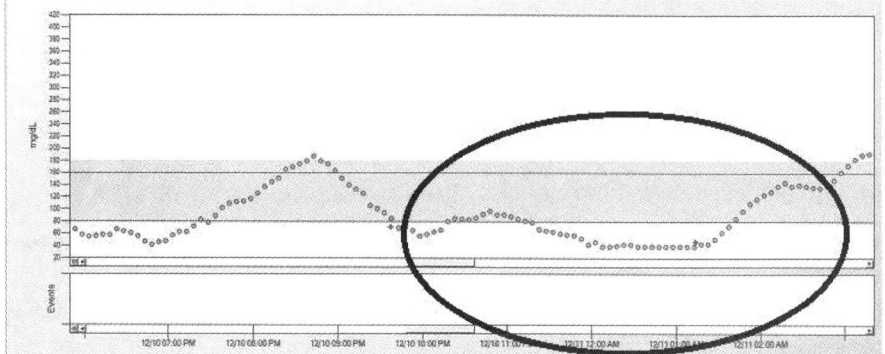

Figure 1. This CGM tracing of a 28-year-old patient with a 15-year history of type 1 diabetes demonstrates the occurrence of hypoglycemia unawareness lasting from 9:00 to 10:30 p.m. The patient experiences a 2-hour episode of hypoglycemia unawareness while sleeping from 11:30 p.m. until 2:00 a.m., when he is finally awakened by his CGM alarm and successfully corrects his hypoglycemia. Reprinted with permission from Unger J: Diabetes Management in Primary Care. *2nd ed. Philadelphia, Pa., Lippincott, Williams, and Wilkins, 2012.*

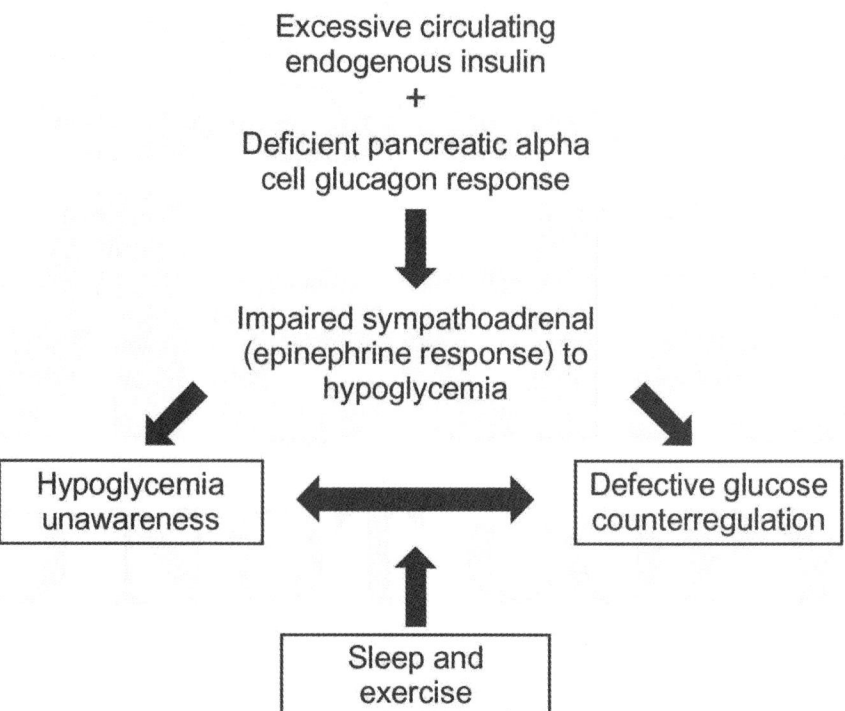

Figure 2. Mechanisms associated with HAAF. Reprinted with permission from Ref. 9.

Patients with type 1 diabetes and HAAF have double the frequency of hypoglycemic events (7.9 vs. 3.7 events in those with normal awareness), seven times the incidence of asymptomatic hypoglycemia (3.7 vs. 0.5 events), and an annual prevalence of severe hypoglycemia of 53 versus just 5% in those with normal awareness.[11] Figures 1 and 2 depict the mechanisms associated with HAAF.

Euglycemic individuals signal glucagon secretion via a reduction in insulin release by pancreatic β-cells, coupled with low glucose stimulation of α-cells. In people with type 1 diabetes, a signaling defect between the α- and β-cells accounts for failure to mount an acceptable counterregulatory response during hypoglycemia. With the autoimmune destruction of glucose-dependent β-cell insulin secretion, signaling pathways between the α- and β-cells become disrupted. Loss of the glucagon secretory response to hypoglycemia is a key feature of HAAF. An attenuated epinephrine response to hypoglycemia completes the syndrome of defective counterregulation. Without glucagon secretion or epinephrine counterregulation, patients are 25 times more likely to experience a severe hypoglycemic event with intensive insulin therapy.[12]

A single hypoglycemic event in patients with type 1 diabetes results in defective counterregulation and delayed reversal of hypoglycemia. Epinephrine secretion and mobilization in response to a subsequent reoccurrence of hypoglycemia in a clinical setting, during which circulating endogenous insulin levels remain elevated and pancreatic α-cell glucagon production is absent, is the hallmark of HAAF. Because both defective glucose counterregulation and HAAF contribute to an increased frequency of hypoglycemia, the incidence of hypoglycemic

induction extends into periods when patients sleep, as well as exercise.[13]

Economic impact of hypoglycemia

A number of health economic studies have evaluated the negative impact of hypoglycemia on society in both the United States and Europe. One study,[5] conducted in the United Kingdom, examined 244 episodes of severe hypoglycemia in 160 patients with diabetes in 1 year. Each episode of hypoglycemia cost ~ $600. The direct and indirect costs of a single severe hypoglycemic event in the United States have been estimated at $1,500, including emergency department evaluation and lost work productivity.[14]

Nocturnal hypoglycemia results in patients arriving late to work or missing entire days at the office. Patients who experience hypoglycemia are likely to use extra test strips for fear of having a recurrence of low blood glucose levels. Calls to doctors for guidance on glucose management are increased after an episode of hypoglycemia, and patients often inappropriately self-titrate their medications to avoid future events.[14]

Clinical characteristics of hypoglycemia in the elderly

Hypoglycemia may have severe consequences in the elderly but is often overlooked by both patients and clinicians. The estimated occurrence of hypoglycemia in patients > 65 years of age is ~ 1.4 episodes/100 patient-years.[15] The risk of hypoglycemia is augmented in elderly patients taking insulin, those with cirrhosis, and those with HAAF or renal insufficiency. Acute and potentially life-threatening consequences of hypoglycemia in elderly patients include acute myocardial infarction, ventricular rhythm disorders, stroke, and injuries from falls.[16]

High-risk hours for hypoglycemia in the elderly population are

toward dinnertime (for patients taking sulfonylureas) or at the end of the morning and afternoon in those taking rapid-acting insulin.[16] Polypharmacy, advanced age, and a recent hospitalization favor hypoglycemia in this high-risk population.[17]

Age-related impairment in counterregulatory hormone responses has been described in elderly patients with respect to glucagon and growth hormone secretion.[18] Declines in renal function and hepatic enzyme activity may also interfere with the metabolism of sulfonylureas and insulin, thereby potentiating their hypoglycemic effects. Hypoglycemia may be prolonged in patients using sulfonylureas, especially those who have chronic renal insufficiency.[19]

Impact of hypoglycemia on pregnancy

Normal plasma glucose levels are ~ 20% lower during pregnancy. Fasting glucose levels average 75 mg/dl, whereas postprandial elevations peak at 110 mg/dl.[20]

Attempts to attain strict glycemic control during pregnancy may be compromised by the risk of inducing severe hypoglycemia, which occurs in 45% of patients with type 1 diabetes. When pregnant women and nonpregnant women are compared using CGM, mild hypoglycemia (defined as blood glucose < 60 mg/dl) is more common in pregnancy.[21]

Women with type 1 diabetes experience three times more hypoglycemia during the first trimester of pregnancy than when they are not pregnant. Hypoglycemia rates tend to decline during the third trimester.[22] Using CGM may help to reduce the number of severe hypoglycemic events in pregnancy.[23,24]

Maternal hypoglycemia generally does not increase risks to the fetus as long as pregnant women avoid injury during hypoglycemic episodes.[25] Table 2 lists the risk factors for hypoglycemia during pregnancy.

Table 2. Risk Factors for Hypoglycemia During Pregnancy and Postpartum[1]

- History of severe hypoglycemia within the preceding year
- History of HAAF
- Low A1C during first trimester
- Glycemic variability
- Insulin stacking when correcting postprandial hyperglycemia
- Breastfeeding

Risks of driving while experiencing hypoglycemia

A meta-analysis of 15 studies[26] suggested that the relative risk (RR) of having a motor vehicle accident for people with diabetes compared to the general population ranges between 1.126 and 1.19%. When compared to patients with other medical conditions such as attention deficit/hyperactivity disorder (RR 4.0) and obstructive sleep apnea (RR 2.4), patients with diabetes are no more likely to be involved in an accident than their euglycemic counterparts.[27,28]

Still, the risk of hypoglycemia-induced motor vehicle accidents is of concern to patients and to government driving regulatory agencies. Driving risk assessment is often overlooked by busy clinicians. Only 62% of health care providers recommend that patients test their blood glucose levels before driving, and 13% of clinicians believe that people can safely operate a motor vehicle when their blood glucose level is < 72 mg/dl.[29] Nearly half of all drivers with type 1 diabetes and 75% of those with type 2 diabetes have never discussed driving guidelines with their physician.[30]

Patients at highest risk for collisions are those with a recent history of hypoglycemia, regardless of the prescribed treatment regimen.[31] Drivers with a history of hypoglycemia-related accidents are at higher risk for having another collision compared to individuals who have been accident free. A hyperinsulinemic clamp study[32] was performed on type 1 diabetes patients with and without a history of hypoglycemia-related accidents who were placed in a driving simulator. As hypoglycemia developed, those who had had previous accidents were observed to drive more recklessly and were noted to release less epinephrine in response to the hypoglycemic induction. This defect in counterregulation would allow patients to slip into a deeper and more prolonged phase of hypoglycemia.[32]

Patients with a history of motor vehicle accidents have been noted to have impaired glucose counterregulation, are more insulin sensitive, and experience difficulty with working memory and speed processing in both euglycemic and hypoglycemic states.[33] Thus, any patients with type 1 diabetes who have been in a recent car accident should be carefully evaluated for HAAF and educated about the effects of driving while hypoglycemic.[31]

Acute insulin-induced hypoglycemia causes significant impairment in spatial cognitive abilities and mental processing.[34] While driving, patients may be able to maintain their grip on the steering wheel, yet become disoriented as to their driving location and direction of navigation. Driving the wrong way on a residential street would be an example of spatial impairment. Table 3 may be used to identify drivers who are potentially at risk and who may require further evaluation and intensive hypoglycemia prevention protocols to minimize their likelihood of motor vehicle accidents.[35]

Having a history of hypoglycemia does not implicate patients as being unsafe drivers. However, patients with a history of severe hypoglycemia should be evaluated to determine the cause, whether it was isolated or recurrent, and how best to mitigate future risks. Recurrent episodes of severe hypoglycemia (defined as two or more events within a 12-month period) may warrant reporting to the appropriate licensing agency indicating that such

Table 3. Drivers Who May Be at Risk for Motor Vehicle Accidents Because of Hypoglycemia

Individuals at risk for motor vehicle accidents include those:
- Who have experienced an episode of severe hypoglycemia within the past 24 months
- Who have had to have others drive on their behalf because of the presence of hypoglycemia
- Who have had a collision in the past 12 months, especially when the accident was attributed to hypoglycemia
- With HAAF
- With coexisting diabetes and obstructive sleep apnea
- Using a sulfonylurea in combination with insulin and benzodiazepines
- Who use insulin and abuse alcohol or drink while skipping meals; alcohol exacerbates the cognitive impairment associated with hypoglycemia[35]
- Using a sulfonylurea and insulin who have chronic kidney disease
- With sensory neuropathy
- With erratic sleep and meal schedules
- On insulin therapies who are nonadherent to SMBG
- Who have limited understanding of how to monitor for and reverse hypoglycemia

patients should not drive until their deficiencies in diabetes self-management are addressed.[31]

High-risk patients should monitor their blood glucose levels before driving and at 1-hour intervals while on long trips. Considerations should be given to factors that may predict a decrease in blood glucose levels, such as insulin dose timing, timing of the last meal, and exercise type and timing. All cars driven by such patients should be equipped with a spare glucose testing meter, as well as a quick source of carbohydrate, which can be stored even in a hot vehicle. Glucose tabs, liquid glucose "shots," and glucose gel may all be placed in the glove compartment and consumed in an emergency. Each 15 g of carbohydrate will raise plasma glucose ~ 75 mg/dl within 15 minutes.

At the first sign of hypoglycemia, individuals should safely exit the road and consume the carbohydrate. Driving should not resume until their blood glucose is safely on the rise > 70 mg/dl and their cognition has recovered.

Reducing the Risk of Hypoglycemia

Patient education
Patient education has been shown to improve outcomes from hypoglycemia, but not to reduce the incidence of events.[36] Medications that are likely to result in hypoglycemia should be reviewed with patients and their family members on a regular basis. Hypoglycemia symptom recognition and management should be discussed at each visit. Written instructions should also be provided to all patients, because caregivers might panic and not remember directions for reversing hypoglycemia in an emergency situation. Patients should be advised to notify their clinicians if they are experiencing hypoglycemic events so that appropriate

adjustments may be made in their treatment regimens.

Some patients with an elevated A1C may experience acute adrenergic symptoms, including lightheadedness, sweating, weakness, fatigue, and palpitations, although their plasma glucose levels remain well above 70 mg/dl. These symptoms are uncomfortable but self-limiting. Dose modifications may be needed as patients adjust to their prescribed therapeutic regimens.

Dietary interventions
Carbohydrates raise blood glucose levels. Patients must understand which carbohydrate choices might be the most appropriate to rapidly

reverse hypoglycemia. Table 4 provides a detailed treatment plan for managing hypoglycemia.[37,38] Patients who are using mixed insulin analogues should also avoid skipping meals because this may trigger hypoglycemia.

Dissociated meal and insulin injection patterns lead to glycemic variability and hypoglycemia. Assuming a premeal glucose level > 80 mg/dl, insulin should be injected 15 minutes before eating so that the rise in insulin concentration will match the time to peak carbohydrate absorption from the gut once the meal is eaten. If the glucose level is < 80 mg/dl, the injection should be given either at mealtime or immediately after eating.[39]

Table 4. A Strategic Approach to Reverse Hypoglycemia[37,38]

- If blood glucose is ≤ 60 mg/dl:
  - Eat or drink 15 g of carbohydrate
  - Recheck blood glucose after 15 minutes. If the reading is ≤ 60 mg/dl, repeat treatment with an additional 15 g of carbohydrate
  - Retest blood glucose after 15 minutes
  - If blood glucose remains ≤ 60 mg/dl, repeat treatment with an additional 15 g of carbohydrate and contact your health care provider
- A useful formula to help patients emerge safely from hypoglycemia without causing rebound hyperglycemia:
  - (100 − blood glucose) 0.2 = g of carbohydrate needed for appropriate blood glucose correction
  - Thus, if blood glucose is 50 mg/dl, consume 100 − 50 = 50; 50 × 0.2 = 10 g of carbohydrate
- Examples of foods containing 15 g of carbohydrate:
  - Glucose tablets (3- to 5-g tablets)
  - 4 oz of juice or regular soda
  - 1 Tbsp of honey or table sugar
  - 1 small box of raisins
  - 1 bottle of glucose "shot" liquid
- Patients with a history of HAAF should have access to a glucagon emergency kit at home and in their work place. Patients with severe hypoglycemia who cannot be aroused should be injected with glucagon, 1 mg intramuscularly, by a family member or associate. This should result in a rapid reversal of hypoglycemia.
- Patients who become hypoglycemic while using α-glucosidase inhibitors (AGIs; acarbose or miglitol) will not respond to sucrose. Oral glucose (dextrose) should be used to treat hypoglycemia because its absorption is not inhibited by AGIs. Glucagon will also effectively reverse hypoglycemia.

Preventing hypoglycemia while exercising

Exercise increases glucose utilization by skeletal muscles and increases the risk of hypoglycemia. The risk factors for exercise-induced hypoglycemia include prolonged physical activity, unaccustomed exercise intensity and mode (e.g., a patient who runs on a treadmill daily but now decides to go cross-country skiing), inadequate carbohydrate intake in relation to ambient insulin "on board" (insulin from a previous dose that is still active), HAAF, and failure to perform SMBG before and during exercise.

The risk of exercise-induced hypoglycemia may be mitigated by performing SMBG before and within 30 minutes of ending exercise sessions. The pre-exercise glucose target should be 120–180 mg/dl. Lower blood glucose levels should be treated before exercise by consuming 15 g of carbohydrate.[40]

Adjusting insulin doses before exercise is prudent. If exercise will be occurring within 4 hours of using prandial insulin, the dose should be reduced by 50%. Programmable insulin pumps allow patients to set a temporary basal rate of insulin delivery while exercising or to stop insulin flow before initiating exercise. Patients who exercise on a regular schedule may also program a lower basal rate to coincide with anticipated exercise sessions each day.[39]

Medication adjustment

Medications should be reviewed at each office visit. If patients appear to be experiencing hypoglycemia, pattern (structured) glucose testing may prove beneficial in determining which therapeutic alterations require active changes.[41] Initially, medications that result in fasting hypoglycemia should be adjusted. The second area of concern would be diurnal hypoglycemia, followed by postprandial hyperglycemia (Figure 3).

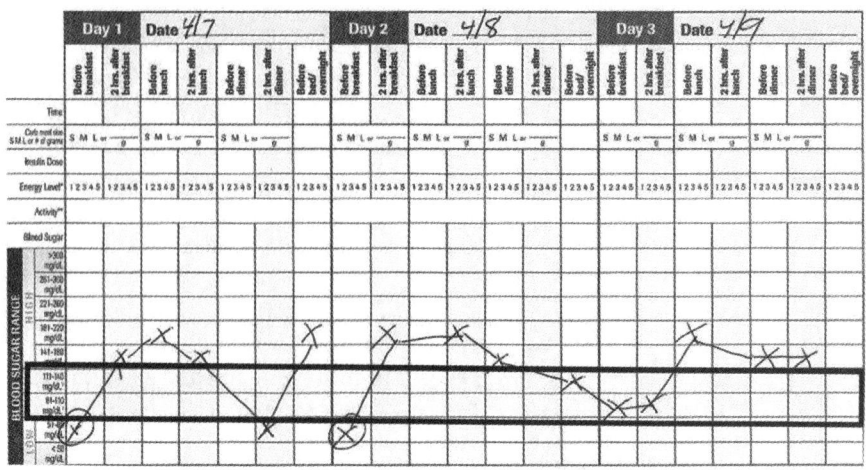

Figure 3. Glucose log of a 51-year-old patient with insulin-requiring type 2 diabetes and an A1C of 7.8% who takes 10 mg of glyburide at bedtime and 25 units of basal insulin at 9:00 p.m. The patient is asymptomatic but noted that she was awakening on two or three mornings with blood glucose values < 70 mg/dl. Her glyburide was discontinued and replaced with a dipeptidyl peptidase-4 inhibitor.

Medication adjustments should be made for patients who have chronic kidney disease (CKD). Most glucose-lowering agents (including metformin, glimepiride, pioglitazone, exenatide, sitagliptin, saxagliptin, pramlintide, insulin, and glinides) undergo some renal clearance. As a consequence, clearance may be delayed, resulting in higher plasma blood levels of these drugs. Patients with advanced CKD (stages 3–5) should have their medications reviewed and doses adjusted when their creatinine clearance is < 50 ml/min/1.73 m^2. The exceptions to this rule are liraglutide and linagliptin, which require no dosing adjustments.[42]

Chronic kidney disease increases patients' risk for both acute hypoglycemia and HAAF. Insulin suppresses glucagon secretion, which, in turn, leads to impaired gluconeogenesis and hypoglycemia counterregulation. Clinicians should consider reducing the total daily dose of insulin by 25% in hospitalized patients with a glomerular filtration rate < 45 ml/min/1.73 m^2 to minimize the risk of hypoglycemia.[43]

Glucose monitoring

Although glucose monitoring is essential in managing diabetes, structured (patterned) glucose testing provides an effective means by which patients may predict impending hypoglycemia.[9] Structured glucose testing allows patients and physicians to identify specific glycemic patterns that may be corrected with pharmacological or lifestyle interventions. The patterns easiest to identify and most often amenable to therapeutic intensification include hypoglycemia, fasting hyperglycemia, and postprandial hyperglycemia. Testing should be performed before and 2 hours after each meal for 3 days before patients' next scheduled appointment.

The difference between the baseline premeal and 2-hour postprandial blood glucose levels is referred to as the Δ (or "delta," a math symbol indicating the difference between two values). A "physiological" response to a meal should result in a positive Δ of 0–50 mg/dl. For example, a patient checks his blood glucose before eating dinner and notes the level as 125 mg/dl. He then determines that

9 units of insulin will be required for that meal. He injects the insulin 15 minutes before eating because his premeal glucose is > 80 mg/dl. His 2-hour postprandial glucose level is 145 (Δ = +20 mg/dl). Thus, the patient gave the correct amount of insulin to cover the amount of carbohydrate consumed in that meal.

The presence of any negative Δ value 2 hours postprandially is worrisome and implies that a mismatch occurred between the insulin bolus dose and the amount of carbohydrate consumed. If the patient's 2-hour postmeal glucose had been 100 mg/dl, his Δ would have been –25 mg/dl. Because rapid-acting insulin has a duration of action of 4 hours, the patient would have known that his blood glucose level is actually decreasing. Performing SMBG again in 1 hour would appear to be a prudent response to the negative Δ value. The patient could then take a corrective action if he continued to show evidence of a decrease in his glucose value.

Using CGM devices

Although SMBG regimens such as before and after meals and periodically in the middle of the night can help predict and may minimize the risk of developing hypoglycemia, CGM technology allows patients to receive real-time notification of impending events, either through preset alarms or simply by looking at the device display.[9] The devices consist of three components: a disposable sensor that measures the current or signal generated by the presence of glucose, a transmitter that is attached to the sensor and powers the electrical chemical glucose reaction in the device, and a receiver that displays and stores glucose information. Using an applicator or insertion device, patients insert a sensor wire under their skin. The transmitter sends a radiofrequency signal to the receiver,

where it is translated into a glucose value. The sensor values are paired to capillary blood glucose values through periodic calibration using capillary blood glucose obtained from a fingerstick to ensure ongoing accuracy of the sensor throughout its wear time (3, 5, or 7 days, depending on the CGM system). CGM devices not only display real-time interstitial glucose values, but also sound auditory alerts for extreme changes in glucose values.

Patients with type 1 diabetes have evidence of dysfunctional glucose counterregulation during sleep and are therefore at greater risk of developing nocturnal hypoglycemia and HAAF.[44] Endogenous concentrations of epinephrine and norepinephrine are reduced during sleep. Other aspects of sympathetic activity, including pulse, blood pressure, and vascular resistance, are mitigated during non-REM sleep in patients with diabetes. Thus, patients who experience nocturnal hypoglycemia are unlikely to reverse the events through normal counterregulatory pathways. Nocturnal hypoglycemia will likely carry over to impair counterregulation during the next day. Patients with a history of HAAF or nocturnal hypoglycemia should be placed on CGM.[9]

Case Discussion: Mrs. B and Hypoglycemia

Let us now analyze the case of Mrs. B, described at the beginning of this article, as it relates to hypoglycemia. This patient had a 15-year history of type 2 diabetes; a long duration of disease increases the likelihood of developing hypoglycemia as a result of defective counterregulation. Mrs. B also has a history of NASH, which decreases insulin clearance and appears to increase the sensitivity of pancreatic β-cells to produce endogenous insulin when exposed to sulfonylureas.[45] In addition, she had a

history of breast cancer and multiple comorbidities.

Mrs. B was referred to an endocrinologist by her PCP for possible intensification of treatment with insulin to address her deteriorating glycemic control. Her family members noted that she had periods of confusion while taking metformin and glyburide, but she did not perform SMBG regularly. A review of her written logs of SMBG within the past 30 days did reveal two worrisome values (55 and 52 mg/dl).

One might argue that a safe A1C target for Mrs. B would have been in the range of 7.5–8%. Nevertheless, her endocrinologist prescribed basal insulin, continued her sulfonylurea, and discontinued her metformin. Mrs. B and her family were not provided with SMBG instructions or education regarding identifying and reversing hypoglycemia.

One month after starting her basal insulin + glyburide regimen, Mrs. B awoke with a blood glucose of 82 mg/dl. Family members do not recall if she ate breakfast that morning. Six hours later, she died in an accident after driving on the wrong side of a street at a high speed.

Sulfonylureas will result in hypoglycemia in the middle of the afternoon, ~ 6–8 hours after they are consumed. Mrs. B's loss of spatial recognition and disorientation secondary to hypoglycemia resulted in her demise.

Future Perspectives

A closed-loop insulin pump-CGM system (also known as a sensor-augmented insulin pump) is being investigated as a means by which intensively managed patients with type 1 diabetes may minimize their risk of treatment-emergent hypoglycemia. Under experimental conditions, closed-loop devices have demonstrated superiority over the current open-loop system in allowing patients to achieve a greater amount of time within a designated glycemic target range while experiencing less hypoglycemia.[46] Sensor-augmented pumps, which are now available in Europe and are under Food and Drug Administration review in the United States, automatically discontinue basal insulin delivery when a pre-set interstitial hypoglycemic threshold is breached.

Conclusions

Iatrogenic hypoglycemia is a substantial barrier to the effective control of blood glucose concentrations in patients with type 1 or type 2 diabetes. Hypoglycemia can have a significant impact on morbidity and mortality, increase the length of hospital stays and health care costs, and negatively affect a person's ability to safely operate a motor vehicle. Patients with diabetes should be educated on ways they can reduce their frequency of hypoglycemic events and reduce their likelihood of developing defective glucose counterregulation.

Physicians should assess medications and SMBG logs at each visit. Appropriate and timely adjustments in medication may reduce patients' risk of experiencing hypoglycemia and HAAF. Structured glucose testing is preferred over random sampling. CGM is recommended for patients who experience HAAF.

Elderly patients should be carefully evaluated for coexisting medical problems such as CKD, liver failure, and coronary artery disease. Hypoglycemia symptoms in elderly patients are often inappropriately attributed to the aging process rather than to actual decline in plasma glucose levels.

REFERENCES

[1]Seaquist ER, Anderson J, Childs B, Cryer P, Dagogo-Jack S, Fish L, Heller SR, Rodriguez H, Rosenzweig J, Vigersky R.: Hypoglycemia and diabetes: a report of a work group of the American Diabetes Association and The Endocrine Society. *Diabetes Care* 36:1384–1395, 2013

[2]U.K. Hypoglycaemia Study Group: Risk of hypoglycaemia in types 1 and 2 diabetes: effects of treatment modalities and their duration. *Diabetologia* 50:1140–1147, 2007

[3]Sherr J, Xing D, Ruedy KJ, Beck RW, Kollman C, Buckingham B, White NH, Fox L, Tsalikian E, Weinzimer S, Arbelaez AM, Tamborlane WV; Diabetes in Children Network: Lack of association between residual insulin production and glucagon response to hypoglycemia in youth with short duration of type 1 diabetes. *Diabetes Care* 36:1470–1476, 2013

[4]Unger J: Uncovering undetected hypoglycemic events. *Diabetes Metab Syndr Obes* 5:57–74, 2012

[5]Leese GP, Wang J, Broomhall J, Kelly P, Marsden A, Morrison W, Frier BM, Morris AD; DARTS/MEMO Collaboration: Frequency of severe hypoglycemia requiring emergency treatment in type 1 and type 2 diabetes: a population-based study of health service resource use. *Diabetes Care* 26:1176–1180, 2003

[6]Zoungas, S, Patel A, Chalmers J, de Galan BE, Li Q, Billot L, Woodward M, Ninomiya T, Neal B, MacMahon S, Grobbee DE, Kengne AP, Marre M, Heller S; ADVANCE Collaborative Group: Severe hypoglycemia and risks of vascular events and death. *N Engl J Med* 263:1410–1418, 2010

[7]Turchin A, Matheny ME, Shubina M, Scanlon JV, Greenwood B, Pendergrass ML: Hypoglycemia and clinical outcomes in patients with diabetes hospitalized in the general ward. *Diabetes Care* 32:1153–1157, 2009

[8]McNay EC, Cotero VE: Mini-review: impact of recurrent hypoglycemia on cognitive and brain function. *Physiol Behav* 100:234–238, 2010

[9]Unger J, Parkin C: Hypoglycemia in insulin-treated diabetes: a case for increased vigilance. *Postgrad Med* 123:81–91, 2011

[10]Whitmer RA, Karter AJ, Yaffe K, Quesenberry CP Jr., Selby JV: Hypoglycemic episodes and risk of dementia in older patients with type 2 diabetes mellitus. *JAMA* 301:1565–1572, 2009

[11]Schopman JE, Geddes J, Frier BM: Frequency of symptomatic and asymptomatic hypoglycaemia in type 1 diabetes: effect of impaired awareness of hypoglycaemia. *Diabet Med* 28:352–355, 2011

[12]White NH, Skor DA, Cryer PE, Levandoski LA, Bier DM, Santiago JV: Identification of type 1 diabetic patients at increased risk for hypoglycemia during intensive therapy. *N Engl J Med* 308:485–491, 1983

[13]Cryer PE: Diverse causes of hypoglycemia-associated autonomic failure in diabetes. *N Engl J Med* 350:2272–2279, 2004

[14]Zhang Y, Wieffer H, Modha R, Balar B, Pollack M, Krishnarajah G: The burden of hypoglycemia in type 2 diabetes: a systematic review of patient and economic perspectives. *J Clin Outcomes Manag* 17:547–557, 2010

[15]Lassmann-Vague V: Hypoglycemia in elderly diabetic patients. *Diabetes Metab* 31 (Suppl. 1):5S53–5S57, 2005

[16]Stepka M, Rogola H, Czyzyk A: Hypoglycemia: a major problem in the management of diabetes in elderly. *Aging (Milano)* 5:117–121, 1993

[17]Shorr RI, Ray WA, Daugherty JR, Griffin MR: Incidence of risk factors for serious hypoglycemia in older persons using insulin or sulfonylureas. *Arch Intern Med* 157:1681–1686, 1997

[18]Meneilly GS, Cheung E, Tuokko H: Counterregulatory hormone responses to hypoglycemia in the elderly patient with diabetes. *Diabetes* 43:403–410, 1994

[19]Seltzer HS: Drug-induced hypoglycemia: a review based on 473 cases. *Diabetes* 21:955–966, 1972

[20]Yogev Y, Ben-Haroush A, Chen R, Rosenn B, Hod M, Langer O: Diurnal glycemic profile in obese and normal weight non-diabetic pregnant women. *Am J Obstet Gynecol* 191:949–953, 2004

[21]Nielsen LR, Pedersen-Bjergaard U, Thorsteinsson B, Johansen M, Damm P, Mathiesen ER: Hypoglycemia in pregnant women with type 1 diabetes: predictors and role of metabolic control. *Diabetes Care* 31:9–14, 2008

[22]Ringholm L, Pedersen-Bjergaard U, Thorsteinsson B, Damm P, Mathiesen ER: Hypoglycemia during pregnancy in women with type 1 diabetes. *Diabet Med* 29:558–566, 2012

[23]Juvenile Diabetes Research Foundation Continuous Glucose Monitoring Study Group, Bode B, Beck RW, Xing D, Gilliam L, Hirsch I, Kollman C, Laffel L, Ruedy KJ, Tamborlane WV, Weinzimer S, Wolpert H: Sustained benefit of continuous glucose monitoring on A1C, glucose profiles, and hypoglycemia in adults with type 1 diabetes. *Diabetes Care* 32:2047–2049, 2009

[24]Worm D, Nielsen LR, Mathiesen ER, Nørgaard K: Continuous glucose monitoring system with an alarm: a tool to reduce hypoglycemic episodes in pregnancy with diabetes. *Diabetes Care* 29:2759–2760, 2006

[25]Middleton P, Crowther CA, Simmonds L: Different intensities of glycaemic control for pregnant women with pre-existing diabetes. *Cochrane Database Syst Rev* 15:8, 2012, CD008540 (doi: 10.1002/14651858.CD008540. pub3)

[26]ECRI: Diabetes and Commercial Motor Vehicle Safety (Federal Motor Carrier Safety Administration). June 2011 Update. Plymouth Meeting, Pa., ECRI, 2011

[27]Jerome L, Habinski L, Segal A: Attention deficit/hyperactivity disorder (ADHD) and driving risk: a review of the literature and a methodological critique. *Curr Psychiatry Rep* 8:416–426, 2006

[28]Tregear S, Reston J, Schoelles K, Phillips B: Obstructive sleep apnea and risk of motor vehicle crash: systematic review and

meta-analysis. *J Clin Sleep Med* 5:573–581, 2009

²⁹Watson WA, Currie T, Lemon JS, Gold AE: Driving and insulin-treated diabetes: who knows the rules and recommendations? *Pract Diabetes Int* 24:201–206, 2004

³⁰Harsch IA, Stocker S, Radespiel-Tröger M, Hahn EG, Konturek PC, Ficker JH, Lohmann T: Traffic hypoglycaemias and accidents in patients with diabetes mellitus treated with different antidiabetic regimens. *J Intern Med* 252:352–360, 2002

³¹American Diabetes Association: Diabetes and driving [Position Statement]. *Diabetes Care* 35 (Suppl. 1):S81–S86, 2012

³²Cox DJ, Kovatchev BP, Gonder-Frederick LA: Type 1 diabetic drivers with and without a history of recurrent hypoglycemia-related mishaps: physiologic and performance differences during euglycemia and the induction of hypoglycemia. *Diabetes Care* 33:2430–2435, 2010

³³Campbell LK, Gonder-Frederick LA, Broshek DK, Kovatchev BP, Anderson S, Clarke WL, Cox DJ: Neurocognitive differences between drivers with type 1 diabetes with and without a recent history of recurrent driving mishaps. *Int J Diabetes Mellit* 2:73–77, 2010

³⁴Wright RJ, Frier BM, Deary IJ: Effects of acute insulin-induced hypoglycemia on spatial abilities in adults with type 1 diabetes. *Diabetes Care* 32:1503–1506, 2009

³⁵Cheyne EH, Sherwin RS, Lunt MJ, Cavan DA, Thomas PW, Kerr D: Influence of alcohol on cognitive performance during mild hypoglycaemia: implications for type 1 diabetes. *Diabet Med* 21:230–237, 2004

³⁶Norris SL, Lau J, Smith SJ, Schmid CH, Engelgau MM: Self-management education for adults with type 2 diabetes: a meta-analysis of the effect on glycemic control. *Diabetes Care* 25:1159–1171, 2002

³⁷Unger J: Insulin pumping and use of continuous glucose sensors in primary care. In Unger J: *Diabetes Management in Primary Care*. 2nd ed. Philadelphia, Pa., Lippincott, Williams, and Wilkins, 2012, p. 491–547

³⁸Unger J: Diagnosis and management of T2DM. In Unger J: *Diabetes Management in Primary Care*. 2nd ed. Philadelphia, Pa., Lippincott, Williams, and Wilkins, 2012, p. 323–412

³⁹Unger J: Type 1 diabetes in adults. In Unger J: *Diabetes Management in Primary Care*. 2nd ed. Philadelphia, Pa., Lippincott, Williams, and Wilkins, 2012, p. 413–452

⁴⁰Unger J: Lifestyle interventions for patients with diabetes. In Unger J: *Diabetes Management in Primary Care*. 2nd ed. Philadelphia, Pa., Lippincott, Williams, and Wilkins, 2012, p. 62–112

⁴¹Rodbard HW, Schnell O, Unger J, Rees C, Amstutz L, Parkin CG, Jelsovsky Z, Wegmann N, Axel-Schweitzer M, Wagner RS: Use of an automated decision support tool optimizes clinicians ability to interpret and appropriately respond to structured self-monitoring of blood glucose data. *Diabetes Care* 35:693–698, 2012

⁴²Unger J: Prevention, diagnosis, and treatment of microvascular complications: Part 2: diabetic nephropathy and diabetic retinopathy. In Unger J: *Diabetes Management in Primary Care*. 2nd ed. Philadelphia, Pa., Lippincott, Williams, and Wilkins, 2012, p. 185–216

⁴³Zander J, Raghu P, Lee H, Molitch M, Glossop V, Smallwood K, Emanuele MA, Munoz C, Baldwin D: Initial insulin doses should be decreased in hospitalized patients with renal insufficiency and type 2 diabetes. Presented at the American Diabetes Association 71st Annual Meeting and Scientific Sessions. San Diego, Calif., 24–28 June 2011 (1081-P)

⁴⁴Jones TW, Porter P, Sherwin RS, Davis EA, O'Leary P, Frazer F, Byrne G, Stick S, Tamborlane WV: Decreased epinephrine response to hypoglycemia during sleep. *N Engl J Med* 338:1657–1662, 1998

⁴⁵Garcia-Compean D, Jaquez-Quintana JO, Gonzalez-Gonzalez JA, Maldonado-Garza H: Liver cirrhosis and diabetes: risk factors, pathophysiology, clinical implications and management. *World J Gastroenterol* 15:280–288, 2009

⁴⁶Bruttomesso D, Farret A, Costa S, Marescotti MC, Vettore M, Avogaro A, Tiengo A, Dalla Man C, Place J, Facchinetti A, Guerra S, Magni L, De Nicolao G, Cobelli C, Renard E, Maran A: Closed-loop artificial pancreas using subcutaneous glucose sensing and insulin deliver and a model predictive control algorithm: preliminary studies in Padova and Montepellier. *J Diabetes Sci Technol* 3:1014–1021, 2009

Jeff Unger, MD, is director of the Catalina Research Institute in Chino, Calif.

Nutrition Therapy Recommendations for the Management of Adults With Diabetes

Alison B. Evert, ms, rd, cde[1]
Jackie L. Boucher, ms, rd, ld, cde[2]
Marjorie Cypress, phd, c-anp, cde[3]
Stephanie A. Dunbar, mph, rd[4]
Marion J. Franz, ms, rd, cde[5]
Elizabeth J. Mayer-Davis, phd, rd[6]

Joshua J. Neumiller, pharmd, cde, cgp, fascp[7]
Robin Nwankwo, mph, rd, cde[8]
Cassandra L. Verdi, mph, rd[4]
Patti Urbanski, med, rd, ld, cde[9]
William S. Yancy Jr., md, mhsc[10]

A healthful eating pattern, regular physical activity, and often pharmacotherapy are key components of diabetes management. For many individuals with diabetes, the most challenging part of the treatment plan is determining what to eat. It is the position of the American Diabetes Association (ADA) that there is not a "one-size-fits-all" eating pattern for individuals with diabetes. The ADA also recognizes the integral role of nutrition therapy in overall diabetes management and has historically recommended that each person with diabetes be actively engaged in self-management, education, and treatment planning with his or her health care provider, which includes the collaborative development of an individualized eating plan (1,2). Therefore, it is important that all members of the health care team be knowledgeable about diabetes nutrition therapy and support its implementation.

This position statement on nutrition therapy for individuals living with diabetes replaces previous position statements, the last of which was published in 2008 (3). Unless otherwise noted, research reviewed was limited to those studies conducted in adults diagnosed with type 1 or type 2 diabetes. Nutrition therapy for the prevention of type 2 diabetes and for the

management of diabetes complications and gestational diabetes mellitus is not addressed in this review.

A grading system, developed by the ADA and modeled after existing methods, was utilized to clarify and codify the evidence that forms the basis for the recommendations (1) (Table 1). The level of evidence that supports each recommendation is listed after the recommendation using the letters A, B, C, or E. A table linking recommendations to evidence can be reviewed at http://professional.diabetes.org/nutrition. Members of the Nutrition Recommendations Writing Group Committee disclosed all potential financial conflicts of interest with industry. These disclosures were discussed at the onset of the position statement development process. Members of this committee, their employers, and their disclosed conflicts of interest are listed in the ACKNOWLEDGMENTS. The ADA uses general revenues to fund development of its position statements and does not rely on industry support for these purposes.

Goals of nutrition therapy that apply to adults with diabetes

■ To promote and support healthful eating patterns, emphasizing a variety of nutrient-dense foods in appropriate portion sizes,

in order to improve overall health and specifically to:

- Attain individualized glycemic, blood pressure, and lipid goals. General recommended goals from the ADA for these markers are as follows:*
  o A1C <7%.
  o Blood pressure <140/80 mmHg.
  o LDL cholesterol <100 mg/dL; triglycerides <150 mg/dL; HDL cholesterol >40 mg/dL for men; HDL cholesterol >50 mg/dL for women.
- Achieve and maintain body weight goals.
- Delay or prevent complications of diabetes.

■ To address individual nutrition needs based on personal and cultural preferences, health literacy and numeracy, access to healthful food choices, willingness and ability to make behavioral changes, as well as barriers to change.
■ To maintain the pleasure of eating by providing positive messages about food choices while limiting food choices only when indicated by scientific evidence.
■ To provide the individual with diabetes with practical tools for day-to-day meal planning rather than focusing on individual macronutrients, micronutrients, or single foods.

*A1C, blood pressure, and cholesterol goals may need to be adjusted for the individual based on age, duration of diabetes, health history, and other present health conditions. Further recommendations for individualization of goals can be found in the ADA Standards of Medical Care in Diabetes (1).

Metabolic control can be considered the cornerstone of diabetes management. Achieving A1C goals decreases the risk for microvascular complications (4,5) and may also be important for cardiovascular disease (CVD) risk reduction, particularly in newly diagnosed patients (6–8). In addition, achieving blood pressure and lipid goals can help reduce risk for CVD events (9,10). Carbohydrate intake has a direct

From the [1]University of Washington Medical Center, Seattle, Washington; the [2]Minneapolis Heart Institute Foundation, Minneapolis, Minnesota; the [3]Department of Endocrinology, ABQ Health Partners, Albuquerque, New Mexico; the [4]American Diabetes Association, Alexandria, Virginia; [5]Nutrition Concepts by Franz, Minneapolis, Minnesota; the [6]Gillings School of Global Public Health and School of Medicine, University of North Carolina at Chapel Hill, Chapel Hill, North Carolina; the [7]Department of Pharmacotherapy, Washington State University, Spokane, Washington; the [8]University of Michigan Medical School and the Center for Preventive Medicine, Ann Arbor, Michigan; [9]pbu consulting, llc., Cloquet, Minnesota; and the [10]Duke University School of Medicine, Durham, North Carolina.
Corresponding authors: Alison B. Evert, atevert@u.washington.edu, and Jackie L. Boucher, jboucher@mhif.org.
DOI: 10.2337/dc13-2042

Table 1—*Nutrition therapy recommendations*

Topic	Recommendation	Evidence rating
Effectiveness of nutrition therapy	Nutrition therapy is recommended for all people with type 1 and type 2 diabetes as an effective component of the overall treatment plan.	A
	Individuals who have diabetes should receive individualized MNT as needed to achieve treatment goals, preferably provided by an RD familiar with the components of diabetes MNT.	A
	o For individuals with type 1 diabetes, participation in an intensive flexible insulin therapy education program using the carbohydrate counting meal planning approach can result in improved glycemic control.	A
	o For individuals using fixed daily insulin doses, consistent carbohydrate intake with respect to time and amount can result in improved glycemic control and reduce risk for hypoglycemia.	B
	o A simple diabetes meal planning approach such as portion control or healthful food choices may be better suited to individuals with type 2 diabetes identified with health and numeracy literacy concerns. This may also be an effective meal planning strategy for older adults.	C
	People with diabetes should receive DSME according to national standards and diabetes self-management support when their diabetes is diagnosed and as needed thereafter.	B
	Because diabetes nutrition therapy can result in cost savings (B) and improved outcomes such as reduction in A1C (A), nutrition therapy should be adequately reimbursed by insurance and other payers. (E)	B, A, E
Energy balance	For overweight or obese adults with type 2 diabetes, reducing energy intake while maintaining a healthful eating pattern is recommended to promote weight loss.	A
	Modest weight loss may provide clinical benefits (improved glycemia, blood pressure, and/or lipids) in some individuals with diabetes, especially those early in the disease process. To achieve modest weight loss, intensive lifestyle interventions (counseling about nutrition therapy, physical activity, and behavior change) with ongoing support are recommended.	A
Optimal mix of macronutrients	Evidence suggests that there is not an ideal percentage of calories from carbohydrate, protein, and fat for all people with diabetes (B); therefore, macronutrient distribution should be based on individualized assessment of current eating patterns, preferences, and metabolic goals. (E)	B, E
Eating patterns	A variety of eating patterns (combinations of different foods or food groups) are acceptable for the management of diabetes. Personal preferences (e.g., tradition, culture, religion, health beliefs and goals, economics) and metabolic goals should be considered when recommending one eating pattern over another.	E
Carbohydrates	Evidence is inconclusive for an ideal amount of carbohydrate intake for people with diabetes. Therefore, collaborative goals should be developed with the individual with diabetes.	C
	The amount of carbohydrates and available insulin may be the most important factor influencing glycemic response after eating and should be considered when developing the eating plan.	A
	Monitoring carbohydrate intake, whether by carbohydrate counting or experience-based estimation remains a key strategy in achieving glycemic control.	B
	For good health, carbohydrate intake from vegetables, fruits, whole grains, legumes, and dairy products should be advised over intake from other carbohydrate sources, especially those that contain added fats, sugars, or sodium.	B
Glycemic index and glycemic load	Substituting low–glycemic load foods for higher–glycemic load foods may modestly improve glycemic control.	C
Dietary fiber and whole grains	People with diabetes should consume at least the amount of fiber and whole grains recommended for the general public.	C
Substitution of sucrose for starch	While substituting sucrose-containing foods for isocaloric amounts of other carbohydrates may have similar blood glucose effects, consumption should be minimized to avoid displacing nutrient-dense food choices.	A
Fructose	Fructose consumed as "free fructose" (i.e., naturally occurring in foods such as fruit) may result in better glycemic control compared with isocaloric intake of sucrose or starch (B), and free fructose is not likely to have detrimental effects on triglycerides as long as intake is not excessive ($>$12% energy). (C)	B, C
	People with diabetes should limit or avoid intake of SSBs (from any caloric sweetener including high fructose corn syrup and sucrose) to reduce risk for weight gain and worsening of cardiometabolic risk profile.	B

Table 1—*Continued*

Topic	Recommendation	Evidence rating
NNSs and hypocaloric sweeteners	Use of NNSs has the potential to reduce overall calorie and carbohydrate intake if substituted for caloric sweeteners without compensation by intake of additional calories from other food sources.	B
Protein	For people with diabetes and no evidence of diabetic kidney disease, evidence is inconclusive to recommend an ideal amount of protein intake for optimizing glycemic control or improving one or more CVD risk measures; therefore, goals should be individualized.	C
	For people with diabetes and diabetic kidney disease (either micro- or macroalbuminuria), reducing the amount of dietary protein below usual intake is not recommended because it does not alter glycemic measures, cardiovascular risk measures, or the course of GFR decline.	A
	In individuals with type 2 diabetes, ingested protein appears to increase insulin response without increasing plasma glucose concentrations. Therefore, carbohydrate sources high in protein should not be used to treat or prevent hypoglycemia.	B
Total fat	Evidence is inconclusive for an ideal amount of total fat intake for people with diabetes; therefore, goals should be individualized (C); fat quality appears to be far more important than quantity. (B)	C, B
MUFAs/PUFAs	In people with type 2 diabetes, a Mediterranean-style, MUFA-rich eating pattern may benefit glycemic control and CVD risk factors and can therefore be recommended as an effective alternative to a lower-fat, higher-carbohydrate eating pattern.	B
Omega-3 fatty acids	Evidence does not support recommending omega-3 (EPA and DHA) supplements for people with diabetes for the prevention or treatment of cardiovascular events.	A
	As recommended for the general public, an increase in foods containing long-chain omega-3 fatty acids (EPA and DHA) (from fatty fish) and omega-3 linolenic acid (ALA) is recommended for individuals with diabetes because of their beneficial effects on lipoproteins, prevention of heart disease, and associations with positive health outcomes in observational studies.	B
	The recommendation for the general public to eat fish (particularly fatty fish) at least two times (two servings) per week is also appropriate for people with diabetes.	B
Saturated fat, dietary cholesterol, and *trans* fat	The amount of dietary saturated fat, cholesterol, and *trans* fat recommended for people with diabetes is the same as that recommended for the general population.	C
Plant stanols and sterols	Individuals with diabetes and dyslipidemia may be able to modestly reduce total and LDL cholesterol by consuming 1.6–3 g/day of plant stanols or sterols typically found in enriched foods.	C
Micronutrients and herbal supplements	There is no clear evidence of benefit from vitamin or mineral supplementation in people with diabetes who do not have underlying deficiencies.	C
	o Routine supplementation with antioxidants, such as vitamins E and C and carotene, is not advised because of lack of evidence of efficacy and concern related to long-term safety.	A
	o There is insufficient evidence to support the routine use of micronutrients such as chromium, magnesium, and vitamin D to improve glycemic control in people with diabetes.	C
	o There is insufficient evidence to support the use of cinnamon or other herbs/supplements for the treatment of diabetes.	C
	It is recommended that individualized meal planning include optimization of food choices to meet recommended dietary allowance/dietary reference intake for all micronutrients.	E
Alcohol	If adults with diabetes choose to drink alcohol, they should be advised to do so in moderation (one drink per day or less for adult women and two drinks per day or less for adult men).	E
	Alcohol consumption may place people with diabetes at increased risk for delayed hypoglycemia, especially if taking insulin or insulin secretagogues. Education and awareness regarding the recognition and management of delayed hypoglycemia is warranted.	C
Sodium	The recommendation for the general population to reduce sodium to less than 2,300 mg/day is also appropriate for people with diabetes.	B
	For individuals with both diabetes and hypertension, further reduction in sodium intake should be individualized.	B

effect on postprandial glucose levels in people with diabetes and is the primary macronutrient of concern in glycemic management (11). In addition, an individual's food choices have a direct effect on energy balance and, therefore, on body weight, and food choices can also impact blood pressure and lipid levels. Through the collaborative development of individualized nutrition interventions and ongoing support of behavior changes, health care professionals can facilitate the achievement of their patients'/clients' health goals (11–13).

Diabetes nutrition

therapy—Ideally, the individual with diabetes should be referred to a registered dietitian (RD) (or a similarly credentialed nutrition professional if outside of the U.S.) for nutrition therapy at—or soon after—diagnosis (11,14) and for ongoing follow-up. Another option for many people is referral to a comprehensive diabetes self-management education (DSME) program that includes instruction on nutrition therapy. Unfortunately, a large percentage of people with diabetes do not receive any structured diabetes education and/or nutrition therapy (15,16). National data indicate that about half of the people with diabetes report receiving some type of diabetes education (17) and even fewer see an RD. In one study of 18,404 patients with diabetes, only 9.1% had at least one nutrition visit within a 9-year period (18). Many people with diabetes, as well as their health care provider(s), are not aware that these services are available to them. Therefore this position statement offers evidence-based nutrition recommendations for all health care professionals to use.

In 1999, the Institute of Medicine (IOM) released a report concluding that evidence demonstrates that medical nutrition therapy (MNT) can improve clinical outcomes while possibly decreasing the cost to Medicare of managing diabetes (19). The IOM recommended that individualized MNT, provided by an RD upon physician referral, be a covered Medicare benefit as part of the multidisciplinary approach to diabetes care (19). MNT is an evidence-based application of the Nutrition Care Process provided by the RD and is the legal definition of nutrition counseling by an RD in the U.S. (20). The IOM also defines nutrition therapy, which has a broader definition than MNT (19). Nutrition therapy is the treatment of a disease or condition through the modification of nutrient or whole-food intake. The

definition does not specify that nutrition therapy must be provided by an RD (19). However, both MNT and nutrition therapy should involve a nutrition assessment, nutrition diagnosis, nutrition interventions (e.g., education and counseling), and nutrition monitoring and evaluation with ongoing follow-up to support long-term lifestyle changes, evaluate outcomes, and modify interventions as needed (20).

Nutrition therapy studies included in this position statement use a wide assortment of nutrition professionals as well as registered and advanced practice nurses or physicians. Health care professionals administering nutrition interventions in studies conducted outside the U.S. did not provide MNT as it is legally defined. As a result, the decision was made to use the term "nutrition therapy" rather than "MNT" in this article, in an effort to be more inclusive of the range of health professionals providing nutrition interventions and to recognize the broad definition of nutrition therapy. However, the unique academic preparation, training, skills, and expertise of the RD make him/her the preferred member of the health care team to provide diabetes MNT (Table 2).

Diabetes self-management
education/support—In addition

to diabetes MNT provided by an RD, DSME and diabetes self-management support (DSMS) are critical elements of care for all people with diabetes and are necessary to improve outcomes in a disease that is largely self-managed (21–26). The National Standards for Diabetes Self-Management Education and Support recognize the importance of nutrition as one of the core curriculum topics taught in comprehensive programs. The American Association of Diabetes Educators also recognizes the importance of healthful eating as a core self-care behavior (27). For more information, refer to the ADA's National Standards for Diabetes Self-Management Education and Support (21).

Effectiveness of nutrition therapy
- Nutrition therapy is recommended for all people with type 1 and type 2 diabetes as an effective component of the overall treatment plan. (A)
- Individuals who have diabetes should receive individualized MNT as needed to achieve treatment goals, preferably provided by an RD familiar with the components of diabetes MNT. (A)

Table 2—*Academy of Nutrition and Dietetics Evidence-Based Nutrition Practice Guidelines*

Academy of Nutrition and Dietetics Evidence-Based Nutrition Practice Guidelines recommend the following structure for the implementation of MNT for adults with diabetes (11)

- A series of 3–4 encounters with an RD lasting from 45–90 min.
- The series of encounters should begin at diagnosis of diabetes or at first referral to an RD for MNT for diabetes and should be completed within 3–6 months.
- The RD should determine whether additional MNT encounters are needed.
- At least 1 follow-up encounter is recommended annually to reinforce lifestyle changes and to evaluate and monitor outcomes that indicate the need for changes in MNT or medication(s); an RD should determine whether additional MNT encounters are needed.

  o For individuals with type 1 diabetes, participation in an intensive flexible insulin therapy education program using the carbohydrate counting meal planning approach can result in improved glycemic control. (A)
  o For individuals using fixed daily insulin doses, consistent carbohydrate intake with respect to time and amount can result in improved glycemic control and reduce the risk for hypoglycemia. (B)
  o A simple diabetes meal planning approach such as portion control or healthful food choices may be better suited to individuals with type 2 diabetes identified with health and numeracy literacy concerns. This may also be an effective meal planning strategy for older adults. (C)
- People with diabetes should receive DSME according to national standards and DSMS when their diabetes is diagnosed and as needed thereafter. (B)
- Because diabetes nutrition therapy can result in cost savings (B) and improved outcomes such as reduction in A1C (A), nutrition therapy should be adequately reimbursed by insurance and other payers. (E)

The common coexistence of hyperlipidemia and hypertension in people with diabetes requires monitoring of metabolic parameters (e.g., glucose, lipids, blood pressure, body weight, renal function) to ensure successful health outcomes (28). Nutrition therapy that includes the development of an eating pattern designed to lower glucose, blood pressure, and alter lipid profiles is important in the management of diabetes as well as lowering the risk of CVD, coronary heart disease, and stroke. Successful approaches should also include regular physical activity and behavioral interventions to help sustain improved lifestyles (11).

Findings from randomized controlled trials (RCTs) and from systematic and Cochrane reviews demonstrate the effectiveness of nutrition therapy for improving glycemic control and various markers of cardiovascular and hypertension risk (13,14,29–46). In the general population, MNT provided by an RD to individuals with an abnormal lipid profile has been shown to reduce daily fat (5–8%), saturated fat (2–4%), and energy intake (232–710 kcal/day), and lower triglycerides (11–31%), LDL cholesterol (7–22%), and total cholesterol (7–21%) levels (47).

Effective nutrition therapy interventions may be a component of a comprehensive group diabetes education program or an individualized session (14,29–38,40–42,44,45). Reported A1C reductions are similar or greater than what would be expected with treatment with currently available pharmacologic treatments for diabetes. The documented decreases in A1C observed in these studies are type 1 diabetes: −0.3 to −1% (13,39,43,48) and type 2 diabetes: −0.5 to −2% (5,14,29–38,40–42,44,45,49).

Due to the progressive nature of type 2 diabetes, nutrition and physical activity interventions alone (i.e., without pharmacotherapy) are generally not adequately effective in maintaining persistent glycemic control over time for many individuals. However, after pharmacotherapy is initiated, nutrition therapy continues to be an important component of the overall treatment plan (2). For individuals with type 1 diabetes using multiple daily injections or continuous subcutaneous insulin infusion, a primary focus for nutrition therapy should be on how to adjust insulin doses based on planned carbohydrate intake (13,39,43,50–53). For individuals using fixed daily insulin doses, carbohydrate intake on a day-to-day basis should be consistent with respect to time and amount (54,55). Intensive insulin management education programs that include nutrition therapy have been shown

to reduce A1C (13). Retrospective studies reveal durable A1C reductions with these types of programs (51,56) and significant improvements in quality of life (57) over time. Finally, nutritional approaches for reducing CVD risk, including optimizing serum lipids and blood pressure, can effectively reduce CVD events and mortality (1).

Energy balance
- For overweight or obese adults with type 2 diabetes, reducing energy intake while maintaining a healthful eating pattern is recommended to promote weight loss. (A)
- Modest weight loss may provide clinical benefits (improved glycemia, blood pressure, and/or lipids) in some individuals with diabetes, especially those early in the disease process. To achieve modest weight loss, intensive lifestyle interventions (counseling about nutrition therapy, physical activity, and behavior change) with ongoing support are recommended. (A)

More than three out of every four adults with diabetes are at least overweight (17), and nearly half of individuals with diabetes are obese (58). Because of the relationship between body weight (i.e., adiposity) and insulin resistance, weight loss has long been a recommended strategy for overweight or obese adults with diabetes (1). Prevention of weight gain is equally important. Long-term reduction of adiposity is difficult for most people to achieve, and even harder for individuals with diabetes to achieve given the impact of some medications used to improve glycemic control (e.g., insulin, insulin secretagogues, and thiazolidinediones) (59,60). A number of factors may be responsible for increasing adiposity in people with diabetes, including a reduction in glycosuria and thus retention of calories otherwise lost as an effect of therapeutic intervention, changes in food intake, or changes in energy expenditure (61–64). If adiposity is a concern, medications that are weight neutral or weight reducing (e.g., metformin, incretin-based therapies, sodium glucose co-transporter 2 [SGLT-2] inhibitors) could be considered. Several intensive DSME and nutrition intervention studies show that glycemic control can be achieved while maintaining weight or even reducing weight when appropriate lifestyle counseling is provided (14,31,35,41,42,44,45,50,65,66).

In interventional studies lasting 12 months or longer and targeting individuals with type 2 diabetes to reduce excess body weight (35,67–75), modest weight losses were achieved ranging from 1.9 to 8.4 kg. In the Look AHEAD trial, at study end (~10 years), the mean weight loss from baseline was 6% in the intervention group and 3.5% in the control group (76,77). Studies designed to reduce excess body weight have used a variety of energy-restricted eating patterns with various macronutrient intakes and occasionally included a physical activity component and ongoing follow-up support. Studies achieving the greatest weight losses, 6.2 kg and 8.4 kg, respectively, included the Mediterranean-style eating pattern (72) and a study testing a comprehensive weight loss program that involved diet (including meal replacements) and physical activity (76). In the studies reviewed, improvements in A1C were noted to persist at 12 months in eight intervention groups within five studies (67,69,72,73,76); however, in one of the studies including data at 18 months, the A1C improvement was not maintained (69). The Mediterranean-style eating pattern reported the largest improvement of A1C at 1 year (−1.2%) (72), and the Look AHEAD study intensive lifestyle intervention reported the next largest improvement (−0.64%) (76). One of these studies included only individuals with newly diagnosed diabetes (72), and the other included predominantly individuals with diabetes early in the disease process (<30% were on insulin) (76). Significant improvements in A1C at 1 year were also reported in other studies using energy-restricted eating plans; these studies used meal replacements (67), or low-fat (72)/high-protein (73), or high-carbohydrate eating patterns (73). Not all weight loss interventions reviewed led to improvements in A1C at 1 year (35,68,70,71,74,75), although these studies tended to achieve less weight loss.

Among the studies reviewed, the most consistently reported significant changes of reducing excess body weight on cardiovascular risk factors were an increase in HDL cholesterol (67,72,73,75–77), a decrease in triglycerides (72,73,76–78), and a decrease in blood pressure (67,70,72,75–77). Despite some improvements in cardiovascular risk factors, the Look AHEAD trial failed to demonstrate reduction in CVD events among individuals randomized to an intensive lifestyle intervention for sustained weight loss (77). Of note, however, those randomized to the intervention experienced statistically significant weight loss, requiring less medication for glycemic control and management of CVD risk factors, and experienced several additional health benefits (e.g., reduced sleep apnea, depression, and urinary incontinence and improved health-related quality of life) (79–82).

Intensive lifestyle programs (ongoing, with frequent follow-up) are required to achieve significant reductions in excess body weight and improvements in A1C, blood pressure, and lipids (76,83). Weight loss appears to be most beneficial for individuals with diabetes early in the disease process (72,76,83). In the Look AHEAD study, participants with early-stage diabetes (shortest duration, not treated with insulin, good baseline glycemic control) received the most health benefits with a small percentage of individuals achieving partial or complete diabetes remission (84). It is unclear if the benefits result from the reduction in excess weight or the energy restriction or both. Long-term maintenance of weight, following weight reduction, is possible, but research suggests it requires an intensive program with long-term support. Many individuals do regain a portion of their initial weight loss (77,85). Factors contributing to the individual's inability to retain maximal weight loss include socioeconomic status, an unsupportive environment, and physiological changes (e.g., compensatory changes in circulating hormones that encourage weight regain after weight loss is achieved) (86).

The optimal macronutrient intake to support reduction in excess body weight has not been established. Thus, the current state of the literature does not support one particular nutrition therapy approach to reduce excess weight, but rather a spectrum of eating patterns that result in reduced energy intake. A weight loss of >6 kg (approximately a 7–8.5% loss of initial body weight), regular physical activity, and frequent contact with RDs appear important for consistent beneficial effects of weight loss interventions (85). In the Look AHEAD study, weight loss strategies associated with lower BMI in overweight or obese individuals with type 2 diabetes included weekly self-weighing, regular consumption of breakfast, and reduced intake of fast foods (87). Other successful strategies included increasing physical activity, reducing portion sizes, using meal replacements (as appropriate), and encouraging individuals with diabetes to eat those foods with the greatest consensus for improving health.

Health professionals should collaborate with individuals with diabetes to integrate lifestyle strategies that prevent weight gain or promote modest, realistic weight loss. The emphases of education and counseling should be on the development of behaviors that support long-term weight loss or weight maintenance with less focus on the outcome of weight loss. Bariatric surgery is recognized as an option for individuals with diabetes who meet the criteria for surgery and is not covered in this review. For recommendations on bariatric surgery, see the ADA Standards of Medical Care (1).

Optimal mix of macronutrients

- Evidence suggests that there is not an ideal percentage of calories from carbohydrate, protein, and fat for all people with diabetes (B); therefore, macronutrient distribution should be based on individualized assessment of current eating patterns, preferences, and metabolic goals. (E)

Although numerous studies have attempted to identify the optimal mix of macronutrients for the meal plans of people with diabetes, a systematic review (88) found that there is no ideal mix that applies broadly and that macronutrient proportions should be individualized. On average, it has been observed that people with diabetes eat about 45% of their calories from carbohydrate, ~36–40% of calories from fat, and the remainder (~16–18%) from protein (89–91). Regardless of the macronutrient mix, total energy intake should be appropriate to weight management goals. Further, individualization of the macronutrient composition will depend on the metabolic status of the individual (e.g., lipid profile, renal function) and/or food preferences. A variety of eating patterns have been shown modestly effective in managing diabetes including Mediterranean-style, Dietary Approaches to Stop Hypertension (DASH) style, plant-based (vegan or vegetarian), lower-fat, and lower-carbohydrate patterns (36,46,72,92,93).

Eating patterns

- A variety of eating patterns (combinations of different foods or food groups) are acceptable for the management of diabetes. Personal preferences (e.g., tradition, culture, religion, health beliefs and goals, economics) and metabolic goals should be considered when recommending one eating pattern over another. (E)

Eating patterns, also called dietary patterns, is a term used to describe combinations of different foods or food groups that characterize relationships between nutrition and health promotion and disease prevention (94). Individuals eat combinations of foods, not single nutrients, and thus it is important to study diet and disease relationships (95). Factors impacting eating patterns include, but are not limited to, food access/availability of healthful foods, tradition, cultural food systems, health beliefs, knowledge of foods that promote health and prevent disease, and economics/resources to buy health-promoting foods (95).

Eating patterns have also evolved over time to include patterns of food intake among specific populations to eating patterns prescribed to improve health. Patterns naturally occurring within populations based on food availability, culture, or tradition and those prescribed to prevent or manage health conditions are important to research. Eating patterns studied among individuals with type 1 or type 2 diabetes were reviewed to evaluate their impact on diabetes nutrition goals. The following eating patterns (Table 3) were reviewed: Mediterranean, vegetarian, low fat, low carbohydrate, and DASH.

The Mediterranean-style eating pattern, mostly studied in the Mediterranean region, has been observed to improve cardiovascular risk factors (i.e., lipids, blood pressure, triglycerides) (11,72,88,100) in individuals with diabetes and lower combined end points for CVD events and stroke (83) when supplemented with mixed nuts (including walnuts, almonds, and hazelnuts) or olive oil. Individuals following an energy-restricted Mediterranean-style eating pattern also achieve improvements in glycemic control (88). Given that the studies are mostly in the Mediterranean region, further research is needed to determine if the study results can be generalized to other populations and if similar levels of adherence to the eating pattern can be achieved.

Six vegetarian and low-fat vegan studies (36,93,101–103,131) in individuals with type 2 diabetes were reviewed. Studies ranged in duration from 12 to 74 weeks, and the diets did not consistently improve glycemic control or CVD risk factors except when energy intake was restricted and weight was lost. Diets often did result in weight loss (36,101–103,131). More research on vegan and vegetarian diets is needed to assess diet

Table 3—*Reviewed eating patterns*

Type of eating pattern	Description
Mediterranean style (96)	Includes abundant plant food (fruits, vegetables, breads, other forms of cereals, beans, nuts and seeds); minimally processed, seasonally fresh, and locally grown foods; fresh fruits as the typical daily dessert and concentrated sugars or honey consumed only for special occasions; olive oil as the principal source of dietary lipids; dairy products (mainly cheese and yogurt) consumed in low to moderate amounts; fewer than 4 eggs/week; red meat consumed in low frequency and amounts; and wine consumption in low to moderate amounts generally with meals.
Vegetarian and vegan (97)	The two most common ways of defining vegetarian diets in the research are vegan diets (diets devoid of all flesh foods and animal-derived products) and vegetarian diets (diets devoid of all flesh foods but including egg [ovo] and/or dairy [lacto] products). Features of a vegetarian-eating pattern that may reduce risk of chronic disease include lower intakes of saturated fat and cholesterol and higher intakes of fruits, vegetables, whole grains, nuts, soy products, fiber, and phytochemicals.
Low fat (98)	Emphasizes vegetables, fruits, starches (e.g., breads/crackers, pasta, whole grains, starchy vegetables), lean protein, and low-fat dairy products. Defined as total fat intake <30% of total energy intake and saturated fat intake <10%.
Low carbohydrate (88)	Focuses on eating foods higher in protein (meat, poultry, fish, shellfish, eggs, cheese, nuts and seeds), fats (oils, butter, olives, avocado), and vegetables low in carbohydrate (salad greens, cucumbers, broccoli, summer squash). The amount of carbohydrate allowed varies with most plans allowing fruit (e.g., berries) and higher carbohydrate vegetables; however, sugar-containing foods and grain products such as pasta, rice, and bread are generally avoided. There is no consistent definition of "low" carbohydrate. In research studies, definitions have ranged from very low-carbohydrate diet (21–70 g/day of carbohydrates) to moderately low-carbohydrate diet (30 to <40% of calories from carbohydrates).
DASH (99)	Emphasizes fruits, vegetables, and low-fat dairy products, including whole grains, poultry, fish, and nuts and is reduced in saturated fat, red meat, sweets, and sugar-containing beverages. The most effective DASH diet was also reduced in sodium.

quality given studies often focus more on what is not consumed than what is consumed.

The low-fat eating pattern is one that has often been encouraged as a strategy to lose weight or to improve cardiovascular health within the U.S. In the Look AHEAD trial (77), an energy-reduced low-fat eating pattern was encouraged for weight loss, and individuals achieved moderate success (76). However, in a systematic review (88) and in four studies (70,71,75,103a) and in a meta-analysis (103b) published since the systematic review, lowering total fat intake did not consistently improve glycemic control or CVD risk factors. Benefit from a low-fat eating pattern appears to be more likely when energy intake is also reduced and weight loss occurs (76,77).

For a review of the studies focused on a low-carbohydrate eating pattern, see the CARBOHYDRATES section. Currently there is inadequate evidence in isocaloric comparison recommending a specific amount of carbohydrates for people with diabetes.

In people without diabetes, the DASH eating plan has been shown to help control blood pressure and lower risk for CVD and is frequently recommended as a healthful eating pattern for the general population (104–106). Limited evidence exists on the effects of the DASH eating plan on health outcomes specifically in individuals with diabetes; however, one would expect similar results to other studies using the DASH eating plan. In one small study in people with type 2 diabetes, the DASH eating plan, which included a sodium restriction of 2,300 mg/day, improved A1C, blood pressure, and other cardiovascular risk factors (46). The blood pressure benefits are thought to be due to the total eating pattern, including the reduction in sodium and other foods and nutrients that have been shown to influence blood pressure (99,105).

The evidence suggests that several different macronutrient distributions/eating patterns may lead to improvements in glycemic and/or CVD risk factors (88). There is no "ideal" conclusive eating pattern that is expected to benefit all individuals with diabetes (88). Total energy intake (and thus portion sizes) is an important consideration no matter which eating pattern the individual with diabetes chooses to eat. Because dietary patterns are influenced by food availability, perception of healthfulness of certain foods and by the individual's preferences, culture, religion, knowledge, health beliefs, and access to food and resources (e.g., budget/income) (95), these factors should be considered when individualizing eating pattern recommendations.

Individual macronutrients

Carbohydrates

- Evidence is inconclusive for an ideal amount of carbohydrate intake for people with diabetes. Therefore, collaborative goals should be developed with the individual with diabetes. (C)
- The amount of carbohydrates and available insulin may be the most important factor influencing glycemic response after eating and should be considered when developing the eating plan. (A)
- Monitoring carbohydrate intake, whether by carbohydrate counting or experience-based estimation, remains a key strategy in achieving glycemic control. (B)
- For good health, carbohydrate intake from vegetables, fruits, whole grains, legumes, and dairy products should be advised over intake from other carbohydrate sources, especially those that contain added fats, sugars, or sodium. (B)

Evidence is insufficient to support one specific amount of carbohydrate intake for all people with diabetes. Collaborative goals should be developed with each person with diabetes. Some published studies comparing lower levels of carbohydrate intake (ranging from 21 g daily up to 40% of daily energy intake) to higher carbohydrate intake levels indicated improved markers of glycemic control and insulin sensitivity with lower carbohydrate intakes (92,100,107–111). Four RCTs indicated no significant difference in glycemic markers with a lower-carbohydrate diet compared with higher carbohydrate intake levels (71,112–114). Many of these studies were small, were of short duration, and/or had low retention rates (92,107, 109,110,112,113).

Some studies comparing lower levels of carbohydrate intake to higher carbohydrate intake levels revealed improvements in serum lipid/lipoprotein measures, including improved triglycerides, VLDL triglyceride, and VLDL cholesterol, total cholesterol, and HDL cholesterol levels (71,92,100,107,109,111,112,115). A few studies found no significant difference in lipids and lipoproteins with a lower-carbohydrate diet compared with higher carbohydrate intake levels. It should be noted that these studies had low retention rates, which may lead to loss of statistical power and biased results (110,113,116). In many of the reviewed studies, weight loss occurred, confounding the interpretation of results from manipulation of macronutrient content.

Despite the inconclusive results of the studies evaluating the effect of differing percentages of carbohydrates in people with diabetes, monitoring carbohydrate amounts is a useful strategy for improving postprandial glucose control. Evidence exists that both the quantity and type of carbohydrate in a food influence blood glucose level, and total amount of carbohydrate eaten is the primary predictor of glycemic response (55,114,117–122). In addition, lower A1C occurred in the Diabetes Control and Complications Trial (DCCT) intensive-treatment group and the Dose Adjustment For Normal Eating (DAFNE) trial participants who received nutrition therapy that focused on the adjustment of insulin doses based on variations in carbohydrate intake and physical activity (13,123).

As for the general U.S. population, carbohydrate intake from vegetables, fruits, whole grains, legumes, and milk should be encouraged over other sources of carbohydrates, or sources with added fats, sugars, or sodium, in order to improve overall nutrient intake (105).

Quality of carbohydrates

Glycemic index and glycemic load

- Substituting low–glycemic load foods for higher–glycemic load foods may modestly improve glycemic control. (C)

The ADA recognizes that education about glycemic index and glycemic load occurs during the development of individualized eating plans for people with diabetes. Some organizations specifically recommend use of low–glycemic index diets (124,125). However the literature regarding glycemic index and glycemic load in individuals with diabetes is complex, and it is often difficult to discern the independent effect of fiber compared with that of glycemic index on glycemic control or other outcomes. Further, studies used varying definitions of low and high glycemic index (11,88,126), and glycemic response to a particular food varies among individuals and can also be affected by the overall mixture of foods consumed (11,126).

Some studies did not show improvement with a lower–glycemic index eating pattern; however, several other studies using low–glycemic index eating patterns have demonstrated A1C decreases of −0.2 to −0.5%. However, fiber intake was not consistently controlled, thereby making interpretation of the findings difficult (88,118,119,127). Results on CVD risk measures are mixed with some showing the lowering of total or LDL cholesterol and others showing no significant changes (120).

Dietary fiber and whole grains

- People with diabetes should consume at least the amount of fiber and whole grains recommended for the general public. (C)

Intake of dietary fiber is associated with lower all-cause mortality (128,129) in people with diabetes. Two systematic reviews found little evidence that fiber significantly improves glycemic control (11,88). Studies published since these reviews have shown modest lowering of preprandial glucose (130) and A1C (−0.2 to −0.3%) (119,130) with intakes of >50 g of fiber/day. Most studies on fiber in people with diabetes are of short duration, have a small sample size, and evaluate the combination of high-fiber and low–glycemic index foods, and in some cases weight loss, making it difficult to isolate fiber as the sole determinant of glycemic improvement (119,131–133). Fiber intakes to improve glycemic control, based on existing research, are also unrealistic, requiring fiber intakes of >50 g/day.

Studies examining fiber's effect on CVD risk factors are mixed; however, total fiber intake, especially from natural food sources (vs. supplements), seems to have a beneficial effect on serum cholesterol levels and other CVD risk factors such as blood pressure (11,88,134). Because of the general health benefits of fiber, recommendations for the general public to increase intake to 14 g fiber/1,000 kcals daily or about 25 g/day for adult women and 38 g/day for adult men are encouraged for individuals with diabetes (105).

Research has also compared the benefits of whole grains to fiber. The *Dietary Guidelines for Americans, 2010* defines whole grains as foods containing the entire grain seed (kernel), bran, germ, and endosperm (105). A systematic review (88) concluded that the consumption of whole grains was not associated with improvements in glycemic control in individuals with type 2 diabetes; however, it may have other benefits, such as reductions in systemic inflammation. Data from the Nurses' Health Study examining whole grains and their components (cereal fiber, bran, and germ) in relation to all-cause and CVD-specific mortality among women with type 2 diabetes suggest a potential benefit of whole-grain intake in reducing mortality and CVD (128). As with the general population, individuals with diabetes should consume at least half of all grains as whole grains (105).

Resistant starch and fructans

—Resistant starch is defined as starch physically enclosed within intact cell structures as in some legumes, starch granules as in raw potato, and retrograde amylose from plants modified by plant breeding to increase amylose content. It has been proposed that foods containing resistant starch or high amylose foods such as specially formulated cornstarch may modify postprandial glycemic response, prevent hypoglycemia, and reduce hyperglycemia. However, there are no published long-term studies in subjects with diabetes to prove benefit from the use of resistant starch.

Fructans are an indigestible type of fiber that has been hypothesized to have a glucose-lowering effect. Inulin is a fructan commonly added to many processed food products in the form of chicory root. Limited research in people with diabetes is available. One systematic review that included three short-term studies in people with diabetes showed mixed results of fructan intake on glycemia. There are no published long-term studies in subjects with diabetes to prove benefit from the use of fructans (135).

Substitution of sucrose for starch

- While substituting sucrose-containing foods for isocaloric amounts of other carbohydrates may have similar blood glucose effects, consumption should be minimized to avoid displacing nutrient-dense food choices. (A)

Sucrose is a disaccharide made of glucose and fructose. Commonly known as table sugar or white sugar, it is found naturally in sugar cane and in sugar beets. Research demonstrates that substitution of sucrose for starch for up to 35% of calories may not affect glycemia or lipid levels (11). However, because foods high in sucrose are generally high in calories, substitution should be made in the context of an overall healthful eating pattern with caution not to increase caloric intake. Additionally, as with all people, selection of foods containing sucrose or starch should emphasize more nutrient-dense foods for an overall healthful eating pattern (105).

Fructose

- Fructose consumed as "free fructose" (i.e., naturally occurring in foods such as fruit) may result in better glycemic control compared with isocaloric intake of sucrose or starch (B), and free fructose is not likely to have detrimental effects on triglycerides as long as intake is not excessive (>12% energy). (C)
- People with diabetes should limit or avoid intake of sugar-sweetened beverages (SSBs) (from any caloric sweetener including high-fructose corn syrup and sucrose) to reduce risk for weight gain and worsening of cardiometabolic risk profile. (B)

Fructose is a monosaccharide found naturally in fruits. It is also a component of added sugars found in sweetened beverages and processed snacks. The term "free fructose" refers to fructose that is naturally occurring in foods such as fruit and does not include the fructose that is found in the form of the disaccharide sucrose, nor does it include the fructose in high-fructose corn syrup.

Based on two systematic reviews and meta-analyses of studies conducted in persons with diabetes, it appears that free fructose (naturally occurring from foods such as fruit) consumption is not more deleterious than other forms of sugar unless intake exceeds approximately 12% of total caloric intake (136,137). Many foods marketed to people with diabetes may contain large amounts of fructose (such as agave nectar); these foods should not be consumed in large amounts to avoid excess caloric intake and to avoid excessive fructose intake.

In terms of glycemic control, Cozma et al. (138) conducted a systemic review and meta-analysis of controlled feeding trials to study the impact of fructose on glycemic control compared with other sources of carbohydrates. Based on 18 trials, the authors found that isocaloric exchange of fructose for carbohydrates reduced glycated blood proteins and did not significantly affect fasting glucose or insulin. However, it was noted that applicability may be limited because most of the trials were less than 12 weeks in duration. With regard to the treatment of hypoglycemia, in a small study comparing glucose, sucrose, or fructose, Husband et al. (139) found that fructose was the least effective in eliciting the desired upward correction of the blood glucose. Therefore, sucrose or glucose in the form of tablets, liquid, or gel may be the preferred treatment over fruit juice, although availability and convenience should be considered.

There is now abundant evidence from studies of individuals without diabetes that because of their high amounts of rapidly absorbable carbohydrates (such as sucrose or high-fructose corn syrup), large quantities of SSBs should be avoided to reduce the risk for weight gain and worsening of cardiometabolic risk factors (140–142). Evidence suggests that consuming high levels of fructose-containing beverages may have particularly adverse effects on selective deposition of ectopic and visceral fat, lipid metabolism, blood pressure, insulin sensitivity, and de novo lipogenesis, compared with glucose-sweetened beverages (142). In terms of specific effects of fructose, concern has been raised regarding elevations in serum triglycerides (143,144). Such studies are not available among individuals with diabetes; however, there is little reason to suspect that the diabetic state would mitigate the adverse effects of SSBs.

Nonnutritive sweeteners and hypocaloric sweeteners

- Use of nonnutritive sweeteners (NNSs) has the potential to reduce overall calorie and carbohydrate intake if substituted for caloric sweeteners without compensation by intake of additional calories from other food sources. (B)

The U.S. Food and Drug Administration has reviewed several types of hypocaloric sweeteners (e.g., NNSs and sugar alcohols) for safety and approved them for consumption by the general public, including people with diabetes (145). Research supports that NNSs do not produce a glycemic effect; however, foods containing NNSs may affect glycemia based on other ingredients in the product (11). An American Heart Association and ADA scientific statement on NNS consumption concludes that there is not enough evidence to determine whether NNS use actually leads to reduction in body weight or reduction in cardiometabolic risk factors (146). These conclusions are consistent with a systematic review of hypocaloric sweeteners (including sugar alcohols) that found little evidence that the use of NNSs lead to reductions in body weight (147). If NNSs are used to replace caloric sweeteners, without caloric compensation, then NNSs may be useful in reducing caloric and carbohydrate intake (146), although further research is needed to confirm these results (147).

Protein

- For people with diabetes and no evidence of diabetic kidney disease, evidence is inconclusive to recommend an ideal amount of protein intake for optimizing glycemic control or improving one or more CVD risk measures; therefore, goals should be individualized. (C)
- For people with diabetes and diabetic kidney disease (either micro- or macro-albuminuria), reducing the amount of dietary protein below the usual intake is not recommended because it does not alter glycemic measures, cardiovascular risk measures, or the course of glomerular filtration rate (GFR) decline. (A)
- In individuals with type 2 diabetes, ingested protein appears to increase insulin response without increasing plasma glucose concentrations. Therefore, carbohydrate sources high in protein should not be used to treat or prevent hypoglycemia. (B)

Several RCTs have examined the effect of higher protein intake (28–40% of total energy) to usual protein intake (15–19% total) on diabetes outcomes. One study demonstrated decreased A1C with a higher-protein diet (148). However, other studies showed no effect on glycemic control (149–151). Some trials comparing higher protein intakes to usual protein intake have shown improved levels of serum triglycerides, total cholesterol, and/or LDL cholesterol (148,150). However, two trials reported no improvement in CVD risk factors (149,151). Factors affecting interpretation of this research include small sample sizes (148,151) and study durations of less than 6 months (148–150).

Several RCTs comparing protein levels in individuals with diabetic kidney disease with either micro- or macroalbuminuria had adequately large sample sizes and durations for interpretation. Four studies reported no difference in GFR and/or albumin excretion rate (152–155), while one smaller study found some potentially beneficial renal effects with a low-protein diet (156). Two meta-analyses found no clear benefits on renal parameters from low-protein diets (157,158). One factor affecting interpretation of these studies was that actual protein intake differed from goal protein intake. Two studies reported higher actual protein intake in the lower protein group than in the control groups. None of the five reviewed studies since 2000 demonstrated malnourishment as evidenced by hypoalbuminemia with low-protein diets, but both meta-analyses found evidence for this in earlier studies.

There is very limited research in people with diabetes and without kidney disease on the impact of the type of protein consumed. One study did not find a significant difference in glycemic or lipid measures when comparing a chicken- or red meat–based diet (156). For individuals with diabetic kidney disease and macroalbuminuria, changing the source of protein to be more soy-based may improve CVD risk factors but does not appear to alter proteinuria (159,160).

For individuals with type 2 diabetes, protein does not appear to have a significant effect on blood glucose level (161,162) but does appear to increase insulin response (161,163,164). For this reason, it is not advised to use protein to treat hypoglycemia or to prevent hypoglycemia. Protein's effect on blood glucose levels in type 1 diabetes is less clear (165,166).

Total fat

- Evidence is inconclusive for an ideal amount of total fat intake for people with diabetes; therefore goals should be individualized (C); fat quality appears to be far more important than quantity. (B)

Currently, insufficient data exist to determine a defined level of total energy intake from fat at which risk of inadequacy or prevention of chronic disease occurs, so there is no adequate intake or recommended daily allowance for total fat (167). However, the IOM did define an acceptable macronutrient distribution range (AMDR) for total fat of 20–35% of energy with no tolerable upper intake level defined. This AMDR for total fat was "estimated based on evidence indicating a risk for CHD [coronary heart disease] at low intake of fat and high intakes of carbohydrate and on evidence for increased obesity and its complications (CHD) at high intakes of fat" (167). These recommendations are not diabetes-specific; however, limited research exists in individuals with diabetes. Fatty acids are categorized as being saturated or unsaturated (monounsaturated or polyunsaturated). *Trans* fatty acids may be unsaturated, but they are structurally different and have negative health effects (105). The type of fatty acids consumed is more important than total fat in the diet in terms of supporting metabolic goals and influencing the risk of CVD (83,105,168); thus more attention should be given to the type of fat intake when individualizing goals. Individuals with diabetes should be encouraged to moderate their fat intakes to be consistent with their goals to lose or maintain weight.

Monounsaturated fatty acids/ polyunsaturated fatty acids

- In people with type 2 diabetes, a Mediterranean-style, monounsaturated fatty acid (MUFA)-rich eating pattern may benefit glycemic control and CVD risk factors and can, therefore, be recommended as an effective alternative to a lower-fat, higher-carbohydrate eating pattern. (B)

Evidence from large prospective cohort studies, clinical trials, and a systematic review of RCTs indicate that high-MUFA diets are associated with improved glycemic control and improved CVD risk or risk factors (70,169–171). The intake of MUFA-rich foods as a component of the Mediterranean-style eating pattern has been studied extensively over the last decade. Six published RCTs that included individuals with type 2 diabetes reported improved glycemic control and/or blood lipids when MUFA was substituted for carbohydrate and/or saturated fats (70,72,83,100,108,172). However, some of the studies also included caloric restriction, which may have contributed to improvements in glycemic control or blood lipids (100,108).

In 2011, the Evidence Analysis Library (EAL) of the Academy of Nutrition and Dietetics found strong evidence that dietary MUFAs are associated with improvements in blood lipids based on 13 studies including participants with and without diabetes. According to the EAL, 5% energy replacement of saturated fatty acid (SFA) with MUFA improves insulin responsiveness in insulin-resistant and type 2 diabetic subjects (173).

There is limited evidence in people with diabetes on the effects of omega-6 polyunsaturated fatty acids (PUFAs). Controversy exists on the best ratio of omega-6 to omega-3 fatty acids; PUFAs and MUFAs are recommended substitutes for saturated or *trans* fat (105,174).

Omega-3 fatty acids

- Evidence does not support recommending omega-3 (EPA and DHA) supplements for people with diabetes for the prevention or treatment of cardiovascular events. (A)
- As recommended for the general public, an increase in foods containing long-chain omega-3 fatty acids (EPA and DHA) (from fatty fish) and omega-3 linolenic acid (ALA) is recommended for individuals with diabetes because of their beneficial effects on lipoproteins, prevention of heart disease, and associations with positive health outcomes in observational studies. (B)
- The recommendation for the general public to eat fish (particularly fatty fish) at least two times (two servings) per week is also appropriate for people with diabetes. (B)

The ADA systematic review identified seven RCTs and one single-arm study (2002–2010) using omega-3 fatty acid supplements and one cohort study on whole-food omega-3 intake. In individuals with type 2 diabetes (88), supplementation with omega-3 fatty acids did not improve glycemic control, but higher-dose supplementation decreased triglycerides.

Additional blood-derived markers of CVD risk were not consistently altered in these trials. In subjects with diabetes, six short-duration (30 days to 12 weeks) RCTs were published after the macronutrient review comparing omega-3 (EPA and DHA) supplements to placebo and reported minimal or no beneficial effects (175,176) or mixed/inconsistent beneficial effects (177–180) on CVD risk factors and other health issues (e.g., depression). Supplementation with flaxseed (32 g/day) or flaxseed oil (13 g/day) for 12 weeks did not affect glycemic control or adipokines (181). Three longer-duration studies (4 months [182]; 40 months [183]; 6.2 years [184]) also reported mixed outcomes. Two studies reported no beneficial effects of supplementation (183,184). In one study, patients with type 2 diabetes were randomized to atorvastatin or placebo and/ or omega-3 supplements (2 g/day) or placebo. No differences on estimated 10-year CVD risks were observed with the addition of omega-3 fatty acid supplements compared with placebo (182). In the largest and longest trial, in patients with type 2 diabetes, supplementation with 1 g/day omega-3 fatty acids compared with placebo did not reduce the rate of cardiovascular events, death from any cause, or death from arrhythmia (184). However, in one study in postmyocardial patients with diabetes, low-dose supplementation of omega-3 fatty acids (400 mg/day) exerted a protective effect on ventricular arrhythmia–related events, and a reduction in mortality was reported (183). Thus, RCTs do not support recommending omega-3 supplements for primary or secondary prevention of CVD despite the strength of evidence from observational and preclinical studies.

Studies in persons with diabetes on the effect of foods containing marine-derived omega-3 fatty acid or the plant-derived omega-3 fatty acid, α-linolenic acid, are limited. Previous studies using supplements had shown mixed effects on fasting blood glucose and A1C levels. However, a study comparing diets with a high proportion of omega-3 (fatty fish) versus omega-6 (lean fish and fat-containing linoleic acid) fatty acids reported both diets had no detrimental effect on glucose measures, and both diets improved insulin sensitivity and lipoprotein profiles (185).

Saturated fat, dietary cholesterol, and *trans* fat

- The amount of dietary saturated fat, cholesterol, and *trans* fat recommended for people with diabetes is the same

as that recommended for the general population. (C)

Few research studies have explored the relationship between the amount of SFA in the diet and glycemic control and CVD risk in people with diabetes. A systematic review by Wheeler et al. found just one small 3-week study that compared a low-SFA diet (8% of total kcal) versus a high-SFA diet (17% of total kcal) and found no significant difference in glycemic control and most CVD risk measures (88,186).

In addition, there is limited research regarding optimal dietary cholesterol and *trans* fat intake in people with diabetes. One large prospective cohort study (171) in women with type 2 diabetes found a 37% increase in CVD risk for every 200 mg cholesterol/1,000 kcal.

Due to the lack of research in this area, people with diabetes should follow the guidelines for the general population. The *Dietary Guidelines for Americans, 2010* (105) recommends consuming less than 10% of calories from SFAs to reduce CVD risk. Consumers can meet this guideline by replacing foods high in SFA (i.e., full-fat dairy products, butter, marbled meats and bacon, and tropical oils such as coconut and palm) with items that are rich in MUFA and PUFA (i.e., vegetable and nut oils including canola, corn, safflower, soy, and sunflower; vegetable oil spreads; whole nuts and nut butters, and avocado). CVD is a common cause of death among individuals with diabetes. As a result, individuals with diabetes are encouraged to follow nutrition recommendations similar to the general population to manage CVD risk factors. These recommendations include reducing SFAs to <10% of calories, aiming for <300 mg dietary cholesterol/day, and limiting *trans* fat as much as possible (105).

Plant stanols and sterols

- Individuals with diabetes and dyslipidemia may be able to modestly reduce total and LDL cholesterol by consuming 1.6–3 g/day of plant stanols or sterols typically found in enriched foods. (C)

Plant sterol and stanol esters block the intestinal absorption of dietary and biliary cholesterol (3). Currently, the EAL from the Academy of Nutrition and Dietetics recommends individuals with dyslipidemia incorporate 2–3 g of plant sterol and stanol esters per day as part of a cardioprotective diet through consumption of

plant sterol and stanol ester–enriched foods (187). This recommendation, though not specific to people with diabetes, is based on a review of 20 clinical trials (187). Furthermore, the academy reviewed 28 studies that showed no adverse effects with plant stanol/sterol consumption (187).

There is a much smaller body of evidence regarding the cardioprotective effects of phytosterol/stanol consumption specifically in people with diabetes. Beneficial effects on total, LDL cholesterol, and non-HDL cholesterol have been observed in four RCTs (188–191). These studies used doses of 1.6–3 g of phytosterols or stanols per day, and interventions lasted 3–12 weeks. Two of these studies were in people with type 1 diabetes (188,189), and one found an added benefit to cholesterol reduction in those who were already on statin treatment (189). In addition, two RCTs compared the efficacy of plant sterol consumption (1.8 g daily) in subjects with type 2 diabetes and subjects without diabetes (191, 192). Neither study found a difference in lipid profiles between the two groups, suggesting that efficacy of this treatment is similar for those with and without diabetes who are hypercholesterolemic (191,192).

A wide range of foods and beverages are now available that contain plant sterols including many spreads, dairy products, grain and bread products, and yogurt. These products can contribute a considerable amount of calories. If used, patients should substitute them for comparable foods they eat in order to keep calories balanced and avoid weight gain (3,187).

Micronutrients and herbal supplements

- There is no clear evidence of benefit from vitamin or mineral supplementation in people with diabetes who do not have underlying deficiencies. (C)
  - o Routine supplementation with antioxidants, such as vitamins E and C and carotene, is not advised because of lack of evidence of efficacy and concern related to long-term safety. (A)
  - o There is insufficient evidence to support the routine use of micronutrients such as chromium, magnesium, and vitamin D to improve glycemic control in people with diabetes. (C)

o There is insufficient evidence to support the use of cinnamon or other herbs/supplements for the treatment of diabetes. (C)

o It is recommended that individualized meal planning include optimization of food choices to meet recommended dietary allowance/dietary reference intake for all micronutrients. (E)

There currently exists insufficient evidence of benefit from vitamin or mineral supplementation in people with or without diabetes in the absence of an underlying deficiency (3,193,194). Because uncontrolled diabetes is often associated with micronutrient deficiencies (195), people with diabetes should be aware of the importance of acquiring daily vitamin and mineral requirements from natural food sources and a balanced diet (3). For select groups of individuals such as the elderly, pregnant or lactating women, vegetarians, and those on calorie-restricted diets, a multivitamin supplement may be necessary (196).

While there has been significant interest in antioxidant supplementation as a treatment for diabetes, current evidence not only demonstrates a lack of benefit with respect to glycemic control and progression of complications, but also provides evidence of potential harm of vitamin E, carotene, and other antioxidant supplements (197–203).

Findings from supplement studies with micronutrients such as chromium, magnesium, and vitamin D are conflicting and confounded by differences in dosing, micronutrient levels achieved with supplementation, baseline micronutrient status, and/or methodologies used. A systematic review on the effect of chromium supplementation on glucose metabolism and lipids concluded that larger effects were more commonly observed in poor-quality studies and that evidence is limited by poor study quality and heterogeneity in methodology and results (204). Evidence from clinical studies evaluating magnesium (205,206) and vitamin D (207–211) supplementation to improve glycemic control in people with diabetes is likewise conflicting.

A systematic review (212) evaluating the effects of cinnamon in people with diabetes concluded there is currently insufficient evidence to support its use, and there is a lack of compelling evidence for the use of other herbal products for the improvement of glycemic control in people with diabetes (213). It is important to consider that herbal products are not standardized and vary in the content of active ingredients and may have the potential to interact with other medications (214). Therefore, it is important that patients/clients with diabetes report the use of supplements and herbal products to their health care providers.

Alcohol

- If adults with diabetes choose to drink alcohol, they should be advised to do so in moderation (one drink per day or less for adult women and two drinks per day or less for adult men). (E)
- Alcohol consumption may place people with diabetes at increased risk for delayed hypoglycemia, especially if taking insulin or insulin secretagogues. Education and awareness regarding the recognition and management of delayed hypoglycemia is warranted. (C)

Moderate alcohol consumption has minimal acute and/or long-term detrimental effects on blood glucose in people with diabetes (215–219), with some epidemiologic data showing improved glycemic control with moderate intake. Moderate alcohol intake may also convey cardiovascular risk reduction and mortality benefits in people with diabetes (220–223), with the type of alcohol consumed not influencing these beneficial effects (221,224). Accordingly, the recommendations for alcohol consumption for people with diabetes are the same as for the general population. Adults with diabetes choosing to consume alcohol should limit their intake to one serving or less per day for women and two servings or less per day for men (105). Excessive amounts of alcohol ($\geq$3 drinks/day) consumed on a consistent basis may contribute to hyperglycemia (221). One alcohol-containing beverage is defined as 12 oz beer, 5 oz wine, or 1.5 oz distilled spirits, each containing approximately 15 g of alcohol. Abstention from alcohol should be advised, however, for people with a history of alcohol abuse or dependence, women during pregnancy, and people with medical conditions such as liver disease, pancreatitis, advanced neuropathy, or severe hypertriglyceridemia (3).

Despite the potential glycemic and cardiovascular benefits of moderate alcohol consumption, use may place people with diabetes at increased risk for delayed hypoglycemia. This is particularly true in those using insulin or insulin secretagogue therapies. Consuming alcohol with food can minimize the risk of nocturnal hypoglycemia (3,225–227). Individuals with diabetes should receive education regarding the recognition and management of delayed hypoglycemia and the potential need for more frequent self-monitoring of blood glucose after consuming alcoholic beverages.

Sodium

- The recommendation for the general population to reduce sodium to less than 2,300 mg/day is also appropriate for people with diabetes. (B)
- For individuals with both diabetes and hypertension, further reduction in sodium intake should be individualized. (B)

Limited studies have been published on sodium reduction in people with diabetes. A Cochrane review of RCTs found that decreasing sodium intake reduces blood pressure in those with diabetes (228). Likewise, a small study in people with type 2 diabetes showed that following the DASH diet and reducing sodium intake to about 2,300 mg led to improvements in blood pressure and other measures on cardiovascular risk factors (46).

Incrementally lower sodium intakes (i.e., to 1,500 mg/day) show more beneficial effects on blood pressure (104,229); however, some studies in people with type 1 (230) and type 2 (231) diabetes measuring urine sodium excretion have shown increased mortality associated with the lowest sodium intakes, therefore warranting caution for universal sodium restriction to 1,500 mg in this population. Additionally, an IOM report suggests there is no evidence on health outcomes to treat certain population subgroups—which includes individuals with diabetes—differently than the general U.S. population (232).

In the absence of clear scientific evidence for benefit in people with combined diabetes and hypertension (230,231), sodium intake goals that are significantly lower than 2,300 mg/day should be considered only on an individual basis. When individualizing sodium intake recommendations, consideration must also be given to issues such as the palatability, availability, and additional cost of specialty low sodium products and the difficulty in achieving both low sodium recommendations and a nutritionally adequate diet given these limitations (233).

While specific dietary sodium targets are highly debated by various health groups, all agree that the current average

Table 4—*Summary of priority topics*

1. Strategies for all people with diabetes:
   - Portion control should be recommended for weight loss and maintenance.
   - Carbohydrate-containing foods and beverages and endogenous insulin production are the greatest determinant of the postmeal blood glucose level; therefore, it is important to know what foods contain carbohydrates—starchy vegetables, whole grains, fruit, milk and milk products, vegetables, and sugar.
   - When choosing carbohydrate-containing foods, choose nutrient-dense, high-fiber foods whenever possible instead of processed foods with added sodium, fat, and sugars. Nutrient-dense foods and beverages provide vitamins, minerals, and other healthful substances with relatively few calories. Calories have not been added to them from solid fats, sugars, or refined starches.
   - Avoid SSBs.
   - For most people, it is not necessary to subtract the amount of dietary fiber or sugar alcohols from total carbohydrates when carbohydrate counting.
   - Substitute foods higher in unsaturated fat (liquid oils) for foods higher in *trans* or saturated fat.
   - Select leaner protein sources and meat alternatives.
   - Vitamin and mineral supplements, herbal products, or cinnamon to manage diabetes are not recommended due to lack of evidence.
   - Moderate alcohol consumption (one drink/day or less for adult women and two drinks or less for adult men) has minimal acute or long-term effects on blood glucose in people with diabetes. To reduce risk of hypoglycemia for individuals using insulin or insulin secretagogues, alcohol should be consumed with food.
   - Limit sodium intake to 2,300 mg/day.
2. Priority should be given to coordinating food with type of diabetes medicine for those individuals on medicine.
   - For individuals who take insulin secretagogues:
     - Moderate amounts of carbohydrate at each meal and snacks.
     - To reduce risk of hypoglycemia:*
       - Eat a source of carbohydrates at meals.
       - Moderate amounts of carbohydrates at each meal and snacks.
       - Do not skip meals.
       - Physical activity may result in low blood glucose depending on when it is performed. Always carry a source of carbohydrates to reduce risk of hypoglycemia.*
   - For individuals who take biguanides (metformin):
     - Gradually titrate to minimize gastrointestinal side effects when initiating use:
       - Take medication with food or 15 min after a meal if symptoms persist.
       - If side effects do not resolve over time (a few weeks), follow up with health care provider.
       - If taking along with an insulin secretagogue or insulin, may experience hypoglycemia.*
   - For individuals who take α-glucosidase inhibitors:
     - Gradually titrate to minimize gastrointestinal side effects when initiating use.
     - Take at start of meal to have maximal effect:
       - If taking along with an insulin secretagogue or insulin, may experience hypoglycemia.
       - If hypoglycemia occurs, eat something containing monosaccharides such as glucose tablets as drug will prevent the digestion of polysaccharides.
   - For individuals who take incretin mimetics (GLP-1):
     - Gradually titrate to minimize gastrointestinal side effects when initiating use:
       - Injection of daily or twice-daily GLP-1s should be premeal.
       - If side effects do not resolve over time (a few weeks), follow up with health care provider.
       - If taking along with an insulin secretagogue or insulin, may experience hypoglycemia.*
       - Once-weekly GLP-1s can be taken at any time during the day regardless of meal times.
   - For individuals with type 1 diabetes and insulin-requiring type 2 diabetes:
     - Learn how to count carbohydrates or use another meal planning approach to quantify carbohydrate intake. The objective of using such a meal planning approach is to "match" mealtime insulin to carbohydrates consumed.
     - If on a multiple-daily injection plan or on an insulin pump:
       - Take mealtime insulin before eating.
       - Meals can be consumed at different times.
       - If physical activity is performed within 1–2 h of mealtime insulin injection, this dose may need to be lowered to reduce risk of hypoglycemia.*
     - If on a premixed insulin plan:
       - Insulin doses need to be taken at consistent times every day.
       - Meals need to be consumed at similar times every day.
       - Do not skip meals to reduce risk of hypoglycemia.
       - Physical activity may result in low blood glucose depending on when it is performed. Always carry a source of quick-acting carbohydrates to reduce risk of hypoglycemia.*
     - If on a fixed insulin plan:
       - Eat similar amounts of carbohydrates each day to match the set doses of insulin.

GLP-1, glucagon-like peptide-1. *Treatment of hypoglycemia: current recommendations include the use of glucose tablets or carbohydrate-containing foods or beverages (such as fruit juice, sports drinks, regular soda pop, or hard candy) to treat hypoglycemia. A commonly recommended dose of glucose is 15–20 g. When blood glucose levels are ~50–60 mg/dL, treatment with 15 g of glucose can be expected to raise blood glucose levels ~50 mg/dL (239). If self-monitoring of blood glucose and about 15–20 min after treatment shows continued hypoglycemia, the treatment should be repeated.

intake of sodium of 3,400 mg/day (excluding table salt) is excessive and should be reduced (105,234–237). The food industry can play a major role in lowering sodium content of foods to help people meet sodium recommendations (233,234).

Clinical priorities for nutrition management for all people with diabetes

—A wide range of diabetes meal planning approaches or eating patterns have been shown to be clinically effective, with many including a reduced energy intake component. There is not one ideal percentage of calories from carbohydrates, protein, or fat that is optimal for all people with diabetes. Nutrition therapy goals should be developed collaboratively with the individual with diabetes and be based on an assessment of the individual's current eating patterns, preferences, and metabolic goals. Once a thorough assessment is completed, the health care professional's role is to facilitate behavior change and achievement of metabolic goals while meeting the patient's preferences, which may include allowing the patient to continue following his/her current eating pattern. If the individual would like to try a different eating pattern, this should also be supported by the health care team. Various behavior change theories and strategies can be used to tailor nutrition interventions to help the client achieve specific health and quality-of-life outcomes (238).

Multiple meal planning approaches and eating patterns can be effective for achieving metabolic goals. Examples include: carbohydrate counting, healthful food choices/simplified meal plans (i.e., the Plate Method), individualized meal planning methods based on percentages of macronutrients, exchange list for meal planning, glycemic index, and eating patterns including Mediterranean style, DASH, vegetarian or vegan, low carbohydrate, and low fat. The meal planning approach or eating pattern should be selected based on the individual's personal and cultural preferences; literacy and numeracy; and readiness, willingness, and ability to change. This may need to be adjusted over time based on changes in life circumstances, preferences, and disease course.

A summary of key topics for nutrition education can be found in Table 4.

Future research directions

—The evidence presented in this position statement concurs with the review previously published by Wheeler et al. (88) that many different approaches to nutrition therapy and eating patterns are effective for the target outcomes of improved glycemic control and reduced CVD risk among individuals with diabetes. Evaluating nutrition evidence is complex given that multiple dietary factors influence glycemic control and CVD risk factors, and the influence of a combination of factors can be substantial. Based on a review of the evidence, it is clear that gaps in the literature continue to exist and further research on nutrition and eating patterns is needed in individuals with type 1 and type 2 diabetes.

For example, future studies should address:

- The relationships between eating patterns and disease in diverse populations.
- The basis for the beneficial effects of the Mediterranean-style eating pattern and approaches to translation of the Mediterranean-style eating pattern into diverse populations.
- The development of standardized definitions for high– and low–glycemic index diets and implementation of these definitions in long-term studies to further evaluate their impact on glycemic control.
- The development of standardized definitions for low- to moderate-carbohydrate diets and determining long-term sustainability.
- Whether NNSs, when used to replace caloric sweeteners, are useful in reducing caloric and carbohydrate intake.
- The impact of key nutrients on cardiovascular risk, such as saturated fat, cholesterol, and sodium in individuals with both type 1 and type 2 diabetes.
- Intake of SFA and its relationship to insulin resistance.

Importantly, research needs to move away from just evaluating the impact of individual nutrients on glycemic control and cardiovascular risk. More research on eating patterns, unrestricted and restricted energy diets, and diverse populations is needed to evaluate their long-term health benefits in individuals with diabetes. Individuals eat nutrients from foods and within the context of mixed meals, and nutrient intakes are intercorrelated, so overall eating patterns must be studied to fully understand how these eating patterns impact glycemic control (88, 240). Eating patterns are selected by individuals based on more than the healthfulness of food and food availability; tradition, cultural food systems, health beliefs, and economics are also important (95). Studies on gene-diet interactions will also be important, as well as studies on potential epigenetic effects that depend on nutrients to moderate gene expression.

Given the benefits of both nutrition therapy and MNT for individuals with diabetes, it is also important to study systematic processes within the context of health care delivery that encourage more individuals with diabetes to receive nutrition therapy initially, upon diagnosis, and long term. Further research is also needed on the best tools and strategies for educating individuals with diabetes (e.g., the Plate Method) and how to improve adherence to healthful eating patterns among individuals with diabetes. This research should include multiple settings that can impact food choices for individuals with diabetes, such as where they live, work, learn, and play. Individuals with diabetes spend the majority of their time outside health care settings so more research on how public health, the health care system, and the community can support individuals with diabetes in their efforts to achieve healthful eating is needed.

In summary—There is no standard meal plan or eating pattern that works universally for all people with diabetes (1). In order to be effective, nutrition therapy should be individualized for each patient/client based on his or her individual health goals; personal and cultural preferences (241,242); health literacy and numeracy (243,244); access to healthful choices (245,246); and readiness, willingness, and ability to change. Nutrition interventions should emphasize a variety of minimally processed nutrient-dense foods in appropriate portion sizes as part of a healthful eating pattern and provide the individual with diabetes with practical tools for day-to-day food plan and behavior change that can be maintained over the long term.

Acknowledgments—This position statement was written at the request of the ADA Executive

Committee, which has approved the final document. The process involved extensive literature review, one face-to-face meeting of the entire writing group, one subgroup writing meeting, numerous teleconferences, and multiple revisions via e-mail communications.

The final draft was also reviewed and approved by the Professional Practice Committee of the ADA. The authors are indebted to Sue Kirkman, MD, for her guidance and support during this process.

The two face-to-face meetings and the travel of the writing group and teleconference calls were supported by the ADA.

During the past 12 months, the following relationships with companies whose products or services directly relate to the subject matter in this document are declared: A.B.E.: no conflicts of interest to report. J.L.B.: research with CDC >$10,000, money goes to institution. M.C.: consultant/advisory board with Becton Dickenson. S.A.D.: no conflicts of interest to report. M.J.F.: no conflicts of interest to report. E.J.M.-D.: research with Abbott Diabetes Care and Eli Lilly >$10,000, money goes to institution. J.J.N.: research with AstraZeneca, Bristol-Myers Squibb, Johnson & Johnson, Novo Nordisk, Merck, and Eli Lilly >$10,000, money goes to institution; consultant/advisory board with Janssen Phamaceuticals; other research support through the National Institutes of Health (NIH) and the Patient-Centered Outcomes Research Institute. R.N.: consultant/advisory board with Boehringer Ingelheim, Eli Lilly, Type Free Inc., NIH/National Institute of Diabetes and Digestive and Kidney Diseases Advisory Council. C.L.V.: no conflicts of interest to report. P.U.: speakers' bureau/honoraria with Eli Lilly and consultant/advisory board with Eli Lilly, Sanofi, Halozyme Therapeutics, Medtronic, YourEncore, Janssen Pharmaceuticals. W.S.Y.: research with NIH and the Veterans Administration >$10,000, money goes to institution; spouse employee of ViiV Healthcare >$10,000. No other potential conflicts of interest relevant to this article were reported.

All the named writing group authors contributed substantially to the document including researching data, contributing to discussions, writing and reviewing text, and editing the manuscript. All authors supplied detailed input and approved the final version. A.B.E. and J.L.B. directed, chaired, and coordinated the input with multiple e-mail exchanges or telephone calls between all participants.

The authors also gratefully acknowledge the following experts who provided critical review of a draft of this statement: Jane Chiang, MD, American Diabetes Association, Alexandria, VA; Joan Hill, RD, CDE, Hill Nutrition Consulting LLC, Boston, MA; Sue Kirkman, MD, University of North Carolina, Chapel Hill, NC; Penny Kris-Etherton, PhD, RD, Penn State, University Park, PA; Melinda Maryniuk, MS, RD, FADA, CDE, Joslin Diabetes Center, Boston, MA; Dariush Mozaffarian, MD, Harvard School of Public Health, Boston, MA; and

Madelyn Wheeler, MS, RD, FADA, Nutritional Computing Concepts, Zionsville, IN.

References

1. American Diabetes Association. Standards of medical care in diabetes—2013. Diabetes Care 2013;36(Suppl. 1):S11–S66
2. Inzucchi SE, Bergenstal RM, Buse JB, et al.; American Diabetes Association (ADA); European Association for the Study of Diabetes (EASD). Management of hyperglycemia in type 2 diabetes: a patient-centered approach: position statement of the American Diabetes Association (ADA) and the European Association for the Study of Diabetes (EASD). Diabetes Care 2012;35:1364–1379
3. Bantle JP, Wylie-Rosett J, Albright AL, et al.; American Diabetes Association. Nutrition recommendations and interventions for diabetes: a position statement of the American Diabetes Association. Diabetes Care 2008;31(Suppl. 1):S61–S78
4. The Diabetes Control and Complications Trial Research Group. The effect of intensive treatment of diabetes on the development and progression of long-term complications in insulin-dependent diabetes mellitus. N Engl J Med 1993;329:977–986
5. UK Prospective Diabetes Study (UKPDS) Group. Effect of intensive blood-glucose control with metformin on complications in overweight patients with type 2 diabetes (UKPDS 34). Lancet 1998;352:854–865
6. Nathan DM, Zinman B, Cleary PA, et al.; Diabetes Control and Complications Trial/Epidemiology of Diabetes Interventions and Complications (DCCT/EDIC) Research Group. Modern-day clinical course of type 1 diabetes mellitus after 30 years' duration: the Diabetes Control and Complications Trial/Epidemiology of Diabetes Interventions and Complications and Pittsburgh Epidemiology of Diabetes Complications Experience (1983-2005). Arch Intern Med 2009;169:1307–1316
7. Holman RR, Paul SK, Bethel MA, Matthews DR, Neil HA. 10-year follow-up of intensive glucose control in type 2 diabetes. N Engl J Med 2008;359:1577–1589
8. Turnbull FM, Abraira C, Anderson RJ, et al.; Control Group. Intensive glucose control and macrovascular outcomes in type 2 diabetes. Diabetologia 2009;52:2288–2298
9. Chobanian AV, Bakris GL, Black HR, et al.; National Heart, Lung, and Blood Institute Joint National Committee on Prevention, Detection, Evaluation, and Treatment of High Blood Pressure; National High Blood Pressure Education

Program Coordinating Committee. The Seventh Report of the Joint National Committee on Prevention, Detection, Evaluation, and Treatment of High Blood Pressure: the JNC 7 report. JAMA 2003; 289:2560–2572
10. Kearney PM, Blackwell L, Collins R, et al.; Cholesterol Treatment Trialists' (CTT) Collaborators. Efficacy of cholesterol-lowering therapy in 18,686 people with diabetes in 14 randomised trials of statins: a meta-analysis. Lancet 2008;371:117–125
11. Franz MJ, Powers MA, Leontos C, et al. The evidence for medical nutrition therapy for type 1 and type 2 diabetes in adults. J Am Diet Assoc 2010;110:1852–1889
12. Al-Sinani M, Min Y, Ghebremeskel K, Qazaq HS. Effectiveness of and adherence to dietary and lifestyle counselling: effect on metabolic control in type 2 diabetic Omani patients. Sultan Qaboos Univ Med J 2010;10:341–349
13. DAFNE Study Group. Training in flexible, intensive insulin management to enable dietary freedom in people with type 1 diabetes: Dose Adjustment For Normal Eating (DAFNE) randomised controlled trial. BMJ 2002;325:746
14. Andrews RC, Cooper AR, Montgomery AA, et al. Diet or diet plus physical activity versus usual care in patients with newly diagnosed type 2 diabetes: the Early ACTID randomised controlled trial. Lancet 2011;378:129–139
15. Siminerio LM, Piatt G, Zgibor JC. Implementing the chronic care model for improvements in diabetes care and education in a rural primary care practice. Diabetes Educ 2005;31:225–234
16. Siminerio LM, Piatt GA, Emerson S, et al. Deploying the chronic care model to implement and sustain diabetes self-management training programs. Diabetes Educ 2006;32:253–260
17. Ali MK, Bullard KM, Saaddine JB, Cowie CC, Imperatore G, Gregg EW. Achievement of goals in U.S. diabetes care, 1999-2010. N Engl J Med 2013;368:1613–1624
18. Robbins JM, Thatcher GE, Webb DA, Valdmanis VG. Nutritionist visits, diabetes classes, and hospitalization rates and charges: the Urban Diabetes Study. Diabetes Care 2008;31:655–660
19. Institute of Medicine. *The Role of Nutrition in Maintaining Health in the Nation's Elderly: Evaluating Coverage of Nutrition Services for the Medicare Population.* Washington, DC, National Academies Press, 2000
20. Lacey K, Pritchett E. Nutrition care process and model: ADA adopts road map to quality care and outcomes management. J Am Diet Assoc 2003;103:1061–1072
21. Haas L, Maryniuk M, Beck J, et al.; 2012 Standards Revision Task Force. National

Standards for Diabetes Self-Management Education and Support. Diabetes Care 2012;35:2393–2401

22. Gary TL, Genkinger JM, Guallar E, Peyrot M, Brancati FL. Meta-analysis of randomized educational and behavioral interventions in type 2 diabetes. Diabetes Educ 2003;29:488–501

23. Norris SL, Lau J, Smith SJ, Schmid CH, Engelgau MM. Self-management education for adults with type 2 diabetes: a meta-analysis of the effect on glycemic control. Diabetes Care 2002;25:1159–1171

24. Renders CM, Valk GD, Griffin SJ, Wagner EH, Eijk Van JT, Assendelft WJ. Interventions to improve the management of diabetes in primary care, outpatient, and community settings: a systematic review. Diabetes Care 2001;24:1821–1833

25. Brown SA, Hanis CL. Culturally competent diabetes education for Mexican Americans: the Starr County Study. Diabetes Educ 1999;25:226–236

26. Deakin T, McShane CE, Cade JE, Williams RD. Group based training for self-management strategies in people with type 2 diabetes mellitus. Cochrane Database Syst Rev 2005;2:CD003417

27. American Association of Diabetes Educators. *Guidelines for the Practice of Diabetes Self-Management Education and Training (DSME/T)*. Chicago, American Association of Diabetes Educators, 2010

28. Karmally W. Nutrition Therapy for Diabetes and Lipid Disorders. In *American Diabetes Association Guide to Nutrition Therapy for Diabetes*. Franz M, Evert A, Eds. Alexandria, VA, American Diabetes Association, 2012, p. 265–294

29. Rickheim PL, Weaver TW, Flader JL, Kendall DM. Assessment of group versus individual diabetes education: a randomized study. Diabetes Care 2002;25:269–274

30. Miller CK, Edwards L, Kissling G, Sanville L. Nutrition education improves metabolic outcomes among older adults with diabetes mellitus: results from a randomized controlled trial. Prev Med 2002;34:252–259

31. Ash S, Reeves MM, Yeo S, Morrison G, Carey D, Capra S. Effect of intensive dietetic interventions on weight and glycaemic control in overweight men with type II diabetes: a randomised trial. Int J Obes Relat Metab Disord 2003;27:797–802

32. Goldhaber-Fiebert JD, Goldhaber-Fiebert SN, Tristán ML, Nathan DM. Randomized controlled community-based nutrition and exercise intervention improves glycemia and cardiovascular risk factors in type 2 diabetic patients in rural Costa Rica. Diabetes Care 2003;26:24–29

33. Ziemer DC, Berkowitz KJ, Panayioto RM, et al. A simple meal plan emphasizing healthy food choices is as effective as an exchange-based meal plan for urban African Americans with type 2 diabetes. Diabetes Care 2003;26:1719–1724

34. Takahashi M, Araki A, Ito H. Development of a new method for simple dietary education in elderly patients with diabetes mellitus. Geriatr Gerontol Int 2004;4:111–119

35. Wolf AM, Conaway MR, Crowther JQ, et al.; Improving Control with Activity and Nutrition (ICAN) Study. Translating lifestyle intervention to practice in obese patients with type 2 diabetes: Improving Control with Activity and Nutrition (ICAN) study. Diabetes Care 2004;27:1570–1576

36. Barnard ND, Cohen J, Jenkins DJ, et al. A low-fat vegan diet improves glycemic control and cardiovascular risk factors in a randomized clinical trial in individuals with type 2 diabetes. Diabetes Care 2006;29:1777–1783

37. Nield L, Moore HJ, Hooper L, et al. Dietary advice for treatment of type 2 diabetes mellitus in adults. Cochrane Database Syst Rev 2007;3:CD004097

38. Davis RM, Hitch AD, Salaam MM, Herman WH, Zimmer-Galler IE, Mayer-Davis EJ. TeleHealth improves diabetes self-management in an underserved community: diabetes TeleCare. Diabetes Care 2010;33:1712–1717

39. Rossi MC, Nicolucci A, Di Bartolo P, et al. Diabetes Interactive Diary: a new telemedicine system enabling flexible diet and insulin therapy while improving quality of life: an open-label, international, multicenter, randomized study. Diabetes Care 2010;33:109–115

40. Huang MC, Hsu CC, Wang HS, Shin SJ. Prospective randomized controlled trial to evaluate effectiveness of registered dietitian-led diabetes management on glycemic and diet control in a primary care setting in Taiwan. Diabetes Care 2010;33:233–239

41. Al-Shookri A, Khor GL, Chan YM, Loke SC, Al-Maskari M. Effectiveness of medical nutrition treatment delivered by dietitians on glycaemic outcomes and lipid profiles of Arab, Omani patients with type 2 diabetes. Diabet Med 2012;29:236–244

42. Coppell KJ, Kataoka M, Williams SM, Chisholm AW, Vorgers SM, Mann JI. Nutritional intervention in patients with type 2 diabetes who are hyperglycaemic despite optimised drug treatment—Lifestyle Over and Above Drugs in Diabetes (LOADD) study: randomised controlled trial. BMJ 2010;341:c3337

43. Laurenzi A, Bolla AM, Panigoni G, et al. Effects of carbohydrate counting on glucose control and quality of life over 24 weeks in adult patients with type 1 diabetes on continuous subcutaneous insulin infusion: a randomized, prospective clinical trial (GIOCAR). Diabetes Care 2011;34:823–827

44. Tan MY, Magarey JM, Chee SS, Lee LF, Tan MH. A brief structured education programme enhances self-care practices and improves glycaemic control in Malaysians with poorly controlled diabetes. Health Educ Res 2011;26:896–907

45. Battista MC, Labonté M, Ménard J, et al. Dietitian-coached management in combination with annual endocrinologist follow up improves global metabolic and cardiovascular health in diabetic participants after 24 months. Appl Physiol Nutr Metab 2012;37:610–620

46. Azadbakht L, Fard NR, Karimi M, et al. Effects of the Dietary Approaches to Stop Hypertension (DASH) eating plan on cardiovascular risks among type 2 diabetic patients: a randomized crossover clinical trial. Diabetes Care 2011;34:55–57

47. Academy of Nutrition and Dietetics. Disorders of lipid metabolism [Internet], 2010. Evidence Analysis Library. Available from http://andevidencelibrary.com/topic.cfm?cat=3582&auth=1. Accessed 1 July 2013

48. Kulkarni K, Castle G, Gregory R, et al.; The Diabetes Care and Education Dietetic Practice Group. Nutrition Practice Guidelines for type 1 diabetes mellitus positively affect dietitian practices and patient outcomes. J Am Diet Assoc 1998;98:62–70

49. Franz MJ, Monk A, Barry B, et al. Effectiveness of medical nutrition therapy provided by dietitians in the management of non-insulin-dependent diabetes mellitus: a randomized, controlled clinical trial. J Am Diet Assoc 1995;95:1009–1017

50. Graber AL, Elasy TA, Quinn D, Wolff K, Brown A. Improving glycemic control in adults with diabetes mellitus: shared responsibility in primary care practices. South Med J 2002;95:684–690

51. Sämann A, Mühlhauser I, Bender R, Kloos Ch, Müller UA. Glycaemic control and severe hypoglycaemia following training in flexible, intensive insulin therapy to enable dietary freedom in people with type 1 diabetes: a prospective implementation study. Diabetologia 2005;48:1965–1970

52. Lowe J, Linjawi S, Mensch M, James K, Attia J. Flexible eating and flexible insulin dosing in patients with diabetes: results of an intensive self-management course. Diabetes Res Clin Pract 2008;80:439–443

53. Scavone G, Manto A, Pitocco D, et al. Effect of carbohydrate counting and medical nutritional therapy on glycaemic control in type 1 diabetic subjects: a pilot study. Diabet Med 2010;27:477–479

54. Wolever TM, Hamad S, Chiasson JL, et al. Day-to-day consistency in amount and source of carbohydrate intake associated with improved blood glucose

control in type 1 diabetes. J Am Coll Nutr 1999;18:242–247

55. Rabasa-Lhoret R, Garon J, Langelier H, Poisson D, Chiasson JL. Effects of meal carbohydrate content on insulin requirements in type 1 diabetic patients treated intensively with the basal-bolus (ultralente-regular) insulin regimen. Diabetes Care 1999;22:667–673

56. McIntyre HD, Knight BA, Harvey DM, Noud MN, Hagger VL, Gilshenan KS. Dose Adjustment For Normal Eating (DAFNE) - an audit of outcomes in Australia. Med J Aust 2010;192:637–640

57. Speight J, Amiel SA, Bradley C, et al. Long-term biomedical and psychosocial outcomes following DAFNE (Dose Adjustment For Normal Eating) structured education to promote intensive insulin therapy in adults with sub-optimally controlled type 1 diabetes. Diabetes Res Clin Pract 2010;89:22–29

58. Nguyen NT, Nguyen XM, Lane J, Wang P. Relationship between obesity and diabetes in a US adult population: findings from the National Health and Nutrition Examination Survey, 1999-2006. Obes Surg 2011;21:351–355

59. UK Prospective Diabetes Study 7. UK Prospective Diabetes Study 7: response of fasting plasma glucose to diet therapy in newly presenting type II diabetic patients, UKPDS Group. Metabolism 1990; 39:905–912

60. Fonseca V, McDuffie R, Calles J, et al.; ACCORD Study Group. Determinants of weight gain in the action to control cardiovascular risk in diabetes trial. Diabetes Care 2013;36:2162–2168

61. Carlson MG, Campbell PJ. Intensive insulin therapy and weight gain in IDDM. Diabetes 1993;42:1700–1707

62. Heller S. Weight gain during insulin therapy in patients with type 2 diabetes mellitus. Diabetes Res Clin Pract 2004; 65(Suppl. 1):S23–S27

63. Jacob AN, Salinas K, Adams-Huet B, Raskin P. Weight gain in type 2 diabetes mellitus. Diabetes Obes Metab 2007;9: 386–393

64. McMinn JE, Baskin DG, Schwartz MW. Neuroendocrine mechanisms regulating food intake and body weight. Obes Rev 2000;1:37–46

65. Banister NA, Jastrow ST, Hodges V, Loop R, Gillham MB. Diabetes self-management training program in a community clinic improves patient outcomes at modest cost. J Am Diet Assoc 2004;104:807–810

66. Barratt R, Frost G, Millward DJ, Truby H. A randomised controlled trial investigating the effect of an intensive lifestyle intervention v. standard care in adults with type 2 diabetes immediately after initiating insulin therapy. Br J Nutr 2008;99: 1025–1031

67. Metz JA, Stern JS, Kris-Etherton P, et al. A randomized trial of improved weight

loss with a prepared meal plan in overweight and obese patients: impact on cardiovascular risk reduction. Arch Intern Med 2000;160:2150–2158

68. Li Z, Hong K, Saltsman P, et al. Long-term efficacy of soy-based meal replacements vs an individualized diet plan in obese type II DM patients: relative effects on weight loss, metabolic parameters, and C-reactive protein. Eur J Clin Nutr 2005;59:411–418

69. West DS, DiLillo V, Bursac Z, Gore SA, Greene PG. Motivational interviewing improves weight loss in women with type 2 diabetes. Diabetes Care 2007;30: 1081–1087

70. Brehm BJ, Lattin BL, Summer SS, et al. One-year comparison of a high-monounsaturated fat diet with a high-carbohydrate diet in type 2 diabetes. Diabetes Care 2009;32: 215–220

71. Davis NJ, Tomuta N, Schechter C, et al. Comparative study of the effects of a 1-year dietary intervention of a low-carbohydrate diet versus a low-fat diet on weight and glycemic control in type 2 diabetes. Diabetes Care 2009;32:1147–1152

72. Esposito K, Maiorino MI, Ciotola M, et al. Effects of a Mediterranean-style diet on the need for antihyperglycemic drug therapy in patients with newly diagnosed type 2 diabetes: a randomized trial. Ann Intern Med 2009;151:306–314

73. Larsen RN, Mann NJ, Maclean E, Shaw JE. The effect of high-protein, low-carbohydrate diets in the treatment of type 2 diabetes: a 12 month randomised controlled trial. Diabetologia 2011;54:731–740

74. Krebs JD, Elley CR, Parry-Strong A, et al. The Diabetes Excess Weight Loss (DEWL) Trial: a randomised controlled trial of high-protein versus high-carbohydrate diets over 2 years in type 2 diabetes. Diabetologia 2012;55:905–914

75. Guldbrand H, Dizdar B, Bunjaku B, et al. In type 2 diabetes, randomisation to advice to follow a low-carbohydrate diet transiently improves glycaemic control compared with advice to follow a low-fat diet producing a similar weight loss. Diabetologia 2012;55:2118–2127

76. Pi-Sunyer X, Blackburn G, Brancati FL, et al.; Look AHEAD Research Group. Reduction in weight and cardiovascular disease risk factors in individuals with type 2 diabetes: one-year results of the Look AHEAD trial. Diabetes Care 2007; 30:1374–1383

77. Look AHEAD Research Group. Cardiovascular effects of intensive lifestyle intervention in type 2 diabetes. N Engl J Med 2013;369:145–154

78. Li TY, Brennan AM, Wedick NM, Mantzoros C, Rifai N, Hu FB. Regular consumption of nuts is associated with a

lower risk of cardiovascular disease in women with type 2 diabetes. J Nutr 2009;139:1333–1338

79. Faulconbridge LF, Wadden TA, Rubin RR, et al.; Look AHEAD Research Group. One-year changes in symptoms of depression and weight in overweight/obese individuals with type 2 diabetes in the Look AHEAD study. Obesity (Silver Spring) 2012;20:783–793

80. Foster GD, Borradaile KE, Sanders MH, et al.; Sleep AHEAD Research Group of Look AHEAD Research Group. A randomized study on the effect of weight loss on obstructive sleep apnea among obese patients with type 2 diabetes: the Sleep AHEAD study. Arch Intern Med 2009;169:1619–1626

81. Phelan S, Kanaya AM, Subak LL, et al.; Look AHEAD Research Group. Weight loss prevents urinary incontinence in women with type 2 diabetes: results from the Look AHEAD trial. J Urol 2012;187: 939–944

82. Williamson DA, Rejeski J, Lang W, Van Dorsten B, Fabricatore AN, Toledo K; Look AHEAD Research Group. Impact of a weight management program on health-related quality of life in overweight adults with type 2 diabetes. Arch Intern Med 2009;169:163–171

83. Estruch R, Ros E, Salas-Salvadó J, et al.; PREDIMED Study Investigators. Primary prevention of cardiovascular disease with a Mediterranean diet. N Engl J Med 2013;368:1279–1290

84. Gregg EW, Chen H, Wagenknecht LE, et al.; Look AHEAD Research Group. Association of an intensive lifestyle intervention with remission of type 2 diabetes. JAMA 2012;308:2489–2496

85. Franz MJ, VanWormer JJ, Crain AL, et al. Weight-loss outcomes: a systematic review and meta-analysis of weight-loss clinical trials with a minimum 1-year follow-up. J Am Diet Assoc 2007;107: 1755–1767

86. Warshaw, HS. Nutrition therapy for adults with type 2 diabetes. In *American Diabetes Association Guide to Nutrition Therapy for Diabetes*. Franz MJ, Evert AB, Eds. Alexandria, VA, American Diabetes Association, 2012, p. 117–142

87. Raynor HA, Jeffery RW, Ruggiero AM, Clark JM, Delahanty LM; Look AHEAD (Action for Health in Diabetes) Research Group. Weight loss strategies associated with BMI in overweight adults with type 2 diabetes at entry into the Look AHEAD (Action for Health in Diabetes) trial. Diabetes Care 2008;31: 1299–1304

88. Wheeler ML, Dunbar SA, Jaacks LM, et al. Macronutrients, food groups, and eating patterns in the management of diabetes: a systematic review of the literature, 2010. Diabetes Care 2012;35: 434–445

89. Delahanty LM, Nathan DM, Lachin JM, et al.; Diabetes Control and Complications Trial/Epidemiology of Diabetes. Association of diet with glycated hemoglobin during intensive treatment of type 1 diabetes in the Diabetes Control and Complications Trial. Am J Clin Nutr 2009;89:518–524

90. Vitolins MZ, Anderson AM, Delahanty L, et al.; Look AHEAD Research Group. Action for Health in Diabetes (Look AHEAD) trial: baseline evaluation of selected nutrients and food group intake. J Am Diet Assoc 2009;109:1367–1375

91. Oza-Frank R, Cheng YJ, Narayan KM, Gregg EW. Trends in nutrient intake among adults with diabetes in the United States: 1988-2004. J Am Diet Assoc 2009;109:1173–1178

92. Stern L, Iqbal N, Seshadri P, et al. The effects of low-carbohydrate versus conventional weight loss diets in severely obese adults: one-year follow-up of a randomized trial. Ann Intern Med 2004; 140:778–785

93. Turner-McGrievy GM, Barnard ND, Cohen J, Jenkins DJ, Gloede L, Green AA. Changes in nutrient intake and dietary quality among participants with type 2 diabetes following a low-fat vegan diet or a conventional diabetes diet for 22 weeks. J Am Diet Assoc 2008;108: 1636–1645

94. Schwerin HS, Stanton JL, Smith JL, Riley AM Jr, Brett BE. Food, eating habits, and health: a further examination of the relationship between food eating patterns and nutritional health. Am J Clin Nutr 1982;35(Suppl.):1319–1325

95. Jones-McLean EM, Shatenstein B, Whiting SJ. Dietary patterns research and its applications to nutrition policy for the prevention of chronic disease among diverse North American populations. Appl Physiol Nutr Metab 2010; 35:195–198

96. Heising ETA. The Mediterranean diet and food culture: a symposium. Eur J Clin Nutr 1993;47:1–100

97. Craig WJ, Mangels AR; American Dietetic Association. Position of the American Dietetic Association: vegetarian diets. J Am Diet Assoc 2009;109:1266–1282

98. National Heart, Lung, and Blood Institute. *Your Guide to Lowering Your Cholesterol With TLC* [Internet]. Available from http://www .nhlbi.nih.gov/health/public/heart/chol/ chol_tlc.pdf. U.S. Department of Health and Human Services, 2005 (NIH Publication No. 06-5235)

99. Harsha DW, Lin PH, Obarzanek E, Karanja NM, Moore TJ, Caballero B; DASH Collaborative Research Group. Dietary Approaches to Stop Hypertension: a summary of study results. J Am Diet Assoc 1999;99(Suppl.):S35–S39

100. Elhayany A, Lustman A, Abel R, Attal-Singer J, Vinker S. A low carbohydrate Mediterranean diet improves cardiovascular risk factors and diabetes control among overweight patients with type 2 diabetes mellitus: a 1-year prospective randomized intervention study. Diabetes Obes Metab 2010;12:204–209

101. Nicholson AS, Sklar M, Barnard ND, Gore S, Sullivan R, Browning S. Toward improved management of NIDDM: a randomized, controlled, pilot intervention using a low fat, vegetarian diet. Prev Med 1999;29:87–91

102. Tonstad S, Butler T, Yan R, Fraser GE. Type of vegetarian diet, body weight, and prevalence of type 2 diabetes. Diabetes Care 2009;32:791–796

103. Kahleova H, Matoulek M, Malinska H, et al. Vegetarian diet improves insulin resistance and oxidative stress markers more than conventional diet in subjects with type 2 diabetes. Diabet Med 2011; 28:549–559

103a. Papakonstantinou E, Triantafillidou D, Panagiotakos DB, et al. A high-protein low-fat diet is more effective in improving blood pressure and triglycerides in calorie-restricted obese individuals with newly diagnosed type 2 diabetes. Eur J Clin Nutr 2010;64: 595–602

103b. Kodama S, Saito K, Tanaka S, et al. Influence of fat and carbohydrate proportions on the metabolic profile in patients with type 2 diabetes: a meta-analysis. Diabetes Care 2009;32:959–965

104. Sacks FM, Svetkey LP, Vollmer WM, et al.; DASH-Sodium Collaborative Research Group. Effects on blood pressure of reduced dietary sodium and the Dietary Approaches to Stop Hypertension (DASH) diet. N Engl J Med 2001;344: 3–10

105. U.S. Department of Health and Human Services and U.S. Department of Agriculture. *Dietary Guidelines for Americans, 2010* [Internet]. Available from www .health.gov/dietaryguidelines/. Accessed 30 June 2011

106. Appel LJ, Moore TJ, Obarzanek E, et al.; DASH Collaborative Research Group. A clinical trial of the effects of dietary patterns on blood pressure. N Engl J Med 1997;336:1117–1124

107. Miyashita Y, Koide N, Ohtsuka M, et al. Beneficial effect of low carbohydrate in low calorie diets on visceral fat reduction in type 2 diabetic patients with obesity. Diabetes Res Clin Pract 2004;65:235–241

108. Shai I, Schwarzfuchs D, Henkin Y, et al.; Dietary Intervention Randomized Controlled Trial (DIRECT) Group. Weight loss with a low-carbohydrate, Mediterranean, or low-fat diet. N Engl J Med 2008;359:229–241

109. Jönsson T, Granfeldt Y, Ahrén B, et al. Beneficial effects of a Paleolithic diet on cardiovascular risk factors in type 2 diabetes: a randomized cross-over pilot study. Cardiovasc Diabetol 2009; 8:35

110. Khoo J, Piantadosi C, Duncan R, et al. Comparing effects of a low-energy diet and a high-protein low-fat diet on sexual and endothelial function, urinary tract symptoms, and inflammation in obese diabetic men. J Sex Med 2011;8:2868–2875

111. Jenkins DJ, Kendall CW, Banach MS, et al. Nuts as a replacement for carbohydrates in the diabetic diet. Diabetes Care 2011;34:1706–1711

112. Daly ME, Paisey R, Paisey R, et al. Short-term effects of severe dietary carbohydrate-restriction advice in type 2 diabetes—a randomized controlled trial. Diabet Med 2006;23:15–20

113. Dyson PA, Beatty S, Matthews DR. A low-carbohydrate diet is more effective in reducing body weight than healthy eating in both diabetic and non-diabetic subjects. Diabet Med 2007;24:1430–1435

114. Wolever TM, Gibbs AL, Mehling C, et al. The Canadian Trial of Carbohydrates in Diabetes (CCD), a 1-y controlled trial of low-glycemic-index dietary carbohydrate in type 2 diabetes: no effect on glycated hemoglobin but reduction in C-reactive protein. Am J Clin Nutr 2008; 87:114–125

115. Kirk JK, Graves DE, Craven TE, Lipkin EW, Austin M, Margolis KL. Restricted-carbohydrate diets in patients with type 2 diabetes: a meta-analysis. J Am Diet Assoc 2008;108:91–100

116. Iqbal N, Vetter ML, Moore RH, et al. Effects of a low-intensity intervention that prescribed a low-carbohydrate vs. a low-fat diet in obese, diabetic participants. Obesity (Silver Spring) 2010;18: 1733–1738

117. Jenkins DJ, Kendall CW, McKeown-Eyssen G, et al. Effect of a low-glycemic index or a high-cereal fiber diet on type 2 diabetes: a randomized trial. JAMA 2008;300:2742–2753

118. Jenkins DJ, Srichaikul K, Kendall CW, et al. The relation of low glycaemic index fruit consumption to glycaemic control and risk factors for coronary heart disease in type 2 diabetes. Diabetologia 2011;54:271–279

119. Jenkins DJ, Kendall CW, Augustin LS, et al. Effect of legumes as part of a low glycemic index diet on glycemic control and cardiovascular risk factors in type 2 diabetes mellitus: a randomized controlled trial. Arch Intern Med 2012;172:1653–1660

120. Thomas D, Elliott EJ. Low glycaemic index, or low glycaemic load, diets for diabetes mellitus. Cochrane Database Syst Rev 2009;1:CD006296

121. Fabricatore AN, Wadden TA, Ebbeling CB, et al. Targeting dietary fat or glycemic

load in the treatment of obesity and type 2 diabetes: a randomized controlled trial. Diabetes Res Clin Pract 2011;92:37–45

122. Brazeau AS, Mircescu H, Desjardins K, et al. Carbohydrate counting accuracy and blood glucose variability in adults with with type 1 diabetes. Diabetes Res Clin Pract 2013;99:19–23

123. Delahanty LM, Halford BN. The role of diet behaviors in achieving improved glycemic control in intensively treated patients in the Diabetes Control and Complications Trial. Diabetes Care 1993;16:1453–1458

124. Mann JI, De Leeuw I, Hermansen K, et al.; Diabetes and Nutrition Study Group (DNSG) of the European Association. Evidence-based nutritional approaches to the treatment and prevention of diabetes mellitus. Nutr Metab Cardiovasc Dis 2004;14:373–394

125. Dyson PA, Kelly T, Deakin T, et al.; Diabetes UK Nutrition Working Group. Diabetes UK evidence-based nutrition guidelines for the prevention and management of diabetes. Diabet Med 2011; 28:1282–1288

126. Franz MJ. Diabetes mellitus nutrition therapy: beyond the glycemic index. Arch Intern Med 2012;172:1660–1661

127. Thomas DE, Elliott EJ. The use of low-glycaemic index diets in diabetes control. Br J Nutr 2010;104:797–802

128. He M, van Dam RM, Rimm E, Hu FB, Qi L. Whole-grain, cereal fiber, bran, and germ intake and the risks of all-cause and cardiovascular disease-specific mortality among women with type 2 diabetes mellitus. Circulation 2010;121:2162–2168

129. Burger KN, Beulens JW, van der Schouw YT, et al. Dietary fiber, carbohydrate quality and quantity, and mortality risk of individuals with diabetes mellitus. PLoS ONE 2012;7:e43127

130. Post RE, Mainous AG 3rd, King DE, Simpson KN. Dietary fiber for the treatment of type 2 diabetes mellitus: a meta-analysis. J Am Board Fam Med 2012;25: 16–23

131. Barnard ND, Cohen J, Jenkins DJ, et al. A low-fat vegan diet and a conventional diabetes diet in the treatment of type 2 diabetes: a randomized, controlled, 74-wk clinical trial. Am J Clin Nutr 2009;89: 1588S–1596S

132. De Natale C, Annuzzi G, Bozzetto L, et al. Effects of a plant-based high-carbohydrate/ high-fiber diet versus high-monounsaturated fat/low-carbohydrate diet on postprandial lipids in type 2 diabetic patients. Diabetes Care 2009;32:2168–2173

133. Wolfram T, Ismail-Beigi F. Efficacy of high-fiber diets in the management of type 2 diabetes mellitus. Endocr Pract 2011;17:132–142

134. Slavin JL. Position of the American Dietetic Association: health implications of dietary fiber. J Am Diet Assoc 2008;108: 1716–1731

135. Bonsu NK, Johnson CS, McLeod KM. Can dietary fructans lower serum glucose? J Diabetes 2011;3:58–66

136. Sievenpiper JL, Carleton AJ, Chatha S, et al. Heterogeneous effects of fructose on blood lipids in individuals with type 2 diabetes: systematic review and meta-analysis of experimental trials in humans. Diabetes Care 2009;32:1930–1937

137. Livesey G, Taylor R. Fructose consumption and consequences for glycation, plasma triacylglycerol, and body weight: meta-analyses and meta-regression models of intervention studies. Am J Clin Nutr 2008;88:1419–1437

138. Cozma AI, Sievenpiper JL, de Souza RJ, et al. Effect of fructose on glycemic control in diabetes: a systematic review and meta-analysis of controlled feeding trials. Diabetes Care 2012;35:1611–1620

139. Husband AC, Crawford S, McCoy LA, Pacaud D. The effectiveness of glucose, sucrose, and fructose in treating hypoglycemia in children with type 1 diabetes. Pediatr Diabetes 2010;11:154–158

140. Schulze MB, Manson JE, Ludwig DS, et al. Sugar-sweetened beverages, weight gain, and incidence of type 2 diabetes in young and middle-aged women. JAMA 2004;292:927–934

141. Malik VS, Popkin BM, Bray GA, Després JP, Willett WC, Hu FB. Sugar-sweetened beverages and risk of metabolic syndrome and type 2 diabetes: a meta-analysis. Diabetes Care 2010;33:2477–2483

142. Stanhope KL, Schwarz JM, Keim NL, et al. Consuming fructose-sweetened, not glucose-sweetened, beverages increases visceral adiposity and lipids and decreases insulin sensitivity in overweight/obese humans. J Clin Invest 2009;119: 1322–1334

143. Dhingra R, Sullivan L, Jacques PF, et al. Soft drink consumption and risk of developing cardiometabolic risk factors and the metabolic syndrome in middle-aged adults in the community. Circulation 2007;116:480–488

144. Nettleton JA, Lutsey PL, Wang Y, Lima JA, Michos ED, Jacobs DR Jr. Diet soda intake and risk of incident metabolic syndrome and type 2 diabetes in the Multi-Ethnic Study of Atherosclerosis (MESA). Diabetes Care 2009;32:688–694

145. U.S. Department of Agriculture. Nutritive and Nonnutritive Sweetener Resources [Internet], 2013. Available from http://fnic .nal.usda.gov/food-composition/nutritive-and-nonnutritive-sweetener-resources. National Agricultural Library, Food and Nutrition Information Center. Accessed 13 August 2013

146. Gardner C, Wylie-Rosett J, Gidding SS, et al.; American Heart Association Nutrition Committee of the Council on Nutrition, Physical Activity and Metabolism, Council on Arteriosclerosis, Thrombosis and Vascular Biology, Council on Cardiovascular Disease in the Young; American Diabetes Association. Nonnutritive sweeteners: current use and health perspectives: a scientific statement from the American Heart Association and the American Diabetes Association. Diabetes Care 2012;35:1798–1808

147. Wiebe N, Padwal R, Field C, Marks S, Jacobs R, Tonelli M. A systematic review on the effect of sweeteners on glycemic response and clinically relevant outcomes. BMC Med 2011;9:123

148. Gannon MC, Nuttall FQ, Saeed A, Jordan K, Hoover H. An increase in dietary protein improves the blood glucose response in persons with type 2 diabetes. Am J Clin Nutr 2003;78:734–741

149. Wycherley TP, Noakes M, Clifton PM, Cleanthous X, Keogh JB, Brinkworth GD. A high-protein diet with resistance exercise training improves weight loss and body composition in overweight and obese patients with type 2 diabetes. Diabetes Care 2010;33:969–976

150. Parker B, Noakes M, Luscombe N, Clifton P. Effect of a high-protein, high-monounsaturated fat weight loss diet on glycemic control and lipid levels in type 2 diabetes. Diabetes Care 2002;25:425–430

151. Brinkworth GD, Noakes M, Parker B, Foster P, Clifton PM. Long-term effects of advice to consume a high-protein, low-fat diet, rather than a conventional weight-loss diet, in obese adults with type 2 diabetes: one-year follow-up of a randomised trial. Diabetologia 2004;47: 1677–1686

152. Pijls LT, de Vries H, van Eijk JT, Donker AJ. Protein restriction, glomerular filtration rate and albuminuria in patients with type 2 diabetes mellitus: a randomized trial. Eur J Clin Nutr 2002;56: 1200–1207

153. Meloni C, Tatangelo P, Cipriani S, et al. Adequate protein dietary restriction in diabetic and nondiabetic patients with chronic renal failure. J Ren Nutr 2004; 14:208–213

154. Hansen HP, Tauber-Lassen E, Jensen BR, Parving HH. Effect of dietary protein restriction on prognosis in patients with diabetic nephropathy. Kidney Int 2002; 62:220–228

155. Dussol B, Iovanna C, Raccah D, et al. A randomized trial of low-protein diet in type 1 and in type 2 diabetes mellitus patients with incipient and overt nephropathy. J Ren Nutr 2005;15:398–406

156. Gross JL, Zelmanovitz T, Moulin CC, et al. Effect of a chicken-based diet on renal function and lipid profile in patients with type 2 diabetes: a randomized

crossover trial. Diabetes Care 2002;25:
645–651

157. Pan Y, Guo LL, Jin HM. Low-protein diet for diabetic nephropathy: a meta-analysis of randomized controlled trials. Am J Clin Nutr 2008;88:660–666

158. Robertson L, Waugh N, Robertson A. Protein restriction for diabetic renal disease. Cochrane Database Syst Rev 2007;4: CD002181

159. Teixeira SR, Tappenden KA, Carson L, et al. Isolated soy protein consumption reduces urinary albumin excretion and improves the serum lipid profile in men with type 2 diabetes mellitus and nephropathy. J Nutr 2004;134:1874–1880

160. Azadbakht L, Atabak S, Esmaillzadeh A. Soy protein intake, cardiorenal indices, and C-reactive protein in type 2 diabetes with nephropathy: a longitudinal randomized clinical trial. Diabetes Care 2008;31:648–654

161. Gannon MC, Nuttall JA, Damberg G, Gupta V, Nuttall FQ. Effect of protein ingestion on the glucose appearance rate in people with type 2 diabetes. J Clin Endocrinol Metab 2001;86:1040–1047

162. Papakonstantinou E, Triantafillidou D, Panagiotakos DB, Iraklianou S, Berdanier CD, Zampelas A. A high protein low fat meal does not influence glucose and insulin responses in obese individuals with or without type 2 diabetes. J Hum Nutr Diet 2010;23:183–189

163. Nordt TK, Besenthal I, Eggstein M, Jakober B. Influence of breakfasts with different nutrient contents on glucose, C peptide, insulin, glucagon, triglycerides, and GIP in non-insulin-dependent diabetics. Am J Clin Nutr 1991;53:155–160

164. Nuttall FQ, Mooradian AD, Gannon MC, Billington C, Krezowski P. Effect of protein ingestion on the glucose and insulin response to a standardized oral glucose load. Diabetes Care 1984;7:465–470

165. Gray RO, Butler PC, Beers TR, Kryshak EJ, Rizza RA. Comparison of the ability of bread versus bread plus meat to treat and prevent subsequent hypoglycemia in patients with insulin-dependent diabetes mellitus. J Clin Endocrinol Metab 1996;81:1508–1511

166. Peters AL, Davidson MB. Protein and fat effects on glucose responses and insulin requirements in subjects with insulin-dependent diabetes mellitus. Am J Clin Nutr 1993;58:555–560

167. Institute of Medicine. *Dietary Reference Intakes for Energy, Carbohydrate, Fiber, Fat, Fatty Acids, Cholesterol, Protein, and Amino Acids.* Washington, DC, National Academies Press, 2002

168. Ros E. Dietary cis-monounsaturated fatty acids and metabolic control in type 2 diabetes. Am J Clin Nutr 2003;78 (Suppl.):617S–625S

169. Schwingshackl L, Strasser B, Hoffmann G. Effects of monounsaturated fatty acids on

glycaemic control in patients with abnormal glucose metabolism: a systematic review and meta-analysis. Ann Nutr Metab 2011;58:290–296

170. Itsiopoulos C, Brazionis L, Kaimakamis M, et al. Can the Mediterranean diet lower HbA1c in type 2 diabetes? Results from a randomized cross-over study. Nutr Metab Cardiovasc Dis 2011;21: 740–747

171. Tanasescu M, Cho E, Manson JE, Hu FB. Dietary fat and cholesterol and the risk of cardiovascular disease among women with type 2 diabetes. Am J Clin Nutr 2004;79:999–1005

172. Brunerova L, Smejkalova V, Potockova J, Andel M. A comparison of the influence of a high-fat diet enriched in monounsaturated fatty acids and conventional diet on weight loss and metabolic parameters in obese non-diabetic and type 2 diabetic patients. Diabet Med 2007;24: 533–540

173. Academy of Nutrition and Dietetics Evidence Analysis Library. Available from http://andevidencelibrary.com/template.cfm?template=guide_summary&key= 2984#supportevidence [Internet], 2011

174. Harris WS, Mozaffarian D, Rimm E, et al. Omega-6 fatty acids and risk for cardiovascular disease: a science advisory from the American Heart Association Nutrition Subcommittee of the Council on Nutrition, Physical Activity, and Metabolism; Council on Cardiovascular Nursing; and Council on Epidemiology and Prevention. Circulation 2009;119:902–907

175. Crochemore IC, Souza AF, de Souza AC, Rosado EL. ω-3 Polyunsaturated fatty acid supplementation does not influence body composition, insulin resistance, and lipemia in women with type 2 diabetes and obesity. Nutr Clin Pract 2012;27:553–560

176. Bot M, Pouwer F, Assies J, Jansen EH, Beekman AT, de Jonge P. Supplementation with eicosapentaenoic omega-3 fatty acid does not influence serum brain-derived neurotrophic factor in diabetes mellitus patients with major depression: a randomized controlled pilot study. Neuropsychobiology 2011; 63:219–223

177. Mas E, Woodman RJ, Burke V, et al. The omega-3 fatty acids EPA and DHA decrease plasma F(2)-isoprostanes: results from two placebo-controlled interventions. Free Radic Res 2010;44:983–990

178. Stirban A, Nandrean S, Götting C, et al. Effects of n-3 fatty acids on macro- and microvascular function in subjects with type 2 diabetes mellitus. Am J Clin Nutr 2010;91:808–813

179. Wong CY, Yiu KH, Li SW, et al. Fish-oil supplement has neutral effects on vascular and metabolic function but improves renal function in patients with type 2 diabetes mellitus. Diabet Med 2010;27:54–60

180. Malekshahi Moghadam A, Saedisomeolia A, Djalali M, Djazayery A, Pooya S, Sojoudi F. Efficacy of omega-3 fatty acid supplementation on serum levels of tumour necrosis factor-alpha, C-reactive protein and interleukin-2 in type 2 diabetes mellitus patients. Singapore Med J 2012;53:615–619

181. Taylor CG, Noto AD, Stringer DM, Froese S, Malcolmson L. Dietary milled flaxseed and flaxseed oil improve n-3 fatty acid status and do not affect glycemic control in individuals with well-controlled type 2 diabetes. J Am Coll Nutr 2010;29:72–80

182. Holman RR, Paul S, Farmer A, Tucker L, Stratton IM, Neil HA; Atorvastatin in Factorial with Omega-3 EE90 Risk Reduction in Diabetes Study Group. Atorvastatin in Factorial with Omega-3 EE90 Risk Reduction in Diabetes (AFORRD): a randomised controlled trial. Diabetologia 2009;52:50–59

183. Kromhout D, Geleijnse JM, de Goede J, et al. n-3 Fatty acids, ventricular arrhythmia-related events, and fatal myocardial infarction in postmyocardial infarction patients with diabetes. Diabetes Care 2011;34: 2515–2520

184. Bosch J, Gerstein HC, Dagenais GR, et al.; ORIGIN Trial Investigators. n-3 Fatty acids and cardiovascular outcomes in patients with dysglycemia. N Engl J Med 2012;367:309–318

185. Karlström BE, Järvi AE, Byberg L, Berglund LG, Vessby BO. Fatty fish in the diet of patients with type 2 diabetes: comparison of the metabolic effects of foods rich in n-3 and n-6 fatty acids. Am J Clin Nutr 2011;94:26–33

186. Rivellese AA, Giacco R, Annuzzi G, et al. Effects of monounsaturated vs. saturated fat on postprandial lipemia and adipose tissue lipases in type 2 diabetes. Clin Nutr 2008;27:133–141

187. Academy of Nutrition and Dietetics Evidence Analysis Library. Disorders of Lipid Metabolism (DLM) and Plant Stanols and Sterols [Internet], 2004. Available from http://andevidencelibrary.com/template.cfm?key=2986&auth=1. Accessed 8 April 2013

188. Hallikainen M, Lyyra-Laitinen T, Laitinen T, Moilanen L, Miettinen TA, Gylling H. Effects of plant stanol esters on serum cholesterol concentrations, relative markers of cholesterol metabolism and endothelial function in type 1 diabetes. Atherosclerosis 2008;199:432–439

189. Hallikainen M, Kurl S, Laakso M, Miettinen TA, Gylling H. Plant stanol esters lower LDL cholesterol level in statin-treated subjects with type 1 diabetes by interfering the absorption and synthesis of cholesterol. Atherosclerosis 2011;217:473–478

190. Lee YM, Haastert B, Scherbaum W, Hauner H. A phytosterol-enriched spread

improves the lipid profile of subjects with type 2 diabetes mellitus—a randomized controlled trial under free-living conditions. Eur J Nutr 2003;42:111–117

191. Lau VW, Journoud M, Jones PJ. Plant sterols are efficacious in lowering plasma LDL and non-HDL cholesterol in hypercholesterolemic type 2 diabetic and nondiabetic persons. Am J Clin Nutr 2005;81:1351–1358

192. Yoshida M, Vanstone CA, Parsons WD, Zawistowski J, Jones PJ. Effect of plant sterols and glucomannan on lipids in individuals with and without type II diabetes. Eur J Clin Nutr 2006;60:529–537

193. Sesso HD, Christen WG, Bubes V, et al. Multivitamins in the prevention of cardiovascular disease in men: the Physicians' Health Study II randomized controlled trial. JAMA 2012;308:1751–1760

194. Macpherson H, Pipingas A, Pase MP. Multivitamin-multimineral supplementation and mortality: a meta-analysis of randomized controlled trials. Am J Clin Nutr 2013;97:437–444

195. Mooradian AD, Morley JE. Micronutrient status in diabetes mellitus. Am J Clin Nutr 1987;45:877–895

196. Franz MJ, Bantle JP, Beebe CA, et al. Evidence-based nutrition principles and recommendations for the treatment and prevention of diabetes and related complications. Diabetes Care 2002;25:148–198

197. Stampfer MJ, Hennekens CH, Manson JE, Colditz GA, Rosner B, Willett WC. Vitamin E consumption and the risk of coronary disease in women. N Engl J Med 1993;328:1444–1449

198. Yochum LA, Folsom AR, Kushi LH. Intake of antioxidant vitamins and risk of death from stroke in postmenopausal women. Am J Clin Nutr 2000;72:476–483

199. Hasanain B, Mooradian AD. Antioxidant vitamins and their influence in diabetes mellitus. Curr Diab Rep 2002;2:448–456

200. Lonn E, Yusuf S, Hoogwerf B, et al.; HOPE Study; MICRO-HOPE Study. Effects of vitamin E on cardiovascular and microvascular outcomes in high-risk patients with diabetes: results of the HOPE study and MICRO-HOPE substudy. Diabetes Care 2002;25:1919–1927

201. Miller ER 3rd, Pastor-Barriuso R, Dalal D, Riemersma RA, Appel LJ, Guallar E. Meta-analysis: high-dosage vitamin E supplementation may increase all-cause mortality. Ann Intern Med 2005;142:37–46

202. Belch J, MacCuish A, Campbell I, et al. The prevention of progression of arterial disease and diabetes (POPADAD) trial: factorial randomised placebo controlled trial of aspirin and antioxidants in patients with diabetes and asymptomatic peripheral arterial disease. BMJ 2008; 337:a1840

203. Kataja-Tuomola MK, Kontto JP, Männistö S, Albanes D, Virtamo JR. Effect of alpha-tocopherol and beta-carotene supplementation on macrovascular complications and total mortality from diabetes: results of the ATBC Study. Ann Med 2010;42:178–186

204. Balk EM, Tatsioni A, Lichtenstein AH, Lau J, Pittas AG. Effect of chromium supplementation on glucose metabolism and lipids: a systematic review of randomized controlled trials. Diabetes Care 2007;30:2154–2163

205. Rodríguez-Morán M, Guerrero-Romero F. Oral magnesium supplementation improves insulin sensitivity and metabolic control in type 2 diabetic subjects: a randomized double-blind controlled trial. Diabetes Care 2003;26:1147–1152

206. de Valk HW, Verkaaik R, van Rijn HJ, Geerdink RA, Struyvenberg A. Oral magnesium supplementation in insulin-requiring type 2 diabetic patients. Diabet Med 1998;15:503–507

207. Jorde R, Figenschau Y. Supplementation with cholecalciferol does not improve glycaemic control in diabetic subjects with normal serum 25-hydroxyvitamin D levels. Eur J Nutr 2009;48:349–354

208. Patel P, Poretsky L, Liao E. Lack of effect of subtherapeutic vitamin D treatment on glycemic and lipid parameters in type 2 diabetes: a pilot prospective randomized trial. J Diabetes 2010;2:36–40

209. Parekh D, Sarathi V, Shivane VK, Bandgar TR, Menon PS, Shah NS. Pilot study to evaluate the effect of short-term improvement in vitamin D status on glucose tolerance in patients with type 2 diabetes mellitus. Endocr Pract 2010;16:600–608

210. Nikooyeh B, Neyestani TR, Farvid M, et al. Daily consumption of vitamin D- or vitamin D + calcium-fortified yogurt drink improved glycemic control in patients with type 2 diabetes: a randomized clinical trial. Am J Clin Nutr 2011;93:764–771

211. Soric MM, Renner ET, Smith SR. Effect of daily vitamin D supplementation on HbA1c in patients with uncontrolled type 2 diabetes mellitus: a pilot study. J Diabetes 2012;4:104–105

212. Leach MJ, Kumar S. Cinnamon for diabetes mellitus. Cochrane Database Syst Rev 2012;9:CD007170

213. Yeh GY, Eisenberg DM, Kaptchuk TJ, Phillips RS. Systematic review of herbs and dietary supplements for glycemic control in diabetes. Diabetes Care 2003; 26:1277–1294

214. Tariq SH. Herbal therapies. Clin Geriatr Med 2004;20:237–257

215. Mackenzie T, Brooks B, O'Connor G. Beverage intake, diabetes, and glucose control of adults in America. Ann Epidemiol 2006;16:688–691

216. Kerr D, Cheyne E, Thomas P, Sherwin R. Influence of acute alcohol ingestion on the hormonal responses to modest hypoglycaemia in patients with type 1 diabetes. Diabet Med 2007;24:312–316

217. Shai I, Wainstein J, Harman-Boehm I, et al. Glycemic effects of moderate alcohol intake among patients with type 2 diabetes: a multicenter, randomized, clinical intervention trial. Diabetes Care 2007; 30:3011–3016

218. Ahmed AT, Karter AJ, Warton EM, Doan JU, Weisner CM. The relationship between alcohol consumption and glycemic control among patients with diabetes: the Kaiser Permanente Northern California Diabetes Registry. J Gen Intern Med 2008; 23:275–282

219. Bantle AE, Thomas W, Bantle JP. Metabolic effects of alcohol in the form of wine in persons with type 2 diabetes mellitus. Metabolism 2008;57:241–245

220. Tanasescu M, Hu FB, Willett WC, Stampfer MJ, Rimm EB. Alcohol consumption and risk of coronary heart disease among men with type 2 diabetes mellitus. J Am Coll Cardiol 2001;38:1836–1842

221. Howard AA, Arnsten JH, Gourevitch MN. Effect of alcohol consumption on diabetes mellitus: a systematic review. Ann Intern Med 2004;140:211–219

222. Beulens JW, Algra A, Soedamah-Muthu SS, Visseren FL, Grobbee DE, van der Graaf Y; SMART Study Group. Alcohol consumption and risk of recurrent cardiovascular events and mortality in patients with clinically manifest vascular disease and diabetes mellitus: the Second Manifestations of ARTerial (SMART) disease study. Atherosclerosis 2010;212:281–286

223. Nakamura Y, Ueshima H, Kadota A, et al.; NIPPON DATA80 Research Group. Alcohol intake and 19-year mortality in diabetic men: NIPPON DATA80. Alcohol 2009;43:635–641

224. Koppes LL, Dekker JM, Hendriks HF, Bouter LM, Heine RJ. Meta-analysis of the relationship between alcohol consumption and coronary heart disease and mortality in type 2 diabetic patients. Diabetologia 2006;49:648–652

225. Richardson T, Weiss M, Thomas P, Kerr D. Day after the night before: influence of evening alcohol on risk of hypoglycemia in patients with type 1 diabetes. Diabetes Care 2005;28:1801–1802

226. Lange J, Arends J, Willms B. Alcohol-induced hypoglycemia in type I diabetic patients. Med Klin (Munich) 1991;86:551–554 [in German]

227. Burge MR, Zeise TM, Sobhy TA, Rassam AG, Schade DS. Low-dose ethanol predisposes elderly fasted patients with type 2 diabetes to sulfonylurea-induced low blood glucose. Diabetes Care 1999;22:2037–2043

228. Suckling RJ, He FJ, Macgregor GA. Altered dietary salt intake for preventing and treating diabetic kidney disease. Cochrane Database Syst Rev 2010;12:CD006763

229. Bray GA, Vollmer WM, Sacks FM, Obarzanek E, Svetkey LP, Appel LJ; DASH Collaborative Research Group. A further subgroup analysis of the effects of the DASH diet and three dietary sodium levels on blood pressure: results of the DASH-Sodium Trial. Am J Cardiol 2004;94:222–227

230. Thomas MC, Moran J, Forsblom C, et al.; FinnDiane Study Group. The association between dietary sodium intake, ESRD, and all-cause mortality in patients with type 1 diabetes. Diabetes Care 2011;34:861–866

231. Ekinci EI, Clarke S, Thomas MC, et al. Dietary salt intake and mortality in patients with type 2 diabetes. Diabetes Care 2011;34:703–709

232. Institute of Medicine. *Sodium Intake in Populations: Assessment of Evidence*. Washington, DC, National Academy of Sciences, 2013

233. Maillot M, Drewnowski A. A conflict between nutritionally adequate diets and meeting the 2010 dietary guidelines for sodium. Am J Prev Med 2012;42:174–179

234. Centers for Disease Control and Prevention. CDC grand rounds: dietary sodium reduction - time for choice. MMWR Morb Mortal Wkly Rep 2012; 61:89–91

235. Appel LJ, Frohlich ED, Hall JE, et al. The importance of population-wide sodium reduction as a means to prevent cardiovascular disease and stroke: a call to action from the American Heart Association. Circulation 2011;123:1138–1143

236. World Health Organization. Guideline: Sodium intake for adults and children, 2012. Geneva, World Health Organization. Available from http://www.who.int/nutrition/publications/guidelines/sodium_intake_printversion.pdf. Accessed 22 September 2013

237. Institute of Medicine. *Strategies to Reduce Sodium Intake in the United States*. Washington, DC, National Academies Press, 2010

238. Spahn JM, Reeves RS, Keim KS, et al. State of the evidence regarding behavior change theories and strategies in nutrition counseling to facilitate health and food behavior change. J Am Diet Assoc 2010;110:879–891

239. Cryer PE, Fisher JN, Shamoon H. Hypoglycemia. Diabetes Care 1994;17:734–755

240. Wirfält E, Drake I, Wallstrom P. What do review papers conclude about food and dietary patterns? Food Nutr Res. 4 March 2013 [Epub ahead of print]

241. Kattelmann KK, Conti K, Ren C. The medicine wheel nutrition intervention: a diabetes education study with the Cheyenne River Sioux Tribe. J Am Diet Assoc 2009;109:1532–1539

242. Mian SI, Brauer PM. Dietary education tools for South Asians with diabetes. Can J Diet Pract Res 2009;70:28–35

243. Schillinger D, Grumbach K, Piette J, et al. Association of health literacy with diabetes outcomes. JAMA 2002;288:475–482

244. Cavanaugh K, Huizinga MM, Wallston KA, et al. Association of numeracy and diabetes control. Ann Intern Med 2008; 148:737–746

245. Pan L, Sherry B, Njai R, Blanck HM. Food insecurity is associated with obesity among US adults in 12 states. J Acad Nutr Diet 2012;112:1403–1409

246. Grimm KA, Foltz JL, Blanck HM, Scanlon KS. Household income disparities in fruit and vegetable consumption by state and territory: results of the 2009 Behavioral Risk Factor Surveillance System. J Acad Nutr Diet 2012;112: 2014–2021

Dietary Supplements for Diabetes Are Decidedly Popular: Help Your Patients Decide

Laura Shane-McWhorter, PharmD, BCPS, BC-ADM, CDE, FASCP, FAADE

According to the National Health and Nutrition Examination Study 2003–2006, about half of all Americans use supplements, spending $14.8 billion annually.[1,2] Various reports describe supplement use by people with diabetes. The National Health Interview Survey reported that 22% of diabetes patients use herbal products.[3] A survey of adult patients with diabetes found that 67% were using some type of vitamin or supplement.[4] Another survey of parents of children with type 1 diabetes found that different modalities and supplements were being used, including aloe vera and cinnamon.[5] Ethnic group differences may partially determine the use of supplements. For example, many Hispanics use herbs such as nopal or aloe vera, and Asians may use other products.[6] A review of medication histories of 459 individuals with diabetes indicated that 55% use a supplement on a daily basis.[7]

Although there may be many explanations for why patients with diabetes take supplements, increased costs of medications and provider visits is one likely reason that individuals may seek more easily accessible supplement products.[7] Other factors may also influence supplement use, including a desire to avoid adverse effects of traditional medications, the belief that supplements are "natural," the realization that traditional treatments are unable to "cure" diseases, and the powerful suggestions of friends, family members, or coworkers.[8] Diabetes severity and duration may also influence supplement use.[9]

Dietary supplements are used to lower glucose or to treat comorbidities such as hypertension and hyperlipidemia. Numerous supplements have been used for diabetes.[10] Widely used and much discussed in the literature are products such as aloe vera, bitter melon, chromium, gymnema sylvestre, fenugreek, ginseng, and nopal. More recently, information has emerged about the use of cinnamon and coenzyme Q10, as well as less well-known but increasingly popular products, including benfotiamine, berberine, hibiscus, mulberry, turmeric, and vinegar.

Diabetes clinicians should become familiar with these products and provide evidence-based information to their patients, but they must also caution patients that long-term safety information is not available. More than half of Class 1 drug recalls in the United States involve supplements. Class 1 recalls are for products for which there is a reasonable probability that use may result in serious adverse health outcomes or possibly death.[11] A report on vitamins and supplements in the September 2012 issue of *Consumer Reports* stated that > 6,300 serious adverse events involving supplements were reported to the U.S. Food and Drug Administration (FDA) between 2007 and 2012; these reports involved emergency room visits, hospitalizations, and 115 deaths.[12]

Benfotiamine (Other Names: Vitamin B1, Allithiamines)
People with neuropathy may have a thiamine deficiency.[13] Different neurological disorders, including diabetes and alcohol-related neuropathy, have been treated with vitamin B1 (thiamine).

Diabetes Spectrum • November 2013 • 26:259-266

Although B1 is sold as a supplement, clinicians are reminded that it is an important vitamin. However, thiamine is not well absorbed, and high doses are needed for successful treatment. Benfotiamine, a fat-soluble form of thiamine, provides much higher blood and tissue levels and thus may be a more effective form.[14] Benfotiamine is also manufactured in combination with other B vitamins as well as alpha lipoic acid. Another name for this group of vitamins is allithiamines because they are found in the Allium vegetable family, including garlic and onions.[14] Benfotiamine has been used for diabetes-related neuropathy in both type 1 and type 2 diabetes.

Some studies of benfotiamine have had an open-label design, whereas others were randomized controlled trials (RCTs). One open-label, 6-week study in 36 patients with type 1 or type 2 diabetes looked at different doses of benfotiamine in combination with B vitamins. Although all groups had beneficial effects, the best results were reported in patients taking the highest dose ($P < 0.01$ for all parameters compared to baseline).[15] Another open-label, 3-month study in 45 people with type 1 or type 2 diabetes compared benfotiamine (combined with other B vitamins) to a conventional B vitamin control group. Although improvement occurred in both groups, the benfotiamine group had significant neuropathic pain relief ($P < 0.001$) and an improved vibration perception threshold.[16] A short, 3-week randomized trial reported improved neuropathy symptoms ($P < 0.05$) in 40 patients with type 1 or type 2 diabetes.[17] A randomized, 6-week study in 133 patients with type 1 or type 2 diabetes compared two doses of benfotiamine to placebo. The neuropathy symptom score was significant in the per protocol population ($P = 0.033$) but not in the intention-to-treat population.[18] A randomized, 12-week study in 24 patients with type 1 or type 2 diabetes comparing a benfotiamine plus a vitamin B6 and B12 combination to placebo used higher benfotiamine doses for 2 weeks and then a lower dose for 10 weeks. The benfotiamine group had improved vibration perception threshold scores in the metacarpal and metatarsal nerves, although the results were not significant. The benfotiamine group also had improved nerve conduction velocity in the peroneal nerve ($P = 0.006$) but not the median nerve.[19]

Study results are not always positive. A 24-month, randomized trial in 67 patients with type 1 diabetes found no benefit with benfotiamine for peripheral nerve function.[20] However, the results of this study have been questioned by other researchers.[21]

Although benfotiamine has been highly studied for neuropathy, it has also been studied for retinopathy[22] and nephropathy.[23,24] There have been numerous studies with varying results, and study designs were not always optimal.

Benfotiamine enhances transketolase activity (the rate-limiting enzyme of the pentose phosphate pathway) and thus may inhibit three major pathways possibly involved in vascular damage (the diacylglycerol-protein kinase C pathway, the advanced glycation end product formation pathway, and the hexosamine pathway).[14,22] Transketolase activation also blocks hyperglycemia-induced activation of nuclear factor κB, a pro-inflammatory transcription factor.[22] It may also diminish or correct cell damage by normalizing cell division rates and decreasing apoptosis.[14]

There are no reports of major side effects, but people who are prone to allergy may experience skin rashes.[14] Certain botanical dietary supplements may decrease thiamine activity, such as betel nuts (Areca), and others, such as horsetail (Equisetum), may cause thiamine deficiency.[13] Antibiotics, oral contraceptives, diuretics, some seizure medications, and chemotherapeutic agents may decrease the body's natural thiamine levels.[13] Interestingly, metformin may also decrease thiamine activity. The doses that have been studied in people with diabetes are 300–600 mg/day, administered in divided doses (e.g., 100 or 150 mg taken three times daily).[15–19]

Berberine (*Coptis chinensis* [*Huanglian or French*])
Berberine is an isoquinoline plant alkaloid that is extracted from many different plants, including the Chinese herb *Coptis chenensis* (*Huanglian or French*), goldenseal, European barberry, tree tumeric, and others. It has been found to lower glucose when used to treat bacterial diarrhea in people with diabetes.[25] It also has lipid-lowering and weight loss effects.[26]

Berberine was compared to placebo in a 3-month study in 116 people with newly diagnosed type 2 diabetes and hyperlipidemia.[26] Subjects took 500 mg twice daily or a placebo, and there was a significant decrease in A1C and fasting and postprandial glucose in the berberine group compared to placebo ($P < 0.0001$ for each parameter). A1C decreased from 7.5 to 6.6% in the berberine group and from 7.6 to 7.3% in the placebo group. There were also significant decreases favoring berberine in LDL cholesterol ($P < 0.0001$), weight ($P = 0.034$), and systolic blood pressure ($P = 0.038$).

Another RCT evaluated two groups with type 2 diabetes, one newly diagnosed and the other poorly controlled.[27] The newly diagnosed group took berberine or metformin for 3 months. In both newly diagnosed groups, there were significant declines from baseline in A1C, fasting glucose, and postprandial glucose ($P < 0.01$ compared to baseline). A1C decreased from 9.5 to 7.5% in the berberine group and from 9.2 to 7.7% in the metformin group. Fasting glucose decreased from 191 to 123 mg/dl in the berberine group and from 179 to 129 mg/dl in the metformin group. Postprandial glucose decreased from 357 to 199 mg/dl in the berberine group and from 370 to 232 mg/dl in the metformin group. The authors did not provide a statistical analysis of the comparison between berberine and metformin, but the numbers were very similar. Patients in the poorly controlled group continued their medications (oral hypoglycemic agents or insulin), adding berberine for 3 months. A1C decreased from 8.1 to 7.3%, fasting glucose decreased from 173 to 137 mg/dl, and postprandial glucose decreased from 266 to 194 mg/dl. Decreases were all statistically significant ($P < 0.001$ for all three parameters).

A different randomized study evaluated 97 type 2 diabetes patients for 2 months.[28] Of these, 50 were randomized to berberine, 26 to metformin, and 21 to rosiglitazone. Fasting glucose and A1C decreased significantly from baseline in all three groups ($P < 0.001$ for berberine and metformin, $P < 0.01$ for rosiglitazone). A1C decreased from 8.3 to 6.8% in the berberine group, from 9.4 to 7.2% in the metformin group, and from 8.3 to 6.8% in the rosiglitazone group. Triglycerides decreased significantly only in the berberine group ($P < 0.01$).

There are a variety of theorized mechanisms for the therapeutic effects of berberine. It may enhance glucose-stimulated insulin secretion, facilitate glucose transporter type 4 translocation, exert α-glucosidase inhibitor activity, enhance adenosine monophosphate–activated protein-kinase, increase insulin receptor expression, and possibly upregulate LDL receptors.[26,28]

The main side effects of berberine are abdominal upset and constipation.[25] However, it should not be used by pregnant or lactating women or in infants because it may result in fatal kernicterus.[13] Berberine may inhibit certain cytochrome P 450 enzymes (CYP3A4) and thus increase levels of cyclosporine or other drugs metabolized by this system (i.e., certain statins and some calcium channel blockers).[13] It may also be involved in CYP2D6 metabolism.[29] Thus, caution is warranted when it is used with other agents.

Berberine was evaluated in a meta-analysis of 14 RCTs involving 1,068 subjects and found to be significantly more effective than placebo and as effective as metformin, sulfonylureas, or glitazones. It was also effective when combined with glucose-lowering agents.[25] Doses studied have been 500 mg two or three times daily.

Cinnamon (Cinnamomum cassia)

Cinnamon is a widely used supplement for diabetes and hyperlipidemia. There have been several studies of cinnamon with varying results. A meta-analysis of five clinical trials involving 282 people with diabetes indicated that doses of 1–6 g/day of cassia cinnamon resulted in decreased fasting glucose and lipids but not A1C.[30] A real-world, 3-month study in 102 people with type 2 diabetes found a significant decrease in A1C of 0.83% using 1 g/day.[31] Another smaller study in 58 people with type 2 diabetes showed a small decrease in A1C of only 0.36% with 2 g/day.[32] A Cochrane Database systematic review evaluating 10 RCTs of 577 people concluded that there is insufficient evidence to support cinnamon use.[33] A different meta-analysis of six clinical trials involving 435 people found that cinnamon improved fasting glucose by 15 mg/dl and only slightly decreased A1C in short-term studies.[34]

There is much controversy regarding the appropriate form of cinnamon, but most studies have used cassia cinnamon. The main active ingredients are procyanidin type-A polymers.[35] Various theorized mechanisms include enhanced insulin action, increased phosphorylation of the insulin receptor, and overall facilitation of the insulin signaling system,[13,35–37] as well as possible α-glucosidase inhibitor activity[38] and possible activation of peroxisome proliferator–activated receptors.[39] Cinnamon also decreases postprandial glucose.[40]

Side effects include topical allergic reactions and possible bleeding or hepatotoxicity because of cinnamon's coumarin content.[13,36] Interactions would include possible hypoglycemia if combined with secretagogues or bleeding if combined with any agent (supplement or medication) that may have anticoagulant properties.[13,36]

The most appropriate form of cinnamon is unknown, and it remains controversial whether supplements should be the whole powdered spice (possibly a combination of different types of cinnamon) or an aqueous extract.[39] Doses have ranged from 1 to 6 g/day. Overall, cinnamon

continues to be widely used and may have more benefits than drawbacks.

Coenzyme Q10 (Ubiquinone)

Coenzyme Q10 (CoQ10) is one of the most frequently used supplements in people both with and without diabetes. CoQ10 is a vitamin-like substance that is thought to be deficient in many diseases, including diabetes.[41,42]

It has been used for a variety of cardiovascular diseases, including hypertension, angina, heart failure, and statin-induced myopathy, as well as other disease states, including Parkinson's disease.[41,43,44] A recent meta-analysis of CoQ10 in heart failure showed improved ejection fraction and a slight improvement in New York Heart Association functional class. However, the analysis included few studies, and many were older evaluations in which patients were not taking agents that are now commonly used to treat heart failure.[45] In combination with selenium, CoQ10 has been shown to decrease biomarkers associated with adverse outcomes and decreased cardiovascular morality.[46]

In 34 patients with type 1 diabetes, CoQ10 resulted in a nonsignificant decline in fasting glucose (from 160 to 145 mg/dl) and A1C (from 8.04 to 7.86%).[47] It has been shown to have a statistically significant benefit in glucose control and blood pressure in 74 patients with type 2 diabetes when combined with fenofibrate (A1C decreased significantly from 7.5 to 7.2%; systolic pressure decreased by 6.1 mmHg; and diastolic pressure decreased by 2.9 mmHg).[48] Another small study in nine type 2 diabetes patients showed that CoQ10 decreased A1C from 7.1 to 6.8% ($P = 0.03$).[49]

Recent study has indicated that CoQ10 supplementation may attenuate hyperglycemia due to reduced glucose transporter type 4 protein levels caused by some statins.[50] One of the main reasons it is used in diabetes is that it reduces endothelial dysfunction.[51]

CoQ10 is produced endogenously. Also known as ubiquinone, it has a 10-carbon side chain and is similar in structure to vitamin K.[13,41] It is an antioxidant that may increase adenosine triphosphate production, scavenge oxygen free radicals, and stabilize membranes.[13,41,43]

CoQ10 does not exhibit serious effects in long-term trials. The most serious drug interaction may occur in patients taking warfarin because CoQ10 may decrease the International Normalized Ratio due to its structural similarity to vitamin K.[13,41] It may also decrease adriamycin-induced cardiotoxicity and potentially produce additive blood pressure–lowering effects with antihypertensives or additive hypoglycemia with secretagogues.[13,41] Overall, doses have ranged from 100 to 600 mg/day.

Although the exact role of CoQ10 in diabetes is unknown, it may benefit the cardiovascular risk factors that plague patients with diabetes. Fortunately, it has demonstrated long-term safety.

Hibiscus (Hibiscus sabdariffa L.)

Hibiscus is a shrub that bears brightly colored flowers. In patients with or without diabetes, its bloom is used to make tea as a treatment for hypertension and hyperlipidemia. This product is known by a variety of names, including "hibiscus tea," "roselle," "agua de Jamaica," "sour tea," and others.[52]

Hibiscus flowers and tea sachets steeped in water have shown blood pressure–lowering effects. In comparison to ACE inhibitors, hibiscus was as effective as captopril, but less effective than lisinopril in lowering blood pressure.[53,54] In a 4-week comparison of hibiscus tea and black tea, 27 people with type 2 diabetes and hypertension who took hibiscus experienced a significant decrease in blood pressure (from 134.4 to 112.7 mmHg), whereas 26 in the comparison group had an increase in blood pressure (from 118.6 to 127.3 mmHg) ($P < 0.001$ for hibiscus versus black tea).[55] In the same 27 people with type 2 diabetes, LDL cholesterol decreased from 137.5 to 128.5 mg/dl, whereas the 26 in the comparison group had an increase in LDL ($P < 0.003$ for hibiscus vs. black tea).[56]

Two reviews of hibiscus have concluded that evidence favoring its use is inconclusive and recommended more study.[54,57]

The active chemical constituents of hibiscus include anthocyanins (including delphinidin-3-sambubioside and cyanidin-3-sambubioside)[52] and polyphenols[53] that may exert the antihypertensive effects through ACE inhibition and vasorelaxation,[52] as well as through diuretic properties. Lipid-lowering effects are attributed to the polyphenol content and may be the result of inhibition of LDL cholesterol oxidation.[53] Possible drug interactions include decreased elimination half-life of diclofenac,[58] increased retention of hydrochlorothiazide when co-administered,[59] and enhanced acetaminophen elimination.[60]

Hibiscus is used as a tea, and there are no standardized doses. Steeping the flowers in boiling water has been described,[53] but there are also commercially available tea bags or sachets that are steeped in water for a few minutes.[13]

Overall, the benefits are mainly for mild hypertension, shown in trials that were small in number of patients, of short duration, and suboptimal in study design. However, better designed trials are emerging,[52] and the glucose-lowering effects of hibiscus are being studied.[61]

When patients report that they use "teas" to treat their diseases, clinicians should ask patients about the specific teas or other products they use because hibiscus may be among them. Hispanic patients often report "agua de Jamaica" as a commonly used beverage, and they may not recognize the term "hibiscus."

Mulberry (Morus alba)

Mulberry leaf tea and extract have been widely used in Asia for diabetes. A 30-day study in 24 people with type 2 diabetes compared mulberry to a sulfonylurea. Mulberry significantly decreased fasting glucose from 153 to 110 mg/dl ($P < 0.01$), LDL cholesterol from 102 to 79 mg/dl ($P < 0.01$), and triglycerides from 200 to 68 mg/dl ($P < 0.01$) and increased HDL cholesterol from 50 to 59 mg/dl ($P < 0.01$).[62] In another small, 30-day study, mulberry leaf was combined with propolis in 12 people with type 2 diabetes and significantly lowered

blood glucose from 202.8 to 129 mg/dl and A1C from 7.8 to 7%.[63] A different cross-over study compared 10 people with type 2 diabetes to 10 people without diabetes who received 1 g mulberry leaf before a 75-g sucrose challenge to evaluate the attenuation of increase in blood glucose. In both groups, mulberry attenuated the increase in blood glucose, and carbohydrate malabsorption was greater in the mulberry group.[64]

A proprietary mulberry leaf extract is used for diabetes. Mulberry leaf contains various active ingredients, including 1-deoxynojirimycin, fagomine, and antioxidants, and its berries contain resveratrol.[13,65] The ingredient 1-deoxynojirimycin has α-glucosidase inhibitor activity,[65] fagomine may induce insulin secretion,[66] and the antioxidants may decrease lipid peroxidation.[65]

Theoretical expected side effects would be gastrointestinal upsets similar to α-glucosidase inhibitors, and theoretical drug interactions may be additive glucose-lowering effects with secretagogues.[13]

Although not well characterized, doses used in studies have ranged from 1 g before an oral glucose tolerance test to 3 g daily. Combinations of black, green, and mulberry tea are also being used.

The overall benefit may be decreased carbohydrate absorption. Thus, mulberry may sometimes be used with a large meal to decrease postprandial glucose levels.

Turmeric (Curcuma longa)

Turmeric is a spice recognized for its anti-inflammatory medicinal properties. Because diabetes is considered an inflammatory disease, it is no surprise that research evaluating turmeric for diabetes and its comorbidities is emerging.[67] Turmeric is a perennial that grows in Southern Asia, and its roots, rhizomes, and bulbs are used. When boiled and dried, these parts turn into a bright yellow powder.[68]

One study evaluated the effect of turmeric on postprandial glucose and insulin levels in people without diabetes who were given a 75-g oral glucose tolerance test. The subjects were given 6 g of Curcuma longa or a placebo, and fingerstick glucose readings and venous samples were obtained every 15 minutes for 120 minutes. The insulin response was higher after 30 minutes ($P = 0.048$) and 60 minutes ($P = 0.033$), but there was no effect on glucose.[69] A recent evaluation determined that turmeric may have benefit in preventing type 2 diabetes. In the 9-month, randomized, double-blind, placebo-controlled trial, 240 patients with prediabetes were given 1,500 mg/day of turmeric or a placebo. At the end of the study, 16.4% of patients on placebo had developed type 2 diabetes, whereas there were no cases in those taking turmeric ($P < 0.001$). Furthermore, turmeric improved β-cell function with higher homeostatic model assessment-β, lower C-peptide, and higher adiponectin levels.[70] In 40 type 2 diabetes patients with nephropathy, a 2-month RCT showed that 1,500 mg of turmeric daily improved urinary protein excretion compared to placebo.[71] Turmeric in a lecithinized system was given to 38 people with diabetes for diabetic microangiopathy and retinopathy.[72] Microangiopathy improved, including improved veno-arteriolar response and decreased peripheral edema. Retinal edema also improved and was associated with improved visual acuity.

Curcumin, is the principal ingredient in turmeric, and is the major constituent of curry powder. The active ingredient is diferuloyl-methane, a hydrophobic polyphenol with a characteristic yellow color.[73] Turmeric exhibits α-glucosidase inhibitor activity[74] and may also exert other effects through improved β-cell function and decreased insulin resistance.[12] Turmeric has anti-inflammatory effects, inhibits nuclear factor κB,[75] and may stimulate glucagon-like peptide 1 secretion.[76] Also, because dietary turmeric is poorly absorbed, it is being manufactured in a unique formulation using nanoparticles and lipid/liposome particles to improve absorption and bioavailability.[75]

Side effects are mostly abdominal upset and allergic dermatitis, and turmeric may increase bleeding when co-administered with antiplatelet

agents such as warfarin, clopidogrel, or aspirin.[13] Also, additive hypoglycemia may occur if taken with secretagogues.[13]

Turmeric has garnered interest for its many potential therapeutic benefits for diabetes. Doses used have ranged from 1,500 mg to 6 g daily. Absorption of the active ingredient may be enhanced if it is taken with food. Because of its antiplatelet activity, patients should be counseled to stop using the supplement 2 weeks before surgery to prevent excessive bleeding.[13]

Vinegar

Many people are interested in adding vinegar to their diet. A small, randomized study of 10 patients with well-controlled type 1 diabetes evaluated the effect of vinegar on postprandial glucose. The study showed that vinegar use significantly decreased postprandial glucose by 20% after a standardized meal ($P = 0.005$).[77] A complicated, randomized, double-blind, crossover study of 38 patients with or without diabetes consisted of four sub-trials.[78] The study found that ~2 tsp of vinegar taken with meals decreased postprandial glucose by about 20%.[78] Another small, randomized trial in 27 patients with type 2 diabetes showed that vinegar resulted in a small decrease in A1C ($P = 0.018$).[79] Yet another small, randomized study in 11 people with well-controlled type 2 diabetes found that vinegar given at bedtime decreased fasting glucose ($P = 0.033$).[80]

Acetic acid is the main active chemical ingredient in vinegar.[79] The mechanism of action of vinegar in diabetes is varied. Vinegar may delay gastric emptying, inhibit disaccharide activity, and promote muscle glucose uptake.[79] It may also alter the glycolysis and hepatic gluconeogenesis cycle, which may benefit individuals who experience the "dawn phenomenon" (an early-morning increase in glucose level).[80]

Most side effects from vinegar are gastrointestinal in nature.[81] However, hypoglycemia has been reported in type 1 diabetes patients with gastroparesis.[82] Oropharyngeal inflammation and caustic esophageal injury have also been reported.[83] A

case report involving ingestion of large amounts of vinegar reported hypokalemia.[84] Drug interactions are mainly theoretical and related to the mechanism of action of vinegar. They could involve additive hypoglycemia with secretagogues or problems when used with agents that pose a hypokalemia risk, such as digoxin.[13,84]

Vinegar has aroused much interest for its potential effects in improving postprandial glucose elevations. Some authors have suggested that as little as 2 tsp of vinegar used in a salad, for example, may attenuate increased postprandial glucose.[78]

Summary

Many dietary supplements are used for diabetes and its comorbidities.[10,85,86] However, there is no exact information regarding how many people with diabetes use supplements or which supplements are most widely used. Consumer habits vary, and the popularity of various supplements may change over time. Variability in dosage forms and inconsistent information, such as the exact botanical parts that are used, as well as a lack of adequate dose-finding studies may be problematic.

Clinicians must realize that patients believe supplements are "natural," but may not know that they contain active chemical constituents with pharmacological activity and may cause adverse effects and drug interactions. There are many instances in which adverse events secondary to supplement use have been reported to the FDA and many supplements have been recalled.[11,12] Furthermore, supplements have not been unequivocally found to decrease the morbidity and mortality associated with diabetes or its comorbidities. However, there is a great amount of ongoing research, and it is important for clinicians to be unbiased and stay informed about this subject.

References

[1] Bailey RL, Gahche JJ, Lentino CV, Dwyer JT, Engel JS, Thomas PR, Betz JM, Sempos CT, Picciano MF: Dietary supplement use in the United States, 2003–2006. *J Nutr* 141:261–266, 2011

[2]Nathin RL, Barnes PM, Stussman BJ, Bloom B: Costs of complementary and alternative medicine (CAM) and frequency of visits to CAM practitioners: United States, 2007. National Health Statistics Report no 18. Hyattsville, Md., National Center for Health Statistics, 2009

[3]Kennedy J: Herb and supplement use in the U.S. adult population. *Clin Ther* 27:1847–1858, 2005

[4]Garrow D, Egede LE: Association between complementary and alternative medicine use, preventive care practices, and use of conventional medical services among adults with diabetes. *Diabetes Care* 29:15–19, 2006

[5]Dannemann K, Hecker W, Haberland H, Herbst A, Galler A, Schafer T, Brahler E, Kiess W, Kapellen TM: Use of complementary and alternative medicine in children with type 1 diabetes mellitus: prevalence, patterns of use, and costs. *Pediatr Diabetes* 9:228–235, 2008

[6]Villa-Caballero L, Morello CM, Chynoweth ME, Prieto-Rosinol A, Polonsky WH, Palinkas LA, Edelman SV: Ethnic differences in complementary and alternative medicine use among patients with diabetes. *Complement Ther Med* 18:241–248, 2010

[7]Odegard PS, Janci MM, Foepppel MP, Beach JR, Trence DL: Prevalence and correlates of dietary supplement use in individuals with diabetes mellitus at an academic diabetes care clinic. *Diabetes Educ* 37:419–425, 2011

[8]Palinkas LB, Kabongo ML, San Diego Unified Practice Research in Family Medicine Network: The use of complementary and alternative medicine by primary care patients: a SURF*NET study. *J Fam Pract* 49:1121–1130, 2000

[9]Nahin RL, Byrd-Clark D, Stussman BJ, Kalyanaraman N: Disease severity is associated with the use of complementary medicine to treat or manage type-2 diabetes: data from the 2002 and 2007 National Health Interview Survey. *BMC Complement Altern Med* 12:193, 2012 (doi: 10.1186/1472-6882-12-193)

[10]Chang CLT, Lin Y, Bartolome AP, Chen Y-C, Chiu S-C, Yang W-C: Herbal therapies for type 2 diabetes mellitus: chemistry, biology, and potential application of selected plants and compounds. *Evid Based Complement Altern Med* Article ID 378657. Available from http://dx.doi.org/10.1155/2013/378657. Accessed 25 May 2013

[11]Harel Z, Harel S, Waid R, Mamdani M, Bell CM: The frequency and characteristics of dietary supplement recalls in the United States. *JAMA Intern Med* 15:1–3, 2013

[12]ConsumerReports.org: 10 surprising dangers of vitamins and supplements: Don't assume they're safe because they're 'all natural.' Consumer Reports September 2012. Available from http://www.consumerreports.org/content/cro/en/consumer-reports-magazine/z2012/September/vitaminsSupplements.print.html. Accessed 25 May 2013

[13]Jellin JM, Gregory PJ: *Pharmacist's Letter/Prescriber's Letter Natural Medicines Comprehensive Database*. 13th ed. Stockton, Calif., Therapeutic Research Faculty, 2013

[14]Head KA: Benfotiamine. *Altern Med Rev* 11:238–242, 2006

[15]Winkler G, Pal B, Nagybeganyi E, Ory I, Porochnavec M, Kempler P: Effectiveness of different benfotiamine dosage regimens in the treatment of painful diabetic neuropathy. *Arzneimittelforschung* 49:220–224, 1999

[16]Simeonov S, Pavlova M, Mitkov M, Mincheva L, Troey D: Therapeutic efficacy of "Milgamma" in patients with painful diabetic neuropathy. *Folia Medica* 39:5–10, 1997

[17]Haupt E, Ledermann H, Kopcke W: Benfotiamine in the treatment of diabetic polyneuropathy: a three-week randomized, controlled pilot study (BEDIP Study). *Int J Clin Pharmacol Ther* 43:71–77, 2005

[18]Stracke H, Gaus W, Achenbach U, Federlin K, Bretzel RG: Benfotiamine in diabetic polyneuropathy (BENDIP): results of a randomised, double blind, placebo-controlled clinical study. *Exp Clin Endocrinol Diabetes* 116:600–605, 2008

[19]Stracke H: A benfotiamine-vitamin B combination in treatment of diabetic polyneuropathy. *Exp Clin Endocrinol Diabetes* 104:311–316, 1996

[20]Fraser DA, Diep LM, Hovden IA, Nilsen KB, Sveen KA, Seljeflot I, Hanssen KF: The effects of long-term oral benfotiamine supplementation on peripheral nerve function and inflammatory markers in patients with type 1 diabetes: a 24-month, double-blind, randomized, placebo-controlled trial. *Diabetes Care* 35:1095–1097, 2012

[21]Ziegler D, Tesfaye S, Kempler P: Comment on: Fraser et al. The effects of long-term oral benfotiamine supplementation on peripheral nerve function and inflammatory markers in patients with type 1 diabetes: a 24-month, double-blind, randomized, placebo-controlled trial. *Diabetes Care* 35:1095–1097, 2012

[22]Hammes H-P, Du X, Edelstein D, Taguchi T, Matsumura T, Ju Q, Lin J, Bierhaus A, Nawroth P, Hannak D, Neumaier M, Bergfeld R, Giardino I, Brownlee M: Benfotiamine blocks three major pathways of hyperglycemic damage and prevents experimental diabetic retinopathy. *Nat Med* 9:294–299, 2003

[23]Rabbani N, Alam SS, Riaz S, Larkin JR, Akhtar MW, Shafi T, Thornalley PJ: High-dose thiamine therapy for patients with type 2 diabetes and microalbuminuria: a randomized, double-blind placebo-controlled study. *Diabetologia* 52:208–212, 2009

[24]Alkhalaf A, Klooster A, van Oeveren W, Achenbach U, Kleefstra N, Slingerland RJ, Mijnhout GS, Bilo HJ, Gans RO, Navis GJ, Bakker SJ: A double-blind, randomized, placebo-controlled clinical trial on benfotiamine treatment in patients with diabetic nephropathy. *Diabetes Care* 33:1598–1601, 2010

[25]Dong H, Wang N, Zhao L, Lu F: Berberine in the treatment of type 2 diabetes mellitus: a systematic review and meta-analysis. *Evid Based Complement Alternat Med* 591654, 2012 (doi:10.1155/2012/591654)

[26]Zhang Y, Li X, Zou D, Liu W, Yang J, Zhu N, Huo L, Wang M, Hong J, Wu P, Ren G, Ning G: Treatment of type 2 diabetes and dyslipidemia with the natural plant alkaloid berberine. *J Clin Endocrinol Metab* 93:2559–2565, 2008

[27]Yin J, Xing H, Ye J: Efficacy of berberine in patients with type 2 diabetes mellitus. *Metabolism* 57:712–717, 2008

[28]Zhang H, Wei J, Xue R, Wu J-D, Zhao W, Wang Z-Z, Wang S-K, Zhou Z-X, Song D-Q, Wang Y-M, Pan H-N, Kong W-J, Jiang J-D: Berberine lowers blood glucose in type 2 diabetes mellitus patients through increasing insulin receptor expression. *Metabolism* 59:285–292, 2010

[29]Guo Y, Li F, Ma X, Cheng X, Zhou H, Klaassen CD: CYP2D plays a major role in berberine metabolism in liver of mice and humans. *Xenobiotica* 41:996–1005, 2011

[30]Baker WL, Gutierrez-Williams G, White CM, Kluger J, Coleman CI: Effect of cinnamon on glucose control and lipid parameters. *Diabetes Care* 31:41–43, 2008

[31]Crawford P: Effectiveness of cinnamon for lowering hemoglobin A1c in patients with type 2 diabetes: a randomized, controlled trial. *J Am Board Fam Med* 22:507–512, 2009

[32]Akilen R, Tsiami A, Devendra D, Robinson N: Glycated haemoglobin and blood pressure-lowering effect of cinnamon in multi-ethnic type 2 diabetic patients in the UK: a randomized, placebo-controlled, double-blind clinical trial. *Diabet Med* 27:1159–1167, 2010

[33]Leach MJ, Kumar S: Cinnamon for diabetes mellitus. *Cochrane Database Syst Rev* 9:CD007170, 2012 (doi:10.1002/14651858.CD007170.pub2)

[34]Akilen R, Tsiami A, Devendra D, Robinson N: Cinnamon in glycaemic control: systematic review and meta analysis. *Clin Nutr* 31:609–615, 2012

[35]Anderson RA, Broadhurst CL, Polansky MM, Schmidt WF, Khan A, Flanagan VP, Schoene NW, Graves DJ: Isolation and characterization of polyphenol type-A polymers from cinnamon with insulin-like biological activity. *J Agric Food Chem* 52:65–70, 2004

[36]Chase CK, McQueen CE: Cinnamon in diabetes mellitus. *Am J Health-Syst Pharm* 64:1033–1035, 2007

[37]Kirkham S, Akilen R, Sharma S, Tsiami A: The potential of cinnamon to reduce blood glucose levels in patients with type 2 diabetes and insulin resistance. *Diabetes Obes Metab* 11:1100–1113, 2009

[38]Kim SH, Huyn SH, Choung SY: Antidiabetic effect of cinnamon extract on blood glucose in db/db mice. *J Ethnopharmacol* 104:119–123, 2006

[39]Rafehi H, Ververis K, Karagiannis TC: Controversies surrounding the clinical

potential of cinnamon for the management of diabetes. *Diabetes Obes Metab* 14:493–499, 2012

[40]Hlebowicz J, Darwiche G, Bjorgell, Almer L-O: Effect of cinnamon on post-prandial blood glucose, gastric emptying, and satiety in healthy subjects. *Am J Clin Nutr* 85:1552–1556, 2007

[41]Pepping J: Alternative therapies: coenzyme Q10. *Am J Health-Syst Pharm* 56:519–521, 1999

[42]Villalba JM, Parrado C, Santos-Gonzalez M, Alcain FJ: Therapeutic use of coenzyme Q10 and coenzyme Q10-related compounds and formulations. *Expert Opin Investig Drugs* 19:535–554, 2010

[43]Bonakdar RA, Guarneri E: Coenzyme Q10: *Am Fam Phys* 72:1065–1070, 2005

[44]Littarru GP, Luca T: Clinical aspects of coenzyme Q10: an update. *Nutrition* 26:250–254, 2010

[45]Fotino AD, Thompson-Paul AM, Bazzano LA: Effect of coenzyme Q10 supplementation on heart failure: a meta-analysis. *Am J Clin Nutr* 97:268–275, 2013

[46]Alehagen U, Johansson P, Bjornstedt M, Rosen A, Dahlstrom U: Cardiovascular mortality and N-terminal-proBNP reduced after combined selenium and coenzyme Q10 supplementation: a 5-year prospective randomized double-blind placebo-controlled trial among elderly Swedish citizens. *Int J Cardiol* 176:1860–1866, 2013

[47]Henriksen JE, Andersen CB, Hother-Nielsen O, Vaag A, Mortensen SA, Beck-Nielsen H: Impact of ubiquinone (coenzyme Q10) treatment on glycaemic control, insulin requirement and well-being in patients with type 1 diabetes mellitus. *Diabet Med* 16:312–318, 1999

[48]Hodgson JM, Watts GF, Playford DA, Burke V, Croft KD: Coenzyme Q10 improves blood pressure and glycaemic control: a controlled trial in subjects with type 2 diabetes. *Eur J Clin Nutr* 56:1137–1142, 2002

[49]Mezawa M, Takemoto M, Onishi S, Ishibashi R, Ishikawa T, Yamaga M, Fujimoto M, Okabe E, He P, Kobayashi K, Yokote K: The reduced form of coenzyme Q10 improves glycemic control in patients with type 2 diabetes: an open label pilot study. *Biofactors* 38:416–421, 2012

[50]Ganesan S, Ito MK: Coenzyme Q10 ameliorates the reduction in GLUT4 transporter expression induced by simvastatin in 3T3-L1 adipocytes. *Metab Syndr Relat Disord* 11:251–255, 2013

[51]Hamilton SJ, Chew GT, Watts GF: Coenzyme Q10 improves endothelial dysfunction in statin-treated type 2 diabetic patients. *Diabetes Care* 32:810–812, 2009

[52]McKay DL, Chen CYO, Saltzman E, Blumberg J: Hibiscus Sabdariffa L. tea (Tisane) lowers blood pressure in prehypertensive and mildly hypertensive adults. *J Nutr* 140:298–303, 2010

[53]Hopkins AL, Lamm MG, Funk JL, Ritenbaugh C: Hibiscus sabdariffa L, in the treatment of hypertension and hyperlipidemia: a comprehensive review of animal and human studies. *Fitoterapia* 85:84–94, 2013

[54]Wahabi HA, Alansary LA, Al-Sabban AH, Glasziuo P: The effectiveness of Hibiscus sabdariffa in the treatment of hypertension: a systematic review. *Phytomedicine* 17:83–86, 2010

[55]Mozaffari-Khosravi H, Jalali-Khanabadi BA, Afkhami-Ardekani M, Fatehi F, Noori-Shadkam M: The effects of sour tea (Hibiscus sabdariffa) on hypertension in patients with type II diabetes. *J Hum Hypertens* 23:48–54, 2009

[56]Mozaffari-Khosravi H, Jalali-Khanabadi BA, Afkhami-Ardekani M, Fatehi F: Effects of sour tea (Hibiscus sabdariffa) on lipid profile and lipoproteins in patients with type II diabetes. *J Alt Compl Med* 15:899–903, 2009

[57]Ngamjarus C, Pattanittum P, Somboonporn C: Roselle for hypertension in adults. *Cochrane Database Syst Rev* 1:CD007894, 2010 (doi: 10.1002/14651858.CD007894.pub2)

[58]Fakeye TO, Adegoke AO, Omoyeni OC, Famakinde AA: Effects of water extract of Hibiscus sabdariffa, Linn (Malvaceae) 'Roselle" on excretion of a diclofenac formulation. *Phytother Res* 21:96–98, 2007

[59]Ndu OO, Nworu CS, Ehiemere CO, Ndukwe NC, Ochiogu IS: Herb-drug interaction between the extract of Hibiscus sabdariffa L. and hydrocholorothiazide in experimental animals. *J Med Food* 14:640–644, 2011

[60]Kolawole JA, Maduenyi A: Effect of zobo drink (Hibiscus sabdariffa water extract) on the pharmacokinetics of acetaminophen in human volunteers. *Eur J Drug Metab Pharmacokinet* 29:25–29, 2004

[61]Venkatesh S, Thilagavathi J, Shyam Sundar D: Anti-diabetic activity of flowers of Hibiscus rosasinensis. *Fitoterapia* 79:79–81, 2008

[62]Andallu B, Suryakanham V, Srikanthi BL, Reddy GK: Effect of mulberry (Morus indica L) therapy on plasma and erythrocyte membrane lipids in patients with type 2 diabetes. *Clin Chim Acta* 314:47–53, 2001

[63]Murata K, Yatsunami K, Fukuda E, Onodera S, Mizukami O, Hoshino G, Kamel T: Antihyperglycemic effects of propolis mixed with mulberry leaf extract on patients with type 2 diabetes. *Altern Ther Health Med* 10:78–79, 2004

[64]Mudra M, Ercan-Fang N, Zhong L, Furne J, Levitt M: Influence of mulberry leaf extract on the blood glucose and breath hydrogen response to ingestion of 75 g sucrose by type 2 diabetic and control subjects. *Diabetes Care* 30:1272–1274, 2007

[65]Hansawasdi C, Kawabata J: α-Glucosidase inhibitory effect of mulberry (Morus alba) leaves on Caco-2. *Fitoterapia* 77:568–573, 2006

[66]Taniguchi S, Asano N, Tomino F, Miwa I: Potentiation of glucose-induced insulin secretion by fagomine, a pseudo-sugar isolated from mulberry leaves. *Horm Metab Res* 30:679–683, 1998

[67]Aggarwal BB: Targeting inflammation-induced obesity and metabolic diseases by curcumin and other nutraceuticals. *Annu Rev Nutr* 30:173–199, 2010

[68]University of Maryland Medical System: Turmeric. Available from http://www.umm.edu/altmed/articles/turmeric-000277.htm. Accessed 25 May 2013

[69]Wickenberg J, Ingemansson SL, Hlebowicz J: Effects of Curcuma longa (turmeric) on postprandial plasma glucose and insulin in healthy subjects. *Nutr J* 9:43–47, 2010

[70]Chuengsamarn S, Rattanamongkolgul S, Luechapudiporn R, Phisalaphong C, Jirawatnotai S: Curcumin extract for prevention of type 2 diabetes. *Diabetes Care* 35:2121–2127, 2012

[71]Khajehdehi P, Pakfetrat M, Javidnia K, Azad F, Malekmakan L, Nasab MH, Dehghanzadeh G: Oral supplementation of turmeric attenuates proteinuria, transforming growth factor-β and interleukin-8 levels in patients with overt type 2 diabetic nephropathy: a randomized, double-blind and placebo-controlled study. *Scand J Urol Nephrol* 45:365–370, 2011

[72]Steigerwalt R, Nebbioso M, Appendino G, Belcaro G, Ciammaichella G, Cornelli U, Luzzi R, Togni S, Dugall M, Cesarone MR, Ippolito E, Errichi BM, Ledda A, Hosoi M, Corsi M: Meriva, a lecithinized curcumin delivery system, in diabetic microangiopathy and retinopathy. *Panminerva Med* 54 (1 Suppl. 4):11–16, 2012

[73]Epstein J, Sanderon IR, MacDonald TT: Curcumin as a therapeutic agent: the evidence from in vitro, animal and human studies. *Br J Nutr* 103:1545–1557, 2010

[74]Lekshmi PC, Arimboor R, Indulekha PS, Menon AN: Turmeric (Curcuma longa L.) volatile oil inhibits key enzymes linked to type 2 diabetes. *Int J Food Sci Nutr* 63:832–834, 2012

[75]Maradana MR, Thomas R, O'Sullivan BJ: Targeted delivery of curcumin for treating type 2 diabetes. *Mol Nutr Food Res* 57:1550–1556, 2013

[76]Takikawa M, Kurimoto Y, Tusda T: Curcumin stimulates glucagon-like peptide-1 secretion in GLUTag cells via Ca2+/calmodulin-dependent kinase II activation. *Biochem Biophys Res Commun* 435:165–170, 2013

[77]Mitrou P, Raptis AE, Lambadiari V, Boutati E, Petsiou E, Spanoudi F, Papakonstantinou E, Maratou E, Economopoulos T, Dimitriadis G, Raptis SA: Vinegar decreases postprandial hyperglycemia in patients with type 1 diabetes. *Diabetes Care* 33:e27, 2010

[78]Johnston CS, Steplewska I, Long CA, Harris LN, Ryals RH: Examination of the antiglycemic properties of vinegar in healthy adults. *Ann Nutr Metab* 56:74–79, 2010

[79]Johnston CS, White AM, Kent SM: Preliminary evidence that regular vinegar ingestion favorably influences hemoglobin A1c values in individuals with type 2 diabetes mellitus. *Diabetes Res Clin Pract* 84:e15–e17, 2009

[80]White AM, Johnston CS: Vinegar ingestion at bedtime moderates waking glucose concentrations in adults with well-controlled type 2 diabetes. *Diabetes Care* 30:2814–2815, 2007

[81]Johnston CS, White AM, Kent SM: A preliminary evaluation of the safety and tolerance of medicinally ingested vinegar in individuals with type 2 diabetes. *J Med Food* 11:179–183, 2008

[82]Hlebowicz J, Darwiche G, Bjorgell O, Almer L: Effect of apple cider vinegar on delayed gastric emptying in patients with type 1 diabetes: a pilot study. *BMC Gastroenterol* 7:46, 2007

[83]Wrenn K: The perils of vinegar and the Heimlich maneuver. *Ann Emerg Med* 47:207–208, 2006

[84]Lhotta K, Hofle G, Gasser R, Finkenstedt G: Hypokalemia, hyperreninemia and osteoporosis in a patient ingesting large amounts of cider vinegar. *Nephron* 80:242–243, 1998

[85]Birdee GS, Yeh G: Complementary and alternative medicine therapies for diabetes: a clinical review. *Clinical Diabetes* 28:147–153, 2010

[86]Shane-McWhorter L: Dietary supplements for diabetes: an evaluation of commonly used products. *Diabetes Spectrum* 22:206–213, 2009

Laura Shane-McWhorter, PharmD, BCPS, BC-ADM, CDE, FASCP, FAADE, is a clinical professor in the Department of Pharmacotherapy at the University of Utah College of Pharmacy in Salt Lake City.

In Brief

Diabetes management has evolved with the presence of smartphones, offering a plethora of applications, or "apps," to assist technologically savvy users. This rapidly growing field of mobile apps has hosted a multifarious selection ranging from novice startup software to programs designed for professional use. This article reviews some crucial factors for consideration when seeking to optimize diabetes management via smartphone.

Evaluation and Evolution of Diabetes Mobile Applications: Key Factors for Health Care Professionals Seeking to Guide Patients

Ryan A. Ristau, BS, Jessica Yang, BA, and John R. White, PA-C, PharmD

According to statistics from 2011, the American Diabetes Association (ADA) estimates that 25.8 million children and adults in the United States have type 1 or type 2 diabetes.[1] Diabetes poses a heavy economic burden on the U.S. health care system, with estimated associated costs in 2007 of $174 billion.[1] Proper patient education and management are pivotal because diabetes is a progressive disease that leads to macro- and microvascular complications, including heart disease, stroke, hypertension, nephropathy, and neuropathy.

With the advent of smartphones, patients are increasingly using mobile technology through automated text messages and various applications, or "apps," to monitor their disease states. Myriad mobile apps with various features for diabetes management are now available, and the growing number of technologically savvy patients with diabetes has ratcheted up the use of these programs.

Several randomized studies have reported on the effectiveness of diabetes management using mobile app interventions.[2] One such study[3] revealed that using a smartphone app for diabetes management resulted in a statistically significant improvement in A1C in adults with type 2 diabetes.

To encourage the efficient management of diabetes and maximize the benefits of mobile apps, it is crucial for health care professionals (HCPs) to recognize and assess the needs of each patient. Patients' age, app cost, and app-specific features are key factors for HCPs to consider when recommending apps for diabetes self-management.

Factors for Consideration

Patient demographics

In 2010, an estimated 10.9 million people > 65 years of age and 215,000 people < 20 years of age in the United States had diabetes.[1] The diversity among people with diabetes imposes a challenge for HCPs to identify and address the needs of each patient, including those related to patients' age.

In the fast-paced and evolving world of technology, younger populations are often highly proficient with and adaptable to smartphones. As a result, mobile apps for Apple iOS (used in the iPhone, iPad, and iPod Touch) and Android operating systems have overwhelming popularity. More than 500 million Apple iOS and Android devices have been activated since 2007.[4]

Many software development agencies have identified the growing market in mobile apps and are developing apps to target individual disease states. A recent study[5] showed that a smartphone glucose monitoring system had significant potential for improving glucose management for adolescents with type 1 diabetes.

However, people with diabetes who are > 55 years of age and did not grow up immersed in advanced technological systems may face challenges in adopting app-based mobile technologies for diabetes management.

Although mobile apps typically are not designed to appeal to older populations, some easy-to-use apps may still be worth considering for older patients.

Technology costs

The initial cost of obtaining and activating a smartphone may be a significant barrier for patients considering mobile apps to aid in managing their diabetes. The latest version of popular smartphones using the Android or Apple iOS operating system, without a wireless service contract, can cost $500–700 per device.[6]

Wireless networks subsidize the cost of smartphones by setting up contracts, alleviating much of the initial burden by offering previous-generation models of popular phones (i.e., phones that are one model earlier than the latest version) for a fraction of their original price. A study by a mobile tracking service[7] reported that the average selling price for smartphones fell to a relatively affordable $135 in 2011. Decreasing phone prices may be one factor contributing to the estimation that nearly one in seven people worldwide are now using a smartphone.

Smartphone owners have access to an extensive selection of mobile apps. Depending on the apps' specific features, app prices vary from free to $50.

Initial fees associated with smartphone devices, service contracts, and apps may seem costly, but such investments could benefit patients by providing daily reminders and motivation for self-managing their health. Managing diabetes via mobile apps can be a practical means of improving patient adherence to glucose targets and health care goals.

Platform varieties

It has been estimated that > 322 million people in the United States owned a smartphone in 2012.[8] Platforms currently available include Apple iOS, Android, RIM BlackBerry, Symbian, and Windows.[9] As of February 2013, Android and Apple iOS are the dominant platforms in the U.S. market. A keyword search for "diabetes" conducted in April 2013 identified > 650 available apps for Apple iOS and > 1,600 for Android.

According to the market research firm Manhattan Research, > 75% of physicians use Apple iOS devices, which had the highest number of

available health-related apps in 2012.[10] Although a majority of physicians prefer Apple iOS apps, it is important to recognize that many of those apps are not available for other platforms. HCPs must explore popular apps for different operating platforms to provide recommendations appropriate for patients' specific smartphones.

Ease of use

Diabetes self-management requires patients to self-monitor medication adherence, carbohydrate intake, exercise, and blood glucose levels. HCPs want to encourage patients to self-manage their health and provide them with tools to help achieve optimal control of their diabetes. For patients to maximize apps as resources, it is crucial that the apps are easy to use.[11]

HCPs should recommend apps that are commensurate with patients' comfort level with technology and tailored to patient-specific needs. Some apps are designed with simple, easy-to-use features, whereas others offer a multitude of features for technologically savvy populations. Ease of navigation, logging, data modification, note-taking, and time-tracking should be considered based on each patient's knowledge of technology. Patients should be encouraged to continue using a new app for at least a couple of weeks before deciding whether it will work for them. Navigating through an app may become easier in time, as proficiency improves with repetition.

App Features

Blood glucose logging

Self-monitoring of blood glucose (SMBG) is recognized as an important tool for guiding management strategies and decision-making for both patients and HCPs.[12] Historically, patients have used paper log books to document their blood glucose values and report their findings to HCPs at their next scheduled appointment. Advances in blood glucose meters and mobile technology have empowered patients to record blood glucose values electronically on the go.

The ADA recommends that patients whose medication regimen includes multiple daily insulin injections or who use insulin pumps test and record their blood glucose ≥ 3 times daily.[1] Recording blood glucose values using an app that logs results may alleviate some of the burden

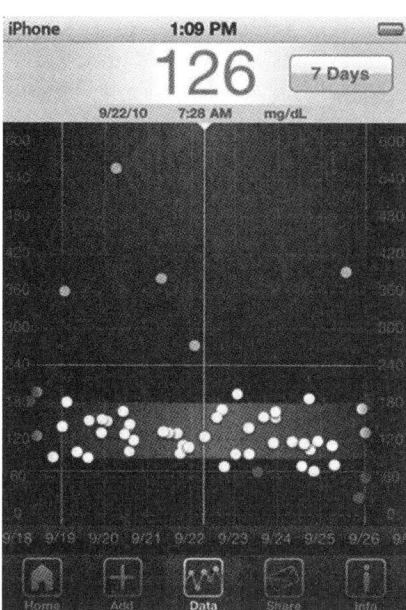

Figure 1. iBGStar's blood glucose tracking trend chart.[13]

of carrying a hard copy recording system. Some apps offer additional advantages, such as graphic displays of SMBG trends to help identify and correct hypoglycemic events linked to medications, food, diet, and exercise (Figure 1).[13]

Nutrition databases and carbohydrate tracking

Monitoring carbohydrate and caloric intake is imperative to maintain optimal glycemic control because food directly affects blood glucose levels and the amount of insulin a person needs.[14] Unhealthy food choices and large portions may lead to out-of-range blood glucose levels. Patients may benefit from using apps to help them improve their nutritional choices and monitor their carbohydrate intake.

Many apps include a feature that allows users to search food databases by typing or scanning bar codes for specific nutritional data that can be saved to the smartphone. For example, apps such as Diabetes Buddy, Diabetes Log, and Track3 offer extensive databases, allowing users to quickly look up nutritional information, including carbohydrate content and calories. Calorie Counter by MyNetDiary offers target-planning and goal-setting to help users manage their weight and caloric intake with advice from a registered dietitian.[15] A comprehensive database is also available specifically to guide people with diabetes in making healthy choices. Nutrition databases put detailed information at users' fingertips, empowering them to take charge of their health and make healthy food choices.

Tracking physical activity and weight

According to the ADA,[1] modest weight loss has been shown to improve insulin resistance and overall health. Apps that allow users to track their activity, count calories, and discover new ideas for fitness may aid weight management efforts. Learning about new fitness activities and visualizing weight loss using a smartphone may be useful as a constant reminder to encourage users to continuing working to achieve their fitness goals. One recent study[16] found that patients using a smartphone to help track their weight loss goals lost on average 8.5 lb more than individuals without a smartphone at each 3-month interval of the study.

These types of apps would be beneficial for patients motivated to self-manage their diabetes through lifestyle modification. HCPs seeking to make recommendations about such apps should consider patients' socioeconomic factors. Also, patients should discuss their fitness goals with their HCP before starting a new fitness regimen because exercise tolerance varies depending on comorbid conditions, usual physical activity, and overall health status.

Data-sharing and social support

Numerous apps have features that enable users to e-mail and export data into a file that can be shared with HCPs. Obvious benefits of this technology are that it can make data-sharing more frequent and is paperless.

Apps such as iBGStar Diabetes Manager App & Glucose Meter (Apple iOS) and OnTrack (Android) allow users to e-mail data to HCPs and family members. Additionally, use of a device such as iBGStar may allow for effective blood glucose measurement and logging with a single multi-use device, reducing the inconvenience associated with using multiple devices.

Monitoring changes in blood glucose using a smartphone may be convenient for patients, but the data collected often do not automatically transfer out of the device. Data synchronization is an important feature because it allows HCPs to have an accurate snapshot of their patients' glycemic control. A 2010 study[11] found that diabetes management apps capable of seamlessly sharing SMBG data with HCPs are likely to benefit patients. HCPs in the study were able to rapidly visualize trends and make adjustments to medication therapy regimens, thereby improving health outcomes.

Telcare, the first U.S. Food and Drug Administration (FDA)–approved, wireless-capable glucose meter, transfers data to a private online database that patients, family members, and HCPs can access. Family members may also receive text messages each time users check their blood glucose levels. Apps such as Diabetes Guardian (Apple iOS) allow parents to closely monitor their child's blood glucose levels from a distance, alleviating the stress of not knowing the state of their child's condition.

Maintaining close communication with HCPs, friends, and family is likely to result in better monitoring and management of diabetes. Likewise, the ability to share data and communicate with friends or other people with diabetes is another feature that may entice patients to use smartphone apps. Apps that offer such features can foster a sense of connection and serve as a virtual social support system, which may further improve diabetes self-management. It has been documented that acquiring new knowledge and information through mutual exchange of experiences occurs more effectively when such exchanges involve peers with whom individuals identify and share common experiences.[17] Through interaction with other app users, patients may become more aware of the importance of diabetes management and learn more pragmatic and efficient ways to control their diabetes.

Short message service and reminders

Short message service (SMS), also known as text messaging, has become an integral form of communication and can be useful in promoting adherence because it does not require a high level of technological expertise. Apps with incorporated SMS are widely used to remind patients when to administer insulin and to encourage regular blood glucose logging. A meta-analysis[2] identified common design elements of text messaging for diabetes data collection, including blood glucose levels, diabetes facts, and tailored messages based on individual characteristics and goals.

For effective diabetes management, apps should also provide the ability to remind users to take medications at appropriate times throughout the day. More than $300 billion are spent annually for complications associated with patients failing to take their medications properly.[18] SMS alerts could potentially reduce such costs.

Guidelines and Regulations

The market for health care–related apps nearly doubled in 1 year, from $718 million in 2011 to $1.3 billion in 2012.[19] This rapid growth of the mobile app industry has raised some concerns regarding the lack of regulation for health monitoring apps. In some cases, apps may not comply with evidence-based guidelines or may contain outdated information.

In 2011, the FDA issued draft guidelines for mobile medical apps, including those used as an accessory to a regulated device, those that transform mobile devices into medical devices, and those intended for use with a medical device connected to a smartphone.[20] In the past few years, the FDA has approved multiple diabetes management apps, including WellDoc, Glooko, and Telcare.

Unfortunately, most apps on the market are not approved by the FDA because they are exempt from regulation as outlined in the draft guidelines. Even so, the FDA has published its intention to monitor the performance of all apps to protect public health.[20] HCPs should review smartphone apps that their patients intend to use because it is likely that the market of new health care apps will be too saturated for close FDA monitoring.

Precautions for Patients

Patients should be advised that smartphone apps may be used as helpful tools but should not be a substitute for regular check-ups or follow-ups with HCPs. Because many apps are developed by programmers who may not be in the health care field, apps sometimes contain outdated or inaccurate information. In addition, patients who use virtual social support features on mobile apps should be warned not to rely heavily on comments or advice from other users.

HCPs may also encourage patients to notify them if they notice any significant fluctuations in weight, blood glucose, or medication tolerance. Patients whose medical care is covered by the Centers for Medicare and Medicaid Services should be advised to continue recording their blood glucose readings on a physical paper copy because electronic copies from beneficiaries are not currently recognized by this payer.

Summary and Conclusion

Diabetes is a chronic illness that requires vigilant monitoring and management of glycemic fluctuations through medication, diet, and exercise. Patients diagnosed with diabetes are often challenged by the need to incorporate these various monitoring components into their daily lives. The recent emergence of mobile technology in the health care field has made diabetes self-management apps available. These smartphone apps can allow for more accurate and convenient self-monitoring. Evidence of the benefits of smartphone apps in health care is mounting as researchers conduct and publish studies evaluating these new tools.

HCPs must evaluate a wide array of factors before recommending mobile apps for their patients with diabetes (Figure 2). First, they should assess their patients' comfort level and proficiency with mobile technology. In general, elderly patients may require a longer period of time and more experience to become accustomed to apps

and may be reluctant to use mobile technology for diabetes management. In contrast, patients with advanced technological proficiency may prefer apps. The cost associated with smartphones and apps is also an integral factor. Not all diabetes management apps are free, and the costs may pose additional financial burdens for patients. HCPs also must be aware of the different types of platforms available to consumers. Most importantly, they should tailor their recommendations to apps that address each patient's particular areas of difficulty in managing diabetes.

It is important to discuss overall goals to gain an understanding of what each patient hopes to gain by using a smartphone app. For example, some apps focus on tracking blood glucose, whereas others also include carbohydrate-tracking features. Patients' expectations should help to guide HCPs in recommending an app that best fits their lifestyle and health condition.

Patients may prefer certain apps to others based on their ease of use. The availability of other important features, such as reminders via text messages, data-sharing with HCPs, and compatibility with medical devices, is also a consideration.

The FDA recently developed draft guidelines for mobile medical apps in three categories: those that are used as an accessory to a regulated device,

those that transform a mobile platform into a medical device, and those that are intended to use with a medical device connected to a smartphone.[20] Unfortunately, most diabetes management apps on the market do not fit into these categories and thus remain unregulated. These could potentially provide inaccurate information that is unsupported by clinical evidence.

The smartphone app market is becoming inundated with hundreds of health care apps as technology advancements continue. As smartphones have become more affordable and user-friendly, the number of smartphone owners has continued to grow in all age-groups. It is incumbent on HCPs to appropriately tailor their app recommendations to individual patients and to guide patients in selecting the most useful and reliable apps to meet their needs.

References

[1]Centers for Disease Control and Prevention: National Diabetes fact sheet: national estimates and general information on diabetes and prediabetes in the United States, 2011. Atlanta, Ga., U.S. Department of Health and Human Services, Centers for Disease Control and Prevention, 2011

[2]Mulvaney SA, Lee RM, Bosslet L: Mobile intervention design in diabetes: review and recommendations. *Curr Diabetes Rep* 11:486–493, 2011

[3]Quinn CC, Clough SS, Minor JM, Lender D, Okafor MC, Gruber-Baldini A: WellDoc mobile diabetes management randomized controlled trial: change in clinical and behavioral outcomes and patient and physician satisfaction. *Diabetes Technol Ther* 10:160–168, 2008

[4]Newark-French C: Mobile app usage further dominates web, spurred by Facebook [article online]. Available from http://blog.flurry.com/bid/80241/Mobile-App-Usage-Further-Dominates-Web-Spurred-by-Facebook. Accessed 10 March 2013

[5]Carroll AE, DiMeglio LA, Stein S, Marrero DG: Contracting and monitoring relationships for adolescents with type 1 diabetes: a pilot study. *Diabetes Technol Ther* 13:543–549, 2011

[6]Weston L: The real costs of a smartphone [article online]. Available from http://money.msn.com/shopping-deals/the-real-costs-of-a-smartphone. Accessed 22 March 2013

[7]NPD Group: As smartphone prices fall, retailers are leaving money on the table, according to The NPD Group [article online]. Available from https://www.npd.com/wps/portal/npd/us/news/press-releases/pr_111114a/. Accessed 5 March 2013

[8]CTIA: The Wireless Association's semi-annual wireless industry survey [article online]. Available from http://files.ctia.org/

Factors to Consider for Diabetes Management Application

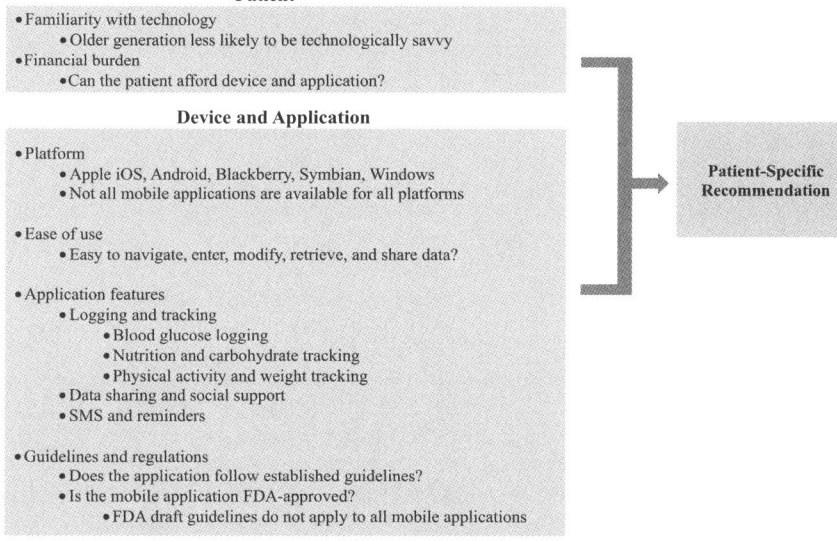

Figure 2. Factors to consider when recommending a diabetes management app to patients.

pdf/CTIA_Survey_MY_2012_Graphics-_final.pdf. Accessed 10 March 2013

[9]Boulos MNK, Wheeler S, Tavares C, Jones R: How smartphones are changing the face of mobile and participatory healthcare: an overview, with example from eCAALYX. *Biomed Eng Online* 10:24, 2011

[10]Hando B: Apple vs. Android in healthcare: who is winning? [article online] Available from http://medicalappjournal.com/medicalblog/2012/10/16/apple-vs-android-in-healthcare-who-is-winning/#.UWTld7Xqlr8. Accessed 5 March 2013

[11]Rao A, Hou P, Golnik T, Flaherty J, Vu S: Evolution of data management tools for managing self-monitoring of blood glucose results: a survey of iPhone applications. *J Diabetes Sci Technol* 4:949–957, 2010

[12]Rodbard HW, Blonde L, Braithwaite SS, Brett EM, Cobin RH, Handelsman Y, Hellman R, Jellinger PS, Jovanovic LG, Levy P, Mechanick JI, Zangeneh F, Parkin CG: American Association of Clinical Endocrinologists medical guidelines for clinical practice for the management of diabetes mellitus. *Endocr Pract* 13:1–68, 2007

[13]Apple iTunes: iBGStar® Diabetes Manager. Available from https://itunes.apple.com/us/app/ibgstar-diabetes-manager/id506018173?mt=8. Accessed 15 March 2013

[14]Souto DL, Rosado EL: Use of carb counting in the dietary treatment of diabetes mellitus. *Nutr Hosp* 25:18–25, 2010

[15]Apple iTunes: Calorie counter and diet tracker by MyNetDiary. Available from https://itunes.apple.com/us/app/calorie-counter-diet-tracker/id287529757?mt=8. Accessed 25 March 2013

[16]Spring B, Duncan JM, Janke EA, Kozak AT, McFadden HG, DeMott A, Pictor A, Epstein LH, Siddique J, Buscemi J, Hedeker D: Integrating technology into standard weight loss treatment: a randomized controlled trial. *JAMA Intern Med* 2:105–111, 2013

[17]Heisler M: Overview of peer support models to improve diabetes self-management and clinical outcomes. *Diabetes Spectrum* 20:214–221, 2007

[18]Council for Affordable Health Coverage: Medication adherence: a $300 billion opportunity [article online]. Available from http://cahc.net/medication-adherence-a-300-billion-opportunity/. Accessed 10 March 2013

[19]Jahns R: US$ 1.3 billion: the market for mHealth applications in 2012 [article online]. Available from http://www.research2guidance.com/us-1.3-billion-the-market-for-mhealth-applications-in-2012/. Accessed 10 March 2013

[20]U.S. Food and Drug Administration: Draft guidance for industry and Food and Drug Administration staff, mobile medical applications [article online]. Available from http://www.fda.gov/downloads/MedicalDevices/DeviceRegulationandGuidance/GuidanceDocuments/UCM263366.pdf. Accessed 10 March 2013

Ryan A. Ristau, BS, and Jessica Yang, BA, are doctorate in pharmacy candidates, and John R. White, Jr., PA-C, PharmD, is a professor and interim chair of the Department of Pharmacotherapy at Washington State University College of Pharmacy in Spokane.